The U.S. RDA (used on food labels)

Nutrient	RDA for an Adult Man (1968)	RDA for an Adult Woman (1968)	U.S. RDA
Nutrients that *must* appear on the label[a]			
Protein (g), PER ≥ casein[b]	(45)	—	45
Protein (g), PER < casein	(65)	55	65
Vitamin A (RE)	(1,000[c])	800[c]	1,000[c]
Vitamin C (ascorbic acid) (mg)	(60)	55	60
Thiamin (vitamin B$_1$) (mg)	1.4	1.0	1.5
Riboflavin (vitamin B$_2$) (mg)	(1.7)	1.5	1.7
Niacin (mg)	18	13	20
Calcium (g)	0.8	0.8	1.0
Iron (mg)	10	(18)	18
Nutrients that *may* appear on the label			
Vitamin D (IU)	—	—	400
Vitamin E (IU)	(30)	25	30
Vitamin B$_6$ (mg)	(2.0)	2.0	2.0
Folate (folic acid, folacin) (mg)	(0.4)	0.4	0.4
Vitamin B$_{12}$ (μg)	(6)	6	6
Phosphorus (g)	0.8	0.8	1.0
Iodine (μg)	120	100	150
Magnesium (mg)	350	300	400
Zinc (mg)	—	—	15
Copper (mg)	—	—	2
Biotin (mg)	—	—	0.3
Pantothenic acid (mg)	—	—	10

[a]Whenever nutrition labeling is required.

[b]PER is an index of protein quality.

[c]1,000 RE was originally expressed as 5,000 IU. 800 RE was originally expressed as 4,000 IU.

Source: Adapted from U.S. Department of Health and Human Services, Public Health Service, Food and Drug Administration, Office of Public Affairs, 5600 Fishers Lane, Rockville, Maryland 20857, HHS publication no. (FDA) 81-2146, revised March 1981.

The U.S. RDA numbers used on labels are those taken from the 1968 RDA. The circled numbers are those chosen for the U.S. RDA from the adult male and female recommendations. In each case, the higher number is chosen.

In the case of thiamin, niacin, iodine, and magnesium, the RDA for an adolescent boy is used, because this is even higher than the adult RDA.

In the case of calcium and phosphorus, 1 gram per day is used, more than the adult RDA. Pregnant and lactating women and rapidly growing teenagers have RDA even higher than this, but 1 gram was considered generous enough for use as a standard for labels.

In the case of the last four nutrients—zinc, copper, biotin, and pantothenic acid—RDA had not been set as of 1968, but these nutrients are known to be essential. The agency set "guestimates" for these so that percent-of-U.S.-RDA labels could include them. These four nutrients are now included in the RDA tables, but the U.S. RDA values have not changed to correspond; they are considered close enough already. The Food and Drug Administration is currently working on a plan to replace the U.S. RDA with a new set of daily nutrient guidelines when they become available. For further discussion, see Nutrition in Practice 5.

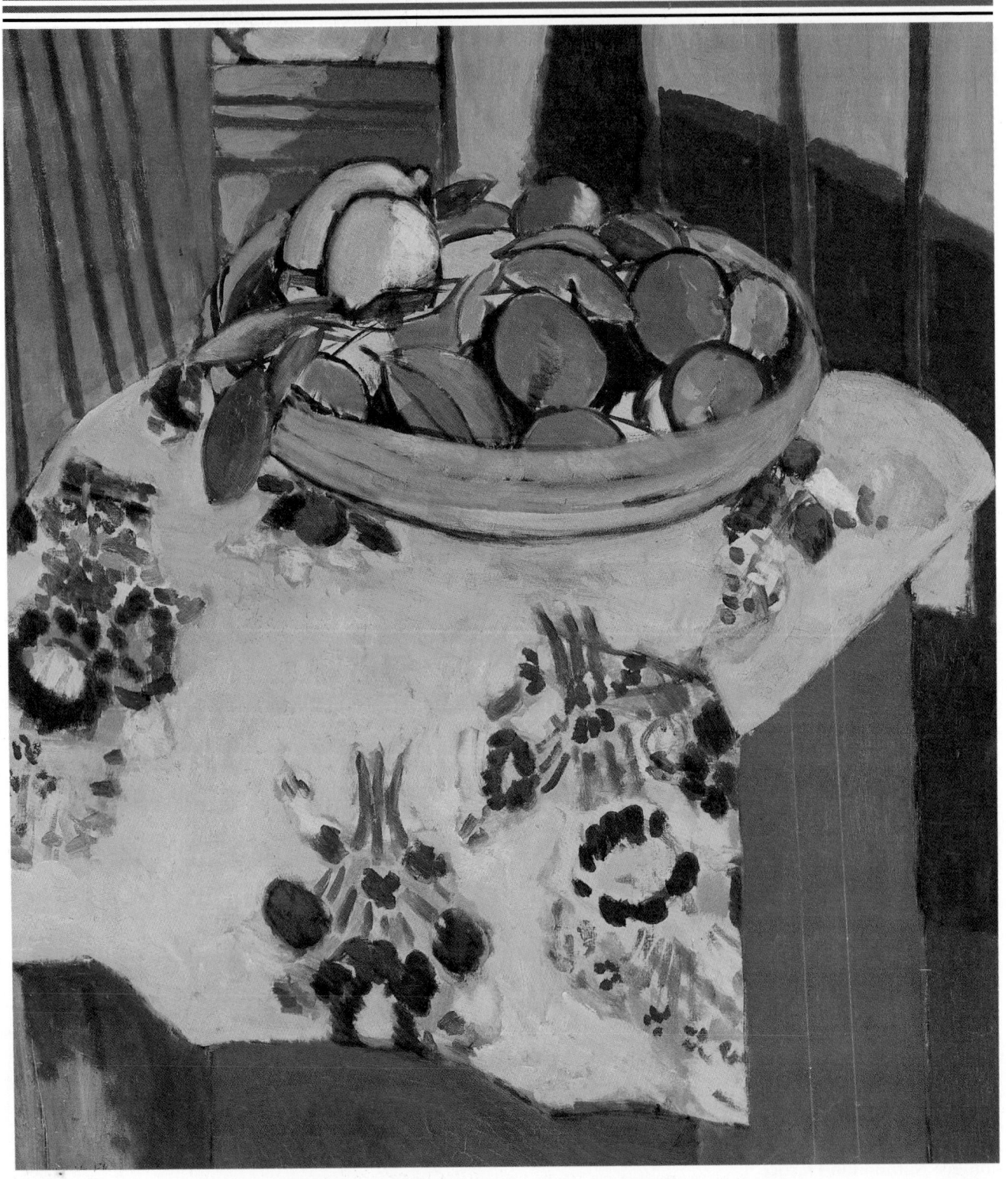

Henri Matisse, Still Life with Oranges, Musée du Louvre, Photo R.M.N.; © 1992 Les Heritiers Matisse, Paris/ARS, N.Y.

THIRD EDITION

Nutrition &
Diet Therapy

PRINCIPLES AND PRACTICE

Corinne Balog Cataldo
Linda Kelly DeBruyne
Eleanor Noss Whitney

WEST PUBLISHING COMPANY

Saint Paul   New York   Los Angeles   San Francisco

Copyediting: Mary Berry, Naples Editing Services
Index: JoAnne Naples, Naples Editing Services
Interior/cover design: K. M. Weber
Page layout: David J. Farr, Imagesmythe, Inc.
Composition: Carlisle Communications, Ltd.
New illustrations: Sandy McMahon and Randy Miyake
Cover image: Henri Matisse, *Still Life with Oranges*, Musée du Louvre, Photo R.M.N.; © 1992 Les
Heritiers Matisse, Paris/ARS, N.Y.

Copyright © 1985, 1989   By WEST PUBLISHING COMPANY
Copyright © 1992   By WEST PUBLISHING COMPANY
                        610 Opperman Drive
                        P.O. Box 64526
                        St. Paul, MN 55164-0526

Printed in the United States of America

99 98 97 96 95 94 93 92   8 7 6 5 4 3 2 1 0

Library of Congress Cataloging-in-Publication Data

Cataldo, Corinne Balog.
   Nutrition and diet therapy : principles and practice / Corinne
Balog Cataldo, Linda Kelly DeBruyne, Eleanor Noss Whitney. — 3rd
ed.
      p.   cm.
   Includes index.
   ISBN 0-314-93359-X (soft)
   1. Diet therapy.   2. Nutrition.   I. DeBruyne, Linda K.
II. Whitney, Eleanor Noss.   III. Title.
RM216.C36 1992
615.8'54 — dc20   92-2595
                                                                 CIP

WEST'S COMMITMENT TO THE ENVIRONMENT

In 1906, West Publishing Company began recycling materials left over from the production of books.
This began a tradition of efficient and responsible use of resources. Today, up to 95 percent of our legal
books and 70 percent of our college texts are printed on recycled, acid-free stock. West also recycles
nearly 22 million pounds of scrap paper annually—the equivalent of 181,717 trees. Since the 1960s,
West has devised ways to capture and recycle waste inks, solvents, oils, and vapors created in the
printing process. We also recycle plastics of all kinds, wood, glass, corrugated cardboard, and batteries,
and have eliminated the use of styrofoam book packaging. We at West are proud of the longevity and
the scope of our commitment to our environment.

Production, Prepress, Printing and Binding by West Publishing Company.

PHOTO CREDITS

Dedication Page: From THE PROPHET by Kahlil Gibran. Copyright 1923 by Kahlil Gibran and
renewed 1951 by Administrators C.T.A. of Kahlil Gibran Estate, and Mary G. Gibran. Reprinted by
permission of Alfred A. Knopf, Inc. **11** Courtesy of USDA; Courtesy of USDA; © Four By Five; ©
Richard Palsey/Stock Boston; Courtesy of USDA; Courtesy of USDA; **28** Ray Stanyard; **28** © Tony
Photo Credits continued after Index

Corinne Balog Cataldo, M.M.Sc., R.D., C.N.S.D., received her B.S. in community health nutrition from Georgia State University in 1976 and her M.M.Sc. in clinical dietetics from Emory University in 1979. She has worked in private practice in Atlanta, as a clinical dietitian and metabolic support nutritionist at Georgia Baptist Medical Center in Atlanta, as a faculty member and dietetic internship coordinator at Emory University, and as a nutritionist with the Infant Formula Council. She has made numerous presentations, and in addition to this book, she has written a manual on tube feeding and the book *Understanding Normal and Clinical Nutrition*. She is a certified nutrition support dietitian and continues to do consulting work.

Linda Kelly DeBruyne, M.S., R.D., received her B.S. in 1980 and her M.S. in 1982 in nutrition and food science at Florida State University. She serves on the board of directors of the Nutrition and Health Associates, an information resource center in Tallahassee, Florida, where her specialty areas are fitness and life cycle nutrition. Her other textbooks include *Life Cycle Nutrition: Conception through Adolescence, Life Span Nutrition: Conception through Life*, and *The Fitness Triad: Motivation, Training, and Nutrition*. Her monographs, published in the *Nutrition Clinics* series, include *Vegetarian Diets during Vulnerable Times, Nutrition and Behavior, Nutrition for Sport, Nutrition and the Aging Brain*, and *Vitamin Supplements*. As a consultant for a group of Tallahassee pediatricians, she teaches infant nutrition classes to parents. She is a member of the American Dietetic Association and the American Alliance for Health, Physical Education, Recreation, and Dance.

Eleanor Noss Whitney, Ph.D., R.D., received her B.A. in biology from Radcliffe College in 1960 and her Ph.D. in biology from Washington University, St. Louis, in 1970. Formerly on the faculty at Florida State University, she now devotes full time to research, writing, and consulting in nutrition, health, and environmental issues. She is president of the Nutrition and Health Associates, an information resource center in Tallahassee, Florida. Her publications include articles in *Science, Journal of Nutrition, Genetics*, and other journals, and the textbooks *Nutrition: Concepts and Controversies, Understanding Nutrition*, and *Life Choices: Health Concepts and Strategies*, among others.

DEDICATION

To Frank Pittman for helping me find myself amid the confusion, to Jeffrey Bogart for helping me like who I found, and especially to Marsha Chassner, a person synonymous with the most important things in life—friendship, laughter, and love.

Corkie

"And in the sweetness of friendship let there be laughter, and sharing of pleasures; For in the dew of little things the heart finds its morning and is refreshed." (Kahlil Gibran)
To my family and friends, whose love and laughter refresh my heart, even when it is aching.

Linda

To Fran, Linda, Sharon, Corkie, and Lori, the finest nutrition and health experts I know.

Ellie

CONTENTS • IN • BRIEF

CONTENTS

Summary of Modified Diets by Organ System

DISORDERS	POSSIBLE DIET MODIFICATIONS	PAGE REFERENCE
CONDITIONS AFFECTING OR INVOLVING THE GI TRACT, LIVER, AND EXOCRINE PANCREAS[a]		
Blind loop syndrome	Low-fat	554
Broken jaw	Mechanical soft	433
Celiac disease	Gluten-restricted	605
Cirrhosis	Protein-restricted, sodium-restricted, fluid-restricted	593
Constipation	High-fiber, increased fluids	443
Cystic fibrosis	Low-fat, high-kcalorie, high-protein	551
Dental caries	Mechanical soft	433
Diarrhea	Liquid, low-fiber, regular, fluid and electrolyte replacement	426
Difficulty swallowing (dysphagia)	Mechanical soft, tube feeding, total parenteral nutrition (TPN)	435
Diverticulitis	Low-fiber	445
Diverticulosis	High-fiber	445
Dry mouth	Mechanical soft	433
Dumping syndrome	Carbohydrate-restricted; no concentrated sugars; small, frequent feedings; fluid and electrolyte replacement	530
Gastritis	Low-fiber, bland	437
Hepatic coma	Protein-restricted, sodium-restricted, fluid-restricted	595
Hepatitis	Regular, high-kcalorie, high-protein	593
Hiatal hernia	Small, frequent feedings; low-fat; bland; kcalorie-restricted	448
Ill-fitting dentures	Mechanical soft	433
Indigestion (dyspepsia)	Low-fiber; bland; small, frequent feedings	446
Inflammatory bowel disease	Low-fiber, low-fat, high-kcalorie, high-protein, fluid and electrolyte replacement, lactose-restricted, tube feeding, TPN	552
Irritable bowel syndrome	Low-fiber	444
Lactose intolerance	Lactose-restricted	534
Malabsorption	Low-fat, high-kcalorie, high-protein, fluid and electrolyte replacement	548
Missing teeth	Mechanical soft	433
Nausea	Low-fiber; bland; small, frequent feedings; no liquids with meals	447
Oral surgery	Mechanical soft	433
Pancreatitis	Low-fat; regular; small, frequent feedings; tube feeding; TPN	550
Peptic ulcer	Bland	440
Periodontal disease	Mechanical soft	433
Plastic surgery of head or neck	Mechanical soft, tube feeding, TPN	433
Reflux esophagitis	Small, frequent feedings; low-fat; bland; kcalorie-restricted	448
Short bowel syndrome	Low-fat, high-kcalorie, high-protein, fluid and electrolyte replacement	555
Ulcers of mouth or gums	Mechanical soft, bland	433
Vomiting	Fluid and electrolyte replacement	447
CONDITIONS AFFECTING THE ENDOCRINE PANCREAS[a]		
Diabetes mellitus	Carbohydrate-controlled, kcalorie-restricted, fat-controlled, high-fiber	513
Hypoglycemia	No concentrated sweets; small, frequent feedings	528

(continued)

Summary of Modified Diets by Organ System—(*continued*)

DISORDERS	POSSIBLE DIET MODIFICATIONS	PAGE REFERENCE
CONDITIONS AFFECTING THE BLOOD VESSELS, HEART, AND LUNGS		
Atherosclerosis	Fat-controlled, kcalorie-restricted, sodium-restricted, high-fiber	564
Congestive heart failure	Sodium-restricted; kcalorie-restricted; low-fiber; bland; small, frequent feedings; fluid-restricted	579
Coronary heart disease	(See *Atherosclerosis* above)	564
Hyperlipidemias	Fat-controlled, kcalorie-restricted, carbohydrate-controlled	564
Hypertension	Low-sodium, kcalorie-restricted, high-potassium, fat-controlled	571
Myocardial infarction	Low-sodium; kcalorie-restricted; low-fiber; bland; small, frequent feedings; moderate-temperature; fat-controlled	574
Pulmonary disease	High-kcalorie, high-protein	478
CONDITIONS AFFECTING THE KIDNEYS		
Acute renal disease	Protein-restricted, high-kcalorie, fluid-controlled, sodium-controlled, potassium-controlled, fat-controlled, carbohydrate-controlled	604
Chronic renal disease	Protein-restricted, low-sodium, fluid-restricted, potassium-restricted, phosphorus-restricted	600
Kidney stones	Increased fluid intake, calcium-controlled, low-oxalate	611
Nephrotic syndrome	Sodium-restricted, high-kcalorie, high-protein, potassium-restricted	580
CONDITIONS AFFECTING MANY ORGAN SYSTEMS		
Acquired immune deficiency syndrome (AIDS)	High-kcalorie, high-protein, low-fat, low-residue, low-fiber, fluid and electrolyte replacement, lactose-restricted, mechanical soft, tube feeding, TPN	473
Burns	High-kcalorie, high-protein, increased fluid intake	463
Cancer	High-kcalorie, high-protein (see also specific related conditions: *Dry mouth, Indigestion (dyspepsia), Malabsorption, Nausea, Plastic surgery of head or neck, Ulcers of mouth or gums, Vomiting,* and so on)	466
Food sensitivities	Elimination of offending substance	299
Galactosemia	Galactose-restricted	536
Obesity, overweight	kCalorie-restricted, high-fiber	494
Phenylketonuria (PKU)	Phenylalanine-restricted	606
Stroke	Mechanical soft, regular, tube feeding	436
Surgery	Regular, high-kcalorie, high-protein, increased fluids	428
Underweight	High-kcalorie, high-protein	458

[a]The pancreas produces both external (exocrine) and internal (endocrine) secretions. The external secretions (enzymes) play an important role in the digestion of food; the internal secretions (insulin and other hormones) play a primary role in the regulation of glucose metabolism.

PREFACE

The third revision of *Nutrition and Diet Therapy* offers its readers concise, accurate nutrition information based on the most recent research available. Because so much new information has surfaced since the second revision was published, each chapter and Nutrition in Practice has been revised to reflect these changes. No doubt in the years before the next revision is published, additional information will continue to become available. To help sort through new information, this book not only provides simple facts and figures but also shows how to judge and interpret new nutrition information.

Each chapter deals with subjects of importance to health care professionals that relate to nutrition. At the end of each chapter, a Nutrition in Practice section deals with practical questions you may have about nutrition, and questions you may be asked by the people you work with. Within the chapters, digressions discuss topics of current or personal interest, to make the subject more relevant to personal lives. Page margins define technical terms and provide notes pertinent to the discussion. This arrangement permits the reader to continue reading if the term is already known, to stop and learn the term if it is new, or to return to the terms for review at a later time. Study Questions at the end of each chapter and Case Studies provide students with an opportunity to apply the information presented in the chapters.

The first eight chapters of the book present nutrition information as it relates to all healthy people. Each chapter has been updated and reorganized to facilitate students' understanding of the topics discussed. Chapter 9 emphasizes the health benefits of physical activity, the nutrients that best fuel physical activity, and the synergistic effect that nutrition and fitness exert on health.

Chapter 10 introduces the reader to nutrition assessment and provides the reader with the newest information about assessing nutrition status. The chapter includes new tables and describes the assessment of nutrition-related anemias. Chapters 11, 12, and 13 discuss the special nutrient needs of people through the life span—pregnant women and infants, children and adolescents, and older adults.

Chapter 14 delves into the relationships between nutrition and illness, including the body's responses to severe stress, to attacks on the immune system, and to drug therapy. A section of the chapter also describes the relationships between nutrition and mental illnesses. Chapter 15 shows how nutrition care providers develop, implement, and evaluate nutrition care plans to meet their clients' needs.

Chapters 16 through 23 address the nutrition concerns of people who are ill or have medical conditions that require dietary modifications. This edition of the text continues to approach diet therapy based on diet rather than on organ systems. Each diet is described once, and disorders for which each diet is used are then discussed so that the rationale for the diet will be understandable.

Some areas of clinical interest that have been extensively revised for this edition of the book include dysphagia, enteral and parenteral nutrition, drug-nutrient interaction tables, acquired immune deficiency syndrome (AIDS), and ethical issues in clinical nutrition.

This edition includes the revised Recommended Dietary Allowances (1989) and the Canadian Recommended Nutrient Intakes (1990). Appendix B provides supplemental information about nutrition assessment and includes an extensively revised table on drug-nutrient interactions and standards for hand grip strength. The presentation of information on enteral formulas in Appendix D has been revised, and many new formulas have been added.

We know that textbooks often present material in a more formal fashion than this one does, but we have found that most readers of our books appreciate the relaxed-sounding pace, and still respect and trust the books' contents for their accuracy. We hope our informal, conversational writing style makes the study of nutrition an enjoyable experience. Nutrition is a fascinating subject, and we hope our enthusiasm for it comes through on every page.

Acknowledgments

The completion of this book would not have been possible without the assistance and support of many individuals who contributed in many ways to its publication. Our sincerest appreciation goes to the many reviewers who have consistently provided us with excellent suggestions for improving the text. The reviewers of this text include:

Alice Bartholomew—Northampton Community College
Jacque Coulson—Iowa Methodist School of Nursing
Judy K. Davidson—Columbus College
Lois Ellis—Indiana Wesleyan University
Catherine Graziano—Salve Regina University
Barbara L'Heureux—Bristol Community College
Patricia Lillis—Medical College of Georgia
Jo Anne Lish—Alcorn State University
Sylvia Nissila—College of St. Catherine
Nancy Shaw—Southeastern Louisiana University
Barbara Troy—Marquette University

Special thanks to our friends and associates Sharon Rolfes, Lori Turner, and Frances Sizer for sharing their expertise on many of the topics in this text; to our editors, Jane Bass, Poh Lin Khoo, and Peter Marshall, for their dedication and expert guidance through this project; and to Bob and Betty Geltz for the extensive and thorough food composition table and the computerized diet analysis program that goes with this text.

Nutrition & Diet Therapy

PRACTICE AND PRINCIPLES

THIRD EDITION

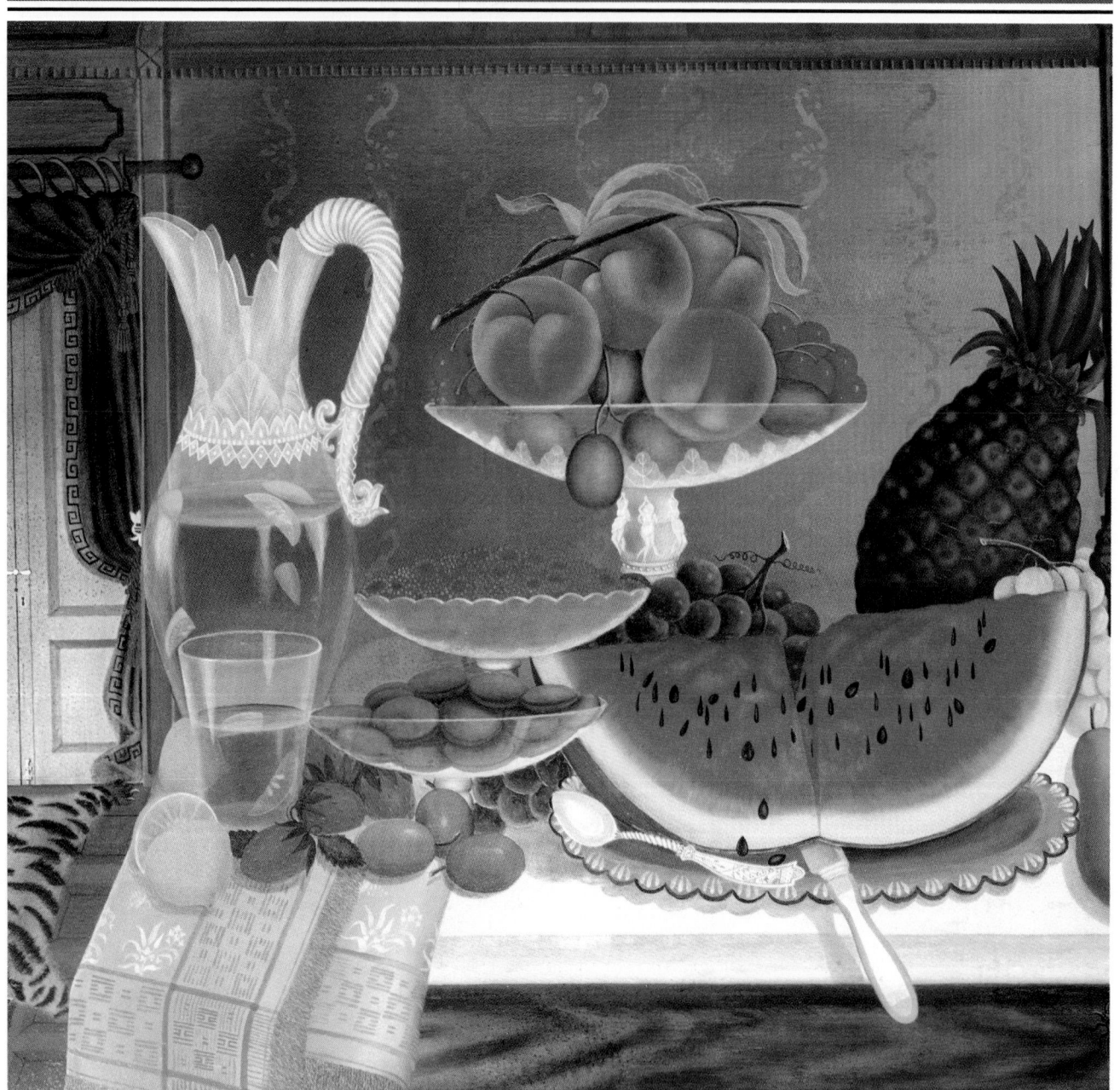

Henry Church, Still Life, The Collection of Frances O. Stem Babinsky.

Perspective on Nutrition

CONTENTS

CHAPTER 1

You are a collection of molecules that move. All these moving parts are arranged into patterns of extraordinary complexity and order—cells, tissues, and organs. Although the arrangement remains constant, the parts are continually changing, using nutrients and energy derived from nutrients. To maintain your "self," therefore, you must continuously replace the *pieces* you lose and replenish the *energy* you burn.

The pieces you are made of and your energy come from the nutrients contained in the food you eat. The science of nutrition is the study of the nutrients in food and the body's handling of these nutrients.

Most people know that the nutrients in food nourish the body and promote health. Despite this knowledge, however, most people choose the foods they eat for reasons other than their nutrient contributions. Food choices are personal and not always sensible, and to a great extent, they resist change. Before undertaking diet planning, the planner must understand the dynamics of food choices, because people will alter their eating habits only if their preferences are honored.

science of nutrition: the study of nutrients and of their ingestion, digestion, absorption, transport, metabolism, interaction, storage, and excretion. A broader definition includes the study of the environment and of human behavior as it relates to these processes.

Food Choices

Why do you choose the particular foods you do? Several reasons come to mind. You may choose the foods you eat for any of the following reasons:

1. Personal preference (you like the taste).
2. Associations (you associate happiness or prestige with them).
3. Habit or tradition (they are familiar; you always eat them).
4. Social pressure (they are offered; you can't refuse).
5. Availability (there are no others to choose from).
6. Convenience (you are too rushed to prepare anything else).
7. Economy (they are within your financial means).
8. Physical ideals (you seek or avoid foods that you expect will improve or impair your physical appearance).
9. Nutritional value (you think they are good for you).
10. Medical reasons (you must follow a special diet for a health problem).

Of these ten possible reasons, only one has to do with nutrition directly. Even people who pride themselves on eating nutritious foods will admit that the other factors also influence their food choices. They may know how to prepare nutritious meals, but they may not actually eat them. People tend to eat the foods they simply like.

Why do you like certain foods? One reason, of course, is your preference for certain tastes. Some of these preferences are widely shared, such as the tastes for fat, sugar, and salt.

People also like foods with which they have happy associations—those they eat in the midst of warm family gatherings on traditional holidays, those given to them as children by someone who loved them, or those eaten by people whom they admire. By the same token, people can attach an intense and unalterable dislike to foods that they ate when they were sick, foods that were forced on them when they weren't hungry, or foods they think are eaten by people they don't respect. Your parents may have taught you to like and dislike certain foods for reasons of their own without even being aware of it.

Every country—and every region of a country—has its own typical foods and ways of combining them into meals. North America embodies people from many different cultural and ethnic backgrounds. The foodways of this continent reflect this intermingling of cultures. Many foods with ethnic origins—tacos, egg rolls, lasagna, and gyros, to name a few—are familiar features on North American menus. Still others, such as pizza, spaghetti, and croissants, are integral in the "American diet." North American regional cuisines like Cajun and TexMex exemplify a gradual blending of cross-cultural foods. Table 1–1 presents characteristics of selected ethnic diets.

Religious beliefs and customs, like ethnic origin, also influence people's food choices. For example, the Jewish laws set forth an extensive set of dietary rules. Many Christians forgo meat during Lent, the period prior to Easter. Other faiths prohibit some dietary practices and promote others. Diet planners can promote sound nutrition practices only if they respect and honor personal, ethnic, and religious food preferences.

Social pressure is another powerful influence on peoples' food choices. How can you refuse when your friends are going out for pizza and beer (or doughnuts and coffee)? Such pressure operates in all circles and across all cultural lines. It is often considered rude not to accept food or drink being shared by a group or offered by a host; you are usually not accepted as a member of the social gathering unless you do.

The influence of availability, convenience, and economy on people's food selections is clear. You cannot eat foods if they are not available, if you cannot prepare them, or if you cannot afford them. (Nutrition in Practice 10 describes how the environment influences food availability). Convenience plays a major role in many people's food selections today. The demand for foods that are ready to eat or can be easily prepared in a microwave oven demonstrates this influence.[1]

Sometimes people associate foods, usually wrongly, with ideals of body image, and these ideals influence their food choices. The fashion and movie industry, not the medical community, have defined what people believe to be the ideal body—an excessively thin body. Whereas other nations view thinness as a sign of malnutrition, our society values thinness, equating it with youth and beauty. Both men and women seek "beautiful bodies," and in doing so, they select or avoid foods that they believe will improve or impair their physical appearance. Such intentions are rational when based on sound nutrition knowledge, but when based on faddism, they undermine good health.

Sometimes medical conditions determine which foods a person can select. The second half of this text discusses diets modified for different medical conditions.

Some people's food preferences present specific challenges to the diet planner. Consider vegetarian diets. People adopt vegetarian diets for a variety of religious, ethical, social, or economic reasons, but to the diet planner,

ethnic diets: foodways and cuisines typical of national origins, races, cultural heritages, or geographic locations.

TABLE 1–1   **Characteristics of Selected Ethnic Diets**

GROUP AND PLACE OF ORIGIN	STAPLE FOODS	FOODS EXCLUDED	STRENGTHS AND WEAKNESSES OF THE DIET
Hispanic Americans from Cuba, Haiti, Puerto Rico	Steamed white rice; many varieties of beans; wheat breads; starchy vegetables such as cassavas, yuccas, yams, breadfruit, plantains, and green bananas; green peppers; tomatoes; garlic; dried, salted fish; chicken; pork; lard; olive oil; sugar; jams and jellies; sweet pastries; sugared fruit juices; coffee	Green leafy vegetables; milk as a beverage for adults; fish other than dried and salted	Provides adequate protein, many other nutrients, and fiber; may provide too much fat, especially animal fat; may lack calcium
Hispanic Americans from Mexico, Central America	Many varieties of beans; steamed rice; corn products such as tortillas made from lime-soaked cornmeal; chili peppers; tomatoes; mangoes; prickly pear fruit; potatoes; meat and sausages; fish; poultry; eggs; cheeses; milk custards and bread puddings; lard; sweet chocolate and coffee drinks; cakes; pastries	Green leafy vegetables; yellow vegetables; milk as a beverage for adults	Is high in kcalories and fat (especially saturated fat) and high in sugar; most nutrients can be obtained, but with many kcalories
Black Americans from the West Indies, Central or South America, and recent African immigrants	Dumplings or gruel made from millet, corn, wheat, rice, or barley; starchy roots such as cassavas, yams, plantains, and bananas; coconuts; peanuts; fresh fruits; hot peppers; tomatoes; onions; okra; palm oil; fruit wine; tea; coffee; honey; molasses	Milk and milk products (meat and fish limited in use)	Is low in calcium, iron, and vitamin B_{12}; is potentially low in protein, depending on availability of foods; is low in fat and salt; is high in fiber
Southern Black Americans from West Africa (many generations in United States)	Hominy grits; biscuits; cornmeal and corn bread; rice; legumes; potatoes; onions; tomatoes; hot peppers; green leafy vegetables; okra; sweet potatoes; squashes; corn; cabbage; melons; peaches; pecans; smoked pork; fresh meats and poultry; fish; thick stews; butter, shortening, and lard; sugar; bread puddings; pies and sweets	Milk and milk products; yeast breads	Provides ample nutrients of meat; provides excess protein; is high in kcalories; provides excess fat, especially saturated fat; is high in salt; is low in calcium
Chinese Americans from China (diets vary sometimes with region)	Rice and rice gruel; wheat noodles; corn; green vegetables, especially from the cabbage family; squashes; cucumbers; eggplant; leafy vegetables; various shoots, including bamboo, mung, and soy; sweet potatoes; radishes; onions; peas and pods; mushrooms; roots; many local seasonal vegetables; pickled vegetables; sea vegetables; plums; peaches; tangerines; kumquats and other citrus fruits; litchis; longans; mangoes; papayas; pomegranates; soybean products such as tofu (soybean curd), soy sauces, bean noodles, and soy milk; tiny portions of meat, fish with bones, or poultry; seafood; soup or tea as beverage; sugar as seasoning	Milk and most milk products	Depending on availability of protein-rich foods, protein and iron may be low; is low in fat; is high in fiber and many nutrients

TABLE 1–1 **Characteristics of Selected Ethnic Diets** (*continued*)

GROUP AND PLACE OF ORIGIN	STAPLE FOODS	FOODS EXCLUDED	STRENGTHS AND WEAKNESSES OF THE DIET
Japanese Americans from Japan	Rice; vegetables; pickled vegetables; soy as miso (soup), tofu, bean paste, and soy sauce; fruits; salads; fish with bones; sugar as seasoning; sea vegetables; seafood; ginseng	Milk and milk products	Provides abundant nutrients with little fat; is high in salt
Korean Americans from South Korea	Rice; noodles; many leafy vegetables; kimchi (extremely hot pickled cabbage); sea vegetables; hot peppers; seasonal fruits; mushrooms, small fish with bones; large servings of grilled beef; chicken; fresh or dried squid, octopus, and lobster; mussels; eggs; lard and vegetable fat for frying; sesame oil; nut and seeds; ginger; sugar as seasoning	Milk and milk products	Is high in fat and adequate in protein; is monotonous in winter (kimchi is served at each meal, to the exclusion of other vegetables); without the traditional small fish with bones, calcium can be lacking
Vietnamese Americans from Vietnam	Rice and rice noodles; French bead and croissants with butter; hot peppers; curries of asparagus and potatoes; salads; tropical fruits and vegetables; lemons and limes; small portions of poultry; eggs; fish pâtés; nuoc nam (a strong, fermented fish sauce); sweets and candies; sweetened drinks; coffee; tea	Milk and milk products	Can be low in iron or calcium
Native Americans (Indians)	*Southeast:* corn; cornmeal; coontie (flour from a palmlike plant); fried breads; swamp cabbage (now illegal to harvest); pumpkins; squashes; papayas; alligator; snake; wild hog; duck; fish; shellfish. *Northeast:* blueberries; cranberries; beans; corn; pumpkins; fish; lobster; wild game; maple syrup. *Midwest:* bison; beans; corn; melons; squashes; tomatoes. *Southwest:* corn (many colors and varieties); beans; squashes; pumpkins; chili peppers; melons; pine nuts; cactus. *Northwest:* salmon; caviar; other fish; otter; seal; whale; bear; elk; other game; wild fruits; acorns and other wild nuts; wild greens	Milk and milk products	Varies with region; may be low in calcium
Italian Americans from Italy	*Northern Italy:* meat; butter; cheese; eggs; cream; egg-based, ribbon-shaped pastas. *Southern Italy:* artichokes, eggplant, peppers, and tomatoes accompanied by beans and olive oil; wheat pastas shaped like macaroni	—	Is adequate in protein and most nutrients, but can be high in fat

all vegetarian diets present similar challenges. A few nutrients in a vegetarian diet deserve careful attention if the diet is to offer nutrition and health benefits to adults.[2] Nutrition in Practice 4 shows how to make vegetarian diets nutritious.

No matter what foods you eat—whether you exclude or include specific foods or subscribe to the diet of a particular ethnic group—you have no guarantee of diet adequacy. Since sound nutrition promotes health and longevity, it is in every person's own best interest to know how to obtain optimal nourishment. Consumers today cite nutrition as a primary concern in making food choices, yet the foods they choose do not always reflect this concern; they need to know more about the nutrients in food.[3]

The Nutrients

Almost any food you eat is composed of dozens or even hundreds of different kinds of materials—atoms and molecules tinier than anything that can be seen with the most powerful microscope. The complete chemical analysis of a food such as spinach shows that it is composed mostly of water (95 percent) and that most of the solid materials are organic compounds—carbohydrate, fat, and protein. If you could remove these materials, you would find a tiny residue of minerals, vitamins, and other items. Water, carbohydrate, fat, protein, vitamins, and some of the minerals are nutrients. Some of the other materials are not.

Four of the six classes of nutrients (carbohydrate, fat, protein, and vitamins) are organic. On being oxidized during metabolism, three of these four (carbohydrate, fat, and protein) provide energy the body can use. The energy-yielding nutrients provide continual replenishment of the energy you spend daily. Without them you would soon die.

Vitamins are organic but do not provide energy to the body. They catalyze the release of energy from the other three organic nutrients. In contrast, minerals and water are inorganic nutrients. Minerals do not yield energy in the human body but, like vitamins, help to regulate the release of energy. As for water, it is the medium in which all of the body's processes take place.

The amount of energy the energy-yielding nutrients release can be measured in calories (or more properly, kilocalories, or kcalories), which are familiar to everyone as a reflection of how fattening a food is. The energy content of a food therefore depends on how much carbohydrate, fat, and protein the food contains. If you know how many grams of each nutrient a food contains, you can derive the number of kcalories in the food. Simply multiply the carbohydrate grams times 4, the fat grams times 9, and the protein grams times 4, and add them together.

If your body doesn't use the energy-yielding nutrients to fuel metabolic and physical activities, it rearranges them (and the energy they contain) into storage compounds, such as body fat, and puts them away for later use. Thus if you take in more energy than you expend, whether from carbohydrate, fat, or protein, the result is a weight gain as body fat. Too much meat (a protein-rich food) is just as fattening as too many potatoes (a carbohydrate-rich food).

---

vegetarian diets: a general term used to describe diets that exclude meat, poultry, fish, or other animal-derived foods. The **lacto-ovo vegetarian** uses milk and eggs (animal products) but excludes meat, fish, and poultry (animal flesh) from the diet. The **vegan** excludes all these foods and uses only plant foods.

nutrient: a substance obtained from food and used in the body to promote growth, maintenance, or repair.

The **essential nutrients** are those the body cannot make for itself in sufficient quantity to meet physiological needs and so has to obtain from food.

The six classes of nutrients are carbohydrate, fat, protein, vitamins, minerals, and water.

organic: carbon containing. The four organic nutrients are carbohydrate, fat, protein, and vitamins.

oxidation: a type of chemical reaction. Oxidation reactions usually result in the release of energy. In chemical oxidation of nutrients, the energy released is largely chemical and mechanical; in oxidative combustion (burning), the energy released is mostly heat and light.

Metabolism—the set of processes by which nutrients are rearranged into body structures or broken down to yield energy—is described in Chapter 6.

The major **energy-yielding nutrients** are carbohydrate and fat. Protein becomes a major fuel only when other fuels are unavailable.

kcalorie: a unit by which energy is measured. Most people speak of these units simply as calories, but on paper the word *calorie* is prefaced by a *k* for *kilocalorie*. We use *kcalories* and *kcal* throughout this book. Food energy can also be measured in kilojoules (kJ). One kcalorie equals 4.2 kJ. The kilojoule is not yet in popular use.

Calculation of the kCalories in Food

Calculate the kcalories in a bread slice that has 1 tsp butter on it (15 g carbohydrate, 2 g protein, 5 g fat).

15 g of carbohydrate at 4 kcal/g = 60 kcal.
2 g of protein at 4 kcal/g = 8 kcal.
5 g of fat at 9 kcal/g = 45 kcal.
Total = 113 kcal.

Alcohol is not a nutrient, because it does not promote growth, maintenance, or repair in the body. Alcohol does share several characteristics with the energy-yielding nutrients, however. The body metabolizes alcohol into energy, just as it metabolizes the other energy-yielding nutrients (alcohol yields 7 kcalories per gram). When taken in excess of energy need, alcohol, too, is converted to body fat and stored. However, when alcohol contributes a substantial portion of the energy in a person's diet, its effects are damaging. Nutrition in Practice 6 discusses alcohol's effects on nutrition.

Practically all foods contain mixtures of the energy-yielding nutrients, although they are sometimes classified by the predominant nutrient. Thus to speak of meat as "a protein" or of bread as "a carbohydrate" is inaccurate. Each is a food rich in a particular nutrient, but a protein-rich food such as beef contains a lot of fat along with protein, and a carbohydrate-rich food such as corn also contains fat (corn oil) and protein. Only a few foods are exceptions to this rule, the common ones being sugar (which is pure carbohydrate) and oil (which is almost pure fat).

To nourish yourself optimally, you need to eat foods that provide adequate amounts of energy and essential nutrients. To see if you have chosen appropriate foods, you need to know how much energy and how much of each nutrient you need, as well as how much the foods contain.

Recommended Nutrient Intakes

Nutrient intake recommendations, such as the Recommended Dietary Allowances (RDA) of the United States, all have the same objective—to offer a rough guideline for diet adequacy. This discussion focuses on the RDA of the United States as an example of recommended intakes; Canadian and other standards are in Appendix A. The main RDA table includes recommendations for protein, eleven vitamins, and seven minerals, while another table specifies energy needs for people of different ages, and still another presents tentative recommendations for ten more vitamins and minerals. The main table is used and referred to so often that it is presented on the inside front cover of this book. It tells you how many kcalories and how much protein, vitamin A, iron, and many other nutrients people similar to you need each day for nutritional health.

The RDA have been much misunderstood. One person, on first learning of their existence, was outraged: "You mean Uncle Sam tells me that I must eat exactly 45 grams of protein every day?" This is not the government's

RDA: Recommended Dietary Allowances. The RDA are daily recommended intakes of nutrients intended to provide for individual variations among most normal, healthy people in the United States under usual environmental stresses. (See the inside front cover.)

The U.S. RDA (see the inside back cover) used on food labels are different and are described in Nutrition in Practice 5.

Different nations and international groups have published different sets of standards similar to the RDA. The Canadian equivalent is called the **RNI, or Recommended Nutrient Intakes for Canadians.** Among the most widely used recommendations is a set developed by two international groups, the Food and Agricultural Organization and the World Health Organization (the FAO/WHO recommendations). (See Appendix A.)

requirement: the minimum amount of a nutrient that will just prevent the development of specific deficiency signs; distinguished from the RDA, which are recommended allowances that include a safety factor to provide for individual variability.

FIGURE 1–1 **Naive versus Accurate Views of Nutrient Needs**
The RDA represent a point within a range of appropriate and reasonable intakes. Nutrient intakes within the range are safe; intakes above or below the ranges may be harmful.

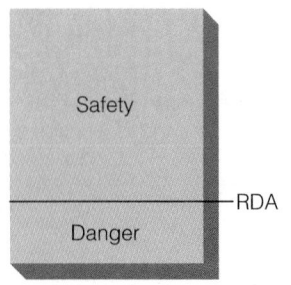

Naive view

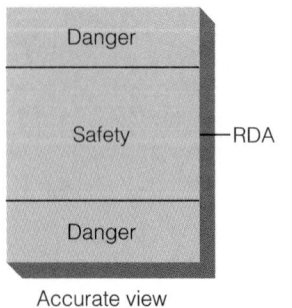

Accurate view

Diet-planning Principles:

- Adequacy.
- Balance.
- kCalorie control.
- Nutrient Density.
- Moderation.
- Variety.

intention, and the RDA are not laws, just suggestions. The following facts will help put the RDA in perspective:

- They are published by the government, but the study group that determines them is composed of highly qualified scientists selected by the National Academy of Sciences.
- The RDA are based on available scientific evidence to the greatest extent possible; they are periodically reviewed and, if necessary, revised.
- The RDA are not absolute requirements. *R* stands for *recommended,* not for *required.* They are allowances, and except for energy (see Figures 1–1 and 1–2), they are generous. Even so, they do not necessarily cover every individual for every nutrient.
- The RDA take into account the differences among individuals and define a range within which most healthy persons' intakes of nutrients probably should fall. Individuals whose needs are higher than the average are included within this range.
- The RDA are for healthy persons only. Medical problems alter nutrient needs.
- Separate recommendations are made for different sets of people: men, women, pregnant women, children, and other groups. Children aged 4 to 6 are distinguished from men and women aged 19 to 24, for example. Each individual can look up the recommendations for his or her own age and sex group.

With the understanding that the RDA are approximate, flexible, and generous, they can be used as a yardstick, not to assess the adequacy of individual diets but to measure the adequacy of diets in entire populations, such as those of the United States. Diets of individuals are often assessed by comparing them to the RDA, but such comparisons provide only rough estimates of adequacy, for individuals' needs differ unpredictably.

To evaluate your own or someone else's diet, you need not only the RDA but also a listing of the foods you or the other person ate over a period of time and a listing of the energy and nutrients in each food. An assessor uses a diet history form to obtain a record of the types and amounts of foods an individual eats (Chapter 10 provides a diet history form). The "Table of Food Composition" in the back of this book lists the energy and nutrients in several thousand foods; many computer diet analysis programs also contain these data.

Diet-Planning Principles

How can people juggle the foods available to them to create a diet that supplies all the needed nutrients in the appropriate amounts for good health? The principle is simple enough: select a variety of foods that present the nutrients your body needs. In practice, how do you do this? It helps to keep in mind six basic diet-planning principles, which are listed in the margin in alphabetical order for ease in remembering them.

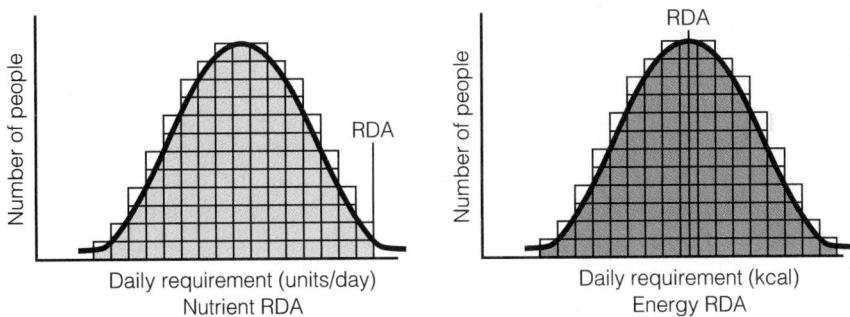

FIGURE 1–2　**The Differences between the Nutrient RDA and the Energy RDA**
The nutrient RDA are set so that nearly all people's requirements will be met by them (squares represent people). The energy RDA are set so that half the population's requirements will fall below and half above them.

The ideal of dietary adequacy has already been touched on. A diet that provides enough energy and enough of every nutrient to meet daily needs is adequate.

As for dietary balance, the essential minerals calcium and iron illustrate its importance. Meats, fish, poultry, and legumes are rich in iron but are poor sources of calcium. Similarly, milk and milk products are rich in calcium but are poor sources of iron. In fact, milk (except breast milk) and milk products are so low in iron that the overuse of these foods can actually cause iron-deficiency anemia (they displace iron-rich foods from the diet). The anemia even has a special name: milk anemia.

Use enough—but not too many—servings of meat and meat alternates for iron; use enough—but not too many—servings of milk and milk products for calcium. Save some space, too, for other foods, for a diet consisting only of milk and meat would be far from adequate. To obtain the other needed nutrients, you have to eat vegetables, fruits, grains, and other foods. In short, balance in the diet helps to ensure adequacy.

While it takes thought and skill to design an adequate, balanced diet, an added challenge is to incorporate kcalorie control—to eat an adequate, balanced diet without overeating. (Energy balance and weight control are discussed in Chapter 19.)

To this end, the concept of nutrient density helps: seek out foods that have high nutrient values per kcalorie cost. Consider foods containing iron: a 3-ounce portion of high-fat beef pot roast or water-packed tuna each provides about the same amount of iron; but the beef supplies over 300 kcalories, the tuna about 100 kcalories (see items 593 and 592 in Appendix C). The tuna, then, is more iron dense: it has the same amount of iron for a smaller number of kcalories. Both beef and tuna are nutritious in the sense that both provide substantial iron, but based on the amount of iron they offer for a given kcalorie amount, tuna has a higher nutrient density than beef.

Moderation in diet planning refers to control of food constituents that are undesirable in excess—fat, sugar, and salt. Since fat and sugar add kcalories to foods, seeking out foods with high nutrient density automatically helps control them. Consider the example of the beef and the tuna once again. The

dietary adequacy: the characteristic of a diet that provides all the essential nutrients and kcalories necessary to maintain health and body weight. Ideally, a diet will be more than just adequate; it will be optimal, providing an assortment and balance of nutrients and kcalories that maintain a favorable body weight and the best possible state of health.

dietary balance: providing foods of a number of types in balance with one another such that foods rich in one nutrient do not crowd out the foods that are rich in another nutrient.

kcalorie control: management of energy intake.

nutrient density: a characteristic of a food. A nutrient-dense food provides a high quantity (relative to need) of one or (preferably) several essential nutrients, with a small quantity (relative to need) of kcalories.

Example of nutrient density: 1 c of cola beverage and a small slice of watermelon. Each provides about 100 kcal, but the watermelon offers a little protein and some vitamins, minerals, and fiber along with its kcalories; the cola beverage does not. Watermelon is a more nutrient-dense food.

moderation: providing no unwanted constituent in excess.

tuna not only offers the same amount of iron for fewer kcalories, but it also contains far less fat than the beef. The cola and watermelon example in the margin shows that although both provide about the same number of kcalories, the watermelon delivers many more nutrients. A person who chooses watermelon over cola will need to eat fewer total kcalories to meet his or her daily nutrient needs. Among different types of fat- and sugar-containing foods, the most nutrient-dense foods are the best choices for moderation's sake.

To control salt intake might seem to require another approach, for salt contains no kcalories, and so added salt doesn't reduce the nutrient density of foods. Still, choosing nutrient-dense, low-fat, low-sugar foods does help keep your salt intake down. Why? Because manufacturers usually add all three—salt, sugar, and fat—together when they dress up foods to make them tasty. Thus pursuing nutrient density helps you keep your salt intake moderate. You may perceive that to follow this recommendation is to seek out mostly *unprocessed* foods. That is true, in the sense that additions of sugar, salt, and fat are forms of processing. But other forms of food processing are beneficial, so wait until you've learned more about processing from Nutrition in Practice 5 before attempting to generalize.

A diet can have all of the characteristics just described but still lack variety if you eat the same foods day after day. Vary your choices within each class of foods from day to day, for two reasons. First, different foods in the same group contain different arrays of nutrients. Among the fruits, for example, strawberries are especially rich in vitamin C, while peaches are rich in vitamin A. Thus variety helps ensure adequacy. Second, no food is guaranteed entirely free of constituents that in excess could harm you. (Contamination of foods is the subject of Nutrition in Practice 14.) By choosing food A today, B tomorrow, and C the day after, you ensure dilution of these contaminants within your total diet.

These diet-planning principles offer a framework of excellence to strive for in planning diets; they are dietary ideals. To plan a diet that achieves these ideals, the planner needs knowledge and skill. It helps to know which kinds of foods offer which nutrients and how many daily servings of the different foods are recommended.

dietary variety: using different foods to obtain the same nutrients on different occasions.

Four Food Group Plan: the original and widely taught eating plan, developed to ensure dietary adequacy. (It calls for a minimum of 2 servings a day of milk/milk products, 2 of meat/meat alternates, 4 of vegetables and fruits, and 4 of breads and cereals.)

Daily Food Choices pattern: a newer, more refined plan for ensuring dietary adequacy that offers five categories of foods to choose from. (It treats vegetables and fruits separately; for recommended servings see Figure 1–3.)

Food Group Plans

About 40 vitamins and minerals are needed altogether. Each nutrient has its own unique pattern of distribution in foods. It might seem quite a challenge, then, to work them all into the meals you eat, and yet people all over the world obtain fine nutrition from an astonishing variety of diets.

For many people, whether they know it or not, food plans such as the Four Food Group Plan they learned in school, or the new Daily Food Choices pattern serve as the basis for planning adequate, balanced diets. Figure 1–3 shows the Daily Food Choices pattern. Adults need to choose numbers of servings daily from each group that fall within the ranges shown. The pattern can help a diet planner design an adequate and balanced diet.

FIGURE 1–3   The Daily Food Choices Pattern

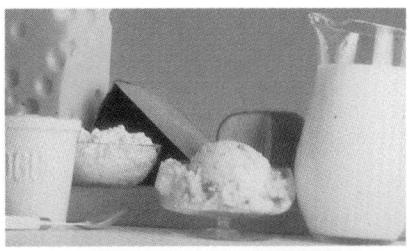

Milk and Milk Products

(These foods supply calcium, riboflavin, protein, and other nutrients.)

2 servings

Serving = 1 c milk or yogurt; 2 oz process cheese food; 1 ½ oz cheese.

■ Nonfat milk, buttermilk, low-fat milk, plain yogurt.

   Whole milk, cheese, fruit-flavored yogurt, cottage cheese.

■ Custard, milk shakes, pudding, ice cream.

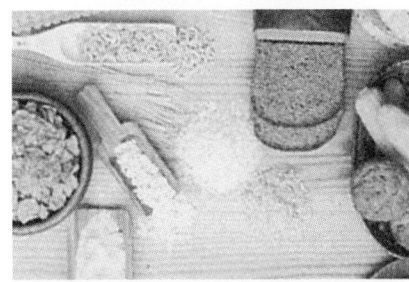

Breads and Cereals

(These foods supply riboflavin, thiamin, niacin, iron, and other nutrients.)

6 to 11 servings per day.

Serving = 1 slice bread; ½ c cooked cereal, rice, or pasta; 1 oz ready-to-eat cereal; ½ bun, bagel or English muffin; 1 small roll, biscuit, or muffin; 3 to 4 small or 2 large crackers.

■ Whole grains (wheat, oats, barley, millet, rye, bulgur), enriched breads, rolls, tortillas.

   Rice, cereals, pastas (macaroni, spaghetti), bagels.

■ Pancakes, muffins, corn bread, biscuits, presweetened cereals.

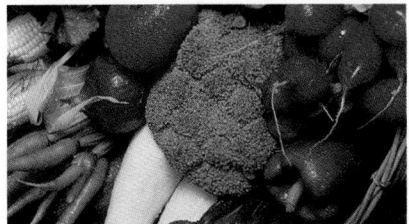

Vegetables

(These foods supply vitamin A, folate, and other nutrients.)

3 to 5 servings

Serving = ½ c cooked or raw vegetables; 1 c leafy raw vegetables.

■ Bean sprouts, broccoli, Brussels sprouts, cabbage, carrots, cauliflower, cucumbers, green beans, green peas, leafy greens (spinach, mustard, collard), lettuce, mushrooms, tomatoes, winter squash.

   Corn, potatoes.

■ Avocados, sweet potatoes.

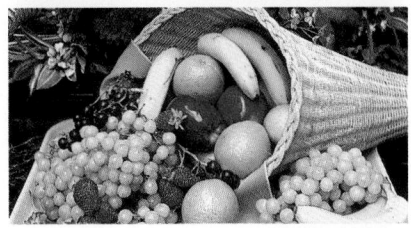

Fruits

(These foods supply vitamin C, vitamin A, potassium, and other nutrients.)

2 to 4 servings

Serving = ½ c or typical portion (1 medium apple, ½ grapefruit); ¾ c juice.

■ Apricots, cantaloupe, grapefruit, oranges, orange juice, peaches, strawberries, watermelon.

   Apples, bananas, canned fruit, pears.

■ Dried fruit.

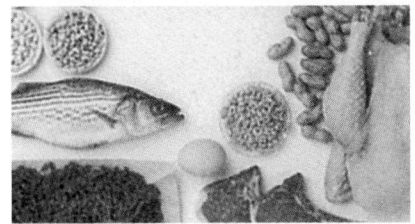

Meat, Poultry, Fish and Alternates

(These foods supply protein, iron, and other nutrients.)

2 to 3 servings

Serving = 2 to 3 oz lean, cooked meat, poultry, or fish.

Note: 1 oz. meat, poultry, or fish = 1 egg, ½ to ¾ c legumes, 2 tbsp. peanut butter.

■ Poultry, fish, lean meat (beef, lamb, pork), dried peas and beans, eggs.

   Beef, lamb, pork, refried beans.

■ Hot dogs, luncheon meats, peanut butter, nuts.

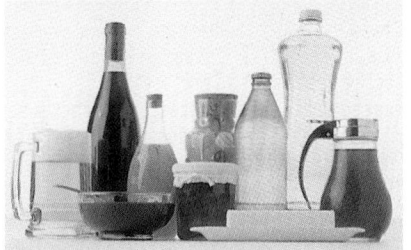

Miscellaneous Group

(These foods are not recommended in the pattern because they provide few nutrients.)

■ Miscellaneous foods not high in kcalories include spices, herbs, coffee, tea, and diet soft drinks.

■ Foods high in fat include margarine, salad dressings, oils, mayonnaise, cream, cream cheese, butter, gravy, and sauces.

■ Foods high in salt include potato chips, corn chips, pretzels, pickles, olives, bouillon, prepared mustard, soy sauce, steak sauce, salt, and seasoned salt.

■ Foods high in sugar include cakes, pies, cookies, doughnuts, sweet rolls, candy, soft drinks, fruit drinks, jelly, syrup, gelatin desserts, sugar, and honey.

■ Alcoholic beverages include wine, beer, and liquor.

KEY:
■ Foods generally highest in nutrient density.
  Foods moderate in nutrient density.
■ Foods generally lowest in nutrient density.

TABLE 1–2   **Daily Food Choices Pattern for Vegetarians**

FOOD GROUP	SERVINGS/DAY (ADULT)
Milk and milk products	2[a]
Breads and cereals (whole-grain only)	6 to 11
Vegetables	3 to 5[b]
Fruits	2 to 4
Protein-rich foods	2[c]
Legumes	2[d]

[a]If not using milk or milk products, use soy milk fortified with calcium and vitamin B_{12}.
[b]Include 1 c dark greens daily to help women meet iron requirements.
[c]Examples of protein-rich foods: cheeses and tofu.
[d]Legumes (2 c daily) should be eaten in addition to protein-rich foods to help women meet iron requirements.

A person can control kcalories while using this pattern. The foods color-coded with green boxes are the lowest in kcalories within each group; those with yellow boxes are intermediate; and those with red boxes are highest in kcalories. A person who chooses the smallest recommended number of servings, all from the green-coded foods, will obtain the needed nutrients and only about 1,200 kcalories. A person choosing the highest number of servings, also from the green-coded foods, raises the kcalorie level to about 2,000 kcalories. Beyond this, a person who needs more food energy, say to support weight gain, may substitute some of the higher-calorie selections suggested by the pattern—that is, yellow and red-coded foods.

The beauty of the Daily Food Choices pattern lies in its simplicity and ease in learning. It may appear quite rigid, but it can be used with great flexibility once its intent is understood. For example, you can substitute cheese for milk, because both supply the same nutrients (protein, calcium, and riboflavin) in about the same amounts (although cheese is generally a much-higher kcalorie, higher-fat choice than milk). Legumes are alternative choices for meats, so the lacto-ovo vegetarian can adapt the pattern by using legumes as meat selections (see Table 1–2).

Dietary Guidelines

Government authorities are now as much concerned about overnutrition as they once were about undernutrition. Several sets of dietary recommendations have originated from the awareness that overnutrition contributes to disease. Research confirms that excess intakes of fat, cholesterol, salt, sugar, and alcohol are contributing factors to many diseases, including heart disease, cancer, diabetes, and liver disease.

Among the sets of recommendations published in the United States have been the *Dietary Goals for the United States* (1977); the *Dietary Guidelines for Americans* (1990); *The Surgeon General's Report on Nutrition and Health*

overnutrition: overconsumption of food energy or nutrients sufficient to cause disease or increased susceptibility to disease; a form of malnutrition.

undernutrition: underconsumption of food energy or nutrients severe enough to cause disease or increased susceptibility to disease; a form of malnutrition.

(1988); and the report of the National Research Council (NRC) titled *Diet and Health: Implications for Reducing Chronic Disease Risk* (1989). These sets of guidelines differ somewhat from one another, but all emphasize prevention of overnutrition and disease. Table 1–3 summarizes the dietary recommendations from the 1989 *NRC Report.*

Unlike the food group plans described earlier, the NRC dietary recommendations focus not on "getting enough" but rather on "not getting too much." The recommendations state not only what people should eat but also what they should avoid. In addition, the recommendations refer to weight

TABLE 1–3   **Dietary Recommendations to the Public**

NUTRIENT AND ENERGY RECOMMENDATIONS	SUGGESTED FOOD CHOICES
Reduce total *fat* intake to 30% or less of kcalories. Reduce saturated fatty acid intake to less than 10% of kcalories and the intake of cholesterol to less than 300 mg daily.	Reduce the intake of fat and cholesterol by substituting fish, poultry without skin, lean meats, and low-fat or nonfat dairy products for fatty meats and whole-milk products; by choosing more vegetables, fruits, cereals, and legumes; and by limiting fats, oils, egg yolks, and fried and other fatty foods.
Increase intake of starches and other *complex carbohydrates.*	Every day eat five or more servings of a combination of vegetables and fruits, especially green and yellow vegetables and citrus fruits, and six or more daily servings of a combination of breads, cereals, and legumes. The committee does not recommend increasing the intake of added sugars, because their consumption is strongly associated with dental caries.
Maintain *protein* intake at moderate levels.	Meet at least the Recommended Dietary Allowances (RDA) for protein; do not exceed twice the RDA.
Balance food intake and physical activity to maintain appropriate *body weight.*	
For those who drink *alcoholic beverages,* the committee recommends limiting consumption to the equivalent of less than 1 oz pure alcohol in a single day. Pregnant women should avoid alcoholic beverages.	The committee does not recommend alcohol consumption. One ounce of pure alcohol is the equivalent of two cans of beer, two small glasses of wine, or two average cocktails.
Limit total daily intake of *salt* (sodium chloride) to 6 g or less.	Limit the use of salt in cooking, and avoid adding it to food at the table. Salty, highly processed salty, salt-preserved, and salt-pickled foods should be consumed sparingly.
Maintain adequate *calcium* intake.	
Avoid taking dietary *supplements* in excess of the RDA in any one day.	
Maintain an optimal intake of *fluoride,* particularly during the years of primary and secondary tooth formation and growth.	

Source: Adapted from the National Academy of Sciences report *Diet and Health: Implications for Reducing Chronic Disease Risk,* which was produced by the Committee on Diet and Health of the Food and Nutrition Board of the National Research Council and partially reprinted in *Nutrition Reviews* 47 (1989); 142–149.

maintenance and exercise. Some people's diets are close to these recommendations, but the typical North American diet, high in meat, needs to be altered.

> The progress of science is marked by the development of a continually changing picture of nutrition and health. Observations that don't quite fit in the old picture keep coming to light. People cannot, therefore, be dogmatic in stating nutrition facts, because observations aren't facts; they are only findings from which to generalize.
>
> Some people are fully aware that science is an evolving process, but many are uncomfortable on the shifting ground and resent having to adjust constantly in order to integrate new information. People need to become comfortable with the tasks of adjusting and integrating, and even enjoy the process, if they are to adopt a realistic attitude toward nutrition information.

How We Rate Nutritionally

Researchers use nutrition surveys to determine what foods people eat and, after calculating the nutrients in these foods, compare their findings with a standard such as the RDA. One of the first nutrition surveys, taken before World War II, suggested that up to a third of the U.S. population might be eating poorly. Programs to correct nutrition problems have been evolving ever since.

During the 1970s, public awareness of the nutrition status of U.S. citizens reached a new high. The Senate's Poverty Subcommittee and the Select Committee on Nutrition and Human Needs held hearings, widely broadcast on national television, that projected pictures of poor families unable to feed their children. Hunger and malnutrition in the United States became a controversial, political issue, disclaimed by some who said the findings were exaggerated and singled out by others who considered them a scandal and a national disgrace. The findings that generated the controversy arose from the Ten-State Survey conducted from 1968 to 1970. Other important nutrition surveys include the Health and Nutrition Examination Survey (HANES) and the Nationwide Food Consumption Survey.

The most recent Nationwide Food Consumption Survey was conducted in 1987 and 1988.[4] One of its major conclusions was that many people are overweight and obese, not so much because they overeat, as because they are extraordinarily inactive. Inactivity makes it hard, especially for women, to eat the foods available, stay within the energy allowance that will maintain appropriate weight, and still meet needs for all nutrients. Indeed, most surveys that have assessed the nutrition status of families in the United States have revealed that obtaining the proper nutrients and sufficient exercise to maintain weight while not overconsuming food energy are real concerns. There is, then, a need for everyone to choose foods intelligently in the interest of optimal health.

Study Questions

1. List five reasons why people choose the particular foods they do.
2. List the six classes of nutrients.
3. Name the energy-yielding nutrients.
4. Define the term *kcalorie*.
5. Explain how alcohol resembles nutrients, and why it is, nevertheless, not considered to be a nutrient.
6. Explain what the RDA are for.
7. List six diet-planning principles and explain the rationale for each.
8. Define the term *nutrient density* and explain why the concept of nutrient density is useful in diet planning.
9. Outline the Daily Food Choices pattern and explain how it accomplishes the objectives of diet planning.
10. Identify the main purpose behind the many different sets of dietary recommendations published since 1977.

How Balanced Is Your Diet?

Make a record of your typical food intake, and analyze it for the nutrients it contains. You will use the results over and over again in succeeding Self-Studies, so invest time and effort now to achieve maximum accuracy. You can undertake this analysis before you have learned about the nutrients; having the results in front of you as you work will help make the reading meaningful.

1. Use three copies of Form 1, and record on them all the foods you eat for a three-day period. If, like most people, you eat differently on weekdays than on weekends, then you should probably record for two weekdays and one weekend day to get a true average, or record your food intake for a week. You will learn the most from these Self-Studies if you select days that are truly typical of your food intake and physical activity.

As you record each food, make careful note of the measure. Estimate the amount to the nearest ounce, quarter cup, tablespoon, or other common measure. In guessing at the sizes of meat portions, it helps to know that a piece of meat the size of the palm of your hand weighs about 3 or 4 ounces. If you are unable to estimate serving sizes in cups, tablespoons, or teaspoons, try measuring out servings in those proportions to see how they look. It also helps to know that a slice of cheese (like sliced American cheese) or a 1½-inch cube of cheese weighs about 1 ounce.

You may have to break down mixed dishes to their ingredients. Many mixed dishes, however, including soups, are listed in the miscellaneous section at the end of Appendix C. Other mixtures are simple to analyze. A ham and cheese sandwich, for example, can be listed as two slices of bread, 1 tablespoon of mayonnaise, 2 ounces of ham, 1 ounce of cheese, and so on. If you can't identify all the ingredients, just estimate the amounts of the major ones, like the beef, tomatoes, and potatoes in a beef-vegetable soup.

You will, of course, make errors in estimating amounts. In calculations of this kind, errors of up to 20 percent are expected and tolerated. Still, your rough approximation will enable you to compare your nutrient intakes with the recommended ones.

Do not record any nutrient supplements you take. It is important for you to discover whether your food choices alone deliver the nutrients you need. If they don't, you'll have the first clues to a solution, perhaps one that involves better food choices rather than supplements.

2. Using Appendix C, calculate for each day your total intakes of kcalories, protein, fat, carbohydrate, calcium, iron, zinc, vitamin A, thiamin, riboflavin, niacin, folate, and vitamin C.

If a food you have eaten does not appear in Appendix C, read the label on the package. If you eat a packaged food in which the nutrient amounts are listed on the label as "percent of U.S. RDA," use the table on the inside back cover of the text to convert to grams, milligrams, micrograms, or retinol equivalents. Suppose a food label states that a serving contains 25 percent of the U.S. RDA of iron, for example. The table shows that the U.S. RDA for iron is 18 milligrams. The food portion therefore contributes 25 percent of 18 milligrams, or 4.5 milligrams of iron.

If a food you eat offers no information on the label, use your ingenuity to guess the composition. Use the most similar food you can find as a guide. For example, if you ate halibut (which is not listed in Appendix C), you would not be far off in using the values for haddock or perch. If you ate cream of celery soup, you might substitute the values for cream of mushroom soup.

Be careful in recording the nutrient amounts in odd-sized portions. For example, if you used ¼ cup of milk, you will have to divide the amount of every nutrient listed for a cup of milk by four. Also, note the units in which the nutrients are measured:

- Energy is measured in kcalories.
- Protein, fat, and carbohydrates are measured in grams (g).
- Calcium, iron, zinc, thiamin, riboflavin, niacin, and vitamin C are measured in milligrams (mg)—thousandths of a gram (0.001 g). Folate is measured in micrograms (µg)—thousandths of a milligram or millionths of a gram (0.001 mg or 0.000001 g). Thus, 800 mg calcium is the same as 0.8 g calcium, and 400 (µg) folate is the same as 0.4 mg folate. Be sure to convert all calcium amounts to milligrams and all folate amounts to micrograms before calculating.
- Vitamin A can be measured in international units (IU) or retinol equivalents (RE). Appendix C lists vitamin A in RE to ease comparison with the recommended intake, which is also in RE. If you eat a packaged food in which vitamin A is listed in IU on the label, be sure to convert to RE before calculating. (For more details, see Chapter 7.)

3. Now total the amount of each nutrient you've consumed for each day, and transfer your totals to Form 2. Form 2 provides a convenient means of deriving an average intake for each nutrient.
4. As a final step, transfer your average intakes to Form 3 for future reference. For comparison, enter the intakes recommended for a person of your age and sex, using either the RDA (on the inside front cover of the text) or the Recommended Nutrient Intakes for Canadians (in Appendix A), whichever you prefer. Note that no recommendations are made for intakes of fat or carbohydrate. Guidelines for these nutrients and for others, like cholesterol and fiber, are presented and discussed later. Succeeding Self-Studies will guide you in focusing on each of the nutrients provided by your diet.

Suspend judgment about the adequacy of your intakes for the moment. You have much to learn about your individuality, the nutrients, and the recommendations before you can reach any reasonable conclusions.

5. Now, check your overall food intake for balance. You can get an indication of whether you are choosing a balanced selection of foods by using the Daily Food Choices Scorecard (Form 4—one copy for each day). How does your diet score using these criteria?
6. Another way to check for balance is to evaluate your diet using the guideline that about 58 percent of your kcalories should come from carbohydrate, about 12 percent from protein, and not more than 30 percent from fat. Use Form 5 to calculate these percentages. What percentage of the food energy you consume comes from protein? _____ percent. Fat? _____ percent. Carbohydrate? _____ percent. Is your diet balanced using these criteria?

FORM 1 **Nutrient Intakes (Use one form for each day.)**

FOOD	APPROXI-MATE MEASURE OR WEIGHT	ENERGY[a] (kcal)	PROTEIN[b] (g)	FAT[b] (g)	CARBO-HYDRATE[b] (g)	CALCIUM[a] (mg)	IRON[c] (mg)	ZINC[b] (mg)	VITAMIN A[a] (RE)	THIAMIN[c] (mg)	RIBOFLA-VIN[c] (mg)	NIACIN[b] (mg)	FO-LATE[a] (μg)	VITA-MIN C[b] (mg)
Total														

[a]Compute these values to the nearest whole number.
[b]Compute these values to one decimal place.
[c]Compute these values to two decimal places.

FORM 2 **Average Daily Energy and Nutrient Intakes**

DAY	ENERGY (kcal)	PROTEIN (g)	FAT (g)	CARBO-HYDRATE (g)	CALCIUM (mg)	IRON (mg)	ZINC (mg)	VITAMIN A (RE)	THIAMIN (mg)	RIBO-FLAVIN (mg)	NIACIN (mg)	FOLATE (μg)	VITAMIN C (mg)
1													
2													
3													
Total													
Average daily intake (divide total by 3)													

FORM 3 **Comparisons with a Standard Intake**

DAY	ENERGY (kcal)	PROTEIN (g)	FAT (g)	CARBO-HYDRATE (g)	CALCIUM (mg)	IRON (mg)	ZINC (mg)	VITAMIN A (RE)	THIAMIN (mg)	RIBO-FLAVIN (mg)	NIACIN (mg)	FOLATE (μg)	VITAMIN C (mg)
Average daily intake (from Form 2)													
Standard[a]	b												
Intake as percentage of standard[c]													

[a]Taken from RDA tables (Inside front cover) or Recommended Nutrient Intakes for Canadians (Appendix A).

[b]Use your calculation for energy from Self-Study 6, the RDA tables, or Recommended Nutrient Intakes for Canadians (Appendix A).

[c]For example, if your intake was 50 g and the standard for a person your age and sex was 46g, you consumed $(50 \div 46) \nabla 100$, or 109% of the standard.

FORM 4   **Food Selection Scorecard**

FOOD GROUP AND RECOMMENDED INTAKE	YOUR INTAKE FROM GROUP (Specify Food and Amount)	YOUR SCORE
MILK AND MILK PRODUCTS— 2 or more servings (serving = 8 oz fluid milk; calcium equivalents would be 1⅓ oz hard cheese, 1⅓ c cottage cheese, 1 pt ice milk or ice cream).		
1 serving = 10 points.		
SUBTOTAL (no more than 20 points allowed).		
BREADS AND CEREALS— 6 or more servings of whole-grain or "enriched" (serving = 1 oz dry-weight cereal or 1-oz slice bread or equivalent grain product).		
1 serving cereal or 2 bread equivalents = 10 points (no more than 10 points allowed).		
Other bread equivalents = 2.5 points each.		
SUBTOTAL (no more than 20 points allowed).		
VEGETABLES— 3 or more servings (½ c cooked edible portion or 3–4 oz [100 g] raw portion).		
1 serving DARK GREEN or DEEP ORANGE—vitamin A source (any food with more than your RDA). 1 serving = 10 points (no more than 10 points allowed).		
Other vegetables = 2.5 points each.		
SUBTOTAL (no more than 20 points allowed).		
FRUITS— 2 or more portions (1 small fruit such as an apple or peach; ½ large fruit such as a banana or grapefruit; or ½ c fruit)		
1 serving VITAMIN C–RICH fruit (any fruit with more than your RDA). 1 serving = 20 points (no more than 10 points allowed.		
Other fruits = 2.5 points each.		
SUBTOTAL (no more than 40 points allowed).		
MEAT AND MEAT ALTERNATES— 2 or more servings (serving = 2–3 oz cooked lean meat, fish, poultry; protein equivalents would be 2 eggs, 2 oz hard cheese, 1 c cooked legume, 4 tbsp peanut butter, 1 oz nuts or sunflower seeds). Count cheese *either* in milk group or in meat group, not both.		
1 serving = 10 points.		
GRAND TOTAL (no more than 100 points).		

The above are FOUNDATION FOODS. ADDITIONAL FOODS are those that do not fit into the above groupings but add flavor, interest, variety, and (often) kcalories. List those eaten.

_____   _____   _____   _____

_____   _____   _____   _____

_____   _____   _____   _____

FORM 5   **Percentage of kCalories from Protein, Fat, and Carbohydrate**

Average daily intakes from Form 2:

Protein: g/day × 4 kcal/g = (P)_____ kcal/day.

Fat: g/day × 9 kcal/g = (F)_____ kcal/day.

Carbohydrate: g/day × 4 kcal/g = (C)_____ kcal/day.

Total kcal/day = (T)_____ kcal/day.

Percentage of kcalories from protein: $\dfrac{(P)}{(T)} \times 100 =$ _____ % of total kcalories.

Percentage of kcalories from fat: $\dfrac{(F)}{(T)} \times 100 =$ _____ % of total kcalories.

Percentage of kcalories from carbohydrate: $\dfrac{(C)}{(T)} \times 100 =$ _____ % of total kcalories.

Note: The three percentages can total 99, 100, or 101, depending on the way in which figures were rounded off earlier.

If you used an alcoholic beverage, you have to add a line for kcalories from alcohol. To find out how many kcalories in the beverage were from alcohol, look the beverage up in Appendix C. Figure out how many kcalories were from carbohydrate (multiply carbohydrate grams times 4), fat (fat grams times 9), and protein (protein grams times 4). The remaining kcalories were from alcohol.

Notes

1. C. Jackson, Today's food consumers: What they are looking for in a supermarket, *Cereal Foods World* 32 (1987): 417–419.

2. Position of the American Dietetic Association: Vegetarian diets—Technical support paper, *Journal of the American Dietetic Association* 88 (1988): 353–355.

3. D. T. Farr, Consumer attitudes and the supermarket, *Cereal Foods World* 32 (1987): 413–415.

4. Federation of American Societies for Experimental Biology, Life Sciences Research Office, *Nutrition Monitoring in the United States: An Update Report on Nutrition Monitoring,* U.S. Department of Health and Human Services (Washington, D.C.: Government Printing Office, 1989).

1

Professionals Who Deal with Nutrition

With nutrition receiving so much attention in the popular press, it is easy to be overwhelmed with conflicting information. In fact, determining whether nutrition information is accurate may be one of your most challenging tasks. It should also be one of the most important, since nutrition affects both your professional and your personal life.

Everyone seems to be giving advice on nutrition. How can I tell whom to listen to?

Registered dietitians (R.D.'s) or nutrition professionals with advanced degrees (M.S., Ph.D.) are experts (see the Miniglossary). These people are probably in the best position to answer your nutrition questions. On the other hand, "nutritionists" may be experts or quacks, depending on the state they are practicing in. Some states require strict credentials for people to use this title; others do not, and a "nutritionist" may be any individual who claims a career connection with the nutrition field.

In contrast, a health food store owner may be in the nutrition business simply because it is a lucrative market. Such a person may have a background in business or sales and no education in nutrition at all. Such a person is not qualified to provide nutrition information to customers. To effectively communicate nutrition information requires a

trained professional with a knowledge of nutrition—an expert in the field of dietetics.

What about other health care professionals?

All members of the health care team share responsibility for helping each client to achieve optimal health, but the registered dietitian (R.D.) remains the primary nutrition expert. Each other team member has a related specialty. Physicians, nurses, and dietetic technicians (D.T.R.'s) often assist dietitians in providing nutrition information and may help to administer direct nutrition care. Nurses play central roles in client care management and client relationships. Visiting nurses and home health care nurses may become intimately involved in clients' nutrition care at home, teaching them both theory and cooking techniques. Physical therapists can provide individualized exercise programs related to nutrition—for example, to help control obesity. Social workers may provide practical and emotional support.

What roles might these health professionals play in nutrition care?

Some of the responsibilities of the health care professional might be:

- Helping people understand why nutrition is important to them.
- Answering questions about food and diet.
- Explaining to clients how modified diets work.
- Collecting information about clients that may influence their nutrition health.
- Spotting clients at risk for poor nutrition status (see Chapter 10) and taking appropriate action.
- Recognizing when clients need more help with nutrition problems (in such cases, the problems should be referred to someone who can help—a dietitian or physician).

Health care professionals might routinely perform these nutrition-related tasks:

- Obtaining diet histories.
- Weighing and measuring height.
- Feeding clients who cannot feed themselves.
- Recording what clients eat or drink.
- Observing clients' responses and reactions to foods.
- Helping clients mark menus.
- Monitoring weight changes.

- Monitoring food and drug interactions.
- Encouraging clients to eat.
- Assisting clients at home in planning their diets and in managing their kitchen chores.

As you can see, although the dietitian assumes the primary role as the nutrition expert on a health care team, other health care professionals play important roles in administering nutrition care.

MINIGLOSSARY

dietetic technician registered (D.T.R.): a trained professional who has earned an associate degree or higher; has completed a dietetic technician program approved by the American Dietetic Association (ADA); has passed a national registration exam; and assists in planning, implementing, and evaluating nutritional care.

dietetics: the practical application of nutrition, including the assessment of nutrition status, recommendation of appropriate diets, nutrition education, and the planning and servicing of meals.

nutritionist: a person who specializes in the study of nutrition.

Some nutritionists are registered dietitians, but others are self-described experts whose training may be minimal or nonexistent. Some states make the term meaningful by allowing it to apply only to people who have master's (M.S.) or doctoral (Ph.D.) degrees from institutions accredited to offer such degrees in nutrition or related fields.

registered dietitian (R.D.): a trained professional in dietetics with a bachelor's (B.S.) degree in nutrition or food science, a year's internship or the equivalent, and a passing score on the four-hour qualifying exam administered by the ADA or the Canadian Dietetic Association (CDA).

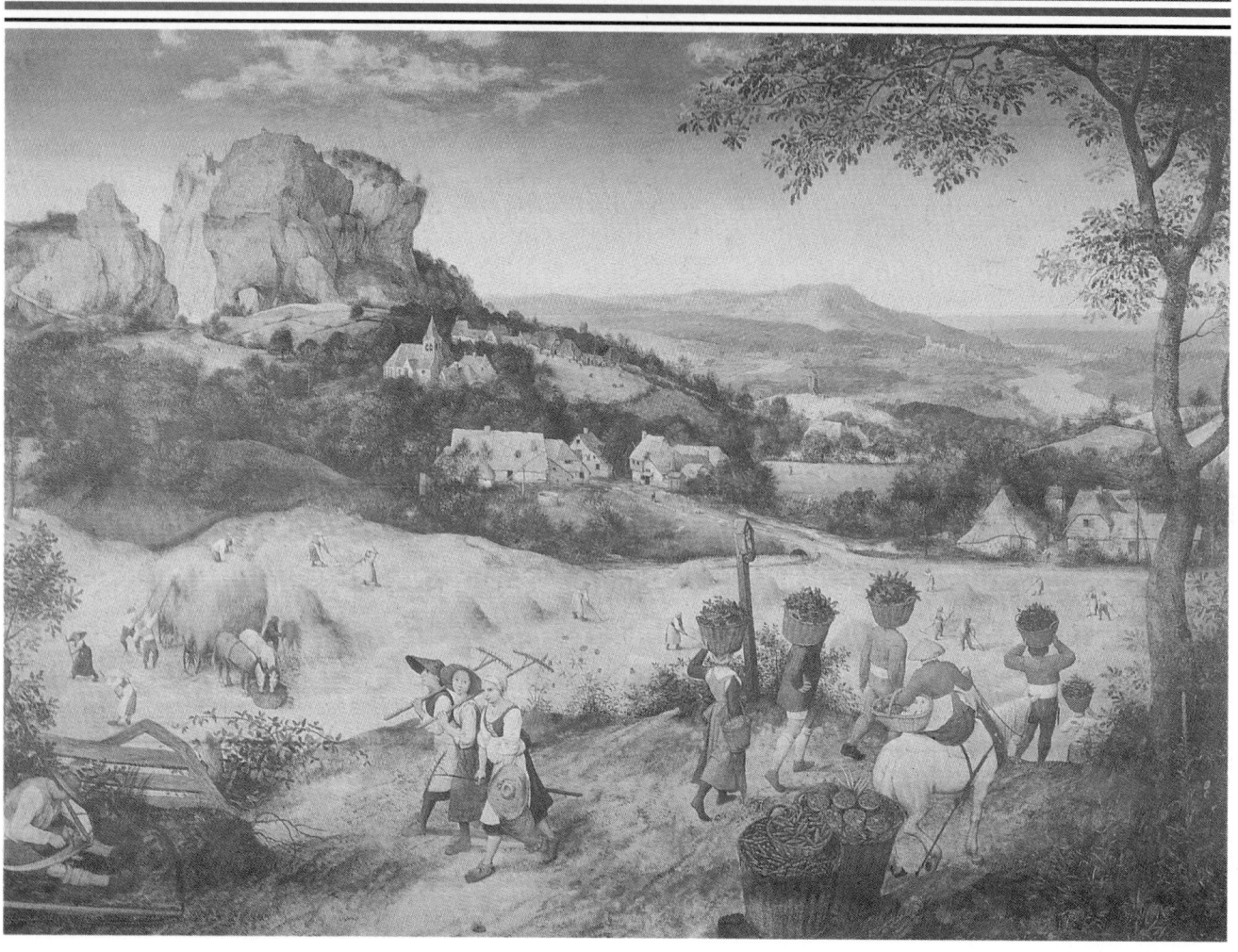

Pieter Brueghel the Elder, La Fenaison; Prague, Narodni Gallery, Giraudon/ Art Resource, N.Y.

2

Carbohydrates

CONTENTS

CHAPTER

2

Most people would like to feel good all the time. The enjoyment available in a day, no matter what the day may bring, can be tremendous when a person's body and mind are tuned for it. The feeling of well-being that comes with energy, alertness, clear thinking, and confidence is so rewarding that if you know how to produce it, you will probably make the necessary effort. Part of the secret of feeling well is keeping your energy supply going, from food. That means (from Chapter 1) choosing foods that contain the energy nutrients—carbohydrate and fat, primarily. But which to choose?

Carbohydrate is the preferred energy source for most of the body's functions; fat is next. The other energy sources available to the body—protein and alcohol—offer no advantage over carbohydrate as energy sources. For example, protein is best left to serve its own diverse functions, as you will see in Chapter 4. Alcohol, of course, has its own well-known undesirable side effects. Carbohydrate is the body's fuel of choice, for even fat has disadvantages: fat is not normally used as fuel by the brain and central nervous system, and diets high in fat are associated with many disease states.

Carbohydrate performs tremendous services for the body. As long as carbohydrate is available to the body, the human brain depends exclusively on it as an energy source. Athletes eat a "high-carb" diet to store as much muscle fuel as possible, and dietary recommendations urge people to eat carbohydrate-rich foods for better health. And where can you find carbohydrate-rich foods? Almost exclusively among the plants; milk is the only animal-derived food that contains significant amounts of carbohydrate.

The Chemist's View of Carbohydrates

Chemists divide the carbohydrates into two categories: simple and complex. The simple carbohydrates (sugars) are:

- Monosaccharides (single sugars).
- Disaccharides (double sugars).

White table sugar is one of the disaccharides. The complex carbohydrates (polysaccharides) are:

- Starch.
- Glycogen.
- Some fibers.

All of these carbohydrates are composed of the simple sugar glucose and other compounds that are much like glucose in composition and structure (see Table 2–1).

Monosaccharides (Single Sugars)

The body's cells almost all use glucose as their chief energy source. Most of the other carbohydrates they convert to glucose for use. The body obtains this glucose from plant foods. Plants capture the sun's radiant energy, and through the process of photosynthesis trap this energy in glucose.

carbohydrate: an energy nutrient composed of monosaccharides.
 carbo = carbon
 hydrate = water

simple carbohydrates: the monosaccharides (glucose, fructose, and galactose) and the disaccharides (sucrose, lactose, and maltose); also called the sugars.

complex carbohydrates: long chains of sugars arranged as starch or fiber; also called polysaccharides.

monosaccharide: a single sugar unit.

disaccharide: a pair of sugar units bonded together.

polysaccharide: another term for complex carbohydrates, compounds of many sugar units bonded together.

glucose: a monosaccharide, the sugar common to all disaccharides and polysaccharides; sometimes known as blood sugar, sometimes as grape sugar; also called dextrose.

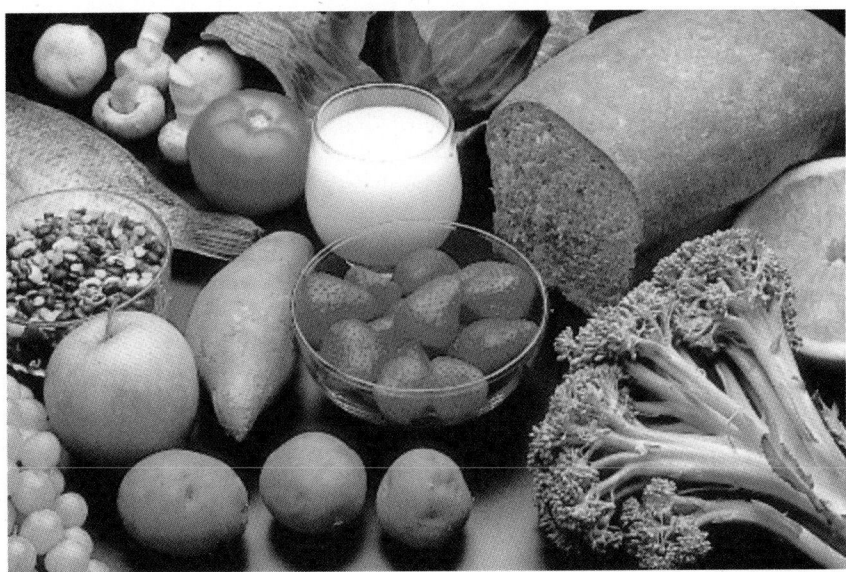

Carbohydrate-rich foods are found almost exclusively among the plants: milk is the only animal-derived food that is rich in carbohydrate.

Another sugar plants make is fructose. Fructose, the sweetest of the sugars, is abundant in fruits, honey, and saps. The body can convert fructose to glucose, or can break it down to fragments from which fat can be made. Glucose and fructose are the most common single sugars in nature. A third single sugar, galactose, does not appear singly in nature, but as part of the double sugar known as milk sugar (lactose), in which it is paired with glucose. During digestion galactose is freed as a single sugar.

fructose: a monosaccharide; sometimes known as fruit sugar. It is abundant in fruits, honey, and saps.
fruct = fruit

galactose: a monosaccharide; part of the disaccharide lactose.

Disaccharides (Double Sugars)

Some sugars, known as disaccharides, come as pairs of single sugars linked together. Lactose is one example, just mentioned, and there are two others. All three have glucose as one of the single sugars in them. The other single sugar is either another glucose (in maltose), or galactose (in lactose), or fructose (in sucrose).

Sucrose (table, or white, sugar) is the most familiar of the three disaccharides. This sugar is usually obtained by refining the juice from sugar beets or sugarcane to provide the brown, white, and powdered sugars available in the supermarket, but it occurs naturally in many fruits and vegetables.

sucrose: a disaccharide composed of glucose and fructose; commonly known as table sugar, beet sugar, or cane sugar.
sucro = sugar

TABLE 2–1   **The Major Sugars**

MONOSACCHARIDES	DISACCHARIDES
Glucose ●	Maltose ●—●
Fructose ▲	Sucrose ●—▲
Galactose ■	Lactose ●—■
(found only as part of lactose)	

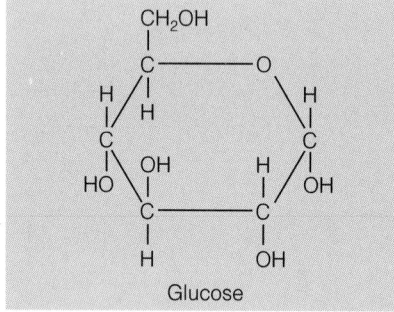

Glucose: the body's principal energy fuel.

Glucose

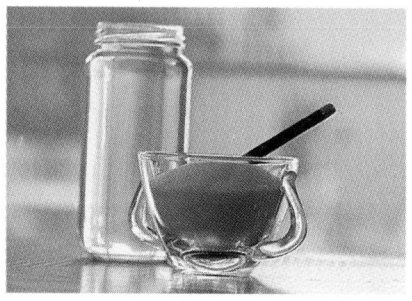

Honey, like sugar, contains glucose and fructose.

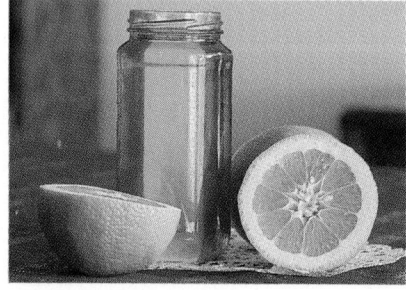

You receive the same sugars from an orange as from honey or sugar, but the packaging makes the difference.

lactose: a disaccharide composed of glucose and galactose; commonly known as milk sugar.
  lact = milk

maltose: a disaccharide composed of two glucose units; sometimes known as malt sugar.

When you eat a food containing sucrose, enzymes in your digestive tract split the sucrose to yield glucose and fructose. One molecule of sucrose can ultimately yield two molecules of glucose.

> What is the difference between honey and white sugar? Is honey more nutritious? Honey, like white sugar, contains glucose and fructose. The difference is that in white sugar, the glucose and fructose are bonded together in pairs, while in honey some of them are and some of them are not. When you eat either white sugar or honey, though, your body breaks the sugars they contain all apart into single sugars. It ultimately makes no difference, then, whether you eat single sugars linked together, as in white sugar, or the same sugars unlinked, as in honey; they will end up as single sugars in your body. True, honey contains trace amounts of a few vitamins and minerals, but to say that honey is nutritious is misleading.
>
> This is not to say that there are no differences between sugar sources. Consider a fruit such as an orange. From an orange you receive the same sugars and about the same energy as from a tablespoon of sugar or honey, but the packaging makes the difference. The fruit's sugars are diluted in a large volume of water that contains valuable vitamins and minerals, and the flesh and skin of the fruit are supported by fibers that also offer health benefits. A cola beverage, containing many teaspoons of sugar, has none of these nutrients either. Table 2–2 shows the vitamin and mineral contents of some sugar sources; note the "0s" and "< 1's" by honey, sugar, and the cola beverage and the substantial numbers by the others. Sucrose is often the principal ingredient of carbonated beverages, candy, cakes, frostings, cookies, and other concentrated sweets.

Lactose is the principal carbohydrate of milk. A human baby is born with the digestive enzymes necessary to split lactose into its two monosaccharide parts, glucose and galactose, so as to absorb it. Breast milk thus provides a simple, easily digested carbohydrate to meet a baby's energy needs; most formulas do too, because they are made from milk.

Some people lose the ability to digest lactose after infancy. This condition, known as lactose intolerance, occurs in about 70 percent of Native American, Asian, African, Mediterranean, and Middle Eastern people. Lactose intolerance is not the same as the commonly observed milk allergy, which is caused by an immune reaction to the protein in milk. Lactose intolerance is discussed further in Chapter 20, and milk allergy in Chapter 12.

The third disaccharide, maltose, is a plant sugar that consists of two glucose units. Maltose is found at only one stage in the life of a plant—when the plant is digesting its stored starch for energy and sprouting.

In summary, then, the major simple carbohydrates, or sugars, are the three single sugars and the three double sugars shown earlier in Table 2–1. Glucose, fructose, maltose, and sucrose are from plants; lactose and galactose, from milk and milk products.

TABLE 2–2 **Sample Nutrients in Sugars and Other Foods**
The indicated portion of any of these foods would provide approximately 100 kcal. Notice what nutrients the eater receives along with the energy.

FOOD	SIZE OF 100-KCAL PORTION	CARBOHYDRATE (g)	Percentage of U.S. RDA[a]				
			PROTEIN	CALCIUM	IRON	VITAMIN A	THIAMIN
Milk, low-fat	¾ c	9	17	26	—	3	5
Kidney beans	½ c	21	12	4	13	< 1	9
Watermelon	4-by-8-inch wedge	23	3	3	12	50	9
Bread, whole wheat	1½ slices	19	7	4	7	—	9
Sugar, white	2 tbsp	24	0	0	0	0	0
Molasses, blackstrap	2 tbsp	22	0	27	35	0	3
Cola beverage	1 c	26	0	0	0	0	0
Honey, strained or extracted	1 ½ tbsp	26	—	< 1	1	0	—

[a]Percentages are rounded to the nearest whole number. A dash means the percentage has not been determined and is not significant. The U.S. RDA are recommended adult intakes (see inside back cover).

Source: Adapted from E. N. Whitney, E. M. N. Hamilton, and S. R. Rolfes, *Understanding Nutrition,* 5th ed. (St. Paul: West, 1990), pp. 82.

Starch and Glycogen (Energy-Yielding Polysaccharides)

The sugars contain three monosaccharides in different combinations. In contrast, the polysaccharides important in nutrition, starch and glycogen, are composed almost entirely of only one monosaccharide—glucose. The differences between starch and glycogen have to do with the bonds that link glucose into the large molecules of starch and glycogen.

Starch is a long, straight, or branched chain of hundreds of glucose units linked together. These giant molecules are packed side by side in the rice grain or potato root—as many as a million per cubic inch of food. When you eat the plant, your body splits the starch to glucose and uses the glucose for energy.

All starchy foods are plant foods. Grains are the richest food source of starch. Most human societies have a staple grain on which their people depend for much of their food energy: rice in Asia; wheat in Canada, the United States, and Europe; corn in much of Central and South America; and millet, rye, barley, and oats elsewhere.

A second important source of starch is the legume (bean and pea) family, including peanuts and "dry" beans such as butter beans, kidney beans,

starch: a plant polysaccharide composed of glucose and digestible by humans.

glycogen (GLY-co-gen): a polysaccharide composed of glucose, made and stored by liver and muscle tissues of human beings and animals as a storage form of glucose. Glycogen is not a significant food source of carbohydrate and is not counted as one of the complex carbohydrates in foods.

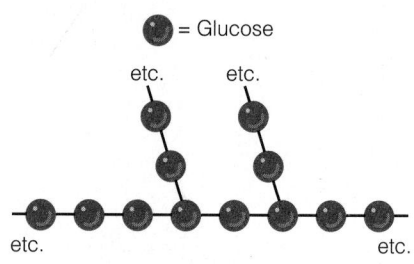

= Glucose

Portion of a starch molecule

Starch can be broken down to shorter chains of glucose units, known as **dextrins**. The word sometimes appears on food labels, because dextrins can be used as thickening agents in foods.

fiber: a general term denoting in plant foods the polysaccharides cellulose, hemicellulose, pectins, gums, and mucilages, as well as the nonpolysaccharide lignins, that are not attacked by human digestive enzymes.

cellulose (CELL-you-loce): a plant polysaccharide composed of glucose, indigestible by humans; one of the fibers.

dietary fiber: the residue of plant food resistant to human digestive enzymes; that is, the fiber that remains from food after digestion in the body.

"baked" beans, black-eyed peas (cowpeas), chick-peas (garbanzo beans), and soybeans. These legumes are not only rich in starch and dietary fiber, but also contain abundant protein. Root vegetables (tubers) such as potatoes and yams are a third major source of starch, and in many non-Western societies, they are the primary starch sources.

Other than forming starch, glucose can be bonded in another way to form chains of glycogen, which are more complex and highly branched than starch is. As starch stores energy for plants, glycogen stores energy for human beings and animals. Because glycogen does not occur in plants, and is found in meats only to a limited extent, it is not important as a nutrient. Its role as a readily available source of glucose in the body is nevertheless an important one.

A third polysaccharide, cellulose, is composed of glucose units, too, but bonded together in still another way. Cellulose is not digestible by humans, so it is classed not as an energy source but as a nonnutritive fiber, discussed next.

The Fibers

Plant foods contain many fibers, predominantly as constituents of the plants' cell walls. These fibers are not digested by the enzymes in people's digestive tracts. Fibers include the polysaccharides cellulose, hemicellulose, gums, pectins, and mucilages, as well as the nonpolysaccharide lignins.

Although cellulose and other fibers are not attacked by human enzymes, some fibers can be digested by bacteria in the human digestive tract and can yield some absorbable products. Food fibers are therefore not totally energy-free, although they vary in energy contribution depending on the extent to which they break down in the body. For the most part, the energy contribution of fibers is considered negligible, although it can be as high as 15 percent of the daily intake on a high-fiber diet.[1]

Dietary fibers are classified according to several characteristics, including their chemical structure, their digestibility by bacterial enzymes, and their solubility in water. These distinctions influence the health effects of fibers. For example, some fibers delay the time it takes materials to pass through the intestine, whereas other fibers accelerate transit time. These and other health effects of fibers are discussed in a later section.

Health Effects and Recommended Intakes of Carbohydrates

Despite dietary recommendations that people should eat generous servings of complex carbohydrate–rich foods for their health, many people still believe that carbohydrate is the "fattening" component of foods. Since carbohydrates contain the same food energy per gram as protein and fewer kcalories than fat, it is erroneous to say that they are more fattening. This point was emphasized by the Senate committee that produced the *Dietary Goals for the United States* when it made the observation that a young man could include as many as 12 slices of bread in a day's meal plan and still lose over a pound a week.[2]

Dietary recommendations state that carbohydrates should contribute 55 to 60 percent of the total daily energy intake. Concentrated sweets, however, should account for only 10 percent or less of total kcalories. For most people this means total carbohydrate intake should increase while sugar intake should decline. Starch- and fiber-rich foods such as vegetables, grains, legumes, and fruits are the carbohydrate-rich foods to emphasize. The sugar in vegetables and fruits, like that in milk, is acceptable because it is accompanied by many nutrients. In contrast, concentrated sweets, accompanied by relatively few nutrients and high in kcalories, should be limited.

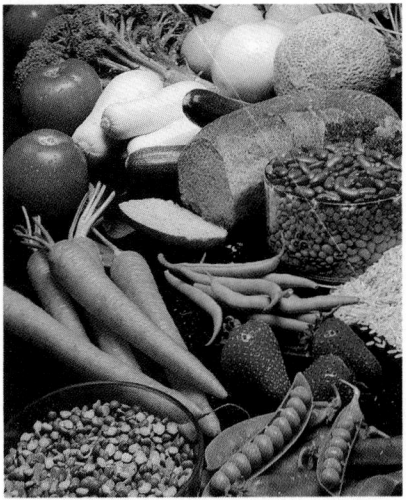

Starch and fiber-rich foods are the foods to emphasize.

Sugar

Many people today eat at least 100 pounds of sugar a year, which represents about 25 percent of the total food energy they consume. Recommendations that people reduce their consumption of concentrated sugar to 10 percent or less of total kcalories stem from widely published research reports during the 1970s.[3] These reports implicated sugar (mainly sucrose) as a possible contributing factor in several diseases. Since then, many accusations have been made against sugar, but the Food and Drug Administration and, more recently, the National Academy of Sciences have concluded that in the amounts people currently consume, sugar carries no proven health risk. Still, the controversy continues.[4] A brief description of accusations pertaining to sugar's effects on health may help clarify the issues. The accusations include:

- Sugar causes obesity.
- Sugar causes diabetes.
- Sugar causes heart disease.
- Sugar causes disruptive behavior (hyperactivity) in children.
- Sugar causes dental caries.

On the first accusation, that sugar causes obesity, the facts are these. Population studies show that obesity rises as sugar consumption increases, but that sugar is not the sole cause. Wherever sugar intakes increase, usually fat and total energy intakes do, too. Simultaneously, physical activity declines. Thus sugar can contribute to obesity, but does not, by itself, cause obesity.

On sugar's relation to diabetes, the evidence is conflicting and interesting. In many parts of the world, as sugar consumption has increased, a profound increase in the incidence of one type of diabetes (Type II) has occurred. Yet in other populations, no relationship has been found between diabetes and sugar consumption. Body fatness seems to be more related to diabetes than diet is: the majority of people with Type II diabetes are overweight or obese, and evidence shows that weight reduction improves the condition. Thus the fairest conclusion is that obesity is a major factor in the causation of Type II diabetes, and that sugar may be a causative factor only if and when it contributes to obesity. Chapter 20 talks more about diabetes.

In relation to heart disease, fat, not sugar, is clearly the major dietary culprit in most people's susceptibility (see Chapter 3). However, in a special subgroup of the population—"carbohydrate-sensitive" individuals—carbohydrate, including sugar, seems to worsen the risk of heart disease.* For most people, moderate sugar intake does not influence the risk of heart disease.

The accusation that sugar causes hyperactive behavior in children stands unproven. Clearly, sugary food, like any energy-containing food, will enable children to do more of whatever they want to do—including misbehave, if they were programmed to misbehave already. If sugar is related to behavior problems in children, it is probably because when sugary foods take the place of nutrient-dense foods in children's diets, nutrient deficiencies are likely. Many different nutrient deficiencies adversely affect behavior. A lack of nutrients in children's diets, not sugar itself, can in some cases contribute to adverse behavior.

On sugar's causing dental caries, the evidence says yes. But any carbohydrate-containing food, including bread, bananas, or milk, as well as sugar, can support the bacterial growth in the mouth that produces the acid that eats away tooth enamel. Nutrition in Practice 2 discusses nutrition and dental health.

In summary, moderate sugar consumption (5 to 10 percent of total kcalories) is recommended—enough for pleasure, but not enough to displace more nutritious foods. Sugar is a delicious, concentrated source of food energy, but it contains no protein, vitamins, or minerals. If you eat it at the expense of nutrient and fiber-rich foods, malnutrition is likely.

People often fail to recognize sugar in all its forms, and so fail to realize how much they consume. To estimate how much sugar you consume, treat all of the following concentrated sweets as equivalent to 1 teaspoon of white sugar:

1 teaspoon brown sugar, candy, jam, jelly, corn sweetener, syrup, honey, molasses, or maple sugar.

1 tablespoon catsup.

1½ ounces carbonated soft drink.

These portions of sugar all provide about the same number of kcalories. Some are closer to 10 kcalories (for example, 14 kcalories for molasses), while some are over 20 (22 kcalories for honey); an average figure of 20 kcalories is an acceptable approximation. The accompanying Miniglossary presents the multitude of names that denote sugar on food labels.** Nutrition in Practice 20 discusses sugar substitutes.

---

*Carbohydrate-sensitive individuals have an abnormally high plasma insulin response to an oral carbohydrate challenge. The ability of insulin to stimulate glucose uptake is reduced in such individuals; the body responds by releasing abnormally high levels of insulin. In carbohydrate-sensitive individuals, high blood lipids are seen when dietary sucrose is increased. Sugar may also worsen the risk of heart disease in people with Type II diabetes.[5]

**New FDA regulations affect the listing of sweeteners on food labels. Once new regulations are in effect, manufacturers must list all sweeteners together in the ingredient list under the collective term "sweeteners." For example, instead of itemizing "sugar, corn syrup, and molasses," the product would list "sweeteners." The term "sweeteners" appears in the order of predominance appropriate for the *sum* of the sweeteners in the product.

MINIGLOSSARY of Sugars

brown sugar: sugar crystals contained in molasses syrup with natural flavor and color; 91 to 96% pure sucrose. (Some refiners add syrup to refined white sugar to make brown sugar.)

confectioners' sugar: finely powdered sucrose; 99.9% pure.

corn sweeteners: corn syrup and sugars derived from corn.

corn syrup: a syrup produced by the action of enzymes on cornstarch, containing mostly glucose. See also *high-fructose corn syrup (HFCS)*.

dextrose: an older name for glucose.

fructose, galactose, glucose: already defined (pp. 26 and 27).

granulated sugar: crystalline sucrose; 99.9% pure.

high-fructose corn syrup (HFCS): the predominant sweetener used in processed foods today. HFCS is mostly fructose; glucose makes up the balance.

honey: sugar formed from nectar (mostly sucrose) gathered by bees. An enzyme splits the sucrose into glucose and fructose. Composition and flavor vary, but honey always contains a mixture of sucrose, fructose, and glucose.

invert sugar: a mixture of glucose and fructose formed by the splitting of sucrose in a chemical process. Sold only in liquid form; sweeter than sucrose; invert sugar is used as an additive to help preserve food freshness and prevent shrinkage.

lactose: already defined (p. 28).

levulose: a name for fructose.

maltitol, mannitol, sorbitol, xylitol: sugar alcohols, which can be derived from fruits or commercially produced from dextrose; absorbed more slowly, and metabolized differently, than other sugars in the human body, and not readily utilized by ordinary mouth bacteria.

maltose: already defined (p. 28).

maple sugar: a sugar (mostly sucrose) purified from concentrated sap of the sugar maple tree. Maple sugar is expensive compared with other sweeteners.

molasses: a thick brown syrup, left over from sugarcane juice during sugar refining. It retains residual sugar and other by-products and a few minerals; blackstrap molasses contains significant amounts of calcium and iron—the iron from the machinery used to process it.

raw sugar: the first crop of crystals harvested during sugar processing. Raw sugar cannot be sold in the United States because it contains too much filth (dirt, insect fragments, and the like). Sugar sold domestically as raw sugar has actually gone through about half of the refining steps.

sucrose: already defined (p. 27).

turbinado (ter-bih-NOD-oh) sugar: raw (brown) sugar from which the filth has been washed; legal to sell in the United States.

white sugar: pure sucrose, produced by dissolving, concentrating, and recrystallizing raw sugar.

Complex Carbohydrates

The health benefits you can expect from a diet high in complex carbohydrate foods and low in concentrated sugar are many and wonderful. Such a diet is inevitably low in fat; low in energy; and high in fiber, vitamins, and minerals. All these factors working together can help reduce the risks of obesity, cancer, cardiovascular disease, diabetes, dental caries, and malnutrition.

There is no RDA for carbohydrate, but there is a recommendation that 55 to 60 percent of total kcalories should come from carbohydrate. For people who eat about 2,000 kcalories a day, the recommended intake would be 1,100 kcalories (55 percent) to 1,200 kcalories (60 percent) from carbohydrate, or, at 4 kcalories per gram, 275 to 300 grams of carbohydrate a day. Consider that most of this carbohydrate should be starch, not sugars, and that a single slice of bread contains 15 grams of starch; you can see that many servings of starchy foods are needed to meet this recommendation. For example, starting with the smallest number of recommended servings from the Daily Food Choices Pattern in Chapter 1 (Figure 1–3) as a core, it takes additional servings of carbohydrate-rich foods to obtain this much carbohydrate. You would need 3 rather than 2 cups of milk, 6 rather than 2 servings of fruits, 6 rather than 3 servings of vegetables, and 8 rather than 6 servings from the bread and cereal group to total about 275 grams of carbohydrate. Figure 2–1 offers a delicious example of meals that provide about 2,000 kcalories and 275 grams of carbohydrate from nutrient-dense, fiber-rich foods. The carbohydrate content of a diet can be determined by using a nutrient composition table such as that found in Appendix C, or by using the exchange list system described in Chapter 19.

It is difficult to sort out which carbohydrates contribute to which health benefits. For example, starch and fiber almost always occur together in foods (except refined foods), so it is hard to distinguish their effects. The next section discusses the health effects that appear to be closely associated with fibers.

Fiber Intake

Fiber benefits health in many ways. Fiber is thought to play a beneficial role in the prevention or management of:

- *Weight control.* Fibrous foods contribute little energy and promote a feeling of fullness as they absorb water. A diet high in fiber-rich foods can promote weight loss if those foods displace concentrated fats and sweets.
- *Constipation, hemorrhoids, and diarrhea.* Fibers that attract water into the digestive tract soften stools and relieve constipation and hemorrhoids. Other fibers help to solidify watery stools.
- *Appendicitis.* Fiber keeps the contents of the intestinal tract moving easily, which helps prevent bacterial infection.
- *Diverticulosis.* Fiber stimulates the muscles of the digestive tract so that they retain their health and tone; this prevents the muscles from becoming weak and bulging out in places, as they do in diverticulosis.
- *Colon cancer.* Fiber speeds up the passage of food materials through the digestive tract, thus helping to prevent exposure of the tissue to cancer-causing agents in food.

FIGURE 2–1   **A Day's Meals That Meet the Carbohydrate Recommendation within 2,000-kCalories (Example)**

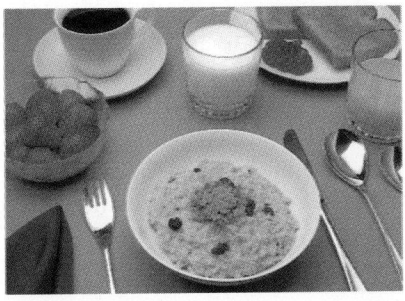

Breakfast

1 c coffee
1 c oatmeal with 2 tbsp raisins
1 c 2% low-fat milk
1¼ c strawberries
1 piece whole-wheat toast
2 tsp jelly
½ c orange juice

■ Total kcal: 2,000
■ 61% kcal from carbohydrate.
■ 24% kcal from fat.
■ 15% kcal from protein.

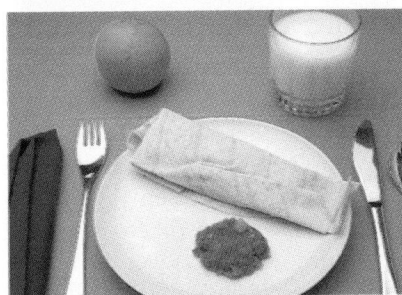

Lunch

1 bean burrito
1 orange
1 c 2% low-fat milk

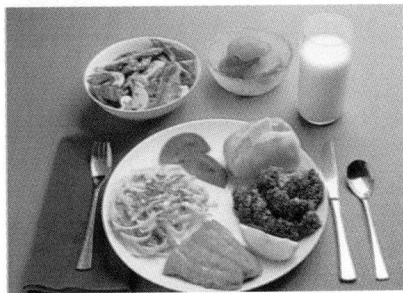

Dinner

A salad made with:
   1 c raw spinach leaves
   1 tbsp sesame seeds
   ¼ c fresh mushroom slices
   ¼ c water chestnuts
   ⅓ c garbanzo beans
   1 tbsp vinaigrette dressing
4 oz shrimp with ⅛ lemon
1 c broccoli

1 tomato
1 dinner roll
2 tsp butter
½ c noodles tossed with 2 tsp butter and
¼ c parsley
½ c sherbet
1 c 2% low-fat milk

■ *Heart disease.* Some fibers bind cholesterol compounds and carry them out of the body with the feces, thus lowering the body's cholesterol concentration and possibly the risk of heart disease.

■ *Diabetes.* Some fibers improve the body's handling of glucose, perhaps by slowing down the digestion or absorption of carbohydrate.

Even with all these advantages, carbohydrate in the form of raw fiber is not a wonder cure. In some cases it can be detrimental. When too much fiber is consumed, essential vitamins and minerals are bound and excreted without ever being available for the body to use. Also, consuming purified fiber such as cellulose may not confer the same health benefits as consuming cellulose from a food source such as whole grains.[6]

Not all fibers have similar effects. For example, wheat bran, which is composed mostly of cellulose, has no cholesterol-lowering effect, whereas oat bran and the fiber of apples (pectin) do lower blood cholesterol. On the other hand, wheat bran seems to be one of the most effective stool-softening fibers, especially if larger particle sizes are used. Fibers that form gels in water (pectin and guar) prolong the time of transit of materials through the intestine, whereas the insoluble fibers (cellulose) tend to reduce the time.

The amounts of dietary fiber in food are hard to estimate. About 20 to 35 grams of dietary fiber daily is a desirable intake.[7] This is two to three times more than the average intake in the United States. The diet can supply that amount, given ample choices of whole foods as shown in Table 2–3. It means consuming more fruits, vegetables, legumes, and grains and fewer meats and dairy products than most people are accustomed to eating, but it is a change with trying, if possible.

Energy Nutrients in Perspective

An uninterrupted flow of energy is so vital to life that other functions are sometimes sacrificed to maintain it. For example, when a child is fed too little food, the food he or she does consume will be used for energy to keep the heart and lungs going, but growth will come to a standstill. To go totally without an energy supply, even for a few minutes, is to die. Over the course of evolution, the urgency of the need for energy has ensured that all creatures have built-in reserves to protect themselves from being deprived of energy. Our provision against this sort of emergency is glycogen, the storage form of glucose.

When you do not eat carbohydrate, your body rapidly devours first its glycogen stores and then its own protein to generate glucose. The body needs its protein, however, for other vital purposes. This protein-sparing effect of carbohydrate is important, for it offers protection against an emergency when the body runs short of glucose: stored glycogen can return glucose to the blood whenever the supply runs short. The liver cells, however, can store only a limited amount of energy as glycogen. Once this supply is depleted, the body must turn to the other energy nutrients—fat and protein—to meet its energy needs.

Unlike the liver, the body's fat mass has a virtually unlimited storage capacity, and fat supplies two-thirds of the body's energy needs. During a prolonged period of food deprivation, fat can provide energy for most tissues. However, fat cannot provide energy in the form of glucose, the substance needed as fuel by the brain and nerves. After a long period of glucose deprivation, brain and nerve cells develop the ability to derive about half of their energy from a special form of fat known as ketones, but they still require glucose as well. With the available glycogen long gone, brain and nerve cells demand this glucose from the only alternative source—protein. Because no protein is coming in from food, the only supply is in the muscles and other lean tissues. These tissues give up their protein and atrophy, bringing on weakness, loss of function, and ultimately, after using half of the body protein, death. Death from loss of lean body tissues will occur even in an obese person who fasts too long. It should be clear, then, that although carbohydrate is an ideal energy source, fat and sometimes protein are extremely important in meeting energy demands.

protein-sparing effect: the effect of carbohydrate and fat in providing energy that allows protein to be used for other purposes.

TABLE 2–3   **Foods to Provide 25 Grams Dietary Fiber per Day**

FRUITS: ABOUT 2 TO 4 G FIBER PER SERVING

Apple, 1 small	Orange, 1 small
Apricots, 3	Peach, 1 medium
Banana, 1 small	Pear ½ small
Blackberries, ½ c	Pineapple, 1 c
Blueberries, ½ c	Plums, 2 small
Cantaloupe, ½	Prunes, 2
Dates, 5	Raspberries, ½ c
Figs, 2	Strawberries, ½ c

GRAINS AND CEREALS: ABOUT 2 TO 4 G FIGER PER SERVING

All-Bran, ½ oz	Raisin Bran, ½ c
Barley, ½ c	Rice, 1 c
Bulgur, ½ c	Rye bread, 1 slice
Cracked-wheat bread, 1 slice	Shredded Wheat, ½ c
Granola, ½ c	Wheat bran, ¼ c
Grape-Nuts, ½ c	Whole-wheat bread, 1 slice
Oatmeal, ½ c	

VEGETABLES: ABOUT 2 TO 4 G FIGER PER SERVING

Artichoke, 1	Green beans, 1 c
Broccoli, ½ stalk	Lettuce, 2 c
Brussels sprouts, ½ c	Potato, 1 small
Carrots, 1 c	Spinach, 1 c
Celery, 1 c	Squash, 1 c
Corn on the cob, 2-inch piece	Tomato, 1 medium

LEGUMES: ABOUT 8 G FIBER PER SERVING

Baked beans, ½ c	Lentils, 1 c
Black beans, ½ c	Lima beans, 1 c
Black-eyed peas, 1 c	Navy beans, ½ c
Garbanzo beans, 1 c	Pinto beans, ½ c
Kidney beans, ½ c	

MISCELLANEOUS: ABOUT 1 G FIBER PER PORTION

Nuts, ½ oz	Peanut butter, 1 tbsp
Olives, 5	Pickle, 1 large

Study Questions

1. What are the simple carbohydrates?
2. What are the complex carbohydrates?
3. What is the chief energy source of the body?
4. What is glycogen?
5. What health benefits does a diet high in complex carbohydrates offer?
6. Describe some of the health benefits of fiber.
7. What is the "protein-sparing" effect of carbohydrate?

SELF-STUDY

How's Your Carbohydrate Intake?

From the forms you filled out for the Self-Study in Chapter 1, answer the following questions and complete Form 6.

1. How many grams of carbohydrate do you consume in an average day (from Form 1). _____ grams
2. How many kcalories does this represent? (Remember, 1 gram of carbohydrate contributes 4 kcalories.) _____ kcalories
3. It is estimated that you should have 125 grams or more of carbohydrate in a day. How does your intake compare with this minimum? _____
4. What percentage of your total kcalories is contributed by carbohydrate (carbohydrate kcalories divided by total kcalories times 100 — or use the answer you obtained on Form 5)? _____ percent
5. How does this figure compare with the dietary goal stating that about 55 to 60 percent of the kcalories in your diet should come from carbohydrate? (Note: If you are on a diet to lose weight, this goal does not apply to you. See Chapter 19.)
6. Another dietary goal is that no more than 10 percent of total kcalories should come from refined and other processed sugars and foods high in such sugars. To assess your intake against this standard, sort the carbohydrate-containing food items you ate into three groups:

    ■■■ *Group A:* Foods containing complex carbohydrate (foods found among the grains, starchy foods, and vegetables in the exchange lists, Chapter 19) contributed _____ kcalories.
    ■■■ *Group B:* Nutritious foods containing simple carbohydrate (foods in the milk and fruit lists) contributed _____ kcalories.
    ■■■ *Group C:* Foods containing mostly concentrated simple carbohydrate (sugar, honey, molasses, syrup, jam, jelly, candy, cakes, doughnuts, sweet rolls, cola beverages, and so on) contributed _____ kcalories.

    Does your concentrated sugar intake (Group C) fall within the recommended maximum of 10 percent of total daily kcalories? _____ If not, what food choices account for the excess sugar? _____

7. Estimate the number of pounds of sugar (concentrated simple carbohydrate) you eat in a year (1 pound = 454 grams):

    _____ kcalories from Group C divided by 4 = _____ grams/day.

    _____ grams/day × 365 days/year = _____ grams/year.

    _____ grams/year divided by 454 grams/pound = _____ pounds/year.

    How does your yearly sugar intake compare with the estimated U.S. and Canadian average of about 75 pounds per person per year? _____
    Comment on this. _____

FORM 6   Carbohydrate and Sugar kCalories

Average daily carbohydrate intake: _____ grams
     Total kcalories from carbohydrate: _____ kcalories (grams × 4)
          Total kcalories from all sources: _____ kcalories

Total kcalories from carbohydrates should equal 60 percent of total kcalories from all sources. Percentage of kcalories from carbohydrate: _____ %

Breakdown of carbohydrate kcalories:
A. _____ complex   B. _____ nutritious simple
C. _____ concentrated simple

kCalories from concentrated simple sugars should equal 10 percent or less of total kcalories from all sources. Percentage of kcalories from concentrated simple sugars: _____ %

Notes

1. M. I. McBurney and L. U. Thompson, Dietary fiber and energy balance: Integration of the human ileostomy and in vitro fermentation models, *Animal Feed Science and Technology* 23 (1989): 261–275.

2. U.S. Senate, Select Committee on Nutrition and Human Needs, *Dietary Goals for the United States,* 2d ed. (Washington, D.C.: Government Printing Office, 1977).

3. B. Szepesi, Carbohydrates, in *Present Knowledge in Nutrition,* 6th ed., ed. M. L. Brown (Washington, D.C.: International Life Sciences Institute — Nutrition Foundation, 1990).

4. Food and Nutrition Board, National Research Council, Committee on Diet and Health, *Implications for Reducing Chronic Disease Risk* (Washington, D.C.: National Academy Press, 1989).

5. G. M. Reaven, Parma symposium: Current controversies in nutrition, *American Journal of Clinical Nutrition* 47 (1988): 1078–1082.

6. J. L Slavin, Dietary fiber: Classification, chemical analyses, and food sources, *Journal of the American Dietetic Association* 87 (1987): 1164–1171.

7. Position of the American Dietetic Association: Health implications of dietary fiber, *Journal of the American Dietetic Association* 88 (1988): 216.

2

Nutrition and Dental Health

The health value of eating complex carbohydrate-rich foods was emphasized throughout Chapter 2. Sound nutrition practices that promote overall health do not necessarily promote dental health—at least not as far as carbohydrates go—unless care is taken to maximize dental health.[1]

Nutrition plays a major role in facilitating the development of healthy teeth. Table NP2–1 shows the effects of nutrient deficiencies on tooth development. Your eating habits and the foods you eat also play a major role in preventing dental caries—a pervasive health problem throughout the world.

What is dental caries?

Dental caries is an infectious oral disease that develops in the tooth enamel. Caries develops when bacteria that reside in the plaque of teeth consume and metabolize carbohydrates, producing acids that attack the tooth enamel. Thus at least two main ingredients are required to make dental caries: bacteria and carbohydrates. In addition, factors such as an individual's heredity, nutrition status during the time of tooth development, dental hygiene practices, and fluoride intake influence a person's susceptibility to caries development.

How do sugar and other carbohydrate-rich foods promote caries development?

The bacteria that promote dental caries thrive on food particles, especially those that contain carbohydrate. Both sugar and starch can support bacterial growth. Equally important is the length of time the food stays in the mouth, and this depends on how soon you brush your teeth after eating and how sticky the food is. The damage sugar does relates to both the amount and the stickiness of the sugar. A

TABLE NP2–1   **Nutrient Deficiencies Affecting Tooth Development**

NUTRIENT DEFICIENCY	EFFECT ON TOOTH DEVELOPMENT
Protein	Small, irregularly shaped teeth; delayed eruption; high caries susceptibility
Vitamin C	Disturbance of collagen matrix of dentin
Vitamin A	Disturbance of keratin matrix of enamel, delayed eruption, poor formation
Vitamin D	Poor mineralization, pitting, striations
Calcium	Poor mineralization
Phosphorus	Poor mineralization
Magnesium	Enamel underdeveloped
Iron	High caries susceptibility
Zinc	High caries susceptibility
Fluoride	High caries susceptibility

sticky, sugary food, such as raisins or granola, causes more caries than a sugary food that is easily rinsed off, such as a sweetened beverage.

You can eat sugar without inviting tooth decay if you remove it from your tooth surfaces promptly. A rule of thumb is that bacterial action is maximal within the first 20 minutes after the first contact. If immediate brushing is not possible, water or other beverages swished in the mouth after a meal can effectively rinse the teeth. Even brushing *before* a meal helps keep caries-causing acid within a safe range for a few hours after eating. Once-a-day flossing may also effectively control formation of caries, regardless of the carbohydrate content of the diet. Some people may never get cavities because they have inherited resistance to them.

Is there anything else about foods that influences the development of caries besides their carbohydrate content or stickiness?

Yes, the ability to stimulate saliva flow. Saliva protects against caries formation because it dilutes the caries-causing acid produced by bacteria, exerts antibacterial action, rinses the mouth, and provides protective minerals.[2] Foods that elicit saliva flow defend against caries formation. But not all foods that stimulate saliva flow are protective, because they may also liberate sugar, which promotes acid formation. Apples are an example: they have both caries-preventing and caries-promoting effects. As you can see, many different factors influence caries development, making it difficult to predict exactly which foods are cariogenic.

Are there any foods that are strictly caries-preventing?

Yes. Some foods stimulate saliva flow and do not contribute to acid formation in the mouth: for example, cheese. Such foods are good choices to eat at the end of a meal. Cheese is a powerful saliva stimulant, does not promote acid formation, and therefore reduces the cariogenicity of a meal. Furthermore, the high calcium and phosphorus content of cheese contributes to dental health.

Some high-fiber carbohydrate foods are anticariogenic. For example, raw vegetables do not stick to the teeth and, because they require vigorous chewing, stimulate saliva flow. Research indicates that cocoa products (including chocolate), coffee, tea, and beer all contain tannin, an acid that prevents caries formation.[3] Table NP2–2 lists some dietary recommendations for controlling dental caries.

What other factors protect against dental caries development?

Research shows that when fluoride is added to the water supply, the children in the community have fewer dental caries than children who drink nonfluoridated water. In fact, water fluoridation is the most effective, least expensive way to provide dental care to everyone. The following recommendations will maximize protection against dental caries:

- Watch for hidden sugars in foods; use low-sugar or sugar-free products whenever possible.
- Restrict sweets to mealtimes.
- Practice oral hygiene after eating between-meal snacks.
- Limit the duration of time that teeth are exposed to sticky foods.
- Brush and floss daily, and visit a dentist regularly.
- Rinse with water after eating if brushing and flossing are not possible.
- Drink fluoridated water; provide infants and children with fluoride supplements when such water is not available.
- Eat a balanced diet composed of a variety of foods that will maintain adequate nutrition status.
- Eat foods that are rich in calcium and phosphorus.
- Eat a variety of firm, fibrous foods that will stimulate saliva flow.

In summary, learning and practicing sound dental hygiene habits, as well as developing eating habits that are consistent with both dental health and nutritional health, will serve a person throughout life.

Notes

1. Parts of this discussion are adapted with permission from E. N. Whitney, E. M. N. Hamilton, and S. R. Rolfes, *Understanding Nutrition,* 5th ed. (St. Paul: West, 1990), pp. 306–313.
2. J. H. Shaw and E. A. Sweeney, Oral Health, in *Nutritional Support of Medical Practice,* 2d ed., eds. H. A. Schneider, C. E. Anderson, and D. B. Coursin (Philadelphia: Harper and Row, 1983), pp. 517–540.
3. University of California School of Dentistry, as cited in Dentists say sweet tooth isn't kiss of death for enamel, *Atlanta Constitution,* 21 March 1991.

TABLE NP2-2   Dietary Recommendations for Controlling Dental Caries

FOOD GROUP	LOW CARIOGENICITY (USE WHEN TEETH CANNOT BE BRUSHED IMMEDIATELY)	HIGH CARIOGENICITY (DO NOT USE UNLESS FOLLOWED BY PROMPT AND THOROUGH DENTAL HYGIENE)
Dairy	Milk, cheese, plain yogurt	Ice cream, ice milk, milk shakes, fruited yogurts, eggnog
Meats/meat alternates	Meat, fish, poultry, eggs, legumes	Peanut butter with added sugar, luncheon meats with added sugar, meats with sugared glazes
Fruits[a]	Fresh, packed in water or juice	Dried, packed in syrup, jams, jellies, preserves, fruit juices and drinks
Vegetables	Most vegetables	Candied sweet potatoes, glazed carrots
Breads/cereals[b]	Popcorn, soda crackers, toast, hard rolls, pretzels, corn chips, pizza	Cookies, sweet rolls, pies, cakes, cereals
Other	Sugarless gum, coffee or tea without sugar, nuts, red licorice[c]	Sugared soft drinks, candy, fudge, caramels, honey, sugars, syrups

[a]Tiny particles of bananas can get lodged between teeth and decompose, increasing risk of caries.
[b]Tiny particles of breads, crackers, and chips can also become lodged in teeth, promoting caries formation.
[c]Red licorice contains glycyrrhizin, a flavoring that inhibits mineral loss.

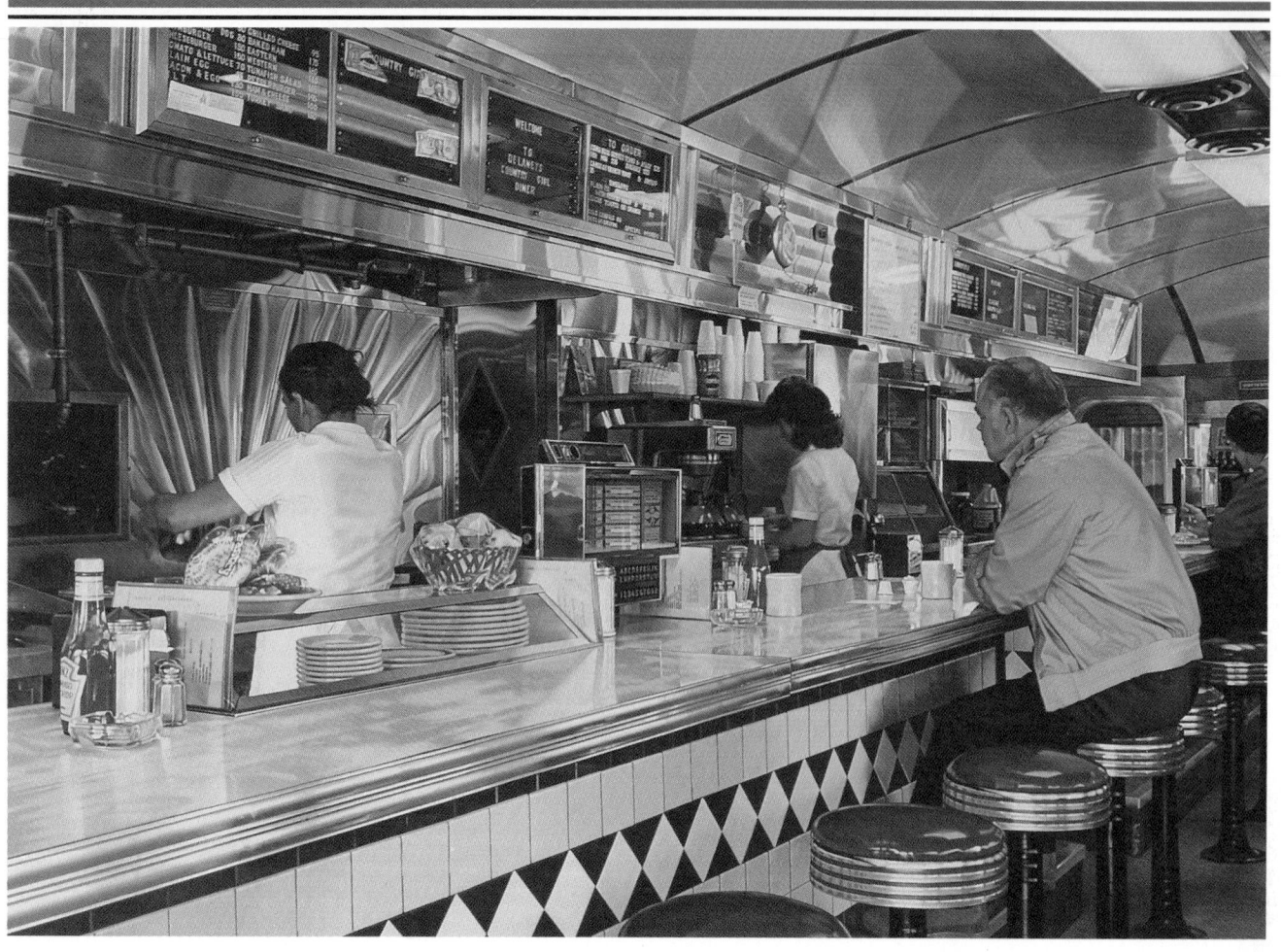

Ralph Goings, Country Girl Diner, 1985; *O.K. Harris Works of Art, New York, N.Y.*

CHAPTER

3

Lipids

CONTENTS

triglyceride (try-GLISS-uh-ride): a compound composed of glycerol with three fatty acids attached to it.

   tri = three

   glyceride = a compound of glycerol

phospholipid: a compound similar to a triglyceride but having choline (or another compound) and a phosphorus-containing acid in place of one of the fatty acids.

sterol: a class of lipids that includes cholesterol, vitamin D, and the sex hormones (such as testosterone).

CHAPTER
3

You probably know that too much fat in the diet imposes health risks, but you may be surprised to learn that too little does, too. It is true, though, that people in the United States are more likely to eat too much fat, rather than too little.

Fat is a member of the class of compounds called lipids. The lipids in foods and in the human body include triglycerides (fats and oils), phospholipids, and sterols.

Lipids in the body perform many tasks, but most important, they provide energy. A constant flow of energy is so vital to life that in a pinch, any other function is sacrificed to maintain it. Chapter 2 described one safeguard against such an emergency—the stores of glycogen in the liver that provide glucose to the blood whenever the supply runs short. The body's stores of glycogen are limited, however. In contrast, the body's capacity to store fat for energy is virtually unlimited, and fat supplies 60 percent of the body's ongoing energy need during rest.[1] During exercise or prolonged periods of food deprivation, fat stores may make an even greater energy contribution.

Fat serves other roles in the body in addition to providing energy. Natural oils in the skin provide a radiant complexion; in the scalp, they help nourish the hair and make it glossy. The layer of fat beneath the skin insulates the body from extremes of temperature. A pad of hard fat beneath each kidney protects it from being jarred and damaged, even during a motorcycle ride on a bumpy road. The soft fat in the breasts of a woman protects the mammary glands from heat and cold and cushions them against shock. The fat that lies embedded in muscle tissue shares with muscle glycogen the task of providing energy when the muscles are active. The phospholipids and the sterol cholesterol are cell membrane constituents that help maintain the structure and health of all cells.

The Chemist's View of Lipids

The diverse and vital functions that lipids play in the body emphasize why eating too little fat can be harmful. As mentioned earlier, though, too much fat in the diet seems to be the bigger problem for most people. To understand both the beneficial and harmful effects that fats exert on the body, a closer look at the structure and function of members of the lipid family is in order.

The Triglycerides

fatty acid: an organic acid composed of a chain of carbon atoms with hydrogens attached and an acid group at one end.

glycerol (GLISS-er-ol): a small compound related to carbohydrates that can form the backbone of triglycerides and phospholipids.

When people talk about fat—for example, "I'm too fat" or "That meat is fatty"—it is triglycerides they are talking about. Among lipids, triglycerides predominate—both in the diet and in the body. The name *triglyceride* almost explains itself: three fatty acids (*tri*) attached to a glycerol "backbone." Figure 3–1 shows how glycerol and three fatty acids combine to make a triglyceride.

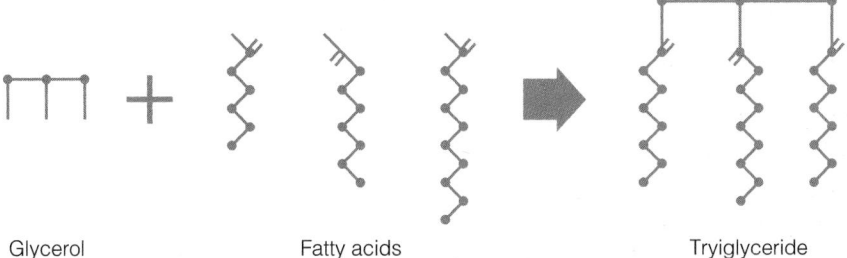

Glycerol   Fatty acids   Tryiglyceride

FIGURE 3–1   **Triglyceride Formation**
Glycerol, a small, water-soluble carbohydrate, plus three fatty acids equals a triglyceride.

The Fatty Acids

When energy from any energy-yielding nutrient is stored as fat, fragments derived from that nutrient are linked together into chains known as fatty acids. Fatty acids are then packaged in threes with glycerol to make triglycerides.

Fatty acids may differ from one another in two ways—in chain length and in degree of saturation. Chain length affects the way the fatty acid is absorbed (see Chapter 5). Saturation refers to the chemical structure—specifically, to the number of hydrogens the fatty acid chain is holding. If every available bond from the carbons is holding a hydrogen, the chain is called a saturated fatty acid, meaning that the chain is filled to capacity with hydrogen. The first zigzag structure in Figure 3–2 represents a saturated fatty acid.

Sometimes, especially in plants and fish, hydrogen atoms are missing in the fatty acid chains. The points where hydrogen atoms are missing are called points of unsaturation, and a chain containing such points is called an unsaturated fatty acid. If there is one point of unsaturation (as in oleic acid), the chain is monounsaturated. The second structure in Figure 3–2 is an example. If there are two or more points of unsaturation, then the fatty acid is polyunsaturated (see the third structure in Figure 3–2). You sometimes see monounsaturated fatty acids abbreviated on food labels as MFA, and polyunsaturated fatty acids such as PUFA.

Any combination of fatty acids can be incorporated into a triglyceride—long chain or short chain, saturated or polyunsaturated. Whether a fat is soft or hard depends on which fatty acids are incorporated into it. Fats that contain shorter-chain fatty acids or the more unsaturated ones are softer and melt more readily (discussed later in the chapter). Each animal species (including human beings) has its own characteristic kinds of triglycerides; but within limits, fats in the diet can affect the types of triglycerides made. For example, animals raised for food can be fed diets with different fats in them to give them softer or harder fat, whichever consumers demand. People, too, incorporate the fatty acids they eat into their own tissues.

The human body can synthesize all the fatty acids it needs from carbohydrate, fat, or protein except for two—linoleic and linolenic acid. These two, which are both polyunsaturated fatty acids, cannot be made from the breakdown of other substances in the body. They must be supplied by the

saturated fatty acid: a fatty acid carrying the maximum possible number of hydrogen atoms (having no points of unsaturation). A saturated fat is a triglyceride that contains three saturated fatty acids.

unsaturated fatty acid: a fatty acid in which one or more points of unsaturation occur (includes monounsaturated and polyunsaturated fatty acids).

monounsaturated fatty acid (MFA): a fatty acid that has one point of unsaturation where hydrogens are missing, for example, oleic acid.

polyunsaturated fatty acid (PUFA): a fatty acid with two or more points of unsaturation. For example, linoleic acid has two such points, and linolenic acid has three. Thus a polyunsaturated fat is composed of triglycerides containing a high percentage of PUFA.

linoleic acid, linolenic acid: polyunsaturated fatty acids, essential for human beings.

essential fatty acids: fatty acids that cannot be synthesized in the body in amounts sufficient to meet physiological need.

omega: the last letter of the Greek alphabet (ω), used by chemists to refer to the position of the last double bond in a fatty acid. The omega-6 fatty acids have their last double bond six carbons back along the chain; the omega-3 acids, three carbons back.

omega-3 fatty acid: relatively newly recognized as important in nutrition, a polyunsaturated fatty acid with its endmost double bond three carbons back from the end of its carbon chain.

DHA, EPA: omega-3 fatty acids made from linolenic acid. The full name for DHA is docosahexaenoic (DOE-cosa-HEXA-ee-NO-ick) acid. The full name for EPA is eicosapentanoic (EYE-cossa-PENTA-ee-NO-ick) acid.

omega-6 fatty acid: long recognized as important in nutrition, a polyunsaturated fatty acid with its endmost double bond six carbons away from the end of its carbon chain.

FIGURE 3–2   **Three Fatty Acids**

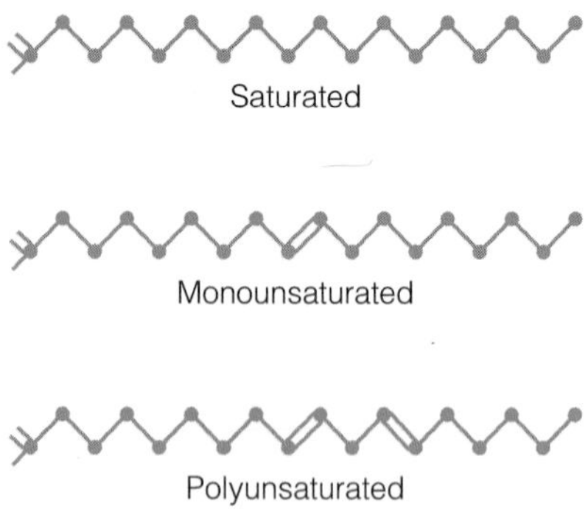

Saturated

Monounsaturated

Polyunsaturated

lecithin: one of the phospholipids.

diet, and they are therefore called *essential* fatty acids. Linoleic and linolenic acids are abundant in plant and fish oils, and the body easily stores them in abundance, so deficiencies are unlikely.

Linolenic acid belongs to a family of polyunsaturated fatty acids known as omega-3 fatty acids, which also includes EPA and DHA, seen on supplement labels. EPA and DHA are found primarily in fish oils. As mentioned, the human body cannot make linolenic acid; but given dietary linolenic acid, it can make EPA and DHA, although this is a slow process.[2] The importance of omega-3 fatty acids is just now being realized. Researchers are studying the effects of omega-3 fatty acids on growth and development, visual function, cancer development, blood clotting, arthritis, heart disease, and hypertension.[3]

Linoleic acid is an omega-6 fatty acid, found in seeds of plants and in oils produced by the seeds. Researchers have long known and appreciated the importance of the omega-6 fatty acid family.

Whenever research suggests that a compound is a protective factor against disease, manufacturers start producing it as a supplement. Omega-3 fatty acid supplements are being aggressively marketed as a cure-all for many different diseases without regard for consumer safety. People are rarely deficient in these fatty acids, and common foods supply them; thus supplements are unnecessary and, in some instances, potentially harmful. Fish oil supplements may contain toxic amounts of fat-soluble vitamins. They may carry pesticide residues as well, and many fail to list the sources of their omega-3 fatty acids, or the presence of other compounds.

The omega-3 and omega-6 fatty acids compete for the same slots in the body. The possible consequences of taking supplements of one is that a deficiency of the other can easily be induced. Another potential problem is that the supplement form may not function the same way as the form available directly from foods. There are still questions about how much is the right amount, and the problem is compounded by the fact that the quantities of omega-3 fatty acids in supplements vary widely from what the labels say they contain. The best way to increase your intake of omega-3 fatty acids is to eat more fish. The darker flesh of fish has the highest fat content, and this is where most omega-3 fatty acids are found.

The Phospholipids

Up to now, this discussion has focused on one of three classes of lipids, the triglycerides, and their component parts, the fatty acids (see Table 3–1). The other two classes of lipids, the phospholipids and sterols, make up only 5 percent of the lipids in the diet, but they are nonetheless worthy of attention. Among the phospholipids, the lecithins are of particular interest.

Like the triglycerides, the lecithins and some other phospholipids have a backbone of glycerol; they are different from the triglycerides in that they have only two fatty acids attached to them. In place of the third fatty acid is

TABLE 3–1   **The Major Lipids**

TRIGLYCERIDES (FATS AND OILS)	PHOSPHOLIPIDS	STEROLS

Glycerol
Fatty acids
  Saturated
  Monounsaturated
  Polyunsaturated
    Omega-6
    Omega-3
	Lecithin (example)	Cholesterol (example)

a molecule of choline or a similar compound. Lecithin is the best-known phospholipid.

Lecithins and other phospholipids are important constituents of cell membranes. They also act as emulsifying agents, helping to keep other fats in solution in the blood and body fluids.

Lecithins periodically receive noisy attention in the popular press and are credited with great deeds. You may have heard that they are a major constituent of cell membranes (true), that the functioning of all cells depends on the integrity of the cells' membranes (true), and that you must therefore purchase bottles of lecithin and give yourself daily doses (false). The body digests lecithins before it absorbs them, so the lecithins you eat do not reach the body tissues intact. The liver then makes from scratch the lecithins you need for building cell membranes. In other words, the lecithins are not essential nutrients. Furthermore, large doses of lecithins have been seen to cause digestive upsets, sweating, salivation, and loss of appetite.[4]

Before buying bottles of lecithin or any other wonder substance, ask yourself, "Do I really need this? What is the evidence that my body is likely to be deficient?"

The Sterols

The sterols are large, complex molecules consisting of interconnected rings of carbon. Cholesterol is the most familiar sterol, but others, such as vitamin D and the sex hormones (for example, testosterone), are important, too.

Like the lecithins, cholesterol can be made by the body, so it is not an essential nutrient. Your liver is manufacturing it now, as you read, at the rate of perhaps 50,000,000,000,000,000 molecules per second. The raw materials that the liver uses to make cholesterol can all be taken from glucose or saturated fatty acids. Another way of saying the same thing is that cholesterol can be made from either carbohydrate or fat. More than nine-tenths of all the body's cholesterol ends up in the cells, where it performs vital structural and metabolic functions.

After being made, cholesterol either leaves the liver or is transformed there into related compounds such as vitamin D. The cholesterol that leaves the liver has three possible destinations:

1. It may be made into bile and move into the intestine, where some may then be excreted in the feces.
2. It may be deposited in the body's cells.
3. It may accumulate in arteries, contributing to arterial disease (athero-sclerosis).

bile: a compound made by the liver from cholesterol and stored in the gallbladder. Bile does not digest fat as enzymes do, but it emulsifies fat, so that the fat can then be split by enzymes for absorption.

Bile, made from cholesterol by the liver, is released into the intestine to aid in the digestion and absorption of fat (see Chapter 5). After doing its job, some of the bile reenters the body with absorbed products of fat digestion. Cholesterol is thus recycled—back to the liver, once again into bile, back to the intestine, again into the body, and once more back to the liver.

On its way around this cycle, during the time it spends out in the intestine, some of the bile can be trapped by certain kinds of dietary fibers or by some medications, which carry it out of the body in feces. The excretion of bile reduces the total amount of cholesterol remaining in the body.

Lipoproteins are made by both the intestine and the liver. Chapter 5 tells the story of lipid transport.

Some cholesterol leaves the liver, packaged with other lipids and protein, for transport to the body tissues. The packages are the lipoproteins. The blood carries lipoproteins through all the body's arteries, and any tissue can extract lipids from the lipoproteins. Some cells take lipoproteins up whole. To pass into the cells, lipids must first cross the artery walls, and some are deposited there. Lipids have been implicated in artery disease because of this association with the artery wall.

Fat in Foods

Not only is fat important in the body, it is also important in foods. Many of the compounds that give foods their flavor and aroma are found in fats and oils. The delicious aromas associated with bacon, ham, and other meats, as well as with onions being fried, come from fats. Four vitamins—A, D, E, and K—are soluble in fat. When the fat is removed from a food, many of the fat-soluble compounds, including these vitamins, are also removed.

Remember, fat is a more concentrated energy source than the other energy nutrients: 1 g carbohydrate or protein = 4 kcal, but 1 g fat = 9 kcal.

Something else is lost when fat is removed: energy (see Figure 3–3). A small pork chop with the fat trimmed to within a half inch of the lean provides 275 kcalories; with the fat trimmed off completely, it provides 165 kcalories. A baked potato with butter and sour cream (1 tablespoon each) has 350 kcalories; a plain baked potato has 220 kcalories. The single most effective step you can take to reduce the energy value of a food is to eat it with less fat. Furthermore, reducing dietary fat is the most important recommendation of almost every nutrition authority. The following five principles can help you meet this recommendation:

- Eliminate fat as a seasoning and in cooking.
- Cut down on your intake of red meat.
- Remove the fat from high-fat foods.
- Substitute high-fat foods with specially manufactured lower-fat versions of those foods (see Table 3–2).
- Replace high-fat foods with natural low-fat alternatives (see Table 3–2).

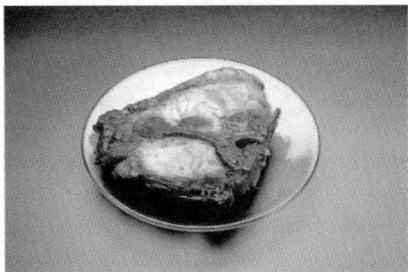

Pork chop with a half inch of fat (275 kcal).

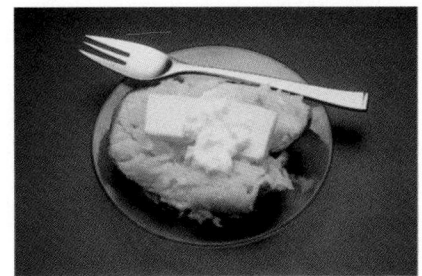

Potato with 1 tbsp butter and 1 tbsp sour cream (350 kcal).

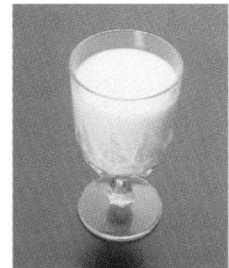

Whole milk, 1 c (150 kcal).

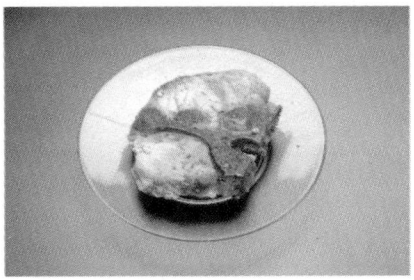

Pork chop with fat trimmed off (165 kcal).

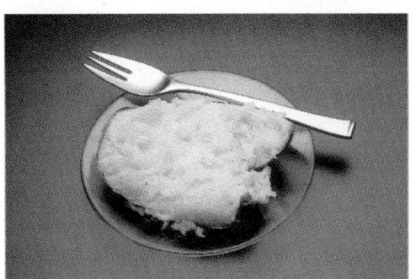

Plain potato (220 kcal).

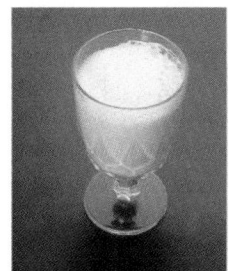

Nonfat milk, 1 c (90 kcal).

Health Effects of Fats and Recommended Intakes

Of all the dietary factors related to diseases prevalent in developed countries, fat is by far the most significant. Many diseases are linked to excessive intakes of dietary fat or to excess body fat. Fat contributes to obesity, diabetes, cancer, hypertension, atherosclerosis, and probably other diseases and disorders. In the interest of good health and disease prevention, the one change that most people should make in their diets is to limit their intakes of total fat, which, as mentioned previously, would moderate energy intake. A second change might be to limit saturated fat and cholesterol specifically, as well. The cholesterol that accumulates in arteries is manufactured largely from fragments derived from saturated fat. Many current recommendations suggest these changes in that priority order: avoid excess fat, saturated fat, and cholesterol.

Dietary guidelines recommend that *total* fat intake should not exceed 30 percent of the day's total energy intake. Saturated fats should contribute less than 10 percent; polyunsaturated fats should not exceed 10 percent; monounsaturates should provide the remaining 10 percent or so. Guidelines for cholesterol intake generally suggest an upper limit of 300 milligrams

Artery disease—atherosclerosis—is discussed in Chapter 22.

TABLE 3–2   **Substitutes for High-Fat Ingredients**

USE	INSTEAD OF
Nonfat milk products	Whole-milk products
Evaporated nonfat ("skim") milk (canned)	Cream
Yogurt[a]	Sour cream
Reduced-kcalorie margarine or butter replacers	Butter
Wine, lemon juice, or broth	Butter
Fruit butters	Butter
Part-skim ricotta or low-fat cottage cheese	Whole-milk ricotta
Part-skim or low-fat cheeses	Regular cheeses
1 tbsp cornstarch (for thickening sauces)	1 egg yolk
Reduced-kcalorie mayonnaise	Regular mayonnaise
Low- or reduced-kcalorie salad dressing (for salads and marinades)	Regular salad dressing
Water-packed canned fish and meats	Oil-packed canned fish and meats
Lean ground meat and grain mixture	Ground beef

[a]If the recipe is to be boiled, the yogurt or cottage cheese must be stabilized with a small amount of cornstarch or flour.

daily. Limiting dietary fat intake to 30 percent of total energy takes careful planning at every meal. According to research on people's food choices, people eat about 37 percent of their energy intake as fat.[5] Even though this is less than in the recent past, it more than at the turn of the century, when foods were less highly processed, and it is more than people need.

Dietary Fat

People who wish to adjust their dietary intake of fat need to know where the fats in foods are found. Most people recognize that butter, margarine, shortening, and oils contain only fat, and many consumers are aware of the high fat content of red meats.

Many people are surprised to learn that an eighth of an avocado, one strip of bacon, or five small olives contain as much fat as a pat of butter (45 kcalories from fat). When you eat these foods, you are eating fat-rich foods.

Other foods that are significant contributors of fat include convenience foods, fried foods, and luncheon and other prepared meats. The fat in these foods is sometimes referred to as invisible fat, because it does not have the obvious appearance of fat. An ounce of lean meat supplies 28 kcalories from its protein and 27 kcalories from its fat. An ounce of a high-fat meat (such as bologna) supplies 28 kcalories from protein and 72 kcalories from fat. Two tablespoons of peanut butter, also with 28 kcalories from protein, supplies 140 kcalories from fat! Thus foods that are usually thought of as protein-rich may actually contain more fat energy than protein energy. Note that the values for meat given here are for 1-ounce portions. An average serving of hamburger is usually 3 or 4 ounces. An average dinner steak may be 6 to 8 ounces or larger.

Surprisingly, abundant fat lurks even on salad bars; you can easily construct a plate of salad bearing 50 percent of its energy as fat. Think about it; not only the salad dressings, but also the mixed salads—potato salad, macaroni salad, coleslaw, and marinated bean salads—are largely fat or oil. This is not to condemn salad bars, but only to remind you to choose your foods with an awareness of the fats they contain. As mentioned, along with the total fat in foods, people need to notice the saturated fat and cholesterol in foods.

The fat in milk is about 62 percent saturated fat; the cholesterol content is 25 milligrams per cup of whole milk or 7 milligrams per cup of nonfat milk. Thus choosing nonfat milk in place of whole milk reduces your intake of saturated fat, as well as your intake of cholesterol.

The fats in meats and eggs are about half saturated; those in poultry and fish are more unsaturated than saturated: a healthier balance. The foods that contain the highest amounts of cholesterol are eggs, organ meats such as liver and kidneys, and high-fat dairy products. Shellfish have been thought to contain high concentrations of cholesterol, but the findings on which this idea was based have been called into question. Shellfish contain sterols, but possibly not the kind that have metabolically negative effects, and they contain much less cholesterol than has been thought in the past.

As a general rule, a person who eats meat and wishes to reduce both saturated fat and cholesterol intake could accomplish these objectives by eating fewer high-fat meats and dairy foods, fewer eggs, and more poultry and fish. A vegetarian who eats dairy products and eggs could shift to nonfat milk and low-fat cheeses and limit butter and egg intake. Vegetarians who omit animal-derived foods eat a diet low in fat and consume no cholesterol, because plant foods do not contain cholesterol.

To the extent that a person does eat fats, the fats to choose are the unsaturated ones. The hardness of fats at room temperature is an indicator: the softer it is, the more unsaturated it is. Chicken fat is softer than pork fat, which is softer than beef tallow. Of the three, chicken fat is the most unsaturated, and beef tallow is the most saturated. Unsaturated fats melt more readily. Generally speaking, vegetable and fish oils are rich in polyunsaturates, olive oil and canola oil are rich in monounsaturates, and the harder fats—animal fats—are more saturated.

If you wish to make choices consistent with current recommendations, you should learn how to read food labels, avoid fat in general, and seek out the polyunsaturated and monounsaturated fats in preference to the saturated ones. But beware: vegetable fat or vegetable oil doesn't always mean

Remember that an ounce of meat is not an ounce of protein. An ounce (30 g) of lean meat contains 7 g protein and 3 g fat. The other 20 g are largely water with associated vitamins and minerals.

Saturated fats are solid at room or body temperature. Polyunsaturated fats are liquid at room or body temperature.

hydrogenation: the process of adding hydrogen to unsaturated fat to make it more solid and resistant to chemical change.

unsaturated fat. Coconut oil and palm oil, for example, are often used in nondairy creamers, and both are saturated fats.

Vegetable oils that are hydrogenated have lost their polyunsaturated character and the health benefits that go along with it. Food producers hydrogenate unsaturated fatty acids to prevent spoilage and make them harder—as when they hydrogenate corn oil to make spreadable margarine. The points of unsaturation in fatty acids are vulnerable to attack by oxygen, which makes them rancid.

Each culture has its own favorite food sources of fats and oils. In Canada, canola oil (also known as rapeseed oil) is widely used. In the Mediterranean area, Greeks, Italians, and Spaniards rely heavily on olive oil. As mentioned, canola oil and olive oil are rich sources of monounsaturated fatty acids. Asians use the polyunsaturated oil of soybeans. Jewish people traditionally employ chicken fat. Everywhere in North America, butter and margarine are widely used.

In the past, the fat that foods were fried in was not a health concern. As research reveals more unhealthy links between saturated fats and heart disease and cancer, however, people have a reason to be concerned about the types of fats used to fry the foods ordered at restaurants. With fast foods becoming a major portion of many people's diets, it is important to know whether the origin of the fats is animal or vegetable. All fats have the same number of kcalories per spoon, but the animal fats are saturated and have increased health risks associated with them. Some popular fast-food establishments continue to use beef tallow, because it is economical, but some are beginning to take consumers' concerns into account. They are frying foods in polyunsaturated vegetable oils as well as offering low-fat alternatives such as raw-vegetable salads. If consumers are concerned enough to avoid foods fried in animal fats, restaurants will change the types of fats they use.

Chapters 2 and 3 looked briefly at the two major energy fuels in the body— carbohydrate and fat. When used for energy, each has desirable characteristics. The glucose derived from carbohydrate is needed by the brain and nerve tissues and is easily used for energy in other cells. Fat is a particularly useful fuel because the body stores it in generous amounts and can use it for energy if carbohydrate is not available. Chapter 4 looks at protein, a nutrient that can be used as fuel, but whose primary role is to provide machinery for getting things done.

Study Questions

1. Name three classes of lipids found in the body and in foods.
2. What are some functions of fat in the body?
3. Describe the general structure of triglycerides.
4. What is the difference between a saturated and an unsaturated fatty acid?
5. Name the essential fatty acids.
6. List some of the ways you can cut down your intake of fat.

SELF-STUDY

How's Your Fat Intake?

From the forms you filled out for the Self-Study in Chapter 1, answer the following questions:

1. How many grams of fat do you consume in an average day (from Form 1)? _____grams
2. How many kcalories does this represent? (Remember, 1 gram of fat contributes 9 kcalories.) _____kcalories
3. What percentage of your total kcalories is contributed by fat? (To figure this, divide fat kcalories by total kcalories, and then multiply by 100, or use the answer you obtained in Chapter 1's Self-Study, Form 5.) _____percent
4. A dietary guideline says that fat should contribute not more than 30 percent of total kcalories. How does your fat intake compare with this recommendation? _____If it is higher, look over your food records. What specific foods could you cut down on or eliminate, and what foods could you add to your diet to bring your total fat intake into line?
5. You may not be aware of how much fat you are eating when you eat meat. Weigh your meat portions for a day or so; then calculate how much fat you derive from meat in a day (use Appendix C). To visualize this amount of fat, weigh out an equal amount from a bottle of oil, a can of cooking fat, or a tub of butter or margarine. Try the same demonstration with a fast-food meal that includes fried foods. How much fat do you eat in a day?

Notes

1. S. M. Hunt and J. L. Groff, *Advanced Nutrition and Human Metabolism* (St. Paul, MN: West, 1990), pp. 405–423.
2. A. P. Simopoulos, ω-3 fatty acids in growth and development and in health and disease, *Nutrition Today,* March/April 1988, pp. 10–19.
3. Simopoulos, 1988; H. R. Knapp and G. A. Fitzgerald, The antihypertensive effects of fish oil, *New England Journal of Medicine* 320 (1989): 1037–1043.
4. J. L. Wood and R. G. Allison, Effects of consumption of choline and lecithin on neurological and cardiovascular systems, *Federation Proceedings* 41 (1982): 3015–3021.
5. Federation of American Societies for Experimental Biology, Life Sciences Research Office, *Nutrition Monitoring in the United States: An Update Report on Nutrition Monitoring,* prepared for the U.S. Department of Health and Human Services (Washington, D.C.: Government Printing Office, 1989).

3

Artificial Fats

Artificial fats are attracting public attention. As people learn more and more about the health consequences of high-fat diets, artificial fats offer hope for the prevention and treatment of heart disease and obesity. One survey found that more than half of the adults in the United States believe there is a need for fat substitutes.[1] This Nutrition in Practice discusses artificial fats, also known as fat substitutes or fat replacements.

What are fat substitutes made of?

Some are processed from substances already in the diet, and some are new substances. Those that are made from substances already in the diet are digested and used by the body in the same way as the substances they originate from; examples are Simplesse and Stellar. The ones made from new substances are undigestible and so contribute no food energy; examples are olestra and Oatrim.

Are these fat substitutes available to consumers?

Yes, Simplesse was declared safe for use in ice cream and frozen desserts by the FDA in 1990.[2] Simplesse is made from protein—either egg white or milk—that is disintegrated into mistlike particles similar in consistency to fat. Because the components of Simplesse have long been used in foods, safety studies are not required. This fat substitute mimics the rich

taste and texture of fat but cuts the kcalorie content up to 80 percent. Since proteins coagulate at high temperatures, this fat substitute cannot be used for frying or cooking, but can be used in ice cream, yogurt, salad dressings, mayonnaise, and butter.

In contrast to Simplesse, the fat substitute Stellar can be heated. Stellar is starch based and derived from corn. Because Stellar is defined as a modified food starch and meets U.S. regulatory requirements, it is approved for use by food manufacturers. Stellar can replace the fat in a wide range of foods, including margarine, salad dressings, ice cream, cheese products, meat products, soups, gravies, and sauces.

What about olestra? And where did sucrose polyester go?

Olestra was formerly known as sucrose polyester (SPE). It was invented in the late 1960s. It is a synthetic combination of sucrose and fatty acids that looks, feels, and tastes like food fat. Unlike either sucrose or fatty acids, olestra is indigestible; the body has no way to take it apart. Olestra can therefore be substituted for fats

without adding kcalories or promoting a rise in a person's blood lipid level.

Olestra is currently awaiting FDA approval. Because oelstra is considered a new structure and does not break down to its component parts during digestion, it must undergo stringent safety tests before approval. Research on animals and human beings seems to support the safety of olestra as a partial replacement for dietary fats and oils.

Researchers at the U.S. Department of Agriculture (USDA) are testing a new extract of oats as a fat substitute.[3] The product, called Oatrim by the USDA researchers, is heat stable and can be used as a fat substitute to reduce the energy content of foods such as frozen desserts, salad dressings, soups, and high-fiber baked goods. Researchers say Oatrim reduces the energy content of frozen desserts like ice cream by half. Unlike Simplesse or other fat substitutes, Oatrim retains its fiber qualities, so it lowers cholesterol not only by replacing saturated fat, but also by providing fiber.

These products sound too good to be true. Are they?

That remains to be seen. Research has not yet shown that fat substitutes promote weight loss or lower blood lipid concentrations. If people use fat substitutes in the most literal sense—as substitutes for fat in their diets—then perhaps potential health benefits will be realized. Some experts are concerned that people may feel at liberty to eat *more* high-fat foods by rationalizing that they obtain fat "credit" when they eat foods containing fat substitutes. Indeed, this seems to be the case with artificial sweeteners. Despite the rising consumption of sugar substitutes since their introduction, sugar consumption has risen as well. Another concern is that people may become so carried away with eating foods containing fat substitutes that they will neglect to eat more nutrient-dense foods such as fresh fruits and vegetables. It seems that with fat substitutes, as with most things in life, moderation is the key.

Notes

1. M. Segal, Fat substitutes: A taste of the future? *FDA Consumer,* December 1990, pp. 25–27.

2. C. L. Rock and A. Coulston, Review: The new fat replacements, *Nutrition and the M.D.,* September 1990, p. 8.

3. Oatrim: New fat substitute (abstract), *Journal of the American Dietetic Association* 91 (1991): p. 738.

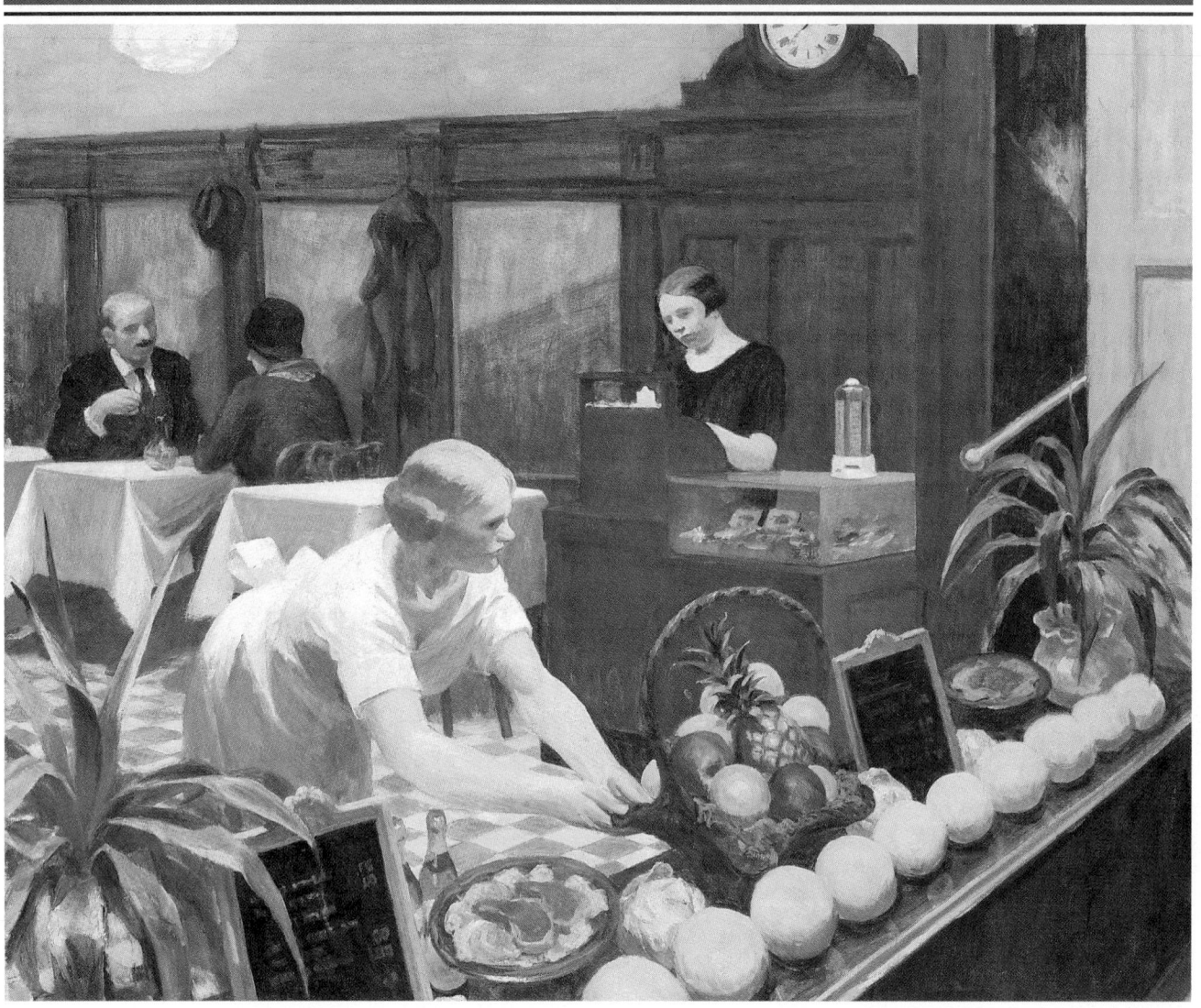

Edward Hopper, Tables for Ladies; *The Metropolitan Museum of Art, George A. Hearn Fund, 1931 (31.62).*

Proteins and Amino Acids

CONTENTS

CHAPTER

4

People think of protein as the body-building nutrient, the material of strong muscles, and rightly so. No new living tissue can be built without it, for protein is part of every cell, every bone, the blood, and every other tissue. Proteins constitute the cells' machinery—they do the cells' work. The energy to fuel that work comes from carbohydrate and fat as they break down.

The Chemist's View of Protein

protein: a compound composed of carbon, hydrogen, oxygen, and nitrogen atoms arranged into amino acids linked in a chain. Some amino acids also contain sulfur atoms.

amino (a-MEEN-oh) **acid:** a building block of protein; a compound containing an amino group and an acid group attached to a central carbon, which also carries a distinctive side chain.
amino = containing nitrogen

dipeptide: two amino acids bonded together.
di = two
peptide = amino acid

tripeptide: three amino acids bonded together.
tri = three

polypeptide: many amino acids bonded together. *Many* refers to ten or more. An intermediate string of between four and ten amino acids is an oligopeptide.
poly = many
oligo = few

A protein is a chemical compound that contains the same atoms as carbohydrate and lipid—carbon (C), hydrogen (H), and oxygen (O)—but protein is different in that it also contains nitrogen (N) atoms. These C, H, O, and N atoms are arranged into amino acids, which are linked into chains to form proteins.

All amino acids share a common chemical "backbone" through which they can be linked together. Each amino acid also carries a side chain, which varies from one amino acid to another. Twenty-two different amino acids may appear in proteins.* The side chains on amino acids are what make proteins so varied in comparison with either carbohydrates or lipids (see Figure 4–1).

The 22 different amino acids can be linked together in a great variety of ways to form proteins. When two amino acids bond together, the resulting structure is known as a dipeptide. Three amino acids bonded together form a tripeptide. As additional amino acids join the chain, a polypeptide is formed. Most proteins are polypeptides, 100 to 300 amino acids long. Because of the different properties of the amino acids in them, polypeptide chains fold and intertwine into intricate coils (see Figure 4–2). The amino acid sequence of a protein determines the specific way the chain will fold.

The 22 amino acids can be linked together in proteins in virtually infinite numbers of sequences. This gives amino acids a tremendous range of possible surface structures, which in turn enables them to perform distinct,

*It is often said that there are 20 amino acids, but if cystine and ornithine are counted, there are 22. Related forms of amino acids occur in nature, and chemists can make others.

FIGURE 4–1 **Examples of Amino Acids**
Note that the side chains are different in each. The asterisk denotes the central carbon.

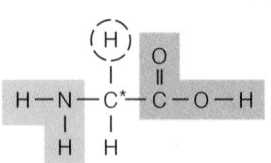

Glycine

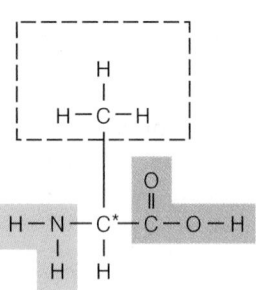

Alanine

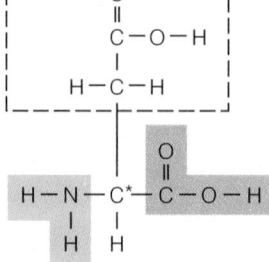

Aspartic acid

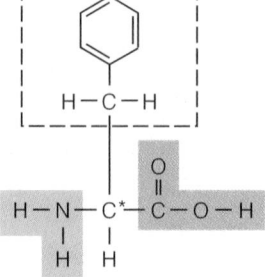

Phenylalanine

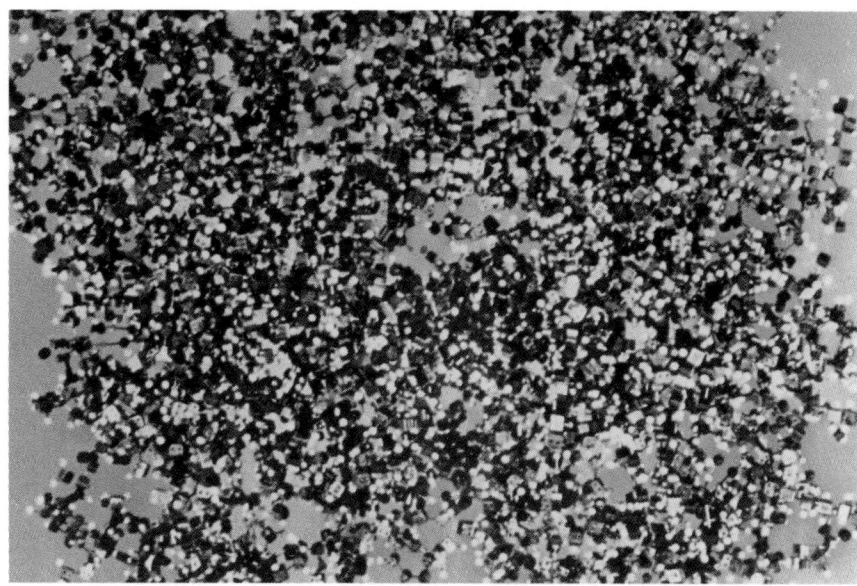

FIGURE 4–2 **Hemoglobin**
This model represents the intricate structure of one molecule of the protein hemoglobin, magnified 27 million times.

individual, and specialized functions. The human body contains an estimated 10,000 to 50,000 different kinds of proteins. The roles of over 1,000 of these proteins are now known.

Proteins in the Body

What distinguishes you chemically from any other human being is minute differences in your particular body proteins (enzymes, antibodies, and others). These differences are determined by the amino acid sequences of your proteins, and these sequences are written into the genes you inherited from your parents and ancestors. The genes direct the making of all the body's proteins. Among the most important of these proteins are the enzymes.

Enzymes

Enzymes are essential to all life processes. All enzymes are proteins. All proteins are made of amino acids. Amino acids have to be put together to make proteins. Enzymes put together the amino acids. In other words, some proteins make other proteins. Enzymes are catalysts that facilitate the building up or breaking down of compounds (both protein and nonprotein) in the body. Enzymes are not themselves altered by the reactions they facilitate.

The protein story moves in a circle. To follow the circle in nutrition, start with a person eating protein. The protein is broken down by proteins (digestive enzymes) into amino acids. The amino acids enter the cells of the body, where proteins (enzymes) put the amino acids together in long chains whose sequences are specified by the genes. The chains fold and twist back

enzyme: a protein that facilitates chemical reactions without itself being changed in the process. A protein catalyst.

catalyst (CAT-uh-list): a compound that facilitates chemical reactions without itself being destroyed in the process.

on themselves to form proteins, and some of these proteins become enzymes themselves. These enzymes may then be used to break apart other compounds or to put other compounds together. Day by day, in billions of reactions, these processes repeat themselves, and life goes on. Only living systems work with such self-renewal. A toaster cannot produce another toaster; a car cannot fix a broken-down car. Only living creatures and the parts they are composed of—the cells—can duplicate and repair themselves.

Fluid and Acid-Base Balance

Proteins help maintain the body's fluid balance. Fluids are present in several body compartments. Chief among them are the spaces inside the blood vessels; the spaces within the cells; and the spaces between the cells (outside the blood vessels). Fluids flow back and forth between these compartments, and proteins in the fluids, together with minerals, help to maintain the needed distribution of these fluids.

The reasons why proteins in fluids can help determine the fluids' distribution in living systems are that proteins are large and attracted to water (hydrophilic). Being large, proteins cannot pass freely across the membranes that separate body compartments. Being hydrophilic, they attract the water molecules near them, which in effect makes them even larger. A cell that "wants" to keep a certain amount of water in its interior space can't move the water around directly, but it can manufacture proteins, and these proteins will hold water. Thus the cell uses protein to help regulate the distribution of water indirectly. Similarly, the body makes proteins for the blood and the intercellular spaces. These proteins help maintain the fluid volume in those spaces.

Proteins also help maintain the balance between acids and bases within the body's fluids. If the body's fluids become too acidic, the structure of vital proteins can be disrupted. When this happens, the proteins lose their shape and can no longer function. A similar situation arises when the balance tips too far toward base. These imbalances are known as acidosis and alkalosis, and either can be fatal.

Proteins such as albumin in plasma help to prevent these imbalances from arising. In a sense, the proteins protect one another by gathering up extra acid (hydrogen) ions when there are too many in the surrounding medium and by releasing them when there are too few. This ability to regulate the acid-base balance of the medium is known as the buffering action of proteins.

Antibodies and Hormones

Other major proteins in the blood—the antibodies—act against viruses, bacteria, and other disease agents. The antibodies work so efficiently that if a million bacterial cells are injected into the skin of a healthy person, fewer than ten are likely to survive for five hours. Without sufficient protein, the body cannot maintain its resistance to disease.

The blood also carries messenger molecules known as hormones, and some are made of amino acids. (Recall that other hormones are sterols.) Among the hormones composed of amino acids are the thyroid hormone

---

The space in the blood vessels is the intravascular space; the space inside the cells is the intracellular space; the space between the cells is the intercellular or interstitial (in-ter-STISH-ul) space.

intra = inside
inter = between
interstice = space between

Minerals are helper nutrients. The attraction of protein and mineral particles to water is due to osmotic pressure (see Chapter 8).

acid-base balance: the balance maintained in the body between too much and too little acid. Blood pH, for example, is regulated normally between 7.38 and 7.42.

pH: the concentration of hydrogen ions. The lower the pH, the stronger the acid. Thus pH 2 is a strong acid; pH 6 is a weak acid; pH 7 is neutral; and a pH above 7 is alkaline.

The change in a protein's shape brought about by heat, acid, or other conditions is known as denaturation (dee-nay-cher-AY-shun). Past a certain point, denaturation is irreversible.

acidosis: too much acid in the blood and body fluids.

alkalosis: too much base in the blood and body fluids.

buffer: a compound that can reversibly combine with hydrogen ions to help control the acidity of a solution.

and insulin. Hormones have many profound effects, which will become evident in subsequent chapters.

Transport Proteins

A specific group of the body's proteins specializes in moving nutrients and other molecules in and out of cells. Transport proteins act as "pumps," picking up compounds on one side of the membrane and depositing them on the other, thereby enabling the cell to "decide" which substances to take up and which to release. Cells can switch the protein machinery of their membranes on or off in response to the body's needs. Often hormones do the switching, with marvelous precision.

Other transport proteins move about in the body fluids, carrying nutrients and other molecules from one organ to another. The protein hemoglobin, which carries oxygen from the lungs to the body's cells, is a prime example. The lipoproteins transport lipids around the body. In addition, special proteins also carry fat-soluble vitamins, water-soluble vitamins, and minerals.

All the body's tissues and organs—muscles, bones, blood, skin, nerves—are made largely of protein. One important protein, collagen, helps make scar tissue, forms the protein matrix of bones and teeth, forms the material of ligaments and tendons, and is a strengthening constituent of artery walls.

The list of protein functions mentioned here is by no means exhaustive, but it does give you some sense of the immense variety and importance of proteins in the body. With this information as background, you are in a position to appreciate the need for protein in the diet.

Protein in Foods

The role of proteins in foods is not to provide body proteins directly but to supply the amino acids from which the body can make its own proteins. The body can make some amino acids for itself; the protein in food does not need to supply these. But there are other amino acids that the body cannot make at all, and some that it cannot make fast enough to meet its needs. The proteins in foods supply these amino acids to the body; they are therefore called the *essential* amino acids. Nine amino acids are essential. The distinction between essential and nonessential amino acids is less clear-cut than it seems, however. For example, histidine has long been known to be an essential amino acid for infants, but only recently has it been added to the list of essential amino acids for adults.[1]

Sometimes a nonessential amino acid can become essential. During illness or conditions of trauma, the need for a nonessential amino acid may be greater than the body's ability to produce it. In such circumstances, an amino acid that is nonessential for healthy people becomes essential for the ill person and is referred to as a "conditionally essential" amino acid. Research suggests that glutamine, normally a nonessential amino acid, may be a conditionally essential amino acid for critically ill people.[2]

antibodies: large proteins of the blood and body fluids, produced in response to invasion of the body by unfamiliar molecules (mostly proteins); antibodies inactivate the invaders and so protect the body. The invaders are called *antigens.*
 anti = against

hormone: a chemical messenger. Hormones are secreted by a variety of glands in the body in response to altered conditions. Each affects one or more target tissues or organs and elicits specific responses to restore normal conditions.

essential amino acid: an amino acid that the body cannot synthesize in amounts sufficient to meet physiological need. Nine amino acids are known to be essential for human adults:
histidine (HISS-tuh-deen)
isoleucine (eye-so-LOO-seen)
leucine (LOO-seen)
lysine (LYE-seen)
methionine (meh-THIGH-oh-neen)
phenylalanine (fee-nul-AL-uh-neen)
threonine (THREE-oh-neen)
tryptophan (TRIP-toe-fane)
valine (VAY-leen)

To make body protein, a cell must have all the needed amino acids available simultaneously. Therefore, the first important characteristic of protein in the diet of a healthy adult is that it should supply at least the nine essential amino acids and enough nitrogen and energy for the synthesis of the other thirteen.

A protein that fits this description is called a complete protein. It contains all the essential amino acids in amounts adequate for human use; it may or may not contain all the others. Generally, proteins derived from animal foods (meats, fish, poultry, eggs, and milk) are complete, although gelatin is an exception. Proteins derived from plant foods (legumes, grains, and vegetables) vary more. Some plant proteins are notoriously incomplete—for example, corn protein. Others are complete—for example, soy protein.[3] The educated vegetarian can design a diet that is adequate in protein, using plant foods alone, by choosing a variety of legumes, grains, and vegetables. (Vegetarian diets are discussed further in Nutrition in Practice 4.) Table 4–1 provides a list of protein-containing foods and shows the energy they provide.

It is desirable that a protein be not only complete, but easily digestible as well, so that sufficient numbers of amino acids reach the body's cells to permit them to make the proteins they need. Such a protein is called a high-quality protein. One of the finest proteins available by these standards is egg protein. Eggs are a highly valued protein source in less developed nations where protein-rich foods are scarce.

complete protein: a protein containing all the amino acids essential in human nutrition in amounts adequate for human use.

high-quality protein: an easily digestible, complete protein.

TABLE 4–1   **Protein-Containing Foods and the Energy They Provide**

Each of the following provides about 7 g of protein.[a]
   1 oz lean meat, poultry, fish—about 55 kcal

And so do these:
   ½ c legumes—80 kcal
   1 c egg noodles—160 kcal
   1 c broccoli or brussels sprouts—50 kcal
   7 oz milk or yogurt—80 kcal
   1 oz cheese[b]—100 kcal
   ¼ c cottage cheese—55 kcal
   2 tbsp peanut butter[b]—200 kcal
   1 to 2 oz nuts or seeds[b]—175 to 250 kcal
   ¼ c tofu—75 kcal

Each of these provides about 3 g protein:
   1 slice bread—80 kcal
   ½ c most cooked cereals and grains—80 kcal
   ⅓ c cooked rice—80 kcal

And these provide about 2 g protein each:
   ½ c cooked vegetables—25 kcal
   1 c raw vegetables—25 kcal

[a]For reference, an adult might need from 40 to 100 g protein in a day.
[b]These are high-fat choices.

Ideally, dietary protein supplies each amino acid in the amount needed for protein synthesis in the body. If one amino acid is supplied in an amount smaller than is needed, then the total amount of protein that can be synthesized will be limited. The body makes only complete proteins. (By analogy, suppose that a sign maker plans to make 100 identical signs, each saying "Left Turn Only." The sign maker needs 200 Ls, 200 Ns, 200 Ts, and 100 of each of the other letters. If only 20 Ls are available, only 10 signs can be made, even if all the other letters are available in unlimited quantities. Suppose further that the sign maker has no place to keep leftover letters—just as the body has no storage place for extra amino acids. If the sign maker doesn't get some additional Ls right away, he will have to throw away all the other letters.)

Dietary protein—no matter how high the quality—will not be used efficiently and will not support growth when energy from carbohydrate and fat is lacking. The body assigns top priority to meeting its energy need and, if necessary, will break down protein to meet this need. After stripping off and excreting the nitrogen from the amino acids, the body will use their carbon skeletons in much the same way it uses those from glucose or from fat. A major reason why people must have ample carbohydrate and fat in the diet is to prevent this wasting of protein.

limiting amino acid: the essential amino acid found in the shortest supply relative to the amounts needed for protein synthesis in the body.

Carbohydrate and fat allow amino acids to be used to build body proteins. This is known as the protein-sparing action of carbohydrate and fat.

Health Effects of Protein

In the short time that scientists have been studying nutrition, no nutrient has been more intensely scrutinized than protein. As you know by now, it is indispensable to life. And it should come as no surprise that protein deficiency can have devastating effects on people's health. But like the other nutrients, too much protein can also be harmful; the end of this section discusses the consequences of protein excess.

Protein-Energy Malnutrition

When people are deprived of food and suffer an energy deficit, they degrade their own body protein for energy and indirectly suffer a protein deficiency, as well as an energy deficiency. Because protein and energy deprivation thus go hand in hand, public health officials have adopted an abbreviation for the overlapping pair: protein-energy malnutrition (PEM). Observed cases of PEM are caused by both extremes—protein deficiency or energy deficiency—and by combinations of both. The classic protein deficiency disease is kwashiorkor, and the classic energy deficiency disease is marasmus. The consequences of PEM as a world malnutrition problem are considered here; the problems associated with PEM in the hospital are described in Chapter 14.

Of all population groups, children are most seriously affected by malnutrition. PEM is the most pervasive form of malnutrition among children in the developing world. PEM takes two forms. Children who are thin for their height may be suffering from acute PEM (recent severe food restriction), whereas children who are short for their age may have experienced chronic

protein-energy malnutrition: a deficiency of protein or food energy or both.
mal = bad, poor

kwashiorkor (kwash-ee-OR-core) or kwash-ee-or-CORE): malnutrition caused by protein deficiency in the presence of adequate food energy.

marasmus (ma-RAZZ-mus): malnutrition caused by simple starvation.

PEM (long-term food restriction). Stunted growth due to PEM is easy to overlook because a small child may look quite normal, but it may be the most common sign of malnutrition in the developing countries.

KWASHIORKOR. The word *kwashiorkor* originally referred to an "evil spirit that infects the first child when the second child is born." If you consider how kwashiorkor often develops, you can easily see how this superstitious belief arose among the Ghanaians who named the disease. When a mother who has been nursing her first child bears a second child, she weans the first child and puts the second one on the breast. The first child, suddenly switched from nutrient-dense, protein-rich breast milk to a starchy, protein-poor gruel, soon begins to sicken and die. The gruel does not supply enough amino acids even to maintain a child's body, much less enough to enable the child to grow.

Kwashiorkor occurs not only in Africa but also in Central America, South America, the Near East, the Far East, and in wealthy and poor countries on every continent. It is probably a mixture of deficiency symptoms from lack of both protein and zinc, and possibly other nutrients as well. Wherever mother's milk is the only reliable and readily available source of protein and zinc for infants, kwashiorkor threatens them at weaning time. It typically sets in at about the age of two. (We'll use a girl as an example here, and a boy for marasmus.) Growth slows down, so that by the age of four, she is no taller than at two. Her hair loses its color; her skin becomes patchy and scaly, sometimes with ulcers and sores that fail to heal. The child's limbs and face become swollen with edema; her belly bulges with a fatty liver; she sickens easily and becomes weak, fretful, and apathetic.

The body follows a priority system when there is not enough protein to meet all its needs. It abandons its less vital systems first. When it cannot obtain enough amino acids from dietary sources, the body switches to a "metabolism of wasting"; it begins to digest its own protein tissues. In this way, it can supply the amino acids needed to continuously maintain the vital internal organs and thus keep itself alive. Hair and skin pigments (which are made of amino acids) are the first to go. They begin to lose their color, and skin sores fail to heal. Many antibodies are also degraded so that their amino acids can be used as building blocks for heart, lung, and brain tissue. A child with a depleted supply of antibodies cannot resist infection and readily contracts dysentery, a disease of the digestive tract. Dysentery causes diarrhea, leading to rapid loss of many nutrients, including amino acids, that the child may be receiving in food. Thus dysentery worsens the protein deficiency, and the protein deficiency in turn increases the likelihood of a second or third or tenth attack of dysentery.

MARASMUS. Whereas kwashiorkor seems to occur in individuals who receive food but too little protein, marasmus occurs in those who receive little or no food at all; it is simple starvation. A marasmic child looks like a wizened little old person—just skin and bones. He is often sick, because his resistance to disease is low. All his muscles are wasted, including the heart muscle, which weakens the heart. Reduced synthesis of key hormones leads to a metabolism so slow that the child's body temperature is subnormal. Unlike the kwashiorkor child, he has no fat accumulation in the liver, and little or no fat under the skin to insulate against cold. Hospital workers find

edema (e-DEE-muh): an accumulation of fluid. In PEM, protein in the blood is depleted, and water cannot be held there. Instead, water seeps into the interstitial space and accumulates. Hormonal imbalances in protein deficiency also contribute to edema.

fatty liver: an accumulation of fat in the liver. In PEM, fat accumulates in the liver because there is no protein available to form the lipoproteins that normally escort fat molecules in the blood.

dysentery (DIS-en-terry): an infection of the gastrointestinal tract caused by an amoeba or bacterium that gives rise to severe diarrhea.
   dys = bad
   entery = intestine

When two variables interact so that each increases the other, **synergism** (SIN-er-jiz-um) is said to be acting. Malnutrition and infection are a deadly combination, because they work in this way.
   syn = with, together
   ergism = work

that the primary need of marasmic victims is to be wrapped up and kept warm.

Unlike the kwashiorkor child, who has been fed milk until weaning, the marasmic child typically has been neglected from early infancy. The disease occurs most commonly in children from 6 to 18 months of age in all the overpopulated city slums of the world and in rural children who have been fed inadequate formulas for too long. Because the brain normally grows to almost its full adult size within the first two years of life, marasmus impairs brain development and so may have a permanent effect on learning ability.

PEM afflicts not only infants but also pregnant and lactating women, just-weaned children, and children in periods of rapid growth. These groups have a great need for protein, and they need ample food energy to protect it. In many cultures, however, these groups are the very ones who are denied nourishing food.

Experts assure us that we possess the knowledge, technology, and resources to end hunger. Some success has rewarded local efforts where programs involved the local people in the process of identifying the problem and devising its solution. To fight the war on hunger, it is going to take the will to do so by those who have the food, technology, and resources.

Protein Excess

While many of the world's people struggle to obtain enough food and enough protein to survive, in the developed nations protein is so abundant that problems of protein excess are seen. There are no benefits, and there are risks associated with the overconsumption of protein. For example, protein-rich foods are often high-fat foods that contribute to obesity with its accompanying health risks. Some studies suggest a link between high-meat diets and colon cancer.[4] The higher a person's intake of protein-rich foods such as meat and milk, the more likely it is that fruits, vegetables, and grains will be crowded out of the diet, making the diet inadequate in other nutrients.

Diets high in protein promote calcium excretion, depleting the bones of their chief mineral.[5] There are evidently no benefits to be gained by consuming a diet that derives more than 15 percent of its energy from protein. The *NRC Recommendations* (Table 1-3, Chapter 1) advise a moderate protein intake—one that falls between the RDA and twice the RDA.

Recommended Protein Intakes

Your body loses protein every day. Skin cells flake off or are rubbed off. Hair and nails (made of protein) grow longer daily and are shed or cut away. People need to eat protein-rich foods every day to replace the protein they lose. If the body is growing, it needs more protein than is necessary just for maintenance. Children end each day with more blood cells, more muscle cells, and more skin cells than they had at the beginning of the day. So protein is needed both for routine maintenance (replacement) and growth (addition).

nitrogen balance: the amount of nitrogen consumed (N in) as compared with the amount of nitrogen excreted (N out) in a given period of time. The laboratory scientist can estimate the protein in a sample of food, body tissue, or excreta by measuring the nitrogen in it. Chapter 10 provides additional information about N balance.

If the body maintains in its tissues the same amount of protein from day to day, it is in nitrogen balance. If the body adds protein, it is in positive nitrogen balance; if it loses protein, it is in negative nitrogen balance.

Normally, healthy adults are in nitrogen balance; that is, they have the same amount of protein in their bodies at all times. They use what nitrogen they need and excrete the excess. Growing children and pregnant women are in positive nitrogen balance, because they are adding protein to their bodies as new blood, bone, and muscle cells. People in negative nitrogen balance are losing body protein. People who are fasting or starving, such as those with anorexia nervosa, or people who are sick or in trauma, such as people with burns (see Chapter 18), are in negative nitrogen balance, because they are forced to use protein for energy.

The Committee on RDA states that a generous daily protein allowance for a healthy adult would be 0.8 gram of high-quality protein per kilogram of appropriate or average body weight for height. Protein RDA for people of average height at all ages are presented in the RDA table (inside front cover). If your height is not average, you can compute your own individualized RDA for protein (see the Self-Study that follows).

In setting the RDA, the committee assumes that the protein eaten will be of high quality, that it will be consumed together with adequate energy from carbohydrate and fat, and that other nutrients in the diet will be adequate. The committee also assumes that the RDA will be applied only to healthy individuals with no unusual metabolic need for protein. Most people in this country already eat this much protein, and more.

Study Questions

1. Chemically, how does protein differ from carbohydrate and fat?
2. What is an enzyme?
3. List and describe at least 3 main functions of proteins in the body.
4. What is an essential amino acid?
5. What is a complete protein?
6. Describe how kwashiorkor differs from marasmus.

Notes

1. P. L. Pellett, Protein requirements in humans, *American Journal of Clinical Nutrition* 51 (1990): 723–727.
2. J. M. Lacey and D. W. Wilmore, Is glutamine a conditionally essential amino acid? *Nutrition Reviews* 48 (1990): 297–309.
3. J. W. Erdman and E. J. Fordyce, Soy products and the human diet, *American Journal of Clinical Nutrition* 49 (1989): 725–737.
4. Pellett, 1990.
5. M. G. Holl and L. H. Allen, Comparative effects of meals high in protein, sucrose, or starch on human mineral metabolism and insulin secretion, *American Journal of Clinical Nutrition* 48 (1988): 1219–1225; M. B. Zemel, Calcium utilization: Effect of varying level and source of dietary protein, *American Journal of Clinical Nutrition* 48 (1988): 880–883.

SELF-STUDY

How's Your Protein Intake?

These exercises make use of the information you recorded on Forms 1 to 5.

1. How many grams of protein do you consume in a day? _____ grams
2. How many kcalories does this represent? (Remember, 1 gram of protein contributes 4 kcalories.) _____ kcalories
3. What percentage of your total kcalories is contributed by protein? _____ percent
4. Dietary guidelines suggest that protein should contribute about 10 to 15 percent of total kcalories. How does your protein intake compare with this recommendation? (Note: If you are on a kcalorie-restricted diet, a higher percentage of your kcalories should come from protein. If your protein intake is out of line, what foods could you consume more or less of to bring it into line?

_____

_____

5. Compare your protein intake (from item 1) with the recommendation for an "average" person of your age and sex as shown in the RDA tables (inside front cover) or in the Canadian recommendations (Appendix A)? _____ If you are not of average height or weight, figure your protein RDA:
   a. Look up the weight for a person your height (inside back cover). Assume this weight is "ideal" for you.
   b. Change pounds to kilograms; 2.2 pounds equals 1 kilogram.
   c. Multiply kilograms by 0.8 grams/kilogram.

   Example (for a medium-frame male 5 feet 10 inches tall):
   a. "Ideal" weight: about 150 pounds.
   b. 150 pounds × 1 kilogram/2.2 pounds = 68 kilograms (rounded off).
   c. 68 kilograms × 0.8 grams/kilogram = 54 grams protein (rounded off).

6. Compare your average daily protein intake with your RDA. About what percentage of that intake are you consuming each day? _____ percent. If you are "average" and healthy, the recommendation is probably generous for you, yet you may be eating more protein than that. This means that you may be spending protein prices for an energy nutrient. What substitutions could you make in your day's food choices for you to derive the kcalories you need for energy from carbohydrate rather than from protein?

_____

_____

7. How many of your protein grams are from animal foods? _____ How many from plant foods? _____ Assuming that the animal protein is of high quality, no more than 20 percent of your total protein has to come from this source. Should you alter the ratio of plant to animal protein in your diet? _____ If you were to do so, what effect would this have on the total fat content of your diet?

_____

_____

4

Vegetarian Diets

Eating patterns all along the continuum of dietary choices—from one end, where people eat no foods of animal origin, to the other end, where they eat generous quantities of meat every day—can support or compromise nutritional health. The quality of the diet depends not on whether it consists of all plant foods or centers on meat, but on whether the eater's food choices are based on sound nutrition principles—adequacy of nutrient intakes; balance and variety of foods chosen; appropriate energy intake; and moderation in intakes of substances such as caffeine, alcohol, sodium, and fat that are harmful in excess.

People choose to exclude meat and other animal-derived foods from their diets for various reasons—health attitudes, taste preferences, philosophies, or religions. Some believe that vegetarianism is ecologically sound, and others believe that it is less costly than the meat-eating alternative. Whatever the reasons, vegetarians and health professionals who work with them should be aware of the nutrition and health implications of the vegetarian diet.

Because vegetarian diets vary in both the types and amounts of animal-derived foods they include, these differences must be considered when evaluating the health status of

vegetarians. The Miniglossary defines kinds of vegetarian diets.

I've been thinking about becoming a vegetarian myself, but I'm still not sure whether vegetarian diets are nutritionally sound. Are they?

The American Dietetic Association acknowledges that well-planned vegetarian diets offer nutrition and health benefits to adults in general.[1] Research suggests that adults who eat vegetarian diets reduce their risks of heart disease, hypertension, diabetes, and obesity.[2]

So what should be my main concerns when planning a nutritionally sound vegetarian diet?

The tasks for a vegetarian diet planner are the same as those for other diet planners—to plan a diet that delivers a variety of foods that provide all the needed nutrients within an energy allowance that maintains a healthy body weight. The challenge is to do so using at least one less food group. Since all vegetarians omit meat, and some omit other animal-derived foods, it is protein, the nutrient that meat is

MINIGLOSSARY

complementary proteins: two or more proteins whose amino acid assortments complement each other in such a way that the essential amino acids missing from each are supplied by the other.

lacto-vegetarians: people who include milk or milk products, but who exclude meat, poultry, fish, seafood, and eggs from their diets.

lacto-ovo vegetarians: people who include milk or milk products and eggs, but who omit meat, fish, and poultry from their diets.

mutual supplementation: the strategy of combining two protein foods in a meal so that each food provides the essential amino acid(s) lacking in the other.

semivegetarians: people who include some, but not all, groups of animal-derived foods in their diets; they usually exclude meat and may occasionally include poultry, fish, and seafood; also called *partial vegetarians*.

vegans: people who exclude all animal-derived foods (including meat, poultry, fish, eggs, cheese, and milk) from their diets; also called *strict vegetarians* or *total vegetarians*.

famous for, that merits the most discussion here.

Yes, I've heard that vegetarian diets are low in protein. Is this true?

No, protein is not the problem it was once thought to be in vegetarian diets. People who include animal-derived foods such as milk and eggs in their diets need not worry at all about protein deficiency. Even for those who eat nothing but plant-derived foods, protein intakes are usually satisfactory as long as energy intakes are adequate and the protein sources varied.[3] A mixture of proteins from whole grains, legumes, seeds, nuts, and vegetables can provide adequate amounts of all the amino acids.

The idea that vegans must carefully combine their plant protein foods in order to obtain the full array of essential amino acids persists despite new knowledge that this is not necessary. Plant foods can provide more than enough of all the essential amino acids, and can sustain people in good health, as long as energy intakes are sufficient and there are not too many empty-kcalorie foods in the diet. It is true, however, that the quality of individual plant proteins can be improved by combining two different ones, each of which supplies amino acids missing from the other. This strategy is called *mutual supplementation*. The two protein foods that mutually supplement each other are called *complementary proteins*. Figure NP4–1 offers mixtures of plant proteins that provide higher-quality protein than the individual foods they are made from.

Tell me more about food energy intakes and vegetarian diets.

Researchers find that vegetarians as a group are closer to a healthy body weight than nonvegetarians. Since obesity impairs health in a number of ways, vegetarians therefore have a health advantage. Vegetarian diets tend to be high in complex carbohydrates

---

FIGURE NP4–1   **Nonmeat Mixtures That Provide High-Quality Protein**

Vegetarians who eat no foods from animal sources select foods from two or more of these columns to create high-quality protein combinations:

GRAINS	LEGUMES	SEEDS AND NUTS	VEGETABLES
Oats	Peanuts	Cashews	Broccoli
Rice	Soy products	Nut butters	Cabbage
Whole-grain breads	Pinto beans	Sesame seeds	Peppers
Pasta	Black beans		Squash
Examples:			Spinach

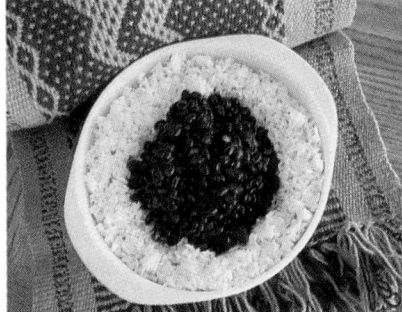

Black beans and rice, a favorite Hispanic combination.

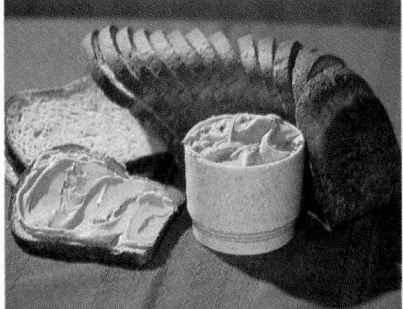

Peanut butter and wheat bread, a North American tradition.

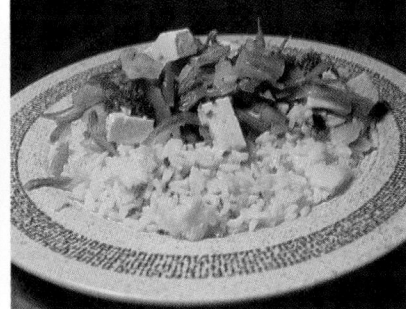

Tofu and stir-fried vegetables with rice, an Asian dish.

and low in fat, characteristics that are consistent with current dietary recommendations aimed at reducing the incidence of obesity and other degenerative diseases in this country.

Not all vegetarians fit the average pattern, though. Obesity does threaten vegetarians who include milk, eggs, and cheese in their diets. They can easily consume both a high-fat diet and excess food energy, and so must be careful to select nonfat and low-fat dairy foods and to avoid relying too heavily on these foods in general.

In contrast, people who exclude all animal-derived foods (vegans) may have trouble obtaining *enough* food energy. This is especially true for children and pregnant and lactating women. Vegan diets can fail to provide adequate food energy to support the growth of a child within a small enough bulk of food for the child to eat.[4] Plant foods that are best suited to meet energy needs in a small volume are cereals, legumes, and nuts; these foods should be emphasized in a vegan child's diet. Table 1–2 in Chapter 1 offers a Daily Food Choices Pattern for vegetarians. Additional servings of vegetables, fruits, and grains and cereals, as well as a serving of nuts and seeds, will help ensure that energy needs are met.

Tell me about vitamins and minerals. If I go on a vegetarian diet, will I need to take vitamin supplements?

That depends on the kind of vegetarian diet you follow. The lacto-ovo vegetarian diet can be complete in all vitamins, but several vitamins may be a problem for the vegan. One such vitamin is B_{12}. Because vitamin B_{12} occurs only in animal-derived foods, supplements are

necessary to prevent deficiency. Women who have adhered to all-plant diets for many years are especially likely to have low vitamin B_{12} stores. The added demands for vitamin B_{12} imposed by pregnancy make it virtually impossible for pregnant women to maintain adequate vitamin B_{12} status without supplementation or the inclusion of a reliable food source of the nutrient. Vitamin B_{12} deficiency can take a long time to develop in adults, because up to four years' worth can be stored in the body. In infants, deficiencies set in more rapidly and can severely damage their nervous systems. All vegan mothers must be sure to use vitamin B_{12}–fortified products or take the appropriate supplements.

What other vitamins do vegans need?

Another vitamin of concern is vitamin D. The milk drinker is protected, provided the milk is fortified with vitamin D, but there is no practical source of vitamin D in plant foods. Regular exposure to the sun will prevent a deficiency, but the homebound or vegan living in a northern climate or smoggy city probably should take vitamin D supplements. Excesses of vitamin D are toxic, and one should not exceed the recommended daily amount of 5 micrograms.

Riboflavin, another vitamin often obtained from milk, is not a problem for the vegan who uses dark greens frequently in ample servings. The vegan who doesn't use a lot of greens, however, may not meet riboflavin needs. Nutritional yeast is a rich source of riboflavin for the vegetarian.

So on a vegan diet, vitamin B_{12}, vitamin D, and riboflavin can be problems if I'm not careful. What about minerals?

Two minerals may be of concern for all vegetarians, not just the vegan. These are iron and zinc. Legumes are an important source of iron in the vegetarian diet. The iron in legumes, however, is not as absorbable as that in meat. In fact, people absorb three times as much iron from a meal that includes meat as from one that does not. Because vitamin C in fruits and vegetables also can triple iron absorption from other foods eaten at the same meal, vegetarian meals should be rich in foods offering vitamin C.

As for zinc, it too may be a problem nutrient for vegetarians. It is widespread in plant foods, but its availability may be hindered by the fibers and other binders found in fruits and vegetables. The zinc needs of vegetarians and the effects of mineral binders are subjects of intensive study at the present time. While research continues, vegetarians are advised to eat varied diets that include whole-grain breads well leavened with yeast, which improves the availability of their minerals.

What about minerals for the vegan? Is calcium a problem?

Good thinking. Yes, of course calcium is of concern. The milk-drinking vegetarian is protected from deficiency, but the vegan must find other sources of calcium. Some good calcium sources are regular and ample servings of stone-ground meal; self-rising flour and meal; legumes; calcium-fortified soy milk; some nuts, such as almonds;

and certain seeds, such as sesame seeds. The choices should be varied, because absorption of calcium from some of these foods may be hindered by binders in them. The vegetarian is urged to use calcium-fortified soy milk in ample quantities regularly. This is especially important for children. Infant formula based on soy is fortified with calcium and can easily be used in cooking foods, even for adults.

It sounds as if I can do well with a vegetarian diet as long as I do a little planning. Are there any nutritional advantages to the vegetarian diet besides how it can help with weight control?

Yes. Vegetarian protein foods are often higher in fiber, richer in certain vitamins and minerals, and lower in fat than meats. Vegetarians can enjoy a nutritious diet very low in fat provided that they limit other high-fat foods such as butter, cream cheese, sour cream, and nuts. If vegetarians follow the guidelines presented here and plan carefully, they can support their health as well as, or perhaps better than, nonvegetarians.

Abundant evidence supports the idea that vegetarians may actually be healthier than meat eaters. Informed vegetarians are not only more likely to be at the desired weights for their heights, but to have lower blood cholesterol levels, lower rates of certain kinds of cancer, better digestive function, and more. Even among people who are health conscious, generally vegetarians experience fewer deaths from cardiovascular diseases than meat eaters do. Since vegetarianism often goes with a clean-living lifestyle (no smoking, abstinence from alcohol, emphasis on supportive family life), it is likely that dietary practices do not alone account for all the aspects of improved health. Clearly, however, they contribute significantly to it.

Notes

1. Position of the American Dietetic Association: Vegetarian diets—Technical support paper, *Journal of the American Dietetic Association* 1988 (88): 353–355.
2. J. T. Dwyer, Health aspects of vegetarian diets, *American Journal of Clinical Nutrition* 48 (1988): 712–738.
3. Dwyer, 1988.
4. C. Jacobs and J. T. Dwyer, Vegetarian children: Appropriate and inappropriate diets, *American Journal of Clinical Nutrition* 48 (1988): 811–818.

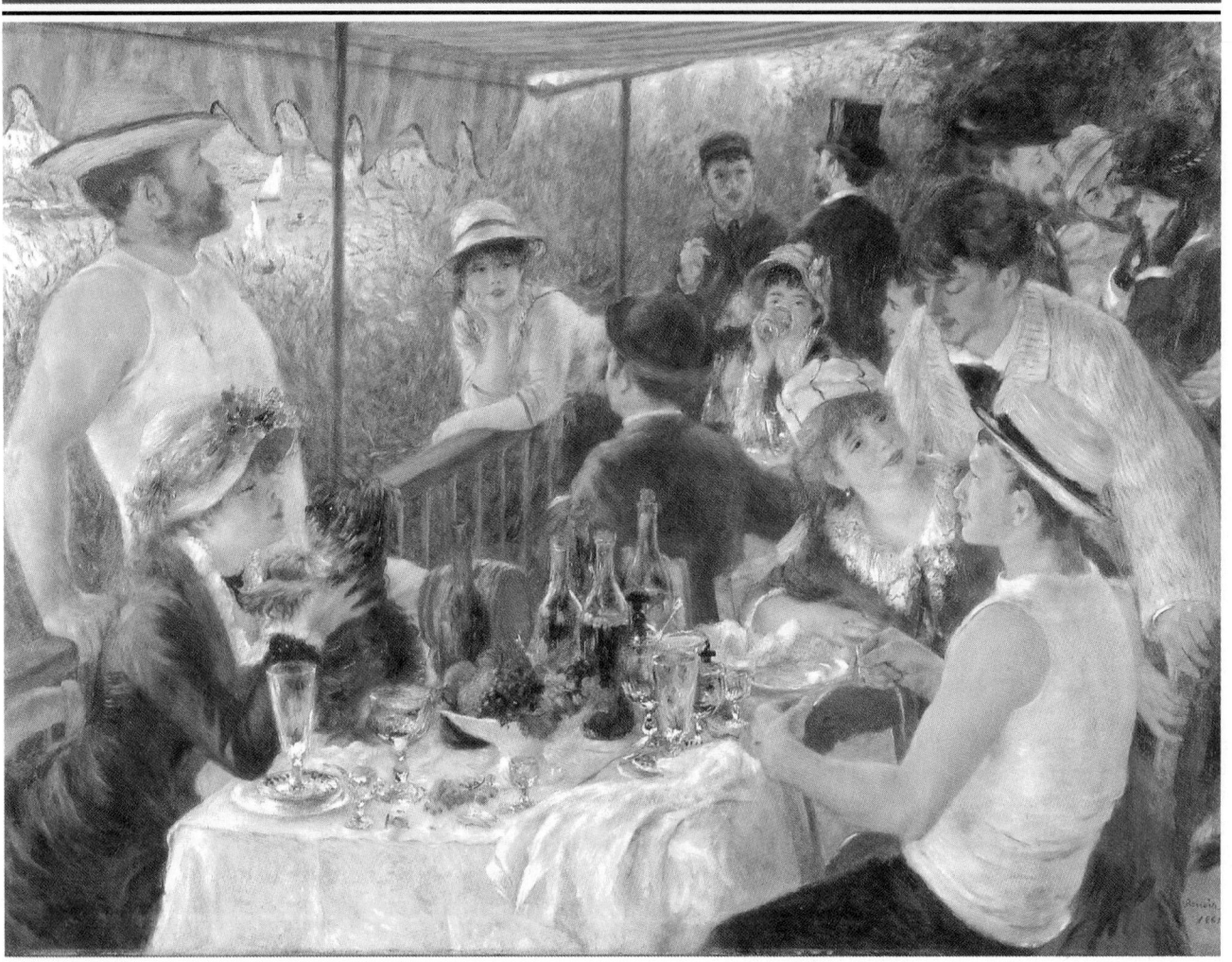

Pierre Renoir, The Luncheon of the Boating Party; © *The Phillips Collection, Washington, D.C.*

CHAPTER

5

Digestion and Absorption

CONTENTS

CHAPTER

5

Your body's ability to transform the foods you eat into the nutrients that fuel your body's work is quite remarkable. Yet most people probably give little, if any, thought to all the body does with food once it is eaten. This chapter offers you the opportunity to learn how the body digests, absorbs, and transports the nutrients in food, and how it excretes the unwanted substances in foods. The next chapter shows you how the body assimilates the nutrients once they are absorbed and traveling in the blood.

One of the beauties of the digestive tract is that it is selective. Materials that are nutritive for the body are broken down into particles that can be absorbed into the bloodstream. Most of the nonnutritive materials are left undigested and pass out the other end of the digestive tract.

Anatomy of the Digestive Tract

The gastrointestinal (GI) tract is a flexible muscular tube measuring about 26 feet in length from the mouth to the anus. Figure 5–1 traces the path followed by food from one end to the other. The Miniglossary on p. 77 defines GI anatomy terms.

The Digestive Organs

GI tract: the gastrointestinal tract or digestive tract; the principal organs are the stomach and intestines.
  gastro = stomach

When you swallow a mouthful of food, it first slides across your epiglottis, bypassing the entrance to your lungs. Whenever you swallow, the epiglottis closes off your air passages so that you do not choke. Once a mouthful of food has been swallowed, it is called a bolus.

bolus (BOH-lus): the portion of food swallowed at one time.

Next, the food slides down the esophagus, which conducts it through the diaphragm to the stomach. The cardiac sphincter, a band of muscle at the stomach's entrance, closes behind the bolus so that it cannot slip back. The stomach retains the bolus for a while, adds water to it, and grinds it into a semiliquid mass called chyme. Then bit by bit, the stomach releases the chyme through another sphincter, the pyloric sphincter, which opens into the small intestine; the pyloric sphincter, too, closes behind the chyme.

chyme (KIME): the semiliquid mass of partly digested food expelled by the stomach into the duodenum.

At the top of the small intestine the chyme bypasses an opening from the common bile duct, which secretes fluids into the small intestine from two organs outside the GI tract—the gallbladder and the pancreas. The chyme travels on down the small intestine through its three segments—the duodenum, the jejunum, and the ileum—a total of 20 feet of tubing coiled within the abdomen.

Having traveled through these segments of the small intestine, the chyme arrives at another sphincter, the ileocecal valve, at the beginning of the large intestine (colon) in the lower right-hand side of the abdomen. Then it travels along the large intestine up the right-hand side of the abdomen, across the front to the left-hand side, down to the lower left-hand side, and finally below the other folds of the intestines to the back side of the body above the rectum.

During chyme's passage to the rectum, the colon withdraws water from it, leaving semisolid waste. The strong muscles of the rectum hold back this

---

MINIGLOSSARY of GI Terms

epiglottis (epp-ee-GLOT-tiss): cartilage in the throat that guards the entrance to the trachea and prevents fluid or food from entering it when a person swallows.
  epi = upon (over)
  glottis = back of tongue

trachea (TRAKE-ee-uh): the windpipe; the passageway from the mouth and nose to the lungs.

esophagus (e-SOFF-uh-gus): the food pipe; the conduit from the mouth to the stomach.

cardiac sphincter (CARD-ee-ack SFINK-ter): the sphincter muscle at the junction between the esophagus and the stomach.
  cardiac = heart

sphincter: a circular muscle surrounding, and able to close, a body opening.
  sphincter = band (binder)

pyloric (pie-LORE-ic) **sphincter**: a sphincter muscle separating the stomach from the small intestine.
  pylorus = gatekeeper

gallbladder: the organ that stores and concentrates bile. When it receives the signal that fat is present in the duodenum, the gallbladder contracts and squirts bile down the bile duct into the duodenum.

pancreas: a gland that secretes digestive juices into the duodenum.

duodenum (doo-oh-DEEN-um or doo-ODD-num): the top portion of the small intestine (about "12 fingers' breadth" long, in ancient terminology).
  duodecim = twelve

jejunum (je-JOON-um): the first two-fifths of the small intestine beyond the duodenum.

ileum (ILL-ee-um): the last segment of the small intestine.

ileocecal (ill-ee-oh-SEEK-ul) **valve**: the sphincter muscle separating the small and large intestines.

colon (COAL-un): the large intestine. Its segments are the ascending colon, the transverse colon, the descending colon, and the sigmoid colon.
  sigmoid = shaped like the letter *S* (*sigma* in Greek)

appendix: a narrow blind sac extending from the beginning of the colon; a vestigial organ with no known function.

rectum: the muscular terminal part of the intestine from the sigmoid colon to the anus.

anus (AY-nus): the terminal sphincter muscle of the GI tract.

Mouth.
Esophagus.
Cardiac sphincter.
Pyloric sphincter.
Duodenum (common bile duct enters here), jejunum, ileum.
Ileocecal valve.
Colon.
Rectum.
Anus.

waste until it is time to defecate. Then the rectal muscles relax, and the last sphincter in the system, the anus, opens to allow the wastes to pass.

In summary, the path followed by food is as shown in the margin. This is a remarkably simple route, considering all that happens on the way.

FIGURE 5–1   **The Gastrointestinal Tract**

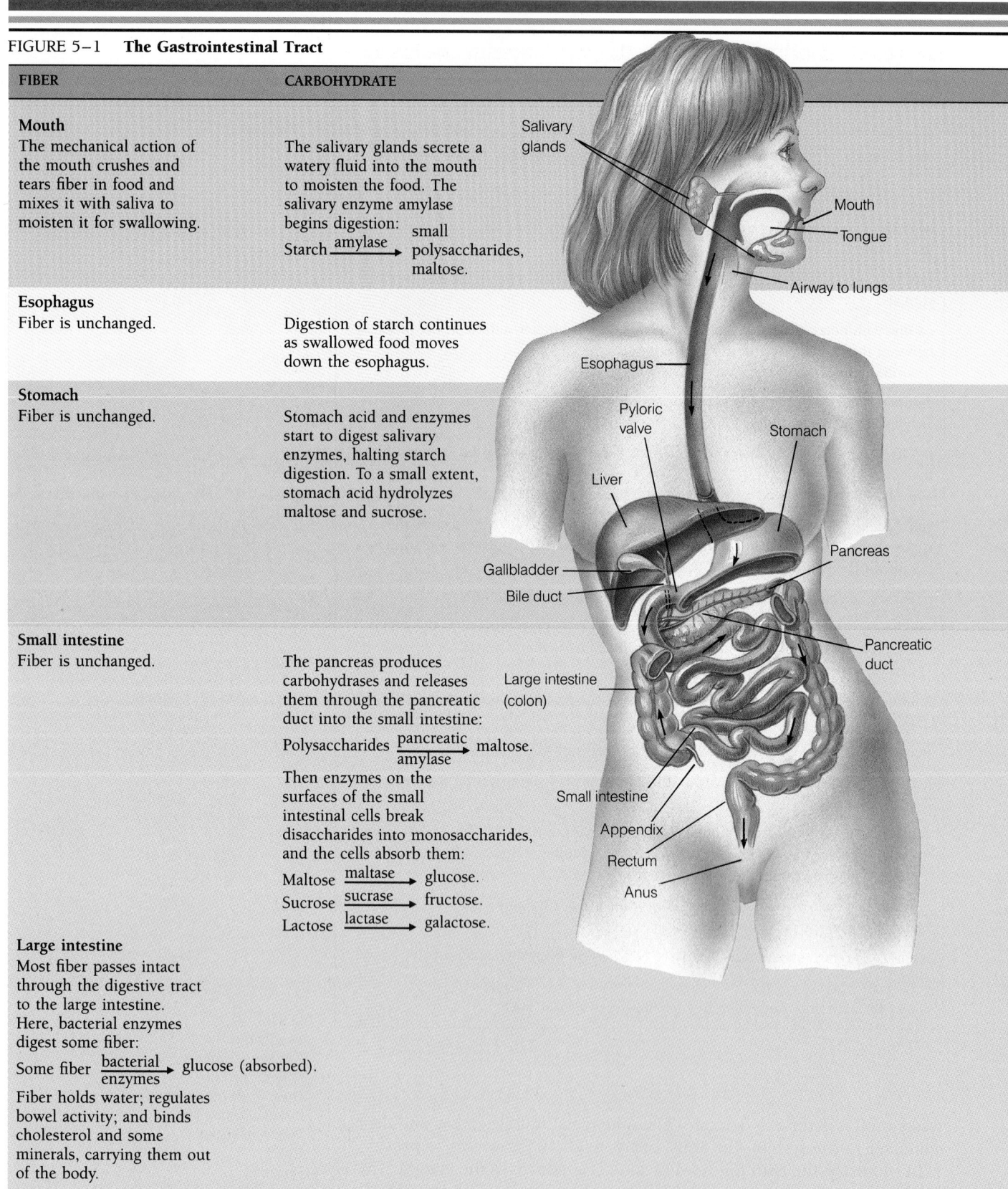

FIBER	CARBOHYDRATE

Mouth

The mechanical action of the mouth crushes and tears fiber in food and mixes it with saliva to moisten it for swallowing.

The salivary glands secrete a watery fluid into the mouth to moisten the food. The salivary enzyme amylase begins digestion:

$$\text{Starch} \xrightarrow{\text{amylase}} \text{small polysaccharides, maltose.}$$

Esophagus

Fiber is unchanged.

Digestion of starch continues as swallowed food moves down the esophagus.

Stomach

Fiber is unchanged.

Stomach acid and enzymes start to digest salivary enzymes, halting starch digestion. To a small extent, stomach acid hydrolyzes maltose and sucrose.

Small intestine

Fiber is unchanged.

The pancreas produces carbohydrases and releases them through the pancreatic duct into the small intestine:

$$\text{Polysaccharides} \xrightarrow[\text{amylase}]{\text{pancreatic}} \text{maltose.}$$

Then enzymes on the surfaces of the small intestinal cells break disaccharides into monosaccharides, and the cells absorb them:

$$\text{Maltose} \xrightarrow{\text{maltase}} \text{glucose.}$$
$$\text{Sucrose} \xrightarrow{\text{sucrase}} \text{fructose.}$$
$$\text{Lactose} \xrightarrow{\text{lactase}} \text{galactose.}$$

Large intestine

Most fiber passes intact through the digestive tract to the large intestine. Here, bacterial enzymes digest some fiber:

$$\text{Some fiber} \xrightarrow[\text{enzymes}]{\text{bacterial}} \text{glucose (absorbed).}$$

Fiber holds water; regulates bowel activity; and binds cholesterol and some minerals, carrying them out of the body.

Labels on figure: Salivary glands, Mouth, Tongue, Airway to lungs, Esophagus, Pyloric valve, Stomach, Liver, Pancreas, Gallbladder, Bile duct, Pancreatic duct, Large intestine (colon), Small intestine, Appendix, Rectum, Anus

FIGURE 5–1   (*continued*)

FAT	PROTEIN	VITAMINS	MINERALS AND WATER
Mouth Glands in the base of the tongue secrete a lipase known as lingual lipase. Some hard fats begin to melt as they reach body temperature.	Chewing and crushing moistens protein-rich foods and mixes them with saliva to be swallowed.	No action.	The salivary glands add water to disperse and carry food.
Esophagus Fat is unchanged.	No action.	No action.	No action.
Stomach Triglycerides are split to produce diglycerides and fatty acids. The degree of hydrolysis of fats is slight for most fats but may be appreciable for milk fats. The stomach's churning action mixes fat with water and acid. A gastric lipase accesses and hydrolyzes a very little fat.	Stomach acid uncoils protein strands and activates stomach enzymes: Protein $\xrightarrow[\text{HC1}]{\text{pepsin}}$ smaller polypeptides.	Intrinsic factor (see Chapter 7) attaches to vitamin B_{12}.	Stomach acid (HC1) acts on iron to reduce it, making it more absorbable (see Chapter 8). The stomach secretes enough watery fluid to turn a moist, chewed mass of solid food into liquid chyme.
Small intestine Bile flows in from the liver (via the common bile duct): Fat $\xrightarrow{\text{bile}}$ emulsified fat. Pancreatic lipase flows in from the pancreas: Emulsified fat $\xrightarrow[\text{lipase}]{\text{pancreatic}}$ monoglycerides, glycerol, fatty acids (absorbed).	Pancreatic and small intestinal enzymes split polypeptides further: Polypeptides $\xrightarrow[\substack{\text{and intestinal} \\ \text{proteases}}]{\text{pancreatic}}$ dipeptides, tripeptides, and amino acids. Then enzymes on the surface of the small intestinal cells hydrolyze these peptides, and the cells absorb them: Peptides $\xrightarrow[\substack{\text{dipeptidases} \\ \text{and tripeptidases}}]{\text{intestinal}}$ amino acids (absorbed).	Bile emulsifies fat-soluble vitamins and aids in their absorption with other fats. Water-soluble vitamins are absorbed.	The small intestine, pancreas, and liver add enough fluid so that the total secreted into the intestine in a day approximates 2 gallons. Many minerals are absorbed. Vitamin D aids in the absorption of calcium.
Large intestine Some fat and cholesterol, trapped in fiber, exits in feces.		Bacteria produce vitamin K, which is absorbed.	More minerals and most of the water are absorbed.

The Involuntary Muscles and the Glands

You are usually unaware of all the activity that goes on between the time you swallow and the time you defecate. As is the case with so much else that goes on in the body, the muscles and glands of the digestive tract meet internal needs without your having to exert any conscious effort to get the work done.

FIGURE 5–2   **Peristalsis**

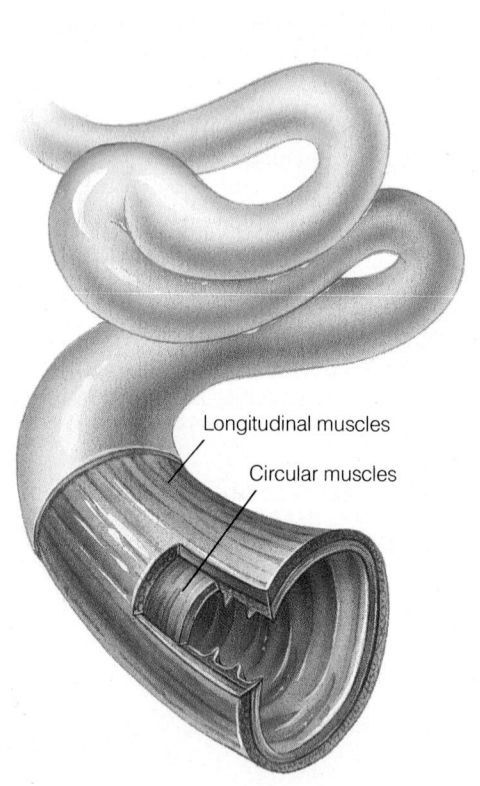

Cross section of the GI tract muscles. Circular muscles are inside; longitudinal muscles are outside. When the inner circular muscles contract, the tube tightens. When the outer longitudinal muscles contract, the circular muscles relax so the tube is loose.

Longitudinal muscles

Circular muscles

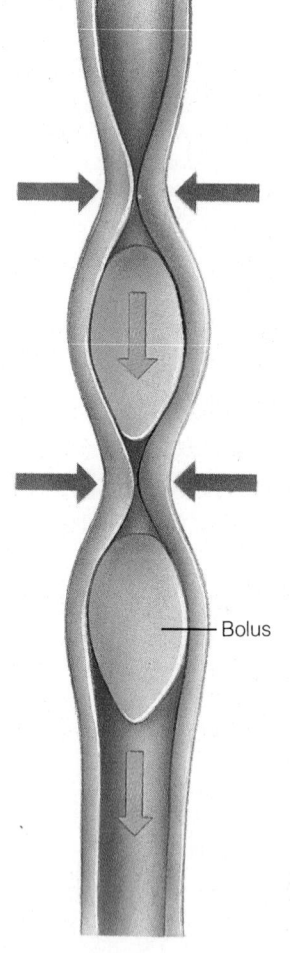

Bolus

The portion of food swallowed at one time is called a *bolus*. Peristalsis, which begins in the esophagus, proceeds.

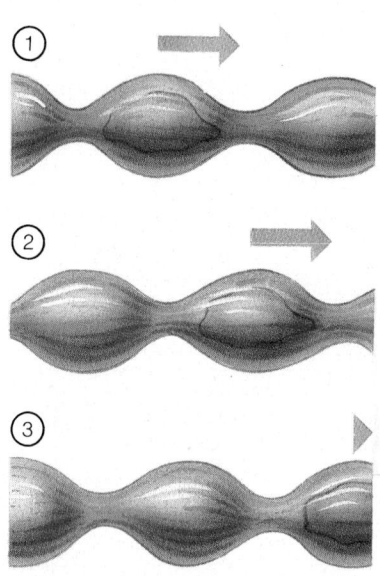

The liquified mass of partly digested food that travels through the intestines is called *chyme*. As the circular and longitudinal muscles tighten and relax, the chyme moves ahead of the constriction.

People consciously chew and swallow, but even in the mouth there are some processes over which you have no control. The salivary glands secrete just enough saliva to moisten each mouthful of food so that it can pass easily down your esophagus.

Peristalsis begins when the bolus enters the esophagus. The entire GI tract is ringed with muscles that can squeeze it tightly. Surrounding these rings of muscle are longitudinal muscles. When the rings tighten and the long muscles relax, the tube is constricted. When the rings relax and the long muscles tighten, the tube bulges. These actions follow each other continuously and push the intestinal contents along. If you have ever watched a bolus of food pass along the body of a snake, you have a good picture of how these muscles work. The waves of contraction ripple through the GI tract at varying rates and intensities depending on the part of the GI tract and on whether food is present. Peristalsis, along with the sphincter muscles that surround the tract at key places, keeps things moving along (see Figure 5–2).

The intestines not only push but also periodically squeeze their contents as if you had put a string around the intestines and pulled it tight. This motion, called segmentation, forces the contents backward a few inches, mixing them and allowing the digestive juices and the absorbing cells of the intestinal walls to make better contact with them.

Besides forcing the bolus along, the muscles of the GI tract help to liquefy it to chyme so that the digestive enzymes will have access to all the nutrients in it. The first step in this process takes place in the mouth, where chewing, the addition of saliva, and the action of the tongue reduce the food to a coarse mash suitable for swallowing. A further mixing and kneading action then takes place in the stomach.

The stomach has the thickest walls and strongest muscles of the parts of the GI tract. In addition to the circular and longitudinal muscles, the stomach has a third layer of diagonal muscles that also alternately contract and relax (see Figure 5–3). While these three sets of muscles are all at work forcing the chyme downward, the pyloric sphincter usually remains tightly closed, preventing the chyme from passing into the duodenum. Meanwhile, the gastric glands release juices that mix with the chyme. As a result, the chyme is churned and forced down, hits the pyloric sphincter, and remains in the stomach. When the chyme is thoroughly liquefied, the pyloric sphincter opens briefly, about three times a minute, to allow small portions through. At this point, the intestinal contents no longer resemble food in the least.

The Process of Digestion

One person eats nothing but vegetables, fruits, and nuts; another, nothing but meat, milk, and potatoes. How is it that both people wind up with essentially the same body composition? It all comes down to the fact that the body renders food—whatever it is to start with—into the basic units that make up carbohydrate, fat, and protein. The body absorbs these units and builds its tissues from them.

gland: a cell or group of cells that secretes materials for special uses in the body. Glands may be *exocrine glands,* secreting their materials "out" (into the digestive tract or onto the surface of the skin), or *endocrine glands,* secreting their materials "in" (into the blood).
   exo = outside
   endo = inside
   krine = to separate

saliva: the secretion of the salivary glands; the principal enzyme is salivary amylase.

peristalsis (peri-STALL-sis): successive waves of involuntary muscular contraction passing along the walls of the intestine.
   peri = around
   stellein = wrap

segmentation: a periodic squeezing or partitioning of the intestine by its circular muscles.

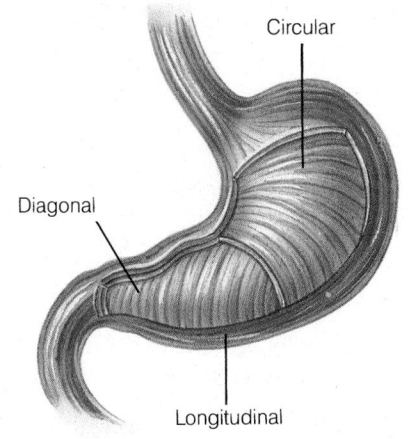

FIGURE 5–3 **Stomach Muscles** The stomach has three layers of muscles.

Circular

Diagonal

Longitudinal

> **MINIGLOSSARY of Digestive Glands and Their Juices**
>
> **amylase** (AM-uh-lace): an enzyme that splits amylose (a form of starch). Amylase is a carbohydrase. The ending *-ase* indicates an enzyme; the root tells what it digests. Other examples: protease, lipase.
>
> **gastric glands:** exocrine glands in the stomach wall that secrete gastric juice into the stomach.
>   *gastro* = stomach
>
> **gastric juice:** the digestive secretion of the gastric glands. The principal enzymes are rennin (curdles the milk protein, casein, and prepares it for pepsin action), pepsin (acts on proteins); and lipase (acts on emulsified fats).
>
> **mucus** (MYOO-cuss): a mucopolysaccharide (relative of carbohydrate) secreted by cells of the stomach wall. The cellular lining of the stomach wall with its coat of mucus is known as the mucous membrane. (The noun is *mucus;* the adjective is *mucous.*)
>
> **pepsin:** a protein-digesting enzyme (gastric protease) in the stomach. It circulates as a precursor, pepsinogen, and is converted to pepsin by the action of stomach acid.
>
> **intestinal juice:** the secretion of the intestinal glands; contains enzymes for the digestion of carbohydrate and protein and a minor enzyme for fat digestion.
>
> **pancreatic** (pank-ree-AT-ic) **juice:** the exocrine secretion of the pancreas, containing enzymes for the digestion of carbohydrate, fat, and protein. Juice flows from the pancreas into the small intestine through the pancreatic duct. The pancreas also has an endocrine function, the secretion of insulin and other hormones.
>
> **bicarbonate:** an alkaline secretion of the pancreas; part of the pancreatic juice. (Bicarbonate also occurs widely in all cell fluids.)
>
> **bile:** an exocrine secretion of the liver (the liver also performs a multitude of metabolic functions). Bile flows from the liver into the gallbladder, where it is stored until needed.

To digest food, five different body organs secrete digestive juices: the salivary glands, the stomach, the small intestine, the liver, and the pancreas. Each of the juices has a turn to mix with the intestinal contents and promote their breakdown to small units that can be absorbed into the body. The accompanying Miniglossary defines some of the digestive glands and their juices.

Digestion in the Mouth

Digestion of carbohydrate begins in the mouth, where the salivary glands secrete saliva, which contains water, salts, and enzymes (including salivary amylase) that break the bonds in the chains of starch. Saliva also protects the tooth surfaces and linings of the mouth, esophagus, and stomach from attack by molecules that might harm them. The enzymes in the mouth do not affect the fats, proteins, vitamins, minerals, and fiber that are present in the foods people eat.

Digestion in the Stomach

Gastric juice is composed of water, enzymes, and hydrochloric acid. The acid is so strong that it burns the throat if it chances to reflux into the upper esophagus and mouth. The strong acidity of the stomach prevents bacterial growth and kills most bacteria that enter the body with food. You might expect that the stomach's acid would attack the stomach itself, but the cells of the stomach wall secrete mucus, a thick, slimy, white polysaccharide that coats the stomach's lining.

Other than being crushed and mixed with saliva, nothing happens to protein until it comes in contact with the gastric juices in the stomach. There, the acid helps to uncoil (denature) the protein's tangled strands so that the stomach enzymes can attack the bonds.

The stomach enzymes work most efficiently in the stomach's strong acid. However, salivary amylase, which is swallowed with food, does not work in acid this strong, so the digestion of starch gradually ceases as the acid penetrates the bolus. In fact, salivary amylase becomes just another protein to be digested. The amino acids in amylase end up being absorbed and recycled into other body proteins.

Note that the strong acidity of the stomach is a desirable condition, TV commercials for antacids notwithstanding. People who overeat or who inhale their food are likely to suffer from indigestion. The muscular reaction of the stomach to being overfilled or to unchewed particles may be so violent as to cause regurgitation (reverse peristalsis). When this happens, the overeater may taste the stomach acid in her mouth and think she is suffering from ''acid indigestion.'' Responding to TV commercials, she may take antacids to neutralize the stomach acid. The consequence of this action is a demand on the stomach to secrete more acid to counteract the neutralizer and enable the digestive enzymes to do their work. The consumer ends up with the same amount of acid in her stomach but has had to work against the antacid to produce it.

Antacids are not designed to relieve the digestive discomfort of the hasty eater. Their proper use is to correct an abnormal condition, such as that of the person with ulcers, whose stomach or duodenal lining has been attacked by acid. To avoid falling into the same trap as our misguided consumer, remember that what such a person needs to do is to chew food more thoroughly, eat it more slowly, and possibly eat less at a sitting.

The major digestive event in the stomach is the initial breakdown of proteins. Both the enzyme pepsin and the stomach acid itself act as catalysts in the process. Minor events are the digestion of some fat by a gastric lipase, the digestion of sucrose (to a very small extent) by the stomach acid, and the attachment of a protein carrier to vitamin B_{12}.

Digestion in the Small and Large Intestines

By the time food leaves the stomach, digestion of all three energy-yielding nutrients has begun, but the process really gains momentum in the small intestine. There, the pancreas and liver contribute three additional digestive juices through ducts leading into the duodenum.

The pancreatic juice contains enzymes that act on fats, proteins, and carbohydrates, and glands in the intestinal wall also secrete digestive enzymes. The pancreatic juice also contains sodium bicarbonate, which neutralizes the acidic chyme as it enters the small intestine. From this point on, the contents of the digestive tract are neutral or slightly alkaline. The enzymes of both the intestine and the pancreas work best in this environment.

Bile is secreted by the liver continuously and is concentrated and stored in the gallbladder. The gallbladder squirts bile into the duodenum whenever fat arrives there. Bile is not an enzyme but an emulsifier that brings fats into suspension in water. After the fats are emulsified, enzymes can work on them, and they can be absorbed. Thanks to all these secretions, all three energy-yielding nutrients are digested in the small intestine.

The rate of digestion of the energy nutrients depends upon the contents of the meal. If the meal is high in simple sugars, digestion proceeds fairly rapidly. On the other hand, if the meal contains a considerable amount of fat, digestion is slower. The fact that fat slows digestion explains why fat increases the satiety value of a meal.

The intestine also contains bacteria that produce a variety of vitamins, including biotin and vitamin K (although bacteria alone cannot meet the need for these vitamins). The GI bacteria also protect people from infections. Provided that the normal intestinal flora is thriving, infectious bacteria have a hard time getting established and launching an attack on the system. In addition, the small intestine, and in fact the entire GI tract, manufactures and maintains a strong arsenal of defenses against foreign invaders. Several different types of defending cells are present there and confer specific immunity against intestinal diseases.

Food evidently needs to be digested completely. The sharing of this task by several organs underscores the body's determination to get the job done. Such distribution of labor is seen in nature whenever the job to be done is absolutely vital, as it is in this case.

---

emulsifier: a substance that mixes with both fat and water and that permanently disperses the fat in the water, forming an *emulsion*.

Mayonnaise, made from vinegar and oil, would separate like some other vinegar and oil salad dressings do if food chemists did not blend the vinegar and oil with a third ingredient—an emulsifier. The emulsifier mixes well with the fatty oil and the watery vinegar. In the case of mayonnaise the emulsifier is lecithin from egg yolks.

satiety (sat-EYE-uh-tee): the feeling of satisfaction and fullness that food brings.

intestinal flora: the bacterial inhabitants of the GI tract.
    flora = plant growth

> Most proteins are broken down into dipeptides, tripeptides, and amino acids before they are absorbed. With this in mind, you will be in a position to refute certain untrue claims made about foods. For instance, ''Don't eat food A. It contains enzyme B, which will harm you.'' Any enzyme you eat becomes but one among thousands of different proteins in your digestive tract. Except for digestive enzymes, whose design prevents them from being digested while they work, enzymes you eat are simply proteins that are broken down to amino acids. Don't be fooled by claims implying that enzymes you eat will act as enzymes in your body.

The story of how food is broken down into nutrients that can be absorbed is now nearly complete. The three energy-yielding nutrients—carbohydrate, fat, and protein—are disassembled to basic building blocks before they are absorbed. Most of the other nutrients—vitamins, minerals, and water—are absorbable as they are. Undigested residues, such as some fibers, are not absorbed but continue through the digestive tract, providing a semisolid mass that helps stimulate the muscles of the GI tract so that they will remain strong and perform peristalsis efficiently. Fiber also retains water, keeping the stools soft, and carries bile acids, sterols, and fat with it out of the body.

The process of absorbing the nutrients into the body is discussed in the next section. For the moment, let us assume that the digested nutrients simply disappear from the GI tract as they are ready. Virtually all are gone by the time the contents of the GI tract reach the end of the small intestine. Little remains but water, a few undissolved salts and body secretions, and undigested materials such as fiber. These enter the large intestine (colon).

In the colon, intestinal bacteria degrade some of the fiber to simpler compounds. The colon itself retrieves from its contents the materials that the body is designed to recycle—water and dissolved salts. The waste that is finally excreted has little or nothing of value left in it. The body has extracted all that it can use from the food.

The Absorptive System

Within three or four hours after you have eaten a meal, your body must find a way to absorb some two hundred thousand, million, million, million amino acid molecules one by one, and an equivalent number of monosaccharide, monoglyceride, glycerol, fatty acid, vitamin, and mineral molecules as well. The absorptive system is ingeniously designed to accomplish this task.

The Small Intestine

The small intestine provides a surface whose extent is comparable to a quarter of a football field in area. Nutrient molecules make contact with this surface and are absorbed. To remove these molecules rapidly and provide room for more to be absorbed, a rush of circulation continuously bathes the underside of the surface, washing away the absorbed nutrients and carrying them to the liver and other parts of the body.

The small intestine is a tube about 20 feet long and an inch or so across. Its inner surface looks smooth and slippery, but viewed through a microscope, it turns out to be wrinkled into hundreds of folds. Each fold is covered with thousands of fingerlike projections as numerous as the hairs on velvet fabric. Each of these small intestinal projections is a villus. A single villus, magnified still more, turns out to be composed of several hundred cells, each covered with microscopic hairs called microvilli (see Figure 5-4).

The villi are in constant motion. Each villus is lined by a thin sheet of muscle so that it can wave, squirm, and wiggle like the tentacles of a sea anemone. Any nutrient molecule small enough to be absorbed is trapped in the microvilli and drawn into the cells beneath them. Some partially digested nutrients are caught in the microvilli, digested further by enzymes there, and then absorbed into the cells.

Once a molecule has entered a cell in a villus, the next problem is to transport it to its destination elsewhere in the body. Everyone knows that

villi (VILL-ee or VILL-eye): fingerlike projections from the folds of the small intestine. The singular form is **villus.**
villus = shaggy hair

microvilli (MY-cro-VILL-ee or MY-cro-VILL-eye): projections from the membranes of the cells of the villi. The singular form is **microvillus.**

FIGURE 5–4   **The Small Intestinal Villi**

A. Five folds in the wall of the small intestine. Each is covered with villi.

B. Two villi (detail of A). Each villus is composed of several hundred cells.

C. Three cells of a single villus (detail of B). Each cell is coated with microvilli.

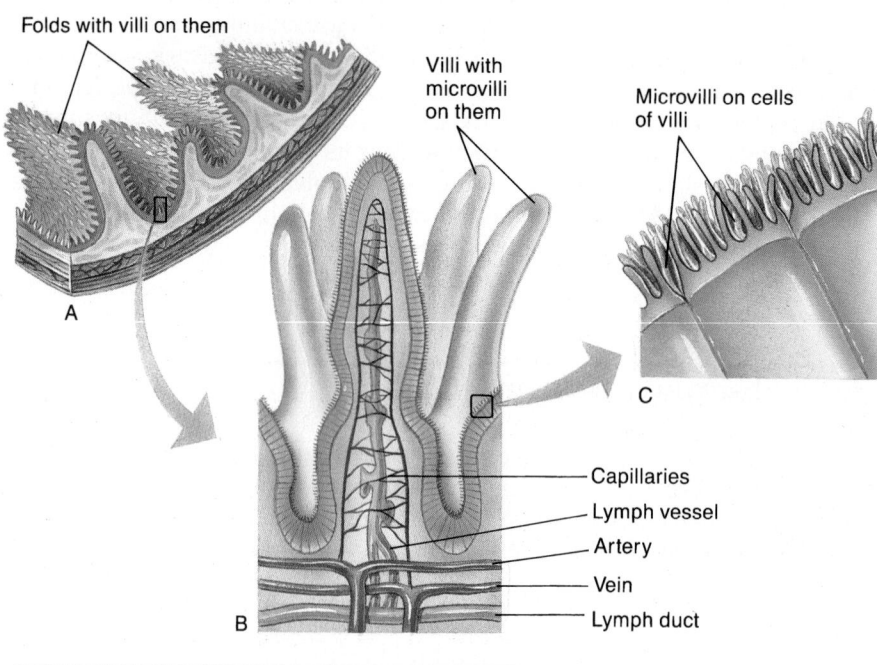

Folds with villi on them

Villi with microvilli on them

Microvilli on cells of villi

A

B

C

Capillaries

Lymph vessel

Artery

Vein

Lymph duct

lymph (LIMF): the body fluid found in lymphatic vessels. Lymph consists of all the constituents of blood except red blood cells. It circulates in a loosely organized system of vessels and ducts known as the *lymphatic system.*

the bloodstream performs this function, but you may be surprised to learn that there is a second transport system—the lymphatic system. Both of these systems supply vessels to each villus, as shown in Figure 5–4. When a nutrient molecule has crossed the cell of a villus, it may enter either the lymph or the blood. In either case, the nutrients end up in the blood, at least for a while.

As you can see, the intestinal tract is beautifully designed to perform its functions. A further refinement of the system is that the cells of successive portions of the tract are specialized to absorb different nutrients. The nutrients that are ready for absorption early on are absorbed near the top of the tract; those that take longer to be digested are absorbed further down. The rate at which the nutrients travel through the GI tract is finely adjusted to maximize their availability to the appropriate absorptive segment of the tract when they are ready. The lowly "gut" turns out to be one of the most elegantly designed organ systems in the body.

Release of Absorbed Nutrients

Once inside the intestinal cells, the products of digestion must be released for transport to the rest of the body. The water-soluble nutrients (including the smaller products of fat digestion) are released directly into the bloodstream by way of the capillaries. The larger fats and the fat-soluble vitamins, however, find access directly into the capillaries impossible, because they are insoluble in water (and blood is mostly water). The intestinal cells assemble the monoglycerides and long-chain fatty acids into larger molecules called triglycerides. These triglycerides, fat-soluble vitamins (when present), and other large lipids (cholesterol and the phospholipids) are then made into bundles with special proteins to form chylomicrons, one kind of lipoprotein (lipoproteins are described beginning on p. 88). Finally, the cells release the chylomicrons into the lymphatic system. They can then glide through the lymph spaces until they move to a point of entry into the bloodstream near the heart.

Chylomicrons are one kind of lipoprotein.

chylomicron (kye-lo-MY-cron): the lipoprotein formed in the intestinal wall cells following digestion and absorption of fat. Released from these cells, chylomicrons transport ingested fats to all cells of the body, which remove the ones they need, leaving chylomicron remnants to be picked up by the liver cells. The liver cells dismantle the chylomicron remnants and construct other lipoproteins for further transport of lipids.

Transport of Nutrients

Once a nutrient has entered the bloodstream or the lymphatic system, it may be transported to any part of the body and thus becomes available to any of the cells, from the tips of the toes to the roots of the hair. The circulatory systems are arranged to deliver nutrients wherever they are needed.

The Vascular System

The vascular or blood circulatory system is a closed system of vessels through which blood flows continuously in a figure eight, with the heart serving as a pump at the crossover point. Blood travels a simple route: heart to arteries to capillaries to veins to heart.

The routing of the blood through the digestive system is different, however. The blood is carried to the digestive system (as it is to all organs) by way of an artery, which (as in all organs) branches into capillaries to reach every cell. Blood leaving the digestive system, however, goes by way of a vein, not back to the heart but to the liver. This vein again branches into capillaries so that every cell of the liver also has access to the blood it carries. Blood leaving the liver then returns to the heart by way of a vein. The route is heart to arteries to capillaries (in intestines) to vein to capillaries (in liver) to vein to heart.

An anatomist studying this system knows there must be a reason for this special arrangement. The liver is placed in the circulation at this point so that it will have the first chance at the materials absorbed from the GI tract. In fact, the liver is the body's major metabolic organ (see Figure 5–5). It must prepare the absorbed nutrients for use by the body and has many jobs to perform in this process. Furthermore, the liver stands as gatekeeper to waylay intruders that might otherwise harm the heart or brain. Chapter 23 offers more information about this noble organ.

artery: a vessel that carries blood away from the heart.

capillary (CAP-ill-ary): a small vessel that branches from an artery. Capillaries connect arteries to veins. Exchange of oxygen, nutrients, and waste materials takes place across capillary walls.

The blood arriving at the intestines flows through the mesentery (MEZ-en-terry), a strong, flexible membrane that surrounds and supports the abdominal organs.
  mes = middle

The vein that collects blood from the mesentery and conducts it to capillaries in the liver is the *portal vein.*
  portal = gateway

The vein that collects blood from the liver capillaries and returns it to the heart is the *hepatic vein.*
  hepat = liver

The Lymphatic System

The lymphatic system is a one-way route for fluid from the tissue spaces to enter the blood. The lymphatic system has no pump; like water in a sponge,

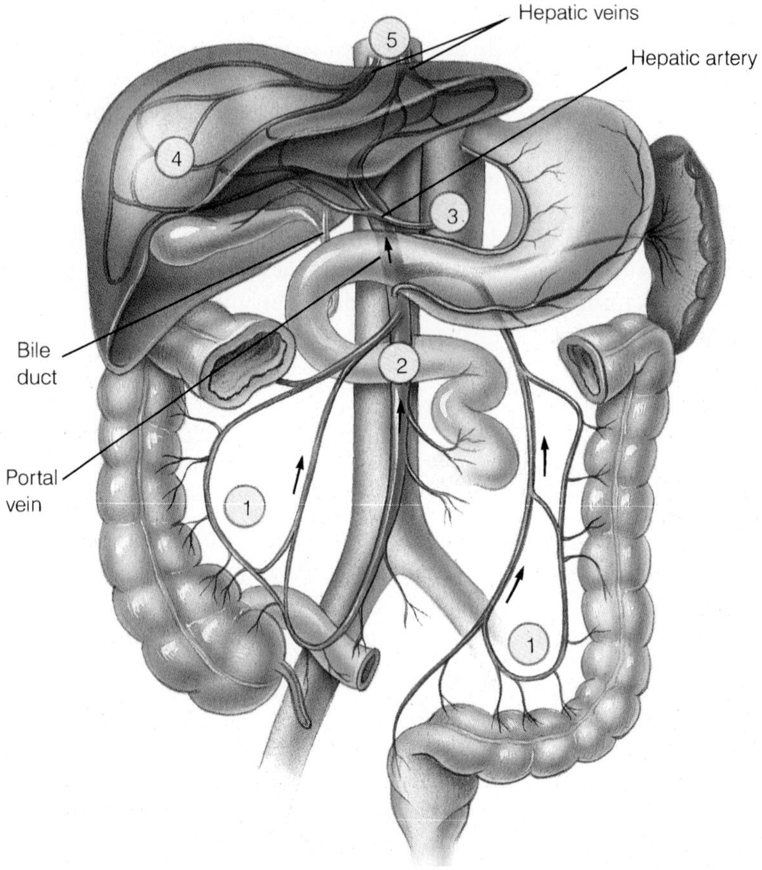

FIGURE 5–5　**The Liver**
The routing of the blood ensures that the liver has first crack at all the nutrients absorbed into the bloodstream from the digestive tract:

1. Vessels gather up nutrients and reabsorbed water and salts from all over the digestive tract.
2. These vessels merge into the portal vein, which conducts all absorbed materials to the liver.
3. The hepatic artery brings a supply of freshly oxygenated blood (not loaded with nutrients) from the lungs, to offer oxygen to the liver's own cells.
4. Capillaries branch out all over the liver, making nutrients and oxygen available to all its cells, and giving the cells access to blood from the digestive system.
5. Hepatic veins gather up blood leaving the liver to return it to the heart.

In contrast, nutrients absorbed into lymph do *not* go to the liver first. They go to the heart, which pumps them to all the body's cells. The cells can remove the nutrients they want, and the liver then has to deal only with the remnants.

The duct that conveys lymph toward the heart is the *thoracic* (thor-ASS-ic) *duct.* The *subclavian vein* connects this duct with the right upper chamber of the heart, providing a passageway by which lymph can be returned to the vascular system.

lymph is squeezed from one portion of the body to another as muscles contract and create pressure here and there. Ultimately, the lymph collects in a large duct behind the heart. This duct terminates in a vein that conducts the lymph into the heart. Thus some materials from the GI tract enter the lymphatic system at first, then later enter the bloodstream.

Transport of Lipids: Lipoproteins

Within the circulatory system, lipids always travel from place to place bundled with protein, that is, as lipoproteins. Lipoproteins are prominent in the medical news these days. In fact, when physicians measure a person's blood lipid profile, they are interested not only in the types of fat present (such as triglycerides and cholesterol) but also in the types of protein they travel with. As mentioned earlier, newly absorbed lipids leaving the intestinal cells are mostly packaged in large lipoproteins known as chylomicrons. As chylomicrons circulate through the body, cells remove their lipid contents, so they get smaller and smaller. The liver picks up and dismantles the chylomicron remnants and assembles new lipoproteins, which are known as very-low-density lipoproteins (VLDL). As the body's cells remove triglycerides from the VLDL, the VLDL become low-density lipoproteins (LDL). Lipids returning to the liver from other parts of the body are packaged in

VLDL: very-low-density lipoprotein; the type of lipoprotein made primarily by liver cells.

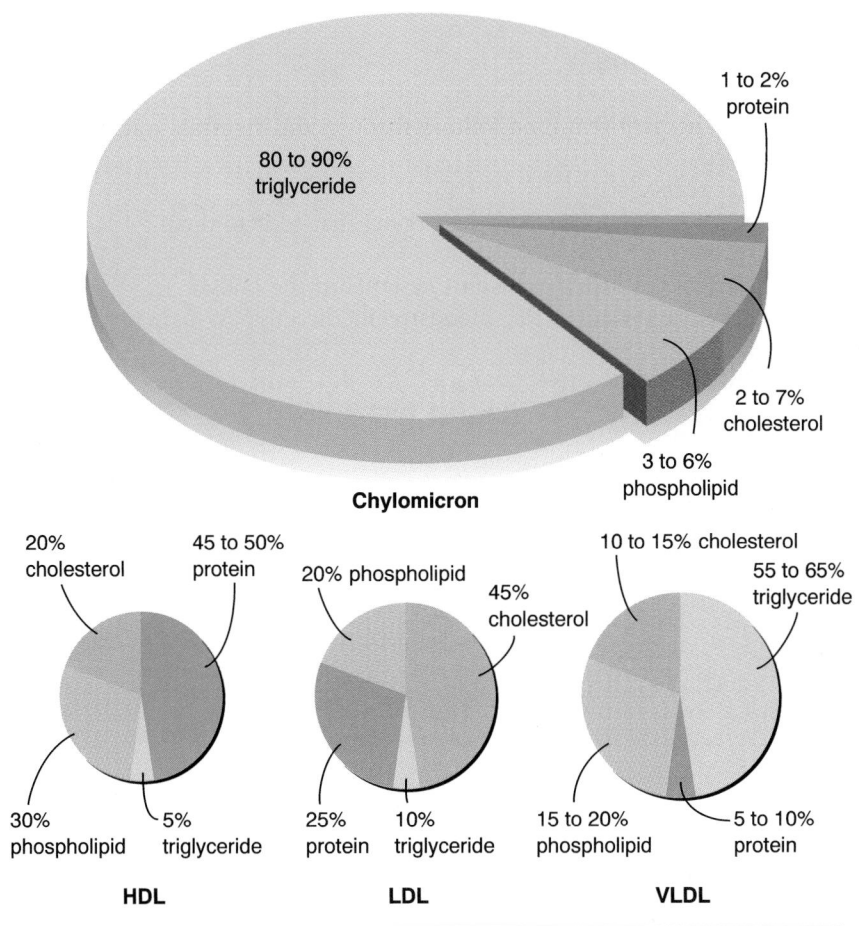

80 to 90%
triglyceride

1 to 2%
protein

2 to 7%
cholesterol

3 to 6%
phospholipid

Chylomicron

20%
cholesterol

45 to 50%
protein

30%
phospholipid

5%
triglyceride

HDL

20% phospholipid

45%
cholesterol

25%
protein

10%
triglyceride

LDL

10 to 15% cholesterol

55 to 65%
triglyceride

15 to 20%
phospholipid

5 to 10%
protein

VLDL

FIGURE 5–6   **The Lipoproteins**
Chylomicron. The density of these
particles is very, very low, because they
contain so little protein and so much
triglyceride. You can see how the
laboratory report that a person has "high
blood triglycerides" might easily reflect a
high concentration of chylomicrons in
the blood.

High-density lipoprotein (HDL). These
particles are denser than the others
because they contain such a high
percentage of protein.

*Very-low-density lipoprotein (VLDL)
and low-density lipoprotein (LDL).*
Compare these particles with the
chylomicrons and HDL. Note that "high
blood cholesterol" might easily reflect a
high LDL concentration.

lipoproteins known as high-density lipoproteins (HDL). The composition of
the lipoproteins is shown in Figure 5–6. Lipoproteins and heart disease are
discussed in Chapter 22.

LDL: low-density lipoprotein; the type of
lipoprotein derived from VLDL as cells
remove triglycerides from them.

HDL: high-density lipoprotein; the type of
lipoprotein that transports cholesterol back
to the liver from peripheral cells.

The System at Its Best

The intricate architecture of the GI tract makes it sensitive and responsive
to conditions in its environment. A condition indispensable to its performance is good health. Such lifestyle factors as sleep, exercise, state of mind,
and nutrition affect the health of the GI tract. For example, in a person
under stress, digestive secretions are reduced, and the blood is routed to the
muscles more than to the digestive tract. This impairs efficient absorption of
nutrients. To digest and absorb food best, one should be relaxed and tranquil
at mealtimes.

Among the characteristics of meals that promote optimal absorption of
nutrients are balance, variety, adequacy, and moderation, because every
nutrient depends on every other. The nutrients all work together, and all are
present in the cells of a healthy digestive tract.

Study Questions

1. Describe the path that food follows through the digestive tract once it is swallowed.
2. Describe peristalsis.
3. List five digestive juices and the organs that secrete them.
4. What does bile do?
5. Name the two nutrient transport systems in the body.
6. Which nutrients enter the bloodstream directly? Which are first absorbed into the lymph?
7. What are chylomicrons?

5

Nutrition Labeling

Today consumers know more about the links between diet and disease than they ever did in the past, and they are demanding still more information on disease prevention. Surveys show that many people rely on food labels to tell them which substances to avoid for health reasons and to provide them with information about nutrition.[1] The same surveys also show that many consumers find food labels confusing and misleading. The Food and Drug Administration (FDA) is in the process of implementing major changes in its food label policy. This discussion describes the information consumers find on food labels, with emphasis on proposed changes in nutrition information and nutrition claims on food labels.

What's the difference between nutrition information and nutrition claims?

Nutrition information on food labels does just what the term implies—informs people about the nutrients in foods. Nutrition *claims* are statements about specific nutrients (for example, "a significant source of vitamin A") or statements designed to appeal to people who want to include more of, or to limit, specific nutrients in their diets. For example, a food label that says "sodium-free" is making a nutrition claim.

What information will I find on food labels?

First of all, according to law, all labels must state the following information:

- The common name of the product.
- The name and address of the manufacturer, packer, or distributor.
- The net contents in terms of weight, measure, or count.

Then, unless the food has a standard of identity (a legally defined recipe for a common product, such as mayonnaise), the label must list:

- The ingredients, in descending order of predominance by weight.

All labels must state at least this much. Even if they say no more, you can learn a lot about the nutritional value of the product from the ingredient list. Consider the following products:

- An orange powder that contains "sugar, citric acid, orange flavor . . ." versus a juice can that contains "water, tomato concentrate, concentrated juices of carrots, celery. . . ."
- A cereal that contains "puffed milled corn, sugar, corn syrup, molasses, salt . . ." versus one that contains "100 percent rolled oats."

By knowing that the first ingredient named is the one that predominates by weight, you can tell what you are getting in the largest quantity. The accompanying miniglossary defines terms that relate to food labels.

Sometimes labels include more than that. Why?

Until the enforcement of recently approved labeling laws, a label that provides any nutrition information or makes any nutrition claim (about 60 percent of labeled foods do) has to meet additional labeling requirements. With the passing of the *Nutrition Labeling and Education Act of 1989,* nutrition labeling is mandatory for most foods. *Voluntary* nutrition labeling guidelines will be provided for 20 varieties of vegetables, fruits, and raw fish that are most frequently consumed within a year.[2] Meats and poultry are exempt from this law. Even though the law was passed in 1990, it will be some time—probably 1993—before consumers see the new labeling on the foods they purchase. Once the new law is enforced, the

MINIGLOSSARY

Daily Values: reference values developed by the FDA specifically for food labels. The Daily Values represent two sets of standards: Reference Daily Intakes (RDI) and Daily Reference Values (DRV).

Reference Daily Intakes (RDI): food labeling values for protein, vitamins, and minerals.

Daily Reference Values (DRV): food labeling values for nutrients and food components (such as fat and fiber) that do not have an RDA value but that do have important relationships with health.

Free: "nutritionally trivial" and unlikely to have a physiological consequence.

High: 20 percent or more of the Daily Value for a given nutrient.

Less: at least 25 percent less of a given nutrient than the comparison food (see individual nutrients below).

Low: an amount that would allow frequent consumption of a food without exceeding the dietary guidelines (see individual nutrients below). A food that is naturally low in a nutrient may make such a claim, but only as it applies to all similiar foods (for example, "fresh cauliflower, a low-sodium food").

More: at least 10 percent more of a given nutrient than the comparison food.

Reduced: must identify the comparison food, the percentage of reduction, and the amount in the comparison food (see individual nutrients below).

Source of: 10 to 19 percent of the Daily Value.

Cholesterol
Note: Foods containing more than 11.5 grams total fat or per 100 grams must indicate those contents immediately after a cholesterol claim. As you will see, all cholesterol claims are prohibited when the food contains more than 2 grams saturated fat per serving.

Cholesterol-free: less than 2 milligrams cholesterol per serving and 2 grams or less saturated fat per serving.

Low in cholesterol: 20 milligrams or less per serving and per 100 grams of food, and 2 grams or less of saturated fat per serving.

Less cholesterol: 25 percent or less cholesterol than the comparison food (reflecting a reduction of at least 20 milligrams per serving), and 2 grams or less saturated fat per serving.

Reduced cholesterol: 50 percent or less cholesterol per serving than the comparison food (reflecting a reduction of at least 20 milligrams per serving), and 2 grams or less saturated fat per serving.

Energy
kCalorie free: fewer than 5 kcalories per serving.

Light: one-third fewer kcalories than the comparison food. Any other use of the term must specify what it is referrring to (for example, "light in color" or "light in texture").

Low kcalorie: less than 40 kcalories per serving and per 100 grams of food.

Reduced kcalorie: at least one-third fewer kcalories than the comparison food.

Fat
Fat free: less than 0.5 grams of fat per serving (and no added fat or oil).

Less fat: 25 percent or less fat than the comparison food.

Less saturated fat: 25 percent or less saturated fat than the comparison food.

Low fat: 3 grams or less fat per serving and per 100 grams of food.

Low saturated fat: 1 gram or less saturated fat per serving, and not more than 15 percent of kcalories from saturated fat.

Percent fat free: may be used only if product meets definition of **low fat**.

Reduced fat: 50 percent or less of the fat in the comparison food *and* reduced by more than 3 grams of fat per serving (for example, "reduced fat, 50 percent less fat than our regular cookies, reduced from 10 grams to 5 grams per serving").

Reduced saturated fat: 50 percent or less of the saturated fat in the comparison food *and* reduced by more than 1 gram.

Fiber
High fiber: 20 percent or more of the Daily Value for fiber; a high-fiber claim made on a food that contains more than 3 grams fat per serving and per 100 grams of food must also declare total fat.

Sodium
Sodium free and salt free: less than 5 milligrams of sodium per serving.

Low sodium: less than 140 milligrams per serving and per 100 grams of food.

Reduced sodium: no more than 50 percent of the sodium of the comparison food.

Very low sodium: less than 35 milligrams per serving and per 100 grams of food.

Sugar
Sugar free: less than 0.5 grams per serving.

following information will be mandatory on food labels:

- Serving or portion size in standard, common household measures.
- Servings or portions per container.
- Total food energy and food energy derived from fat (kcalories) per serving.
- Total carbohydrate per serving.
- Complex carbohydrates per serving.
- Total sugar per serving.
- Total fat per serving.
- Saturated fat per serving.
- Cholesterol per serving.
- Sodium per serving.
- Total protein per serving.
- Dietary fiber per serving.
- Vitamins A (RE), vitamin C (milligrams), and the minerals calcium (milligrams) and iron (milligrams) per serving as percentages of the U.S. RDA. (No claim may be made that a food is a significant source of a nutrient unless it provides at least 10 percent of the U.S. RDA of that nutrient in a serving.) This listing will be renamed "Daily Value" in order to dispel consumer confusion about the RDA and the U.S. RDA (see below).

In creating Daily Values, the FDA first established two set of reference values. The first set, the Reference Daily Intakes (RDI), are for protein, vitamins, and minerals, and reflect average allowances based on the RDA. They represent intakes to achieve; for example, the RDI for zinc is 13 milligrams—an amount to aim for daily. The RDI will serve a role similar to that currently provided by the U.S. RDA.

The second set of reference values established by the FDA for labels is the Daily Reference Values (DRV). The DRV serve as food labeling values for nutrients and food components, such as fat and fiber, that do not have an established RDA but that do have important relationships with health. The FDA strongly believes that the RDI and DRV serve different purposes and prefers to treat them separately. For example, the RDI will serve as standards for federal policies and assistance programs whereas the DRV will not. But the FDA also recognizes that on labels one set of values—called Daily Values—will limit consumer confusion. These Daily Values represent both the RDI and DRV.

There are exemptions for foods sold in restaurants; infant formula; foods with insignificant amounts of the nutrients required to be listed on the label, such as spices; and a few other minor exemptions. Table NP5–1 compares the current nutrition label format with the newly passed label format.

What is the U.S. RDA?

The U.S. Recommended Daily Allowances (U.S. RDA) table is shown on the inside *front* cover of this book. The U.S. RDA are a set of figures designed specifically for use on food labels. They are derived from the RDA tables, already discussed, which appear on the inside *front* cover.

The idea behind the U.S. RDA was to develop single sets of standards for generalized sets of adult human beings whose nutrient needs are high—as high as people's needs generally go. A food label would be most meaningful to you as an individual if it expressed the food's nutrient contents as a percentage of your personal need, but of course it can't do that. The makers of the product don't know who you are: a 10-year-old boy, a 70-year-old woman, or a pregnant teenage girl. Even if they did, they wouldn't know your particular requirements. To standardize labels, four sets of U.S. RDA were developed for different groups of people—infants, children, adults, and pregnant and lactating women. The most commonly used of these is the U.S. RDA for adults. If you read on a label that a serving of cereal provides 10 percent of the U.S. RDA of a nutrient, you can be fairly sure that it will also provide at least a tenth of *your* RDA for that nutrient.

The U.S. RDA are about equal to the highest numbers for each nutrient found in the RDA table. For most nutrients, they are the same as the RDA for adolescent boys or adult men, whichever are higher. For iron, the women's RDA is greater than the men's, so the women's RDA is used. The U.S. RDA have not been revised to agree exactly with new editions of the RDA since 1968, because they still would be judged generous by any standard.

How can I use a label to see how well a food meets my nutrient needs?

If you just want to know generally what amounts of nutrients are in the package, the percentage of the U.S. RDA will tell you that without your having to do any calculating. If you read, for example, that a serving of breakfast cereal provides "25 percent" of the U.S. RDA of calcium, you can be sure it provides at least a quarter of your calcium allowance for a day (unless you are pregnant or lactating). If you want to know exactly how many grams of calcium are in a serving, you can look at the U.S. RDA table, find out that the U.S. RDA is 1 gram

TABLE NP5-1 Present and Future Nutrition Labels

The Nutrition Labeling and Education Act was signed into law by President Bush on November 8, 1990. The left side of the table represents food labels prior to the enforcement of the new labeling law in May 1993. As of May 1993, manufacturers must comply with the new labeling law and present the information shown on the right side of the table.

TO BE OMITTED (−)		TO BE ADDED (+)	
Present Label		**Proposed Label**	
Nutrition Information		Nutrition Information	
Serving size	1/4 pizza	Serving size	1/4 pizza
Servings per container	4	Servings per container	4
kCalories	240	kCalories	240
Protein	9 g	kCalories from fat	63 +
Carbohydrate	35 g	Protein	9 g
Fat	7 g	Carbohydrate	35 g
Sodium	640 mg	Dietary fiber	2 g +
		Fat	7 g
Percent of U.S. Recommended Daily Allowances		Saturated fat	4 g +
		Cholesterol	15 mg +
Protein	20 −	Sodium	640 mg
Vitamin A	15		
Vitamin C	8		
Thiamin	8 −	Percent of Daily Value	
Riboflavin	10 −		
Niacin	10 −	Vitamin A	17
Calcium	10	Vitamin C	8
Iron	6	Calcium	8
		Iron	6

Source: Adapted from Plans for food label changes announced by HHS Secretary Sullivan, *FDA Consumer,* May 1990, p. 2.

of calcium, and figure that 25 percent of that is 0.25 gram (or 250 mg). For the nutrients included in the RDA tables, then, all the information that most consumers might want is listed there.

I have to watch my weight, so I look for foods labeled "low in calories." Are these foods really low in kcalories?

Foods labeled "low in calories" must state the absolute number of kcalories on the label and must contain no more than 40 kcalories per serving. Any food calling itself a "reduced-calorie food" must be at least a third lower in kcalories than the food it most closely resembles and must carry a nutrition label. The Miniglossary of Terms on Food Labels defines the meanings of other terms on food labels.

From what you've said, I think I can deal with nutrition labels on foods like

breakfast cereals. But what about foods that simply say "TV dinner" or "macaroni and cheese"?

The FDA has devised nutritional quality guidelines for the nutrient contents of many kinds of convenience foods: frozen dinners, breakfast cereals, certain beverages, and prepared main dishes such as pizza or macaroni and cheese. If a product complies with the guidelines, it may carry on its label a statement that says so without spelling out the details. The new labeling law requires that these foods, too, provide the mandatory nutrition labeling information.

For some items, the law provides standards of identity and excuses manufacturers from the requirement of listing ingredients. Standards of identity exist for such foods as bread and mayonnaise—common foods that at one time were often prepared at home, so the basic recipes were understood by almost everyone. Certain ingredients must be present in a specific percentage before the food may use the standard name. The new labeling law does away with standards of identity. These foods must provide the mandatory nutrition labeling information.

Another class of foods that concerns consumers is made up of inferior foods developed in imitation of, and as substitutes for, familiar foods. Regulations require that the word *imitation* be used on the label if the product is a substitute for and resembles another food but is nutritionally inferior to the food imitated. Nutritional inferiority is defined as a reduction in the content of an essential vitamin, an essential mineral, or protein that amounts to 10 percent or more of the U.S. RDA. Thus if you read *imitation* on a label, you may conclude that the food is a poor imitation nutritionally.

Many of the convenience foods I use are either enriched or fortified. Does this mean that they are more nutritious than ordinary foods?

Not necessarily. A fortified breakfast cereal may have such large quantities of nutrients added that one serving provides 100 percent of the U.S. RDA for all of them. Yet the shrewd consumer will realize that the word *fortified* sometimes conveys an emptiness of other nutrients. The nutrients named on the label are added, yes, but others may be missing altogether (see Chapter 7). Fruit *juice* is more nutritious than fortified fruit *drink,* even though the drink may be higher in vitamin C content. The fruit juice is likely to contain important trace minerals, fiber, and vitamins other than vitamin C that are not found in the fortified fruit drink.

To distinguish between nourishing foods (those that provide some nutrients besides kcalories) and nutritious foods, you have to apply the concept of nutrient density. Consider these two questions:

1. How much of each nutrient does a serving of this food supply in relation to my need?
2. How many kcalories does a serving supply in relation to my need?

If the food is of high nutrient density—for example, if it supplies half your daily allowance for a vitamin and at the same time only one-tenth of

your daily allowance for kcalories—it is a good source of that vitamin. You could obtain a substantial quantity of the vitamin from it at a low kcalories cost, and it is a nutritious food.

Is there anything else I should know about labels?

Yes, you need to know how to see through misleading claims. As they presently appear, food labels provide useful information, but the law still allows some loopholes. You might be interested in trying your skill at detecting misleading claims by taking the Nutrition Label Quiz.

When a package with an artificially constituted food or dietary supplement claims that the food contains all the vitamins and minerals known to be essential in human nutrition, it is also misleading, because the claim implies a completeness that may be overestimated. We really do not know everything that should be included in such foods.

Finally, consumers may be misled by a label that claims that a breakfast bar or drink has the same amounts of protein, fat, carbohydrate, vitamins, and minerals as those found in a breakfast of milk, egg, toast, and orange juice. The label fails to mention that the carbohydrate is sugar (versus the complex carbohydrate in toast), that the fat is saturated fat (versus the polyunsaturated oil in which the egg might have been fried), or that the salt content is considerable. Furthermore, there are other nutrients in milk, egg, toast, and orange juice that the breakfast bar does not contain. Consumers are putting pressure on

Nutrition Label Quiz

All three of the label claims below are true. Which two claims are misleading?

1. A label says one serving of a food provides "35 times as much iron as an 8-ounce glass of whole milk."
2. A label says a fortified product contains "more vitamin C than fresh orange juice."
3. A label says a brand of instant nonfat dry milk has "all the calcium, protein, and B vitamins of whole milk."

The answers are:
1. True but misleading, because milk is a poor source of iron.
2. True but misleading, because orange juice contains so many other nutrients not provided by the fortified drink.
3. True and responsible.

legislators to provide labeling laws that will make such misleading claims illegal.

Notes

1. Department of Health and Human Services, *A Consumer's Guide to Food Labels,* publication no. 88-2083 (Washington, D.C.: Government Printing Office, 1988); Food label importance, *FDA Consumer,* May 1990, p. 3.
2. Wrap-up of ADA's issues in the 101st Congress, *Journal of the American Dietetic Association* 90 (1990): 1653–1655.

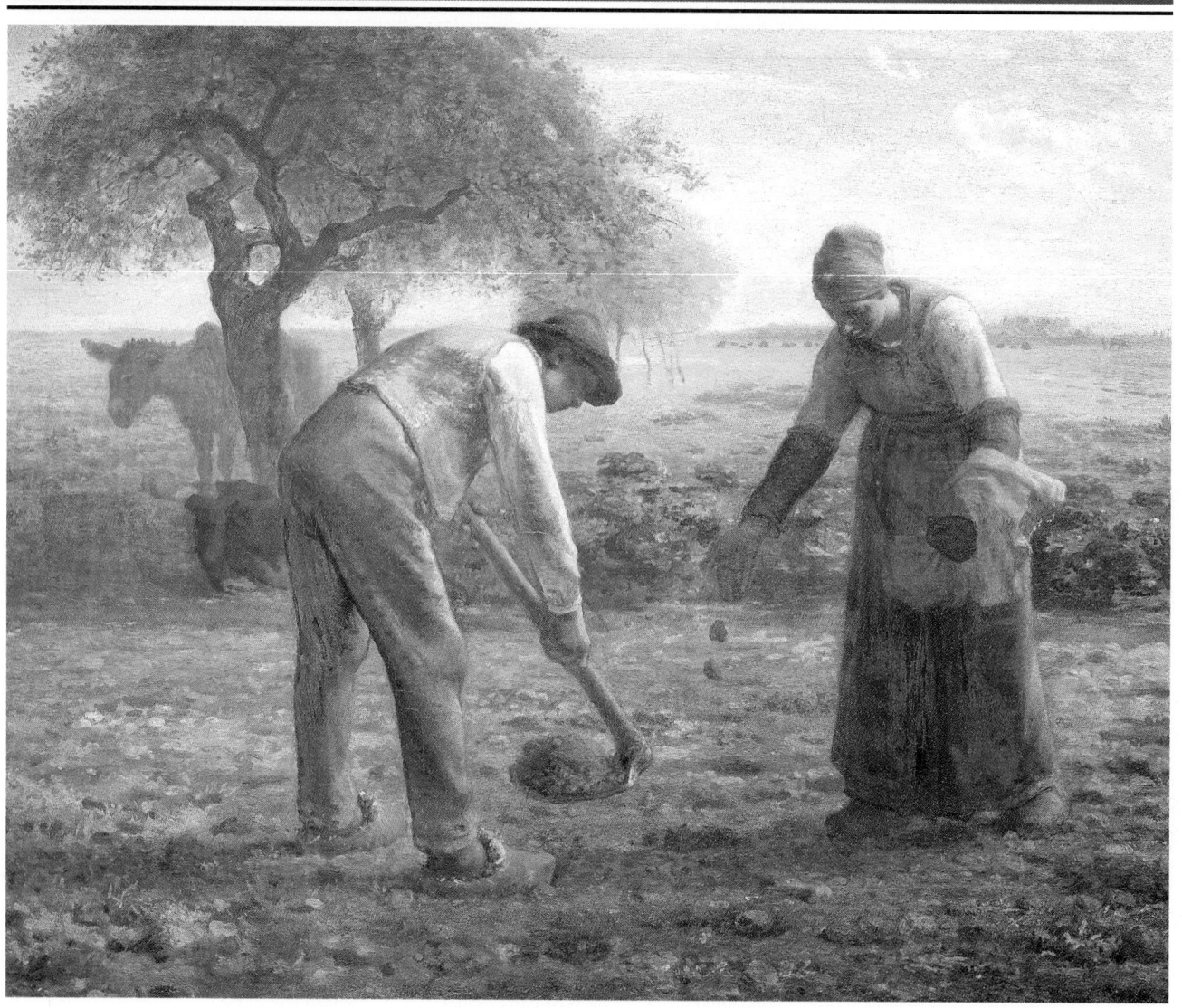

Jean Francois Millet, Potato Planters; *Gift of Quincy Adams Shaw through Quincy A. Shaw, Jr., and Mrs. Marian Shaw Haughton, Courtesy of Musuem of Fine Arts, Boston.*

Metabolism and Energy Balance

CONTENTS

CHAPTER

6

The way the body manages its energy supply is amazing. Consider, for example, that a 1 percent error in energy intake can cause a person to become more than 200 pounds overweight in a lifetime. Yet most people maintain their weight, fluctuating only about 10 or 20 pounds, throughout life. This miraculous energy maintenance system is puzzling in many ways. For instance, how does a person's body defend its weight so consistently day after day? How do people who go without food for long periods of time manage to keep going? Are fat-rich foods more fattening than carbohydrate-rich foods? Is fasting dangerous? Are low-carbohydrate diets dangerous? What's the best way to lose weight? The answers to these and many other questions lie in an understanding of metabolism.

metabolism: the sum total of all the chemical reactions that go on in living cells. *Energy metabolism* includes all the reactions by which the body obtains and uses energy from food or body stores.

  meta = among
  bole = change

Metabolism is defined as the sum total of all the chemical reactions that go on in the body. Energy metabolism includes all the ways in which the body obtains and uses energy from food. The body can use the energy-yielding nutrients in food to build new energy-storage compounds, or to use as fuel for activities.

Earlier chapters introduced the energy-yielding nutrients—carbohydrate, fat, and protein—that are found in food. These compounds are broken down during digestion into basic units that are absorbed into the blood. This chapter focuses on what becomes of the energy nutrients within the body. The basic units on which metabolism centers are:

- From carbohydrate: glucose.
- From lipids: glycerol.
- From lipids: fatty acids.
- From protein: amino acids.

Building Body Compounds

anabolism (an-ABB-o-lism): reactions in which small molecules are put together to build larger ones. Anabolic reactions consume energy.

When the basic units are not needed by the cells for energy, they can be used to build body compounds. These building reactions, in which simple compounds are put together to form larger, more complex structures, involve doing work, and so require energy. They are called anabolic reactions. Glucose units can be strung together to make glycogen chains. Glycerol and fatty acids can be assembled into triglycerides. Amino acids can be used to make proteins. These larger compounds have many uses, and they can be used as fuel if energy is needed later.

Breaking Down Nutrients for Energy

catabolism (ca-TAB-o-lism): reactions in which large molecules are broken down to smaller ones; catabolic reactions usually release energy.

If the body needs energy, it may break apart any or all of the basic units into smaller fragments. The breakdown reactions release energy and are called catabolic reactions. Glucose is broken down first to pyruvate and then to a smaller compound, acetyl CoA. In a series of metabolic reactions called the tricarboxylic acid (TCA) cycle, acetyl CoA splits and donates its energy to storage compounds, or to do the body's work, or to produce heat.

Like glucose, glycerol can be converted to pyruvate and then acetyl CoA, finally releasing energy through the TCA cycle. Fatty acids are not converted to pyruvate; instead they are converted directly into acetyl CoA.

The sequence

$$\text{Glucose} \leftrightarrow \text{pyruvate} \rightarrow \text{acetyl CoA} \rightarrow \text{energy}$$

is central to an understanding of metabolism. Notice the two-way arrow between glucose and pyruvate and the one-way arrows after pyruvate. They show that pyruvate can be reconverted to glucose but acetyl CoA cannot. Anything that can be converted to pyruvate can be used to make glucose. Anything broken down to acetyl CoA cannot be used to make glucose. Fat cannot be converted to glucose, for the most part, because it consists mostly of triglycerides, and they in turn consist mostly of fatty acids, with only a little glycerol.

When fatty acids are broken down, they are converted to acetyl CoA, and for this reason, they cannot be used to make glucose. Glycerol, because it is interconvertible with pyruvate, can yield glucose, but glycerol represents only about 5 percent of the weight of a triglyceride molecule. Thus fat is a poor and inefficient source of glucose. About 95 percent of it cannot be converted to glucose at all; therefore fat, for the most part, cannot normally provide energy for the organs (brain and nervous system) that require glucose as fuel. This leaves mostly to protein and carbohydrate the task of fueling the brain's activities.

Ideally, amino acids will be used to replace needed body proteins and will not be used for energy. If they are needed for energy, or if they are consumed in excess, they are first stripped of their nitrogen—which can be used to make other compounds, including the nonessential amino acids, or can be excreted. With nitrogen removed, about half of the amino acids can be converted to pyruvate and can therefore provide glucose. The other amino acids are converted to acetyl CoA directly or enter the TCA cycle at another point. Thus protein, unlike fat, is a fairly good source of glucose when carbohydrate is not available.

Carbohydrate is, of course, an ideal source of glucose, because it is composed mostly of that substance. The few other sugars in the body's carbohydrates, galactose and fructose, are readily convertible to glucose. Figure 6–1 depicts the metabolic pathways involving these compounds.

pyruvate (PIE-roo-vate): pyruvic acid, a three-carbon compound derived from glucose and certain amino acids in metabolism. The term *pyruvate* means a salt of pyruvic acid. (Throughout this book the ending *-ate* is used interchangeably with *-ic acid;* for our purposes they mean the same thing.)

The metabolic breakdown of glucose to pyruvate is *glycolysis* (gligh-COLL-uh-sis).
  glyco = glucose
  lysis = breakdown

CoA (coh-AY): nickname for a small molecule that participates in metabolism. As pyruvate breaks down to the smaller compound acetic acid, a molecule of CoA is attached to it, making acetyl CoA (ASS-uh-teel or uh-SEET-ul co-AY).

The reactions by which the complete oxidation of acetyl CoA is accomplished are those of the TCA cycle, or Krebs cycle, and oxidative phosphorylation. The net result is that acetyl CoA splits, and the energy it contained is made available for the body's use.

Removal of the amino (NH_2) group from a compound, such as an amino acid, is called **deamination.**

The principal nitrogen-excretion product of metabolism is **urea** (you-REE-uh).

The making of glucose from protein or fat is **gluconeogenesis** (gloo-co-nee-o-JEN-uh-sis). About 5% of fat (the glycerol portion of triglycerides) and about 50% of protein (the glycogenic amino acids) can be converted to glucose.
  gluco, glyco = glucose
  neo = new
  genesis = making

The Economics of Feasting

Everyone knows that when you consume more energy than you expend, much of the excess is stored as body fat. Fat can be made from an excess of any energy-yielding nutrient that you eat. Fat cells enlarge as they fill with fat, and the body's fat-storing capacity seems to be able to expand indefinitely, as Figure 6–2 shows.

Surplus carbohydrate (glucose) is first stored as glycogen, but the glycogen-storing cells have limited capacity. Once glycogen stores are filled,

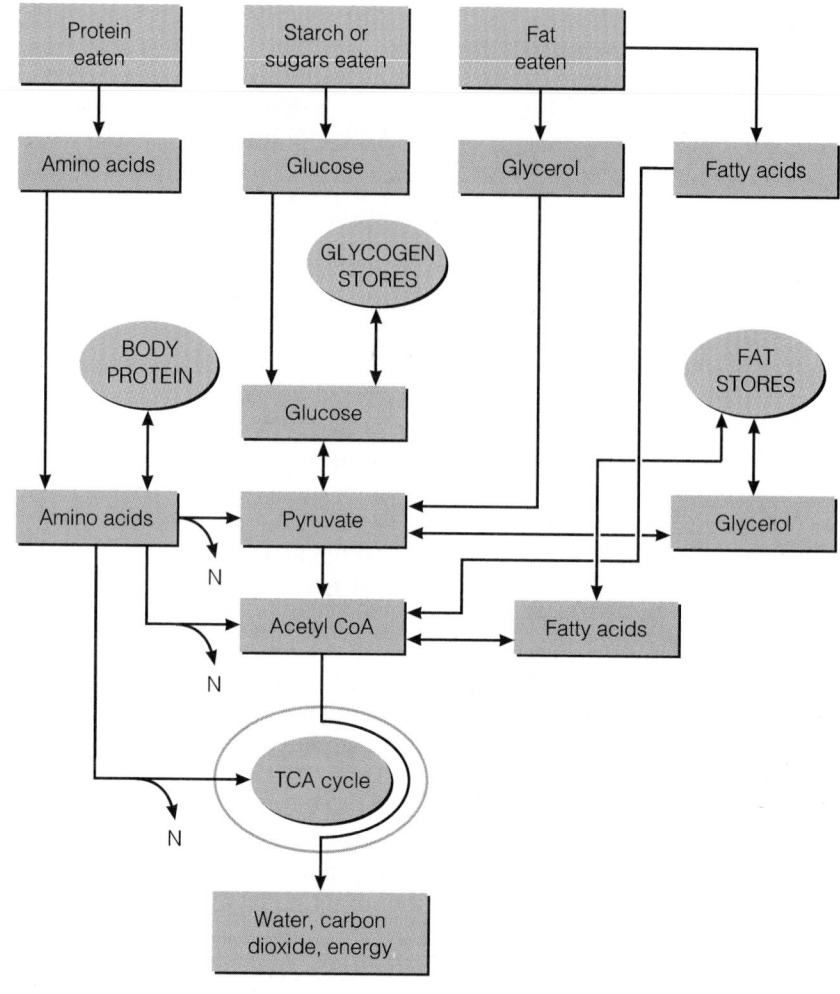

FIGURE 6–1   **The Central Pathways of Energy Metabolism**
Carbohydrate via glucose yields glycogen, fat, or energy. Some amino acids via pyruvate can yield glucose/glycogen. The glycerol from fat (5% of total fat) can also yield glucose/glycogen. The remainder of energy stores are found in body fat.

FIGURE 6–2   **Fat Cell Enlargement**
Fat cells enlarge when you eat too much of any energy-yielding nutrient—carbohydrate, fat, or protein.

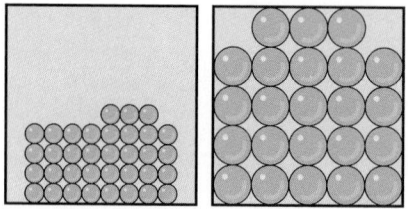

the overflow is routed to fat. Thus excess carbohydrate can contribute to obesity.

Surplus dietary fat contributes easily to the body's fat stores. During digestion and metabolism, fat may break down into fragments, such as acetyl CoA, but if the flow of these fragments is rapid enough to meet the body's need for energy, and if excess fragments are donated by fat, not all will be broken down further. Instead, some will be routed to the assembly of fatty acids and attached to glycerol to be stored as triglycerides in the fat cells.

Finally, surplus protein may encounter the same fate. If protein is consumed in excess of the body's need or is not needed as fuel to meet energy needs, amino acids will lose their nitrogens and will be converted through the intermediates, pyruvate and acetyl CoA, to triglycerides. These, too, swell the fat cells and increase body weight. Figure 6–3 shows the metabolic events of feasting.

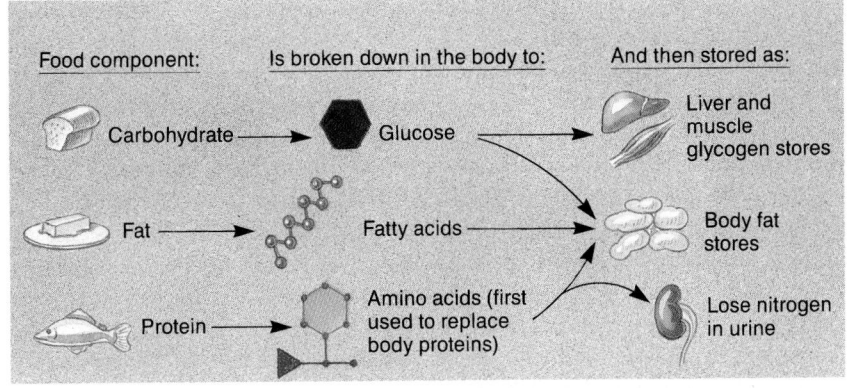

Food component: Is broken down in the body to: And then stored as:

Carbohydrate → Glucose → Liver and muscle glycogen stores

Fat → Fatty acids → Body fat stores

Protein → Amino acids (first used to replace body proteins) → Lose nitrogen in urine

FIGURE 6–3   **Feasting**
When people overeat, they store energy.

The Economics of Fasting

Even when you are asleep and totally relaxed, the cells of many organs are hard at work spending energy. In fact, this work, which you are unaware of, represents about two-thirds of the total energy you spend in a day. (The other one-third is the work that you do with your voluntary muscles during waking hours.)

The body's top priority is to meet the energy needs for this ongoing activity. Its normal way of doing so is by periodic refueling, that is, by eating. When food is not available, the body must find other fuel sources in its own tissues. If people choose not to eat, we say they are fasting; if they have no choice (as in a famine), we say they are starving; but no metabolic difference exists between the two. In either case, the body is forced to switch to a wasting metabolism by drawing on its reserves of carbohydrate and fat and, within a day or so, on its vital protein tissues as well.

As a fast or period of starvation begins, glucose from the liver's stored glycogen and fatty acids from the body's stored fat are both flowing into cells, delivering fuel to power the cells' work. Several hours later, however, most of the glucose is used up—liver glycogen is exhausted. Low blood glucose concentrations serve as a signal to further promote fat breakdown.[1]

At this point, most of the cells are depending on fatty acids to continue providing their fuel. But the nervous system and brain cells cannot use fatty acids; they still need glucose. Even if other energy fuel is available, glucose has to be present to permit the brain's energy-metabolizing machinery to work. Normally, the nervous system (brain and nerves) consumes about two-thirds of the total glucose used each day—about 400 to 600 kcalories' worth.

Because fat stores cannot provide the glucose needed by the brain, body protein tissues (such as liver and muscle) always break down to some extent during fasting. In the first few days of a fast, body protein provides about 90 percent of the needed glucose, and glycerol provides about 10 percent. If body protein loss were to continue at this rate, death would ensue within

The liver releases glucose, and the fat cells release fat to be used as fuel by the body's cells, but the brain can use only glucose.

Fasting = living on the body's fat and protein.

In fasting, muscle and lean tissue atrophy to supply amino acids for conversion to glucose. This glucose, with ketones produced from fat, fuels the brain's activities.

about three weeks. However, as the fast continues, the body finds a way to use its fat to fuel the brain. It adapts by condensing together acetyl CoA fragments derived from fatty acids to produce an alternate energy source, ketone bodies. Normally produced and used only in small quantities, ketones can serve as fuel for some brain cells. Ketone body production rises until, at the end of several weeks of fasting, it is meeting about half or more of the nervous system's energy needs. Still, many areas of the brain rely exclusively on glucose, and body protein continues to be sacrificed to produce it. Figure 6–4 shows the metabolic events that occur during fasting.

As fasting continues and the body is shifting to partial dependence on ketones for energy, the body simultaneously reduces its energy output and conserves both its fat and lean tissue. Because of the slowed metabolism, the loss of fat falls to a bare minimum. Thus, although *weight* loss during fasting may be quite dramatic, *fat* loss may actually be less than when at least some food is supplied.

The body's adaptations to fasting are sufficient to maintain life for a long period. Mental alertness need not be diminished. Even physical energy may remain unimpaired for a surprisingly long time. Still, fasting is not without its hazards. Among the many changes that take place in the body are:

- Wasting of lean tissues.
- Impairment of disease resistance.
- Lowering of body temperature.
- Disturbances of the body's salt and water balance.

Similar alterations are seen in low-carbohydrate dieting (discussed in the next section). Renewed food intake, especially of carbohydrate, results in

FIGURE 6–4 **Fasting**
When people are fasting, they draw on stored energy.

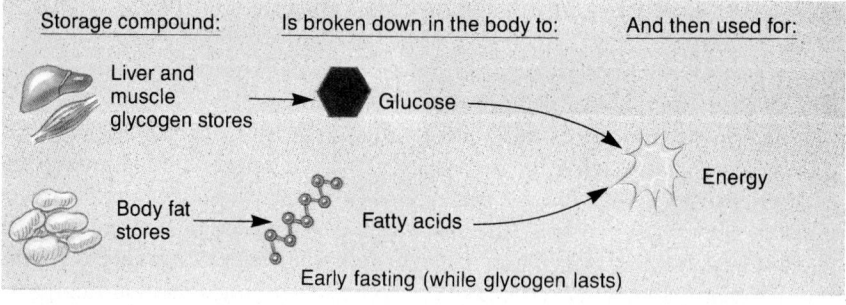

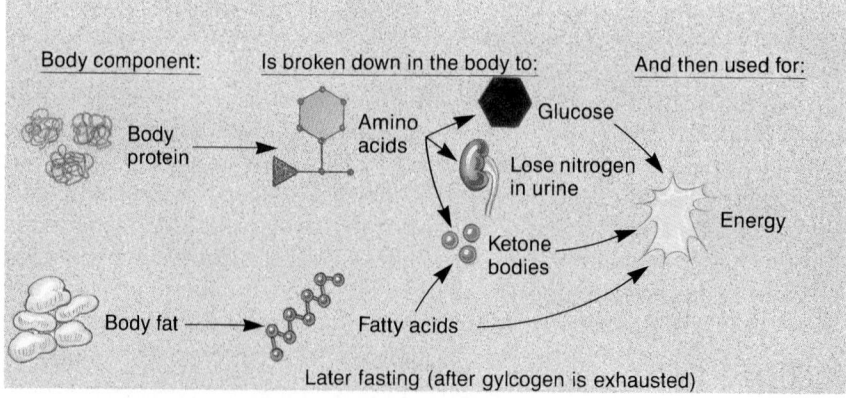

dramatic changes in the body's salt and water balance, accounting for most of the wide swings in body weight seen in people on fasts or low-carbohydrate diets.

The Low-Carbohydrate Diet

An economy similar to that of fasting prevails in a person who consumes a low-carbohydrate diet; ketosis occurs. Advocates of the low-carbohydrate diet would have you believe there is something magical about ketosis, something that promotes faster weight loss than a regular low-kcalorie diet. In fact, however, the low-carbohydrate diet presents the body with the same problem as a fast. Once the available glycogen reserves are spent, the only significant remaining source of glucose is protein. Most low-carbohydrate diets provide some protein from food, but some is still taken from body tissue. The onset of ketosis is the signal that this wasting process has begun.

Low-carbohydrate diet = living on (dietary and body) fat and protein almost exclusively.

Low-kcalorie diet = living on limited food and body fat.

People are attracted to the low-carbohydrate diet because of the dramatic weight loss it brings about within the first few days. They would be disillusioned if they realized that much of this weight loss is a loss of glycogen and protein accompanied by large quantities of water and important minerals. A dieter who boasts of losing 7 pounds in two days on a low-carbohydrate diet must be unaware that a pound or two, at best, are fat and that 5 or 6 pounds are lean tissue, water, and minerals. Once off the diet, the dieter's body avidly devours and retains these needed materials, and weight zooms back to within a few pounds of the starting point.

A warning is suggested by these facts. Beware of those who promote quick-weight-loss schemes. Learn to distinguish between loss of fat and loss of weight.

The Protein-Sparing Fast

A variant on fasting is the protein-sparing fast—the technique of eating only protein. The hope is that the protein will spare lean tissue and provide needed glucose, and that the person will break down body fat at a maximal rate to meet other energy needs. The protein-sparing idea sounded good when it was first advanced, but it has met with mixed results.

Two approaches have been used with protein-sparing fasting: the medical approach and the popular approach. The first has been safe, but the second has been dangerous. The medical approach allows only carefully screened people to participate. They consume 400 to 600 kcalories a day of protein-rich foods, such as lean meat, fish, or a high-quality complete amino acid preparation supplemented with vitamins and minerals, and their progress is accompanied by conscientious monitoring, especially of critical water and mineral balances. This fast has been successful in promoting large weight losses in people who might not otherwise lose weight, although it is not an ideal approach. It seems to become effective only after considerable lean tissue has already been lost, at which time the body may be conserving itself quite efficiently anyway. The protein-sparing fast has not been shown more effective than a diet containing a mixture of protein and carbohydrate.

Protein-sparing fast = eating only protein.

Furthermore, it doesn't seem to "stick" very well; that is, most people regain the lost weight.

The popular use of the protein-sparing fast has been an entirely different matter. Liquid protein-modified fast formulas promoted during the 1970's were linked to more than 60 deaths.[2] Dieters, usually without any medical supervision, drank these liquid protein potions prepared from poor-quality sources. Some of the people who died while on these diets had underlying diseases that may have been a factor in their deaths. The FDA has since ruled that liquid protein and other protein products promoted for use in weight reduction or as dietary supplements have to carry warning labels.

The term *protein-sparing* has also been used in another connection. Hospital clients enduring severe physical stresses, such as certain diseases or major surgery, also lose body protein. Such losses are especially likely to occur, and are especially dangerous, if the person is simultaneously fighting infection. Physicians make every effort to prevent the loss of vital lean tissue by supplying amino acids as well as glucose in some form—through a vein if the person can't eat. The effort to provide protein-sparing therapy in such circumstances should not be confused with the profiteering of faddists who promote protein-sparing fasts.

Moderate Weight Loss

Someone who wants to lose body fat must be reconciled to the hard fact that there is a limit to the rate at which this fat will break down. The maximum rate, except for a very large, very active person, is 1 to 2 pounds a week. The most effective means to achieve weight loss that actually reflects body fat loss is to adopt a balanced, low-kcalorie diet supplying all three energy nutrients in reasonable amounts while adjusting energy expended on physical activity to a reasonable level. In effect, this means adjusting the energy budget so that energy intake is 500 to 1,000 kcalories per day less than energy output. Energy output is the focus of the next section. Guidelines to reduce energy intake by way of safe and effective weight reduction diets are provided in Chapter 19.

Energy Balance

If a person's weight is within the appropriate range for height, the person has a balanced energy budget. Deposits of fat made at one time have been compensated for by withdrawals made at another: food energy intake has equaled energy expenditure. In other words, body fat is similar to a savings account; it differs from money only in that more is not better; there is an optimum. A day's energy balance can be stated like this:

Change in body fat stores (kcalories) = food energy taken in (kcalories) − energy spent on metabolic and other activities (kcalories).

TABLE 6–1 **Factors That Affect the BMR**

FACTOR	EFFECT ON BMR
Age	In youth, the BMR is higher; age brings less lean body mass and slows the BMR.
Height	Tall, thin people have higher BMRs.
Growth	Children and pregnant women have higher BMRs.
Body composition	The more lean tissue, the higher the BMR. The more fat tissue, the lower the BMR.
Fever	Fever raises the BMR.
Stress	Stress hormones raise the BMR.
Environmental temperature	Both heat and cold raise the BMR.
Fasting/starvation	Fasting/starvation hormones lower the BMR.
Malnutrition	Malnutrition lowers the BMR.
Thyroxin	The thyroid hormone thyroxin is a key BMR regulator; the more thyroxin produced, the higher the BMR.

More simply:

Change in fat stores (kcalories) = energy in (kcalories) − energy out (kcalories).

You know about the "energy in" side of this equation. An apple gives you about 100 kcalories; a candy bar contains about 300 kcalories. (Energy amounts for several hundred foods are listed in Appendix C.) On the "energy out" side, if you are physically active for an hour, you may spend 100, 300, or even 500 kcalories or more. For each 3,500 kcalories you eat in excess of expenditures, you store 1 pound of body fat.*

The body spends energy in two major ways: to fuel its basal metabolism and to fuel its voluntary activities. You can change your voluntary activities to spend more or less energy in a day, and over time you can also change your basal metabolism, as explained in Chapter 9.

The basal metabolism supports the work that goes on all the time without conscious awareness. The beating of the heart, the inhaling and exhaling of air, the maintenance of body temperature, and the sending of nerve and hormonal messages to direct these activities are the basal processes that maintain life. Basal metabolic needs are surprisingly large. A person whose total energy needs are 2,000 kcalories a day spends 1,200 to 1,400 of them to support basal metabolism. The hormone thyroxin directly controls basal metabolism—the less secreted, the lower the energy requirements for basal functions. Many other factors affect the BMR (Table 6–1). The accompanying box shows you how to estimate your energy expenditure for basal metabolism.

basal metabolism: the sum total of all the involuntary chemical activities of the cells necessary to sustain life. Basal metabolism, sometimes called *basal metabolic rate (BMR),* is normally the largest component of a person's daily energy expenditure. It is measured while lying down, while awake, and at least 12 hours after eating.

voluntary activities: the component of a person's daily energy expenditure that involves conscious and deliberate muscular work—walking, lifting, climbing, and other physical activities. Voluntary activities normally account for a smaller component of daily energy expenditure than basal metabolism does.

*Pure fat is worth 9 kcalories per gram. A pound of it (450 grams), then, would store 4,050 kcalories. A pound of body fat is not pure fat, though; it contains water, protein, and other materials, and thus has only about 3,500 kcalories per pound.

Estimation of Energy Output

Basal Metabolism. Convert your body weight from pounds to kilograms, and then use the factor 1.0 kcalorie per kilogram of body weight per hour for men, or 0.9 for women.* Example (for a 150-pound man):

1. Change pounds to kilograms:
   150 pounds $\div$ 2.2 pounds/kilogram = 68 kilograms.
2. Multiply weight in kilograms by the BMR factor:
   68 kilograms $\times$ 1 kcalorie/kilogram/hour = 68 kcalories/hour.
3. Multiply kcalories used in 1 hour by hours in a day:
   68 kcalories/hour $\times$ 24 hours/day = 1,632 kcalories/day.

Energy for BMR equals 1,632 kcalories/day.

Voluntary Muscular Activity. The following figures are crude approximations of energy expended, based on the amounts of muscular work people typically perform in a day. To select the category appropriate for you, remember to think in terms of the amount of *muscular* work performed; don't confuse being *busy* with being *active*. Calculate your energy need for activities using both percentages given for your gender and activity level. This will give you the range of energy needs appropriate for people similar to you.†

- Sedentary (mostly sitting): men, 25 to 40 percent; women, 25 to 35 percent.
- Light activity (moving around some of the time, such as a teacher might do): men, 50 to 70 percent; women, 40 to 60 percent.
- Moderate activity (some exercise or physical work): men, 65 to 80 percent; women, 50 to 70 percent.
- Heavy activity (much physical work, such as a roofer might do): men, 90 to 120 percent; women 80 to 100 percent.
- Exceptional activity (intense physical training, such as a football player might undergo): men, 130 to 145 percent; women, 110 to 130 percent.

Suppose the man we are using as an example is a student who bikes about 10 minutes a day, walks to classes, but otherwise sits and studies. To estimate the energy he needs for physical activities (light), first multiply his BMR kcalories per day by 50 percent and then by 70 percent:
Example: 1,632 kcalories/day $\times$ 50 percent = 816 kcalories/day.
          1,632 kcalories/day $\times$ 70 percent = 1,142 kcalories/day.
Energy for activities equals between 816 and 1,142 kcalories/day.
Total: The man in our example spends, in a day:
1,632 kcalories/day + 816 kcalories/day = 2,448 kcalories/day.
1,632 kcalories/day + 1,142 kcalories/day = 2,774 kcalories/day.

Because the exact figure is based on several estimates, express the man's energy expenditure as a range: 2,448 to 2,774 kcalories/day.

*Men's metabolic energy needs are assumed to be higher than women's, because their hormones induce them to develop more lean tissue than do most women, and lean tissue burns more energy per hour.
†Percentages are derived from the RDA (1990) formula for energy expenditure within about 20 percent of total kcalories.

The number of kcalories spent on voluntary activities depends on three factors. The larger the muscle mass required, the heavier the weight of the body part being moved, and the longer the activity takes, the more kcalories are spent. How much an activity costs also depends on several other things. One is the intensity of the activity: the more intense, the more kcalories are spent per minute. Another is the person's style: the streamlined moves of an expert swimmer, for example, cost less in energy than the movements of the untrained swimmer.

Some energy expenditure not taken into account in the estimate above is that required for the body to manage food. When food is taken into the body, many cells that have been dormant begin to be active. The muscles that move the food through the intestinal tract speed up their rhythmic contractions; the cells that manufacture and secrete digestive juices begin their tasks. All these and other cells need extra energy as they come alive to participate in the digestion, absorption, and metabolism of food. This stimulation of cellular activity is called diet-induced thermogenesis, and is generally thought to represent about 6 to 10 percent of the total food energy taken in. For purposes of rough estimates, diet-induced thermogenesis can be ignored; the 10 percent it might contribute to total energy output is smaller than the probable errors involved in estimating energy input from food or output for activities.

Diet-induced thermogenesis is also sometimes called the specific dynamic effect (SDE) or specific dynamic activity (SDA) of food.

In summary, the energy you spend in a day is the sum of two components—your basal metabolic energy and your activity energy. The Self-Study and accompanying Form 7 take you through the steps for computing the range of total energy you spend in a day. This expenditure represents your approximate energy need, which you meet by eating food. If you eat more than this, you will store the excess energy in your body, mostly as fat. If you eat less than this, you will use up body tissue as fuel to make up the deficit.

SELF-STUDY

How Much Energy Do You Spend in a Day?

Use the "Estimation of Energy Output" box in this chapter to estimate the energy you spend in a day. Form 7 will help you record your calculations.

FORM 7   **Estimating Energy Output**

1. BASAL METABOLISM.

Step 1. My weight in pounds (_____ lb) divided by 2.2 lb/kg equals my weight in kilograms: _____kg.

Step 2. My weight in kilograms (_____ kg) times 1.0 kcal/kg/hr for men or 0.9 kcal/kg/hr for women equals the number of kcalories I spend on basal metabolism in an hour: _____kcal/hr.

Step 3. My energy expenditure per hour (_____ kcal/hr) times the hours in a day (24) equals the number of kcalories I spend on basal metabolism in a day: _____kcal/day.

2. ACTIVITIES (CHECK ONE).

Men:

_____I am sedentary, so my activities cost 25 to 40% of my basal metabolic energy each day.

25% of my basal metabolic energy (step 3) equals _____kcal/day.
40% of my basal metabolic energy (step 3) equals _____kcal/day.

_____I am lightly active, so my activities cost 50 to 70% of my basal metabolic energy each day.

50% of my basal metabolic energy (step 3) equals _____kcal/day.
70% of my basal metabolic energy (step 3) equals _____kcal/day.

_____I am moderately active, so my activities cost 65 to 80% of my basal metabolic energy each day.

65% of my basal metabolic energy (step 3) equals _____kcal/day.
80% of my basal metabolic energy (step 3) equals _____kcal/day.

_____I am very active (heavy activity), so my activities cost 90 to 120% of my basal metabolic energy each day.

90% of my basal metabolic energy (step 3) equals _____kcal/day.
120% of my basal metabolic energy (step 3) equals _____kcal/day.

_____I am exceptionally active, so my activities cost 130 to 145% of my basal metabolic energy each day.

130% of my basal metabolic energy (step 3) equals _____kcal/day.
145% of my basal metabolic energy (step 3) equals _____kcal/day.

Study Questions

1. What are the basic units of metabolism in the body?
2. Define metabolism, anabolism, and catabolism.
3. Why do body protein tissues break down during fasting?
4. Describe ketosis.
5. List some of the hazards of fasting.
6. List two ways the body spends energy.
7. Describe basal metabolism.
8. List some factors that affect a person's basal metabolic rate.

FORM 7   **Estimating Energy Output** (*continued*)

2. ACTIVITIES (continued)

Women:

_____I am sedentary, so my activities cost 25 to 35% of my basal metabolic energy each day.

    25% of my basal metabolic energy (step 3) equals _____kcal/day.

    35% of my basal metabolic energy (step 3) equals _____kcal/day.

_____I am lightly active, so my activities cost 40 to 60% of my basal metabolic energy each day.

    40% of my basal metabolic energy (step 3) equals _____kcal/day.

    60% of my basal metabolic energy (step 3) equals _____kcal/day.

_____I am moderately active, so my activities cost 50 to 70% of my basal metabolic energy each day.

    50% of my basal metabolic energy (step 3) equals _____kcal/day.

    70% of my basal metabolic energy (step 3) equals _____kcal/day.

_____I am very active (heavy activity), so my activities cost 80 to 100% of my basal metabolic energy each day.

    80% of my basal metabolic energy (step 3) equals _____kcal/day.

    100% of my basal metabolic energy (step 3) equals _____kcal/day.

_____I am exceptionally active, so my activities cost 110 to 130% of my basal metabolic energy each day.

    110% of my basal metabolic energy (step 3) equals _____kcal/day.

    130% of my basal metabolic energy (step 3) equals _____kcal/day.

3. TOTAL ENERGY SPENT IN A DAY.

Energy for basal metabolism: _____kcal/day.

Range of energy for activities: _____to _____kcal/day.

Total range: _____kcal/day to _____kcal/day.

Notes

1. S. Klein and coauthors, Effect of plasma glucose concentration on the lipolytic response to fasting (abstract), *American Journal of Clinical Nutrition* 45 (1987): 856.

2. J. U. Doherty and coauthors, Long-term evaluation of cardiac function in obese patients treated with a very-low-calorie diet: A controlled clinical study of patients without underlying cardiac disease, *American Journal of Clinical Nutrition* 53 (1991): 854–858.

6

Nutrition and the Alcohol Abuser

Like all drugs, alcohol offers both benefits and hazards. Wine, beer, and other fermented beverages have given pleasure and relaxation to people for more than 5,000 years. People have always known that these beverages affected their moods, sensations, and behavior. Taken in moderation, alcohol can relax people, reduce their inhibitions, and encourage social interactions. The term *moderation* is important in the statement above. Because people differ in their tolerance levels, it is impossible to name an exact amount of alcohol per day that is appropriate for everyone, but authorities have attempted to set limits that are acceptable for most healthy adults. The Dietary Recommendations to the Public (Table 1–3 in Chapter 1) suggest limiting alcohol to less than 1 ounce of pure alcohol in a single day, which is equivalent to two cans of beer, two small glasses of wine, or two average cocktails. This amount is supposed to be enough to produce euphoria without incurring any long-term harm to health. Unfortunately, many people who choose to drink alcoholic beverages do incur long-term harm to health because they drink excessively. This discussion focuses on the nutrition implications of alcohol *abuse*.

Alcohol is the most widely abused drug in the world. Alcohol abuse exerts a heavy toll on the health of the 10 million adults and 3.3 million

teenagers who are considered problem drinkers in the United States.[1] Alcoholism is a serious and debilitating disease that frequently results in illness, disability, and death. Furthermore, the effects of alcohol on nutrition and metabolism—both as a direct effect and as a consequence of alcohol-related diseases—are significant. Every alcohol abuser should be considered at risk for poor nutrition status.

Would you please clarify exactly what alcoholism is.

That's an important starting point, because even the experts can't agree on a precise definition of alcoholism, and many people have misconceptions about it. Most people can take alcohol or leave it, but about one in every ten drinkers, for unknown reasons, becomes addicted to alcohol and develops a risky relationship with it.* The American Medical Association defines alcoholism as a disease, briefly described as an addiction to alcohol. It

*Alcohol *addiction* means the same thing as alcohol *dependence*. This book uses the term *addiction*, because it is more self-explanatory.

is chronic, progressive, and potentially fatal, characterized by tolerance and physical dependency or organ damage caused directly or indirectly by alcohol consumption.

Although alcohol-addicted people may be able to drink moderately on some occasions, on others they drink far more than they intend to, losing control. These occasions occur unpredictably at first, but more and more often the first drink becomes the first of too many—an episode of uncontrolled drinking.

The alcohol-addicted person's craving for alcohol becomes marked by several features. The person thinks about alcohol a lot *(obsession)*, drinks in spite of resolving not to *(broken promises)*, and then suffers *remorse*. Such strong feelings about any substance should signify addiction, but note that these feelings reflect no personal inferiority. The person is simply someone whose internal makeup reacts in a special way to alcohol.

Some misconceptions about alcoholism can be dangerous and demand correction. For example, some people believe that alcoholism is related to the type of alcohol-containing beverage a person drinks. Not true. People who drink only beer and wine can become alcohol addicts just as readily as people who drink hard liquors. Another common misconception is that only morally degenerate people become addicted. Alcohol addiction does not single out people of low moral character or people of any particular age, race, education, social class, or income. It is true, however, that people of certain races and cultures tend to be more susceptible to alcohol addiction than others. Environment and heredity, or perhaps both, can contribute to such differences.

Why do you say that all alcohol abusers are at risk for poor nutrition status?

Alcohol produces euphoria, which depresses appetite, so heavy drinkers tend to eat poorly. Since much of their energy fuel comes from the empty kcalories of alcohol, heavy drinkers consume too few essential nutrients. Nutrient deficiencies are an almost inevitable result of alcohol abuse, not only because the person who drinks obtains fewer nutrients from food but also because alcohol interferes with the body's use of nutrients, making them ineffective even if they are present.

Even if a person eats well, large amounts of alcohol will impair nutritional health, because alcohol itself impairs the ingestion, digestion, absorption, metabolism, and excretion of nutrients. Since alcohol can affect virtually every organ, other complications frequently develop that also change nutrient requirements. Some of these include:

- Anemia (Chapter 8).
- Gastritis and ulcers (Chapter 17).
- Pancreatitis (Chapter 21).
- Liver disease (Chapter 23).

Explain specifically how alcohol alters nutrient metabolism.

Major changes occur in the way the body metabolizes many nutrients, particularly carbohydrate, fat, and protein. Dietary glucose and dietary fat can't be metabolized as they normally are. Instead, they are diverted into making fat, and this fat may accumulate in the liver. Fatty liver, the first stage of liver deterioration in the heavy drinker (which can be reversed by abstinence from alcohol), can progress to cirrhosis (which is irreversible).

Large doses of alcohol inhibit protein synthesis in the brain. In the liver, alcohol has been shown to inhibit the release of proteins, causing them to accumulate in liver cells.[2] Protein deficiency can develop, both from the depression of protein synthesis in the cells and from a poor diet. Alcohol also interferes with amino acid metabolism. The absorption and transport of several amino acids are impaired by high concentrations of alcohol, so that even the amino acids that a person eats are not used efficiently.

Does alcohol affect vitamin and mineral metabolism, too?

Yes. Alcohol impairs absorption of thiamin, folate, and other nutrients, as Figure NP6–1 shows. Alcohol-induced liver injury impairs the activity of the liver enzyme that activates thiamin to its active form.

Alcohol's effect on folate is dramatic. When alcohol is present, it is as though the body were actively trying to expel folate from all its sites of action and storage. The liver, which normally contains enough folate to meet all needs, leaks folate into the blood. As the blood folate concentration rises, the kidneys are deceived into excreting it, as though it were in excess. The intestine normally releases and retrieves folate continuously, but it becomes damaged by folate deficiency and alcohol toxicity, so it fails to retrieve its own folate and misses out on any that may trickle in from food as well. Alcohol abuse causes a folate deficiency that devastates digestive system function.

Alcohol abuse alters the metabolism of many other vitamins—including vitamin B_6, vitamin B_{12}, and vitamin A. One of the products of alcohol metabolism dislodges vitamin B_6 from its protective binding protein so that it is destroyed. Alcohol inhibits vitamin B_{12} absorption—both directly and indirectly—by suppressing the secretion of the factor that facilitates the vitamin's absorption from the intestine to the bloodstream. Alcohol does not impair absorption of vitamin A, but reduces the storage of the vitamin in the liver. Even moderate amounts of alcohol have been shown to deplete liver stores of vitamin A.[3]

Alcohol also promotes water excretion by the kidneys. With it important minerals such as zinc, magnesium, and potassium are lost. So you see, alcohol profoundly affects nutrition status.

I see. What about alcohol's effect on body weight? I thought alcohol had a lot of kcalories, but I had an uncle who abused alcohol and became thinner and thinner.

It is true that the energy contribution of alcohol is relatively high. Alcohol yields about 7 kcalories per gram—more than protein and carbohydrate (4 kcalories per gram), and only slightly less than fat (9 kcalories per gram). In some cases, drinking too much alcohol can contribute to obesity, but chronic alcohol ingestion seems to have the opposite effect. Research explains this observation as follows: although low doses of alcohol (less than 30 percent of total kcalories) do indeed yield about 7 kcalories per gram, when people consume higher doses of alcohol, they may not receive its maximum kcaloric value.[4] In one study, people consuming 50 percent of total kcalories as alcohol lost weight. Some researchers attribute the incomplete energy utilization of large doses of alcohol to an alternate metabolic pathway for alcohol that consumes energy rather than generating it. Subsequent research results do not lend support to this theory, but they do support the idea that large doses of alcohol impair other metabolic processes, which in turn may contribute to the weight loss associated with chronic alcohol abuse.

What are the long-term nutrition effects of alcohol abuse?

Long-term alcohol abuse damages different organs in different individuals, but always affects all organs and organ systems to various extents.

The most common damage is to the liver, where the function of affected cells may be lost forever unless abstinence from alcohol and sound nutrition intervene in time to reverse the damage. The injury to the liver results in many side effects; one is high blood pressure, which may lead to heart damage and stroke. The protein deficiencies that develop contribute to increased susceptibility to infection. As the synthesis of fat speeds up, fat is deposited in the heart, arteries, and liver. Although alcohol was at one time believed to reduce heart disease risk, the lipoproteins that are elevated by alcohol use are not the same ones that are protective against heart disease.[5]

The central nervous system is particularly sensitive to alcohol. The brain shrinks even in people who drink only moderately, but the extent of damage from alcohol is proportional to the amount drunk. The following are a few of the other effects of alcohol:

- Inflammation of the intestines; ulcers of the stomach and intestines.
- Deterioration of the muscles, including the heart muscle.
- Reduced capacity for exercise; heart discomfort sooner during exercise.
- Kidney damage, bladder damage, prostate gland damage.
- Reduced resistance to disease.
- Loss of function of the testicles and damage to the adrenal glands, leading to feminization and sexual impotence in men.
- Failure of the ovaries and early menopause in women.

FIGURE NP6–1 Alcohol's Effect on Vitamin Absorption (Example)

In the presence of alcohol, intestinal cells fail to absorb thiamin, except at very high concentrations.

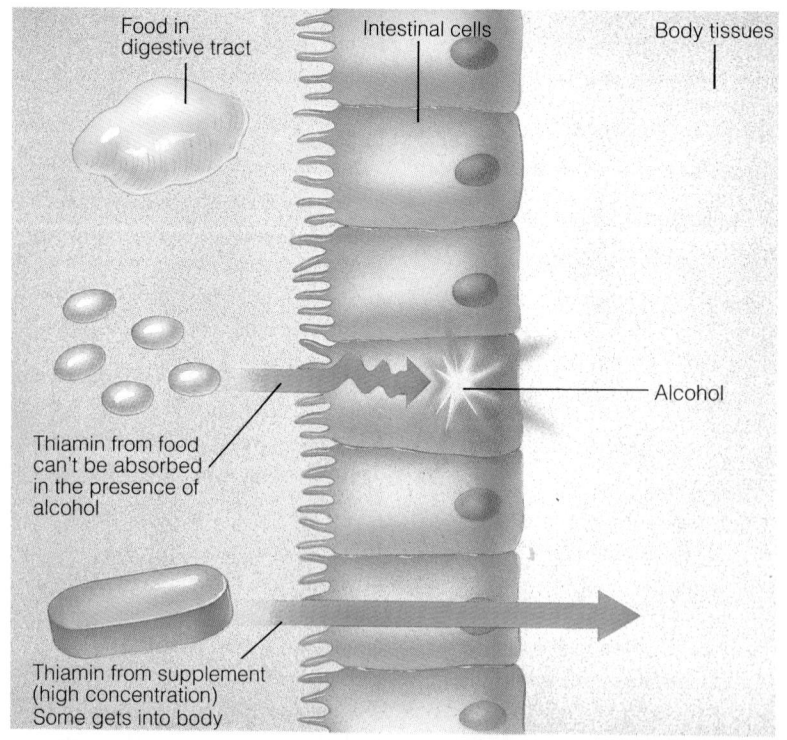

Food in digestive tract

Intestinal cells

Body tissues

Thiamin from food can't be absorbed in the presence of alcohol

Alcohol

Thiamin from supplement (high concentration) Some gets into body

■ Increased susceptibility to lung infections.

The effects of alcohol are frightening. Eating well or even taking supplements of protein, vitamins, and minerals will not protect the drinker. There is no set level of safe drinking where no adverse effects take place. Even just a couple of drinks set in motion the processes described, but the next day's abstinence reverses them. Some place between abstinence and alcoholism, there may be alcohol intakes moderate enough not to harm health, but the more a person drinks, the closer to a dangerous extreme that person comes.

Notes

1. Do you drink too much? *University of Texas Lifetime Health Letter,* September 1989, pp. 1, 5.
2. M. C. Mitchell, Alcohol, in *Present Knowledge in Nutrition,* 6th ed., ed. M. L. Brown (Washington, D.C.: International Life Sciences Institute, Nutrition Foundation, 1990), pp. 457–462.
3. D. H. Barch and S. Mobarhan, Vitamin deficiencies in the alcoholic patient, *Nutrition and the M.D.,* October 1987, pp. 1–3.
4. J. F. Reinus and coauthors, Ethanol: Relative fuel value and metabolic effects *in vivo, Metabolism* 38 (1989): 125–135, as cited in Mitchell, 1990.
5. National Academy of Sciences, Food and Nutrition Board, Committee on Diet and Health, *Diet and Health: Implications for Reducing Chronic Disease Risk* (Washington, D.C.: National Academy Press, 1989), pp. 443–444.

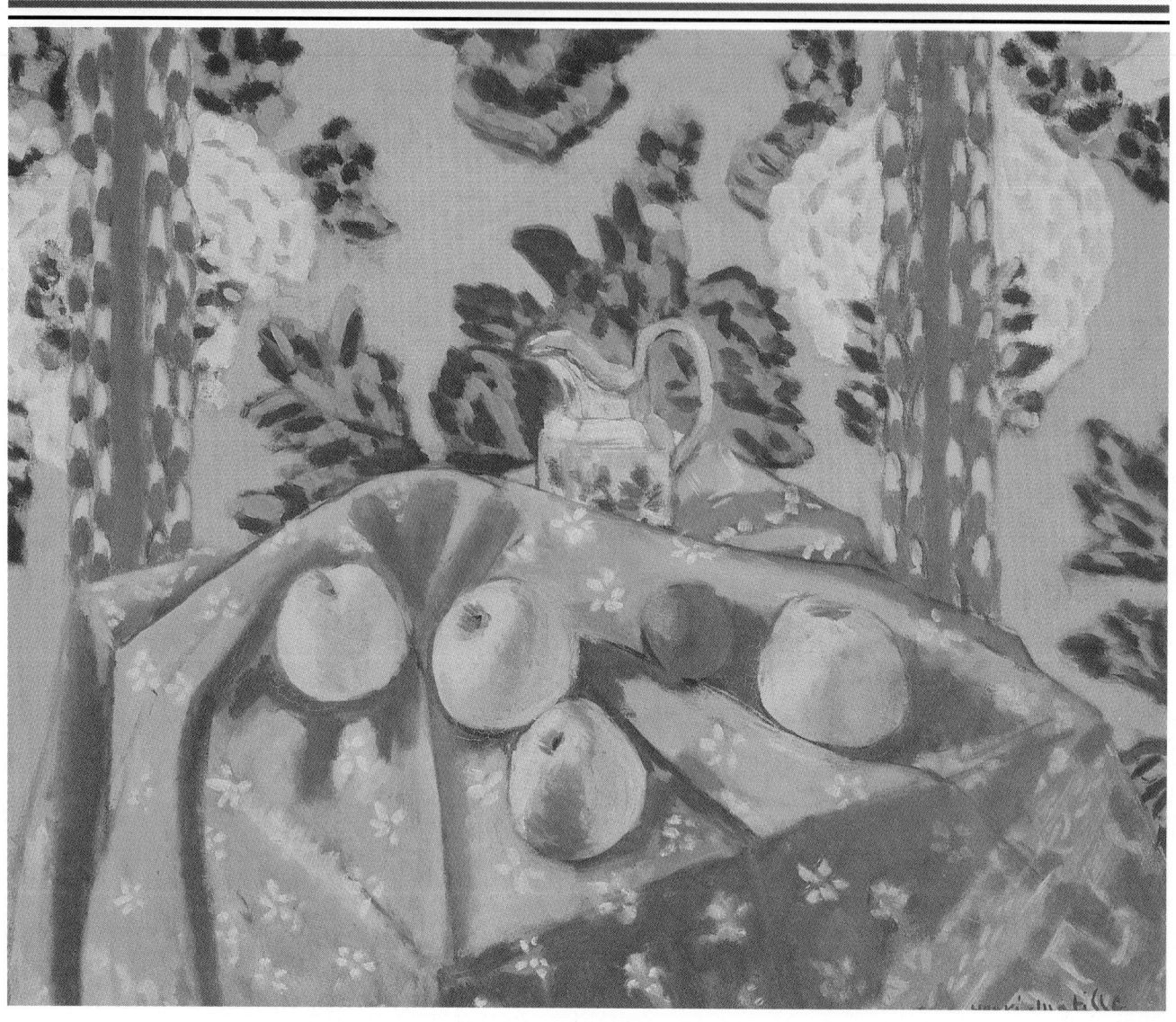

Henri Matisse, Still Life with Apples on Pink Tablecloth; *National Gallery of Art, Washington; Chester Dale Collecton.*

The Vitamins

CONTENTS

The last five chapters focused primarily on the energy-yielding nutrients—carbohydrate, fat, and protein. This chapter and the next one discuss the nutrients everyone thinks of when thinking about nutrition—the vitamins and minerals.

The vitamins occur in foods in much smaller quantities than do the energy-yielding nutrients, and they make no contribution of energy to the body themselves. Instead, they serve mostly as helpers, or facilitators, of body processes. They are, nonetheless, a powerful group of substances, as their absence attests. Vitamin A deficiency can cause blindness; a lack of niacin can cause symptoms of mental illness; and a lack of vitamin D can cause growth retardation. The consequences of deficiencies are so dire and the effects of restoring the needed nutrients so dramatic that they make wonderful stories for faddists to tell: Are you bald? Impotent? Tired? Do you have pimples? Are you nearsighted? The right vitamin will cure whatever ails you. Vitamins certainly contribute to sound nutritional health, but they do not cure all ills. Actually, a vitamin can cure only the disease caused by a deficiency of that vitamin.

vitamins: essential, noncaloric, organic nutrients needed in tiny amounts in the diet.

The only disease a vitamin will cure is the one caused by a deficiency of that vitamin.

Definition and Classification of Vitamins

A child once defined vitamins as "what, if you don't eat, you get sick." The description is both insightful and accurate. A less ingenious definition is that a vitamin is a potent, essential, noncaloric, organic nutrient needed in tiny amounts in the diet. Vitamins perform specific and individual functions to promote growth or reproduction or to maintain health and life. Two characteristics distinguish vitamins from energy nutrients:

1. Vitamins do not yield energy when broken down, but assist the enzymes that release energy from carbohydrate, fat, and protein.
2. Vitamins are needed in much smaller amounts than the energy nutrients.

As the individual vitamins were discovered, they were named or given letters, numbers, or both. This led to the confusion that still exists today. This chapter uses the names shown in Table 7–1; alternative names are given in Tables 7–2, 7–3 and 7–4.

Vitamins fall naturally into two classes—fat soluble and water soluble. The solubility of a vitamin confers on it many characteristic behaviors and determines how it is absorbed and transported, whether it can be stored, and how easily it is lost from the body. This discussion of vitamins begins with the fat-soluble vitamins.

TABLE 7–1   **Vitamin Names**

Fat-soluble vitamins
  Vitamin A
  Vitamin D
  Vitamin E
  Vitamin K
Water-soluble vitamins
  B vitamins
    Thiamin
    Riboflavin
    Niacin
    Vitamin B_6
    Folate
    Vitamin B_{12}
    Pantothenic acid
    Biotin
  Vitamin C

The Fat-Soluble Vitamins

The fat-soluble vitamins—A, D, E, and K—usually occur together in the fats and oils of foods. The body absorbs the fat-soluble vitamins from the GI tract in the same way as it absorbs lipids. Therefore, any condition that interferes with fat absorption can precipitate a deficiency of the fat-soluble vitamins. Once absorbed, fat-soluble vitamins are stored in the liver and fatty tissues until the body needs them. They are not as readily excreted as water-soluble substances are, and unlike most of the water-soluble vitamins, they can build up to toxic concentrations.

The capacity to store vitamins affords a person some flexibility as to dietary intakes of the fat-soluble vitamins. When a person consumes them in excess of immediate need, the body stores the excess. Later, when blood concentrations begin to decline, the body can retrieve the vitamins from storage. Thus a person need not replenish the supply of fat-soluble vitamins every single day, but need only make sure the diet as a whole provides average amounts that approximate the RDA. In contrast, the body does not store the water-soluble vitamins to any great extent, so they must be consumed more regularly.

Vitamin A

Vitamin A has the distinction of being the first fat-soluble vitamin to be recognized. It is clearly one of the most versatile, with roles in several important body processes, the best known of which is vision.

For a person to see, light reaching the eye must be transformed into nerve impulses that the brain interprets to produce visual images. The transformers are molecules of pigment in the cells of the retina (see Figure 7–1). A portion of each pigment molecule is retinal, a compound the body can synthesize only if vitamin A or certain of its relatives are supplied by the diet. When vitamin A is lacking, the eye has difficulty adapting to changing light levels. A lag occurs before the eye can see again after a flash of bright light at night (after the eye has adapted to darkness). This lag in the recovery of night vision is known as night blindness. Because night blindness is easy to test, it aids in the diagnosis of vitamin A deficiency. Night blindness is only a symptom, however, and may indicate a condition other than vitamin A deficiency.

pigment: a molecule capable of absorbing certain wavelengths of light, so that it reflects only those that we perceive as a certain color.

retina (RET-in-uh): the layer of light-sensitive cells lining the back of the inside of the eye; consists of rods and cones.

retinal (RET-in-al): the aldehyde form of vitamin A, active in the pigments of the eye.

night blindness: slow recovery of vision after flashes of bright light at night; an early symptom of vitamin A deficiency.

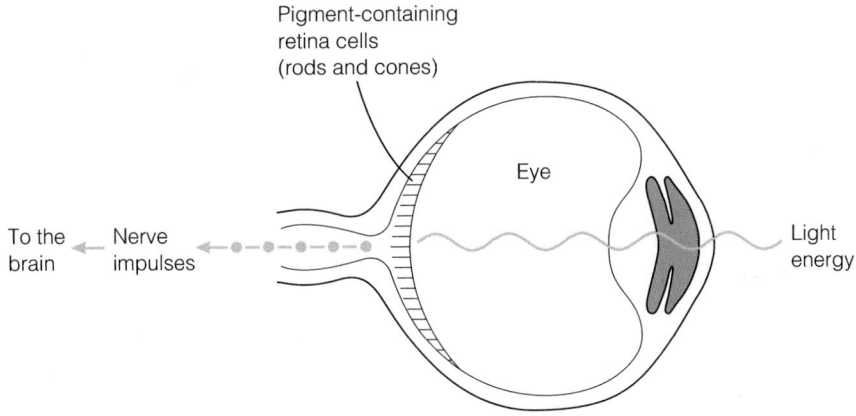

Pigment-containing
retina cells
(rods and cones)

Eye

To the ← Nerve
brain   impulses

Light
energy

FIGURE 7–1   **The Visual Process**
As light enters the eye, pigments within the cells of the retina absorb the light and generate nerve impulses that travel into the brain. Each pigment contains retinal, the active form of vitamin A.

The role that vitamin A plays in vision is undeniably important, but only one-thousandth of the body's vitamin A is in the retina. Much more is in skin and linings of organs, where it helps maintain the integrity of the epithelial cells. It is important that each of these surfaces be smooth: the linings of the mouth, stomach, and intestines; the linings of the lungs and the passages leading to them; the lining of the bladder; the linings of the uterus and vagina; the linings of the eyelids and sinus passageways. The cells lining the surfaces of these and other organs secrete a smooth and slippery substance (mucus) that coats and protects them from invasive microorganisms and other harmful particles. The mucosal lining of the stomach also shields its cells from digestion by gastric juices.

As you may expect from its role in these defensive barriers, vitamin A plays an integral role in fighting infection.[1] Research confirms that this is true not only in theory but in practice: when children with measles complicated by infections such as pneumonia, diarrhea, or both were given vitamin A supplements, their recovery times and hospital stays were shorter, and their overall survival rates significantly greater, than those of similar children who did not receive vitamin A.[2]

In vitamin A deficiency, the epithelial cells flatten and begin to produce keratin—the hard, inflexible protein of hair and nails. In the eye, this process leads to drying and hardening of the cornea, which may progress to permanent blindness. Vitamin A deficiency is the major cause of childhood blindness in the world—more than a half million children lose their sight every year. More than 5 million children worldwide endure less severe forms of vitamin A deficiency, making them vulnerable to infectious diseases.[3]

In the mouth, a vitamin A deficiency results in drying and hardening of the salivary glands, making them susceptible to infection. Mucous secretion in the stomach and intestines is reduced, hindering normal digestion and absorption of nutrients. Infections of other mucous membranes also become likely.

All body surfaces, both inside and out, maintain their integrity with the help of vitamin A. When vitamin A is lacking, cells of the skin harden and flatten, making it dry, rough, scaly, and hard. An accumulation of hard material makes a lump around each hair follicle.

Vitamin A serves many other purposes in the body. It supports normal bone growth, reproduction, and cell membrane stability.

Three different forms of vitamin A are active: retinol, retinal, and retinoic acid. A zinc-containing protein transports vitamin A via the blood from the liver, where it is stored, to sites where it is needed. For this reason, a zinc deficiency can mimic the symptoms of vitamin A deficiency.

Up to a year's supply of vitamin A can be stored in the body, 90 percent of it in the liver. If a healthy adult were to stop eating vitamin A–rich foods, deficiency symptoms would not begin to appear until after stores were depleted, which would take one to two years. Then, however, the consequences would be profound and severe. Table 7–2, later in this chapter, itemizes some of them.

Because the body stores excess vitamin A, toxicity is possible. Normally, toxicity symptoms are likely only when animal-derived foods or supplements are the source of the excess amounts of vitamin A, for in these sources the vitamin is already active; it is called *preformed* vitamin A. Plant foods

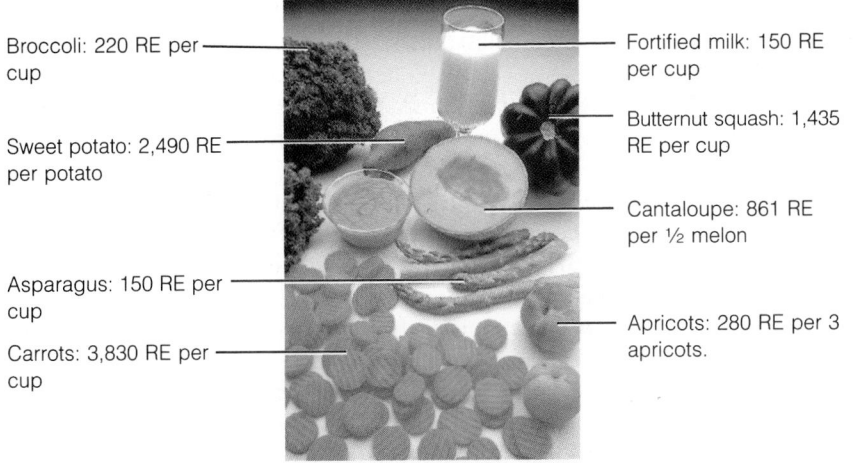

Broccoli: 220 RE per cup

Sweet potato: 2,490 RE per potato

Asparagus: 150 RE per cup

Carrots: 3,830 RE per cup

Fortified milk: 150 RE per cup

Butternut squash: 1,435 RE per cup

Cantaloupe: 861 RE per ½ melon

Apricots: 280 RE per 3 apricots.

FIGURE 7–2   **A Sampling of Vitamin A–Rich Foods**
A man's RDA for vitamin A is 1,000 RE; a woman's is 800 RE. A 3-ounce portion of beef liver (not shown) contains 9,120 RE.[a] See also Appendix C.
[a] Vitamin A recommendations have been expressed in retinol equivalents (RE) since 1980, but food contents of vitamin A are sometimes still expressed using an older terminology, international units (IU). Until this discrepancy is corrected in food tables, you will have to convert from one form to the other if you want to compare your vitamin A intake with recommendations. A rule of thumb is that 1 RE = 5 IU on the average, given a diet composed of both animal and plant sources of vitamin A. Thus, for example, 10,000 IU of vitamin A converts to 2,000 RE.

preformed vitamin A: vitamin A in its active form.

precursor: a compound that can be converted into another compound. For example, carotene is a precursor of vitamin A.

beta-carotene: an orange pigment found in plants.

contain the vitamin only in a precursor form, as beta-carotene, which does not convert to vitamin A rapidly enough to cause toxicity. Beta-carotene taken in excess is stored in fat depots as carotene, rather than as active vitamin A, and causes no toxic symptoms. When large amounts of carotene-rich foods (such as tomato juice and carrot juice) or daily beta-carotene supplements are consumed, however, carotene may accumulate under the skin to such an extent that the overdoser actually turns yellow.

Research suggests that beta-carotene helps defend the body against some types of cancer.[4] Although other forms of vitamin A have not proven effective against cancer, people still tend to take large doses of both beta-carotene and vitamin A in the hopes of preventing cancer. Foods rich in beta-carotene contain many other nutrients, fiber, and possibly undiscovered anticancer factors that supplements do not offer. Foods are always a better choice than supplements for needed nutrients. The best way to ensure a safe vitamin A intake is to eat generous servings of vitamin A–rich foods (see Figure 7–2). Well-nourished, healthy people need no supplements.

Overdoses of vitamin A damage the same body systems that exhibit symptoms in vitamin A deficiency (see Table 7–2, later in the chapter). Children are most vulnerable to vitamin A toxicity, because they need less than adults, they are smaller, and it is easy to give them too much in pill form. The availability of breakfast cereals, instant meals, fortified milk, and chewable candylike vitamins, each containing 100 percent or more of the recommended daily intake of vitamin A, makes it possible for a well-meaning parent to provide several times the daily allowance of the vitamin to a child within a few hours.

Certain relatives of vitamin A, available by prescription, have been used to relieve the symptoms of acne when applied directly to the skin surface. Acne sufferers should be warned, however, that taking massive doses of vitamin A internally will not cure acne and may cause the miseries itemized in Table 7–2.

In the United States about half of the vitamin A activity consumed in foods comes from fruits and vegetables, and half of this comes from the dark leafy greens (like spinach—not iceberg lettuce or green beans) and the rich yellow or deep orange vegetables (such as winter squash, cantaloupe, carrots, and sweet potatoes—not corn). These plant foods supply the vitamin as its precursor, carotene, as mentioned. The other half of vitamin A activity consumed in foods comes from performed vitamin A supplied in milk, cheese, butter, and other dairy products; eggs; and meats. Figure 7–2 shows a sampling of vitamin A–rich foods. Because vitamin A is fat soluble, it is lost when milk is skimmed. Nonfat milk is thus often fortified with vitamin A to compensate. Margarine is usually fortified so as to provide the same amount of vitamin A as butter.

Fast foods are notable for their *lack* of vitamin A. Anyone who dines frequently on fast foods is advised to emphasize vegetables heavily—and not just salads—at other meals.

Liver is an excellent source of preformed vitamin A. In fact, Arctic explorers who have eaten large quantities of polar bear liver have become ill with symptoms suggesting vitamin A toxicity. This problem, however, has never been observed in connection with the frequent use of other kinds of liver.

1 RE = 3.33 IU from animal foods or 10 IU from plant foods. (On the average, 1 RE = about 5 IU.)

Vitamin D

Vitamin D is different from all the other nutrients in that the body can synthesize it with the help of sunlight. Therefore, in a sense, vitamin D is not an essential nutrient. Given enough sun, you need consume no vitamin D at all in the foods you eat. Research suggests that the photosynthesis of vitamin D may be important in enhancing resistance to tuberculosis (TB).[5] This finding helps provide a scientific explanation for the observation that sunshine seems to benefit those with TB.

Another unique feature of vitamin D is that it acts very much like a hormone—a compound manufactured by one organ of the body that has effects on another. As you will see, the classic vitamin D target organs are the intestine, the kidneys, and the bones. Only recently have scientists discovered many other vitamin D target tissues, including the brain, the pancreas, the skin, the reproductive organs, and some cancer cells.[6] The abundance of these discoveries suggests the possibility that numerous additional functions for vitamin D will surface, including the regulation of the immune system.[7]

The liver manufactures a vitamin D precursor, which migrates to the skin and is there converted to vitamin D with the help of the ultraviolet rays from the sun. Regardless of whether your body manufactures vitamin D or obtains it from food, two more steps occur before the vitamin becomes fully active. First the liver alters the molecule, and then the kidneys alter it further to produce the active vitamin. The biologic activity of the active vitamin is 500- to 1,000- fold higher than that of its precursor.[8] Diseases that affect either the liver or the kidneys may impair the transformations of inactive vitamin D to active vitamin D and therefore produce symptoms of vitamin D deficiency.

Vitamin D is a member of a large and cooperative bone-making and maintenance team composed of nutrients and other compounds, including

Sunlight promotes vitamin D formation in the skin.

The precursor of vitamin D made in the liver is 7-dehydrocholesterol, which is made from cholesterol. This is one of the body's many "good" uses for cholesterol.

The shorthand name for the final, active vitamin is dihydroxy vitamin D.

vitamin C; the hormones parathormone and calcitonin; the protein collagen; and the minerals calcium, phosphorus, magnesium, and fluoride. The special function of vitamin D in bone making is to promote normal bone mineralization. Its actions help to make calcium and phosphorus available in the blood that bathes the bones, to be deposited as the bones harden.

Vitamin D acts in three ways to maintain blood concentrations of calcium and phosphorus: it stimulates their absorption from the GI tract; it mobilizes calcium and phosphorus from bones into the blood; and it stimulates their retention by the kidneys.

The symptoms of an inadequate intake of vitamin D are those of calcium deficiency, shown in Table 7−2. The bones fail to calcify normally and may grow so weak that they become bent when they have to support the body's weight. A child with rickets who is old enough to walk characteristically develops bowed legs, often the most obvious sign of the disease. Worldwide, rickets afflicts a large number of children.

Adult rickets, or osteomalacia, occurs most often in women who have low calcium intakes and little exposure to sun and who go through repeated pregnancies and periods of lactation. The bones of the legs may soften to such an extent that a young woman who is tall and straight at 20 may be condemned by repeated pregnancies to become bent, bowlegged, and stooped before she is 30.

Vitamin D deficiency depresses calcium absorption and results in low blood calcium concentrations and abnormal mineralization of bone. An excess of vitamin D does the opposite, as shown in Table 7−2. It enhances calcium absorption, leading to abnormally high concentrations of the mineral in the blood; it promotes return of bone calcium into the blood as well. Excess calcium in the blood tends to precipitate in the soft tissue, forming stones. This is especially likely to happen in the kidneys, which concentrate calcium as they excrete it. Calcification or hardening of the blood vessels may also occur and is especially dangerous in the major arteries of the heart and lungs, where it can cause death.

Vitamin D in excess is the most toxic of all the vitamins. Half the recommended intake is too little, but over a few times the recommended intake may be too much. The amounts of vitamin D found in foods available in the United States and Canada are well within these limits, but pills containing the vitamin in concentrated form are not. Adults should use vitamin D supplements with caution and keep them out of the reach of children.

Most of the world's population relies on natural exposure to sunlight to maintain adequate vitamin D nutrition.[9] The sun imposes no risk of toxicity; prolonged exposure to sunlight degrades the vitamin D precursor in the skin, preventing its conversion to the active vitamin. Even lifeguards on southern beaches are safe from vitamin D toxicity from the sun. No one is safe from vitamin D toxicity from supplements; supplements bypass the body's safeguards and can easily induce toxicity.

Prolonged sunlight exposure does have other, undesirable consequences, such as premature wrinkling of the skin and the increased risk of skin cancer. These risks may be reduced by using sunscreens. Unfortunately, sunscreens with sun protection factors (SPFs) of 8 and above also prevent vitamin D synthesis.[10] A strategy to avoid this dilemma is to apply sunscreen after enough time has elapsed to provide sufficient vitamin D synthesis. For most people, exposing hands, face, and arms on a clear summer day for 10

rickets: the vitamin D–deficiency disease in children.

osteomalacia (os-tee-o-mal-AY-shuh): the vitamin D–deficiency disease in adults.
  osteo = bone
  mal = bad (soft)

Osteomalacia can also occur in calcium deficiency (see Chapter 8).

Sunlight promotes vitamin D synthesis in the skin. Exposure to the sun should be reasonable, however; excessive exposure may cause skin cancer.

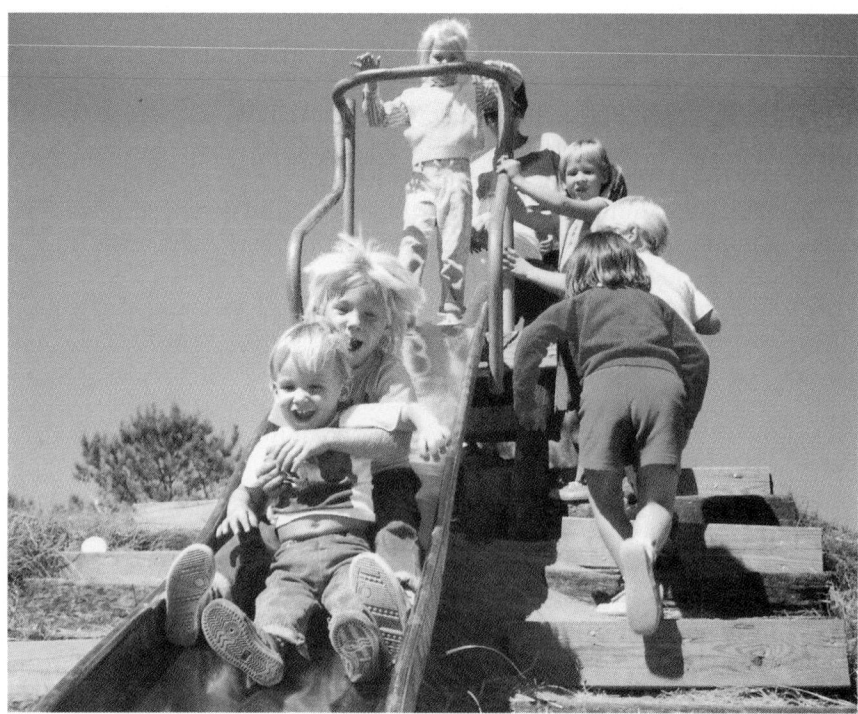

Vitamin D activity was previously expressed in international units (IU), but as of 1980, it is expressed in micrograms of cholecalciferol. To convert, use the following factor:

   100 IU = 2.5 μg.
   400 IU = 10 μg.

to 15 minutes, a few times a week, should be sufficient for maintaining vitamin D nutrition.[11] Dark-skinned people require longer sunlight exposure than light-skinned people do to maximize vitamin D synthesis. By three hours of exposure, however, vitamin D synthesis in heavily pigmented skin arrives at the same plateau as that at 30 minutes in fair skin.

The ultraviolet rays of the sun that promote vitamin D synthesis may be filtered out by heavy clouds, smoke, or smog. These differences (skin pigmentation and smog) probably account for the fact that dark-skinned people in northern, smoggy cities are prone to rickets. For these people, and for those who are unable to go outdoors frequently, dietary vitamin D is important.

Rapidly growing children require daily intakes of close to 10 micrograms of vitamin D; mature adults need half as much. Only a few animal foods supply significant amounts of the vitamin, notably eggs, liver, and some fish. Even in these foods, the vitamin D content varies greatly, depending on the animal's exposure to sun and on its consumption of the vitamin in its foods. Neither cow's milk nor human breast milk supplies enough vitamin D to meet human needs reliably; hence cow's milk is fortified. Infant formulas are fortified with vitamin D in amounts adequate for daily intake. Breast milk is notoriously low in vitamin D, so vitamin D supplements are routinely prescribed for breastfed infants in the United States and Canada. These sources, plus any exposure to the sun, provide babies with more than enough of this vitamin. Well-meaning parents who give their infants extra vitamin drops are risking vitamin D toxicity symptoms, including increased calcium withdrawal from the bones, an effect just the opposite of the desired outcome of strong bones. The fortification of milk with vitamin D is the best guarantee that children will meet their vitamin D needs and underscores the importance of milk in children's diets.

Most adults, especially in sunny regions, need not make special efforts to obtain vitamin D in food. People who are not outdoors much or who live in northern or predominantly cloudy or smoggy areas, however, are advised to make sure their milk is fortified with vitamin D, to drink at least 2 cups a day, and to make frequent use of eggs and periodic use of liver in menu planning.

Smog filters out ultraviolet rays of the sun.

Vitamin E

Vitamin E is one of the body's primary defenders against oxidation. Vitamin E is a fat-soluble antioxidant; it protects other substances from oxidation by being oxidized itself. If there is plenty of vitamin E in the membranes of cells exposed to an oxidant, chances are this vitamin will take the brunt of any oxidative attack, protecting the lipids and other vulnerable components of the membranes. Vitamin E is especially effective in preventing the oxidation of the polyunsaturated fatty acids (PUFA), but it protects all other lipids (for example, vitamin A) as well. Table 7–2 summarizes important information about vitamin E.

oxidation: a type of chemical reaction so named because oxygen is one of the agents that often brings it about.

antioxidant: a compound that protects other compounds from oxidation by being oxidized itself.

oxidant: a compound (such as oxygen itself) that oxidizes other compounds.

Vitamin E exerts an especially important antioxidant effect in the lungs, where the cells are exposed to high concentrations of oxygen. Vitamin E also protects the lungs from air pollutants that are strong oxidants.

When vitamin E intake is deficient and the blood concentration falls below a certain critical level, the red blood cells tend to break open and spill their contents, probably because of oxidation of the PUFA in their membranes. The role of vitamin E in protecting red blood cell membranes has led researchers to ask whether the vitamin might protect white blood cells as well and perhaps participate in the body's immune defenses. Indeed, vitamin E supplements significantly enhance the immune response of the elderly.[12]

The breaking open of red blood cells is **erythrocyte** (eh-REETH-ro-cite) **hemolysis** (he-MOLL-uh-sis), the vitamin E–deficiency disease in human beings.

erythrocyte: red blood cell.
  erythro = red
  cyte = cell

hemolysis: bursting of red blood cells.
  hemo = blood
  lysis = breaking

Abnormal environmental conditions such as air pollution can increase people's vitamin E needs, and so can some diseases, especially those that impair fat absorption. The following individuals can benefit from vitamin E supplementation:

- Premature infants, because the transfer of vitamin E across the placenta becomes maximal only right before full-term delivery.
- Infants, children, or adults who can't absorb fats and oils because of liver, pancreas, or gallbladder disease, GI surgery; or inherited diseases.
- Individuals with certain blood disorders, including sickle-cell anemia, beta thalassemia, and a red blood cell enzyme deficiency (glucose-6-phosphate dehydrogenase deficiency).

Two other conditions seen in human beings appear to respond to vitamin E therapy. One is a nonmalignant breast disease, and the other is an abnormality of blood flow that causes cramping in the legs.

Although researchers have revealed possible roles for vitamin E, they have also shown clearly that some extravagant claims made for vitamin E are unfounded. Vitamin E does not improve athletic endurance or skill, increase

Both diseases have unwieldy names. One is **fibrocystic breast disease;** the other is **intermittent claudication.**
  fibr = fibrous lumps
  cystic = in sacs
  intermittent = at intervals
  claudicare = to limp

Caution: Other serious conditions can cause lumps in the breast and pain in the legs. Don't self-diagnose; see a physician.

muscular dystrophy (DIS-tro-fee): a hereditary disease in which the muscles gradually weaken; its most debilitating effects arise in the lungs. This disease should not be confused with *nutritional* muscular dystrophy, a vitamin E–deficiency disease of animals characterized by gradual paralysis of the muscles.

On vitamin bottles, vitamin E activity is often expressed as IU. One IU is the same as 1 mg of the active form of vitamin E.

sexual potency, enhance sexual performance, prolong the life of the heart, or reverse the damage caused by atherosclerosis and heart attacks. Vitamin E also does not prevent or cure hereditary muscular dystrophy, nor does it slow or prevent processes of aging, such as graying of the hair, wrinkling of the skin, or reduced activity of body organs. An immense amount of experimentation has discredited these and many other similar claims.

Despite the fact that many vitamin E claims have been discredited, people continue to take vitamin E supplements for a variety of reasons. As a result, signs of toxicity are now known or suspected, although toxicity is not nearly as common, and its effects are not as serious, as with vitamins A and D. According to the American Medical Association's Council on Scientific Affairs, the most significant toxic effects of vitamin E at doses ten times the RDA are interference with the blood-clotting action of vitamin K and enhancement of the action of anticoagulant drugs, leading to hemorrhage.[13] In some people, megadoses of vitamin E may reduce serum concentrations of thyroid hormone, resulting in muscle weakness and fatigue. In short, vitamin E supplements beyond the RDA carry some risks and offer no benefits.

Vitamin E is widespread in foods. About 20 percent of the vitamin E in the diet comes directly or indirectly from vegetable oils and the products made from them, such as margarine, salad dressings, and shortenings. Another 20 percent comes from fruits and vegetables. Fortified cereals and other grain products contribute about 15 percent of the vitamin E in the diet, and smaller percentages come from meats, poultry, fish, eggs, nuts, and seeds.[14] Soybean oil and wheat germ oil have especially high concentrations of vitamin E. Cottonseed, corn, and safflower oils rank second, with a tablespoon of any of these supplying more than 10 milligrams (more than the RDA) of the vitamin. Other oils contain less; for example, peanut oil supplies about half as much per tablespoon. Animal fats, such as butter and milk fat, have negligible amounts of vitamin E. Vitamin E is readily destroyed by heat processing and oxidation, so fresh or lightly processed foods are the most desirable sources of this vitamin.

People's needs for vitamin E are higher if the amounts of PUFA they consume are higher. Fortunately, vitamin E and PUFA tend to occur together in the same foods.

People take vitamin supplements for many reasons. Many people rationalize that even if vitamin E supplements do not do all that supplement advocates claim they will, megadoses won't do any harm. This is false. You now know that excessive amounts of vitamin E may interfere with the action of vitamin K in blood clotting and may reduce thyroid hormone concentrations, bringing on fatigue and muscle weakness.

Vitamin K

Vitamin K acts primarily in blood clotting, where its presence can make the difference between life and death. At least 13 different proteins and the mineral calcium are involved in making a blood clot. Vitamin K is essential

K stands for the Danish word *koagulation* ("coagulation" or "clotting").

for the synthesis of at least four of these proteins, among them prothrombin, the precursor of the protein thrombin. Long known for its role in blood clotting, vitamin K is now known to participate with vitamin D in synthesizing a bone protein.[15] Without vitamin K, the bones produce an abnormal protein that cannot bind to the mineral crystal deposits that normally accumulate in bone. Table 7–2 provides additional information about vitamin K.

When any of the blood-clotting factors is lacking, hemorrhagic disease results. If an artery or vein is cut or broken, bleeding goes unchecked. Of course, this is not to say that the cause of hemorrhaging is always a vitamin K deficiency.

Like vitamin D, vitamin K can be obtained from a nonfood source. Bacteria in your intestinal tract can synthesize vitamin K that you can absorb, although you cannot depend on bacterial synthesis alone for your vitamin K.

Vitamin K deficiency is seldom seen except when unusual combinations of circumstances conspire to bring it about. When it does occur, however, it can be fatal. The scenario goes like this: a hospital client with marginal vitamin K stores is given antibiotics to prevent or overcome infection, and is fed a formula diet that does not include vitamin K. The antibiotics kill intestinal bacteria, and vitamin K stores are depleted. During surgery, the blood fails to clot normally, and the client bleeds to death. The combination of antibiotics, inadequate vitamin K intake, and surgery raises a warning flag and requires that clotting time be checked before surgery is performed.[16]

New babies are commonly susceptible to vitamin K deficiency, for two reasons. First, a baby is born with a sterile digestive tract. Second, a baby may not be fed a good source of vitamin K at the outset. Breast milk is a poorer source of vitamin K than cow's milk. A dose of vitamin K, usually in a water-soluble form, may therefore be given at birth to prevent hemorrhagic disease in the newborn. It must be administered carefully to avoid toxic overdosing. People taking sulfa drugs, which destroy intestinal bacteria, may also become deficient in vitamin K.

On the other hand, a high intake of vitamin K can reduce the effectiveness of drugs used to prevent the blood from clotting. People taking anticoagulants should use moderation in eating foods high in vitamin K. Vitamin K-toxicity symptoms include red cell hemolysis, jaundice, and brain damage (see Table 7–2).

Many foods contain ample amounts of the vitamin, notably green leafy vegetables, members of the cabbage family, and liver. Milk, meats, eggs, cereal, fruits, and vegetables provide smaller, but still significant, amounts.

hemorrhagic (hem-o-RAJ-ik) **disease:** the vitamin K–deficiency disease in which blood fails to clot.

Vitamin K can be made within your GI tract, but not by you.

The bacterial inhabitants of the digestive tract are known as the **intestinal flora.**
  flora = plant inhabitants

sterile: free of microorganisms, such as bacteria.

The synthetic substitute usually given for vitamin K is **menadione** (men-uh-DYE-own).

jaundice: yellowing of the skin due to spillover of bile pigments from the liver into the general circulation.

The Water-Soluble Vitamins

The B vitamins and vitamin C are the water-soluble vitamins. These vitamins are found in the watery compartment of foods, and they are distributed into water-filled compartments of the body. They are easily absorbed into the bloodstream and are just as easily excreted if their blood concentration rises too high. Thus, compared with the fat-soluble vitamins, the water-soluble vitamins are less likely to reach toxic concentrations. Nevertheless, most of the water-soluble vitamins can be toxic when taken in large doses.[17]

TABLE 7–2   **The Fat-Soluble Vitamins—A Summary**

VITAMIN NAMES AND RDA FOR HEALTHY ADULTS[a]	CHIEF FUNCTIONS IN THE BODY	DEFICIENCY DISEASE NAME	DEFICIENCY SYMPTOMS	TOXICITY SYMPTOMS	SIGNIFICANT SOURCES
Vitamin A (retinol, retinal, retinoic acid); precursor is provitamin A carotenoids such as beta-carotene RDA: Females: 800 RE Males: 1,000 RE	Vision; maintenance of cornea, epithelial cells, mucous membranes, skin; bone and tooth growth; reproduction; hormone synthesis and regulation; immunity; cancer protection	Hypovitaminosis A	*Bones/Teeth* Cessation of bone growth, painful joints; impaired enamel formation, cracks in teeth, tendency to decay	Bone pain; growth retardation; increase of pressure inside skull, mimicking brain tumor	Retinol: fortified milk, cheese, cream, butter, fortified margarine, eggs, liver Beta-carotene: spinach and other dark, leafy greens; broccoli; deep orange fruits (apricots, cantaloupe) and vegetables (winter squash, carrots, sweet potatoes, pumpkin)
			Blood/Circulatory System Anemia (small-cell type)[b]	Red blood cell breakage, nosebleeds	
			Digestive System Diarrhea, general discomfort	Abdominal cramps and pain, nausea, vomiting, diarrhea, weight loss	
			Immune System Depression of immune reactions; frequent respiratory, digestive, bladder, vaginal, and other infections	Overreactivity	
			Nervous/Muscular Systems Night blindness (retinal)	Blurred vision, pain in calves, fatigue, irritability, loss of appetite	
			Skin and Cornea Keratinization, corneal degeneration leading to blindness,[c] rashes	Dry skin, rashes, loss of hair	
			Other Kidney stones, impaired growth	Cessation of menstruation, liver and spleen enlargement	

[a]The RDA used in this table are for adults from 25 to 50 years old. For other age groups, see the inside front cover.
[b]Small-cell anemia is termed *microcytic anemia*; large-cell type is *macrocytic* or *megaloblastic anemia.*
[c]Corneal degeneration progresses from *keratinization* (hardening) to *xerosis* (drying) to *xerophthalomia* (thickening, opacity, and irreversible blindness).

TABLE 7–2 (*continued*)

VITAMIN NAMES AND RDA FOR HEALTHY ADULTS	CHIEF FUNCTIONS IN THE BODY	DEFICIENCY DISEASE NAME	DEFICIENCY SYMPTOMS		TOXICITY SYMPTOMS	SIGNIFICANT SOURCES
Vitamin D (calciferol, cholecalciferol, dihydroxy-vitamin D); precursor is the body's own cholesterol RDA: 5 μg	Mineralization of bones (raises calcium and phosphorus blood levels by increasing absorption from digestive tract, withdrawing calcium and phosphorus from bones, stimulating retention by kidneys)	Rickets, osteomalacia	*Bones/Teeth* Abnormal growth, misshapen bones (bowing of legs), joint pain; teeth not well formed			Self-synthesis with sunlight; fortified milk, fortified margarine, eggs, liver, small fish (sardines)
			Blood/Circulatory System		Raised blood calcium and phosphorus	
			Digestive System		Constipation, weight loss	
			Nervous System	Muscle spasms	Excessive thirst, headaches, irritability, loss of appetite, weakness, nausea	
			Other		Kidney stones, stones in arteries, mental and physical retardation	
Vitamin E (alpha-tocopherol, tocopherol) RDA: Females: 8 mg Males: 10 mg	Antioxidant (detoxification of strong oxidants), stabilization of cell membranes, regulation of oxidation reactions, protection of PUFA and vitamin A	(No name)	*Blood/Circulatory System* Red blood cell breakage, anemia		Augmented effects of anticlotting medication	Polyunsaturated plant oils (margarine, salad dressings, shortenings), green and leafy vegetables, wheat germ, whole-grain products, nuts, seeds
			Digestive System		General discomfort	
			Nervous/Muscular Systems Degeneration, weakness, difficulty walking, leg cramps			
			Other Fibrocystic breast disease			
Vitamin K (phylloquinone, naphthoquinone) RDA: Females: 65 μg Males: 80 μg	Synthesis of blood-clotting proteins and a blood protein that regulates blood calcium	(No name)	*Blood/Circulatory System* Hemorrhaging		Interference with anticlotting medication, jaundice caused by vitamin K analogues, brain damage	Bacterial synthesis in the digestive tract; liver, green leafy vegetables, cabbage-type vegetables, milk

The B Vitamins

Despite advertisements that claim otherwise, the B vitamins do not give you energy. Carbohydrate, fat, and protein—the *energy-yielding* nutrients—are used for fuel. The B vitamins help to burn that fuel, but do not serve as fuel themselves.

The eight B vitamins are thiamin, riboflavin, niacin, vitamin B_6, folate, vitamin B_{12}, pantothenic acid, and biotin. Table 7–3 lists other names used for these vitamins.

Each of the eight B vitamins is a part of an enzyme helper known as a coenzyme. Each B vitamin has other important functions in the body as well, but the roles these vitamins play as parts of coenzymes are the best understood. A coenzyme is a small molecule that combines with an enzyme to make it active. With the coenzyme in place, the substance to be worked on is attracted to the enzyme, and the reaction proceeds instantaneously. Figure 7–3 illustrates coenzyme action.

Thiamin, niacin, riboflavin, and pantothenic acid are each a part of distinct coenzymes necessary for the production of energy from glucose, amino acids, and fats. A coenzyme containing vitamin B_6 is necessary for synthesizing nonessential amino acids. The making of new cells depends on a folate coenzyme, and the making of this coenzyme depends on vitamin B_{12}. Folate and vitamin B_{12} together are involved in duplicating genetic material when cells divide. (They serve other functions as well.) Biotin serves as a coenzyme in fatty acid synthesis and in energy metabolism.

These eight B vitamins play many specific roles in helping the enzymes to perform thousands of different molecular conversions in your body. They

coenzyme (co-EN-zime): a small molecule that works with an enzyme to promote the enzyme's activity. Many coenzymes have B vitamins as part of their structure.

   co = with

TABLE 7–3   **B Vitamin Terminology**

Many of the vitamins have both names and numbers, a mixture of terminologies that confuses newcomers to the study of nutrition. A single set of names for the vitamins has been agreed on and published, and those names are used in this book.[a] Still, to read the many worthwhile writings published prior to this nomenclature policy, you have to be aware of the alternative names.

STANDARD VITAMIN NAME	OTHER NAMES COMMONLY USED
Thiamin	Vitamin B_1
Riboflavin	Vitamin B_2
Niacin	Nicotinic acid, nicotinamide, niacinamide, vitamin B_3
Vitamin B_6	Pyridoxine, pyridoxal, pyridoxamine
Folate	Folacin, folic acid, pteroylglutamic acid
Vitamin B_{12}	Cobalamin
Pantothenic acid	(None)
Biotin	(None)

[a]The vitamin names used here are those agreed on, and published by, the International Union of Nutritional Sciences Committee on Nomenclature, in Nomenclature policy: Generic descriptors and trivial names for vitamins and related compounds, *Journal of Nutrition* 117 (1987): 7–15.

must be present in every cell continuously for the cells to function as they should.

B Vitamin Deficiency

Although we know a great deal about their individual molecular functions, we are unable to say precisely why a deficiency of one B vitamin produces one disease, whereas the deficiency of another produces a different disease. We do know, however, that with the deficiency of any B vitamin, many body systems become deranged, and similar symptoms may appear.

A deficiency of a B vitamin seldom shows up in isolation. After all, people do not eat nutrients one by one; they eat foods containing mixtures of nutrients. If a major class of foods is missing from the diet, the nutrients contributed by that class of foods will all be lacking to various extents. In only two cases have dietary deficiencies associated with single B vitamins been observed on a large scale in human populations. Diseases have been named for these deficiency states. One of them, beriberi, was first observed in the Far East when the custom of polishing rice became widespread. Rice contributed 80 percent of the energy intake of the people in those areas, and rice hulls were their principal source of thiamin. When the hulls were removed to make the rice whiter, beriberi spread like wildfire.

The niacin-deficiency disease, pellagra, became widespread in the southern United States in the early part of this century among people who subsisted on a low-protein diet with a staple grain of corn. This diet was unusual in that it supplied neither enough niacin nor enough of its amino acid precursor tryptophan to make the niacin intake adequate.

Even in cases of beriberi and pellagra, the deficiencies were not pure. When foods were provided containing the one vitamin known to be needed, the other vitamins that may have been in short supply came as part of the package.

Table 7–4, at the end of this chapter, sums up a few of the better established facts about B vitamin deficiencies. A look at the table will make another generalization possible. Different body systems depend to different extents on these vitamins. Processes in nerves and in their responding tissues, the muscles, depend heavily on glucose metabolism and hence on thiamin. Thus paralysis sets in when this vitamin is lacking. Because the replacement of red blood cells and GI tract cells occurs at a rapid pace, two of the first symptoms of a deficiency of folate are a type of anemia and GI deterioration. Again, each nutrient is important in all systems, and the list of symptoms in Table 7–4 is far from complete.

Major deficiency diseases such as pellagra and beriberi no longer occur in the United States and Canada, but lesser deficiencies of nutrients, including the B vitamins, sometimes are observed. When they do occur, it is usually in people whose food choices are poor because of poverty, ignorance, illness, or poor health habits such as alcohol abuse. If the staple grain food is refined, vitamin B deficiencies are especially likely.

One way to protect people from deficiencies is to add nutrients to their staple food, a process known as fortification or enrichment. The enrichment of refined breads and cereals has drastically reduced the incidence of iron and B vitamin deficiencies.

beriberi: the thiamin-deficiency disease; it pointed the way to the first discovery of a B vitamin, thiamin.

pellagra (pell-AY-gra): the niacin-deficiency disease.
  pellis = skin
  agra = seizure

FIGURE 7–3   **Coenzyme Action**

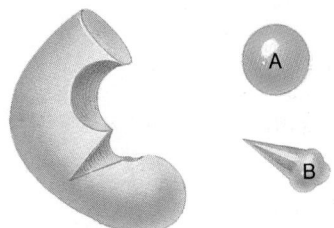

Without the coenzyme, compounds A and B don't respond to the enzyme.

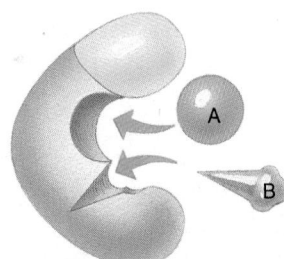

With the coenzyme in place, A and B are attracted to the active site on the enzyme, and they react.

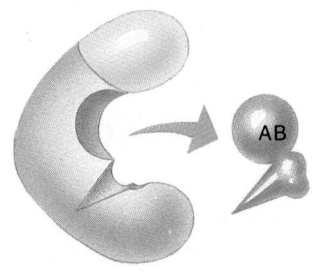

The reaction is completed.

fortification: the addition of nutrients to a food to correct or prevent a widespread nutrient deficiency, to balance the total nutrient profile of a food, or to restore nutrients lost in processing. Often, the added nutrients were not originally present and have been added in amounts greater than might be found there naturally.

enrichment: now considered synonymous with fortification; previously, the addition of four specific nutrients—iron, thiamin, riboflavin, and niacin—to refined breads and cereals in amounts approximately equivalent to those originally present in the whole grain.

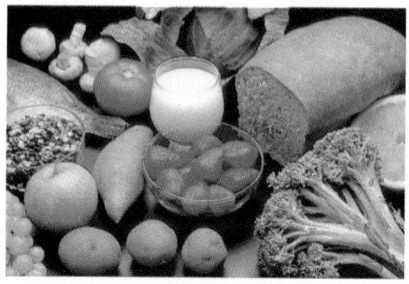

Thiamin: most nutritious foods contribute about 10% of daily needs per serving.

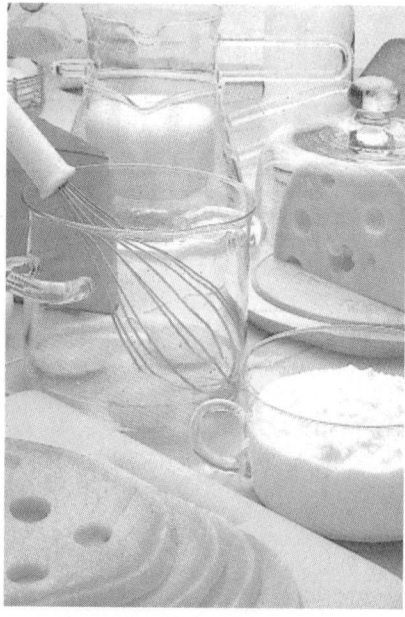

Milk and milk products supply much of the riboflavin in people's diets.

The preceding discussion has shown both the great importance of the B vitamins in promoting normal, healthy functioning of all body systems and the severe consequences of deficiency. Now you may want to know how to be sure you are getting enough of these vital nutrients.

Before reading further, keep in mind that foods can provide all the nutrients you need; supplements are a poor second choice. Some supplements are inexpensive, and others are absurdly costly; but either way, most people don't need them. Overdosing with water-soluble vitamins has no benefit other than to increase the dollar value of your urine. Besides, overdoses are dangerous. Nutrition in Practice 7 discusses uses and choices of supplements in more detail.

Thiamin

Thiamin facilitates energy production; therefore, more is needed when energy expenditure is high. Provided that you are consuming enough food energy to meet your needs—and obtaining that energy from thiamin-containing foods—your thiamin intake will adjust to your need. However, people who derive a large proportion of their energy from empty-kcalorie items, like sugar or alcohol, risk thiamin deficiency. For the most part, thiamin deficiency had virtually disappeared in the United States until recently. It seems to be reappearing as the population of malnourished and homeless people rises.[18] A person who is fasting or who has adopted a very-low-kcalorie diet still needs to obtain the same amount of thiamin as when on a diet that meets energy needs, for thiamin needs are proportional to the energy a person expends, not to energy intake.

Thiamin occurs in small quantities in virtually all nutritious foods, but it is concentrated in only a few foods, of which pork and ham are the most commonly eaten. A useful guideline for meeting thiamin needs is to keep empty-kcalorie foods to a minimum in your diet and to include ten or more different servings of nutritious foods each day, assuming that each serving will contribute, on the average, about 10 percent of your needs. Foods chosen from the bread and cereal group should be either whole grain or enriched. Thiamin is not stored in the body to any great extent, so daily intake is important.

Riboflavin

Like thiamin, riboflavin facilitates energy production in the body. Riboflavin recommendations are stated in terms of milligrams per 1,000 kcalories. Differences in the riboflavin RDA for different age-sex groups primarily reflect differences in energy intakes. Infants', children's, and pregnant women's needs rise rapidly during periods of active growth.

Unlike thiamin, riboflavin is not evenly distributed among the food groups. The major contributors of riboflavin to people's diets are milk, milk products, meats, and green vegetables (broccoli, turnip greens, asparagus, and spinach). The riboflavin contribution of milk and milk products is a good reason to include these foods in every day's meals. No other commonly eaten food can make such a substantial contribution. People who omit milk and milk products from their diets can substitute generous servings of dark green, leafy vegetables. Among the meats, liver and heart are the richest sources, but all lean meats, as well as eggs, offer some riboflavin.

Riboflavin is light sensitive; it can be destroyed by the ultraviolet rays of the sun or of fluorescent lamps. For this reason, milk is seldom sold in transparent glass or translucent plastic containers. Cardboard or opaque plastic containers protect the riboflavin in the milk from light. In contrast, riboflavin is heat stable, so ordinary cooking does not destroy it.

Riboflavin: milk contributes about 50%; meat, about 25%; whole-grain or enriched breads and cereals, additional amounts. The person who does not drink milk should substitute large amounts of dark green vegetables.

Niacin

Niacin is unique among the B vitamins because the body can make it from protein. The amino acid tryptophan can be converted to niacin in the body: 60 milligrams of tryptophan yields 1 milligram of niacin. Recommended niacin intakes are stated in "equivalents," reflecting the body's ability to convert tryptophan to niacin.

Meat, poultry, and fish contribute about half the niacin equivalents most people consume; enriched breads and cereals contribute about a fourth. Vegetarians are advised to emphasize nuts and legumes in their diets, as these are good sources of niacin and protein. Among the vegetables, mushrooms, asparagus, and green leafy vegetables are the richest niacin sources.

niacin equivalents: the amount of niacin present in food, including the niacin that can theoretically be made from its precursor tryptophan present in the food.

A food containing 1 mg niacin and 60 mg tryptophan contains the equivalent of 2 mg niacin, or 2 mg equivalents.

Vitamin B$_6$

Vitamin B$_6$ has been called the "sleeping giant" of vitamins.[19] A surge of research interest in the last decade has revealed not only new roles for the vitamin, but many new questions about it as well. For example, unlike other water-soluble vitamins, researchers now know that vitamin B$_6$ is stored extensively in muscle tissue.[20] Tentative research findings suggest that this vitamin B$_6$ reservoir becomes available to the rest of the body under conditions of intensified energy use, such as physical activity.

Vitamin B$_6$ has long been known to play roles in protein and amino acid metabolism. Research suggests new roles for vitamin B$_6$ in immune function, hormone response, and possibly in the origins and treatments of some diseases.[21]

Vitamin B$_6$'s many roles in amino acid metabolism are reflected in dietary needs that are roughly proportional to protein intakes. The RDA for vitamin B$_6$ is more than adequate to handle average protein intakes of 100 grams per day for men and 60 grams per day for women.[22]

Data on the amounts of vitamin B$_6$ in foods are not extensive enough to permit including the vitamin in the table of food composition in Appendix C. Averaged amounts of vitamin B$_6$, derived from the available data, reveal that the richest food sources are liver, fish, poultry, potatoes, a few other vegetables, fruits, and whole-grain cereals.

For years it was believed that vitamin B$_6$, like other water-soluble vitamins, could not reach toxic concentrations in the body. Toxic effects of vitamin B$_6$ became known when a physician reported them in seven different women who had been taking more than 2 grams of vitamin B$_6$ daily for two months or more. Most of these women had been attempting to cure symptoms of premenstrual syndrome (PMS), the cluster of physical, emotional, and psychological symptoms that some women experience prior to menstruation. The first symptom of toxicity was numb feet; then the women lost sensation in their hands; then they became unable to walk. Since then other researchers have reported neurological symptoms in more than 100 women who took supplements for as long as five years.[23] The women recovered after they discontinued the supplements.

The specific cause or causes of PMS remain undefined, although researchers agree that the hormonal changes of the menstrual cycle must be responsible. Despite a lack of conclusive evidence that vitamin B_6 is an effective treatment for PMS, the vitamin and many other unproven remedies remain popular among PMS sufferers. Nutrition in Practice 8 offers a discussion of nutrition and PMS.

When a normal dose of a nutrient clears up a deficiency condition, the effect is a physiological one. When a megadose (100 times larger) overwhelms some system and acts like a drug, the effect is a pharmacological one.

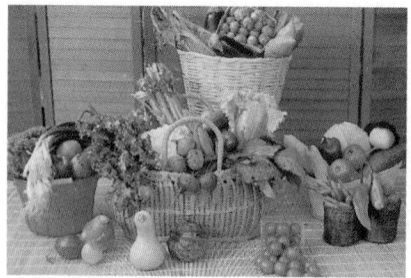

Green leafy vegetables such as broccoli and leafy lettuce are folate-rich.

Folate

The B vitamin folate is active in cell division. When a deficiency occurs, the rapidly dividing cells of the blood and the GI tract stop dividing and begin to deteriorate (see Table 7–4). During periods of rapid growth and cell division, such as pregnancy and adolescence, folate needs increase, and deficiency is especially likely.

Alcohol-addicted people are at risk of folate deficiency, because alcohol impairs folate's absorption and increases its excretion.[24] Furthermore, as people's alcohol intakes rise, their folate intakes decline.[25] Many medications, including aspirin, oral contraceptives, and anticonvulsants, impair folate status; and smoking, too, exerts a negative effect on folate status.

The best food sources of the vitamin are liver; legumes; seeds; green leafy vegetables (the name of the vitamin is related to the word *foliage*); beets; and members of the cabbage family, such as cauliflower, broccoli, and Brussels sprouts. Among the fruits, oranges, orange juice, and cantaloupe are the best sources; among the starchy vegetables, corn, lima beans, parsnips, green peas, pumpkin, and sweet potatoes are good sources.

Vitamin B_{12}

Vitamin B_{12} and folate share a special relationship: vitamin B_{12} assists folate in its cell division work. Their roles intertwine, but each performs a specific task that the other cannot perform. Vitamin B_{12} (in coenzyme form) stands by to accept carbon groups from folate as folate removes them from other compounds. The passing of these carbon groups from folate to vitamin B_{12} regenerates the active form of folate so it can continue its dismantling tasks. In the absence of vitamin B_{12}, folate is trapped in its inactive, metabolically useless form, unable to do its job. When folate is either trapped due to vitamin B_{12} deficiency or unavailable due to a deficiency of folate itself, cells that are growing most rapidly are the first to be affected. Thus a deficiency of either nutrient—vitamin B_{12} or folate—impairs maturation of the rapidly growing blood cells first and produces an anemia characterized by large, immature red blood cells.

Either vitamin B_{12} or folate will clear up the anemia, but if folate is given when vitamin B_{12} is needed, the result is disastrous, because vitamin B_{12} also functions in maintaining nerve fibers. Devastating neurological symptoms, undetectable by a blood test, can ultimately result from an undetected vitamin B_{12} deficiency. A deceptive folate "cure" of the blood symptoms in vitamin B_{12} deficiency allows the nerve symptoms to progress, leading to paralysis and permanent nerve damage.

The way folate masks vitamin B_{12} deficiency underlines a point already made several times: it takes a skilled diagnostician to make a correct diagnosis. The risk you take when you diagnose yourself on the basis of a single observed symptom is clearly intolerable.

Vitamin B_{12} is unique among the nutrients in that it is found almost exclusively in animal-derived foods. People who eat meat are guaranteed an adequate intake, and lacto-ovo vegetarians (who use milk, cheese, and eggs) are also protected from deficiency. It is a myth that fermented soy products such as miso (a soybean paste), or sea algae such as spirulina, provide vitamin B_{12} in its active form. Extensive research shows that the amounts of vitamin B_{12} listed on the labels of these plant products are inaccurate and misleading, because the vitamin B_{12} in these products occurs in an inactive, unavailable form.[26] Strict vegetarians must take vitamin B_{12} supplements or find other sources of the active vitamin B_{12}.

Another unique characteristic of vitamin B_{12} is that it requires an "intrinsic factor"—a compound inside the body—for absorption from the intestinal tract into the bloodstream. The intrinsic factor is made in the stomach, where it attaches to the vitamin; the complex then passes to the small intestine and is gradually absorbed.

In some cases, intrinsic factor production becomes inadequate or ceases altogether—for example, after surgical removal of the stomach. Because vitamin B_{12} deficiency in the body may be caused either by a lack of the vitamin in the diet or by the body's inability to absorb the vitamin, a change in diet alone may not correct it. When an absorption failure is the problem, vitamin B_{12} must be supplied by injection to prevent vitamin B_{12}–deficiency symptoms from developing. The vitamin B_{12} deficiency caused by lack of intrinsic factor is known as pernicious anemia.

Strict vegetarians are at special risk for undetected vitamin B_{12} deficiency for two reasons: first, because they receive none in their diets, and second, because they consume large amounts of folate in the vegetables they eat. Because the amount of vitamin B_{12} that can be stored in the body is 1,000 times the amount used each day, it may take years for a deficiency to develop in a new vegetarian. When it does, though, it may progress to a dangerous extreme, because the deficiency of vitamin B_{12} may be masked by the high folate intake.

Pantothenic Acid and Biotin

The six best-known B vitamins have already been discussed. Two others—pantothenic acid and biotin—are needed for the synthesis of coenzymes that are active in a multitude of body systems. Although they are just as important as the vitamins discussed so far, both pantothenic acid and biotin are widespread in foods. There seems to be no danger that people who consume a variety of foods will suffer deficiencies. Claims that pantothenic acid and biotin are needed in pill form to prevent or cure disease conditions are at best unfounded and at worst intentionally misleading.

Biotin deficiencies have been reported in human adults fed artificially by vein. Even then, however, deficiencies are unlikely, because intestinal bacteria may be able to synthesize enough biotin to meet the host's needs.

Vitamin B_{12} is found exclusively in animal-derived foods.

intrinsic: inside the system. The intrinsic factor necessary to prevent pernicious anemia is now known to be made in the stomach and to aid in the absorption of vitamin B_{12}. The extrinsic factor necessary to prevent pernicious anemia is vitamin B_{12} itself, which must be obtained outside the system from food.

Biotin deficiency becomes likely only when a person is receiving both intravenous feedings and antibiotics.

Non-B Vitamins

A trio of compounds sometimes inappropriately called B vitamins are inositol, choline, and lipoic acid. These are not essential nutrients for human beings. Like the true B vitamins, they serve as coenzymes in metabolism. Even if they were essential, supplements would be unnecessary, because they are abundant in foods.

Numerous false claims have been made about choline and its relative, lecithin (which contains choline as part of its structure). Consequently, many people rush to buy and consume bottles of them.

Physicians have witnessed and reported on the effects of overdoses of these compounds. Overdoses can cause not only short-term discomforts, such as GI distress, sweating, salivation, and anorexia, but also long-term health hazards from the disturbance of the nervous and cardiovascular systems.

Other substances have also been mistaken for essential nutrients. They include para-aminobenzoic acid (PABA), bioflavonoids (vitamin P or hesperidin), and ubiquinone. Other names you may hear are "vitamin B_5" (another name for pantothenic acid), "vitamin B_{15}" (a hoax), "vitamin B_{17}" (laetrile, a fake cancer-curing drug and not a vitamin by any stretch of the imagination), "vitamin B_T" (carnitine, an important piece of cell machinery but not a vitamin), and more. There is, however, one other water-soluble vitamin of great interest and importance—vitamin C.

Vitamin C

scurvy: the vitamin C–deficiency disease.

antiscorbutic factor: the original name for vitamin C.
anti = against
scorbutic = causing scurvy

ascorbic acid: one of the two active forms of vitamin C. Many people consistently and incorrectly refer to all vitamin C by this name.
a = without
scorbic = having scurvy

Two hundred years ago, any man who joined the crew of a seagoing ship knew he had only half a chance of returning alive—not because he might be slain by pirates or die in a storm, but because he might contract the dread disease scurvy. In 1747, the first nutrition experiment conducted on human beings was devised to find a cure for scurvy. Dr. James Lind, a British physician, found that sailors with scurvy who received citrus fruits could be cured of the disease within a short time. Eventually all ships were required to carry lime juice for every sailor. (This is why British sailors are still called "limeys" today.) The antiscurvy "something" in citrus fruits and other foods was dubbed the antiscorbutic factor. Nearly 200 years later, the factor was isolated from lemon juice and found to be a compound similar to glucose. It was named ascorbic acid. Shortly thereafter, it was synthesized, and today hundreds of millions of vitamin C pills are produced in pharmaceutical laboratories.

Vitamin C is the subject of much controversy among experts. Questions about how much people need, and what the risks of taking large doses are, continue to be debated. It is difficult to sort out what is known, what is likely to be shown true, and what claims are clearly unfounded. This section deals with the vitamin's known roles and debunks the obvious myths.

Metabolic Roles of Vitamin C

Vitamin C defies a simple, tidy description of its action. It plays many different important roles in the body, and its modes of action differ in different situations (see Table 7–4). The best-understood metabolic role of vitamin C is the vitamin's function in helping to form the protein collagen, the single most important protein of connective tissue. Collagen serves as the matrix on which bone is formed and is an important part of the tissue that holds cells together. When you are wounded, collagen glues the separated tissues together, forming scars. Cells are held together largely by collagen; this is especially important in the artery walls, which must expand and contract with each beat of the heart, and in the walls of the capillaries, which are thin and fragile.

Another major role of vitamin C in the body is as an antioxidant. Recall from the discussion on vitamin E that antioxidants protect the body from damaging oxidizing agents. This protective function of vitamin C is twofold: by being oxidized itself, vitamin C regenerates already-oxidized substances such as iron and copper to their original, active form and, in the process, removes the damaging oxidizing agent.[27] In the intestines, it protects iron from oxidation. In the cells and body fluids, it helps to protect other molecules, including the fat-soluble compounds vitamin A, vitamin E, and the polyunsaturated fatty acids.

Vitamin C is also involved in the metabolism of several amino acids. Some of these amino acids may end up being converted to hormones of great importance in body functioning, among them norepinephrine and thyroxin.

During stress, the adrenal glands release large quantities of vitamin C together with the stress hormones epinephrine and norepinephrine. What the vitamin has to do with the stress reaction is unclear, but it is known that stress increases vitamin C needs somewhat.

Newspaper headlines touting vitamin C as a cure for colds and cancer have appeared frequently over the years. Some research suggests that vitamin C (2 grams per day for two weeks) may reduce the severity and duration of cold and allergy symptoms by reducing blood histamine concentrations.[28] In other words, vitamin C acts as an antihistamine. If further research confirms vitamin C's antihistamine effect, it may permit people to rely less heavily on antihistamine drugs when suffering from cold and allergy symptoms.

The role of vitamin C in the prevention of, or therapy for, cancer is still being studied. Large-scale studies of populations offer strong support for a protective effect of vitamin C for certain types of cancer.[29]

Vitamin C Deficiency

With an inadequate intake, the body's vitamin C pool dwindles in size, and latent scurvy appears. Two of the earliest signs of a vitamin C deficiency relate to its role in maintaining the integrity of blood vessels. The gums begin to bleed easily around the bases of the teeth, and capillaries under the skin break spontaneously, producing pinpoint hemorrhages. If the vitamin C pool continues to shrink, the symptoms of overt scurvy appear. Muscles, including the heart muscle, may degenerate. The skin becomes rough,

collagen: the characteristic protein of connective tissue.
kolla = glue
gennan = to produce

latent: the period in the course of a disease when the conditions are present but the symptoms have not begun to appear.
latens = lying hidden

overt: out in the open, full-blown.
ouvrire = to open

brown, scaly, and dry. Wounds fail to heal because scar tissue will not form. Bone rebuilding falters; the ends of the long bones become softened, malformed, and painful, and fractures appear. The teeth may become loose in the jawbone, and fillings may loosen and fall out. Anemia is frequently seen, the infections are common. Sudden death is likely, perhaps because of massive bleeding into the joints and body cavities.

Once diagnosed, scurvy is readily reversible with doses of vitamin C. Moderate amounts, in the neighborhood of 100 milligrams per day, are all that are needed. The latest food intake information for the United States shows that nearly all people's vitamin C intakes either meet or exceed the RDA.[30]

Recommended Intakes of Vitamin C

The RDA for vitamin C is 60 milligrams for adults, with an extra 10 milligrams recommended for pregnant women and an additional 35 milligrams for lactating women. This amount is midway between two extremes. At one extreme is the requirement, 10 milligrams per day, which is all you need to prevent the symptoms of scurvy from appearing. At the other extreme is the amount at which the body's pool of vitamin C would be full to overflowing: about 100 milligrams per day.

As is true of all nutrients, unusual circumstances may raise vitamin C needs. Among the stresses known to do so are infections; burns; surgery; extremely high or low temperatures; toxic doses of heavy metals, such as lead, mercury, and cadmium; and the chronic use of certain medications, including aspirin, barbiturates, and oral contraceptives. Smoking, too, has adverse effects on vitamin C status.[31] Accordingly, the vitamin C recommendation for people who smoke is 100 milligrams per day.

Vitamin C Toxicity

The easy availability of vitamin C in pill form and the publication of books recommending vitamin C to prevent colds and cancer have led thousands of people to take megadoses of vitamin C. Not surprisingly, instances have surfaced of vitamin C's causing harm.

Some of the suspected toxic effects of vitamin C megadoses have not been confirmed. Among these are formation of stones in the kidneys; upset of the body's acid-base balance; destruction of vitamin B_{12}, resulting in a deficiency; and interference with the action of vitamin E. Research and reasoning have demonstrated that these effects are theoretically possible, but no cases of their actual occurrence in human beings have yet been seen with intakes as high as 3 grams a day.

Other toxic effects, however, have been seen often enough to warrant concern. Nausea, abdominal cramps, and diarrhea are often reported. Several instances of interference with medical regimens are known. The large amounts of vitamin C excreted in the urine obscure the results of tests used to detect diabetes. People taking anticoagulants may unwittingly abolish the effect of these medicines if they also take massive doses of vitamin C. Vitamin C megadoses can enhance iron absorption too much, resulting in iron overload (see Chapter 8).

Remember the distinction between the requirement and the recommended allowance or standard (see p. 8).

Doses of 10 to 30 or more times the recommended intake of a nutrient are termed megadoses. In the case of vitamin C, any amount over 1 g (1,000 mg) is considered a megadose.

When vitamin C is inactivated and degraded, a product along the way is oxalate, which can form stones in the kidneys (see Nutrition in Practice 23). People can also have oxalate crystals in their kidneys that are not due to vitamin C overdoses.

The anticoagulants with which vitamin C interferes are warfarin and dicumarol.

Some black Americans and Africans, Sephardic Jews, Asians, and certain other ethnic groups have an inherited enzyme deficiency that makes them more likely than others to be harmed by vitamin C megadoses. Megadoses of vitamin C can make these people's red blood cells burst, causing hemolytic anemia. Those with sickle-cell anemia may be especially vulnerable to megadoses of vitamin C. And those who have a tendency toward gout, as well as those who have a genetic abnormality that alters the way they metabolize vitamin C, are more prone to forming stones if they take megadoses of vitamin C.

The body of a person who has taken large doses of vitamin C for a long time adjusts by limiting absorption and destroying and excreting more of the vitamin than usual.[32] If the person then suddenly reduces intake to normal, the accelerated disposal system can't put on its brakes fast enough to avoid destroying too much of the vitamin. Some case histories have shown that adults who discontinue megadosing develop scurvy on intakes that would protect a normal adult. An innocent victim of this kind of error is the newborn baby of a megadoser, because the baby has adjusted to high levels of vitamin C in the mother's womb. Once born into an environment providing much smaller amounts, the baby develops scurvy, a withdrawal reaction.

gout (GOWT): a metabolic disease in which crystals of uric acid precipitate in the joints.

The temporary condition manifested by withdrawal symptoms and experienced by the person who stops overdosing is vitamin C dependency. The body has adjusted to a high intake and so "needs" a high intake until it can readjust.

withdrawal reaction: a reaction to the withdrawal of a drug revealing, in most cases, that the user has become dependent.

> The experience of a person who stops megadosing and then manifests vitamin C–deficiency symptoms on a normal intake may lead the person to the wrong conclusion. ''I took 3 grams a day,'' the person may say, ''and then when I stopped, my gums started to bleed, and I knew I was vitamin C deficient. That proves I need very high doses.''
>
> In reality, this person deceived herself. To see whether the recommended, moderate intake of vitamin C is sufficient, she will have to taper off, reducing her large intakes gradually and allowing her body to ease back into its normal state. The emergence of withdrawal symptoms after drug doses of vitamin C does not prove a need, any more than the emergence of withdrawal symptoms in a person giving up heroin or alcohol proves that the person needs heroin or alcohol.

Few instances warrant the taking of more than 100 to 300 milligrams a day. Adults may not be exposing themselves to severe risks if they choose to dose themselves with 1 to 2 grams a day. Those taking more than 2 grams, and especially those taking above 8 grams per day, should be aware of the distinct possibility of harm.

Vitamin C in Foods

The inclusion of intelligently selected fruits and vegetables in the daily diet guarantees a generous intake of vitamin C. Even those who wish to ingest amounts well above the recommended 60 milligrams can easily meet their goals by eating certain foods. Citrus fruits are rightly famous for their

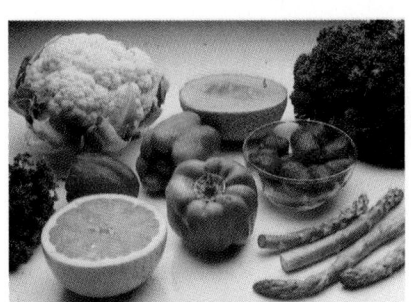

Many fruits and vegetables are vitamin C–rich.

vitamin C contents. Some other fruits and certain vegetables are also rich sources: cantaloupe, strawberries, broccoli, and brussels sprouts. A single serving of any of these provides more than 30 milligrams of the vitamin. No animal foods other than organ meats, such as liver and kidneys, contain vitamin C.

The humble potato is an important source of vitamin C in Western countries, because potatoes are eaten so frequently that they make substantial vitamin C contributions overall. They provide about 20 percent of all the vitamin C in the diet.

Eating foods containing vitamin C at the same meal with foods containing iron can double or triple the absorption of the iron from those foods. This strategy is highly recommended for women and children, whose energy intakes are not large enough to guarantee that they will get enough iron from the foods they eat. Table 7−4 summarizes functions, deficiency and toxicity symptoms, and food sources of the water-soluble vitamins.

By way of conclusion, a summary of the key points about vitamins—both fat soluble and water soluble—seems in order:

- Vitamins are essential, noncaloric, organic nutrients needed in tiny amounts in the diet.
- The only disease a vitamin will cure is the one caused by a deficiency of that vitamin.
- Vitamins yield no energy for the body when broken down, but they facilitate the release of energy from carbohydrate, fat, and protein.
- Vitamins A, D, E, and K are the fat-soluble vitamins. The B vitamins and vitamin C are the water-soluble vitamins.
- Nutritious foods, not supplements, are the best sources of vitamins.

TABLE 7–4   **The Water-Soluble Vitamins—A Summary**

VITAMIN NAMES AND RDA FOR HEALTHY ADULTS[a]	CHIEF FUNCTIONS IN THE BODY	DEFICIENCY DISEASE NAME	DEFICIENCY SYMPTOMS		TOXICITY SYMPTOMS	SIGNIFICANT SOURCES
Thiamin (vitamin B$_1$) RDA: Females: 1.1 mg Males: 1.5 mg	Part of a coenzyme used in energy metabolism; supports normal appetite and nervous system function	Beriberi	*Blood/Circulatory System*			In all nutritious foods in moderate amounts; pork, ham, bacon, liver, whole grains, legumes, nuts
			Edema, enlarged heart, abnormal heart rhythms, heart failure		Rapid pulse	
			Nervous/Muscular Systems			
			Degeneration, wasting, weakness, pain, low morale, difficulty walking, loss of reflexes, mental confusion, paralysis		Weakness, headaches, insomnia, irritability	
Riboflavin (vitamin B$_2$) RDA: Females: 1.3 mg Males: 1.7 mg	Part of a coenzyme used in energy metabolism; supports normal vision and skin health	Ariboflavinosis	*Mouth, Gums, Tongue*			Milk, yogurt, cottage cheese, meat, leafy green vegetables, whole-grain or enriched breads and cereals
			Cracks at corners of mouth,[b] magenta tongue		(No symptoms reported)	
			Nervous System and Eyes			
			Hypersensitivity to light,[c] reddening of cornea			
			Other			
			Skin rash		Interference with anticancer medication	
Niacin (nicotinic acid, nicotinamide, niacinamide, vitamin B$_3$; precursor is dietary tryptophan) RDA: Females: 15 mg Males: 19 mg	Part of a coenzyme used in energy metabolism; supports health of skin, nervous system, and digestive system	Pellagra	*Digestive System*			Milk, eggs, meat, poultry, fish, whole grain and enriched breads and cereals, nuts, and all protein-containing foods
			Diarrhea		Diarrhea, heartburn, nausea, ulcer irritation, vomiting	
			Mouth, Gums, Tongue			
			Black, smooth tongue[d]			*(continued)*

[a]The RDA used in this table are for adults from 25 to 50 years old. For other age groups, see inside front cover.

[b]Cracks at the corners of the mouth are termed *cheilosis* (kee-LOH-sis).

[c]Hypersensitivity to light is *photophobia*.

[d]Smoothness of the tongue is caused by loss of its surface structures and is termed *glossitis* (gloss-EYE-tis).

TABLE 7–4 *(continued)*

VITAMIN NAMES AND RDA FOR HEALTHY ADULTS	CHIEF FUNCTIONS IN THE BODY	DEFICIENCY DISEASE NAME	DEFICIENCY SYMPTOMS	TOXICITY SYMPTOMS	SIGNIFICANT SOURCES
Niacin (continued)			*Nervous System*		
			Irritability, loss of appetite, weakness, dizziness, mental confusion progressing to psychosis or delirium	Fainting, dizziness	
			Skin		
			Flaky skin rash on areas exposed to sun	Painful flush and rash ("niacin rush"), sweating	
			Other		
				Abnormal liver function, low blood pressure	
Vitamin B$_6$ (pyridoxine, pyridoxal, pyridoxamine) RDA: Females: 1.6 mg Males: 2.0 mg	Part of a coenzyme used in amino acid and fatty acid metabolism; helps convert tryptophan to niacin; helps make red blood cells	(No name)	*Blood/Circulatory System*		Green and leafy vegetables, meats, fish, poultry, shellfish, legumes, fruits, whole grains
			Anemia (small-cell type)[e]	Bloating	
			Digestive System		
			Mouth, Gums, Tongue		
			Smooth tongue[d]		
			Nervous/Muscular Systems		
			Abnormal brain wave pattern, irritability, muscle twitching, convulsions	Depression, fatigue, impaired memory, irritability, headaches, numbness, damage to nerves, difficulty walking, loss of reflexes, weakness, restlessness	

[e]Small-cell anemia is termed *microcytic anemia*; large-cell type is *macrocytic* or *megaloblastic anemia*.

TABLE 7-4   (*continued*)

VITAMIN NAMES AND RDA FOR HEALTHY ADULTS	CHIEF FUNCTIONS IN THE BODY	DEFICIENCY DISEASE NAME	DEFICIENCY SYMPTOMS		TOXICITY SYMPTOMS	SIGNIFICANT SOURCES
			Skin			
			Irritation of sweat glands, rashes, greasy dermatitis		"Pins and needles" sensation	
			Other			
			Kidney stones		Bone pain	
Folate (folic acid, folacin, pteroylglutamic acid) RDA: Females: 180 μg Males: 200 μg	Part of a coenzyme used in new cell synthesis	(No name)	*Blood/Circulatory System* Anemia (large-cell type)[e]			Leafy green vegetables, legumes, seeds, liver
			Digestive System Heartburn, diarrhea, constipation		Diarrhea	
			Immune System Depression of immune reactions, frequent infections			
			Mouth, Gums, Tongue Smooth red tongue[d]			
			Nervous System Depression, mental confusion, fainting		Insomnia, irritability	
			Other		Masking of vitamin B_{12}–deficiency symptoms	
Vitamin B_{12} (cyanocobalamin) RDA: Females: 2.0 μg Males: 2.0 μg	Part of a coenzyme used in new cell synthesis; helps maintain nerve cells	(No name)[f]	*Blood/Circulatory System* Anemia (large-cell type)[e]		(No toxicity symptoms known)	Animal products (meat, fish, poultry, shellfish, milk, cheese, eggs)
			Mouth, Gums, Tongue Smooth tongue[d]			

(*continued*)

[f]The name *pernicious anemia* refers to the vitamin$_{12}$ deficiency caused by lack of intrinsic factor, but not to that caused by inadequate dietary intake.

TABLE 7–4   *(continued)*

VITAMIN NAMES AND RDA FOR HEALTHY ADULTS	CHIEF FUNCTIONS IN THE BODY	DEFICIENCY DISEASE NAME	DEFICIENCY SYMPTOMS	TOXICITY SYMPTOMS	SIGNIFICANT SOURCES
Vitamin B_{12} (continued)			*Nervous System* Fatigue, degeneration progressing to paralysis *Skin* Hypersensitivity		
Pantothenic acid	Part of a coenzyme used in energy metabolism	(No name)	*Digestive System* Vomiting, intestinal distress *Nervous System* Insomnia, fatigue *Other*	Occasional diarrhea Water retention (infrequent)	Widespread in foods
Biotin	Part of a coenzyme used in energy metabolism, fat synthesis, amino acid metabolism, and glycogen synthesis	(No name)	*Blood/Circulatory System* Abnormal heart action *Digestive System* Loss of appetite, nausea *Nervous/Muscular Systems* Depression, muscle pain, weakness, fatigue *Skin* Drying, rash, loss of hair	(No toxicity symptoms reported)	Widespread in foods

TABLE 7–4   (continued)

VITAMIN NAMES AND RDA FOR HEALTHY ADULTS	CHIEF FUNCTIONS IN THE BODY	DEFICIENCY DISEASE NAME	DEFICIENCY SYMPTOMS	TOXICITY SYMPTOMS	SIGNIFICANT SOURCES
Vitamin C (ascorbic acid) RDA: Females: 60 mg Males: 60 mg	Collagen synthesis (strengthens blood vessel walls, forms scar tissue, matrix for bone growth); antioxidant; thyroxin synthesis; amino acid metabolism; strengthens resistance to infection; helps in absorption of iron	Scurvy	*Blood/Circulatory System* Anemia (small-cell type),[e] atherosclerotic plaques, pinpoint hemorrhages	Blood cell breakage in certain racial groups[g]	Citrus fruits, cabbage-type vegetables, dark green vegetables, cantaloupe, strawberries, peppers, lettuce, tomatoes, potatoes, papayas, mangoes
			Digestive System	Nausea, abdominal cramps, diarrhea, excessive urination	
			Immune System Depression of immune reactions, frequent infections		
			Mouth, Gums, Tongue Bleeding gums, loosened teeth		
			Muscular/Nervous Systems Muscle degeneration and pain, hysteria, depression	Headache, fatigue, insomnia	
			Skeletal System Bone fragility, joint pain		
			Skin Rough skin, blotchy bruises	Rashes	
			Other Failure of wounds to heal	Interference with medical tests; aggravation of gout symptoms; deficiency symptoms may appear at first on withdrawal of high doses	

[g]Groups susceptible to vitamin C toxicity are Sephardic Jews, Africans, and Asians.

SELF-STUDY

How Are Your Vitamin Intakes?

Compare your intakes of vitamins with the RDA (inside front cover) or the Recommended Nutrient Intakes for Canadians (Appendix A). Express each intake as a percentage of the recommended intake. For example, suppose you ingested 0.9 milligram thiamin, and your RDA is 1.1 milligrams. You ingested (0.9/1.1 × 100), or 82 percent of your RDA. If you had ingested 1.4 milligrams of thiamin, you would have ingested (1.4/1.1 × 100), or 127 percent of your RDA. Use Form 8 to record your findings.

Comment on your intakes. Look closely at any vitamins for which your intakes fell below 80 percent of the recommendations. What are your best food sources of those vitamins? Could you eat more of these foods to bring your intake up to the recommended level? If not, what food or foods could you eat to improve your intake?

Study Questions

1. How do the vitamins differ from the energy nutrients?
2. Describe some general differences between fat-soluble vitamins and water-soluble vitamins.
3. List one major function of vitamins A, D, E, and K.
4. Why is vitamin D unique among the vitamins?
5. What is a coenzyme?
6. Name two B vitamin-deficiency diseases.
7. What do vitamin B_{12} and folate have in common?
8. What is a major function of vitamin C?
9. What are the risks associated with vitamin C megadoses?

FORM 8.   **Vitamin Intakes Compared with Recommended Intakes**

	VITAMIN A	VITAMIN C	THIAMIN	RIBOFLAVIN	NIACIN	FOLACIN
My intake Recommended intake[a] My intake as a percentage of the recommended intake						

[a]RDA or RNI (Appendix A).

Notes

1. K. P. West, G. R. Howard, and A. Sommer, Vitamin A and infection: Public health implications, *Annual Review of Nutrition* 9 (1989): 63–86.

2. Vitamin A administration reduces mortality and morbidity from severe measles in populations nonendemic for hypovitaminosis A, *Nutrition Reviews* 49 (1991): 89–91.

3. J. C. Bauernfeind, Vitamin A deficiency: A staggering problem of health and sight, *Nutrition Today,* March/April 1988, pp. 34–37.

4. T. V. Ringer and coauthors, Beta-carotene's effects on serum lipoproteins and immunologic indices in humans, *American Journal of Clinical Nutrition* 53 (1991): 688–694.

5. R. Weiss, Study sheds light on TB resistance, *Science News,* 133 (1988): p. 60.

6. A. W. Norman, Intestinal calcium absorption: A vitamin D–hormone–mediated adaptive response, *American Journal of Clinical Nutrition* 51 (1990): 290–300.

7. Norman, 1990.

8. H. Reichel, P. Koeffler, and A. W. Norman, The role of the vitamin D endocrine system in health and disease, *New England Journal of Medicine* 320 (1989): 980–991.

9. A. R. Webb and M. F. Holick, The role of sunlight in the cutaneous production of vitamin D_3, *Annual Review of Nutrition* 8 (1988): 375–399.

10. L. Y. Matsuoka and coauthors, Sunscreens suppress cutaneous vitamin D_3 synthesis, *Journal of Clinical Endocrinology and Metabolism* 64 (1987): 1165–1168, as cited in Webb and Holick, 1988.

11. Webb and Holick, 1988.

12. S. N. Meydani and coauthors, Vitamin E supplementation enhances cell-mediated immunity in healthy elderly subjects, *American Journal of Clinical Nutrition* 52 (1990): 557–563.

13. American Medical Association, Council on Scientific Affairs, Vitamin preparations as dietary supplements and therapeutic agents, *Journal of the American Medical Association* 257 (1987): 1929–1936, as cited in C. W. Marshall, Vitamin E supplementation (letter), *American Journal of Clinical Nutrition* 49 (1989): 701–702.

14. S. P. Murphy, A. F. Subar, and G. Block, Vitamin E intakes and sources in the United States, *American Journal of Clinical Nutrition* 52 (1990): 361–367.

15. P. A. Price, Role of vitamin K–dependent proteins in bone metabolism, *Annual Review of Nutrition* 8 (1988): 565–583.

16. Vitamin K deficiency causes coagulopathy (abstract), *Journal of the American Dietetic Association* 88 (1988): 267.

17. C. Henderson, Toxic effects of water-soluble vitamins, *ACSH News and Views* (publication of the American Council on Science and Health), January/February 1987, p. 14.

18. Thiamin deficiency, *Nutrition and the M.D.,* May 1990, p. 3.

19. J. E. Leklem, Vitamin B_6: Of reservoirs, receptors, and requirements, *Nutrition Today,* September/October 1988, pp. 4–10.

20. S. P. Coburn and coauthors, Human vitamin B_6 pools estimated through muscle biopsies, *American Journal of Clinical Nutrition* 48 (1988): 291–294.

21. M. C. Talbott, L. T. Miller, and N. I. Kervliet, Pyridoxine supplementation: Effect on lymphocyte responses in elderly persons, *American Journal of Clinical Nutrition* 46 (1987): 659, as cited in Leklem, 1988; J. E. Leklem and R. D. Reynolds, eds., *Clinical and Physiological Applications of Vitamin B₆* (New York: Alan R. Liss, 1987).

22. National Academy of Sciences, Food and Nutrition Board, *Recommended Dietary Allowances,* 10th ed. (Washington, D.C.: National Academy Press, 1989), pp. 142–149.

23. K. Dalton and M. J. T. Dalton, Characteristics of pyridoxine overdose neuropathy syndrome, *Acta Neurologica Scandinavica* 76 (1987): pp. 8–11, as cited in National Academy of Sciences, 1989.

24. L. B. Bailey, The role of folate in human nutrition, *Nutrition Today,* September/October 1990, pp. 12–19.

25. P. F. Jacques and coauthors, Moderate alcohol intake and nutritional status in nonalcoholic elderly subjects, *American Journal of Clinical Nutrition* 50 (1989): 875–883.

26. V. Herbert, Vitamin B_{12}: Plant sources, requirements, and assay, *American Journal of Clinical Nutrition* 48 (1988): 852–858; P. C. Dagnelie, W. A. van Staveren, and H. van den Berg, Vitamin B_{12} from algae appears not to be bioavailable, *American Journal of Clinical Nutrition* 53 (1991): 695–697.

27. H. Padh, Vitamin C: Newer insights into its biochemical functions, *Nutrition Reviews* 49 (1991): 65–70.

28. Vitamin C suppresses histamine (Newsbreaks), *Nutrition Today,* May/June 1991, p. 4.

29. G. Block, Vitamin C and cancer prevention: The epidemiologic evidence, *American Journal of Clinical Nutrition* 53 (Supplement, 1991): 270–285.

30. H. S. Wright and coauthors, The 1987–88 Nationwide Food Consumption Survey: An update on the nutrient intake of respondents, *Nutrition Today,* May/June 1991, pp. 21–27.

31. G. Schectman, J. C. Byrd, and H. W. Gruchow, The influence of smoking on vitamin C status in adults, *American Journal of Public Health* 79 (1989): 158–162.

32. S. T. Omaye, J. H. Skala, and R. A. Jacob, Rebound effect with ascorbic acid in adult males (letter), *American Journal of Clinical Nutrition* 48 (1988): 379–380.

7

Vitamin Supplements

As many as half of the people in the United States take vitamin supplements, collectively spending billions of dollars on them each year.[1] As scientists discover more and more links between nutrition and disease prevention, the trend toward vitamin supplement use in this country gains momentum. You may use vitamin supplements yourself. Or perhaps, after studying nutrition in health and disease, you are wondering if you should. Nutrition in Practice 7 is intended to provide you with some general information about vitamin and mineral supplements and help you make that decision. The main message, though, is that people can get the nutrients they need from food only.

Can they really?

Emphatically, yes! Foods contain enough vitamins and minerals to supply all that most people need. Healthy adults and children can nourish themselves perfectly adequately by choosing a variety of foods in moderation.[2] The food group plans described in Chapter 1 are the guides to follow to achieve adequate intakes.

Most people do not need to take supplements to meet their nutrient needs. People who meet their nutrient needs from foods, rather than supplements, reduce their risks of toxicity as well as deficiency.

You said most healthy people do not need supplements. Are there some people who do?

Yes, some people may be at risk of marginal nutrient deficiencies due to predisposing conditions such as illness or alcohol or drug addiction, as well as other conditions that inhibit food intake. The American Institute of Nutrition (AIN), the American Society for Clinical Nutrition (ASCN), and the American Dietetic Association (ADA) have issued a statement regarding supplement use. People who may be at risk of marginal deficiencies, and who may therefore benefit from nutrient supplements in amounts consistent with the RDA, include the following:

- People with low energy intakes, such as habitual dieters.
- People with illnesses that take away the appetite.
- People with illnesses that impair nutrient absorption, such as diseases of the liver, gallbladder, pancreas, and digestive system.
- People taking medications that interfere with nutrient metabolism.
- Women who bleed excessively during menstruation (iron supplements).
- Women who are pregnant or lactating (iron, folate, and calcium).
- Strict vegetarians (calcium, iron, zinc, and vitamin B$_{12}$).
- Newborn infants (a single dose of vitamin K at birth under the direction of a physician).

A few other special cases exist:

- People who have infections or injuries, or who have undergone surgery resulting in increased metabolic needs.
- Infants, depending on whether they are receiving breast milk or formula and on whether their water contains fluoride (see Chapter 11). The AIN, ASCN, and ADA caution that nutrients are potentially toxic when taken in large doses and that individual tolerances vary depending on health and age. They urge that whenever a health care professional reviews a person's diet and finds it to be inadequate, the action to take is not to begin supplementation, but to improve the person's food choices and eating patterns.

If only a few situations merit the use of supplements, why do so many people take them?

People frequently take supplements for the wrong reasons, such as "They give me energy" or "They make me strong."[3] Other invalid reasons why people may take supplements include:

- Their feeling of insecurity about the nutrient content of the food supply.
- Their belief that extra vitamins and minerals will help them cope with stress.
- Their desire to prevent, treat, or cure symptoms or diseases ranging from the common cold to cancer.

Ironically, at least one study showed that supplement users eat more nutrient-dense diets than nonusers and therefore need the supplements the least. In addition, little relationship exists between the nutrients people need and the ones they take in supplements.[4] In fact, an argument against supplements is that they may lull people into a false sense of security. A person might eat irresponsibly, thinking, "My supplement will cover my needs."

When I do need a vitamin-mineral supplement, what kind should I use?

Whenever a health care professional prescribes one, you should carefully follow directions as to the type and number of supplements to take. When you are selecting one yourself, a single, balanced vitamin-mineral supplement should suffice. Generally, most people who need supplements should choose the kind that provides all the RDA nutrients in amounts that are equal to, or very close to, the RDA. Remember, you will still be getting some nutrients from foods. Avoid preparations that are in excess of the RDA. Ignore claims such as "stress formula" or "formulated especially for active people." Avoid preparations that contain items not needed in human nutrition, such as choline or inositol.

Appendix D lists the nutrients in several vitamin-mineral supplements. The Miniglossary defines a variety of nutrient preparations.

A good friend of mine religiously takes several different kinds of nutrient supplements and preparations. He says they make him feel better, but I am worried that some of his practices are dangerous. What should I say?

What supplements does your friend take? *My friend takes 500 milligrams of vitamin C, 1,000 units of vitamin E, several tablespoons of nutritional yeast, some kelp tablets, capsules of vitamins A and D, a spirulina tablet, some green pills, and assorted other pills containing trace minerals before breakfast, and then sprinkles desiccated liver, powdered bone, bonemeal, wheat germ, and powdered skim milk on his granola.* You have a good reason to worry about a person with a huge stockpile of nutrient preparations. Some people really do such things, and continue with more of the same for lunch and dinner. If your friend is behaving like this, you should be very concerned.

Such a person is trying to obtain all the nutrients he needs. He feels that he can't do this using ordinary foods. This belief is typical of nutritional faddism, which is born of inadequate knowledge applied with sincere interest. The faddist cares profoundly

---

MINIGLOSSARY

desiccated liver: dehydrated liver; a powder sold in health food stores that is supposed to contain all the nutrients found in liver in concentrated form. This supplement has no particular nutritional merit, even though it may not be dangerous, and grocery store liver is considerably less expensive. Desiccated means "totally dried."

granola: a cereal mixed from rolled oats and other grains.

green pills: pills containing dehydrated, crushed vegetable matter. One pill contains nutrients equal to those in one small forkful of fresh vegetables—minus losses incurred in processing. Sixty pills cost $15.00 and deliver vegetable matter worth about $1.50.

kelp: a kind of seaweed used by the Japanese as a foodstuff. Kelp tablets are made from dehydrated kelp.

nutritional yeast: a preparation of yeast cells, often praised for its high nutrient content. Yeast is a concentrated source of B vitamins, as are many other foods. The type of yeast used is brewer's not baker's, yeast.

powdered bone, bonemeal: two among many nutrient supplements intended to supply calcium and other bone minerals. Some bonemeal has been found to contain high levels of lead.

spirulina: a kind of alga ("blue-green manna") said to contain large amounts of vitamin B_{12} and to suppress appetite. It does neither.

wheat germ: a part of the wheat grain, rich in nutrients.

about his health, which is commendable, but unfortunately, he is misguided.

To avoid alienating your friend while trying to reach him with valid information, you can adopt several strategies. For one thing, you can always acknowledge the validity of the feelings and values that underlie the faddist's practices. Then, distinguish between practices that are dangerous and those that are merely neutral. Ignore the neutral ones, and confront only the dangerous ones. Finally, make yourself responsible for learning the facts of the matter as thoroughly as you can, getting them all in perspective, and communicating them clearly.

In counseling the user, you might praise the value system that puts such a high premium on health and express support of the desire to take good care of the body. Then, in the example given, you might reinforce the use of wheat germ and powdered skim milk, agreeing that these foods are nutritious, reasonable in cost, and delicious. When you are sure of your listener's openness to whatever else you might have to say, you might offer a caution about the use of the potent supplements (the A and D capsules and the minerals), but keep your own counsel about the remaining ones unless you are asked. This way you probably won't lose a friend, and you might provide a substantial boost to exactly what he treasures most—his good health.

Finally, remind your friend that all the nutrients people need can come from food. Foods have so much more to offer than supplements do. The nutrients in foods come with water, fiber, and a host of other beneficial and interesting substances. They offer energy, pleasure, and opportunities for socializing, too. Supplements can do none of these things.

Notes

1. $2.9 billion for vitamins, *FDA Consumer,* April 1987, p. 4.
2. Recommendations concerning supplement usage: ADA statement (commentary), *Journal of the American Dietetic Association* 87 (1987): 1342–1343.
3. P. A. Thomsen, R. D. Terry, and R. J. Amos, Adolescents' beliefs about the reasons for using vitamin/mineral supplements, *Journal of the American Dietetic Association* 87 (1987): 1063–1065.
4. A. Looker and coauthors, Vitamin-mineral supplement use: Association with dietary intake and iron status of adults, *Journal of the American Dietetic Association* 88 (1988): 808–814.

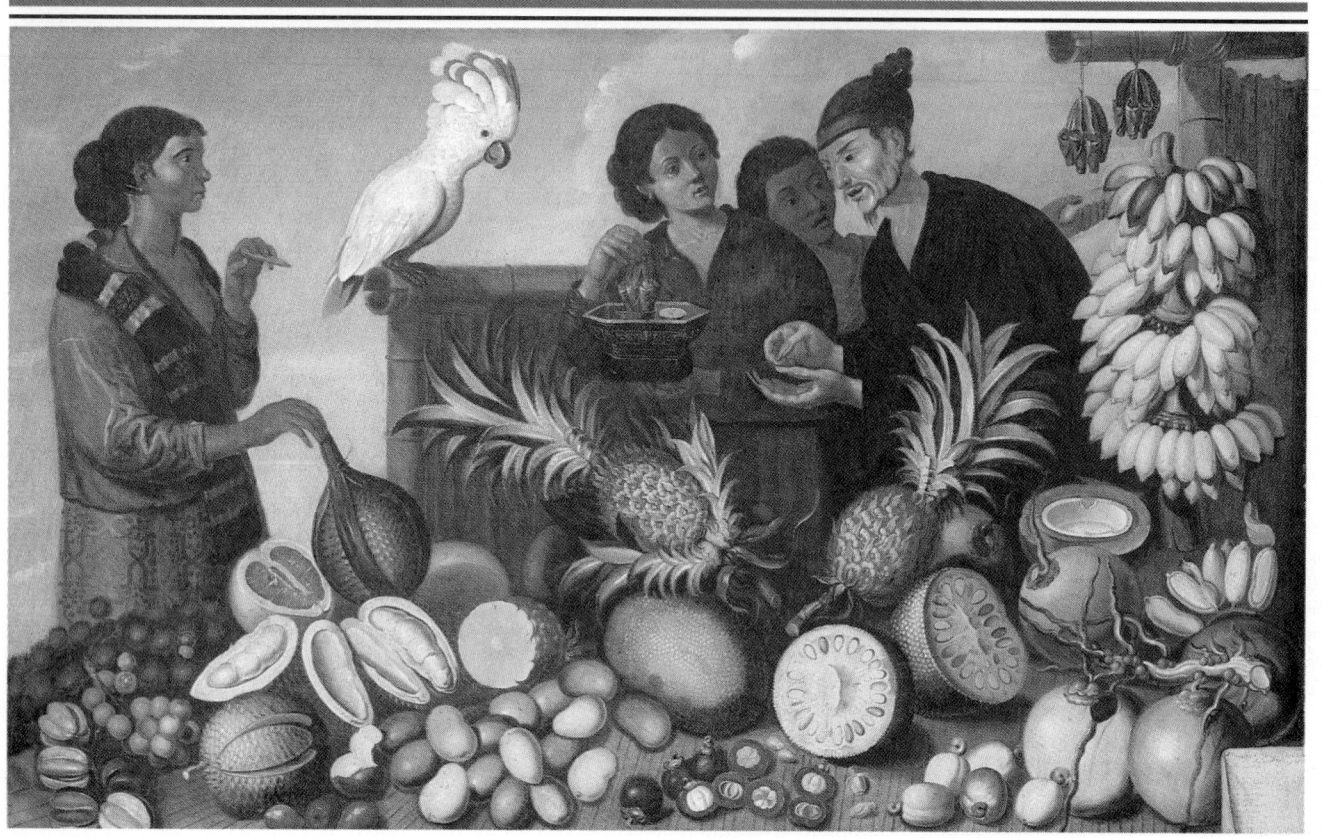

A. Eeckhout, Marktstalletje in Oost-Indië, *A 4070; Rijksmusuem, Amsterdam.*

CHAPTER

8

Water and Minerals

CONTENTS

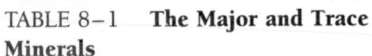

TABLE 8–1   **The Major and Trace Minerals**

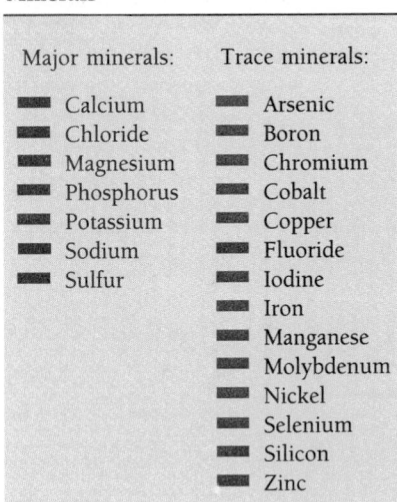

Major minerals:	Trace minerals:
Calcium	Arsenic
Chloride	Boron
Magnesium	Chromium
Phosphorus	Cobalt
Potassium	Copper
Sodium	Fluoride
Sulfur	Iodine
	Iron
	Manganese
	Molybdenum
	Nickel
	Selenium
	Silicon
	Zinc

CHAPTER

8

The body's water cannot be considered separately from the minerals dissolved in it. A person can drink pure water, but in the body, that water mingles with minerals to become fluids in which all life processes take place. This chapter begins by discussing water and the minerals that characterize the body's fluids and regulate their distribution within the body. The chapter's focus then shifts to other functions of the body's minerals.

The body fluids provide the medium in which all of the cells' chemical reactions occur. Every cell in the body is bathed in a fluid with the exact composition that is best for it. These special fluids regulate the functioning of cells. The cells in turn regulate the composition and amount of fluids within and surrounding them. The entire system of cells and fluids remains in a delicate but firmly maintained state of dynamic equilibrium.

Water constitutes about 55 to 60 percent of an adult's body weight and a higher percentage of a child's. Table 8–1 lists the major and trace minerals in the body; Figure 8–1 shows the amounts of minerals found in the body. As you can see, the most prevalent minerals are calcium and phosphorus, the chief minerals of bone (discussed later). The distinction between the major and the trace minerals does not mean that one group is more important than the other. A deficiency of the few micrograms of iodine needed daily by the body is just as serious as a deficiency of the several hundred milligrams of calcium. However, the major minerals (those to the left of the line), because of their larger total quantities, exert a greater influence on the body fluids.

Water and Body Fluids

Water brings to each cell the exact ingredients it requires and carries away the end products of the life-sustaining reactions that take place within the cells' boundaries. But water in the body is not simply a river coursing through the arteries, capillaries, and veins. Some of the water is part of the chemical structure of compounds that form the cells, tissues, and organs of the body. For example, proteins hold water molecules within them. Water also:

- Actively participates in many chemical reactions.
- Serves as the solvent for minerals, vitamins, amino acids, glucose, and a multitude of other small molecules.
- Acts as a lubricant and cushion around joints.
- Serves as a shock absorber inside the eyes, spinal cord, and amniotic sac surrounding a fetus in the womb.
- Aids in the body's temperature maintenance.

The body can survive a deficiency of all other nutrients for long periods of time, but it can survive for only a few days without water. No matter how little water a person consumes, the body must excrete a minimum amount each day as urine—enough to carry away the waste products generated by a day's metabolic activities. Above this amount (a minimum of about 500 milliliters a day), the water you excrete adjusts to balance your intake. If you drink more water than you need, the urine merely becomes more dilute.

500 ml = about ½ qt.

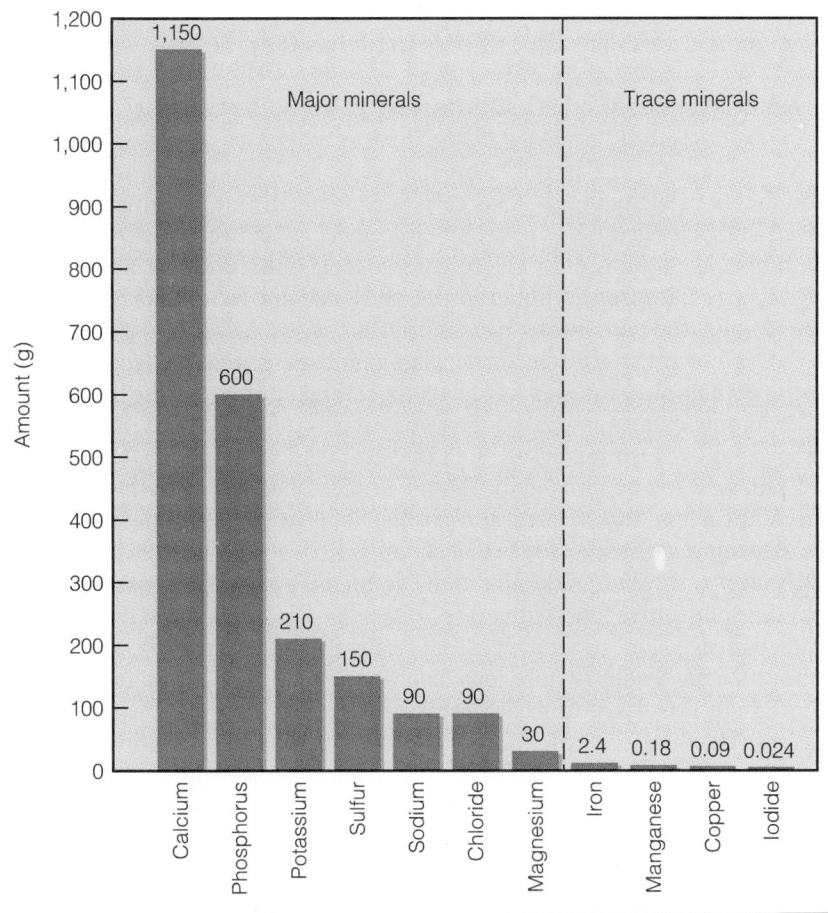

FIGURE 8–1   **The Amounts of Minerals in a 60-Kilogram Human Body**
A line separates the major minerals from the trace minerals. The major minerals are those present in amounts larger than 5 g (1 tsp). One pound is about 454 g; thus only calcium and phosphorus appear in amounts larger than a pound. There are more than a dozen trace minerals (see Table 8–1), although only four are shown here.

This is why drinking plenty of water is one guideline for the person seeking a balanced diet.

In addition to drinking water itself, nearly all foods contain water. Water is also generated from the energy nutrients in foods during metabolism. A person's daily water intake from water, foods, and metabolism totals about 2½ liters (about 2½ quarts) on the average. As for water excretion, it takes four major routes: some water is excreted via the kidneys, some is lost from the lungs as vapor, some is excreted in feces, and some evaporates from the skin. A person's water losses from these routes also total about 2½ liters a day on the average. Table 8–2 shows how fluid intake and urine output naturally balance out.

Water and Electrolyte Balance

The body uses minerals, among other constituents of body fluids, to regulate the distribution of those fluids. This regulation is vital to the life of the cells, for all cells must be bathed in fluids both within and without. The major

TABLE 8–2   **Water Balance**

WATER SOURCE	AMOUNT (ml)
Liquids	550 to 1,500
Foods	700 to 1,000
Metabolic water	200 to 300
	1,450 to 2,800

WATER OUTPUT	
Kidneys	500 to 1,400
Lungs	350
Feces	150
Skin	450 to 900
	1,450 to 2,800

salt: a compound composed of charged particles (ions). An example is potassium chloride (K^+Cl^-). Exceptions: a compound in which the positive ions are hydrogen ions (H^+) is an acid (example: hydrochloric acid, or H^+Cl^-); a compound in which the negative ions are hydroxyl ions (OH^-) is a base (example: potassium hydroxide, or K^+OH^-).

dissociation: physical separation of the ions in an ionic compound. A salt that partly dissociates in water is an electrolyte.

cation (CAT-eye-un): a positively charged ion.

anion (AN-eye-un): a negatively charged ion.

Na = sodium.
Cl = chlorine.

chloride: the ionic form of chlorine (CL^-).

electrolyte solution: a solution that can conduct electricity.

This force is known as the **osmotic pressure** of a solution. Water flows toward the higher osmotic pressure. The substances that create this pressure are the **solutes** (SOLL-yutes) dissolved in the water.

Other terms used to describe electrolyte solutions are *isotonic,* having the same osmotic pressure as a reference solution; *hypertonic,* having a higher osmotic pressure than a reference solution; and *hypotonic,* having a lower osmotic pressure than a reference solution. Standard saline (salt) solutions used in a hospital are made isotonic to human blood.
 iso = equal
 hyper = too much
 hypo = too little

semipermeable: more permeable to some substances (such as water) than to others (such as sodium and potassium). This condition is necessary for osmotic pressure to operate.
 semi = half

minerals form salts that dissolve in the body fluids; the cells direct where the salts go; and this determines where the fluids flow, because water follows salts.

When mineral (or other) salts dissolve in water, they separate (dissociate) into positively and negatively charged particles known as ions. The positive ions are cations; the negative ones are anions. Unlike pure water, which conducts electricity poorly, ions carry electrical current. For this reason, the electrically charged ions are called *electrolytes.* A salt that partly dissociates in water, as sodium chloride (common table salt) does, is known as an electrolyte. Because the fluids of the body contain water and partly dissociated salts, they are electrolyte solutions.

The body must use electrolytes to regulate its fluid balance, because without them water moves freely across cell membranes. Cells have no way to hold onto water molecules; they flow in and out of cells all the time. The cells can move electrolytes around, however, and water follows them, so the cells move water by moving the dissolved salts (electrolytes) around, relying on the principle that water follows salt. The cells sort out the mineral ions so that some of them reside primarily outside the cells (notably sodium and chloride), and some predominate inside the cells (notably potassium, magnesium, phosphate, and sulfate).

Electrolyte solutions are always electrically neutral. There is no such thing as a test tube filled with sodium ions. Sodium ions are always positively charged and cannot exist apart from negatively charged ions. Any fluid with dissolved electrolytes, therefore, will always have the same number of positive and negative ions. If an anion enters the cell, a cation must accompany it or another anion must leave so that electroneutrality will be maintained.

As mentioned, water follows salt. More precisely, a force moves water into a place where a solute, such as sodium chloride, is concentrated. This force can operate only if the divider separating the two fluid solutions is permeable to water but holds the solute back. Figure 8–2 shows this force in operation. In the top compartment, equal amounts of solute on either side of the divider cause the amounts of water also to be equal. In the bottom compartment, the presence of more solute on side B has drawn water across the divider so that the *concentration* of solute on either side becomes equal. The total amount of water is now greater on side B.

The cellular mechanism that regulates fluid distribution is the divider between the water inside and outside the cell, the cell membrane. Proteins in the membrane can attach to ions and move them from one side to the other. When the sodium pumps are active, for example, they pump sodium out of cells faster than the sodium can diffuse in. Water follows the sodium. When potassium pumps are active, they pump potassium into cells, and water follows the potassium ions. By maintaining a certain amount of sodium outside and potassium inside, the cell can regulate exactly the amounts of water inside and outside its boundaries.

The Constancy of Total Body Water

Besides balancing the fluids within and around its cells, the body keeps its total contents of water and salt delicately balanced. Thirst and satiety govern water intake. Thirst in healthy people is finely adjusted to ensure a water

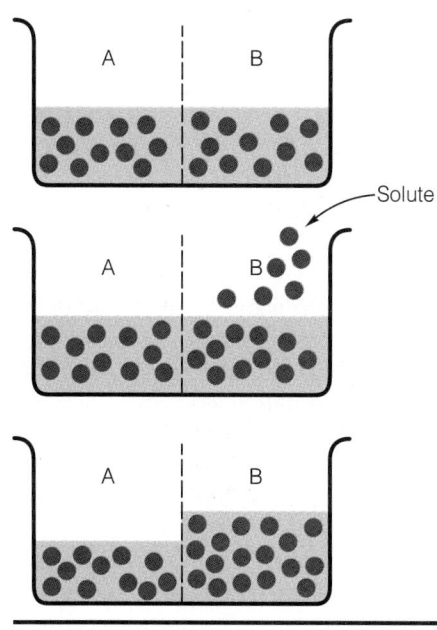

A. With equal numbers of solute particles on both sides, there are equal amounts of water.

B. Now additional solute is added to side B. Solute cannot flow across the divider.

—Solute

C. Water can flow across the divider. It moves both ways, but has a greater tendency to remain on side B, where there is more solute. The volume of water becomes greater on side B, and the concentrations on sides A and B become equal.

FIGURE 8−2 **Osmotic Pressure**
Water flows in the direction of the higher concentration of solute.

intake that meets the body's needs. Thirst itself does not remedy a water deficiency in the body; you have to notice that you are thirsty and take the time to get a drink.[1]

The mechanism of water excretion involves the brain and the kidneys. The cells of the brain's hypothalamus, which monitor salt concentration in the blood, stimulate the pituitary gland to release antidiuretic hormone (ADH) whenever the body's salt concentration is too high. The ADH stimulates the kidneys to hold back (actually, to reabsorb) water so that the water recirculates rather than being excreted. Thus the more water you need, the less you excrete. Cells in the kidney itself respond to the salt concentration in the blood passing through the kidney. When the cells sense a high salt concentration, they too release a substance. By a roundabout route, this substance also causes the kidneys to retain more water. Again, the effect is that when more water is needed, less is excreted.

The kidneys regulate the body's sodium, as well as its water, with remarkable precision. Sodium is absorbed defenselessly by the intestinal tract and travels freely in the blood, so it falls to the kidneys to excrete unneeded amounts. The kidneys actually filter all of the sodium out of the blood; then, with great precision, they return to the bloodstream the exact amount the body needs to retain. Thus the body's total electrolytes remain constant, while the electrolyte composition of the urine fluctuates according to what is eaten.

Normally, the body is well protected from imbalances of water and electrolytes. However, a person may be thrown into situations of imbalance for which the thirst instinct, cell membranes, and kidneys cannot compensate. This is the case when large amounts of fluid and electrolytes are suddenly lost. Vomiting, diarrhea, heavy sweating, fever, burns, wounds, and the like may incur such great fluid and electrolyte losses that a medical emergency results.

The **hypothalamus** (high-poh-THALL-uh-mus) is a part of the brain that helps regulate many body balances, including fluid balance. The **pituitary** (pit-TOO-ih-tary) gland, also in the brain, is the "king gland" that regulates the operation of many other glands.

ADH (antidiuretic hormone): a hormone released by the pituitary gland in response to high osmotic pressure of the blood. The kidney responds by reabsorbing water.

This substance is the enzyme **renin** (REEN-in), released by the kidney in response to a high salt concentration. The mechanism by which renin aids the kidneys in retaining water is the **renin-angiotensin mechanism.**

Technically, these imbalances are known as fluid and electrolyte imbalances.

The details of electrolyte balance are among the most important ones that medical professionals must learn. For the purposes here, it is necessary only to appreciate the importance of this balance and the principles by which it is maintained, and to be aware of the situations that threaten it. Water and salts, which people take for granted and usually ignore, are more vital to life than any of the other nutrients considered in this book.

Acid-Base Balance

The body uses its ions not only to help maintain water balance but also to help regulate the acidity (pH) of its fluids. Electrolyte mixtures in the body fluids, as well as proteins, protect the body against changes in acidity by acting as buffers—substances that can accommodate excess acids or bases.

The body's buffer systems serve as a first line of defense against changes in the fluids' acid-base balance. The lungs, skin, GI tract, and kidneys provide other defenses. Of these organ systems, the kidneys play a primary role in maintaining acid-base balance.

Disorders of the kidney, therefore, impair the body's ability to regulate its fluid and electrolyte, as well as its acid-base, balance. For a person with renal disease, the physician may order, in addition to many medical procedures, adjustment of the electrolyte intake from food. Chapter 23 gives more information about renal disease.

All the major minerals help maintain fluid and electrolyte balance in the body, as just described. Each mineral has other important functions as well, as the next sections describe. Table 8–7, at the end of this chapter, offers a summary of the minerals and their functions.

buffer: a substance or mixture in a solution that is capable of neutralizing both acids and bases and thereby capable of maintaining the original concentration of hydrogen ions (pH) in the solution.

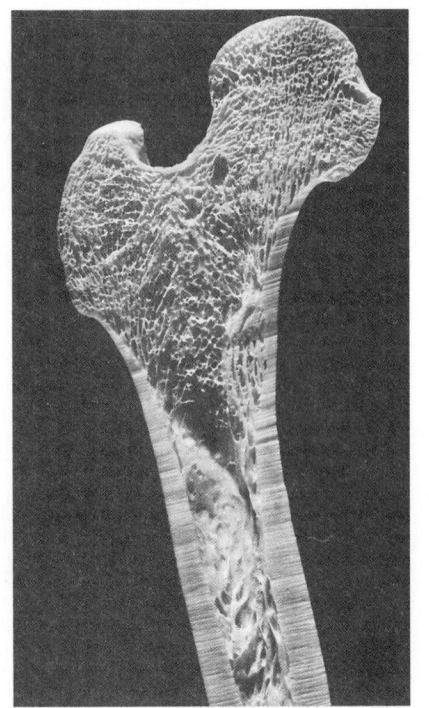

FIGURE 8–3   **Cross Section of Bone**
The lacy structural elements are **trabeculae** (tra-BECK-you-lee), which can be drawn on to replenish blood calcium.

The Major Minerals

The major minerals—calcium, phosphorus, magnesium, sodium, potassium, chloride, and sulfur—are so named because they are the minerals present in the largest amounts in the body. As you will see, their functions are many and diverse.

Calcium

Calcium owns the distinction of being the most abundant mineral in the body. Ninety-nine percent of the body's calcium is stored in the bones, where it plays two important roles. First, it is an integral part of bone structure. Second, it serves as a calcium bank, offering a readily available source of the mineral to the body fluids should even the slightest drop in blood calcium concentration occur. Many people have the idea that calcium, once deposited in bone, stays there forever—that once a bone is built, it is inert, like a rock. Not so. Bones are in a state of constant flux, with formation and dissolution taking place every minute of the day and night. Figure 8–3 shows the lacy network of calcium-containing crystals in the bone.

Only about 1 percent of the body's calcium circulates in the fluids as ionized calcium, but this circulating calcium is vital to life. The calcium ion participates in such diverse processes as the regulation of muscle contraction; the transmission of nerve impulses; and the secretion of hormones, digestive enzymes, and neurotransmitters. Calcium acts as a cell messenger, conveying signals received at the cell surface to the inside of the cell.[2] Calcium must also be present if blood clotting is to occur, because it is one of the many factors directly involved in the process. Calcium is a cofactor for several enzymes as well.

Because blood calcium is so important, its concentration is tightly controlled. Whenever the blood calcium concentration rises too high, a system of hormones and vitamin D promote its deposit into bone. Whenever the blood calcium concentration falls too low, the regulatory system acts in three locations to correct the imbalance:

- *Intestine*. Stimulates calcium absorption.
- *Bone*. Stimulates calcium release.
- *Kidney*. Slows calcium excretion.

Thus blood calcium rises to normal.

The calcium found in bone provides a nearly inexhaustible source of calcium for the blood. Even in calcium deficiency, blood concentration remains normal. Food calcium never affects blood calcium, but this is not to say that blood calcium never changes. Blood calcium does change, but in response to changed regulatory control, not to diet. When blood calcium does rise above normal, the resulting condition is known as calcium rigor: the muscles contract and cannot relax. Similarly, blood calcium concentration may fall below normal, causing calcium tetany—also characterized by uncontrolled muscle contraction. These conditions do not reflect a dietary lack or excess of calcium; they are caused by a lack of vitamin D or by abnormal concentrations of hormones that regulate calcium homeostasis.

On the other hand, a chronic *dietary* deficiency of calcium or a chronic deficiency due to poor absorption over the course of years can diminish the savings account in the bones. Because this is an important concept, we repeat: it is the bones, not the blood, that are depleted by calcium deficiency.

Calcium deficiencies are widespread in human societies. Research suggests that calcium deficiency during the growing years impairs acquisition of peak bone mass and density.[3] A high bone mass at the time of skeletal maturity (about age 30) is the best protection against accelerated age-related bone loss and fracture. All adults lose bone as they grow older, beginning between the ages of 30 and 40, but when bone loss is excessive to the point that bones fracture even under common, everyday stresses, the condition is known as osteoporosis. Osteoporosis afflicts as many as 20 million people, mostly women 45 years of age and older.

Both genetic and environmental factors contribute to osteoporosis. Table 8–3 summarizes risk factors for osteoporosis. Osteoporosis is eight times more prevalent in women than men, for several reasons. First, women consume less dietary calcium than men. In fact, men consume up to twice as much calcium as women do. Second, at all ages, women's bone mass is lower than men's, because women generally have a smaller body size. Finally, bone loss begins earlier in women than in men, and it accelerates in women after menopause.

Many minerals and vitamins are required to form and stabilize the structure of bones, including magnesium, fluoride, and vitamin A. Any or all of

cofactor: a mineral element that, like a coenzyme, works with an enzyme to facilitate a chemical reaction.

The regulators are hormones from the thyroid and parathyroid glands, as well as vitamin D. One, parathormone, raises blood calcium. Others, calcitonin and thyrocalcitonin, lower blood calcium by inhibiting release of calcium from bone. The hormonelike vitamin D raises blood calcium by acting at the three sites listed.

calcium rigor: hardness or stiffness of the muscles caused by high blood calcium.

calcium tetany: intermittent spasms of the extremities due to nervous and muscular excitability, which is caused by low blood calcium.

TABLE 8–3   **Risk Factors for Osteoporosis**

Age
Gender
Race
Family history of osteoporosis
Low calcium intake
Excessive caffeine use
Excessive fiber in the diet
Menopause
Never having given birth
Inactivity or extreme activity with cessation of menstruation
Low body weight
Lean body composition
Short stature, small frame size
Heavy alcohol use
Stomach or intestine surgery (surgery can reduce calcium absorption)
Disease states or long-term medications (consult a physician)

Source: Adapted from B. L. Riggs and L. J. Melton, Involutional osteoporosis, *New England Journal of Medicine* 314 (1986): 1676–1686; L. W. Turner and E. N. Whitney, Nature versus nurture: The calcium controversy, *Nutrition Clinics,* September/October 1989.

rickets: the calcium-deficiency (or vitamin D–deficiency) disease in children.

Altered composition of the bones is reflected in **osteomalacia,** the condition in which the bones become soft. Osteomalacia is sometimes called **adult rickets.** Reduced density of the bones results in **osteoporosis** (oss-tee-oh-pore-OH-sis)—literally, porous bones. Osteomalacia is related to vitamin D deficiency. The causes of osteoporosis are multiple.

osteo = bone

these elements may be essential for preventing osteoporosis. One obvious line of defense, however, is to maintain a lifelong adequate intake of calcium. Moderate weight-bearing exercise, such as walking, running, or dancing, is also necessary, for bones lay down minerals in response to the demands of bearing weight.

The disease rickets was mentioned in Chapter 7 because vitamin D deficiency is the most common cause of rickets. Dietary calcium is often adequate in a person with rickets, but the calcium passes through the intestinal tract without being absorbed into the body, leaving the bones undersupplied. Vitamin D deficiency, by depressing the production of the calcium-binding protein, causes rickets. (The symptoms of rickets are listed in Table 7–2.) The failure to deposit sufficient calcium in the bones of a child causes growth retardation, bowed legs, and other skeletal abnormalities. In an adult, the disease may set in after a normal childhood during which calcium intake and absorption were adequate and after the skeleton has become fully calcified.

Studies of populations at high risk of developing hypertension show that low dietary calcium correlates with a high prevalence of hypertension.[4] Reports that calcium supplements can lower blood pressure in people with and without hypertension further support an association between calcium and hypertension.[5] Some researchers remain skeptical about the relationship between calcium and hypertension, while others look for metabolic explanations or mechanisms of action. As mentioned earlier, calcium is involved in regulating muscle contraction. Some researchers speculate that calcium's effect on blood pressure is related to its action on the smooth muscle surrounding blood vessels.

The calcium RDA for adults is 800 milligrams, although actual intakes vary widely. Adult women consume an average of 200 milligrams less than recommended intakes, and one woman in four consumes less than 300 milligrams of calcium per day.[6] Some authorities advocate calcium recommendations as high as 1,500 milligrams per day for women over 50 to guard against bone loss.

Calcium is found almost exclusively in a single class of foods—milk and milk products. Dietary recommendations advise daily consumption of low-fat or nonfat milk products to help maintain an adequate calcium intake. A cup of milk provides almost 300 milligrams of calcium, so an adult who drinks 2 cups of milk a day is well on the way to meeting daily calcium needs. Pregnant, lactating, and older women need more (see Table 8–4). The other dairy food that contains comparable amounts of calcium is cheese. One slice of cheese (1 ounce) contains about two-thirds as much calcium as a cup of milk. Cottage cheese, however, is a poor source of calcium. Figure 8–4 shows foods that are rich in calcium.

Among the vegetables, mustard greens, kale, parsley, watercress, and broccoli are good sources of available calcium. Some dark green, leafy vegetables—notably spinach and Swiss chard—appear to be calcium-rich but actually provide very little, if any, calcium to the body. These foods contain binders that prevent calcium absorption.

TABLE 8–4 **Recommended Fluid Milk Intakes**

AGE	RECOMMENDED INTAKE
Children	2 c
Teenagers	3 c
Adults	2 c
Pregnant women	3 c
Lactating women	3 c
Older women	3 c

Apparently, all fibers in plant foods—cellulose, hemicellulose, pectin, and others—bind calcium to some extent, as do phytic, oxalic, and uronic acids.

Two cups of milk supply the following percentages of the nutrients an adult man needs:
Calcium: 75%.
Vitamin D: 50%.
Protein: 25%.
Vitamin A: 30%.
Thiamin: 13%.
Riboflavin: 50%.
Plus 24 g carbohydrate in the form of lactose.

People may think that taking a calcium supplement is preferable to getting calcium from food, but as you know by now, foods offer important fringe benefits. For example, drinking 2 cups of milk fortified with vitamins A and D will supply substantial percentages of the nutrients listed in the margin. Furthermore, calcium absorption is enhanced by vitamin D, lactose, fat, and possibly other nutrients in the milk. A calcium supplement supplies only calcium—in a less absorbable form.

People who dislike milk may find it helpful to learn how to conceal it in foods. Powdered nonfat milk, an excellent and inexpensive source of calcium, can be added to many foods (such as baked products and meat loaf) during preparation. Yogurt and kefir (fermented dairy products), as well as cheese, are acceptable substitutes for regular milk. Puddings, custards, and baked goods can be prepared in such a way that they also contain appreciable amounts of milk. Strict vegetarians or people who are either allergic to milk or are lactose intolerant must obtain calcium from calcium-rich substitutes such as calcium-fortified soy milk or tofu (bean curd). Small fish such as canned sardines, or other canned fish prepared with their bones, such as canned salmon, are also rich in calcium.

Some foods offer large amounts of calcium because of fortification. Calcium-fortified orange juice, high-calcium milk (milk with extra calcium added), and calcium-fortified bread are examples.

The word *daily* should be stressed with respect to food sources of calcium. Because of the body's limited ability to absorb calcium, it cannot handle massive doses periodically but instead needs frequent opportunities to take in small amounts.

milk allergy: the most common food allergy; caused by the protein in raw milk. Milk allergy is sometimes overcome by cooking the milk to denature the protein and is sometimes cured by abstinence from, and gradual reintroduction to, milk (see Chapter 12). (See also the discussion of lactose intolerance in Chapter 20.)

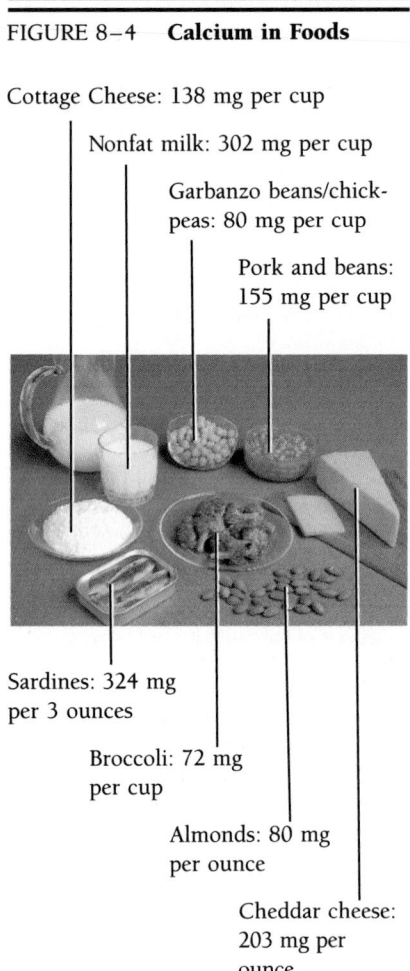

FIGURE 8–4   **Calcium in Foods**

Cottage Cheese: 138 mg per cup

Nonfat milk: 302 mg per cup

Garbanzo beans/chick-peas: 80 mg per cup

Pork and beans: 155 mg per cup

Sardines: 324 mg per 3 ounces

Broccoli: 72 mg per cup

Almonds: 80 mg per ounce

Cheddar cheese: 203 mg per ounce

Some factors enhance calcium absorption. The body is able to regulate its absorption of calcium by altering its production of the calcium-binding protein aided by vitamin D; more of this protein is made if more calcium is needed. The lactose in milk seems to facilitate calcium absorption by a mechanism as yet unknown. Also, calcium seems to be better absorbed if accompanied by an approximately equal amount of phosphorus.

Phosphorus

Phosphorus is the second most abundant mineral in the body. About 85 percent of it is found combined with calcium in the crystals of the bones and teeth.

The concentration of phosphorus in the blood is less than half that of calcium. But as part of one of the body's major buffers (phosphoric acid), phosphorus is found in all body cells. Phosphorus is a part of DNA and RNA, the genetic code material present in every cell. Thus phosphorus is necessary for all growth.

Phosphorus also plays many key roles in energy transfers occurring during cellular metabolism. Many enzymes and the B vitamins become active only when a phosphate group is attached. The energy carrier of the cells, adenosine triphosphate (ATP), contains three phosphate groups and uses them to do its work.

Lipids containing phosphorus as part of their structures help to transport other lipids in the blood; phospholipids also reside in cell membranes, where they affect transport of nutrients into and out of the cells.

Animal protein is the best source of phosphorus, because phosphorus is so abundant in the cells of animals. Recommended intakes for phosphorus are the same as those for calcium, except during infancy. Deficiencies are unknown. A summary of facts about phosphorus appears in Table 8–7.

Magnesium

Magnesium barely qualifies as a major mineral. Only about 1¾ ounces of magnesium is present in the body of a 130-pound person, most of it in the bones. Bone magnesium seems to be a reservoir to ensure that some will be on hand for vital reactions regardless of recent dietary intake.

Magnesium also acts in all the cells of the soft tissues, where it forms part of the protein-making machinery and where it is necessary for the release of energy. Magnesium helps relax muscles after contraction and promotes resistance to tooth decay by holding calcium in tooth enamel.

Dietary intakes of magnesium average about three-quarters of the RDA for both men and women in the United States.[7] Dietary intake data, however, do not assess the nutrient contribution of water. In various parts of the country, the water contains both calcium and magnesium and is known as "hard" water. Hard water can contribute significantly to magnesium intakes.

Despite average intakes below the RDA, the development of deficiency symptoms in the absence of disease is unlikely.[8] Magnesium deficiency may occur as a result of vomiting, diarrhea, alcohol abuse, or protein malnutrition; after surgery in people who have been fed incomplete fluids into a vein for too long; or in people using diuretics. A severe deficiency causes tetany, an extreme and prolonged contraction of the muscles much like the reaction of the muscles when calcium levels fall. Magnesium deficiencies are also thought to cause the hallucinations experienced during withdrawal from alcohol intoxication.

Magnesium-rich food sources include dark green, leafy vegetables; nuts; legumes; whole-grain breads and cereals; seafood; chocolate; and cocoa. Magnesium is easily lost from foods during processing, so unprocessed foods are the best choices.

Sodium

Sodium is the principal electrolyte in the extracellular fluid and the primary regulator of extracellular fluid volume. When the blood concentration of sodium rises, as when a person eats salted foods, thirst ensures that the person will drink water until the appropriate sodium-to-water ratio is restored. Sodium also helps maintain acid-base balance and is essential to muscle contraction and nerve transmission.

Diets rarely lack sodium. For this reason, no RDA is set; instead, the Committee on RDA estimated the *minimum* sodium requirement for adults to be 500 milligrams. The *NRC Recommendations* (Table 1–3 in Chapter 1), which emphasize moderation, not adequacy, set a maximum intake of *salt* at 6 grams (2,400 milligrams of sodium). The most recent food intake survey in the United States estimates that men consume an average of 3,300 milligrams of sodium a day.[9]

Sodium intakes vary widely, but foods usually supply more sodium than the body needs. In general, people who eat diets that emphasize processed foods have the highest sodium intakes, while those who emphasize whole foods, such as fresh fruits and vegetables, have the lowest intakes.[10] In fact, as much as 75 percent of the sodium in people's diets comes from salt added to foods during processing and manufacturing; about 15 percent of daily sodium comes from salt added during cooking and at the table; only 10 percent comes from the natural salt content of foods.[11] Table 8–5 offers suggestions for avoiding excessive sodium intakes.

The connection between sodium and high blood pressure is well known, and many people have reduced their sodium intakes. As researchers began to take a closer look at the sodium-hypertension connection, however, their attention turned to sodium's partner, chloride. Now, it is *salt,* not just sodium, that is suspect as a factor in hypertension among salt-sensitive people.[12] Chapter 22 describes the relationship of these and other factors to blood pressure.

Diets that are low in sodium are invariably high in potassium, which is another nutrient of interest in relation to hypertension. It may be that high potassium intakes, rather than low sodium intakes, offer some people protection against hypertension.

Estimated minimum requirement for sodium: 500 mg/day.
5 g salt is about 2 g sodium.
1 g salt = 1/5 tsp salt.

Potassium

Potassium is the principal positively charged ion inside the body cells. It plays a major role in maintaining fluid and electrolyte balance and cell integrity. It is also critical to maintaining the heartbeat. The sudden deaths

TABLE 8–5   **Suggestions for Avoiding Excessive Sodium Intake**

Learn to enjoy the unsalted flavors of foods.
Cook with only small amounts of added salt.
Add little or no salt to food at the table.
Read labels with an eye open for salt.
Cut down on:
   Foods prepared in brine, such as pickles, olives, and sauerkraut.
   Salty or smoked meats, such as bologna, corned or chipped beef, frankfurters,
   ham, luncheon meats, salt pork, sausage, and smoked tongue.
   Salty or smoked fish, such as anchovies, caviar, salted and dried cod, herring,
   sardines, and smoked salmon.
   Snack items such as potato chips, pretzels, salted popcorn, and salted nuts and
   crackers.
   Bouillon cubes; seasoned salts (including sea salt); and soy, Worcestershire,
   and barbecue sauces.
   Cheeses, especially processed types.
   Canned and instant soups.
   Prepared horseradish, catsup, and mustard.

that occur in severe diarrhea and in children with kwashiorkor are likely due to heart failure caused by potassium loss. Potassium also assists in carbohydrate and protein metabolism.

A dietary deficiency of potassium is unlikely in healthy people, although low potassium intakes are possible with diets low in fresh fruits and vegetables. Because potassium is found inside of all living cells, both plant and animal, and because cells remain intact unless foods are processed, the richest sources of potassium are *fresh* foods of all kinds—especially fruits, vegetables, and legumes.

As with sodium, no RDA is set for potassium; the estimated minimum requirement is 2,000 milligrams for adults. Surveys show wide variations in potassium intakes in the United States; people who emphasize fresh fruits and vegetables in their diets have intakes as high as 11 grams per day.[13]

As mentioned earlier, population studies show a relationship between dietary potassium and hypertension. For instance, primitive populations worldwide eat diets that are low in sodium and high in potassium; hypertension among such people is virtually nonexistent. Conversely, among populations who eat diets that are low in potassium, the incidence of cardiovascular diseases such as hypertension and stroke is abnormally high.[14] Evidence of potassium's influence on blood pressure continues to mount. One long-term study in California showed that people with a high dietary potassium intake had a significantly lower risk of stroke. For some, the risk reduction was as great as 40 percent.[15] In the United States, where strokes are a leading killer, the potential exists for people to reap substantial health benefits simply by emphasizing more potassium-rich fresh fruits, vegetables, and juices in their diets. A reminder is important here: these findings are based on food intakes of potassium, not supplements. Potassium toxicity from foods is not a problem, because healthy kidneys excrete the excess amounts. Potassium supplements can be toxic and can be fatal.

Estimated minimum requirement for potassium: 2000 mg/day.

Potassium deficiency occurs more as a result of excessive losses rather than deficient intake. In abnormal conditions such as diabetic acidosis, dehydration, or prolonged vomiting or diarrhea, potassium deficiency can occur. Furthermore, potassium deficiencies can result from regular use of certain drugs, including diuretics, steroids, and cathartics. One of the earliest symptoms is muscle weakness.

Other Major Minerals

The chloride ion is the major negative ion of the fluids outside the cells, where it occurs primarily in association with sodium. Chloride can move freely across cell membranes and so is also found inside the cells in association with potassium. Like sodium, chloride is critical to maintaining fluid, electrolyte, and acid-base balance in the body. In the stomach, the chloride ion is part of hydrochloric acid, which maintains the strong acidity of the stomach.

Salt is a major food source of chloride, and processed foods are a major contributor of this nutrient, like sodium, in people's diets. The Committee on RDA has not established an RDA for chloride, but has provided an estimated minimum requirement for adults, as for sodium.

Sulfur is present in all proteins and plays its most important role in helping strands of protein to assume a particular shape and hold it—and thus to do the proteins' specific jobs, such as enzyme work. Skin, hair, and nails contain some of the body's more rigid proteins, and they have a high sulfur content.

There is no recommended intake for sulfur, and no deficiencies are known. Only a person who lacks protein to the point of severe deficiency will lack the sulfur-containing amino acids.

The Trace Minerals

Figure 8–1, at the beginning of this chapter, shows how tiny the quantities of trace minerals in the human body are. If you could remove all of them from your body, you would have only a bit of dust, hardly enough to fill a teaspoon. Yet each of the trace minerals performs some vital role for which no substitute will do. A deficiency of any of them can be fatal, and an excess of many can be equally deadly.

The Committee on RDA has established recommended dietary intakes for the best-known trace elements—iron, zinc, iodine, and selenium. Tentative ranges for safe and adequate daily intakes of others are also published. Still others are recognized as essential nutrients for some animals, but not proven to be required for human beings (see Table 8–6). Many others are under study to determine whether they, too, perform indispensable roles in the body.

Iron

Every living cell—both plant and animal—contains iron. Most of the iron in the body is a component of the proteins hemoglobin in red blood cells and

diuretic (dye-yoo-RET-ic): a drug that promotes the excretion of water through the kidneys. Only some diuretics increase the urinary loss of potassium. Others, called potassium-sparing diuretics, are less likely to result in a potassium deficiency.

steroid (STARE-oid): a drug used to reduce tissue inflammation, to suppress the immune response, or to replace certain steroid hormones in people who cannot synthesize them.

cathartic (ca-THART-ic): a strong laxative.

Estimated minimum requirement for chloride: 750 mg/day.

Amino acids containing sulfur are methionine and cysteine. Cysteine in one part of a protein chain can bind to cysteine in another part of the chain by way of a sulfur-sulfur bridge.

hemoglobin: the oxygen-carrying protein of the red blood cells.
  hemo = blood
  globin = globular protein

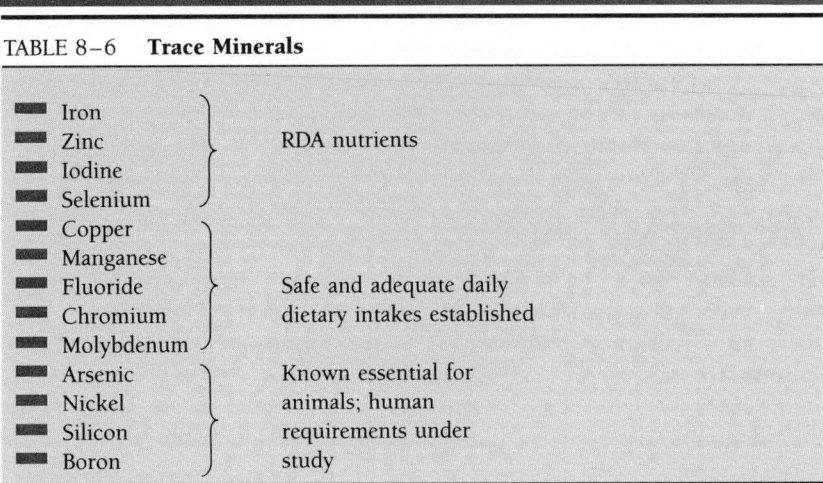

TABLE 8–6   **Trace Minerals**

Iron Zinc Iodine Selenium	RDA nutrients
Copper Manganese Fluoride Chromium Molybdenum	Safe and adequate daily dietary intakes established
Arsenic Nickel Silicon Boron	Known essential for animals; human requirements under study

myoglobin in muscle cells. Hemoglobin in the blood carries oxygen from the lungs to tissues throughout the body. Myoglobin carries and stores oxygen for the muscles when they contract. Both hemoglobin and myoglobin use iron to help carry and hold oxygen and then release it. As part of many enzymes, iron is vital to the processes by which cells generate energy. Iron is also needed to make new cells, amino acids, hormones, and neutrotransmitters.

Iron clearly is the body's gold, a precious mineral to be hoarded and closely guarded. The number of special provisions for its handling shows how vital it is. When a red blood cell dies, the liver saves the iron from its hemoglobin and returns it to the bone marrow to be used for new red blood cells. Thus only tiny amounts of iron are lost, principally in urine, sweat, shed skin, and blood (if bleeding occurs). The chief storage site for iron held in reserve is the liver.

The body also has special provisions for obtaining iron. At the receiving end in the intestines, only about 10 to 15 percent of dietary iron is normally absorbed; but if the body's supply is diminished or if the need increases for any reason, absorption increases. This regulation is provided by a blood protein, transferrin, which captures iron from food and carries it to tissues throughout the body. When more iron is needed, more transferrin is produced so that more than the usual amount of iron can be absorbed. Should there be a surplus of iron, special storage proteins in the bone marrow and other organs store it.

If absorption cannot compensate for a reduced supply and stores are used up, iron deficiency sets in. Because so much of the body's iron is in the blood, iron losses are greatest whenever blood is lost. Women's menstrual losses make a woman's iron needs twice as great as a man's, but anyone who loses blood loses iron. Women are especially prone to iron deficiency, because they not only lose more iron than men but also are, on average, smaller than men; they eat less food. Pregnancy places iron demands on women as well. The information about iron in foods, which appears later in this section, is especially important for women. Iron needs of physically active people are discussed in Chapter 9.

The most common tests for iron deficiency measure the number and size of the red blood cells and the cells' hemoglobin content. Before these levels fall, at the very beginning of an iron deficiency, the transferrin concentration *rises*. A sensitive test that will detect a developing iron deficiency, before it is full-blown, measures the amount of transferrin in the blood and the amount of iron it is carrying. Other tests measure iron stores.

If iron stores are exhausted, the body cannot make enough hemoglobin to fill its new red blood cells. A sample of iron-deficient blood examined under the microscope shows smaller cells that are a lighter red than normal (Figure 8–5). The undersized cells can't carry enough oxygen from the lungs to the tissues, so energy release in the cells is hindered. Every cell of the body feels the effect; the result is fatigue, weakness, headaches, and apathy.

Long before the mass of the red blood cells is affected and anemia is diagnosed, people feel the impact of iron deficiency. A developing iron deficiency affects behavior. Even at slightly lowered iron levels, the complete oxidation of pyruvate is impaired, reducing physical work capacity and productivity. Children deprived of iron become irritable and restless due to abnormal levels of the stress hormones in their systems. These symptoms are among the first to appear when the body's iron level begins to fall and among the first to disappear when iron intake is increased again.

A curious symptom seen in some iron-deficient individuals is an appetite for ice, clay, paste, and other nonnutritious substances. Such people have been known to eat as many as eight trays of ice in a day, for example. This

One common test for iron deficiency is measurement of the **hemoglobin concentration** of blood.
Norms for adults:
—Men: 13 to 16 g/100 ml.
—Women: 12 to 16 g/100 ml.

Norms for children:
—Ages 2 to 5: 11 g/100 ml.
—Ages 6 to 12: 11.5 g/100 ml.

Note that hemoglobin is measured in grams per 100 milliliters, but often just the number of grams alone is used in speaking of it: "hemoglobin, 14."

Another common test, the **hematocrit,** represents the percentage of red blood cells in a whole blood sample.

Norms for adults:
—Men: 40 to 54%.
—Women: 37 to 47%.

Norms for children:
—Ages 2 to 5: 34%.
—Ages 6 to 12: 37%.

FIGURE 8–5 Normal and Anemic Blood Cells

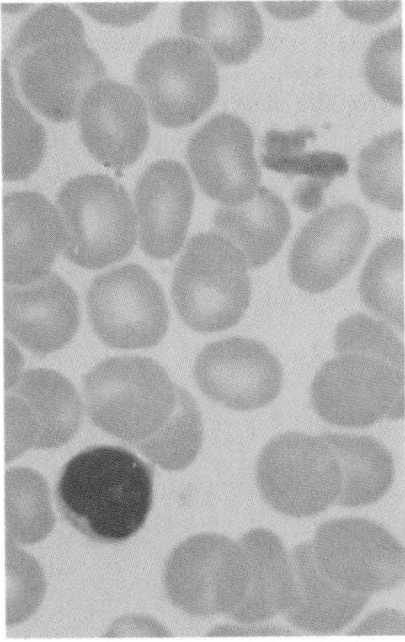

Normal blood cells. Both size and color are normal. The one large, purple cell is a normal white blood cell, stained purple.

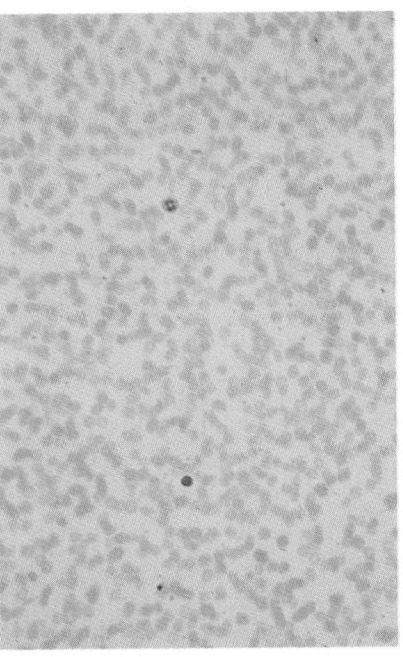

Blood cells in microcytic hypochromic anemia such as that caused by iron deficiency. These cells are small and pale because they contain less hemoglobin.

Transferrin can be measured directly or estimated by measuring the **total iron-binding capacity (TIBC)** and the **transferrin saturation.**

In all people, including those who are dark skinned, a sign of iron deficiency can be observed by looking in the corner of the eye. The eye lining, normally pink, will be very pale, even white. The skin of a fair person who is anemic may be noticeably pale.

microcytic (my-cro-SIT-ic) **hypochromatic** (high-po-KROME-ic) **anemia:** iron-deficiency anemia.

   micro = small
   cytic = cells
   hypo = too little
   chrom = color

There is more about the effects of iron deficiency on children's behavior in Chapter 12.

pica (PIE-ka): a craving for nonfood substances; also known as **geophagia** (jee-oh-FAY-jee-uh) when referring to the clay-eating behavior.

   picus = woodpecker or magpie
   geo = earth
   phagein = to eat

iron deficiency: the state of being without iron stores.

iron-deficiency anemia: the condition in which there are small, pale, blood cells resulting from an iron deficiency.

The provision of binding proteins (ferritin and a transferrin-like protein) in the mucosal cells to capture and hold unneeded iron to be shed with the cells is called the **mucosal block** to iron absorption.

iron overload: toxicity from iron overdose. There are two types, hemochromatosis and hemosiderosis.

behavior, which has been named pica, has been observed for years, especially in women and children of low-income groups who are deficient in either iron or zinc. Pica clears up dramatically within days after iron is given, long before the red blood cells respond.

A low hemoglobin level may represent a dietary iron deficiency, and if it does, the physician may prescribe iron supplements. However, any nutrient deficiency, or disease, or agent that interferes with hemoglobin synthesis, disrupts hemoglobin function, or causes a loss of red blood cells can precipitate anemia. Nutrient deficiencies other than iron that can cause anemia include, among others, those of protein, vitamin B_6, folate, vitamin B_{12}, vitamin C, vitamin A, vitamin E, and copper. Nonnutritional causes of anemia include excessive blood loss, infections, and some chronic diseases.

Feeling fatigued, weak, and apathetic is a sign that something is wrong, but it does not indicate that a person should take iron supplements. It means that (you guessed it!) the person should consult a physician. In fact, taking iron supplements may be the worst possible thing a person can do, because such supplements can mask a serious medical condition, such as hidden bleeding from cancer or an ulcer. Furthermore, a person can waste precious time in not seeking treatment. Once again—the caution deserves repeating—don't self-diagnose.

Worldwide, iron deficiency is the most common nutrient deficiency.[16] The distinction between iron deficiency and anemia is an important one. Iron deficiency and anemia are not one and the same, though they often go hand in hand. People may be iron deficient without being anemic. The term *iron deficiency* refers to depleted body iron stores without regard to the degree of depletion or the presence of anemia. The term *anemia* refers to the hematologic state resulting in a severe deficiency, with lowered hemoglobin concentration.

Iron-deficiency anemia is a major health problem in both the United States and Canada and even more so in developing nations. It is especially common in infants (six months old or older), children, women of childbearing age, and people in low-income and minority groups. But no segment of society is free of iron-deficiency anemia, and the groups mentioned are not the only ones affected.

The cause of iron deficiency is usually nutrition—that is, inadequate intake, from ignorance of what foods to choose, from sheer lack of food altogether, or from high consumption of iron-poor foods. In the Western world, high sugar and fat intakes are often responsible for low iron intakes. Among nonnutritional causes, blood loss is the primary one.

Iron toxicity is rare but not unknown. Normally the body protects itself against absorbing too much iron by setting up a block in the intestinal cells. The system can be overwhelmed, however, and iron overload is the result.

Two kinds of iron overload are known. One is caused by a hereditary defect, the other by the ingestion of too much iron, usually in combination with excessive alcohol consumption. The alcohol abuser is particularly prone to iron overload, because alcohol enhances the absorption of iron. In addition, certain wines contain substantial amounts of iron. Regardless of the cause, tissue damage, especially to the liver, results. Infections are likely, because bacteria thrive in iron-rich blood.

Iron overload occurs more in men than in women. An argument against the fortification of foods with iron to protect women is that it might put more men at risk of overload. Indeed, some evidence from Sweden, where foods are generously fortified with iron, indicates that food fortification has increased the incidence of iron overload in men.

The rapid ingestion of massive amounts of iron can cause sudden death. The second most common cause of accidental poisoning in small children (after aspirin overdose) is ingestion of iron supplements or vitamins with iron. As few as 6 to 12 tablets have caused death in a child. A child suspected of iron poisoning should be rushed to the hospital to have the stomach pumped. Thirty minutes can make a crucial difference.

The usual Western mixed diet provides only about 6 to 7 milligrams of iron in every 1,000 kcalories. The recommended daily intake for an adult man is 10 milligrams; most men easily eat more than 2,000 kcalories, so a man can meet his iron needs without special effort. The recommendation for women during childbearing years, however, is 15 milligrams.[17] Because women have higher iron needs and typically consume fewer than 2,000 kcalories per day, they have trouble achieving an appropriate iron intake. On the average, women receive only 10 to 11 milligrams of iron per day. A woman who wants to meet her iron needs from foods must emphasize the most iron-rich foods in every food group.

Several factors significantly influence the absorption of iron. Iron occurs in two forms in foods: as heme iron, bound into the iron-carrying proteins hemoglobin and myoglobin in meats, poultry, and fish; and as nonheme iron. Heme iron contributes a smaller portion of the iron consumed by most people, but healthy people absorb it at a fairly constant rate of about 23 percent. People absorb nonheme iron at a lower rate (2 to 20 percent); its absorption depends on dietary factors and iron stores. Most of the dietary iron consumed is nonheme iron from vegetables, grains, eggs, meat, fish, and poultry.

Dietary enhancing factors include MFP and vitamin C. Meat, fish, and poultry contain a factor (MFP factor) other than heme that promotes the absorption of iron, even of the iron from other foods eaten at the same time. Vitamin C eaten in the same meal also doubles or triples iron absorption (except heme iron). Tea and coffee interfere with iron absorption.

The following set of guidelines, then, can be used for planning an iron-rich diet:

- *Milk and cheese.* Don't overdo foods from the milk group; they are poor sources of iron. But don't omit them either, because they are rich in calcium. Drink nonfat milk to free kcalories to be invested in iron-rich foods.
- *Meats.* Use liver and other organ meats frequently, perhaps every week or two. Meat, fish, and poultry are excellent iron sources.
- *Meat substitutes.* Don't forget legumes. A cup of peas or beans can supply up to 7 milligrams of iron.
- *Breads and cereals.* Use only whole-grain, enriched, and fortified products (iron is one of the enrichment nutrients).

hemochromatosis (heem-oh-crome-a-TOE-siss): iron overload characterized by deposits of iron-containing pigment in many tissues, with tissue damage. Hemochromatosis is a hereditary defect in iron metabolism.

hemosiderosis (heem-oh-sid-er-OH-sis): iron overload characterized by excessive iron deposits in hemosiderin, the normal iron-storage protein.

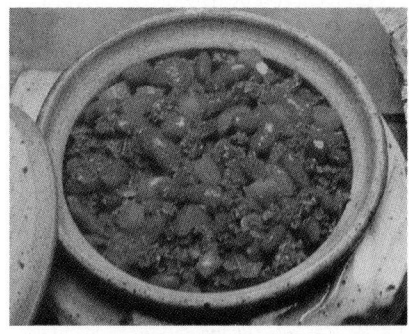

The meat and tomatoes in this chili help the eater to absorb iron from the beans.

About 40% of the iron in meat, fish, and poultry is bound into molecules of heme (HEEM), the iron-holding part of the hemoglobin and myoglobin proteins. This heme iron is much more absorbable (23%) than nonheme iron.

Overconsumption of milk is a common cause of iron deficiency in children; the resulting anemia is known as milk anemia.

Enrichment and fortification are defined on p. 130.

FIGURE 8–6   **Iron in Foods**

Half a liverwurst, whole-wheat sandwich: 2.34 mg

5 steamed clams: 6.30 mg

½ c black beans: 1.80 mg

½ c spinach: 3.21 mg

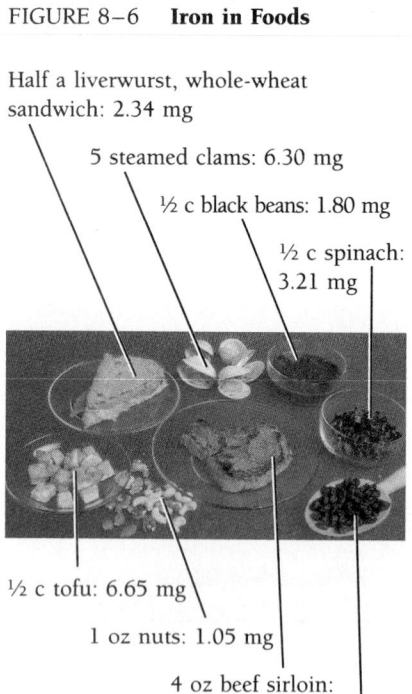

½ c tofu: 6.65 mg

1 oz nuts: 1.05 mg

4 oz beef sirloin: 2.80 mg

¼ c raisins: 0.86 mg

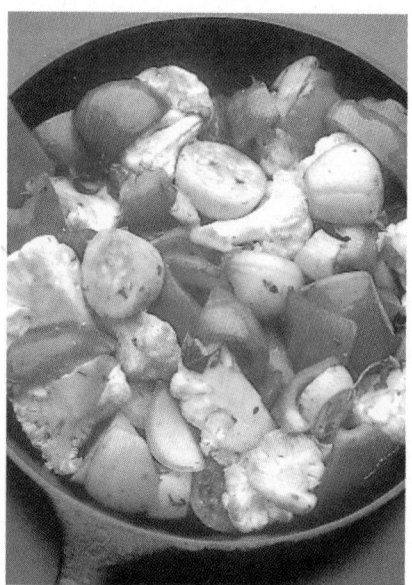

The old-fashioned iron skillet adds additional iron to foods.

■ *Vegetables.* The dark green, leafy vegetables are rich in vitamin C and iron. Eat vitamin C–rich vegetables often to enhance absorption of the iron from foods eaten with them.

■ *Fruits.* Dried fruits, such as raisins, apricots, peaches, and prunes, are high in iron. Eat vitamin C–rich fruits often with iron-containing foods.

Figure 8–6 shows the iron found in usual serving sizes of different foods. Some foods are better choices than others for the person with a limited energy allowance. For example, in the figure, both the half cup of black beans and the ounce of nuts offer about 1 milligram of iron. The black beans offer that much iron for an energy cost of about 100 kcalories, while the nuts cost 200 kcalories for the same amount of iron. Additionally, cooking with iron skillets can contribute iron to the diet.

Zinc

Zinc is a versatile, active trace element; more than 70 enzymes require zinc as a cofactor. These zinc-requiring enzymes perform tasks in the eyes, liver, kidney, muscles, skin, bones, and male reproductive organs. Wherever protein is, zinc is, and it helps with the jobs that proteins do. Zinc is necessary for normal metabolism of protein, carbohydrate, fat, and alcohol. It is associated with the hormone insulin in the pancreas, interacts with platelets in blood clotting, affects thyroid hormone function, and affects behavior and learning performance. Zinc assists proteins involved in the synthesis of the genetic materials DNA and RNA, cell replication, immune reactions, the cells' production and disposal of carbon dioxide, utilization of vitamin A, taste perception, wound healing, the making of sperm, and the development of the fetus.

The body's handling of zinc differs from that of iron, but with some interesting similarities. For example, like iron, extra zinc that enters the body is held within the intestinal cells, and only the amount needed is released into the bloodstream. Like iron, the zinc status of the individual influences the percentage of zinc absorbed from the diet; if more is needed, more is absorbed.

Zinc's main transport vehicle in the blood is the protein albumin. Research suggests that circulating albumin is a main determinant of zinc absorption.[18] This may account for observations that zinc absorption declines in conditions that lower plasma albumin concentrations—for example, pregnancy and malnutrition.

Zinc deficiency in human beings was first reported in the 1960s from studies of growing children and male adolescents in Egypt, Iran, and Turkey. The diets were typically low in zinc and high in fiber and phytates. Diets high in phytates impair zinc absorption. The zinc deficiency was marked by dwarfism or severe growth retardation, as well as arrested sexual maturation—symptoms that were responsive to zinc supplementation.

Since that time, zinc deficiency has been recognized elsewhere and is known to affect more than growth. It drastically impairs immune function; causes loss of appetite; and during pregnancy, may lead to developmental disorders.[19] A detailed list of symptoms of zinc deficiency is presented in Table 8–7, later in the chapter. Conditions other than poor diet that contribute to the development of zinc deficiency include loss of blood due to parasitic infections, climates that increase sweat losses, and clay eating.

Clay eating: see **pica,** p. 166.

Pronounced zinc deficiency is not widespread in developed countries, but deficiencies do occur in the most vulnerable groups of the U.S. population—pregnant women, young children, the elderly, and the poor. Survey data indicate that zinc intakes of adults in the United States fall short of the RDA.[20] The zinc RDA for men is 15 milligrams per day; for women, 12 milligrams. Research shows that even mild zinc deficiency can result in metabolic changes such as impaired immune response, abnormal taste, and abnormal dark adaptation (zinc is required to produce the active form of vitamin A, retinal, in visual pigments).[21]

Pregnant teenagers are at particular risk, because they need zinc for their own ongoing growth, as well as for the developing fetus. Persons on limited food intakes, such as those on weight-control regimens, may also be at risk. A warning to those following very-low-kcalorie or starvation diets: such diets cause not only a low zinc intake but also a loss of zinc from body tissues being broken down as a source of energy. Older people who eat little food may also have limited zinc intakes. People in the hospital with poor appetites or those receiving inadequate nutrition support (Chapter 15) are at risk. Certain drug therapies can impair zinc absorption (see Appendix B).

Vegetarians, especially pregnant vegetarians, who consume large amounts of fiber, phytate, and dairy foods or low levels of protein need to have their diets scrutinized for possible zinc deficiency. Populations dependent on food staples or cultural foods high in phytate and fiber content need to be evaluated as well for zinc status.

Zinc is highest in foods with high protein content, such as shellfish (especially oysters), meats, and liver. As a rule of thumb, two ordinary servings a day of animal protein provide most of the zinc a healthy person needs. Milk, eggs, and whole-grain products are good sources of zinc if large quantities are eaten. For the infant, breast milk is a good source of zinc and is more efficiently absorbed from human milk than from cow's milk. Commercial infant formulas are fortified with zinc, of course. Figure 8–7 shows zinc-rich foods.

FIGURE 8–7   **Zinc in Foods**

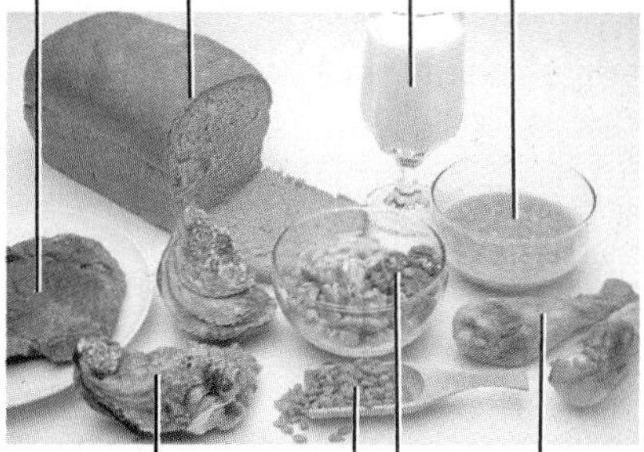

Pork chop: 1.7 mg

Whole-wheat bread: 0.5 mg per slice

Milk: 0.9 mg per cup

Pea soup: 1.3 mg per cup

6 large oysters: 25 mg

Peanuts: 1.9 mg per ounce

Cooked legumes: 2.4 mg per cup

Drumstick: 1.7 mg

Whole-grain breads and cereals contain zinc, but they also contain phytate and fiber. Refined breads and cereals are stripped of their phytate and fiber, but they also contain less zinc. Which is a better zinc source, the whole-grain or the refined product? The answer has to do with the numbers of molecules of zinc and zinc binder present in the grain. Whole grains contain phytate and fiber, yes, but they contain relatively more zinc—enough so that the excess zinc is greater per serving of whole-grain bread than the amount available from a comparable serving of refined bread. Even though whole grains do contain some bound, unavailable zinc, they are still preferred to refined products as a zinc source.

This example illustrates a principle that may well have occurred to you many times. Nutrition "facts" are often more complicated than they may at first seem.

Zinc is a relatively nontoxic element; however, it can be toxic if consumed in large enough quantities. A high zinc intake is known to produce copper-deficiency anemia. Accidental consumption of high levels of zinc can cause vomiting, diarrhea, fever, exhaustion, and a host of other symptoms (see Table 8–7, later in the chapter). Large doses can even be fatal.

Zinc supplements are not recommended except for an accurately diagnosed zinc deficiency or when needed for use as a drug to displace other ions in unusual medical circumstances. Normally, it should be possible to obtain enough zinc from the diet.

Selenium

selenium (se-LEEN-ee-um)

The enzyme of which selenium is a part is glutathione peroxidase, which destroys oxidative compounds that could otherwise oxidize other compounds in the cell.

The heart disease caused by selenium deficiency is named Keshan disease, for one of the provinces of China where it was studied.

Selenium is a trace element that functions as part of an antioxidant enzyme. Selenium has a sparing effect on vitamin E and can substitute for vitamin E in some of that vitamin's antioxidant activities. Selenium's function as an antioxidant was, at first, the only evidence of its essentiality for human beings. The discovery that selenium deficiency was the cause of heart disease in hundreds of thousands of children in China spurred greater interest in selenium and intensified research efforts to learn more about this mineral. The question of whether selenium protects against the development of some cancers is currently under investigation. So far, the results are inconclusive.

High doses of selenium are toxic. Selenium toxicity causes vomiting, diarrhea, loss of hair and nails, and lesions of the skin and nervous system. The inappropriate use of selenium supplements as an anticancer agent increases the possibility of selenium overdose.[22]

Iodine

Iodine occurs in the body in minuscule amounts, but its principal role in human nutrition is well known, and the amount needed is well established. Iodine is an integral part of the thyroid hormones, which regulate body temperature, metabolic rate, reproduction, growth, the making of blood cells, nerve and muscle function, and more.

The ocean is the world's major source of iodine. In coastal areas, seafood, water, and even iodine-containing sea mist are important iodine sources. Further inland, the amount of iodine in the diet is variable and generally reflects the amount present in the soil in which plants are grown or on which animals graze. In areas of the United States where the soil is iodine-poor (most notably in the Plains states), the use of iodized salt has largely wiped out the iodine deficiency that once was widespread.

People sometimes wonder whether sea salt, made by drying ocean water, is preferable to purified sodium chloride for use in the salt shaker. Sea salt does contain trace minerals, but it loses its iodine during the drying process. Thus in regions where goiter is a risk, iodized sodium chloride is the salt to choose.

When the iodine concentration in the blood is low, the cells of the thyroid gland enlarge in an attempt to trap as many particles of iodine as possible. If the gland enlarges until it is visible, the swelling is called a simple goiter. As many as 800 million people are at risk of developing iodine deficiency.[23]

Goiter is estimated to affect 200 million people the world over. In all but 4 percent of these cases, the cause is iodine deficiency. As for the 4 percent (8 million), those people have goiter because they overconsume plants of the cabbage family and others that contain an antithyroid substance whose effect is not counteracted by dietary iodine.

In addition to causing sluggishness and weight gain, an iodine deficiency may have serious effects on the development of an infant in the uterus. Severe thyroid undersecretion during pregnancy causes the extreme and irreversible mental and physical retardation known as cretinism. A cretin has an IQ as low as 20 (100 is normal) and a face and body with many abnormalities. Much of the mental retardation associated with cretinism can be averted if the pregnant woman's deficiency is detected and treated in time.

The need for iodine is easy to meet by consuming seafood, vegetables grown in iodine-rich soil, and (in iodine-poor areas) iodized salt. In the United States, you have to read the label to find out whether salt is iodized; in Canada, all table salt is iodized.

Excessive intakes of iodine can also cause an enlargement of the thyroid gland, just as a deficiency can. In infants, the goiterlike condition can be so severe as to block the airways and cause suffocation.

Iodine intakes in the United States rose dramatically for several decades but are presently on the decline. The emphasis on salt-restricted diets to control high blood pressure is no doubt a contributing factor to declining intakes. The RDA for both men and women is 150 micrograms per day. The U.S. Food and Drug Administration's Total Diet Study found the typical intake for men to be about 250 micrograms and for women, about 170 micrograms, excluding intakes from iodized salt; thus deficiency is not a problem.[24]

goiter (GOY-ter): an enlargement of the thyroid gland due to an iodine deficiency, malfunction of the gland, or overconsumption of a goitrogen. Goiter caused by iodine deficiency is *simple goiter.*

goitrogen: a thyroid antagonist found in food, which causes toxic goiter.

cretinism (CREE-tin-ism): an iodine-deficiency disease characterized by mental and physical retardation.

Copper

The body contains about 75 to 100 milligrams of copper, which performs several vital roles. Copper is part of several enzymes. As a catalyst in the formation of hemoglobin, it helps to make red blood cells. It is involved in the manufacture of the protein collagen, in the healing of wounds, and in the maintenance of sheaths around nerve fibers. One of copper's most vital roles is to ensure the proper utilization of iron.

Copper deficiency is rare but not unknown. It has been seen in children with kwashiorkor and iron-deficiency anemia, and it can severely disturb growth and metabolism. Excess zinc interferes with copper absorption and can cause deficiency. No RDA is set for copper, but the estimated safe and adequate daily dietary intake is 1.5 to 3 milligrams per day.

The best food sources of copper include organ meats, seafood, nuts, and seeds. About a third of the copper taken in food is absorbed, and the rest is eliminated in feces.

Estimated sale and adequate dietary intake for copper: 1.5 to 3.0 mg/day.

Manganese

Animal studies suggest that manganese cooperates with many enzymes, helping to facilitate dozens of different metabolic processes. Deficiencies of

Estimated safe and adequate dietary intake for manganese: 2.5 to 5.0 mg/day.

manganese have not been seen in people, but toxicity may be severe. Miners who inhale large quantities of manganese dust on the job over prolonged periods show many symptoms of a brain disease, with frightening abnormalities in appearance and behavior.

The example of manganese underscores the fact that it is as important not to overdose as it is to have an adequate intake. The Committee on RDA underscores this point by adding a special warning to its trace mineral table: "not to exceed the upper end of the range of recommended intakes." Now that more trace minerals are known, the National Nutrition Consortium also is concerned that these trace minerals will be added to vitamin-mineral pills, making toxic overdoses more likely. Since the FDA is not permitted to enforce limits on the amounts of trace minerals added to supplements, this is an area in which consumers themselves have to be careful. Beware of supplements containing trace minerals. It is a safer bet to consume a diet that provides foods from a variety of sources than to try to put together a combination of pills that will meet all your needs without causing toxicity.

Fluoride

Only a trace of fluoride occurs in the human body, but research demonstrates that where diets are high in fluoride during the time of tooth development, the crystalline structure of teeth is altered such that the enamel is more resistant to caries-producing acid. Once teeth have erupted, the topical application of fluoride by way of toothpaste or mouth rinse, for example, continues to exert a caries-reducing effect.[25]

All normal diets include some fluoride, but drinking water is usually the most significant source. Fish and tea may supply substantial amounts. Where fluoride is lacking in the water supply, the incidence of dental decay is high. Dental problems are of great concern, because they can lead to a multitude of other health problems affecting the whole body. Thus fluoridation of community water where needed is an important public health measure. Despite fluoride's value, violent disagreement often surrounds the introduction of fluoride to a community.

In some areas, the natural fluoride concentration in water is high, and children's teeth develop with mottled enamel. Although this condition, called fluorosis, may not be harmful, it violates some people's prejudice that teeth should be white. In fact, such children's teeth may be extraordinarily decay resistant. Fluorosis does not usually occur in communities where fluoride is added to the water supply.

In communities where fluoride in the water supply falls short of 1 part per million, individual consumers who want the protection provided by fluoride can take other measures. They can use fluoride toothpaste or tablets and can make sure their children have fluoride applied directly to their teeth as part of dental care.

fluorosis (floor-OH-sis): mottling of the tooth enamel from ingestion of too much fluoride during tooth development.

Estimated safe and adequate dietary intake for fluoride: 1.5 to 4.0 mg/day.

Chromium

Chromium is an essential mineral that participates in carbohydrate and lipid metabolism. Experiments on animals have shown that chromium works closely with the hormone insulin, facilitating the uptake of glucose into cells. One form of chromium occurs in association with several different complexes in foods. Best absorbed and most active is a small organic compound named the glucose tolerance factor (GTF). This compound has been purified from brewer's yeast, but its complete structure and function continue to elude researchers.

Chromium deficiency is unlikely, given the small amount required and its presence in a variety of foods.[26] The more people eat refined foods, the less chromium they obtain from their diets. Unrefined foods such as liver, brewer's yeast, whole grains, nuts, and cheeses are the best sources.

Chromium deficiency is difficult to detect, but the effectiveness of insulin is severely impaired when chromium is lacking in the diet. A diabetes-like condition results. Chromium has been shown to remedy impaired carbohydrate metabolism in several groups of older people in the United States. Depleted tissue concentrations have been linked to growth failure in children with protein-energy malnutrition. Chromium toxicity from eating food sources of this element is unknown.

GTF (glucose tolerance factor): a small organic compound containing chromium, which enhances insulin's action.

Estimated safe and adequate dietary intake for chromium: 50 to 200 μg/day.

Molybdenum

Molybdenum has also been recognized as an important mineral in human and animal physiology. It functions as a working part of several metal-containing enzymes, some of which are giant proteins. Deficiencies or toxicities of molybdenum are unknown in human beings.

molybdenum (mo-LIB-duh-num)

Estimated safe and adequate dietary intake for molybdenum: 75 to 250 μg/day.

Other Trace Minerals

The trace minerals have been known for decades, but their role as nutrients is a recent surprise. Nickel is now recognized as important for the health of many body tissues. Nickel deficiencies harm the liver and other organs. Silicon is known to be involved in bone calcification, at least in animals. Tin is necessary for growth in animals, and probably in people also. Cobalt is recognized as the mineral in the large vitamin B_{12} molecule. In the future, we may discover that other trace minerals also play key roles: silver, mercury, lead, barium, and cadmium, for example. Even arsenic—famous as the death potion in many murder mysteries and known to be a carcinogen—may turn out to be an essential nutrient in tiny quantities.

In summary, the body requires trace minerals in tiny amounts, and they function in similar ways—assisting enzymes all over the body. Eating a diet that consists of a variety of foods is the best way to ensure an adequate intake of these important nutrients. Many dietary factors, including the trace minerals themselves, affect the absorption and availability of these nutrients.

Like the vitamins, the minerals perform a multitude of functions throughout the body. Table 8–7 offers a summary of facts about minerals in the body.

TABLE 8–7   **The Minerals—A Summary**

MINERAL NAME AND RDA FOR HEALTHY ADULTS[a]	CHIEF FUNCTIONS IN THE BODY	DEFICIENCY SYMPTOMS	TOXICITY SYMPTOMS	SIGNIFICANT SOURCES
		Major Minerals		
Calcium, phosphorus RDA: Calcium: 800 mg Phosphorus: 800 mg	The principal minerals of bones and teeth. Calcium also acts in normal muscle contraction and relaxation, nerve functioning, blood clotting, blood pressure, and immune defenses. Phosphorus is important in cells' genetic material, in cell membranes as phospholipids, in energy transfer, and in buffering systems.	Calcium: stunted growth in children, adult bone loss (osteoporosis). Phosphorus deficiency unknown.	Excess calcium is excreted except in hormonal imbalance states (not caused by nutritional deficiency). Excess phosphorus may cause calcium excretion.	Calcium: milk and milk products, small fish (with bones), tofu (bean curd), greens, legumes. Phosphorus: all animal tissues.
Magnesium RDA: Females: 350 mg Males: 280 mg	Another factor involved in bone mineralization, the building of protein, enzyme action, normal muscular contraction, transmission of nerve impulses, and maintenance of teeth.	Weakness; confusion; depressed pancreatic hormone secretion; if extreme, convulsions, bizarre movements (especially of eyes and face), hallucinations, and difficulty in swallowing; in children, growth failure.	Not known; large doses have been taken in the form of the laxative Epsom salts, without ill effects except diarrhea.	Nuts, legumes, whole grains, dark green vegetables, seafood, chocolate, cocoa.
Sodium	Sodium, chloride, and potassium (electrolytes): maintain cells' normal fluid balance and acid-base balance in the body. Sodium is critical to nerve impulse transmission.	Muscle cramps, mental apathy, loss of appetite.	Hypertension.	Salt, soy sauce, processed foods.

[a]The RDA used in this table are for adults age 25–50. For other age groups see inside front cover.

TABLE 8–7 *(continued)*

MINERAL NAME AND RDA FOR HEALTHY ADULTS	CHIEF FUNCTIONS IN THE BODY	DEFICIENCY SYMPTOMS	TOXICITY SYMPTOMS	SIGNIFICANT SOURCES
Chloride	Part of the hydrochloric acid found in the stomach, necessary for proper digestion.	Growth failure in children, muscle cramps, mental apathy, loss of appetite, can cause death (uncommon).	Normally harmless (the gas chlorine is a poison but evaporates from water); can cause vomiting.	Salt; soy sauce; moderate quantities in whole, unprocessed foods; large amounts in processed foods.
Potassium	Facilitates reactions, including the making of protein, the maintenance of fluid and electrolyte balance, the support of cell integrity, the transmission of nerve impulses, and the contraction of muscles (including the heart).	Deficiency accompanies dehydration; causes muscular weakness, paralysis, and confusion; can cause death.	Causes muscular weakness; triggers vomiting; if given into a vein, can stop the heart.	All whole foods: meats, milk, fruits, vegetables, grains, legumes.
Sulfur	A component of certain amino acids; part of the vitamins biotin and thiamin and the hormone insulin; combines with toxic substances to form harmless compounds; as part of proteins, stabilizes their shape by forming sulfur-sulfur bridges.	None known; protein deficiency would occur first.	Would occur only if sulfur amino acids were eaten in excess; this (in animals) depresses growth.	All protein-containing foods.
Trace Minerals				
Iodine RDA: 150 µg	A component of the thyroid hormone thyroxin, which helps to regulate growth, development, and metabolic rate.	Goiter, cretinism.	Depressed thyroid activity, goiterlike thyroid enlargement.	Iodized salt, seafood, plants grown in most parts of the country and animals fed those plants.

TABLE 8–7   (*continued*)

MINERAL NAME AND RDA FOR HEALTHY ADULTS	CHIEF FUNCTIONS IN THE BODY	DEFICIENCY SYMPTOMS	TOXICITY SYMPTOMS	SIGNIFICANT SOURCES
Iron RDA: Females: 15 mg Males: 10 mg	Part of the protein hemoglobin, which carries oxygen in the blood; part of the protein myoglobin in muscles, which makes oxygen available for muscle contraction; necessary for the utilization of energy.	Anemia: weakness, pallor, headaches, reduced resistance to infection, inability to concentrate, lowered cold tolerance.	Iron overload: infections, liver injury, acidosis, bloody stools, shock.	Red meats, fish, poultry, shellfish, eggs, legumes, dried fruits.
Selenium RDA: Females: 55 μg Males: 70 μg	Part of an enzyme that breaks down reactive chemicals that harm cells; works with vitamin E.	Muscle discomfort, weakness, pancreas damage, heart disease (cardiomyopathy).	Nausea, abdominal pain, nail and hair changes, nerve damage, fatigue, irritability, diarrhea.	Seafoods; organ meats; other meats; grains and vegetables, depending on soil conditions.
Zinc RDA: Females: 12 mg Males: 15 mg	Part of the hormone insulin and many enzymes; involved in making genetic material and proteins, immune reactions, transport of vitamin A, taste perception, wound healing, the making of sperm, the normal fetal development.	Growth failure in children, sexual retardation, loss of taste, poor wound healing.	Fever, nausea, vomiting, diarrhea, muscle incoordination, dizziness, anemia, accelerated atherosclerosis, kidney failure.	Protein-containing foods: meats, fish, poultry, grains, vegetables.

SELF-STUDY

How Are Your Mineral Intakes?

1. Compare your intakes of minerals with the RDA (inside front cover) or the RNI (Appendix A). Express each intake as a percentage of the recommended intake. For example, suppose you ingested 640 milligrams calcium, and your RDA is 800 milligrams. You ingested 80 percent (640/800 × 100) of your RDA. If you had ingested 1,400 milligrams calcium, you would have ingested 175 percent (1,400/800 × 100) of your RDA. Use Form 9 to record your findings.

   Comment on your mineral intakes. For any mineral for which your intake fell below 80 percent of the recommendation, what were your best food sources? Could you eat more of them to bring your intake up to the recommended level? If not, what food or foods could you eat to increase your intake?

2. Compute your iron absorption from a meal of your choosing. Three factors go into the calculation. First, how much of the iron in the meal was heme iron and how much was nonheme iron? Second, how much vitamin C was in the meal? Third, how much total meat, fish, and poultry (MFP) was consumed? Here's how it works. Begin by answering these six questions:
   a. How much iron was from animal tissues (MFP)? _____milligrams
   b. Forty percent of this is heme iron. _____milligrams heme iron
   c. How much iron was from other sources? _____milligrams
   d. This, plus 60 percent of the iron from animal tissues (MFP), is nonheme iron. _____milligrams nonheme iron
   e. How much vitamin C was in the meal? _____Less than 25 milligrams is low; 25 to 75 milligrams is medium; more than 75 milligrams is high.
   f. How much MFP was in the meal? _____Less than 1 ounce lean MFP is low; 1 to 3 ounces is medium; more than 3 ounces is high.

Now you're ready to calculate your total iron absorption. You absorbed 23 percent of the heme iron (see step b), or _____milligrams heme iron. Now take your best response from step e or f. If either vitamin C or MFP was high, the availability of your nonheme iron was high. If neither was high but either was average, the availability of your nonheme iron was medium. If both were low, your nonheme iron had poor availability. You absorbed:

▬ High availability: 8 percent of the nonheme iron.
▬ Medium availability: 5 percent of the nonheme iron.
▬ Poor availability: 3 percent of the nonheme iron.
▬ Your availability: _____milligrams nonheme iron absorbed.

Now compare your iron absorption by adding the two together:
   _____ milligrams heme iron absorbed.
   _____ milligrams nonheme iron absorbed.
Total = _____ milligrams iron absorbed.

FORM 9   **Mineral Intakes Compared with Recommended Intakes**

	CALCIUM	IRON	ZINC
My intake			
Recommended intake[a]			
My intake as a percentage of the recommended intake			

[a]RDA or RNI (Appendix A).

Study Questions

1. Describe some of the functions of water in the body.
2. List three sources of water intake and four routes for water excretion in the body.
3. How does the body use electrolytes to regulate fluid balance?
4. Describe osmotic pressure.
5. What is ADH? Where does it exert its action?
6. List the major minerals, and describe a role for each one.
7. Describe osteoporosis, and list some of its risk factors.
8. Where does most of the sodium in the diet come from?
9. Describe some of the body's special provisions for iron.
10. Why is the risk of iron deficiency greater for women than for men?
11. What is a pica?
12. Why might pregnant vegetarian women be at risk for zinc deficiency?
13. What do selenium and vitamin E have in common?
14. Describe goiter.
15. How is fluoride important to the body?

Notes

1. P. H. Baylis, Osmoregulation and control of vasopressin secretion in healthy humans, *American Journal of Physiology* 235 (1987): 671–678.
2. H. Rasmussen, The cycling of calcium as an intracellular messenger, *Scientific American,* October 1989, pp. 66–73.
3. V. Matkovic, Calcium metabolism and calcium requirements during skeletal modeling and consolidation of bone mass, *American Journal of Clinical Nutrition* 54 (Supplement, 1991): 245–260.
4. D. A. McCarron and coauthors, Dietary calcium and blood pressure: Modifying factors in specific populations, *American Journal of Clinical Nutrition* 54 (Supplement 1991): 215–219.
5. K. Clark, Calcium and hypertension: Does a relationship exist? *Nutrition Today,* July/August 1989, pp. 21–26; J. T. Repke and J. Villar,

Pregnancy-induced hypertension and low birth weight: The role of calcium, *American Journal of Clinical Nutrition* 54 (Supplement, 1991): 237–241.

6. H. S. Wright and coauthors, The 1987–88 Nationwide Food Consumption Survey: An update on the nutrient intake of respondents, *Nutrition Today,* May/June 1991, pp. 21–27; R. P. Heaney, J. A. Creighton, and M. J. Barger-Lux, Calcium nutrition and prevention of disease, *Food and Nutrition News,* March/April 1991, pp. 7–9.

7. Wright and coauthors, 1991.

8. P. O. Wester, Magnesium, *American Journal of Clinical Nutrition* 45 (1987): 1305–1312; National Academy of Sciences, Food and Nutrition Board, *Recommended Dietary Allowances,* 10th ed. (Washington, D.C.: National Academy Press, 1989), pp. 190–191.

9. Wright and coauthors, 1991.

10. National Academy of Sciences, Food and Nutrition Board, 1989, pp. 250–255.

11. National Academy of Sciences, Food and Nutrition Board, 1989.

12. T. W. Kurtz, H. A. Al-Bander, and R. C. Morris, "Salt-sensitive" essential hypertension in men: Is the sodium ion alone important? *New England Journal of Medicine* 317 (1987): 1043–1048.

13. National Academy of Sciences, Food and Nutrition Board, 1989, pp. 255–257.

14. L. Tobian, Potassium and hypertension, *Nutrition Reviews* 8 (1988): 282–283.

15. K. T. Khaw and E. Barrett-Connor, Dietary potassium and stroke-associated mortality: A 12-year prospective population study, *New England Journal of Medicine* 316 (1987): 235–240.

16. P. R. Dallman, Iron, in *Present Knowledge in Nutrition,* 6th ed., ed. M. L. Brown (Washington, D.C.: International Life Sciences Institute, Nutrition Foundation, 1990), pp. 241–250.

17. National Academy of Sciences, Food and Nutrition Board, 1989.

18. R. A. DiSilvestro and R. J. Cousins, Physiological ligands for copper and zinc, *Annual Review of Nutrition* 3 (1983): 261–288.

19. National Academy of Sciences, Food and Nutrition Board, 1989, pp. 205–211.

20. Wright and coauthors, 1991.

21. A. S. Prasad, Therapeutic role of zinc in disease states, *Nutrition and the M.D.,* May 1991, pp. 1–2.

22. Acute and chronic selenium toxicity (Diet Therapy/Obesity Update), *Nutrition and the M.D.,* January 1991, p. 7.

23. B. S. Hetzel, The iodine deficiency disorders: Their nature and prevention, *Annual Review of Nutrition* 9 (1989), pp. 21–38.

24. J. A. T. Pennington, B. E. Young, and D. B. Wilson, Nutritional elements in U.S. diets: Results from the Total Diet Study, 1982–1986, *Journal of the American Dietetic Association* 89 (1989): 659–664.

25. The impact of fluoride on dental health (position paper of the American Dietetic Association), *Journal of the American Dietetic Association* 89 (1989): 971–974.

26. E. G. Offenbacher and F. X. Pi-Sunyer, Chromium in human nutrition, *Annual Review of Nutrition* 8 (1988): 543–563.

NUTRITION • IN • PRACTICE

8

Nutrition and Premenstrual Syndrome

For the millions of women who suffer symptoms of premenstrual syndrome (PMS), the idea that a vitamin-mineral supplement or a slight change in diet might bring relief is inviting. And no wonder. Surveys show that as many as one in three women suffers one or more symptoms of PMS. Over 100 symptoms—including mood swings, bloating, headaches, breast tenderness, anxiety, and food cravings—have been reported.[1] In about 5 percent of women, at least one physical or psychological symptom can reach such severity as to be temporarily disabling.[2] So far, the prevention or alleviation of PMS remains a challenge. Many nutrition-based remedies have been advocated over the years, and new claims continue to surface. Are they valid?

The scientific literature on PMS and nutrition is inconclusive, conflicting, and confusing. One obstacle researchers encounter in their efforts to find a treatment is that many women with PMS respond favorably to placebo treatments. Despite the uncertainties, to the millions of women afflicted each month with symptoms of PMS, and to the people they live and work with, studies to determine nutrition's role in PMS are no doubt interesting. This Nutrition in Practice reviews possible connections between nutrition and PMS.

How is nutrition related to menstruation and PMS?

The hormones that regulate the menstrual cycle are powerful, and they affect other hormones, neurotransmitters, and many body organs. They alter metabolic rate, glucose tolerance, appetite, and food intake. Many women find that they are hungrier than usual during the week or two prior to menstruation. Research confirms that three things happen during that time:

- Basal metabolic rate speeds up.[3]
- Appetite and food energy intake increase.[4]
- Carbohydrate intake increases.[5]

These findings suggest that eating more food prior to menstruation may be appropriate at that time, because the rise in basal metabolic rate that occurs raises energy need. If any harm comes from eating extra food, it comes from failing to reduce intakes to go with the postmenstrual decline in metabolic rate. Unfortunately, many women attempt to fight their increased appetites in an effort to control their weight. During the two weeks *following* menstruation, this may be relatively easy to do. During the two weeks *prior* to menstruation, however, it may be extremely difficult; women are fighting a natural, hormone-governed increase in metabolic rate and appetite, and possibly even a built-in craving for carbohydrates. It is possible that the stress of responding inappropriately to cyclic changes in appetite and basal metabolic rate contributes to symptoms such as fatigue and tension in women prior to menstruation. In fact, in the above study of women who ate more carbohydrates prior to menstruation, the researchers fed the women a high-carbohydrate meal. An hour later, women with severe PMS

MINIGLOSSARY

placebo (plah-SEE-bow): an inert, harmless substance that resembles medicine; used in research to distinguish the effects of faith and hope from the effects of medicine.

premenstrual syndrome (PMS): a cluster of physical, psychological, and behavioral symptoms that some women experience prior to menstruation; the symptoms diminish during or after menstruation.

reported significant alleviation of the following symptoms: depression, confusion, fatigue, tension, and anger.[6] The high-carbohydrate meal had no effect on women in the control group or on the women with PMS during their postmenstrual week. As in other PMS research, it is possible that the women felt better because they *expected* to (the placebo effect). In any case, the researchers suggest that instead of avoiding carbohydrates, as many women do, they should eat more of them—especially complex carbohydrates such as pasta, whole-grain cereals, and breads—along with vegetables and fruits, especially during the time prior to menstruation. This advice squares with the *NRC Recommendations* of Chapter 1.

Furthermore, when more than 600 women who said they had PMS symptoms were surveyed, one-fourth said they had "changed their diets" to help relieve their symptoms. The most common dietary changes recommended to help relieve PMS discomfort include reducing consumption of sugar, fat, salt, alcohol, and caffeine. Diets that emphasize complex carbohydrates are generally lower in simple sugar, fat, and salt than diets that do not. For this and many other reasons, everyone—including those with PMS—would be wise to eat more complex carbohydrates every day.

You mentioned that common dietary changes recommended to relieve PMS include reducing alcohol and caffeine intake. Is there proof that these changes are beneficial?

Recommendations for women with PMS to reduce their alcohol intakes are based on the knowledge that improvements in general health and well-being are advantageous. Furthermore, alcohol is a depressant. Alcohol can worsen symptoms of mood change and depression in some women. As for caffeine, research shows a dose-dependent relationship between caffeine consumption and PMS prevalence and severity.[7] In other words, premenstrual syndrome is more prevalent among women who consume caffeine than among those who do not. Furthermore, the prevalence and severity of symptoms increase with increasing amounts of caffeine. Thus women who consume caffeine and suffer PMS symptoms may find some relief by reducing their caffeine consumption, especially prior to menstruation.

What about taking vitamin-mineral supplements for PMS? Is PMS caused by vitamin or mineral deficiencies?

No evidence supports nutrient deficiencies as a cause of PMS, and in fact, one study using biochemical tests of nutrition status found no significant difference between women with and without PMS.[8] Despite this, unproven nutrient treatments for PMS continue to be advocated by supplement proponents. Over the years, various nutrients have captured media attention as treatments for PMS. Among the most popular nutrients proposed to treat PMS are vitamin B_6, vitamin E, and most recently, zinc.

Vitamin B_6 has been popularized as a prime candidate for relieving PMS, but trials of vitamin B_6 in PMS have resulted in contradictory findings. One study in which the researchers attempted to use vitamin B_6 to relieve premenstrual depression found that while vitamin B_6 may improve premenstrual symptoms related to autonomic reactions (such as dizziness and vomiting) and behavioral changes (such as poor performance and a tendency to withdraw from social activities), a significant number of physical symptoms remained during the premenstrual phase.[9] In another study, women with PMS symptoms received nutrition counseling, dietary instruction, and vitamin B_6 supplements (250 milligrams per day), or nutrition counseling and dietary instruction only, to see what effects the diet instructions or supplements would have on the severity of PMS symptoms.[10] The researchers found no significant improvement in symptom severity with diet modification or vitamin B_6 supplements. The researchers concluded that evidence of a significant role for vitamin B_6 in PMS is still lacking. Besides, doses of vitamin B_6 as low as 50 milligrams (which is within the range of doses suggested for treatment of PMS) are potentially toxic. For these reasons, any possible benefits derived from this type of therapy must be weighed against the possible detrimental effects of megadoses.

The vitamin B_6–PMS research can be summed up by saying that the vitamin may help remedy symptoms only if a relative or absolute deficiency of the vitamin has caused them. The old lesson of basic nutrition is reinforced here: a vitamin will clear up symptoms caused by a deficiency of that vitamin.

What about vitamin E?

Vitamin E is another popular candidate for treatment of PMS—in fact, many extravagant claims have been made for vitamin E over the years. One condition that may sometimes be caused by vitamin E deficiency is fibrocystic breast disease, as mentioned in Chapter 7. One creditable attempt has demonstrated that vitamin E helps relieve breast pain and tenderness, which is often experienced in PMS. The research involved 41 women in a double-blind, placebo-controlled study. The results suggested that vitamin E (400 IU) brought relief, while the placebo did not. Vitamin E had little effect on many other symptoms of PMS, and until further research is done, the evidence for vitamin E as a treatment for PMS remains inconclusive.[11] Possibly the correct logic is that vitamin E deficiency can cause sore breasts and that the menstrual cycle can make them worse, but not that vitamin E deficiency causes PMS.

What about zinc and PMS?

Because tiny amounts of zinc help regulate the secretion of hormones involved in the menstrual cycle, researchers decided to compare blood zinc concentrations of women with and without PMS.[12] The women with PMS had significantly lower blood zinc concentrations than the women without PMS. The researchers speculate that low blood zinc might impair the secretion of menstrual hormones such as progesterone, as well as the natural opiates, or endorphins, which are the body's own painkillers. Even if zinc deficiency does contribute to PMS, it may affect only some women with the condition. Zinc is toxic in excess. Women should not self-diagnose zinc deficiency or self-prescribe zinc as treatment for PMS. Further research is needed to confirm a relationship between zinc deficiency and PMS. In the meantime, women who suspect their diets may be low in zinc are advised to eat (you guessed it) zinc-rich foods such as those suggested in Chapter 8.

How would you suggest that the person with PMS manage her diet?

The same advice holds for women with PMS as for women or men with any other health problem or need. Be sure to get adequate sleep and adequate exercise. Eat well, and be sensible about intakes of sugar, caffeine, salt, alcohol, and any other "abuse-able" substances. If you have reason to think your nutrient intake is inadequate and you can't rectify it by eating foods, fall back on a daily supplement for a while. But avoid megadoses. Stay with the moderate amounts available in an ordinary multivitamin-mineral supplement (see Nutrition in Practice 7). And be skeptical when someone who wants to pocket your money in return for goods tells you that a product will relieve your symptoms. Watch out for snake-oil salespeople; there are a lot of them out there.

Notes

1. B. Liebman, PMS: Proof or promises? *Nutrition Action,* May 1990, pp. 1, 5–7.
2. R. L. Rein, Premenstrual syndrome, *New England Journal of Medicine* 324 (1991): 1208–1210.
3. P. Webb, 24-hour energy expenditure and the menstrual cycle, *American Journal of Clinical Nutrition* 44 (1986): 614–619.
4. E. J. Gong, D. Garrel, and D. H. Calloway, Menstrual cycle and voluntary food intake, *American Journal of Clinical Nutrition* 49 (1989): 252–258.
5. J. J. Wurtman and coauthors, Effect of nutrient intake on premenstrual depression, *American Journal of Obstetrics and Gynecology* 161 (1989): 1228–1234.
6. Wurtman and coauthors, 1989.
7. A. M. Rossignol and H. Bonnlander, Caffeine-containing beverages, total fluid consumption, and premenstrual syndrome, *American Journal of Public Health* 80 (1990): 1106–1110; A. M. Rossignol and coauthors, Tea and premenstrual syndrome in the People's Republic of China, *American Journal of Public Health* 79 (1989): 67–69.
8. M. Mira, P. M. Stewart, and S. F. Abraham, Vitamin and trace element status in premenstrual syndrome, *American Journal of Clinical Nutrition* 47 (1988): 636–641.
9. K. E. Kendall and P. P. Schnurr, The effects of vitamin B_6 supplementation on premenstrual symptoms, *Obstetrics and Gynecology* 2 (1987): 145–149.
10. M. K. Berman, M. L. Taylor, and E. Freeman, Vitamin B_6 and premenstrual syndrome, *Journal of the American Dietetic Association* 90 (1990): 859–861.
11. R. S. London and coauthors, Efficacy of alpha-tocopherol in the treatment of the premenstrual syndrome, *Journal of Reproductive Medicine* 32 (1987): 400–404.
12. PMS: Hint of a link to lunchtime and zinc, *Science News* 27 October 1990, p. 263.

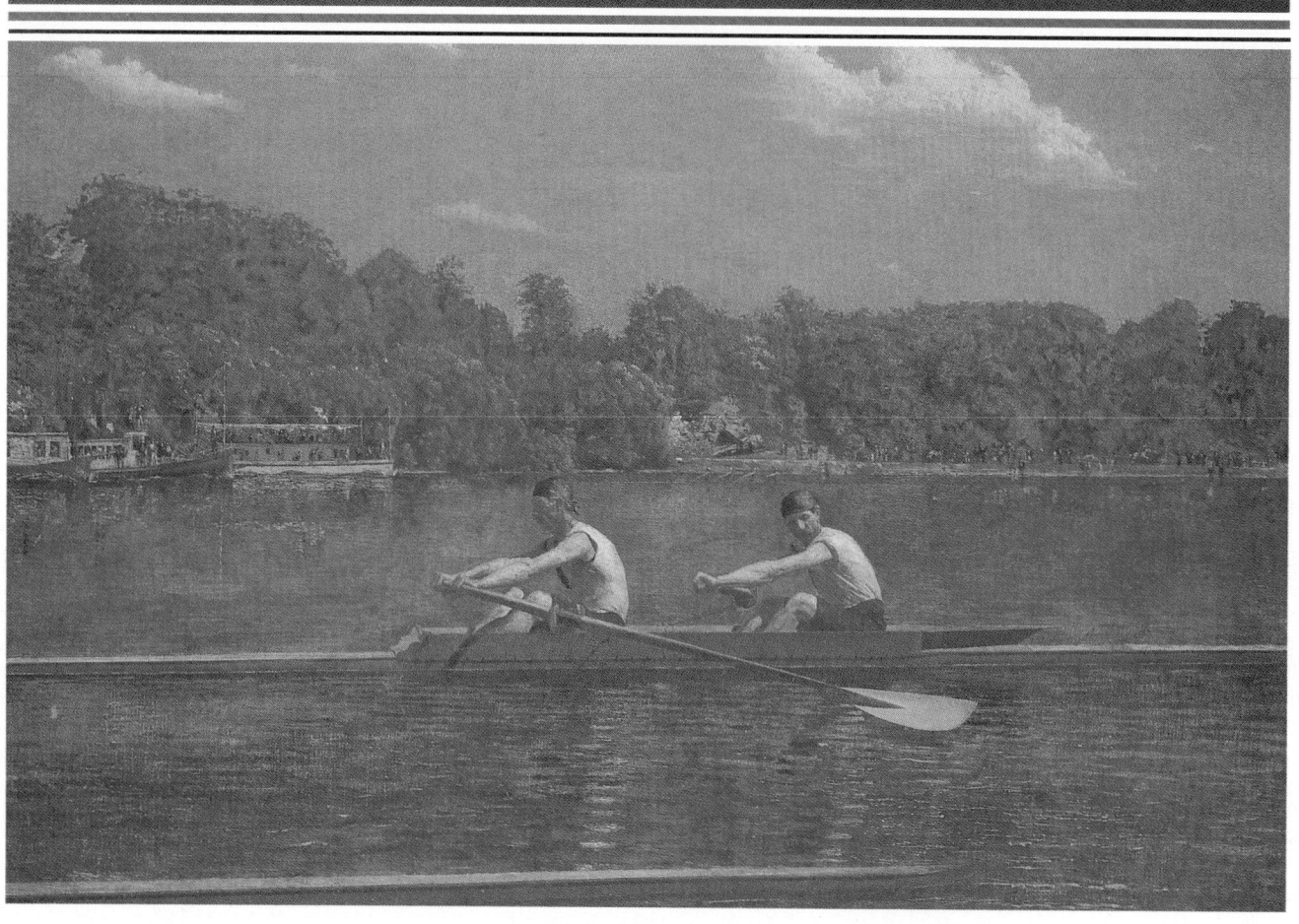

Thomas Eakins, The Biglin Brothers Racing; *National Gallery of Art, Washington; Gift of Mr. and Mrs. Cornelius Vanderbilt Whitney.*

Fitness and Nutrition

CONTENTS

CHAPTER

9

Extensive evidence confirms that regular physical activity promotes health and prevents disease. Still, despite an increasing awareness of the health benefits that physical activity confers, as many as 60 percent of adults in the United States are either irregularly active or completely inactive.[1]

Physical inactivity is linked to the major degenerative diseases—heart disease, cancer, stroke, and hypertension—that are the primary killers of adults in developed countries.[2] Therefore, one of the most important challenges health care professionals face is to motivate more people to become physically active. To motivate others, health care professionals must first become more physically active themselves, thereby enhancing their own health. Second, they can include regular physical activity as a component of therapy for their clients. Even those who make only modest improvements in their fitness can realize health benefits from regular physical activity. In other words, people don't have to run marathons to reap the health rewards of physical activity. Researchers who conducted an extensive study on physical fitness and mortality concluded that "moderate levels of physical fitness that are attainable by most adults appear to be protective against early mortality."[3] Table 9–1 shows that regular physical activity protects against many diseases and conditions.

TABLE 9–1   **Regular Physical Activity Helps to Protect against These Physical Conditions**

- Backaches
- Cancer (colon cancer, breast cancer, and others)[a]
- Diabetes[b]
- Digestive disorders (ulcers, constipation, diarrhea, and others)
- Growth failure in children
- Headaches
- Heart and blood vessel disease (heart attacks and strokes)[c]
- High blood cholesterol, high blood pressure
- Infections (colds, flu, and many others)
- Infertility (some forms)
- Kidney disease[d]
- Menstrual irregularities
- Obesity
- Osteoporosis (adult bone loss)[e]

[a]R. E. Frisch and coauthors, Lower lifetime occurrence of breast cancer and cancers of the reproductive system among former college athletes, *American Journal of Clinical Nutrition* 45 (1987): 328–335; E. R. Eichner, Exercise and cancer prevention, *Sports Medicine Digest,* January 1991, p. 5.

[b]M. J. Franz, Exercise and the management of diabetes mellitus, *Journal of the American Dietetic Association* 87 (1987): 872–880.

[c]L. G. Ekelund and coauthors, Physical fitness as a predictor of cardiovascular mortality in asymptomatic North American men, *New England Journal of Medicine* 319 (1988): 1379–1384.

[d]K. C. Light and coauthors, Psychological stress induces sodium and fluid retention in men at high risk for hypertension, *Science* 220 (1982): 429–431.

[e]B. Krolner and coauthors, Physical exercise as prophylaxis against involutional vertebral bone loss: A controlled trial, *Clinical Science* 64 (1983): 541–546, as cited in M. E. Nelson and coauthors, Diet and bone status in amenorrheic runners, *American Journal of Clinical Nutrition* 43 (1986): 910–916.

This chapter begins by defining fitness and presenting its benefits. The chapter describes the elements of fitness and conditioning, shows how fuel is used during physical activity, and describes how nutrition supports fitness. The chapter closes by showing the relationships between fitness, body composition, and weight control.

Fitness

Perhaps you are already physically fit. If so, the following description applies to you. You are graceful and move with ease. You are strong and meet physical challenges without strain. You have endurance, and your energy lasts for hours. You can meet normal physical challenges with ease and have plenty of energy in reserve to handle emergencies. What is more, you are likely to be well able to meet mental and emotional challenges, too—for physical fitness undergirds mental and emotional, as well as physical, energy and resilience.

If these statements do not describe you as you are today, then you can gain fitness through practice. Activities that promote fitness are themselves enjoyable, and they quickly lead to rewards in terms of physical improvements. Feeling fit can build your confidence in other areas of life, too: social, academic, professional—you name it.

Three Definitions of Fitness

Narrowly defined, the term fitness describes *the characteristics of the body that enable it to perform physical activity.* These characteristics include flexibility of the joints; strength and endurance of the muscles, including the heart muscle; and a healthy body composition. A broader definition of fitness is *the ability to meet routine physical demands, with enough reserve energy to rise to a sudden challenge.* This definition shows how fitness relates to everyday life: ordinary tasks such as carrying heavy suitcases, opening a stuck window, or climbing four flights of stairs, which might strain an unfit person, can be well within the capacity of the fit person. Still another definition is *the body's ability to withstand stress,* meaning stress of all kinds, including psychological stress. There is no contradiction among these three definitions; they are three different descriptions of the same wonderful condition of the body.

A person who practices a physical activity *adapts* by becoming better able to perform it after each session—more flexible, stronger, more enduring. Moreover, a person who gains physical fitness also gains in abilities to take exams in school and to take on major responsibilities in society or on the job. Activity promotes fitness; fitness promotes stress resistance in general; and stress resistance benefits health and life in many, many ways.[4]

Fitness is the reward of a person who leads a physically active life. The opposite of such a life is a sedentary life, which means, literally, "sitting down a lot." Today's world permits many people to lead inactive lives, and even rewards them for it. It provides elevators, escalators, cars, and golf carts

fitness: the characteristics of the body that enable it to perform physical activity; more broadly, the ability to meet routine physical demands with enough reserve energy to rise to a sudden challenge; or the body's ability to withstand stress of all kinds.

sedentary: physically inactive (literally, "sitting down a lot").

so that people can exert a minimum of physical effort. Unfortunately, people are attracted to labor-saving devices, but the more they use them, the more weak and unfit they become, and the less well they feel. The body responds to inactivity by losing muscle and skill, just as it responds to activity by gaining them.

Benefits of Fitness

Physical activity produces fitness; fitness in turn makes activity easy, a beneficial cycle. Activity and fitness are so closely connected that the rest of this chapter makes no distinction between them. The benefits of fitness are the benefits of physical activity, and vice versa.

Fitness contributes to all aspects of health, but most obviously to physical health. Physical health is part of health in general—a large realm that also includes mental, emotional, social, and spiritual health—and fitness enhances these as well (see Figure 9–1). This chapter focuses on physical health, particularly on nutrition and weight control, but as Figure 9–1 shows, fitness benefits every aspect of health. Table 9–2 summarizes the benefits of fitness.

health: a range of states with physical, mental, emotional, social, and spiritual components. At a minimum, health means freedom from negative states in these realms. At a maximum, it means the highest attainable states in these realms.

FIGURE 9–1 **Fitness Contributes to All Aspects of Health**

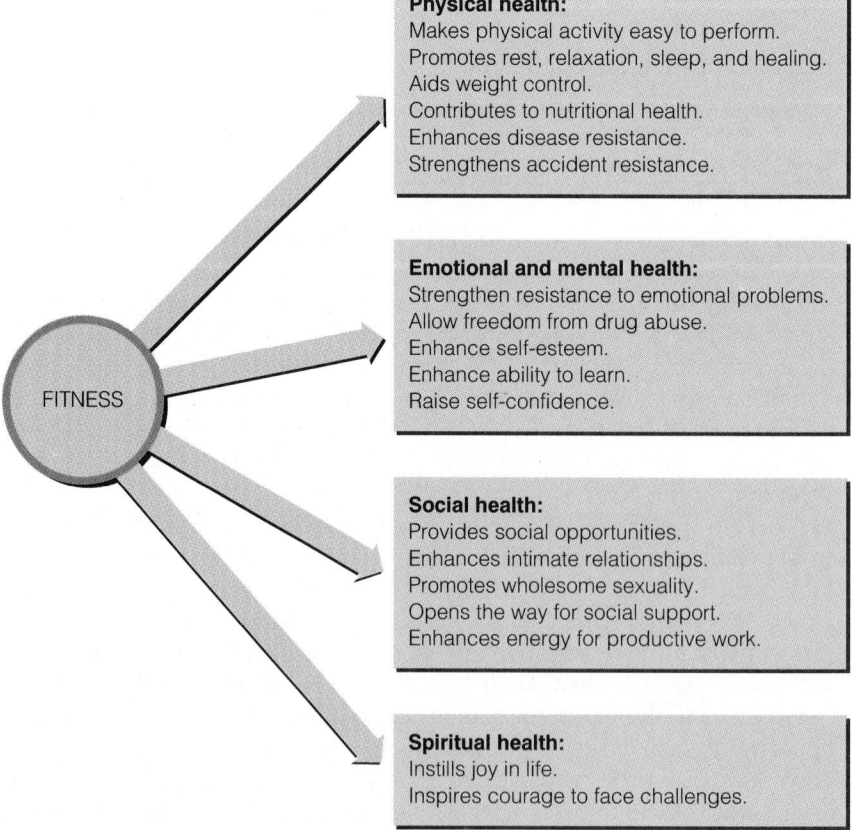

Physical health:
Makes physical activity easy to perform.
Promotes rest, relaxation, sleep, and healing.
Aids weight control.
Contributes to nutritional health.
Enhances disease resistance.
Strengthens accident resistance.

Emotional and mental health:
Strengthen resistance to emotional problems.
Allow freedom from drug abuse.
Enhance self-esteem.
Enhance ability to learn.
Raise self-confidence.

Social health:
Provides social opportunities.
Enhances intimate relationships.
Promotes wholesome sexuality.
Opens the way for social support.
Enhances energy for productive work.

Spiritual health:
Instills joy in life.
Inspires courage to face challenges.

TABLE 9–2   **Benefits of Exercise and Fitness (Summary)**

- Sound, beneficial rest and sleep
- Improved nutritional health
- Reduced fatness and increased lean body tissue
- Improved resistance to colds, other infectious diseases, and cancer
- Reduced risk of heart and blood vessel disease, diabetes, and other diseases
- Reduced probability of accidents; fewer and less severe injuries
- Reduced incidence and severity of anxiety and depression
- Freedom from drug (including alcohol) abuse
- Improved self-image and self-confidence
- Better learning ability
- Greater interpersonal, social, and spiritual strengths
- Improved quality of life in the later years
- Longer life

To be physically fit does not mean you have to be an elite athlete. Rather, you need to develop enough flexibility, muscular strength, and endurance to meet the everyday demands life places on you, plus some to spare, and to achieve a reasonable body weight and body composition.

Components of Fitness

Physical fitness expresses itself in body characteristics. Some are health related; some are skill related. One of the health-related characteristics is flexibility, which is important to the joints. Muscle endurance and strength are important to the muscles. Endurance is also important to the heart and lungs: this type of endurance is called cardiovascular endurance. Fitness also expresses itself in body composition—the proportions of muscle, fat, bone, and other tissue that make up a person's total body weight. Physical activity augments desirable lean body tissue and eliminates excess body fat. As you become physically fit, improving your body composition, flexibility, muscle strength and endurance, and cardiovascular endurance, you improve the health of your entire body.

The person who wants to go beyond general health and enhance athletic *performance* in specific sports will also value *skill-related* components of fitness such as agility, balance, coordination, power, speed, and reaction time. The importance of each characteristic varies widely with individual sports, and athletes practice endless hours to develop them. The miniglossary of Skill-Related Fitness Components describes these characteristics.

flexibility: the ability to bend and recover without injury; it depends on the elasticity of muscles and tendons and on the condition of the joints.

muscle endurance: the ability of a muscle to contract repeatedly within a given time without becoming exhausted.

muscle strength: the ability of muscles to work against resistance.

cardiovascular endurance: the ability of the cardiovascular system to sustain its oxygen-delivery work over a long time.

body composition: the proportions of muscle, bone, fat, and other tissue that make up a person's total body weight.

Principles of Conditioning

Whatever component of fitness you seek to develop—flexibility, strength, or endurance—the principles of conditioning apply. During conditioning, your body adapts microscopically to perform the work you ask of it. The way to achieve conditioning is by training, primarily by applying overload—that is, by asking a little more of yourself in each training session.

conditioning: the physical effect of *training;* improved flexibility, strength, and endurance.

training: practicing an activity, which leads to conditioning. Training is what you do; conditioning is what you get.

Miniglossary of Skill-Related Fitness Components

agility: the ability to move the entire body quickly.

balance: the ability to maintain equilibrium in a fixed position or in motion.

coordination: the harmonious functioning of the senses and the muscles to accurately perform complex movements, such as hitting a baseball or juggling two or more objects.

power: the combination of strength and speed that allows a person to move quickly and forcefully, such as in jumping, shot-putting, or spiking a ball.

speed: the ability to move fast, as in running or swimming.

reaction time: the amount of time between a stimulus and a response to the stimulus, such as when starting a race.

---

overload: an extra physical demand placed on the body; an increase in the *frequency, duration,* or *intensity* of exercise.

progressive overload principle: the training principle that a body system, in order to improve, must be worked at frequencies, durations, or intensities that increase by increments over time.

frequency: the number of occurrences per unit of time (for example, the number of exercise sessions per week).

intensity: the degree of exertion while exercising (for example, the amount of weight lifted or the speed of running).

duration: length of time (for example, the length of time spent in each exercise session).

You can achieve overload by using the progressive overload principle in several different ways. You can perform the activity more often—that is, increase its frequency; you can perform the activity more strenuously—that is, increase its intensity; or you can do it for longer times—that is, increase its duration. All three strategies work well, and you can pick one or a combination, depending on your preferences. For example, if you really love your workout, do it more often. If you do not have much time, increase intensity. If you hate hard work, take it easy and go longer. If you desire continuous improvements, remember to overload progressively as you gain higher levels of fitness.

When you are increasing the frequency, intensity, or duration of your workout, exercise to a point that only *slightly* exceeds your comfortable capacity to work. It is better to progress too slowly than to risk serious injury by overexertion. And, before you begin any fitness program, make sure it is safe to do so. Table 9–3 offers cautions for beginning any exercise program. Allow enough, but not too much, time for recovery between periods of similar exercise (at least, but not more than, 24 to 48 hours). It does not make sense to start with activities so demanding that pain stops you within two days. Learn to enjoy your small steps toward improvement. Fitness builds slowly.

Here are other pointers about applying overload:

- Exercise regularly.
- Train hard only once or twice a week, not every time you work out. Between times, do light workouts.
- Listen to your body, and cooperate. If you feel energetic, work hard; but if you are tired or in pain, go lightly or stop, even if that was not in your original plan.

Training, if done properly, overloads the system without undue strain, as already described. Within training sessions, too, gradualness is a key to success. Sudden intense activity can cause injury, and abrupt discontinu-

TABLE 9–3   **Cautions on Starting Training**

If you answer yes to any of the questions that follow, consult with a health care provider trained in fitness before beginning an exercise program.

- Are you over 35?
- If you are over 35, have you been sedentary for a long time?
- Are you more than 20 lb heavier than you should be?
- Do you now smoke more than a pack and a half of cigarettes per day?
- Do you have any chronic illness?
- Has a health care provider ever said you had heart trouble?
- Did you ever have, or do you now have, a heart murmur?
- Have you ever had a diagnosed or suspected heart attack?
- Do you have chest pains at any time?

ance can hamper recovery, so it is best to ease into and out of activity sessions. The body needs fair warning of physical activity ahead, and after activity, it needs an easy transition into inaction. All strenuous workouts should therefore be fitted inside a frame composed of warm-up and cool-down activities.

A warm-up facilitates gradual warming of the body and also begins the hormonal changes that liberate the needed fuels from storage. Most important, the onset of exercise stimulates the release of the hormone epinephrine, which mobilizes fuels needed for the exercise to come.

Cool-down activity eases the transition from exercising to normal functioning. A few minutes of light activity facilitates the relaxation of tight muscles and enhances the circulation of blood through them. The circulation in turn brings accumulated heat from the body's core to the surface, where it can radiate away. As you approach the end of your workout, gradually ease up on the intensity of the activity (for example, if you are running, begin to slow to a light jog), reaching a minimum intensity over five to ten minutes. Stretching exercises to promote flexibility are particularly well-suited to the end of the cool-down.

Cool-down activities can also help to prevent symptoms—dizziness, for example—that you may experience if you abruptly stop exercising. A cool-down facilitates a gradual drop in blood pressure; an abrupt drop would stress the heart. It can also help to prevent muscle cramps that might otherwise occur.

Your body does physical work every day. The stronger and more fit you are, the less strain it takes to do that work. If your body is weak, you cannot trade it in as you might trade in a car too small to do its job—and fortunately, you do not need to. Unlike a small car, which will break down when consistently overloaded, your body responds to overload in a positive way—it gets itself into better shape to meet the demand next time. As the next section shows, the overload principle applies to the heart muscle in the same way that it does to the other muscles of the body: the heart becomes stronger.

warm-up: five to ten minutes of light exercise, such as easy jogging or cycling, to warm up the body in preparation for vigorous exercise.

epinephrine (ep-ih-NEFF-rin): one of the stress hormones. It is secreted whenever emergency action is called for; it readies body systems for fast action and mobilizes fuel to support that action.

cool-down: five to ten minutes of light exercise following a vigorous workout to gradually cool the body's core to near-normal temperature.

Cardiovascular Endurance

As you know, the heart beats faster during exercise than during rest. The period of time a person can keep exercising with an elevated heart rate—that is, the ability of the heart, lungs, and blood to sustain a given demand—defines the person's cardiovascular endurance. Training can improve ability to sustain a vigorous activity such as running, brisk walking, or swimming. Cardiovascular endurance training enhances the ability of the heart, lungs, and blood to deliver oxygen to, and remove waste from, the body's cells.

Working muscles need oxygen to produce energy. Cardiovascular endurance training requires the heart and lungs to work extra hard to deliver oxygen to the muscle cells for a sustained period. Cardiovascular endurance training, therefore, is *aerobic* (oxygen requiring). As the cardiovascular system gradually adapts to the demands of aerobic exercise, the body delivers oxygen more efficiently.

Muscle cells are not alone in their need for oxygen. All of the cells in the body require oxygen to function. When the cells of the body receive more oxygen more readily, both the body and mind benefit.

The changes gained from aerobic workouts that enhance cardiovascular endurance are called cardiovascular conditioning. Among its components, the total blood volume increases, so the blood can carry more oxygen. The heart becomes larger and stronger, and each beat pumps more blood. As the heart pumps more blood with each beat, fewer beats are necessary, and the pulse rate slows down. The average resting pulse rate for adults is around 70 beats per minute. Thanks to cardiovascular conditioning, active people can have resting pulse rates of 50 or even lower. The muscles that work the lungs become stronger, too, so breathing becomes more efficient. Circulation through the body's arteries and veins improves. Blood moves easily, and blood pressure falls. Cardiovascular endurance is the physical achievement that many people appropriately prize the most highly, because it reflects the health of the heart and circulatory system, on which all other body systems depend. Figure 9–2 shows the major relationships between the heart, circulatory system, and lungs.

To improve your cardiovascular endurance, you must train at an intensity that elevates your heart rate a certain amount beyond its resting level. Your target heart rate zone describes the boundaries within which you should exercise to achieve and maintain cardiovascular fitness. Exercising below your target zone will not condition your cardiovascular system; exercising above it is dangerous and unnecessary.

You can calculate your target heart rate zone from your age and resting heart rate. The older you are, the lower it will be. Figure 9–3 shows how to take your pulse. Table 9–4 shows how to calculate your target heart rate zone.

Once you calculate your target heart rate zone, you have a gauge of how intensely to exercise in order to build cardiovascular fitness. As your cardiovascular fitness improves, you will have to exercise more intensely to reach the same target rate. Be proud; this means you are making progress.

---

cardiovascular endurance: a component of fitness; the ability of the cardiovascular system to sustain effort over a long time.

aerobic (air-ROE-bic): refers to energy-producing processes involving the immediate use of oxygen.
aero = air

cardiovascular conditioning: improvements in the heart and lung function and increased blood volume, brought about by aerobic training.

Training for cardiovascular conditioning:

- Increases blood volume and oxygen delivery.
- Increases heart strength and stroke volume.
- Slows resting pulse.
- Increases breathing efficiency.
- Improves circulation.
- Reduces blood pressure.

stroke volume: the amount of oxygenated blood the heart ejects toward the tissues at each beat.

target heart rate zone: the range of the heartbeat rate that will achieve cardiovascular conditioning for a person—fast enough to push the heart, but not so fast as to strain it.

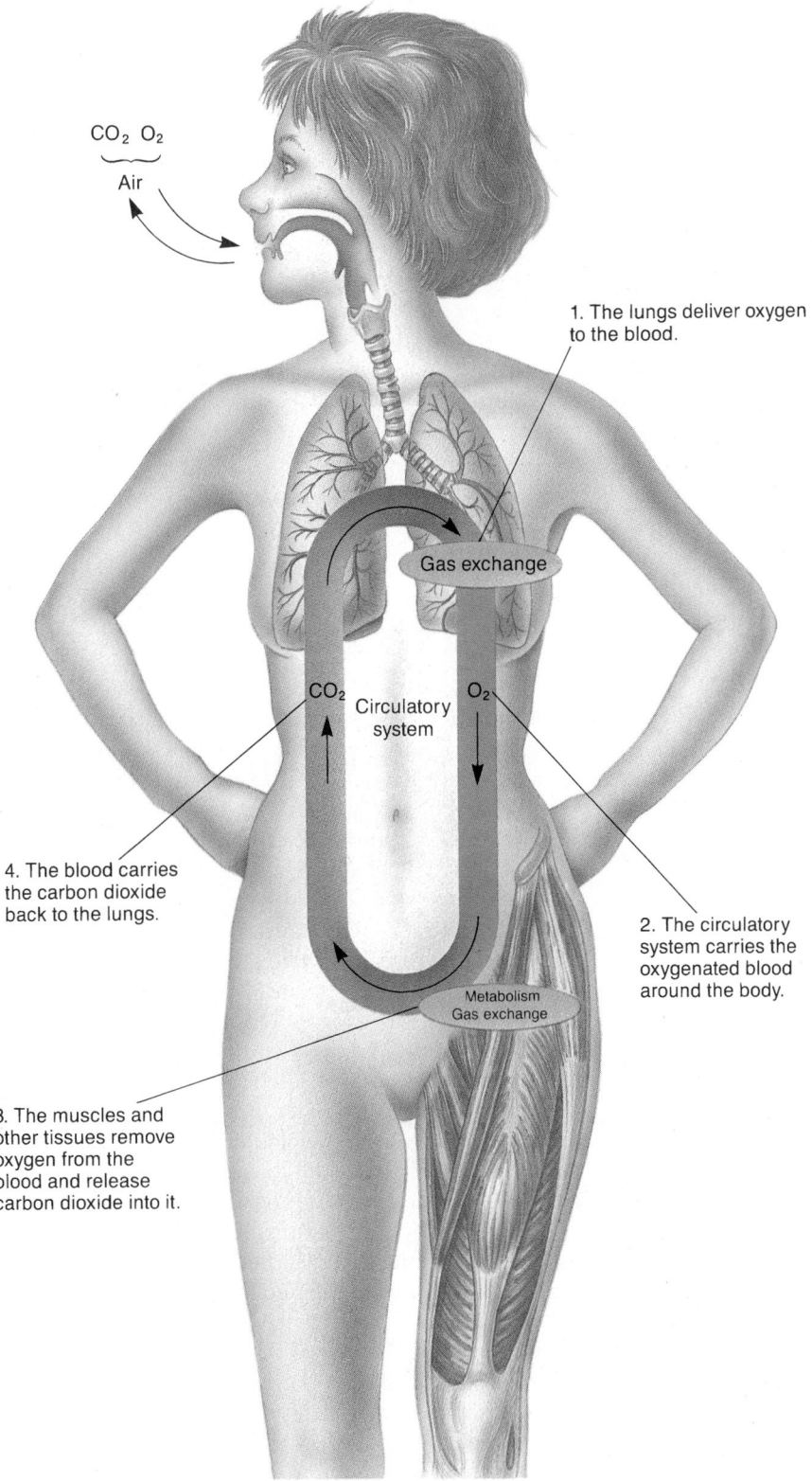

CO_2 O_2

Air

1. The lungs deliver oxygen to the blood.

Gas exchange

CO_2 Circulatory system O_2

4. The blood carries the carbon dioxide back to the lungs.

2. The circulatory system carries the oxygenated blood around the body.

Metabolism Gas exchange

3. The muscles and other tissues remove oxygen from the blood and release carbon dioxide into it.

FIGURE 9–2   **Delivery of Oxygen by the Heart and Lungs to the Muscles**
The more fit a muscle is, the more oxygen it draws from the blood. That oxygen is drawn from the lungs, so the person with more fit muscles extracts from the inhaled air more oxygen than a person with less fit muscles. The cardiovascular system responds to the demand for oxygen by building up its capacity to deliver oxygen. Researchers can measure cardiovascular fitness by measuring the amount of oxygen a person consumes per minute while working out, a measure called VO_2 max.

FIGURE 9–3   **How to take Your Pulse**

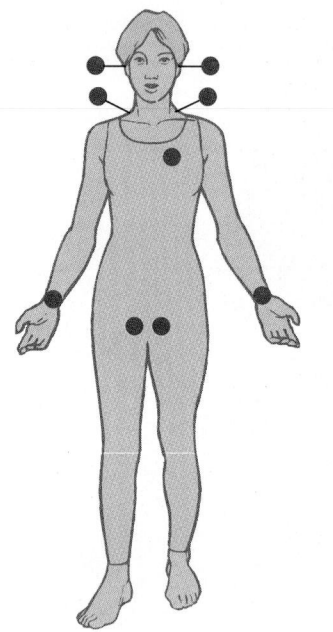

Get a watch or clock with a second hand. Rest a few minutes for a resting pulse. Place your hand over you heart or your finger firmly over an artery in any pulse location that gives a clear rhythm. Start counting your pulse at a convenient second, and continue counting for ten seconds. If a heartbeat occurs exactly on the tenth second, count it as one-half beat. Multiply by 6 to obtain the beats per minute. To ensure a true count:

■ Use only fingers, not your thumb, on the pulse point (the thumb has a pulse of its own).

■ Press just firmly enough to feel the pulse. Too much pressure can interfere with the pulse rhythm.

Admittedly, it is inconvenient to check your pulse constantly, but this need not hinder your exercise program. Once you compute your target heart rate zone and check your pulse a few times while exercising, you will begin to get a "feel" for whether you are exercising in that zone and will need to take your pulse only occasionally as a spot check. As you become more and more conditioned, periodic checking will suffice to tell you when to increase your workload if further conditioning is desired. People with heart disease or hypertension need to monitor their heart rates more carefully and frequently for safety's sake, and competitive athletes may want to do so to maximize the improvement yield of each session.

The American College of Sports Medicine (ACSM) has issued new recommendations for developing and maintaining cardiovascular fitness.[5] Table 9–5 lists these recommendations.

A fringe benefit of aerobic training is its effect on muscles. The more fit a muscle is, the more oxygen it draws from the blood. That oxygen is drawn from the lungs, so the person with more fit muscles extracts from the inhaled air more oxygen than a person with less fit muscles. This improves the efficiency of the cardiovascular system still further, reducing the heart's workload. An added bonus is that muscles that can use more oxygen can burn fat longer—a plus for body composition and weight control.

In contrast to aerobic activity, anaerobic activity generally does not bring about cardiovascular conditioning but develops strength and bulk of muscles. Anaerobic activity involves sudden, all-out exertions of muscles that last less than 90 seconds. Examples include sprinting, jumping a fence, doing push-ups, or lifting weights.

As important as cardiovascular conditioning is, it is only one facet of conditioning. For balanced fitness, stretching enhances flexibility, and

TABLE 9–4   **How to Calculate Your Target Heart Rate Zone**[a]

Follow along with David Williams, age 25, as he calculates his target heart rate zone.

1. *Find your resting heart rate* (pulse) as described in Figure 9–3.
   Example: David takes his resting pulse and finds it is 62.
2. *Estimate your maximum heart rate.* Subtract your age from 220 (205 if you are using swimming as your form of aerobic exercise). This provides an estimate of the absolute maximum heart rate possible for a person your age. Never exercise at this rate.
   Example: David's maximum heart rate is 220 − 25 = 195.
3. *Subtract your resting rate (1) from your maximum rate (2).*
   Example: 195 − 62 = 133.
4. *Find 50% of this figure.*
   Example: 0.50 × 133 = 67 (rounded off).
5. *Add the resulting number (4) to your resting heart rate (1).*
   Example: 67 + 62 = 129.

This number defines the bottom end of your target heart rate zone. Your heart should beat at least this fast when you work aerobically.

6. *Now repeat steps 4 and 5, but use 85%.*
   Example: 0.85 × 133 = 113 (rounded off). 113 + 62 = 175.

This number defines the top end of your target heart rate zone. Your heart should not beat faster than this when you work aerobically.

Example (conclusion): David's target zone is between 129 and 175 beats per minute.

[a]All calculations are in beats per minute.

weight training or calisthenics develops muscle strength and endurance, while aerobic activity improves cardiovascular fitness. Table 9–6 shows a sample fitness program.

The Active Body's Use of Fuels

The body responds to physical activity by adjusting its fuel use. When a person begins to exercise, hormones, including epinephrine and norepinephrine, are released into the bloodstream. These hormones signal the liver and fat cells to liberate their stored energy nutrients, primarily glucose and fatty acids, with a few amino acids mixed in.

During rest, the body derives a little more than half of its energy from fatty acids and most of the rest from glucose, along with a small percentage from amino acids. How much of which fuels the muscles use during physical activity depends on an interplay among the fuels available, the intensity and duration of the exercise, and the degree to which the body is conditioned to perform that activity.

TABLE 9–5   **American College of Sports Medicine Guidelines for Cardiovascular and Muscular Fitness**

- **Frequency of training:** three to five days per week.
- **Intensity of training:** 50 to 85% of maximum heart rate.
- **Duration of activity:** 20 to 60 minutes of continuous activity.
- **Mode of activity:** any activity that uses large muscle groups.
- **Resistance training:** strength training of moderate intensity at a minimum of two times per week.

Note: The ACSM notes that duration and intensity are interrelated, so that 40 to 50 minutes of brisk walking may be needed to gain the same result as 20 to 30 minutes of jogging.

Carbohydrate and Performance

The body's carbohydrate glucose, stored in the liver and muscles as glycogen, is vital to physical activity. During exertion, the liver releases its glucose into the bloodstream. The muscles pick up this glucose and use it in addition to glucose from their own glycogen stores. Although glycogen supplies are ample to support everyday activity, they are less abundant than body fat stores; in other words, glycogen is limited.

The body constantly uses and replenishes its glycogen. How much glycogen a body stores depends partially on the amount of carbohydrate in the diet. How much carbohydrate a person eats affects how much glycogen is stored, which in turn influences how much will be used during activity.[6] Thus diet bears on performance, because the more glycogen you store, the longer the stores will last as you work. Training also affects how much glycogen muscles store—muscles that deplete their glycogen through work adapt to store greater amounts of glycogen to support that work. The more

TABLE 9–6   **Sample Fitness Program (45 Minutes a Day)**

Monday, Wednesday, Friday:

- 10 minutes of warm-up activity and stretching.
- 25 minutes of aerobic exercise.
- 10 minutes of cool-down activity.

Tuesday, Thursday:

- 10 minutes of warm-up activity and stretching.
- 25 minutes of weight training
- 10 minutes of cool-down activity.

Saturday or Sunday:

- Softball, walking, hiking, biking, or swimming.

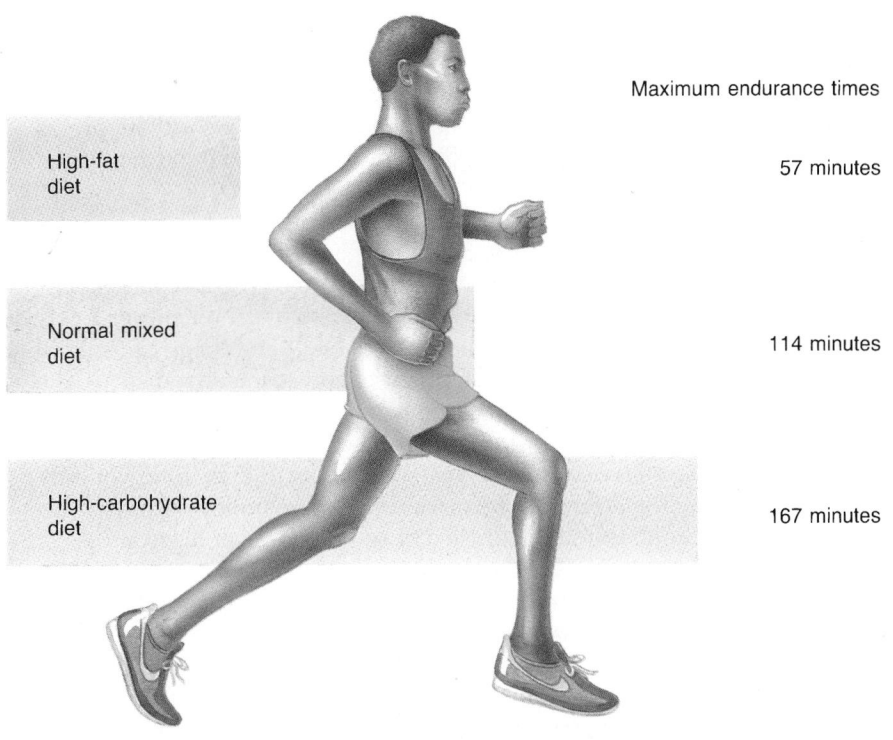

Maximum endurance times

High-fat diet — 57 minutes

Normal mixed diet — 114 minutes

High-carbohydrate diet — 167 minutes

FIGURE 9–4 **The Effect of Diet on Physical Endurance**
A high-carbohydrate diet can triple an athlete's endurance.

glycogen the muscles store, the longer the stores last during physical activity. Muscles make still another adaptation to training that affects glycogen use during activity—conditioned muscles rely less on glycogen and more on fat for energy, so that the rate of glycogen breakdown in trained individuals is lower than in untrained individuals at the same intensity of work.

A classic study compared fuel use during exercise among three groups of runners, each on a different diet. For several days before testing, one of the groups consumed a normal mixed diet (55 percent of kcalories from carbohydrate), the second group consumed a high-carbohydrate diet (83 percent of kcalories from carbohydrate), and the third group consumed a high-fat diet (94 percent of kcalories from fat). Figure 9–4 shows that the high-carbohydrate diet allowed the athletes to keep going longer before exhaustion. This study and many others that followed suggest that a high-carbohydrate diet enhances endurance by promoting the storage of ample glycogen. A later section of this chapter describes how to choose a performance diet, paying special attention to carbohydrate.

How long an exercising person's glycogen lasts depends not only on diet, but also partly on the intensity of the exercise. The most intense activities—the kind, such as sprinting, that make it difficult to "catch your breath"—quickly use up glycogen. Other, less intense activities, such as jogging, during which breathing is steady and easy, use glycogen more slowly. But joggers still use it, and if they run long enough, eventually they run out of it. Glycogen depletion usually occurs within less than two hours from the onset of moderately intense exercise.

The relationship between exercise intensity and glycogen use involves the availability of oxygen. Muscles use glycogen especially rapidly during high-intensity exercise because they can derive glucose from it—and glucose from glycogen can serve as a fuel even when oxygen is in short supply, as when a person is "out of breath." Glucose can "burn" without oxygen; it can serve as an anaerobic fuel.

During *moderate* exercise, the lungs and circulatory system have no trouble keeping up with the muscles' need for oxygen—the exercise is aerobic. During aerobic exercise, energy derives from both glucose and fatty acids.

Intense exercise presents a different metabolic situation. Whenever a person exercises at a rate that exceeds the rate the heart and lungs can supply oxygen to the muscles—that is, whenever energy demand outstrips the oxygen supply—aerobic metabolism cannot meet energy needs. The muscles must instead draw more heavily on glucose for energy.

lactic acid: a compound produced in muscles when they break down glucose anaerobically; it can cause burning pain if not promptly drained away.

The way that muscles use glucose anaerobically is to break it down only partway to a compound known as lactic acid. This acid builds up and causes burning pain in the muscles. Lactic acid accumulation can lead to muscle exhaustion within seconds if it is not cleared away. A strategy for dealing with lactic acid buildup is to relax the muscles at every opportunity so that the circulating blood can carry it away to the liver, which can reconvert it to glucose. Tired mountain climbers can ascend the final peak by relaxing their leg muscles at each step (the "mountain rest step").

Glycogen use during exercise depends not only on the *intensity,* but also on the *duration,* of the exercise—how long it continues. Within the first 20 minutes or so of moderate exercise, a person uses mostly glycogen for fuel. A person who continues exercising moderately for longer than 20 minutes begins to use less and less glycogen and more and more fat. Still, glycogen use continues, and if the activity is long and hard enough, glycogen stores run out almost completely. Exercise can continue for a short time thereafter only because the liver scrambles to produce from available lactic acid and amino acids the minimum amount of glucose needed to briefly forestall total depletion. When glycogen and glucose depletion hits, it brings nervous system function almost to a halt, making continued exertion almost impossible.

These factors affect glucose use in exercise:

- Dietary and stored carbohydrate.
- Intensity of the exercise.
- Duration of the exercise.

Since glucose depletion brings on fatigue, people who compete try to maintain their blood glucose concentrations. Some eat sugary foods or drink liquids that provide glucose. This extra glucose may indeed be of value to endurance athletes, who often run short of glucose at the end of competition. Taken at such times, glucose can slowly make its way from the digestive tract to the muscles. The glucose in dilute drinks can augment the body's supply just enough to forestall exhaustion.

Before concluding that sugar might be good for your own performance, though, consider whether you engage in *endurance* activity. Do you run, swim, bike, or ski nonstop at a steady pace for more than an hour and a half at a time? If not, the sugar picture changes. For an everyday jog, swim, or game match, sugar will not help performance, and unless the timing is right, it may actually hinder it. Taking a moderate sugar dose (300 kcalories) 30 minutes before exercise accelerates glycogen depletion. This is because insulin is secreted in response to a rise in blood glucose. Insulin impairs fat use by the muscles, thereby causing greater reliance on glycogen for fuel.[7]

Fat and Performance

Unlike glycogen stores, which are limited, body fat stores can fuel hours of activity without running out, as long as the activity is not too intense. Fat is a virtually unlimited source of energy. Early in an activity, the muscles draw on and use the fatty acids already available to them from the blood. If the activity continues for more than a few minutes, the fat cells get the message that more fat is needed for energy, and they begin rapidly breaking down their stored fat to keep the supply going. After about 20 minutes of sustained, moderate exercise, the fat cells are significantly shrinking in size as they empty out their lipid stores.

In addition to duration, intensity also affects fat use. As intensity increases, fat makes less and less of a contribution to the total fuel used. Fat can be broken down for energy in one way only—aerobically. Thus, for fat to fuel exercise, oxygen is indispensable. (Remember, if you are breathing easily during exercise, your muscles are getting all the oxygen they need and are able to burn fat.)

The body adapts in response to aerobic activity. For one thing, the trained person's heart and lungs become stronger and better able to deliver oxygen at high exercise intensities. For another, as already mentioned, the muscles cells develop greater capacity to use fat as fuel. For still another, the trained person's hormones slow glucose release from the liver and encourage fat use instead. The person who wishes to burn fat by exercising can conclude that patient, persistent training is worthwhile, and that steady, long-duration activity works best. The intensity to choose depends on your present conditioning level: work so that you breathe faster than usual but not so fast as to feel out of breath.

The key to burning fat is steady, long-duration exercise.

Unlike carbohydrate, fat is not recommended in large quantities in the diets of active people. Your body can supply your fat for you, and it will make more when it needs to as long as food energy is adequate. High-fat diets do promote fat use during exercise, but at the expense of performance, and at the risk of heart disease.

Table 9–7 summarizes fuel use during exercise as discussed so far. You may wonder why the third energy-yielding nutrient, protein, is not listed in

TABLE 9–7   Carbohydrate and Fat Use during Activity

FUEL USED[a]	PERFORMANCE TIME	OXYGEN NEEDED?	EXERCISE INTENSITY	ACTIVITY EXAMPLES
Carbohydrate	30 seconds to 3 minutes	No	Very high	¼-mile sprint, a football play
Mostly carbohydrate (and some fat)	3 to 20 minutes	Yes	High	Distance swimming or running
Mostly fat (and some carbohydrate)	More than 20 minutes	Yes	Moderate	Distance running or jogging, cross-country skiing

[a]All of these fuels are converted to ATP for use as energy. The ATP pool already available donates the first 30 seconds of energy.

Source: Adapted in part from M. H. Williams, Human energy, in *Nutritional Aspects of Human Physical Performance,* 2d ed. (Springfield, Ill.: Charles C. Thomas, 1985), pp. 21–57; E. L. Fox, Sports activities and the energy continuum, in *Sports Physiology,* 2d ed. (New York: Saunders, 1984), pp. 26–39.

the table. The reason is that protein is not a major donor of energy to exercise. However, it does donate some energy, and it provides the structural material of muscle tissue, so it is still important to active people.

Protein and Physical Activity

The body handles protein differently during activity than at rest. Synthesis of body proteins is suppressed during exercise and for several hours afterwards. In the hours following this period, though, protein synthesis rebounds beyond normal resting levels.[8] The body must adapt and build the tissues it needs for the next period of exercise. Whenever the body remodels a part of itself, it must tear down old structures to make way for new ones. Repeated exercise, with just a slight overload, triggers the equipment of each muscle cell to do so—that is, the muscle cells adapt.

The physical work of each muscle cell acts as a signal to its protein-building systems to begin producing the kinds of proteins that best support that work.[9] Take jogging, for example. In the first difficult sessions, the body is not yet fully equipped to perform—the muscle fibers have not adapted to producing the energy needed for aerobic work. But with each session, the cells get the message that an overhaul is needed. In the hours that follow the session, muscle cells get busy breaking down any unneeded protein structures and begin producing the needed new structures. This does not appreciably affect the muscles in just one or two exercise sessions, but within a few weeks, remodeling occurs, and jogging becomes easier.

The factors that modify how much protein is used during an activity seem to be the same ones that modify the use of fat and carbohydrate. Among them are the intensity and duration of the activity.[10] For example, endurance athletes who train for over an hour a day may deplete their glycogen stores and become more dependent on body protein for energy. In fact, despite widely held beliefs to the contrary, research suggests that endurance athletes' protein needs exceed those of bodybuilders and weight lifters.[11] Protein needs of bodybuilders and weight lifters are slightly higher than those of sedentary people but not as high as some recommendations, and certainly not as high as the protein intakes many bodybuilders consume.[12]

Another factor that influences a person's protein use during physical activity is the person's degree of training. As you might expect, the better trained a person is, the less protein the person uses during an activity.

You might also guess, correctly, that diet modifies the amount of protein used as fuel. People who consume diets rich in *carbohydrate* burn less protein than those who eat protein- and fat-rich diets.[13] This could be related to the protein-sparing effect of carbohydrate first mentioned in Chapter 2.

All athletes, as well as those who work like athletes, probably need a little more protein than do sedentary people. How much protein should an active person consume? The American Dietetic Association (ADA) recommends about 25 percent over the recommendation for sedentary people.[14] Typically, people's diets in the United States contain about 12 percent protein. For a man who weighs 70 kilograms (154 pounds), this translates into a protein intake of about 75 grams per day, or a little more than 1 gram of protein per kilogram of body weight. Most active people eat more food than sedentary people do; as long as protein provides 12 percent or more of food energy, dietary protein will be ample. How this translates into diet is a question answered in a later section. As you will see, no one needs protein supplements, or even large servings of meat, to obtain the highest recommended protein intakes.

Vitamins and Performance

Popular belief has it that vitamin supplements have something to offer those who work out, both in health benefits and in physical performance. It goes without saying that active people need adequate vitamins and minerals to do what they do, as Table 9–8 shows. But research confirms that nutrient supplements do not enhance the performance of well-nourished people. In a well-controlled study of 30 runners, substantial nutrient supplementation for three months did not improve performance.[15] Active people do not need supplements—they can get the nutrients they need from food.

Minerals and Performance

Like the vitamins, the nutrient minerals are essential to exercise—all of them. Three are of special current interest: chromium, zinc, and copper, which people excrete in their urine in larger amounts when they exercise

TABLE 9–8   **Roles of Vitamins and Minerals in Exercise**

VITAMIN OR MINERAL	FUNCTION
Thiamin, riboflavin, niacin, magnesium	Energy-releasing reactions
Vitamin B_6, zinc	Building of muscle protein
Folate, vitamin B_{12}	Building of red blood cells to carry oxygen
Vitamin C	Collagen formation for joint and other tissue integrity; hormone synthesis
Iron	Transport of oxygen in blood and in muscle tissue; energy transformation reactions
Calcium	Building of bone structure; muscle contractions; nerve transmissions
Phosphorus	ATP component
Sodium, potassium, chloride	Maintenance of fluid balance; transmission of nerve impulses for muscle contraction
Chromium	Assistance in insulin's energy-storage function
Magnesium	Cardiac and other muscle contraction

Note: This is just a sampling. Other vitamins and minerals play equally indispensable roles in exercise.

than when they are sedentary.[16] So far, though, it is too early to say whether these added losses increase people's nutrient needs. In general, the minerals are probably like the vitamins in that active people do not need them in supplement form. For the most part, active people who choose foods with care can be sure of meeting their vitamin and mineral needs without supplements.

Iron and Performance

Iron is an exception to the rule just stated. Physically active young women, especially those who engage in endurance activities such as distance running, are prone to iron deficiency. Research studies show that as many as 45 percent of female runners of high school age have low iron stores.[17] Habitually low intakes of iron-rich foods, combined with iron losses aggravated by exercise, may cause iron deficiency in physically active young women. Iron is in every cell, so growing children have high needs; the blood is especially rich in iron, so bleeding (or excessive menstrual losses) increases iron needs.

Iron deficiency impairs physical performance, because iron is crucial to the body's handling of oxygen. Iron is the key ingredient of hemoglobin, the protein in the red blood cells that carries oxygen to all the tissues, including the muscles. Without adequate oxygen transport to the muscles, as you know already, you cannot combust fat as fuel; you cannot perform aerobic activity; and you will tire easily. People with iron-deficiency anemia can do less work less well, and even think less well, than people with adequate iron status. Even marginal iron deficiency without obvious symptoms of anemia is known to impair physical performance to some extent.[18]

sports anemia: a transient condition of low hemoglobin in the blood, associated with the early stages of sports training or other strenuous activity.

The condition known as sports anemia is not a true iron-deficiency condition. Sports anemia manifests itself in a temporary decrease in hemoglobin concentration after a sudden increase in aerobic exercise. Strenuous aerobic exercise promotes destruction of the red blood cells that are fragile and older, and the resulting cleanup work reduces the blood's iron content, although it may not reduce its *effective* iron by much. Strenuous aerobic exercise also prompts the body to increase its blood volume. The body does this by adding fluid to the blood supply, thereby diluting its contents and making a blood sample seem to have less iron. Again, this may not diminish the working iron much, if at all. The exact causes of sports anemia remain controversial. Marginal iron intakes may contribute to it, but most people seem to think it is just an adaptive, temporary response to endurance training. Iron-deficiency anemia requires iron-supplementation therapy; sports anemia goes away by itself.

runner's anemia: an apparent or real iron-deficiency condition in runners.

Another term that people use to describe iron status in athletes is *runner's anemia,* which refers to an apparent or real iron-deficiency condition in high-mileage runners. Some people consider this term synonymous with sports anemia; others use it to refer to a true iron-deficiency condition. When you read *runner's anemia,* be sure to notice which meaning is ascribed to it.

Because true iron deficiency is a real possibility for all people, and especially for active people and athletes, it is important to keep track of your own iron status. (All routine physical examinations that include blood work check you for the extreme deficiency state, anemia, but you should also be aware that such tests will not tell you if your iron stores are low.) Consider your individual needs. Many young menstruating women probably border on iron deficiency even without the additional iron losses incurred through exercise. Active teens of both sexes, because they are growing, have high iron needs, too. Especially for women and teens, then, supplements may be needed to maintain iron stores or to correct a deficiency of iron.

Iron supplements are available over the counter, and because the absorption of iron from them is poor, it may take a dose as high as twice the RDA or more for several weeks to deliver an amount of iron sufficient to replenish depleted stores. Taking a self-prescribed supplement may mask symptoms of a dangerous condition such as gastrointestinal bleeding from ulcers or cancer, though, so anyone considering this course of action should consult a health care professional before adopting it.

Electrolytes and Performance

Electrolytes, the charged minerals sodium, potassium, chloride, and magnesium, are lost from the body in sweat. People who are just beginning an exercise regimen lose electrolytes to a much greater extent than do trained people; as the body adapts to exercise, it becomes better at conserving most electrolytes. People normally need make no special effort to replenish lost electrolytes. A regular diet that meets their energy and nutrient needs also supplies all the electrolytes they need.

During exercise, electrolyte replacement is also not necessary, unless a person works up a drenching sweat amounting to the loss of 5 to 10 pounds or more each day (3 percent of body weight) for several consecutive days. In that case, drinking plain water and relying on food to replace lost electrolytes may not suffice, and a commercial "sweat replacer" beverage, diluted by half with water, may be drunk for fluid and electrolyte replacement. A homemade mixture of ⅓ teaspoon of table salt and 1 cup of fruit juice added to each quart of water will also serve the purpose. Avoid electrolyte or salt tablets; they can irritate the stomach and cause vomiting, and they always cause water to flow into the digestive tract from the tissues at first, thereby temporarily worsening dehydration and impairing performance. As for potassium, avoid potassium supplements unless prescribed by a physician; while they better some conditions, they worsen others.

Food for Fitness

No one diet best supports physical performance. Many different diets can be excellent for active people. However, food choices must be made within the framework of rules for diet planning presented in Chapter 1.

First of all, remember that water is the most important nutrient. Exercise blunts the thirst mechanism, especially in cold weather. During exercise, thirst signals too late, after fluid stores are depleted, so don't wait to feel thirsty before drinking. To find out how much water you need to replenish exercise losses, weigh yourself before and after the activity—the difference is all water. One pound equals roughly 2 cups of fluid. You will feel better and your workout will seem easier if you consistently tend to your body's

TABLE 9–9   **Schedule of Hydration before, during, and after Exercise**

WHEN TO DRINK	TOTAL AMOUNT OF FLUID (CONSUME IN 1-c SERVINGS)
2 hours before exercise	About 3 c
10 to 15 minutes before exercise	About 2 c
Every 60 to 90 minutes during exercise	About 1 qt (or 1 liter)
After exercise	Replace each pound of body weight lost with 2 c (½ liter) fluid

Source: Adapted from J. B. Marcus, ed., *Sports Nutrition* (Chicago: American Dietetic Association, 1986), p. 57; American College of Sports Medicine position stand on the prevention of thermal injuries during distance running, *Medicine and Science in Sports and Exercise* 19 (1987): 529–533.

fluid needs. Plain, cool water is the best fluid for the exercising body for two reasons: it rapidly leaves the digestive tract to enter the tissues, and it cools the body. Table 9–9 offers a schedule of hydration for exercise.

As for food, the active person needs a diet composed mostly of nutrient-dense foods, the kind that supply a maximum of vitamins and minerals for the energy they provide. When active people eat mostly refined, processed foods that have suffered nutrient losses and that contain added sugar and fat, nutrient status suffers.[19]

Active people need to eat both for adequacy and for energy. Active people are not immune to heart disease and cancer and so must limit fats. A diet that is high in carbohydrate (60 percent of total kcalories or more), low in fat (25 percent or less), and adequate in protein (12 to 15 percent) ensures full glycogen and other nutrient stores. Such a diet helps to control weight (thus reducing risks of diabetes and other diseases) and provides adequate fiber while supplying abundant nutrients. Table 9–10 shows some sample diet plans for people who wish to increase their energy and carbohydrate intakes.

Glycogen stores can be depleted when an exerciser eats a diet that is high in protein and low in carbohydrates. Glycogen stores may be used up during the first few days of exercise. If generous servings of carbohydrate-rich foods are not eaten, the exerciser may start to feel burned out and sluggish. The exerciser may attribute these symptoms to vitamin deficiencies, but they indicate a need not for increased vitamins but for increased energy in the form of glycogen, which comes from a carbohydrate-rich diet. A low-carbohydrate diet may be responsible for the discouragement and tiredness a person feels a few days after beginning a fitness program.

On certain occasions the active person's high-carbohydrate, fiber-rich diet may require temporary adjustment. One occasion is during intensive training, when energy needs outstrip the capacity to eat enough kcalories from food, in which case added sugar and fat may be needed. Another special occasion is the pregame meal, in which case fiber-rich, bulky foods are best avoided. Carbohydrate-rich foods such as pasta and fruit juices—low in fat, protein, and fiber—are the basis of the pregame meal. Both of these excep-

TABLE 9–10   Examples of High-Carbohydrate Food Patterns for Various Energy Levels

		kCalories Provided					
		1,500	2,000	2,500	3,000	4,000	5,000
TYPE OF FOOD	REPRESENTATIVE SERVING SIZE	Number of Servings					
Low-fat (2%) milk	1 c	2	3	3	4	6	8
Vegetable	½ c	5	6	7	10	12	14
Fruit	½ c	5	7	10	11	14	20
Starchy vegetable or grain	½ c or 1 slice	6	7	9	10	14	18
Meat or meat alternate	2½ oz	2	2	2	4	4	4
Fat	1 tsp	2	3	4	5	6	8

These plans provide 55 to 61% of total energy as carbohydrate, 17 to 22% as protein, and 21 to 25% as fat.

tions deal with training for competition rather than fitness. Both diet and fitness influence the next topics of discussion, body composition and weight control.

Body Composition and Weight Control

A fit body differs in composition from an unfit body in many ways. For one thing, a fit body contains more muscle tissue, and muscle tissue burns more kcalories than other tissues. Thus fitness improves body composition and contributes to weight control. A balanced program of physical activity can reduce fat tissue and augment lean tissue.

Your body's weight reflects its composition—the total mass of its bone, muscles, fat, fluids, and other tissues. The more of any of these you have, the more you weigh. All of your body components can vary in quantity and quality—the bones can be dense or porous; the muscles can be well developed or underdeveloped; fat can be abundant or scarce; and so on. One tissue, though, stands out as by far the most variable: your body fat. Fat is the material in which the body can store the most food energy; it is fat that responds most to changes in food intake and exercise; and it is fat that is usually the target of efforts at weight control.

Determining Body Fatness

Techniques for estimating body fat percentage include underwater weighing, measuring electrical impedance, and determining fatfold thickness. These techniques vary in complexity. For example, underwater weighing, recognized as one of the most accurate ways to measure body composition, requires considerable time, expensive equipment, and skilled technicians.

Underwater weighing determines body density, from which you can calculate body fat percentage (lean tissue is denser than fat tissue). Measuring electrical impedance requires expensive equipment. Electrodes are placed on a person's hand and foot on the same side of the body, and a small current is transmitted. This method is based on the principle that lean tissues are full of electrolyte-containing fluids that readily conduct an electrical current. Fat, on the other hand, is a poor conductor. A direct and practical method for estimating body fatness is to use a fatfold caliper—a device that measures the thickness of a fold of fat on the back of the arm or elsewhere. These techniques for assessing body composition are discussed further in Chapter 10. Other simple techniques such as the pinch test permit a ballpark estimate of whether a person is too fat or not. Table 9–11 provides rules of thumb to assess body fatness.

Most experts agree that a body fat content of 10 to 25 percent for men and 18 to 32 percent for women is optimal for health.[20] Men and women pursuing higher levels of fitness will seek body fat percentages closer to the bottom of the optimal range. The minimum amount of body fat recommended for men is 5 percent; the minimum for women is between 12 and 20 percent. Below a certain threshold, some individuals develop symptoms such as infertility, depression, or abnormal hunger regulation. The threshold differs according to an individual's characteristics and may vary for each symptom even within an individual. Much remains to be learned about the hazards of extremely low levels of body fat.

Controlling Weight

Physical activity makes many contributions to weight control. For one thing, it directly increases energy output by the muscles and cardiovascular system. A 150-pound person walking a brisk 4 miles per hour for 30 minutes spends an extra 185 kcalories on that activity. A football player in training may spend several thousand extra kcalories on a day of heavy training.

pinch test: an informal means of measuring body fatness by lifting a fold on the back of one arm with the fingers and estimating its thickness.

TABLE 9–11   **Rules of Thumb to Assess Body Fatness**

These methods for estimating how much body fat you have are just for fun:

- A crude measure of body fatness is the pinch test (this is a fatfold measure without the equipment to make it accurate). Pick up the skin and fat at the back of either arm with the thumb and forefinger of the other hand. Keep your fingers still, so as not to lose the "measurement" when you pull them away from your arm. Measure the thickness on a ruler. A fatfold over an inch thick reflects obesity.
- Another shortcut method is to compare your waist and chest (not bust) measurements. Every inch by which your waist measurement exceeds your chest measurement is said to take two years off your life.
- Another crude measure is to lie down, relax, and place a ruler across your abdomen from one hipbone to the other. If the ruler does not easily touch both bones while you're relaxing, you're too fat.

Activity also contributes to energy output in an indirect way—by increasing basal metabolism. It does this in two ways—today, and over the long term. Today, if you exercise vigorously (for an hour, for example), your metabolism may stay speeded up for several hours afterwards. That may add a few dozen kcalories to your output, and so will make a small contribution toward the loss of the pound you are currently working to lose. Over the long term, if you keep repeating such vigorous activity daily for many weeks, your body composition will gradually change to favor more lean tissue. Your metabolic rate will rise accordingly, because lean tissue is more active metabolically than fat tissue—and that, over still more time, will make a contribution toward continued weight loss or maintenance of a healthy weight. The more lean tissue you develop, the more kcalories you spend, and the more you can afford to eat. Eating more brings you both pleasure and nutrients. Exercise continues to maintain your raised metabolic rate for as long as you keep your body conditioned.

Another thing activity helps with is appetite control. People think that exercising will make them hungry, but this is not entirely true. Yes, active people do have healthy appetites, but immediately after a good workout, most people do not feel like eating. They want to shower; they may be thirsty; but they are not hungry. The reason is that the body has responded to the stress of exercise by mobilizing fuels from storage—glucose and fatty acids are abundant in the blood. (A physiologist would say you are in a "fed state.") At the same time, the body has suppressed its digestive functions. Hard physical work and eating are not compatible. You must calm down, put your fuels back in storage, and relax before you eat. Thus exercise helps curb appetite, especially the inappropriate appetite accompanying boredom, anxiety, or depression that might prompt you to eat when you really do not need to. (Weight-control programs encourage you to go out and exercise when you're tempted to eat, but not really hungry. It will fill your time, improve your mood, and curb your misleading appetite. Later, when true hunger comes, it will be appropriate to eat.)

Activity also helps reduce stress. Since stress, too, is a cue to inappropriate eating behavior for many people, activity can help here, too.

Activity offers still more psychological benefits. The fit person looks and feels healthy, and high self-esteem accompanies these benefits. High self-esteem, in turn, tends to support a person's resolve to persist in a weight-control effort.

Weight loss *without* exercise can have a negative effect on body composition. A person who diets without exercising loses both lean and fat tissue. Now suppose the person then regains weight without exercising; the gain will be mostly fat. Finally, suppose the person eats the same amount as before. Because fat tissue burns fewer kcalories to maintain itself, the person will not stay at an even weight or at the old weight plateau but will gain additional fat and weight. This is the so-called ratchet effect, or yo-yo effect, of dieting without exercise (Figure 9–5).

Clearly, then, physical activity is a beneficial part of a weight-control program. What kind of physical activity is best? For the person seeking to *lose* weight, the activities that burn the most *fat,* not necessarily the ones that burn the most *kcalories,* are the ones to choose. Intense exercise burns a lot of kcalories, but many of them come from glycogen, not fat. In any one person, the amount of fat burned is about the same above a certain threshold of intensity—that is, you burn more and more fat per minute up to a certain

Benefits of physical activity in a weight-control program:

- Increased expenditure of energy today (including metabolic energy).
- Long-term increase (slight) in resting metabolic rate.
- Control of inappropriate eating urges.
- Stress reduction.
- Physical, and therefore psychological, well-being.
- High self-esteem.

ratchet effect or **yo-yo effect:** the effect of repeated rounds of dieting without exercise; the person rebounds to a higher weight and higher body fat content at the end of each round.

Thinness is not the same as fitness.

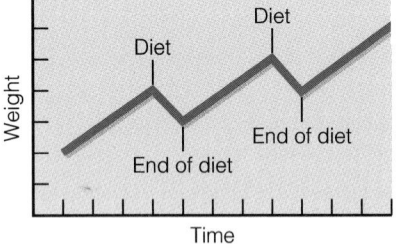

FIGURE 9–5　The Ratchet Effect of Dieting without Exercise
Each round of dieting, without physical activity, is followed by a rebound of weight to a higher level than before. The body fat content increases, and kcaloric needs fall after each round, making the next round of weight loss harder.

threshold, but above that threshold, your fat use continues unchanged or will even decline, and only your glycogen use increases. That is because above a certain intensity level, you can use only anaerobic fuel. Aerobic exercises or cardiovascular endurance exercises, therefore, are best to promote weight loss.

This brings us to another point in favor of regular physical activity in weight control. The body that trains to do aerobic work develops greater and greater ability to use fat as an energy source, even at higher intensities. (In other words, it raises the threshold, mentioned earlier, that limits fat-burning ability.) The conditioned athlete burns fat at an intensity level where the unconditioned person would be burning mostly glycogen. Therefore, training leads to the highly prized goal of being able to get the maximum fat-burning benefit of activity—to burn more kcalories and to burn more of them as fat.

People sometimes ask about "spot reducing." Can you lose fat in particular locations? Unfortunately, muscles do not "own" the fat that surrounds them. Fat cells release fat not into the underlying muscles but into the blood, and the fat is shared by all the muscles. Spot-reducing exercises, therefore, do not work to take the fat from particular areas—and incidentally, neither do massage machines that claim to break up fat on trouble spots. Being moved passively by machines or pounded by massages takes off neither fat nor kcalories. You have to move your muscles, so choose active exercises.

Exercise can help with trouble spots in another way, though. Strengthening loose muscles in a trouble area can help to improve their condition; stretching to gain flexibility can help with associated posture problems. Thus not only aerobic but also strength and flexibility workouts have their place in a weight-control routine.

This all adds up to a recommendation you might have guessed by now: to enhance weight control, adopt a balanced program of physical activity. Do it all—cultivate flexibility, strength, and endurance together with proper nutrition, and the desired body composition will follow.

SELF-STUDY

How Physically Active Are You?

Record your answers on Form 1. (follows this questionaire)

"The road to fitness is physical activity." How physically active are you? For each question answered yes, give yourself the number of points indicated. Then total your points to determine your score. Don't take this quiz too seriously; it is intended only to help make you aware of opportunities that your life offers you to develop your capacity for fitness.

A. Formal, Vigorous Exercise Routines

1. I participate in active recreational sports such as tennis or handball for an hour or more:
   a. About once a week. (*2 points*)
   b. About twice a week. (*4 points*)
   c. Three times a week. (*6 points*)
   d. Four times a week. (*8 points*)

(Adjust your point score if your answer is less or more than these. For example, if you play sports *six* days a week, give yourself more points— say, 12 points. If you play once a week for only 30 minutes, give yourself 1 point. Note: Any session of less than 20 minutes counts as zero.)

2. At least once a week, I participate in vigorous fitness activities like aerobic dancing, jogging, or swimming (at least 20 continuous minutes each session):
   a. About once a week. (*3 points*)
   b. About twice a week. (*6 points*)
   c. Three times a week. (*9 points*)
   d. Four times a week. (*12 points*)

(Adjust your point score upward or downward if your answer is slightly different from these. For example, if you work out *six* days a week, give yourself more points—say, 18 points.)

B. Other Formal Exercise Routines

3. At least two times a week, I perform floor workouts (sit-ups, push-ups) for at least ten minutes:
   a. Two sessions a week. (*2 points*)
   b. Three sessions a week. (*3 points*)
   c. Four or more sessions a week. (*4 points*)

(No points for a session of less than ten minutes; no points for only one session a week; maximum is 4 points.)

4. At least two times a week, I participate in yoga or perform stretching exercises for at least ten minutes:
   a. Two sessions a week. (*2 points*)
   b. Three sessions a week. (*3 points*)
   c. Four or more sessions a week. (*4 points*)

(*continued*)

SELF-STUDY

(No points for a session of less than ten minutes; no points for only one session a week; maximum is 4 points.)

5. At least two times a week, I work out with weights for at least ten minutes:
    a. Two sessions a week. (*2 points*)
    b. Three sessions a week. (*3 points*)
    c. Four or more sessions a week. (*4 points*)

(No points for a session of less than ten minutes; no points for only one session a week; maximum is 4 points.)

C. Occupation and Daily Activities

6. I walk to and from school, work, and shopping (½ mile or more each way), two or three times a week or more. (*1 point*)
7. I climb stairs rather than using elevators or escalators, every other day or more. (*1 point*)
8. My school, job, or household routine involves physical activity that fits the following description:
    a. It is mostly desk work or light physical activity. (*0 points*)
    b. It is mostly farm activities, moderate physical activity, brisk walking, or the like. (*4 points*)
    c. Many of my typical days include several hours of heavy physical activity (shoveling, lifting, or the like). (Don't include sports practice here. See part A.) (*2 points per day*)

(Section C maximum: 12 points.)

D. Leisure Activities

9. I do several hours of gardening, lawn work, or equally active hobby work each week. (*1 point*)
10. I fish or hunt once a week or more on the average. (This must involve active work such as rowing a boat or tracking game. Dock and truck sitting don't count.) (*1 point*)
11. At least once a week I dance vigorously (folk or square dance) for an hour or more. (*1 point*)

(Section D maximum: 4 points.)

12. In season, I play 9 to 18 holes of golf at least once a week, and I do not use a power cart. (*2 points*)
13. I walk for exercise or recreation:
    a. One to two hours a week. (*1 point per hour*)
    b. Three to four hours a week. (*2 points*)
    c. Five hours or more a week. (*3 points*)

14. In *addition* to the above, I choose to engage in other forms of physical activity:
    a. One to two hours a week. (*1 point*)
    b. Three to four hours a week. (*2 points*)
    c. Five hours or more a week. (*3 points*)

(For Section D, don't count sports practice. See Part A.)

FORM 1   **Record your point scores here for the Self-Study.**

Category	Score	
A. Formal, Vigorous Exercise Routines	_____	(A high score would be 20.)
B. Other Formal Exercise Routines	_____	(A high score would be 12.)
C. Occupation and Daily Activities	_____	(A high score would be 12.)
D. Leisure Activities	_____	(A high score would be 14.)
Total:	_____	(A high score would be 50.)

Evaluation of total score (circle one):

• Inactive (0 to 5 points).
• Moderately active (6 to 11 points).
• Active (12 to 20 points).
• Very active (21 points or over).

If your score categorized you as inactive or only moderately active, return to parts A through D, reread the questions, and choose some activities that you would like and could realistically undertake to raise your score to "Active" (12 points or more). List these activities below. You are not committing yourself to doing these things, just acknowledging that you could.

A. Formal, Vigorous Exercise Routines

I could:_____
_____
_____
_____

State for how long and how many times a week:_____
_____

B. Other Formal Exercise Routines

I could:_____
_____
_____
_____

State for how long and how many times a week:_____
_____

C. Occupation and Daily Activities

I could:_____
_____
_____
_____

State for how long and how many times a week:_____
_____

(continued)

FORM 1   **Record your point scores here for the Self-Study.**

D. Leisure Activities

I could:_____

_____

_____

State for how long and how many times a week:_____

_____

Study Questions

1. Define fitness in three ways.
2. Explain how fitness benefits physical health.
3. Describe the health-related components of fitness.
4. Discuss the differences between conditioning and training.
5. Describe the progressive overload principle.
6. Why are warm-up and cool-down activities important to fitness?
7. Describe some of the conditioning effects of cardiovascular endurance training.
8. Describe the relationship between glycogen use during exercise and the intensity of the exercise.
9. What is sports anemia?
10. Why is plain, cool water the best fluid for the exercising body?
11. What kinds of foods should active people emphasize in their diets?
12. What are the positive effects of physical activity in terms of body composition and weight control?

Notes

1. U.S. Department of Health and Human Services, Public Health Service, *Year 2000 Health Objectives for the Nation* (Washington, D.C.: Government Printing Office, 1990), as cited in D. C. Nieman, *Fitness and Sports Medicine: An Introduction* (Palo Alto, Calif.: Bull Publishing, 1990), pp. 3–25.
2. K. E. Powell and coauthors, Physical activity and chronic diseases, *American Journal of Clinical Nutrition* 49 (1989): 999–1006.
3. S. N. Blair and coauthors, Physical fitness and all-cause mortality, *Journal of the American Medical Association* 262 (1989): 2395–2401.
4. Parts of this discussion are based on L. K. DeBruyne, F. S. Sizer, and E. N. Whitney, *The Fitness Triad: Motivation, Training, and Nutrition* (St. Paul: West, 1991).

5. ACSM revised position on fitness in healthy adults, *Sports Medicine Digest,* July 1990, p. 3.

6. W. M. Sherman, Carbohydrate, muscle glycogen, and improved performance, *Physician and Sportsmedicine* 15 (1987): 157–164.

7. Sugar use and abuse, *Sports Medicine Digest* (Special Report on Nutrition and the Athlete), 1989, p. 7.

8. M. J. Zackin, Protein requirements for athletes, *Sports Medicine Digest,* March 1990, pp. 1–2.

9. P. Babij and F. W. Booth, Biochemistry of exercise: Advances in molecular biology relevant to adaptation of muscle to exercise, *Sports Medicine* 5 (1988): 137–143.

10. Zackin, 1990.

11. M. A. Tarnopolsky, J. D. MacDougall, and S. A. Atkinson, Influence of protein intake and training status on nitrogen balance and lean body mass, *Journal of Applied Physiology* 64 (1988): 187–193.

12. Tarnopolsky, MacDougall, and Atkinson, 1988.

13. P. W. R. Lemon, Protein and exercise: Update 1987, *Medicine and Science in Sports and Exercise* 19 (1987): S179–S188.

14. Position of the American Dietetic Association: Nutrition for physical fitness and athletic performance for adults, *Journal of the American Dietetic Association* 87 (1987): 933–939.

15. L. M. Weight, K. H. Myburgh, and T. D. Noakes, Vitamin and mineral supplementation: Effect on the running performance of trained athletes, *American Journal of Clinical Nutrition* 47 (1988): 192–195.

16. W. W. Campbell and R. A. Anderson, Effects of aerobic exercise and training on the trace minerals chromium, zinc, and copper, *Sports Medicine* 4 (1987): 9–18.

17. T. W. Rowland, S. A. Black, and J. F. Kelleher, Iron deficiency in adolescent endurance athletes, *Journal of Adolescent Health Care* 8 (1987): 322–326; H. J. Nickerson, M. C. Holubets, and B. R. Weiler, Causes of iron deficiency in adolescent athletes, *Journal of Pediatrics* 114 (1989): 657–663.

18. W. B. Strong and coauthors, The effect of iron therapy on the exercise capacity of nonanemic iron-deficient adolescent runners, *American Journal of Diseases of Children* 142 (1988): 165–169.

19. S. A. Tilgner and M. R. Schiller, Dietary intakes of female college athletes: The need for nutrition education, *Journal of the American Dietetic Association* 89 (1989): 967–969.

20. T. G. Lohman, Body composition assessment in sports medicine, *Sports Medicine Digest,* September 1990, pp. 1–2.

9

Athletic Hocus-pocus: Ergogenic Aids Athletes Use

In a world where body condition and skill are hard won, athletes gravitate to promises that they can easily improve their performance by taking pills or potions. Athletes too often hear well-intended, but unsubstantiated, advice from their coaches and peers that they should use special nutrients, drugs, or procedures to enhance performance. The wish to win is strong, but no amount of wishing can change the fact that an overwhelming majority of supplements sold for athletes are frauds. If the products that are tried have no effect and are harmless, they are only a waste of money; when the products are harmful or actually impair performance, they are a waste of athletic potential. This Nutrition in Practice looks at some of the so-called magical potions that promise to improve physical performance.

What does ergogenic **mean?**

Ergogenic means work enhancing or work producing. In connection with athletic performance, ergogenic aids are substances or treatments that are theoretically designed to improve athletic performance above and beyond that which is possible through normal training. Most of the time, research findings do not support the claims made by those who promote ergogenic aids. When you hear a claim that a product is ergogenic, remember to consider the source of the claim and to ask who may gain from the sale.[1]

My coach told me to take protein supplements. Should I take them?

Protein and amino acid supplements are advocated to improve both strength and endurance. Valid nutrition supports of fitness were discussed in Chapter 9. Well-nourished, active people and athletes do not need protein supplements. Extra protein cannot be forced into the muscles to make them grow. Cells don't respond to what's given to them by helplessly accepting it. They respond to the hormones that regulate them and to the demands put upon them, and they select the nutrients they need from what is offered. The way to make muscle cells grow is to put a demand on them—that is, to make them work. They will respond by taking up nutrients—amino acids included—so that they can grow. The only role for diet in this process is to make protein available, and good diets always do. Although the protein needs of some endurance and strength athletes may be slightly higher than those of sedentary people, the additional protein is easily obtained from foods, as Chapter 9 described.

What about vitamin-mineral supplements for athletes? I have a friend who is a bodybuilder. She always takes several vitamin pills right before she competes. What should I tell her?

Tell your friend that this practice is pointless, although probably harmless. For one thing, vitamins taken right before competition have no effect, because they are still waiting in the blood during the event; they have not been assembled into working molecules.

Besides, research shows that most bodybuilders' diets provide adequate amounts of vitamins and minerals, and that when a nutrient is lacking, the supplements chosen are seldom the ones needed to remedy the deficiencies. In one study, researchers noted that the diets of the women bodybuilders were so deficient in calcium that supplementation by itself could probably not compensate fully. The women omitted all dairy products from their diets as early as four months before competition.[2] The researchers also noted that all of the women and 90 percent of the men in this study used supplements, that these supplements did not supply calcium, and that many of the supplements did not carry standard nutrient label information. If a diet lacks nutrients, it should be modified to provide the needed nutrients. In the case of a clinical nutrient deficiency identified by a health professional, the appropriate nutrient supplements may be prescribed—in addition to dietary modification.

An ordinary multivitamin and mineral supplement might be prudent when an athlete's need for energy outstrips the ability to eat the quantity of food required to supply it. In this case, many athletes must turn to concentrated energy sources, such as candies and fats. While such foods supply abundant energy, they lack vitamins and minerals. The energy they supply, though, requires processing by vitamin- and mineral-containing enzymes. Consequently, the need for these nutrients is greater in proportion to that energy. Thus, for a short time during the heaviest training, a supplement might be appropriate. Chapter 9 described the other instance when supplementation is justified: iron deficiency in endurance athletes, especially women athletes, for which iron supplements may help provide a remedy.

I have heard of a technique for improving endurance called glycogen loading. What is glycogen loading?

The fuel for intense muscular activity is carbohydrate, stored in the muscles as glycogen. Athletes who compete in long-distance endurance events naturally want to have as much stored energy in their muscles as they can. Various techniques, called glycogen loading, have been used in the past to trick muscles into storing more glycogen than normal. These techniques involved sudden, drastic changes in diet that caused nausea or cramping in some athletes. Other athletes experienced more dangerous effects, such as abnormal heart and kidney function.

Exercise physiologists now recommend a modified plan of glycogen loading that confers benefits without such side effects. First, about two or three weeks before competition, the athlete increases exercise intensity while eating a normal, high-carbohydrate diet. Then during the last week before competition, the athlete does two things. With respect to exercise, the athlete gradually cuts back on exercise, and on the day before, rests completely. Meanwhile, with respect to foods, the athlete eats carbohydrate as usual until three days before competition, and then eats a very-high-carbohydrate diet.[3] Endurance athletes who follow this plan can keep going longer than their competitors without ill effects. In a hot climate, extra glycogen confers an additional advantage: as glycogen breaks down, it releases water, which helps to meet the athlete's fluid needs.

Extra glycogen benefits only those who exercise long (90 minutes or more) and hard enough to deplete their stores; the regular, everyday exerciser will not benefit from having larger stores. What that person does need, though, is *adequate* glycogen from eating a diet high in complex carbohydrates.

I have heard that steroids are dangerous, but I have a friend who takes them. His mother is a physician, and she constantly monitors his blood pressure when he is taking steroids. Are they safe in his case?

Steroids have serious side effects and are illegal. Anabolic steroid drugs are derivatives of the androgenic-anabolic male sex hormone testosterone. Testosterone promotes the development of male characteristics (androgenic) and lean body mass (anabolic). Athletes take steroids to stimulate muscle bulking. Steroids are not safe in your friend's case or in any case. The American College of Sports Medicine and the American Academy of Pediatrics condemn the use of steroids by athletes, and their use is banned by the International Olympic Committee.[4] The International Olympic Committee members support their position by citing the known toxic side effects and by stating their belief that steroid use is a form of cheating. Competitors who use the drugs put other athletes in the difficult position of either conceding an unfair advantage to abusing competitors or taking steroids themselves and accepting the risk of untoward side effects.

The list of hazards and adverse reactions from steroids continues to grow amid only a slight decline in use of the drugs. Among the side effects and adverse reactions that steroids produce are cancerous liver tumors that impair liver function, causing it to rupture and hemorrhage; testicular shrinkage in men and masculinization of women; cardiovascular problems; and sterility.[5]

Steroid users also experience a sharp change in their blood lipid profiles to that associated with a high risk of heart disease. In one study, at the peak of steroid use, all users had blood lipid profiles indicative of a very high risk of heart disease. Even six months after cessation of steroid use, the users demonstrated an increased risk.[6] Your friend is sure to develop side effects no matter how closely a trainer or physician monitors him. Table NP9–1 lists side effects and adverse reactions to anabolic steroids.

Health care providers can play a critical role in educating athletes who seek their counsel about steroid use. The dangers of steroid use cannot be overemphasized. To convey this

MINIGLOSSARY

amino acids: isolated components of protein promoted to athletes on the mistaken notion that the body prefers single chemicals to those combined naturally in foods.

astragalus: see *herbal steroids.*

bee pollen: a product sold with the claim that it aids in weight loss and boosts athletic performance, but that in reality has no such effects.

branched-chain amino acids: amino acids that are burned for energy by muscle tissue; athletes do not need supplements of these, because the liver liberates exactly the right amounts with exactly the right timing to support exercise; leucine, isoleucine, and valine.

brewer's yeast: a preparation of yeast cells promoted because it contains high concentrations of B vitamins; falsely promoted as an energy booster.

damiana: see *herbal steroids.*

DNA (deoxyribonucleic acid): a necessary chemical in protein synthesis; falsely promoted as an energy booster.

dong quai: see *herbal steroids.*

fo ti teng: see *herbal steroids.*

gelatin: protein used to thicken foods; sometimes falsely claimed to be a strength enhancer.

ginseng: a plant whose extract has been inappropriately promoted as an energy booster. See also *herbal steroids.*

ginseng root: see *herbal steroids.*

glandular products: extracts and concentrates of glands and tissues from cows, pigs, and sheep; falsely promoted as providing specific nutrition to the athlete's glands and organs.

glycine: see *amino acids.*

growth hormone releasers: a product falsely promoted as enhancing athletic performance.

herbal steroids: curious mixtures of "adaptogens" and "aphrodisiacs"; marketed with false claims that these herbs contain and enhance hormonal activity.[a]

licorice root: see *herbal steroids.*

octacosanol: an alcohol isolated from wheat germ; often falsely promoted as enhancing athletic performance.

palmetto berries: see *herbal steroids.*

pangamic acid: also called vitamin B_{15} (but it is not a vitamin); falsely promoted as an energy booster.

RNA (ribonucleic acid): a necessary chemical in protein synthesis; falsely promoted as enhancing athletic performance.

royal jelly: the substance produced by worker bees and fed to the queen bee. If it often falsely promoted as an ergogenic aid to athletes.

sarsaparilla: see *herbal steroids.*

sarsaparilla leaf: see *herbal steroids.*

schizandra: see *herbal steroids.*

superoxide dismutase (SOD): an enzyme that protects the body from oxidative damage; inappropriately marketed to athletes in tablet form as an energy booster.

unicorn root: see *herbal steroids.*

wheat germ oil: the oil from the wheat kernel; often falsely promoted as an energy booster.

yohimbe bark: see *herbal steroids.*

yucca: see *herbal steroids.*

[a]V. E. Tyler, "Bodybuilding" herbs, *Nutrition Forum,* March 1988, p. 23.

TABLE NP9–1   Anabolic Steroids: Side Effects and Adverse Reactions

ESTABLISHED SIDE EFFECTS AND ADVERSE REACTIONS:

Acne
Cancer
Cholesterol increase
Clitoris enlargement
Death
Edema (water retention in tissue)
Fetal damage
Frequent or continuing erections
HDL (which helps reduce cholesterol) decrease
Heart disease
Hirsutism (hairiness in women—irreversible)
Increased risk of coronary artery disease (heart attack, stroke)
Jaundice

Liver disease
Liver tumors
Male pattern baldness (in women—irreversible)
Oily skin (females only)
Peliosis hepatitis (a liver disease)
Penis enlargement (young boys)
Priapism (painful, prolonged erections)
Prostate enlargement
Sterility (reversible)
Stunted growth
Swelling of feet or lower legs
Testicular atrophy
Yellowing of the eyes or skin

OTHER POSSIBLE SIDE EFFECTS AMD ADVERSE REACTIONS:

Abdominal or stomach pains
Aggressive, combative behavior ("roid rage")
Anaphylactic shock (from injections)
Black, tarry, or light-colored stools
Bone pain
Breast development (sore or swelling—male)
Chills
Dark-colored urine
Depression
Diarrhea
Fatigue
Feeling of abdominal or stomach fullness
Feeling of discomfort
Fever
Frequent urge to urinate (mature males)
Gallstones
Headache
High blood pressure
Hives
Hypercalcemia (too much calcium)
Impotence
Increased chance of injury to muscles, tendons and ligaments, plus longer recovery period from injuries

Insomnia
Kidney disease
Kidney stones (from hypercalcemia)
Listlessness
Menstrual irregularities
Muscle cramps
Nausea or vomiting
Purple- or red-colored spots on body, inside of mouth, or nose
Rash
Septic shock (blood poisoning from injections)
Sexual problems
Sore tongue
Unexplained darkening of skin
Unexplained weight loss
Unnatural hair growth
Unpleasant breath odor
Unusual bleeding
Unusual weight gain
Urination problems
Vomiting blood

Source: R. W. Miller, Athletes and steroids: Playing a deadly game, *FDA Consumer,* November 1987, pp. 17–21, adapted from information in B. Goldman, P. Bush, and R. Katz, *Death in the Locker Room* (South Bend, Ind.: Icarus, 1984).

message, professionals must speak simply and emphatically: the price for the potential competitive edge that steroids confer is high—sometimes the cost is life itself. The commissioner for the Food and Drug Administration (FDA) warns that steroids are not a simple material that builds bigger muscles. They are complex chemicals that the body does not handle easily, particularly in the large amounts that bodybuilders or other athletes frequently use.[7] The safest effective way to build muscle has always been through hard training, and—despite popular misconceptions—it still is.

What about caffeine? I've heard that it can improve endurance performance.

Although some research findings support the use of caffeine to enhance endurance, other findings suggest that caffeine has no effect on endurance.[8] If caffeine does enhance endurance, it is probably because it stimulates fatty acid release, thereby slowing glycogen use.

What is certain is that caffeine is a drug that acts as a stimulant to the nervous system. It elicits a number of physiological and psychological effects in users. The possible benefits must be weighed against caffeine's adverse effects—stomach upset, nervousness, irritability, headache, and diarrhea. Caffeine induces fluid losses that can be potentially hazardous if caffeine-containing fluids are used in place of other fluids by athletes competing in hot environments.[9] The use of caffeine is banned by the International Olympic Committee when it exceeds a dosage equivalent to 5 or 6 cups of coffee in a two-hour period prior to competition.[10]

I've heard that among endurance athletes, blood doping is gaining popularity as a way to enhance performance. What is it, and how does it work?

Blood doping involves removing about 1 liter of blood from an athlete approximately two or three months before competition, freeze-storing the blood, and then reinfusing it back into the athlete a few days before competition. During the time the blood is stored, training resumes as usual, and the athlete's body gradually regenerates new red blood cells. Once the athlete's red blood cells return to normal, which should be timed to occur a few days before competition, the stored blood cells are infused back into the athlete's blood. This causes a 5 to 10 percent rise in hemoglobin concentration, which temporarily increases the oxygen-carrying capacity of the blood and improves cardiovascular endurance.[11] Blood doping does seem to temporarily improve aerobic performance, but not without risks. For endurance athletes competing in hot weather, dehydration increases the relative volume of red blood cells; blood doping augments this further, enhancing the possibility that blood clots may develop. Besides the health hazard, blood doping is considered unethical and illegal; it is forbidden by the International Olympic Committee.

OK, protein supplements and vitamin supplements are ineffective performance enhancers, except when used to treat a true deficiency. Glycogen loading works, but it is unnecessary unless a person works out hard for longer than 90 minutes at a

time. Caffeine may or may not be effective, but can have adverse side effects. Steroids pose serious health risks, and blood doping is risky as well. Caffeine, steroids, and blood doping are also illegal for competition. What about all the other substances athletes use to boost performance? Do they work?

In short, no. Many of these substances have been studied and found to be worthless. The accompanying Miniglossary describes them.

Health professionals can positively influence athletes and others interested in boosting athletic performance by stressing the measures that do help to enhance performance. They are, of course, regular training and sound nutrition.

Notes

1. Adapted in part from E. N. Whitney, E. M. N. Hamilton, and S. R. Rolfes, *Understanding Nutrition,* 5th ed. (St. Paul: West, 1990), pp. 425–428, and E. M. N. Hamilton, E. N. Whitney, and F. S. Sizer, *Nutrition: Concepts and Controversies,* 5th ed. (St. Paul: West, 1991), pp. 345–349.

2. S. M. Kleiner, T. L. Bazarre, and M. D. Litchford, Metabolic profiles, diet, and health practices of championship male and female bodybuilders, *Journal of the American Dietetic Association* 90 (1990): 962–967.

3. W. M. Sherman, Carbohydrate, muscle glycogen, and improved performance, *Physician and Sportsmedicine* 15 (1987): 157–161, 164.

4. P. G. Dyment and B. Goldberg, An-

abolic steroids and the adolescent, *Nutrition* 49 (1989): 1066–1069.

5. H. Haupt and G. D. Rovere, Anabolic steroids: A review of the literature, *American Journal of Sports Medicine* 12 (1984): 469–484.

6. S. M. Kleiner and coauthors, Dietary influences on cardiovascular disease risk in anabolic steroid using and nonusing bodybuilders, *Journal of the American College of Nutrition* 8 (1989): 109–119.

7. R. W. Miller, Athletes and steroids: Playing a deadly game, *FDA Consumer,* November 1987, pp. 17–21.

8. G. I. Wadler and B. Hainline, *Drugs and the Athlete* (Philadelphia: F. A. Davis Co., 1989), pp. 107–113, as cited in J. A. Work, Are java junkies poor sports? *Physician and Sportsmedicine* 19 (1991): 83–88.

9. F. T. O'Neil, M. T. Hynak-Hankinson, and J. Gorman, Research and application of current topics in sports nutrition, *Journal of the American Dietetic Association* 86 (1986): 1007–1015.

10. M. H. Williams, Nutritional ergogenic aids and athletic performance, *Nutrition Today,* January/February 1989, pp. 7–14.

11. D. C. Nieman, *Fitness and Sports Medicine: An Introduction* (Palo Alto, Calif.: Bull Publishing, 1990), pp. 221–268.

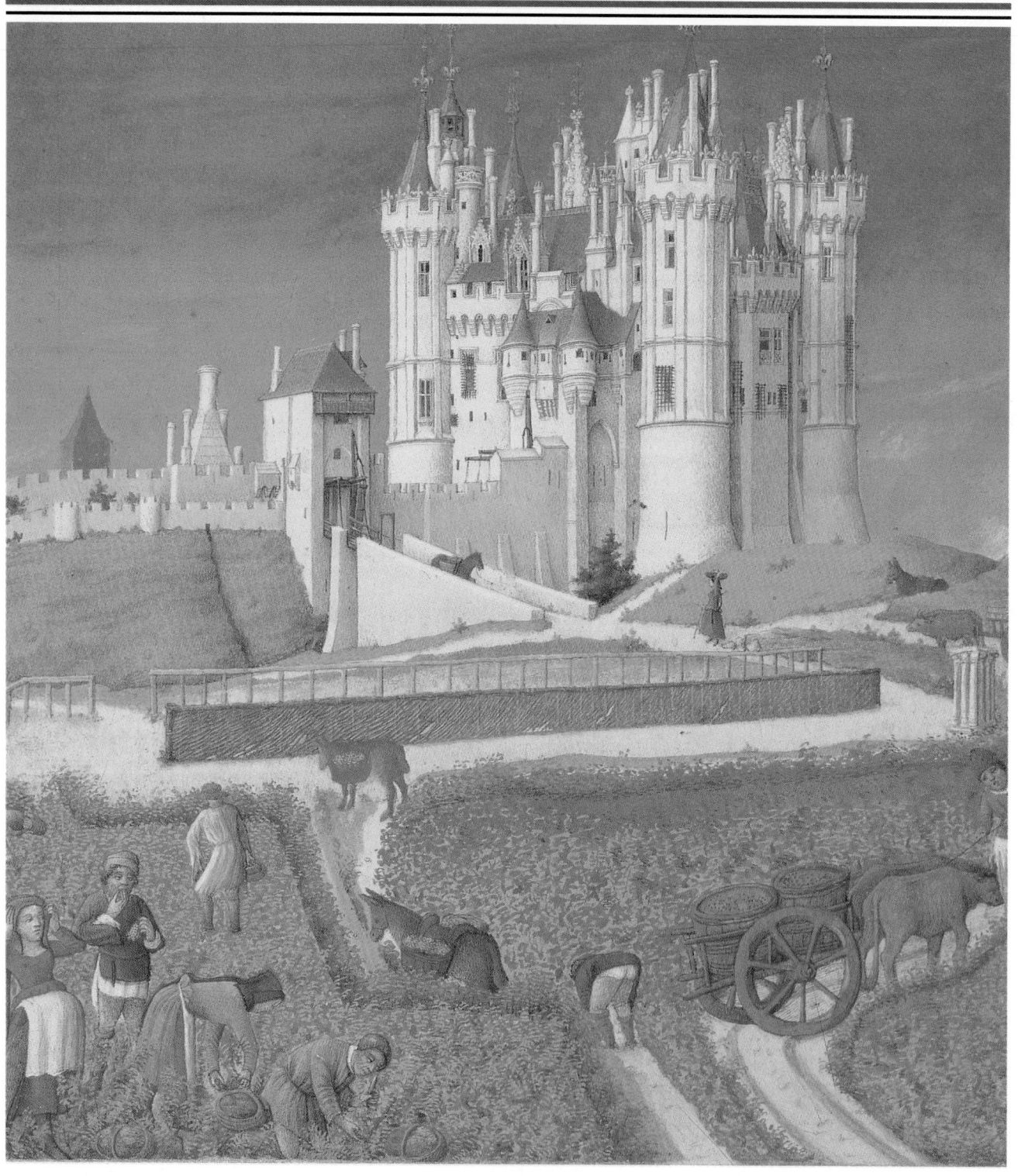

Tres Riches du Duc de Berry, *September, Grape Harvest, Chateau de Saumer, Musee Conde, Giraudon/Art Resource, N.Y.*

Nutrition Assessment

CONTENTS

CHAPTER 10 A finely tuned body and mind depend on the availability and interaction of the essential nutrients. Deficiency, excess, or imbalance of these nutrients upsets the body's metabolic environment and can exert a wide range of effects, depending on the nutrients involved and on the imbalance. Throughout the earlier chapters of this book, the impacts of the various nutrient imbalances have been described. Now it's time to see how health care professionals determine how well people's nutrient needs are being met. Nutrition assessments, the subject of this chapter, provide foundations upon which to build plans for maintaining optimal nutrition status or correcting nutrition problems. The plans themselves, known as nutrition care plans, are described in Chapter 15.

This chapter will make clear that nutrition assessment, correctly performed, is a far cry from the kind of experience the person on the street may encounter in a "nutrition clinic" where a "nutritionist" offers "nutrition assessment." People today are easily led to believe that "computer diet analysis," "hair analysis," or urine tests will accurately determine their nutrition status. They do not understand all the processes involved in doing such tests. They see, however, that the "experts" seem to know a lot and that the systems being used are complicated, so they think there must be some validity to the "results." The tests described in this chapter are those used routinely in standard nutrition assessments, responsibly performed. The section on screening, at the end of this chapter, shows how a rapid, cursory nutrition assessment is correctly performed.

Defining Nutrition Status

Health care professionals perform nutrition assessments to evaluate people's health from a nutrition perspective. For healthy people, nutrition assessments identify nutrition factors that can be improved to achieve optimal health. For people who are ill, nutrition assessments alert health care professionals to nutrition factors that may hinder responses to medical treatment and recovery from illness. Nutrition assessments performed at regular intervals provide ways to monitor changes in nutrition status.

The person conducting a nutrition assessment is usually a skilled dietitian or other qualified health care professional. The assessor gathers information from many sources, including:

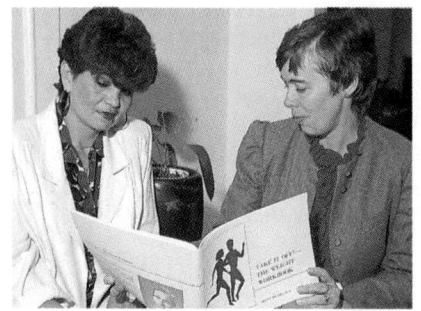

Nutrition assessments define a person's nutrition status.

■ Historical data.
■ Anthropometric measurements.
■ Biochemical analyses (laboratory tests).
■ Physical examinations.

The assessor uses many techniques to collect information from these sources and interprets each finding in relation to the others in order to create a complete picture of a client's nutrition status. The accurate gathering of this information and its careful interpretation provide the basis for a meaningful evaluation. The following sections describe each method in detail.

Historical Data

Clues about present nutrition status become evident with a review of a person's historical data (see Table 10–1). Even when data are subjective, they reveal important facts about a person. A thorough history provides a sense of the whole person.

An adept history taker uses the interview not only to gather facts, but also to establish rapport, exploring a person's life from several angles: health, socioeconomic status, drug use, and diet. The evaluation of histories identifies risk factors associated with poor nutrition status (see Table 10–2, p. 224). Form 10–1 (p. 225) shows the kinds of questions asked to collect information on the many aspects of a person's life that influence nutrition status and to provide clues to possible problems. This discussion briefly reviews the major areas in a person's history that are relevant to nutrition.

Health History

The assessor can obtain health histories from records completed by attending physicians, nurses, or other health care providers. In addition, conversations with the client can uncover valuable health-related information previously overlooked because no one thought to ask or because the client was too upset to think clearly or had simply forgotten to mention it.

An accurate, complete health history can reveal conditions that place a client at risk for malnutrition (review Table 10–2, p. 224). Disorders and their therapies can exert either immediate or long-term effects on nutrition status by interfering with ingestion, digestion, absorption, metabolism, or excretion of nutrients.

Traditionally, histories have been called *medical histories*. However, given that their contents describe a person's health status and that current trends in the medical profession are emphasizing health promotion and disease prevention, the term *health histories* seems more appropriate.

Socioeconomic History

Socioeconomic factors profoundly affect nutrition status. A person's ethnic background and educational level, as well as those of other household

---

TABLE 10–1   **Historical Data Used in Nutrition Assessments**

TYPE OF HISTORY	WHAT IT IDENTIFIES
Health history	Health-related factors that affect nutrition status
Socioeconomic history	Personal, financial, and environmental influences on food intake
Drug history	Medications that affect nutrition status
Diet history	Nutrient intake excesses or deficiencies
24-hour recall	
Usual intake	
Food frequency checklist	
Food diary	

TABLE 10–2 **Risk Factors for Poor Nutrition Status**

HEALTH HISTORY		
Acquired immune deficiency syndrome (AIDS)	Diseases of the GI tract	Pancreatic insufficiency
Alcoholism	Drug addiction	Paralysis
Anorexia	Fever	Physical disability
Cancer	Heart disease	Pregnancy
Chewing or swallowing difficulties (including poorly fitted dentures, dental caries, and missing teeth)	Hormonal imbalance	Radiation therapy
	Hyperlipidemia	Recent major illness
	Hypertension	Recent major surgery
Chronic obstructive pulmonary disease	Infection	Recent weight loss or gain
	Kidney disease	Smoking of cigarettes
Circulatory problems	Liver disease	Surgery of the GI tract
Constipation	Lung disease	Trauma
Crohn's disease	Mental retardation or deterioration	Ulcerative colitis
Dementia	Multiple pregnancies	Ulcers
Diabetes	Nausea	Underweight
Diarrhea	Neurologic disorders	Vomiting
	Overweight	

SOCIOECONOMIC HISTORY		
Eating alone	Inadequate food storage facilities	Poor self-concept
Inadequate food budget	Poor education	Unavailability of transportation
Inadequate food preparation facilities		

DRUG HISTORY		
Analgesics	Antidiarrheal agents	Immunosuppressants
Antacids	Antihyperlipemic agents	Laxatives
Antibiotics	Antihypertensive agents	Oral contraceptives
Anticancer agents	Antiulcer agents	Sulfonylurea agents
Anticonvulsant agents	Catabolic steroids	Vitamin and other nutrient preparations
Antidepressant agents	Diuretics	

DIET HISTORY		
Anorexia nervosa	Inadequate food intake	No intake for ten or more days
Bulimia	Intravenous fluids (other than total parenteral nutrition) for ten or more days	Poor appetite
Excessive food intake		Restricted or fad diets
Frequent eating out		

members, influence food availability and food choices. An understanding of the community customs and resources also helps the assessor evaluate nutrition status. For example, knowing the food habits of the major ethnic groups within the locale, regional food preferences, and nutrition resources and programs available in the community prepares the interviewer with

FORM 10-1 **History**

Name _____   Date _____

Address _____   Date of last medical checkup _____

_____   Age _____ Sex _____

_____   Height _____ Weight _____

Phone _____   Usual weight _____

Reason for admission _____   Ideal weight _____

HEALTH HISTORY

1. Have you been told that you have any of the following (check any that apply)?

____ Diabetes   ____ Heart disease   ____ Ulcers

____ GI disorders   ____ Lung disease   ____ Cancer

____ High blood pressure ____ Kidney disease   ____ Other

____ Hardening of arteries ____ Liver disease   _____

2. Do you have complaints about any of the following?

____ Lack of appetite   ____ Diarrhea   ____ Nausea

____ Difficulty chewing or swallowing ____ Indigestion   ____ Vomiting

____ Constipation   ____ Fever   ____ Other

3. For females:

Are you pregnant? _____ How many months? _____

How many pregnancies have you carried to term? _____

When was your last child born? _____

Are your menstrual periods normal? _____ If not, please explain: _____

SOCIOECONOMIC HISTORY

1. Last grade of school completed _____ Still in school? _____
2. Are you employed? _____ Occupation _____
3. Does someone else live with you? _____ Who? _____
4. Do you use tobacco in any way? _____ How much? _____
5. Where do you eat most of your meals? _____
6. Do you have a refrigerator? _____ Stove? _____
7. How often do you shop for food? _____

DRUG HISTORY

1. Do you take medication, either prescribed by a doctor or over-the-counter?

Name of drug	Reason for taking	Dose	Frequency	Duration of intake
_____	_____	_____	_____	_____
_____	_____	_____	_____	_____
_____	_____	_____	_____	_____

2. Have you noticed any side effects from taking these medications? ____ If so, please explain: _____
3. Do you take vitamins or any kind of supplements? _____ Which ones? _____

How often? _____ For what reason? _____

(continued)

FORM 10–1   *(continued)*

DIET HISTORY

1. Have you recently lost or gained more than 10 lb? _____ If yes, explain the surrounding circumstances (including associated illness, dietary changes, and time frame): _____

2. Do you eat at regular times each day? _____ How many times per day? _____

3. Do you usually eat snacks? _____ When? _____

4. What foods do you particularly like? _____ Dislike? _____

5. Are there foods you don't eat for other reasons? _____

6. Do you have difficulty eating? _____

7. How would you describe your feelings about food? _____

8. How do your eating habits change when you are emotionally upset? _____

9. Are you, or is any member of your family, on a special diet? ____ If yes, who and what kind? _____

10. Do you drink alcohol? _____ How much? _____ How often? _____

11. How would you describe your exercise habits? _____ Type of exercise _____
    Intensity _____ Duration _____ Frequency _____

12. Are there any other facts about your lifestyle that you think might be related to your nutritional health? _____
    Explain _____

Note: Use the appropriate form to record food intake data (Form 10–2, 10–3, or 10–4).

needed background information. Local health departments and social agencies often can help provide such information.

Level of income also influences the diet. In general, the quality of the diet declines as income falls, and an inadequate income puts an adequate diet out of reach. Agencies use poverty indexes to identify people at risk for poor nutrition and to qualify people for government food assistance programs.

Low income affects not only the power to purchase foods but also the ability to shop for, store, and cook them. A skilled assessor will note whether a person has transportation to a grocery store that sells a sufficient variety of low-cost foods, and whether the person has access to clean running water, a refrigerator, and a stove.

Drug History

The interactions of foods and drugs require that special attention be paid to any client who takes drugs routinely. Hundreds of drugs interact with nutrients, making imbalances or deficiencies likely. Nausea and vomiting, common side effects of many drugs, interfere with food intake. Table B = ref in Appendix B contains an extensive list of drug-nutrient interactions.

If a person is taking any drug, the assessor records the name of the drug; the dose, frequency, and duration of intake; the reason for taking the drug; and signs of any adverse effects. Chapter 14 discusses nutrient-drug interactions in more detail.

Diet History

A diet history provides a record of a person's food intake. The accurate recording of such data requires skill. Skilled dietitians often use food

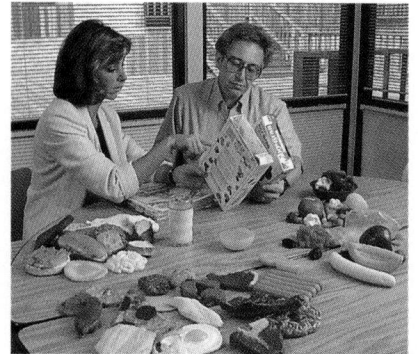

Plastic food models and measuring devices help clients visualize portion sizes.

models or photos and measuring devices to help clients identify the types of foods and quantities consumed. The assessor also needs to know how the foods are prepared. In addition to foods, assessors must ask about consumption of beverages, including those containing alcohol or caffeine. Food choices are an important part of the lifestyle and often represent an expression of personal philosophy. The assessor who asks nonjudgmental, open-ended questions about food intake encourages trust and can then gather accurate information.

Tools for obtaining food intake data include the 24-hour recall, the usual intake record, the food frequency checklist, and the food diary. After obtaining food intakes, the assessor compares them with standards, usually nutrient recommendations or food guides. The question the assessor is preparing to answer is how closely the person's diet meets the recommendations. Are the types and amounts of proteins, carbohydrates, and fats (including cholesterol) appropriate? Is caffeine or alcohol consumption excessive? Are intakes of any vitamins or minerals (including sodium and iron) excessive or deficient?

Besides identifying possible nutrient imbalances, diet histories provide valuable clues about how people will accept diet changes should they be necessary. Information about what and how a person eats facilitates the setting of realistic and attainable nutrition goals.

24-HOUR RECALL. The 24-hour recall provides data for one day only and is commonly used in nutrition surveys to obtain estimates of the typical food intakes of large numbers of people in given populations. The assessor asks each client to recount everything eaten or drunk in the past 24 hours or for the previous day. (Form 10–2 on p. 228 shows a typical 24-hour recall form.) The recall's usefulness is limited in that it does not provide enough accurate information to allow generalizations about an individual's usual food intake. This limitation is partially overcome when 24-hour recalls are collected on several nonconsecutive days, including both weekdays and weekend days.[1]

An advantage of the 24-hour recall is that it is easy to obtain. It is also more likely to provide accurate data, at least about the past 24 hours, than a person's estimates of average intakes over long times. However, the previous day's intake may not be typical; the person may be unable to report portion sizes accurately; and the person may even conceal or forget facts about foods eaten. As a result, sometimes the information gathered in a 24-hour recall does not truly reflect a person's usual intake.

USUAL INTAKE. To obtain data about a person's usual intake, an inquiry might begin with, "What is the first thing you usually eat or drink during the day?" Similar questions follow until a typical daily intake pattern emerges. This method is similar to the 24-hour recall and uses the same form (Form 10–2). A person's usual intake pattern can provide much useful information, especially in verifying food intake when the past 24 hours have been atypical. A person whose intake varies widely from day to day, however, may find it difficult to answer such general questions, and in such a case, the data may be useless in estimating nutrient intake.

Judgmental responses express an opinion about something that is said. For example:

INTERVIEWER: Do you ever use milk?

CLIENT: Only a half-cup about once a week when I eat dry cereal.

JUDGMENTAL RESPONSE: You know you should be drinking at least 2 glasses of milk each day.

NONJUDGMENTAL RESPONSE: Is there any reason why you don't use milk more often?

Open-ended questions allow the client a choice of answers to the question. For example:

OPEN-ENDED QUESTION: How do you prepare your sliced turkey sandwich?

CLOSED-ENDED QUESTION: Do you put lettuce, tomato, and mayonnaise on your sliced turkey sandwich?

FORM 10–2   **24-Hour Recall or Usual Intake Pattern**

Name and address _____   Date _____

_____

_____

Did you take a vitamin/mineral supplement? _____

If yes, what kind? _____   Dose _____

Please record the amount and type of foods and beverages consumed today. [Or: Please record the amount and type of foods and beverages you typically consume each day.]

FOOD	AMOUNT (c, tbsp, or piece)	DESCRIPTION (how cooked, how served)

FOOD FREQUENCY CHECKLIST. Another approach is to use a food frequency checklist. The purpose of this record is to ascertain how often an individual eats a specific type of food per day, week, or month. The assessor uses a long list of foods or types of foods, asking clients to state how often they eat each one. This information helps pinpoint food groups, and therefore nutrients, that may be excessive or deficient in the diet. That a person ate no vegetables yesterday may not seem particularly significant, but that the person never eats vegetables should ring a bell warning of possible nutrient deficiencies. If used together with the usual intake or 24-hour recall approach, the food frequency checklist permits cross-checking the information obtained to improve accuracy. Form 10–3 (p. 229) is a food frequency checklist.

FOOD RECORDS. Food records taken over several days or even weeks provide a valuable tool for gathering food intake data. The assessor instructs the person keeping the record to write down all foods consumed, as well as the amounts of foods consumed and the way the foods are prepared. The information should be recorded as promptly after eating each meal or snack as possible.

FORM 10-3　**Food Frequency Checklist**

The following information will help us to understand your regular eating habits so that we may offer you the best service possible. If you have any doubt about some items, be sure to underestimate the "goodness" of your habits rather than to overestimate.

1. How many times *per week* do you eat the following foods? Circle the appropriate number:　　　PER WEEK

Poultry	0 <1 1 2 3 4 5 6 7 8 9 >9
Fish	0 <1 1 2 3 4 5 6 7 8 9 >9
Hot dogs	0 <1 1 2 3 4 5 6 7 8 9 >9
Bacon	0 <1 1 2 3 4 5 6 7 8 9 >9
Luncheon meat	0 <1 1 2 3 4 5 6 7 8 9 >9
Sausage	0 <1 1 2 3 4 5 6 7 8 9 >9
Pork or ham	0 <1 1 2 3 4 5 6 7 8 9 >9
Salt pork	0 <1 1 2 3 4 5 6 7 8 9 >9
Liver	0 <1 1 2 3 4 5 6 7 8 9 >9
Beef or veal	0 <1 1 2 3 4 5 6 7 8 9 >9
Other meats (which?) _____	0 <1 1 2 3 4 5 6 7 8 9 >9
Cooked dried beans or peas	0 <1 1 2 3 4 5 6 7 8 9 >9
Eggs	0 <1 1 2 3 4 5 6 7 8 9 >9
Fast foods	0 <1 1 2 3 4 5 6 7 8 9 >9

2. How many times *per day* do you eat the following foods? Circle the appropriate number:　　　PER DAY

Bread, toast, rolls, muffins	0 <1 1 2 3 4 5 6 7 8 9 >9
Milk (including on cereal)	0 <1 1 2 3 4 5 6 7 8 9 >9
Yogurt or tofu	0 <1 1 2 3 4 5 6 7 8 9 >9
Cheese or cheese dishes	0 <1 1 2 3 4 5 6 7 8 9 >9
Sugar, jam, jelly, syrup, honey	0 <1 1 2 3 4 5 6 7 8 9 >9
Butter or margarine	0 <1 1 2 3 4 5 6 7 8 9 >9

3. How many times *per week* do you eat the following foods? Circle the appropriate number:　　　PER WEEK

Fruits or fruit juices	0 <1 1 2 3 4 5 6 7 8 9 >9
Vegetables other than potatoes	0 <1 1 2 3 4 5 6 7 8 9 >9
Potatoes and other starchy vegetables	0 <1 1 2 3 4 5 6 7 8 9 >9
Salads or raw vegetables	0 <1 1 2 3 4 5 6 7 8 9 >9
Cereal (which kind?) _____	0 <1 1 2 3 4 5 6 7 8 9 >9
Pancakes or waffles	0 <1 1 2 3 4 5 6 7 8 9 >9
Rice or other cooked grains	0 <1 1 2 3 4 5 6 7 8 9 >9
Noodles (macaroni, spaghetti)	0 <1 1 2 3 4 5 6 7 8 9 >9
Crackers or pretzels	0 <1 1 2 3 4 5 6 7 8 9 >9
Sweet rolls or doughnuts	0 <1 1 2 3 4 5 6 7 8 9 >9
Peanut butter or nuts	0 <1 1 2 3 4 5 6 7 8 9 >9
Milk or milk products	0 <1 1 2 3 4 5 6 7 8 9 >9
TV dinners, pot pies, other prepared meals	0 <1 1 2 3 4 5 6 7 8 9 >9
Sweet bakery goods (cake, cookies)	0 <1 1 2 3 4 5 6 7 8 9 >9
Snack foods (potato or corn chips)	0 <1 1 2 3 4 5 6 7 8 9 >9

(continued)

FORM 10-3   *(continued)*

	PER WEEK
Candy	0 <1 1 2 3 4 5 6 7 8 9 >9
Soft drinks (which?) _____	0 <1 1 2 3 4 5 6 7 8 9 >9
Coffee or tea	0 <1 1 2 3 4 5 6 7 8 9 >9
Frozen sweets (which?) _____	0 <1 1 2 3 4 5 6 7 8 9 >9
Instant meals such as breakfast bars or diet meal beverages (which?) _____	0 <1 1 2 3 4 5 6 7 8 9 >9
Wine	0 <1 1 2 3 4 5 6 7 8 9 >9
Beer	0 <1 1 2 3 4 5 6 7 8 9 >9
Whiskey, vodka, rum, etc.	0 <1 1 2 3 4 5 6 7 8 9 >9

4. What specific kinds of the following foods do you eat most often? Include the name of the food; whether it is fresh, canned, or frozen; and how it is prepared.

Fruits and fruit juices _____

Vegetables _____

Milk and milk products _____

Meats and meat alternates _____

Breads and cereals _____

Desserts _____

Snack foods _____

5. Please list the names of any liquid, powder, or pill forms of vitamin or mineral products you take, and state how often you take them. Please list also any diet supplement you use (such as protein milk shakes or brewer's yeast), how much you use, and how often you use it. _____

6. Is there anything else we should know about your food/nutrient intake? _____
_____

Food records work especially well with cooperative people but require considerable time and effort on their part. A prime advantage of the food record is that the record keeper assumes an active role and may for the first time become aware of personal food habits and begin to assume responsibility for them. Food records can be particularly valuable for overweight people trying to lose weight. Researchers found that among 2000 individuals in a weight-loss program, their faithfulness in keeping food records was a better predictor of their weight loss than their initial body mass indexes, exercise habits, or ages.[2]

One type of food intake record is the food diary, which includes not only the foods eaten, but time of day, place, others present, and mood. (Form 10–4 on p. 231 provides an example.) A food diary can help both the assessor and the client to determine factors associated with eating that may affect dietary balance and adequacy. The food diary also provides the assessor with an accurate picture of the diary keeper's lifestyle and factors that affect food intake. For these reasons, a food diary can be particularly useful in outpatient counseling for such nutrition problems as overweight, underweight, or food allergy.

The major disadvantages of food records stem from poor compliance in recording the data. Additionally, conscious or unconscious changes in eat-

FORM 10-4   **Food Diary**

Time	Place	With Whom	Emotional State	Hungry or Not Hungry	Food Eaten (amount)
Name				Date	

(etc.)

ing habits may occur while the person is keeping the record, distorting the assessment of the person's food habits.

ANALYSIS OF FOOD INTAKE DATA. After collecting food intake data, the assessor estimates nutrient intakes, either informally or by using food composition tables. An informal estimate is quick and can be used to get a general picture of an individual's diet.

Informal estimates require a general knowledge of the nutrients in the different food groups. Table 1-1 shows the major nutrient contributions of the four food groups. If an individual consistently failed to use dairy products of any kind, for example, the assessor might suspect possible deficiencies of protein, calcium, vitamin D, riboflavin, or zinc. If the assessor then determined that the individual made up for lack of these nutrients through suitable food choices from the other groups, no concern would be indicated. If, however, the nutrients were not being consumed, this would warn the assessor of a possible deficiency.

The formal calculation can be performed either manually (by looking up each food in a table of food composition, recording its nutrients, and adding them up) or by using a computer diet analysis program. The assessor then compares the intakes with standards such as the RDA.

Used with skill, diet histories can be superbly informative about a client's nutrient intakes. The skillful assessor uses them with their limitations in mind. For example, a computer diet analysis tends to imply an accuracy greater than is possible to obtain from data as uncertain as those that provide the starting information. Nutrient contents of foods listed in tables of food composition or stored in computer databases are averages, and for some nutrients, complete data are not available. In addition, the available data on nutrient contents of foods do not reflect the amounts of nutrients a person actually absorbs. Iron is a case in point: its availability from a given meal may vary from as high as 50 percent to less than 2 percent. Chapter 8 explains how to calculate iron absorption from a meal.

> Although computers are invaluable for doing rapid calculations on valid data that have been assembled with care, they turn out nonsense when used to process data that are meaningless from the start ("garbage in, garbage out"). A computer program using arbitrary values for nutrients or a program assembled hastily and carelessly cannot accurately compute nutrient intakes.

Furthermore, there is uncertainty about portion sizes. The person who reports eating "a serving" of greens may not distinguish between ¼ cup and 2 whole cups. Thus there are many opportunities for error when comparing reported nutrient intakes with nutrient needs.

An estimate of nutrient intakes from a diet history provides clues only. It is a starting point, and must be combined with other sources of information to allow the assessor to confirm or eliminate the possibility of suspected nutrition problems. The assessor must constantly remember that a sufficient *intake* of a nutrient does not guarantee adequate nutrient *status* for an individual. Likewise, insufficient intake does not always indicate deficiency, but it does alert the assessor to a possible problem. Each person is in a unique state of health, and each digests, absorbs, metabolizes, and excretes nutrients in a unique way. Individual needs vary; intakes of nutrients identified by diet histories are only pieces of a puzzle that must be put together with other indicators of nutrition status to extract meaning.

primary deficiency: a nutrient deficiency caused directly by lack of that nutrient in the diet. A nutrient deficiency caused by the body's inability to digest, absorb, or utilize a nutrient in the normal fashion, or by excess destruction or excretion of the nutrient, is a **secondary deficiency.**

Anthropometric Measurements

anthropometric measurements: measurements of physical characteristics of the body, such as height, weight, and various girths.

Anthropometric measurements are physical measurements that provide an indirect assessment of body composition and development (see Table 10–3). They serve two primary purposes: first, to evaluate the progress of growth in pregnant women, infants, children, and adolescents; and second, to detect undernutrition and obesity in all age groups.

In using anthropometry, health care providers compare measurements taken on an individual with standards specific for gender and age or with previous measurements of the individual. Measurements taken periodically and compared with previous measurements reveal changes in an individual's status.

Anthropometric measurements require minimal equipment, but mastering the correct techniques requires proper instruction and practice to ensure reliability. Height and weight are well-recognized anthropometrics; others include fatfold measurements and various measures of lean tissue. Some

TABLE 10–3   **Anthropometric Measurements Used in Nutrition Assessments**

TYPE OF MEASUREMENT	WHAT IT REFLECTS
Abdominal girth measurement	Abdominal fluid retention
Height-weight	Overnutrition and undernutrition; growth in children
%IBW, %UBW,[a] recent weight change	Overnutrition and undernutrition
Head circumference	Brain growth and development in infants and children under two
Midarm circumference	Muscle mass and subcutaneous fat
Fatfold	Subcutaneous fat and total body fat
Midarm muscle circumference	Muscle mass (i.e., protein status)

[a]%IBW = percent ideal body weight; %UBW = percent usual body weight. These concepts are discussed in the text.

measurements are useful in specific situations. For example, a head circumference measurement may help to assess brain development in an infant, and an abdominal girth measurement supplies information about abdominal fluid retention in individuals with liver disease.

Measures of Growth and Development

Height and weight are among the most common and useful anthropometric measurements. Length measurements for infants and height measurements for children are particularly valuable in assessing growth, and therefore nutrition status. For adults, height measurements alone are not critical but help to estimate desirable weight and to interpret other assessment data. Once adult height has been reached, changes in body weight provide useful information in assessing overnutrition and undernutrition.

HEIGHT. For infants or children who cannot stand erect, health care professionals measure length using special equipment. The assessor lays the barefoot infant on a measuring board that has a fixed headboard and movable footboard attached at right angles to the surface. Often it takes two people to obtain an accurate measurement: one to hold the infant's head against the headboard and keep the legs straight, and the other to do the measuring. This method provides the most accurate measure possible, but many health care providers use a less exacting method. They may simply hold the infant straight, with its head against the headboard or other vertical support; then mark the blanket with a chalk or pen at the infant's heel; and then measure the distance from the headboard to the mark. Even more informally and less accurately, with the infant lying on a flat surface, they may extend a nonstretchable measuring tape along the side of the infant from the top of the head to the heel of the foot.

The procedure for measuring a child who can stand erect and cooperate is the same as for an adult. The best way to measure standing height is with

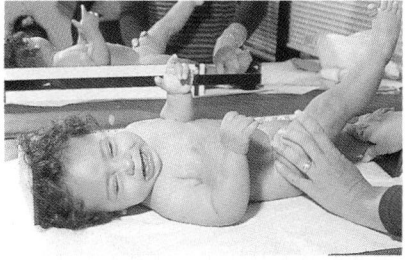

A measuring board with a fixed headboard and movable footboard provides the most accurate tool for measuring an infant's length.

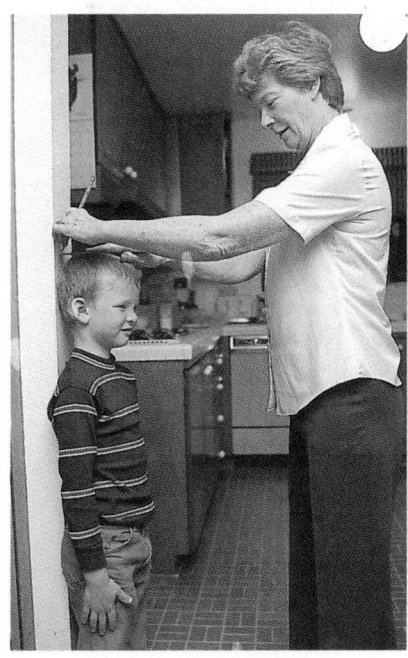

Accurate height measurements are obtained in children and adults using a measuring tape affixed to a flat wall.

the person's back against a flat wall alongside an affixed, nonstretchable measuring tape or stick. The person stands erect, without shoes, with heels together. The person's line of sight should be horizontal, with the heels, buttocks, shoulders, and head touching the wall. The assessor uses a block, book, or other square-cornered object to ensure that the top of the head is measured at an exact right angle to the wall. The assessor carefully checks the height measurement and immediately records the result in either inches or centimeters. (Immediate recording prevents forgetting the measurement.)

The measuring rod of a scale is an acceptable tool, but because of its movability, it provides a less accurate measurement of height. The assessor follows the same general procedure, asking the person to face away from the scale and to take extra care to stand erect. Accuracy improves if the assessor keeps an eye on the rod to make sure it doesn't bend up or down from a true right angle to the vertical.

Unfortunately, many health care providers merely ask clients how tall they are rather than measuring their height. Self-reported height is often inaccurate and should be used only as a last resort when measurement is impractical (in the case of an uncooperative client, an emergency admission, or the like).

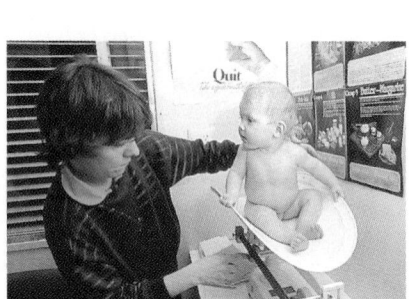

Infants are measured on special scales designed to hold them.

WEIGHT. For measuring weight, beam balance and electronic scales are most accurate. To measure infants' weights, assessors use special scales that allow infants to lie or sit. Weighing infants naked, without diapers, is standard procedure. To weigh children who can stand, health care providers use the same procedure as for adults. To make repeated measures useful, standardized conditions are necessary. Each weighing should take place at the same time of day (preferably before breakfast), in the same amount of clothing (without shoes), after the person has voided, and on the same scale. Special scales are available for weighing people who are bedridden. Bathroom scales are inaccurate and inappropriate in a professional setting. As with all measurements, the assessor records observed weight immediately, in either pounds or kilograms.

HEAD CIRCUMFERENCE. Assessors may also measure head circumference to confirm that infant growth is proceeding normally or to help detect protein-energy malnutrition (PEM) and evaluate the extent of its impact on brain size. To measure head circumference, the assessor places a nonstretchable tape so as to encircle the largest part of the infant's or child's head: just above the eyebrow ridges, just above the point where the ears attach, and around the occipital prominence at the back of the head. For accuracy in recording, the assessor immediately notes the measure in either inches or centimeters.

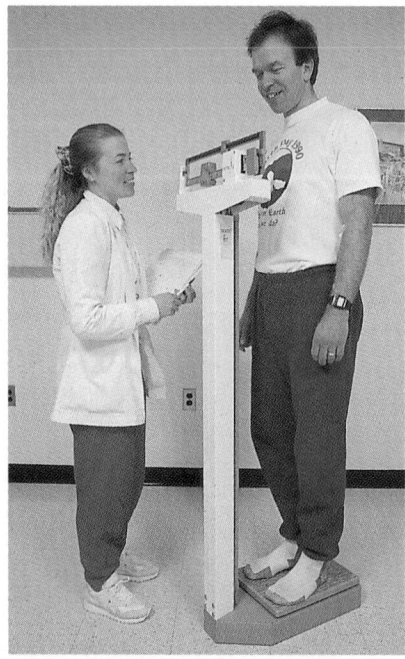

Beam balance scales provide accurate weight measurements for children and adults.

ANALYSIS OF MEASURES. Growth retardation indicated by measurements below standard for height, weight, or head circumference in infants and young children is an important sign of poor nutrition status. Health professionals generally evaluate physical development by comparing a child's growth rate with standard charts. Standard charts compare weight to age, height to age, and weight to height; ideally, height and weight are within the same or neighboring percentiles. Although individual growth patterns may vary, in general, a child's growth curve will stay at about the same percentile throughout childhood. In children whose growth has been retarded, nutrition rehabilitation will ideally induce height and weight to increase to higher percentiles. In overweight children, the goal is for weight to remain stable as height increases, until weight becomes appropriate for height. Appendix B provides growth charts and describes how they are used.

Head circumference is a useful measure in children under two years of age. Since the brain is rapidly growing before birth and during early infancy, malnourished children may have fewer brain cells and smaller head circumferences. The assessor plots head circumference measurements on a percentile growth chart; head circumference percentile should be similar to the child's weight and height percentiles. Small head circumference can reflect both nutrition- and nonnutrition-related factors.[3] Extreme and chronic malnutrition, as well as medical disorders and genetic variation, represent some of these factors.

For adults, health care providers typically compare weights with weight-for-height tables (such as Table 10–4), which are specific for height, gender, and frame size. To use the height-weight table, the assessor refers to a table

TABLE 10–4   **Metropolitan Height and Weight Tables**

MEN					WOMEN				
Height		Frame			Height		Frame		
Feet	Inches	Small	Medium	Large	Feet	Inches	Small	Medium	Large
5	2	128–134	131–141	138–150	4	10	102–111	109–121	118–131
5	3	130–136	133–143	140–153	4	11	103–113	111–123	120–134
5	4	132–138	135–145	142–156	5	0	104–115	113–126	122–137
5	5	134–140	137–148	144–160	5	1	106–118	115–129	125–140
5	6	136–142	139–151	146–164	5	2	108–121	118–132	128–143
5	7	138–145	142–154	149–168	5	3	111–124	121–135	131–147
5	8	140–148	145–157	152–172	5	4	114–127	124–138	134–151
5	9	142–151	148–160	155–176	5	5	117–130	127–141	137–155
5	10	144–154	151–163	158–180	5	6	120–133	130–144	140–159
5	11	146–157	154–166	161–184	5	7	123–136	133–147	143–163
6	0	149–160	157–170	164–188	5	8	126–139	136–150	146–167
6	1	152–164	160–174	168–192	5	9	129–142	139–153	149–170
6	2	155–168	164–178	172–197	5	10	132–145	142–156	152–173
6	3	158–172	167–182	176–202	5	11	135–148	145–159	155–176
6	4	162–176	171–187	181–207	6	0	138–151	148–162	158–179

Note: Weights at ages 25 to 29 based on lowest mortality. Weights in pounds according to frame (in indoor clothing weighing 5 lb for men or 3 lb for women; shoes with 1-inch heels). For frame size standards, see Appendix B.

Source: Reproduced courtesy of Metropolitan Life Insurance Company. Source of basic data. Society of Actuaries and Association of Life Insurance Medical Directors of America, *1979 Build Study,* 1980.

TABLE 10–5   **Quick Estimation of Ideal Body Weight**

MEN

For 5 ft, consider 106 lb a reasonable weight.
For each inch over 5 ft, add 6 lb.
Subtract 6 lb for each inch under 5 ft.
Add 10% for a large-framed individual; subtract 10% for a small-framed individual.
Example: A man 5 ft 8 inches tall (medium frame) would start at 106 lb, add 48,
   and arrive at a reasonable weight of 154 lb.

WOMEN

For 5 ft, consider 100 lb a reasonable weight.
For each inch over 5 ft, add 5 lb.
Subtract 5 lb for each inch under 5 ft.
Add 10% for a large-framed individual; subtract 10% for a small-framed individual.
Example: A woman 5 ft 6 inches tall (medium frame) would start at 100 lb, add
   30, and arrive at a reasonable weight of 130 lb.

of frame sizes, such as the one based on wrist circumference provided in Appendix B. The height and weight tables suggest an appropriate weight range, rather than pinpointing one ideal weight. This is a good reminder that there is no perfect weight for anyone. A quick method of estimating ideal body weight frequently used by health care professionals is shown in Table 10–5.

The height-weight tables are useful for identifying both undernutrition and overnutrition. A standard derived from height and weight, which is especially useful for estimating the risk to health associated with overnutrition, is the body mass index (BMI). Appendix B presents a nomogram for determining the BMI, and the inside back covers show height and weight ranges based on the BMI.

The table of average weights for height is less useful in cases where a person has weighed much more or much less than the average throughout life. To assess such a person's weight, it may be more informative to compare the present weight not with an "ideal" body weight (IBW), but with the person's usual body weight (UBW). Deviations from ideal or usual body weight may indicate malnutrition (Table 10–6).

To calculate the percent ideal body weight (%IBW), an assessor compares a person's actual weight with the ideal weight. This provides a rough estimate of the degree of overnutrition or undernutrition. A %IBW greater than 115 to 120 indicates obesity; less than 90 indicates undernutrition.

A more valuable parameter for assessing weight measurements is the percent usual body weight (%UBW), which considers what is normal for a particular individual. The client, family, friends, and older medical records can provide such information. A health care provider can pick up malnutrition in an obese person by using %UBW, not by using %IBW.

TABLE 10–6 **Weight as an Indicator of Nutrition Status**

%IBW	%UBW	NUTRITION STATUS
>120	—	Obese
110–120	—	Overweight
80–90	85–95	Mildly undernourished
70–79	75–84	Moderately undernourished
<70	<75	Severely undernourished

To determine any recent weight change, the assessor compares the %UBW with the time period over which a change, if any, has occurred. A 5 percent weight loss might be significant if it occurred within a month, yet might be insignificant if it occurred over five months. The accompanying box describes how to estimate %IBW and %UBW.

How to Estimate %IBW and %UBW

To estimate %IBW and %UBW, compare the individual's current weight with the ideal body weight from standard height-weight tables. For example, to calculate %IBW and %UBW in a 45-year-old man of medium frame who is 5 feet 8 inches tall, weighs 115 pounds, and has lost 15 pounds in the last month, follow these steps:

1. $\%IBW = \dfrac{\text{actual weight}}{\text{ideal weight}} \times 100$.

   For ideal weight, use the midpoint of the weight range. In this example, the ideal weight is 153 lb.

2. $\%IBW = \dfrac{115 \text{ pounds}}{153 \text{ pounds}} \times 100 = 76$ percent.

   The man in this example is at 76 percent of his ideal body weight.

3. $\%UBW = \dfrac{\text{actual weight}}{\text{usual weight}} \times 100$.

   Calculate the usual weight (130 pounds) by adding the weight loss (15 pounds) to the current body weight (115 pounds).

4. $\%UBW = \dfrac{115 \text{ pounds}}{130 \text{ pounds}} \times 100 = 89$ percent.

   The man is at 89 percent of his usual body weight. The recent weight change is significant; he has lost weight at a rate of almost 4 pounds per week.

Weight measurements in hospitalized clients are sometimes difficult to evaluate. Diseases or therapy can cause fluid retention and mask significant weight loss. In fact, starvation itself is accompanied by an expanded extracellular fluid volume. Very ill people may also be difficult to weigh if they are bedridden. Bed scales are useful in such cases. State-of-the-art hospital beds equipped with built-in scales are also available.

One of the most important anthropometric measures predictive of the birthweight of a child is the mother's amount and pattern of weight gain or loss during pregnancy (see Chapter 11 for more information). Appendix B provides a prenatal weight gain grid.

Measures of Body Fat and Lean Tissue

Significant weight changes in both children and adults can reflect overnutrition and undernutrition with respect to energy and protein. To estimate the degree to which various body compartments (fat stores or lean tissues) are affected by overnutrition or undernutrition, the measurements listed in Table 10–3 (p. 233) are useful.

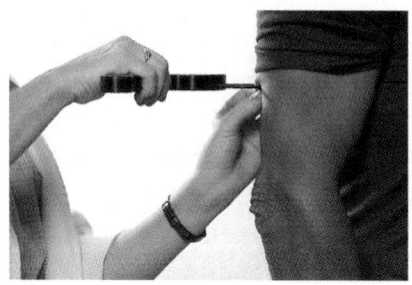

Fatfold measures provide an estimate of body fat.

FATFOLD MEASURES. Approximately half the fat in the body is located directly beneath the skin (subcutaneous), and its thickness reflects total body fat. In some parts of the body, this fat is loosely attached; a person can pull it up between the thumb and forefinger. These sites provide an ideal place to measure fatfold thickness. In the hands of a skilled person, the fatfold test is a valuable and practical diagnostic procedure. Body fat calculations determined by fatfold measures correlate well with calculations based on other, more sophisticated methods, such as underwater weighing, obtaining radioactive potassium counts, or determining total body water. Training in the use of fatfold calipers is critical to obtaining accurate measurements, however.

A major limitation of the fatfold test is that fat may be thicker under the skin in one area than in another. A pinch at the side of the waistline may not yield the same measurement as a pinch on the back of the arm. This limitation can be overcome by taking fatfold measurements at several (often three) different places on the body. However, multiple measures are not always practical in clinical settings, and the triceps fatfold measurement alone is used most often, because the triceps are easily accessible. To measure fatfold, a skilled technician follows a standard procedure using reliable calipers. The technique for measuring triceps fatfold, as well as triceps fatfold percentiles, is given in Appendix B.

MIDARM MUSCLE CIRCUMFERENCE. Taking both the triceps fatfold measurement and the midarm circumference enables an assessor to derive the midarm muscle circumference. The assessor measures midarm circumference with a nonstretchable tape around the arm midway between the shoulder and the elbow (see Appendix B). The midarm circumference measures the diameter of the arm, which includes muscle mass, subcutaneous fat, and bone. This measurement is then used to estimate the midarm muscle circumference, using a mathematical equation. Because the derived midarm muscle circumference permits an estimate of muscle mass, it reflects protein nutrition status. Appendix B shows how to derive the midarm muscle circumference and includes an alternative method using a nomogram.

ANALYSIS OF MEASURES. The accuracy and value of anthropometric measurements are limited by the skills of the measurer, the accuracy of the equipment used for measurement, changes in body composition related to different disorders (such as fluid retention or dehydration), and skill in interpretation of measurements. Triceps fatfold and midarm muscle circumference measurements can be difficult to determine for people who are obese or for elderly individuals with loose skin hanging on the upper arm. Significant changes in measurements occur slowly in adults. When changes do occur, they represent prolonged alterations in nutrient intake. Therefore, anthropometrics cannot be used to describe small changes in body composition that occur over short periods of time.[4]

Fatfold measurements and derived midarm muscle circumferences must be interpreted with extreme caution for people who are under severe stress (see Chapter 14). Further research is needed to determine if internal fat stores change at the same rate as the triceps fatfold or if changes in total body water markedly influence fatfold measurements during severe stress. It is conceivable that fatfold measurements may remain constant at first, even while internal fat stores are rapidly dwindling. Any error in the fatfold measurement would produce an error in the derived midarm muscle circumference as well, rendering this estimate of protein nutrition erroneous. Furthermore, independently of nutrition factors, exercise influences muscle size, and lack of exercise may alter muscle mass.[5]

Fatfolds, midarm circumferences, and the derived midarm muscle circumferences are reproducible measurements when standard procedures are followed. Accurately following standard procedure requires practice, however. Generally, the same person should measure the same subject routinely for best results.

Hydrodensitometry and bioelectrical impedance techniques are two additional methods for assessing body composition. Both of these techniques are popularly used among athletes and in health clubs.

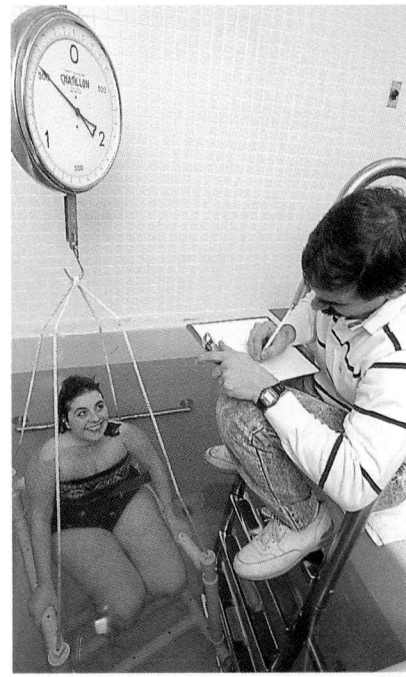

Underwater weighing is the "gold standard" for estimating percent body fat.

HYDRODENSITOMETRY. Underwater weighing, or hydrodensitometry, measures body density. The person is weighed on a standard scale, to obtain weight. Then the person is submerged in water, and the amount of water displaced is measured to obtain volume. A mathematical expression using the two measurements (weight divided by volume) provides the body's density and allows the assessor to determine the percent body fat. The assessor then uses sex-specific reference standards for men and women to evaluate the body fat measurement.

Underwater weighing generates an excellent estimate of body fat, although the technique has drawbacks. Underwater weighing requires bulky, expensive, and nonportable equipment. Furthermore, it is impractical to submerge some people (especially those who are ill or fearful) under water. Errors can result from the mathematical equation used to translate body density into an estimate of percent fat. Underwater weighing is therefore not widely used in typical clinical settings, but is valuable in research.

hydrodensitometry: the measurement of body density by submerging the person underwater.

BIOELECTRICAL IMPEDANCE. Bioelectrical impedance techniques to determine body composition are rapidly gaining popularity. The techniques are less

bioelectrical impedance: a method for estimating body fat using very-low-intensity electrical current.

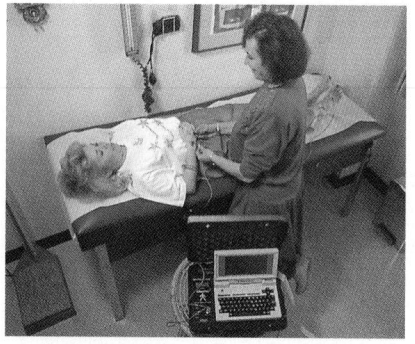

Bioelectrical impedance is gaining popularity as a simple and painless technique for estimating body fat.

Isotope studies, ultrasonography, and computerized axial tomography (CAT scan) are other methods that have been used to determine body composition. The expense and impracticality of these tests limit their clinical value, although they are useful in research.

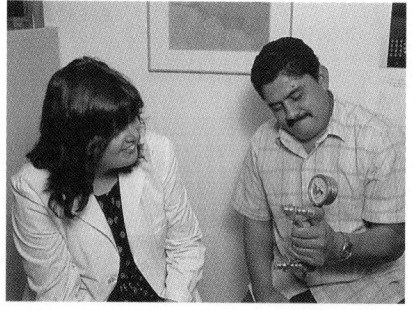

A dynamometer measures hand grip strength.

The automated measurement of several blood components from a single blood sample is referred to as an **SMA (simultaneous multiple analysis)**. SMA is followed by a number (for example, SMA-12) that indicates how many tests will be run.

expensive than underwater weighing, the equipment is portable, and the procedure is painless. To measure body fat using the bioelectrical impedance technique, a very-low-intensity electrical current is briefly sent through the body by way of electrodes placed on the wrist and ankle. Since electrolyte-containing fluids are found primarily in lean body tissues, and they readily conduct electrical currents, the leaner the person, the less resistance to the electrical current. The measurement of electrical resistance is then used in a mathematical equation to yield an estimate of the percent body fat.

In healthy adults, the bioelectrical impedance technique compares favorably in accuracy with other measures of body composition. Additional research to define the technique's proper application and refine its interpretation is needed before it will become a useful clinical tool for assessing all individuals. For example, when compared to hydrodensitometry, bioelectrical impedance may underestimate body fat in obese people.[6]

OTHER ANTHROPOMETRIC MEASUREMENTS. The techniques described up to this point have traditionally helped to define body composition. Recently, investigators and clinicians also have begun to relate changes in body composition to organ function. One such technique, the measurement of hand grip strength, relates grip strength to muscle function and provides a practical and inexpensive way of assessing nutrition status. The assessor asks the person to grip an instrument (called a dynamometer) as tightly as possible and reads the grip strength from a scale on the dynamometer. Low grip strength (weak muscle function) indicates risk for poor nutrition status. In a study of people with cancer who needed to undergo surgery, grip strength measurements accurately predicted postoperative complications.[7] Age- and sex-specific standards for evaluating hand grip strength have been published.[8] Appendix B provides more information on the hand grip strength measurement and standards.

Biochemical Analyses

Most of the approaches to nutrition assessment discussed so far are external approaches. Biochemical analyses, or laboratory tests, help to determine what is happening to the body internally. Most tests are based on analysis of blood and urine samples, which contain nutrients, enzymes, and metabolites that reflect nutrition status. Other tests, such as serum glucose, help pinpoint problems that require nutrition-related solutions. Tests that define fluid and electrolyte balance, acid-base balance, and organ function also have nutrition implications. Table 10–7 lists some common lab tests valuable in nutrition assessments and shows how these tests are used. Tests important in specific circumstances will be discussed in Chapters 16 through 23 wherever appropriate.

The interpretation of biochemical data requires skill. Long metabolic sequences lead to the production of the end products and metabolites seen in blood and urine. No test reflects nutrition status alone, because many nonnutritional factors influence laboratory tests. The low blood concentration of a nutrient may reflect a primary deficiency of that nutrient, but it

TABLE 10-7   **Selected Laboratory Tests and Their Uses**

TEST	USES
Hematology	
Hemoglobin (Hg)	To detect anemia and determine state of hydration
Hematocrit (Hct)	To detect anemia and determine state of hydration
White blood cells (WBC)	To detect infection and determine total lymphocyte count
Mean corpuscular volume (MCV)	To detect anemia and determine its causes
Mean corpuscular hemoglobin (MCH)	To detect anemia and determine its causes
Mean corpuscular hemoglobin concentration (MCHC)	To detect anemia and determine its causes
Blood Chemistry	
Electrolytes	
Sodium	To check state of hydration
Potassium	To monitor acid-base balance, renal function, and response to diuretics
Chloride	To monitor acid-base balance and detect GI losses of chloride (from vomiting or nasogastric suctioning)
Carbon dioxide	To monitor acid-base balance
Other	
Glucose	To detect diabetes mellitus, glucose intolerance, stress, and pancreatic tumors
Blood urea nitrogen	To monitor renal function and determine state of hydration
Calcium	To detect hormonal imbalances, certain malignancies, and steatorrhea (malabsorption)
Phosphorus	To detect hormonal imbalances, PEM, and cirrhosis
Magnesium	To monitor renal function and detect PEM
Total protein[a]	To detect PEM and various nutrient imbalances
Albumin	To detect PEM and determine state of hydration
Cholesterol	To assess risk of heart disease and possibility of obstructive jaundice
Uric acid	To detect gout and determine state of hydration
Serum creatinine	To monitor renal function and determine state of hydration
Serum enzymes	
Creatinine phosphokinase (CPK)	To monitor heart function
Lactic dehydrogenase (LDH)	To monitor heart and renal function
Alanine transaminase (ALT, formerly SGPT)	To monitor heart and liver function
Aspartate transaminase (AST, formerly SGOT)	To monitor heart and liver function
Alkaline phosphatase	To monitor liver function
Serum amylase	To monitor pancreatic function
Serum lipase	To monitor pancreatic function

Note: This table presents a partial listing of the major uses of certain commonly performed lab tests that have implications for nutrition. [a]More than half of the total protein is albumin.

may also be secondary to the deficiency of one or several other nutrients or to a disease. However, taken together with other assessment data, laboratory test results help to make a total picture that becomes clear with careful interpretation. They are especially useful in helping to detect subclinical malnutrition by uncovering early signs of malnutrition before the clinical signs of a classic deficiency disease appear.

Laboratory tests used to assess vitamin and mineral status (see Table 10-8, p. 242) are useful, particularly when combined with health histories

TABLE 10–8   **Biochemical Tests Useful for Assessing Nutrition Status**

NUTRIENT	ASSESSMENT TESTS
Protein	Urinary creatinine excretion, serum albumin, serum prealbumin, serum transferrin, retinol-binding protein, total lymphocyte count, nitrogen balance
Vitamins	
Vitamin A	Retinol-binding protein, serum carotene
Thiamin	Erythrocyte (red blood cell) transketolase activity, urinary thiamin
Riboflavin	Erythrocyte glutathione reductase activity, urinary riboflavin
Vitamin B_6	Urinary xanthurenic acid excretion after tryptophan load test, urinary vitamin B_6, erythrocyte transaminase activity
Niacin	Urinary metabolites NMN (N-methyl nicotinamide) or 2-pyridone, or preferably both expressed as a ratio
Folate	Free folate in the blood, erythrocyte folate (reflects liver stores), urinary formiminoglutamic acid (FIGLU), vitamin B_{12} status (because folate assessment tests alone do not distinguish between the two deficiencies)
Vitamin B_{12}	Serum vitamin B_{12}, erythrocyte vitamin B_{12}, urinary methylmalonic acid synthesis or DUMP test (from the abbreviation for the chemical name of DNA's raw material, deoxyuridine monophosphate)
Biotin	Serum biotin, urinary biotin
Vitamin C	Serum or plasma vitamin C,[a] leukocyte vitamin C, urinary vitamin C
Vitamin D	Serum alkaline phosphatase
Vitamin E	Serum tocopherol, erythrocyte hemolysis
Vitamin K	Blood clotting time (prothrombin time)
Minerals	
Potassium	Serum potassium
Magnesium	Serum magnesium
Iron	Hemoglobin, hematocrit, serum ferritin, total iron-binding capacity (TIBC), transferrin saturation, erythrocyte protoporphyrin, serum ferritin, serum iron
Iodine	Serum protein-bound iodine, radioiodine uptake
Zinc	Plasma zinc, hair zinc

[a]Vitamin C shifts unpredictably between the plasma and the white blood cells known as leukocytes; thus a plasma or serum determination may not accurately reflect the body's pool. The appropriate clinical test may be a measurement of leukocyte vitamin C. A combination of both tests may be more reliable than either one alone.
Source: Adapted from A. Grant and S. DeHoog, *Nutritional Assessment and Support,* 3d ed. (available from Anne Grant and Susan DeHoog, Box 25057, Northgate Station, Seattle, WA 98125).

and physical findings. Vitamin and mineral levels present in the blood and urine sometimes reflect recent intakes, however, rather than long-term intakes. If recent intakes have been adequate, they may mask long-term subclinical deficiencies, concealing depleted nutrient stores or impaired metabolic processes. Furthermore, many nutrients interact; therefore, the amounts of some nutrients in the body can alter lab values for other nutrients. It is also important to remember that nonnutrient conditions influence biochemical measures.

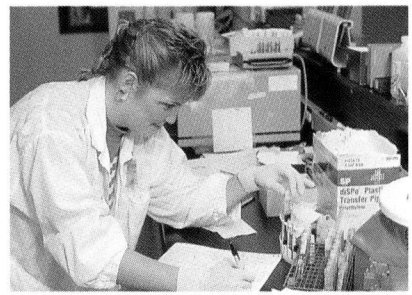

Blood samples offer valuable clues in assessing nutrition status.

Hair analyses are sometimes advocated by unscrupulous practitioners to assess vitamin and mineral status. However, hair analyses are still being studied to determine what their validity and usefulness may be. In several instances, hair contents of minerals have been demonstrated *not* to reflect body content of minerals in any consistent way. Too many confounding variables interfere: air and water pollution, shampoos and dyes, and water hardness, among others. Hair analyses may reflect exposures to toxic heavy metals, but that is a toxicological, not a nutritional, matter.

It is beyond the scope of this text to describe all laboratory tests and their relationships to nutrition status. Instead, the emphasis is on lab tests used to detect two common conditions: protein-energy malnutrition and nutrition-related anemias.

Assessment of Protein-Energy Malnutrition

Tests available to determine protein status include serum albumin, serum transferrin, other serum proteins, and total lymphocyte count and other tests of immune function. Of these, serum albumin and total lymphocyte count are most commonly used. Physicians may also order additional tests, such as nitrogen balance studies and urinary creatinine, under special circumstances.

SERUM ALBUMIN. The protein albumin accounts for over 50 percent of total serum proteins. When protein status degenerates, serum albumin concentrations tend to decline slowly, in part because albumin is plentiful in the body and in part because it can shift from the cells to the blood when blood concentrations begin to fall. Additionally, albumin breaks down slowly, so it is slow to reflect changes in nutrition status. Therefore, when low serum albumin levels associated with malnutrition are seen, they are known to represent prolonged protein depletion. Serum albumin levels appear to correlate well with survival among people in the hospital.[9] Conversely, albumin concentrations increase slowly with appropriate nutrition support, so measuring albumin as an indicator of early response to nutrition therapy is of limited value. Appendix B provides standards for determining the severity of low serum albumin concentrations.

Many other conditions besides malnutrition can depress albumin concentrations, including liver disease, advanced kidney disease (nephrotic syndrome), infection, cancer, burns, certain gastrointestinal disorders, and eclampsia. Therefore, as is true for all other nutrition assessment parameters, albumin cannot alone determine protein status, but rather serves as one indicator among many.

The **serum** is the watery portion of the blood that remains after removal of the cells and clot-forming material; **plasma** is the fluid that remains when unclotted blood is centrifuged. In most cases, serum and plasma concentrations are similar. Lab technicians usually prefer serum samples, because plasma samples are more likely to clog mechanical blood analyzers.

The protein found in the blood and internal organs is also called **visceral protein.** The protein of skeletal muscle is called **somatic protein.**

SERUM TRANSFERRIN. Transferrin is a protein that transports iron between the intestine and sites of hemoglobin synthesis and degradation. Researchers consider transferrin a more sensitive indicator of protein malnutrition than albumin, because its body pool is smaller, and it respond more promptly to changes in protein intake.

The liver synthesizes most of the body's transferrin. Transferrin levels are inversely related to iron stores: levels are high in iron deficiency and low when iron storage is excessive. Therefore, when an iron deficiency is present, assessors may have difficulty using transferrin as an indicator of protein status. Liver disease, nephrotic syndrome, and burns lower the transferrin levels; pregnancy and blood loss elevate them. Standards for determining the severity of transferrin depletion are given in Appendix B.

OTHER SERUM PROTEINS. Many other serum proteins have been studied as indicators of protein status. Prealbumin and retinol-binding protein are sensitive indicators of protein status. These proteins promptly reflect incipient PEM and rapidly respond with appropriate refeeding. These sensitive tests are most likely to be ordered in institutions with active nutrition support programs. Other serum proteins that may be useful in nutrition assessment include serum somatomedin-C, fibronectin, fibrinogen, haptoglobin, and C-reactive protein. Unfortunately, these indicators of protein status are less practical and more expensive to measure than albumin and transferrin and are not in common use.

TOTAL LYMPHOCYTE COUNT AND OTHER TESTS OF IMMUNE STATUS. Various forms of PEM and individual nutrient deficiencies depress the immune system (see Chapter 14). Lymphocytes are important participants in the immune response. Their numbers are reduced as protein depletion occurs, so the total lymphocyte count is one useful index in nutrition assessment. White blood cell (WBC) volume and WBC counts are routinely measured in hospital tests, so the total lymphocyte count can be easily derived (see Appendix B).

Another test of immune function is antigen skin testing. Organisms (usually three or four kinds) to which most people are immune are injected just under the skin. After 48 hours, the sites of the injections are inspected for raised, hardened areas (induration). In general, such areas will be apparent in the well-nourished person, but in the malnourished person, hardened areas will not appear or will be very small.

Many factors other than nutrition, including infections; uremia (Chapter 23); cirrhosis and hepatitis (Chapter 23); trauma, surgery, and burns (Chapter 18); and several drugs can interfere with the immune response.[10] For these reasons the value of skin testing as an index of nutrition status in people who are ill has been questioned.

NITROGEN BALANCE AND URINARY CREATININE EXCRETION. Because the element nitrogen is present in protein and not in carbohydrate or fat, its ingestion and excretion balance whenever body protein is constant. Studies of the balance of nitrogen entering and leaving the body help to estimate the degree to which protein is being depleted or repleted in the body and provide a measure of the adequacy of protein intake. Ideally, nitrogen balance is determined by measuring total urinary nitrogen excretion and com-

refeeding: providing adequate nutrients after a period of inadequate nutrient intake.

induration: a raised, hardened area of skin.
dirus = hard

Nitrogen balance:
    Nitrogen intake = nitrogen output.

Positive nitrogen balance:
    Nitrogen intake > nitrogen output.

Negative nitrogen balance:
    Nitrogen intake < nitrogen output.

paring the amount of nitrogen excreted with the amount of nitrogen ingested in the diet.[11] However, traditional methods of determining total urinary nitrogen are impractical in most clinical settings, and this method is not widely available. More recently, a newer, more practical method of determining total urinary nitrogen has been developed, and as laboratories become familiar with the technique, estimating nitrogen balance using total urinary nitrogen may become more widespread.

Nitrogen excretion is frequently estimated from the urinary urea nitrogen (UUN). Urinary urea nitrogen measured from a 24-hour urine collection is compared with the client's protein (nitrogen) intake during the same 24-hour period. (Appendix B provides an example.)

Nitrogen balance studies provide a prime example of the need for communication and cooperation between health care professionals and various hospital departments. A nitrogen balance study is invalid if even one urine specimen is discarded or one meal's protein intake not accurately recorded; the whole procedure would need to be repeated, at great inconvenience to the client and staff. Appendix B describes the proper technique for collecting a 24-hour urine specimen.

Another substance measured from a 24-hour urine collection is creatinine. Urinary creatinine excretion reflects the body's skeletal muscle mass. Appendix B describes how urinary creatinine determinations are used in nutrition assessments.

Assessment of Nutritional Anemias

Anemia, a symptom of a wide variety of nutrition- and nonnutrition-related disorders, is characterized by a reduced number of red blood cells. A low hemoglobin or hematocrit level most frequently alerts the health care professional to the presence of anemia. Iron, folate, and vitamin B_{12} deficiencies caused by inadequate intake, poor absorption, or abnormal metabolism of these nutrients most often account for nutritional anemias. Some nonnutrition-related causes of anemia include massive blood loss, infections (see Chapter 18), hereditary blood disorders such as sickle-cell anemia, and chronic liver disease.

To help differentiate between different types of anemias, laboratory tests determine the size and color of the red blood cells. Further tests are ordered to pinpoint the cause of anemia as appropriate.

Distinguishing folate-deficiency anemia from vitamin B_{12}–deficiency anemia is particularly important, for these two types of anemia present similar clinical pictures, but their treatments differ. Giving folate to a person with vitamin B_{12} deficiency improves many of the lab test results indicative of vitamin B_{12} deficiency but is a dangerous error, for a vitamin B_{12} deficiency also causes nerve damage that folate cannot correct. Thus inappropriate folate administration masks vitamin B_{12}–deficiency anemia, and nerve damage worsens. Table 10–9 shows laboratory tests that are helpful in distinguishing among the three most common nutrition-related anemias.

Red blood cells that are larger than normal are **macrocytic. Microcytic** cells are smaller than normal.

The pigmentation of red blood cells comes from the amount of hemoglobin the cells contain. **Hypochromic cells** contain less hemoglobin than **normochromic cells.**

TABLE 10–9   **Laboratory Tests Useful in Evaluating Nutrition-Related Anemia**

TEST OR TEST RESULT	WHAT IT REFLECTS
General Tests for Anemia	
Hemoglobin (Hg)	Total amount of hemoglobin in the red blood cells (RBC)
Hematocrit (Hct)	Percentage of RBC in the total blood volume
Red blood cell (RBC) count	Number of RBC
Mean corpuscular volume (MCV)	RBC size; helps to determine if anemia is microcytic or macrocytic
Mean corpuscular hemoglobin concentration (MCHC)	Hemoglobin concentration within the average RBC; helps to determine if anemia is hypochromic or normochromic
Bone marrow aspiration	The manufacture of blood cells in different developmental states
Iron-Deficiency Anemia	
↓ Serum ferritin	Early deficiency state with depleted iron stores
↓ Transferrin saturation	Progressing deficiency state with diminished transport iron
↑ Erythrocyte protoporphyrin	Later deficiency state with limited hemoglobin production
Folate-Deficiency Anemia	
↓ Serum folate	Progressing deficiency state
↓ RBC folate	Later deficiency state
Vitamin B_{12}–Deficiency Anemia	
↓ Serum vitamin B_{12}	Progressing deficiency state
Schilling test	Absorption of vitamin B_{12}

Physical Examinations

The assessor can also use a physical examination to search for signs of nutrient deficiencies or toxicities. Like the other assessment methods, such an examination requires skill in the performance and knowledge in the interpretation. Many physical signs are nonspecific; they can reflect any of several nutrient deficiencies, as well as conditions not related to nutrition (see Table 10–10, p. 247). For example, cracked lips can result from sunburn, windburn, dehydration, or any of several B vitamin deficiencies, to name only a few causes. For this reason, physical findings are especially unreliable, by themselves, for diagnosis of nutrition problems. Instead, their value is in revealing possible problems for other assessment techniques to confirm, or in confirming the findings of other assessment measures.

With this limitation understood, physical symptoms can be most informative; they communicate much information about nutritional health. Many tissues and organs can reflect signs of malnutrition.

Physical signs of malnutrition appear most rapidly in parts of the body where cell replacement occurs at a high rate, such as in the hair, skin, and digestive tract (including the mouth and tongue). The summary tables in Chapters 7 and 8 list physical signs of vitamin and mineral malnutrition.

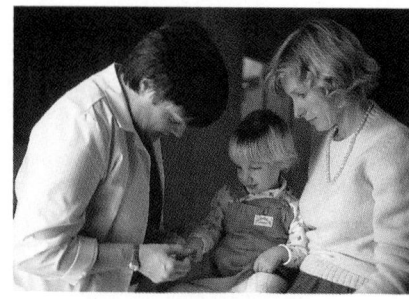

A physical examination provides valuable clues about a person's nutrition status.

TABLE 10–10   **Physical Findings Useful in Nutrition**

BODY SYSTEM	ACCEPTABLE FINDINGS	MALNUTRITION FINDINGS	WHAT FINDINGS REFLECT
Hair	Shiny, firm in the scalp	Dull, brittle, dry, loose; falls out	PEM
Eyes	Bright, clear pink membranes that adjust easily to light	Pale membranes; spots; redness; adjust slowly to darkness	Status of vitamin A, the B vitamins, zinc, and iron
Teeth and gums	No pain or caries, gums firm, teeth bright	Missing, discolored, decayed teeth; gums bleed easily and are swollen and spongy	Mineral and vitamin C status
Face	Clear complexion without dryness or scaliness	Off-color, scaly, flaky, cracked skin	PEM; vitamin A and iron status
Glands	No lumps	Swollen at front of neck, cheeks	PEM; iodine status
Tongue	Red, bumpy, rough	Sore, smooth, purplish, swollen	B vitamin status
Skin	Smooth, firm, good color	Dry, rough, spotty; "sandpaper" feel or sores; lack of fat under skin	PEM; status of vitamin A, the B vitamins, and vitamin C
Nails	Firm, pink	Spoon-shaped, brittle, ridged	Iron status
Internal systems	Regular heart rhythm with a heart rate between 60 and 100 and blood pressure below 140/90; no impairment of digestive function, reflexes, or psychological development	Abnormal heart rate, heart rhythm, or blood pressure; enlarged liver, spleen; abnormal digestion; burning, tingling of hands, feet; loss of balance, coordination	PEM; mineral status
Muscles and bones	Muscle tone; posture, long bone development appropriate for age	"Wasted" appearance of muscles; swollen bumps on skull or ends of bones; small bumps on ribs; bowed legs or knock-knees	PEM; vitamin D status

Note: See Table = ref in Appendix B for a summary of symptoms of vitamin and mineral deficiencies and toxicities.

Classifying Protein-Energy Status

Assessment of PEM is often indispensable to the development of an appropriate nutrition care plan (see Chapter 15), and the plan may well be indispensable to recovery. Once health care providers recognize the signs of PEM, they classify it as either kwashiorkor, marasmus, or kwashiorkor-marasmus mix.

The person with kwashiorkor has normal or above-standard anthropometric measurements with below-normal indexes of blood and organ proteins. Because the individual with kwashiorkor may be obese, malnutrition may easily be overlooked. Such a case illustrates clearly why the various components of nutrition assessment (historical data, anthropometric measurements, biochemical analyses, and physical examinations) cannot be used singly to define nutrition status.

Marasmus takes on an appearance opposite that of kwashiorkor. The individual with marasmus has blood and organ protein levels that appear to be adequate, while skeletal muscle and subcutaneous fat are depleted.

Kwashiorkor-marasmus mix malnutrition presents signs of depleted blood, organ, and skeletal muscle proteins, as well as signs of depleted subcutaneous fat. The individual with this type of malnutrition has virtually no energy reserves and is in grave danger, especially if also confronted with other severe stresses, such as from trauma or infection (see Chapter 14).

In addition to uncovering PEM, nutrition assessments help pinpoint energy overnutrition, vitamin and mineral deficiencies and toxicities, poor dietary practices, possible drug-nutrient interactions, and a host of other risk factors that alert the assessor that nutrition and health status may be deteriorating. Nutrition status can change at any time. One person, previously healthy, may develop a disorder that affects nutrition status; another person may correct poor nutrition practices; still another may develop poor eating habits. Therefore, nutrition assessment repeated at regular intervals is an important tool in assisting people to maintain or recover their health.

Nutrition Screening

As you can tell from the many previous pages of text, thorough nutrition assessment requires much time and money—both limited commodities in health care today. (Nutrition in Practice 15 discusses many of the issues surrounding nutrition and cost containment.) One way to help reduce the costs of nutrition assessment is to use nutrition screening techniques.

nutrition screening: the use of preliminary nutrition assessment techniques to identify people who are malnourished or who are at risk for malnutrition.

Collecting detailed information on each person entering the hospital may not be practical or even essential. A strategic compromise is to screen clients by collecting preliminary data and observing each client for signs of problems that may affect nutrition status. A basic nutrition screening includes the following:

- Reviewing the individual's diet, drug, and health history. Does the person's history reveal risk factors for poor nutrition status (review Table 10–2)?
- Weighing each person on admission and at regular intervals during the hospital stay. Is the person's weight for height adequate, but not excessive? Has the person been losing or gaining weight? How much? How fast?
- Checking the available laboratory reports. Do serum albumin, total lymphocyte count, hemoglobin, and hematocrit suggest malnutrition? Are additional tests indicated?
- Looking at the person. Are there obvious signs of malnutrition (see Table 10–10)? Is the client emaciated? Obese? Extremely pale?

In addition to the above nutrition assessment procedures, take the opportunity to:

▬ Check the client's tray to see if food is being eaten. If the client is to receive no food or is unable to eat, how long has it been since the client has eaten? Is the client expected to be able to eat soon? Are adequate nutrients being delivered by vein? (Chapter 16 explains how nutrients are delivered intravenously.)

▬ Most important, communicate any problems that you discover, and follow up to make sure the problems are being handled. Always record problems in the medical record to ensure that whoever cares for a particular client will be alert to the problem. Alert a dietitian to perform a more in-depth nutrition assessment if you detect a problem. Be persistent if you suspect that a problem is being ignored.

Nutrition screening identifies common problems that place clients at risk for malnutrition. It is especially important in health care settings where nutrition assessments are not routinely performed on each client.

To know what is wrong with a person's nutrition status is not to remedy it. All the effort expended in evaluating a person's nutrition problems will be for naught if it is not used to formulate a plan of action that will correct nutrition problems. In the chapters ahead, the many ways that age and illness influence nutrition status will be obvious. This knowledge will help clarify why specific nutrition strategies are implemented to maintain or improve nutrition status.

CASE STUDY

Nutrition Assessment and Care

Ms. Green, a 38-year-old computer scientist, was admitted to the hospital for testing following a car accident. Her injuries included several broken bones and a collapsed left lung. Her lab report revealed a mildly depleted serum albumin and a moderately depleted total lymphocyte count. After reviewing her medical record, the health care team decided that a complete nutrition assessment was necessary. The following significant information resulted.

Health History
Increased nutrient requirements due to injuries sustained in the car accident.

Socioeconomic History
Lives alone; her busy schedule seldom leaves time for her to prepare meals, so she often eats at fast-food restaurants. Money for food and food preparation facilities are adequate.

(continued)

Nutrition Assessment and Care (continued)

Drug History

One standard multivitamin-mineral tablet daily.

No other drugs.

Diet History

Weight-loss intentional.

Very-low-kcalorie (700 kcalories/day), low-carbohydrate diet over the past six weeks.

Dairy products used only about once or twice a month.

Anthropometric Measurements

Height: 5 feet 7 inches.

Weight: 150 pounds.

Usual weight: 175 pounds.

Frame size: medium.

Biochemical Analysis

Serum albumin: 3 grams/100 milliliters.

Total lymphocyte count: 1,000 cubic millimeters (moderately depleted).

Physical Examination

Hair: dull, easily plucked.

Other: none noted.

Determine Ms. Green's ideal body weight, and calculate percent ideal body weight. Consider Ms. Green's recent weight change. What is a safe rate of weight loss? How does Ms. Green's weight loss compare with the safe rate? Does her recent weight change increase her risk of poor nutrition status?

What do Ms. Green's lab values indicate with respect to her protein status? Are there any other factors in Ms. Green's health, diet, socioeconomic, or drug history or physical findings suggestive of malnutrition?

Based on Ms. Green's nutrition assessment, you determine that she is at risk for PEM. When you have learned more about PEM and the effects of severe stress on nutrition status, you will be ready to devise a nutrition care plan for Ms. Green.

Study Questions

1. Describe the four components of nutrition assessment and what each can reveal.
2. Describe the purpose of obtaining food intake data.
3. What are the advantages and disadvantages of the 24-hour recall, usual food intake, food frequency checklist, and food record?
4. How do anthropometric measurements help define nutrition status? What anthropometric measurements are frequently used in nutrition assessments?
5. How do lab tests help define nutrition status? Describe the lab tests used to uncover PEM.
6. What is anemia? What are the major nutrition-related causes of anemia? What lab tests are useful in detecting anemia?
7. What is the purpose of nutrition screening? List screening techniques.

Notes

1. K. J. Morgan and coauthors, Collection of food intake data: An evaluation of methods, *Journal of the American Dietetic Association* 87 (1987): 888–896.
2. K. J. Streit, N. H. Stevens, and V. J. Stevens, Food records: A predictor and modifier of weight change in a long-term weight loss program, *Journal of the American Dietetic Association* 91 (1991): 213–216.
3. R. S. Gibson, *Principles of Nutritional Assessment* (New York: Oxford University Press, 1990), p. 172.
4. S. B. Heymsfield and K. Casper, Anthropometric assessment of the adult hospitalized patient, *Journal of Parenteral and Enteral Nutrition* 11 (Supplement, 1987): 36–41.
5. K. N. Jeejeebhoy, A. S. Detsky, and J. P. Baker, Assessment of nutrition status, *Journal of Parenteral and Enteral Nutrition* 14 (Supplement, 1990): 193–196.
6. F. Kalfarentzos and coauthors, Comparison of forearm muscle dynamometry with nutritional prognostic index as a preoperative indicator in cancer patients, *Journal of Parenteral and Enteral Nutrition* 13 (1989): 34–36.
7. A. E. Webb and coauthors, Hand-grip dynamometry as a predictor of postoperative complications: Reappraisal using age standardized grip strengths, *Journal of Parenteral and Enteral Nutrition* 13 (1989): 30–33.
8. N. S. Burgess, Effect of a very-low-calorie diet on body composition and resting metabolic rate in obese men and women, *Journal of the American Dietetic Association* 91 (1991): 430–434.
9. J. P. Doweiko and D. J. Nompleggi, The role of albumin in human physiology and pathophysiology, Part III: Albumin and disease states, *Journal of Parenteral and Enteral Nutrition* 15 (1991): 476–483.
10. Jeejeebhoy, Detsky, and Baker, 1990.
11. F. N. Konstantinides and coauthors, Urinary urea nitrogen: Too insensitive for calculating nitrogen balance studies in surgical clinical nutrition, *Journal of Parenteral and Enteral Nutrition* 15 (1991): 189–193.

10

The Food Supply: Environmental Impact

The availability of food is a substantial determinant of food intake and, therefore, nutrition status. Chapter 10 addressed many socioeconomic factors that influence food availability for the individual. However, the world's food supply is a critical determinant of food availability and, therefore, food intake and nutrition well-being throughout the world. This Nutrition in Practice describes the effect of the environment on the world's food supply.

The well-being of every human being depends on an environmental balance. Densely populated urban areas must be balanced by rural agricultural areas and wilderness. The populated areas depend on the agricultural areas to supply food, and on the wilderness areas to generate oxygen, produce rain, and renew the soils upon which the human food supply demands. Disruption of this environmental balance is threatening our food supply, as well as human health in general.

I can see why we need farming and wilderness areas to support our population, but we have farms and wilderness areas. So what exactly is the problem?

At the heart of the problem is our growing population and the way our population uses its natural resources. There is an optimal population size for the earth to bear—that size at which the air, water, and wilderness can

renew themselves and support human life indefinitely. This optimal population size depends, in part, on how people behave. The more resources each person demands, the fewer people there can be. For example, if everyone on earth must own and drive a car every day, then each requires much more of the earth's support than if he or she walked or rode a bicycle.

It is not possible to say exactly what number of people might be ideal for our well-being, but the earth's population size may well exceed that number by now. There are currently over 5 billion people in the world, and each year, the number of people added to the population is greater than the number added the year before.[1] Furthermore, by the year 2000, half of all the people on earth will be living in cities. A growing population spreads across the land, converting forests to pastures, pastures to parking lots, and parking lots to industrial developments. The process might have been beneficial to people so long as

elsewhere on earth, there was enough rural and forested land to continue replenishing the resources on which everyone depends: air, food, and water. Now, however, the spread of the human population is not beneficial, for we are eating into the few remaining "elsewheres"—the rural and forested lands that are vital to sustain our lives.

Whenever I go to the grocery store, I find it hard to believe there even is a problem with the world's food supply. I am amazed at how many foods are available and how many varieties of new foods I see.

Those of us living in wealthy, industrialized nations may have difficulty believing that a world food problem exists or that the problem will affect us. But many indicators are simultaneously revealing that the problem is very real and that everyone should be concerned. One of the primary indicators is the sudden, recent downturn in the world's food supply.

The world's food supply is often measured in grain output, for grain is the world's single largest crop. Between 1950 and 1984, the world's grain supply increased tremendously. Then in 1984 the picture changed. Grain output leveled off, and in 1987 it began to fall off sharply, as shown in Figure NP10–1. Whereas at the start of 1987, stored grain surpluses were sufficient to feed the world for 101 days, at the end of 1988, they were sufficient to feed the world for only 54 days.[2]

In the past, when grain supplies have fallen short, two options eased the problem: dip into the world's stored surpluses, or increase grain outputs. Now the stored grain surpluses are dwindling, and outputs cannot increase much more. Grain outputs have been increased in the past by farming more land, but now nearly all of the land that is suitable for farming is already under cultivation. Farming *unsuitable* land (such as the land on steep, erodible mountainsides or in rain forests) results in losses of soil and water to an extent that cannot be sustained for more than a few years. Furthermore, human habitation and industrial development are claiming the very same land, labor, and water that might be recruited for agricultural development. Thus remedies for grain shortages that have worked in the past are now failing, because they are based on the fallacy that the world's resources are infinite. The world's multiplying people are demanding more resources per year than the earth can replenish.

FIGURE NP10–1 **World Grain Output, 1950 to 1988**
There was a steep decline in grain output after 1984. The statistics used are per capita, but total grain output also fell equally steeply.
Source: U.S. Department of Agriculture, as presented by L. R. Brown, *The Changing World Food Prospect: The Nineties and Beyond,* Worldwatch paper 85 (Washington, D.C.: Worldwatch Institute, 1988), Figure 10.

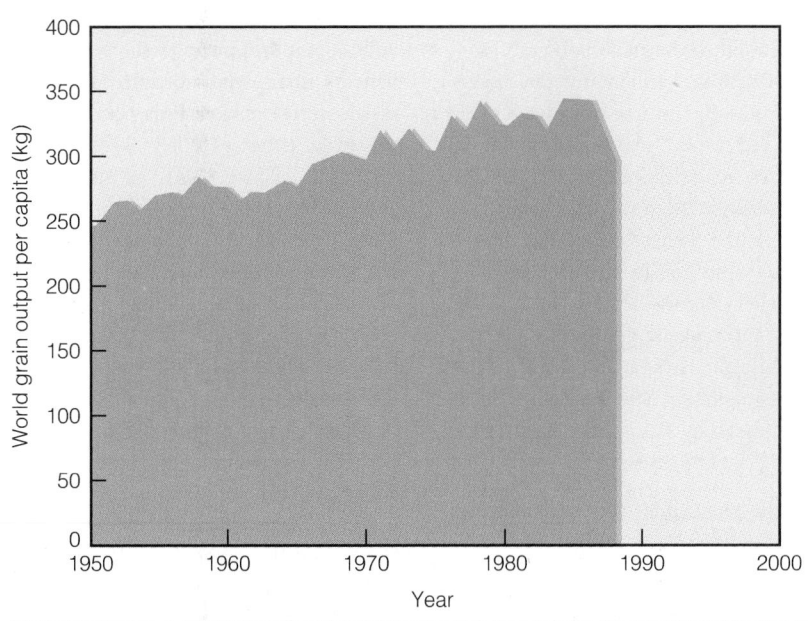

Is it too late to stop the process, or can something be done?

There is a way to stop this process, and it is urgent that we learn about it and implement it as soon as possible. Since the world population is growing whether we want it to or not, development will continue. However, there is a type of development we cannot live with and another type we can live with, at least until we get our numbers under control. The kind of development we cannot live with is exploitative development, which uses up resources such as soil, water, and trees without restoring them. The kind of development that will tide us over is sustainable development, which involves the use of renewable resources at a pace equal to the pace of their return.

It's easy to see how cutting down trees or using up water supplies could be a problem, but how can soil be used up?

Soil forms a thin layer around the earth. It is both created and lost all the time. Soil is created from the erosion of rocks, initiated through the action of wind and water. It is lost by being blown away by the wind or washed down slopes by waterways, ultimately sinking irretrievably into the ocean. Soil creation is slow, and in recent times, losses have predominated.

Not all plants must have soil to grow in; some trees, for example, may be able to gain a footing on bare rock or thin soil. Trees then protect the soil from erosion by sheltering it from wind and water. Grasses and agricultural crops do need soil—the thicker the better. Beneath the soil lie rock and clay, in which such plants cannot grow. When trees are removed to plant grasses or crops, the soil is left unprotected from the erosive action of winds and water. The soil is eventually lost, leaving behind bare rock or clay that no longer can support new vegetation.

Soil loss amounts to 25 billion tons a year, enough to fill Yankee Stadium 175,000 times.[3] Soil loss due to human misuse of the land is taking place so fast that *a quarter of the world's once-farmable land is fated to become permanent wasteland.*

What can be done to prevent further losses?

The only sustainable way of reversing this problem is by returning vulnerable areas to forest and grassland. Reforestation reduces the amount of land presently being farmed, but with a difference: the plants and trees are preserved, and they help to replenish clean air and water.

How do trees and plants replenish clean air?

Trees have covered much of the earth since prehistoric times. They provide a deep layer of vegetation in which many processes take place that support and renew the environment. They help replenish clean air, thanks to their capacity for photosynthesis, a process by which plants use the sun's energy to manufacture carbohydrates. During the process, the plant consumes carbon dioxide and releases oxygen into the atmosphere. People, on the other hand, require oxygen to obtain the energy they need to support their lives. While using oxygen, they exhale carbon dioxide; and they depend on green plants to consume the carbon dioxide and return oxygen to the air. People's fuel-burning processes such as

cooking, heating homes, and running cars or factories do the same thing: they consume oxygen and release carbon dioxide. The more people there are, and the more intense our use of fossil fuels, the more plants (especially forests) we need to surround us and compensate for our production of carbon dioxide with their consumption of it.

The oxygen that trees produce is essential to our existence, but their consumption of carbon dioxide is also important to our atmosphere and food supply. Carbon dioxide blocks the escape of heat into the outer atmosphere, and it helps to keep the earth warm. In the years between 1958 and 1988, however, the concentration of carbon dioxide in the earth's air has increased by 25 percent, mostly as the result of increased burning of oil and coal. The result is that the earth appears to be warming up—the so-called greenhouse effect.[4]

The greenhouse effect is expected to increase the earth's average temperature by 3 to 8 degrees Fahrenheit in the next half-century (before 2050)—an amount that may not sound like much, but that is expected to have major effects. Rainfall appears to be declining across the corn and wheat belts in the United States, Europe, the Soviet Union, and the rest of Asia, resulting in more frequent droughts than in the past, with loss of crops and rangelands. Forests and agricultural crops, adapted for thousands of years to a certain climate, are stressed by rising temperatures and are yielding to diseases and pests.

How do plants and trees replenish water supplies?

Trees play a major role in replenishing fresh water. By preserving soil, they

help the earth hold moisture; but more than that, they return vast amounts of underground water to the atmosphere by a process known as evapotranspiration. Transpired water is pure, and it forms clouds that will fall again as rain.

I guess this is why you hear so much in the news about the destruction of the rain forests. How is this destruction related to our food supply?

The trees in a rain forest provide an excellent example of how trees help us preserve the environment and protect our food supply. Rain forest trees may be more than 100 feet tall, and measure 20 feet across at the base. They support a mass of vegetation and animal life. They create shade and hold moisture. By evapotranspiration they create rain clouds, which frequently release drenching torrents. The rain forest trees generate oxygen by photosynthesis, permitting all living things in the forest to breathe. They drop tons of leaf litter, bark, branches, and animal droppings to the ground beneath them, where quantities of molds, fungi, and bacteria break down this litter as fast as it falls, keeping the system in balance. (Only an inch of soil lies below the litter, and beneath that is often impermeable clay. That is why tropical forestlands are so unsuitable for clearing and agricultural use.) The rain forest is most useful, from the point of view of basic human needs, to generate oxygen and rain.

When an acre of forest is cleared—for example, to plant grass and grow beef—its soil's fertility is used up within about eight years. Unprotected by tree cover, the soil quickly washes or blows away, leaving bare clay. When a whole region's forest is gone, rain ceases to fall, and the land becomes uninhabitable—not only for cattle, but for all other life.

Eight years of supposed value to human beings is a short time, compared with the hundreds of thousands of years it took for that rain forest system to evolve. Within that eight-year time span, the acre will produce only 50 pounds of cattle per year—400 pounds total. Of that, 200 pounds is usable meat, enough to yield 800 four-ounce hamburgers. The trade-off: 55 square feet of forest, representing half a ton of forest life, lost permanently for each hamburger.[5] This is a prime example of exploitative development. Some 27 million acres of tropical forests and other woodlands are being cleared each year.[6]

The rain forests can support human agriculture indefinitely if handled in the age-old ways developed by the forests' original people. The natives of such an area, living on small, cleared patches beneath the undisturbed forest canopy, were able to grow 5000 pounds of shelled corn and 4000 pounds of root and vegetable crops each year on each acre for five to seven years. Then they would allow the plots to return to forest and clear others. They rotated their crops of citrus, rubber, cacao, avocado, and papaya in a system known as agroforestry, which could be continued indefinitely. Food production systems practiced by traditional rain forest Indians are, without exception, more productive than the pasturelands that often replace them.[7]

If this is true, why are the rain forests still being cleared?

The rain forests are being cleared mostly by large-scale "development" projects.[8] These projects make sense only from the point of view of a very few people who make money from them in the short term. They do not help the people they displace, for as the land's richness degenerates beyond supporting even basic food crops, the people are forced to cut deeper and deeper into the forest to cultivate new lands while continuing to live in poverty and desperation.

Are there other environmental problems threatening our food supply?

There are many environmental factors with potential to disrupt the food supply. They are often interrelated with other environmental problems and cannot be described fully here. But three important environmental factors that can affect the food supply are:

1. The water supply.
2. The ozone layer.
3. Acid rain.

All plants and animals must have water to exist. The water supply is threatened by the demands of our ever-increasing population both in terms of the water we consume directly and the water needed to grow and process our food. Cities use water for domestic and industrial use. Industry uses water for transporting, dissolving, washing, rinsing, cooling, flushing away wastes, and many other purposes. Human overpopulation is also threatening the purity of the water supply. Fertilizers, pesticides, radioactive wastes, acid rain, and human waste materials all contribute to the pollution of the water supply. Other pollutants affect our atmosphere and, thus, can affect the food supply.

The depletion of the ozone layer is one example of an atmospheric condition caused by pollution that can affect our food supply. The ozone layer is a protective layer of gas in the outer atmosphere that filters out 99 percent of the ultraviolet rays of the sun, allowing just enough through to support plant growth. Air pollution from human activities all over the world is eating away at the ozone layer. As a result, more ultraviolet radiation is reaching the earth's surface each year. Ultraviolet rays in excess of the norm disrupt the genetic material in all living tissues, damaging all future generations of forests, agricultural crops, grasslands, gardens, and animal life on land and in the seas, as well as causing skin cancers in animals and people.

Another problem arising from air pollution that affects our food supply is acid rain. Each time it rains, the air is scrubbed of its pollutants; they fall to the earth. Many of them, when combined with water, form acids, which affect living things profoundly. Whatever compound forms the acid, the effects are similar, because the acid part is always the same: a tiny, charged particle of hydrogen. This chemical busybody disrupts cell membranes, distorts the proteins that do the work of living cells, and changes the characteristics of fluids so that they cannot support normal life processes. Millions of acres in many areas of the world, including U.S. mountain ranges, the Black Forest in Germany, and many parts of China, have been deforested by acid rain. In the soil, acid particles promote the release of toxic compounds into water supplies; in the air, they damage human lungs directly.

The Earth *before* Human Impact

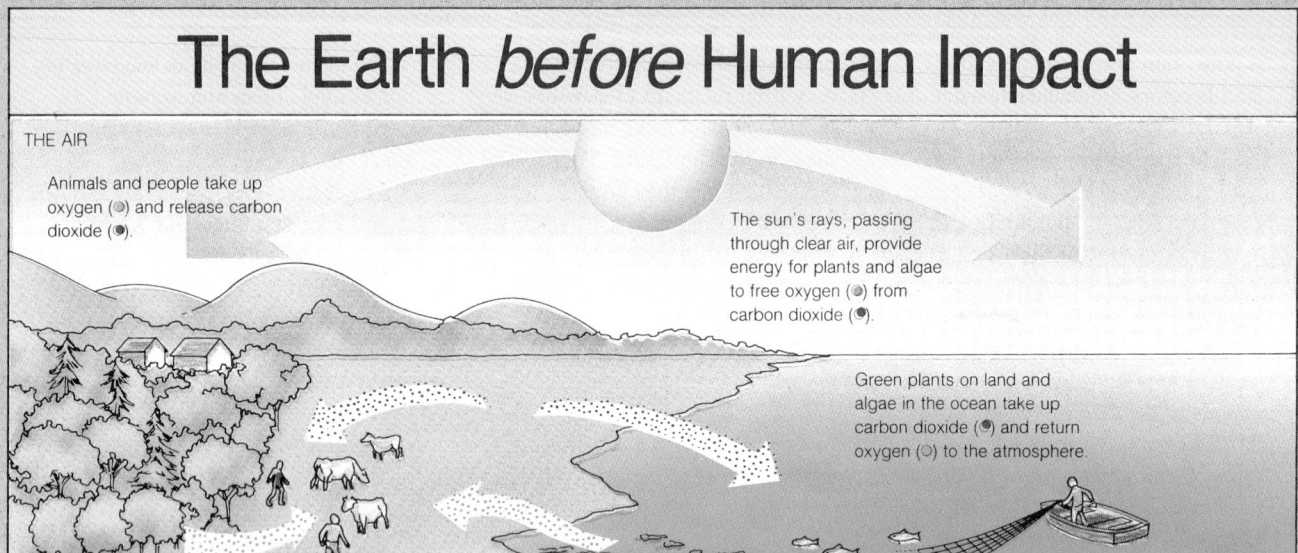

THE AIR

Animals and people take up oxygen (◉) and release carbon dioxide (●).

The sun's rays, passing through clear air, provide energy for plants and algae to free oxygen (◉) from carbon dioxide (●).

Green plants on land and algae in the ocean take up carbon dioxide (●) and return oxygen (○) to the atmosphere.

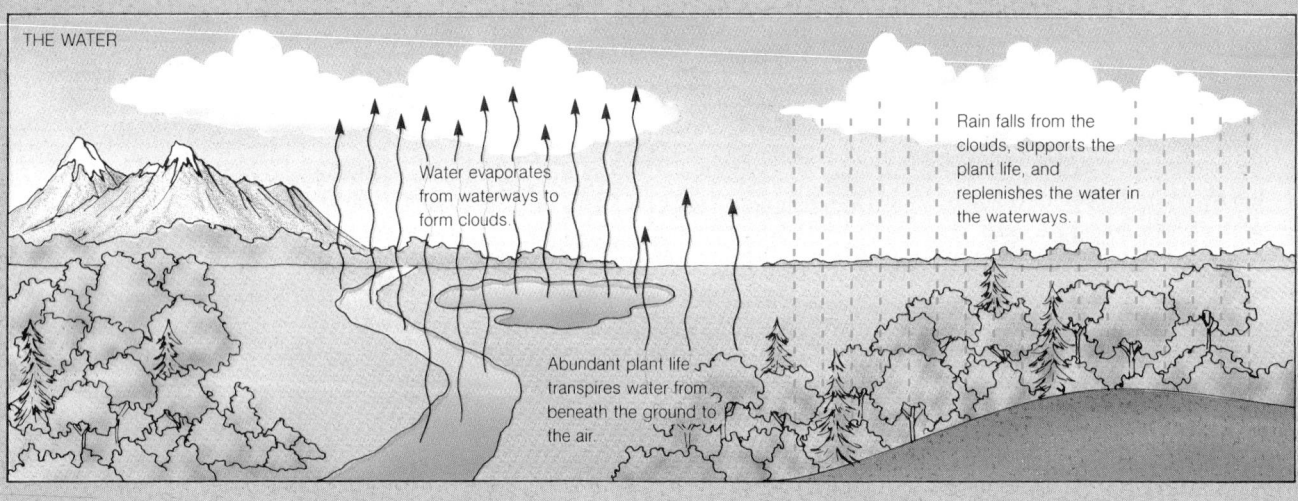

THE WATER

Water evaporates from waterways to form clouds.

Rain falls from the clouds, supports the plant life, and replenishes the water in the waterways.

Abundant plant life transpires water from beneath the ground to the air.

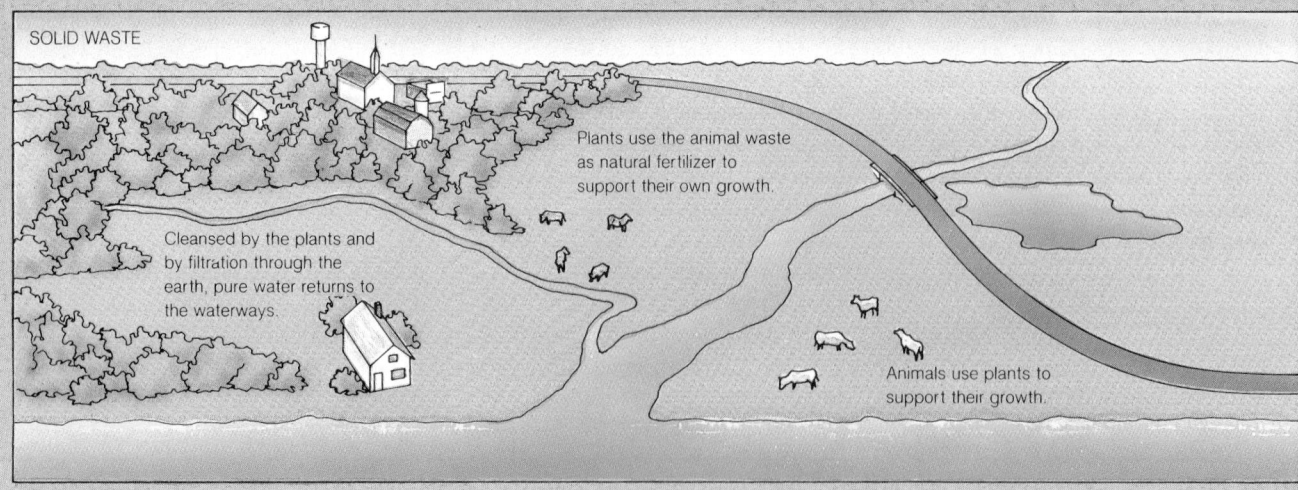

SOLID WASTE

Plants use the animal waste as natural fertilizer to support their own growth.

Cleansed by the plants and by filtration through the earth, pure water returns to the waterways.

Animals use plants to support their growth.

The Earth *with* Human Impact

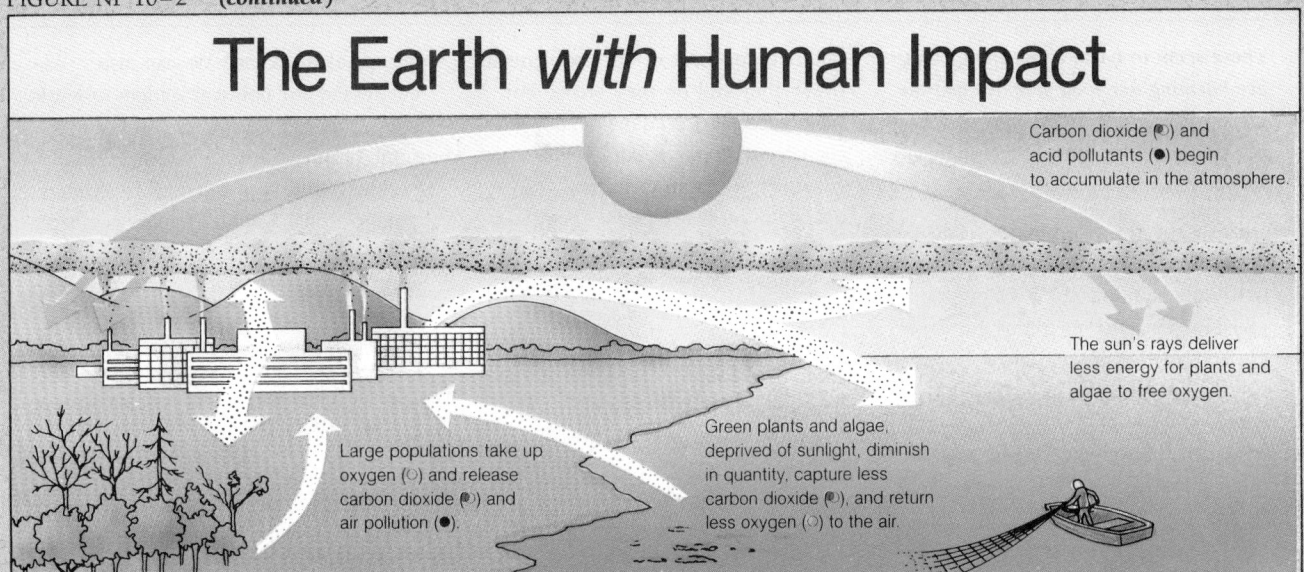

Carbon dioxide (◉) and acid pollutants (●) begin to accumulate in the atmosphere.

The sun's rays deliver less energy for plants and algae to free oxygen.

Large populations take up oxygen (○) and release carbon dioxide (◉) and air pollution (●).

Green plants and algae, deprived of sunlight, diminish in quantity, capture less carbon dioxide (◉), and return less oxygen (○) to the air.

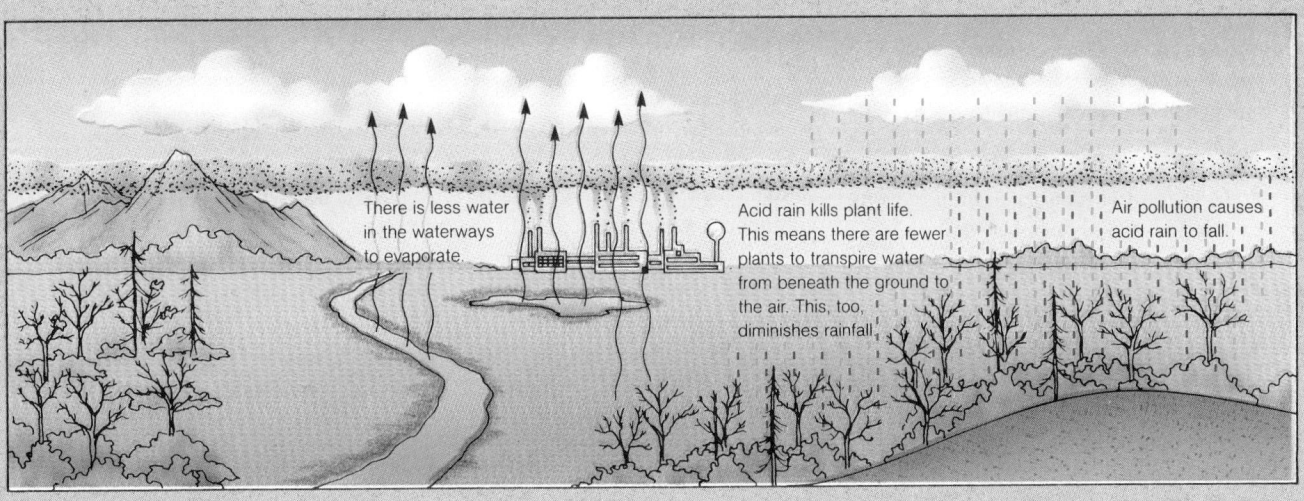

There is less water in the waterways to evaporate.

Acid rain kills plant life. This means there are fewer plants to transpire water from beneath the ground to the air. This, too, diminishes rainfall.

Air pollution causes acid rain to fall.

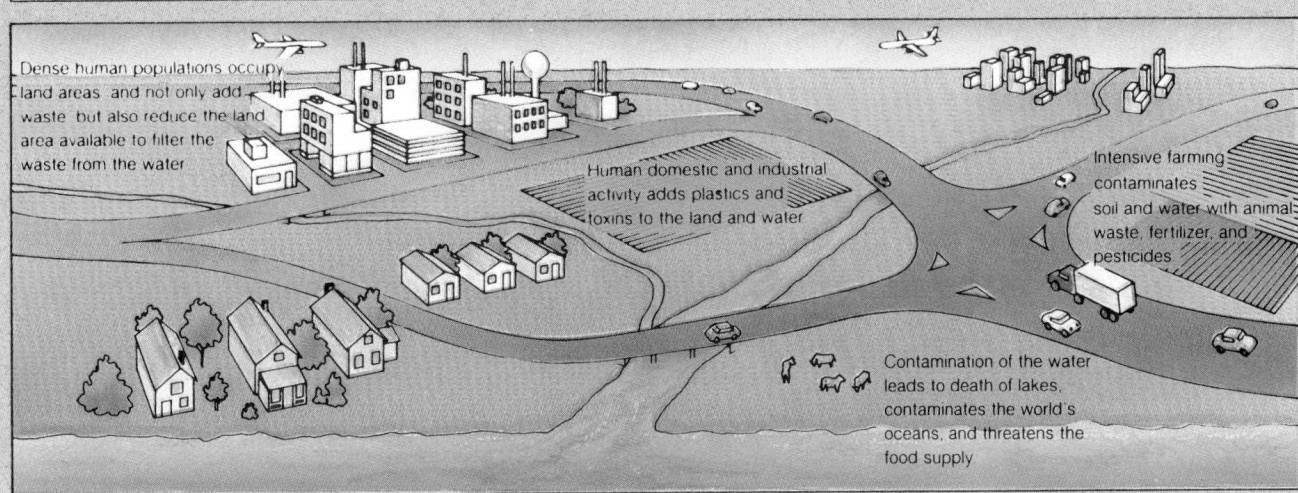

Dense human populations occupy land areas and not only add waste but also reduce the land area available to filter the waste from the water.

Human domestic and industrial activity adds plastics and toxins to the land and water.

Intensive farming contaminates soil and water with animal waste, fertilizer, and pesticides.

Contamination of the water leads to death of lakes, contaminates the world's oceans, and threatens the food supply.

There seem to be so many things that are harming our food supplies and the quality of life in general. It's hard to put it into perspective. Is there any way to put it in a nutshell?

You're right. It's a complicated and confusing subject. But it is also so vital that understanding the problems and reversing the current trends are imperative. Basically, to grow food we need land areas rich in fertile soil with adequate water and sun. To hold and replenish the soil and recycle the water into rain, we need forests. The forests need soil and water, too, and all need oxygen and protection by the ozone layer from the damaging rays of the sun. The earth's balance among these elements, which has made life possible for millennia, is now threatened by three simultaneous trends:

1. The spread of industrialization.
2. The destruction of natural resources.
3. The multiplication of people.

The effects of each trend compound those of the others, because every person in an industrialized society devours the earth's resources and pollutes the environment much more heavily than a person in a primitive society. Figure NP10–2 shows a simplified picture of the burdens we human beings place on the earth.

The problems seem so overwhelming. What can we do before it's too late?

The good news is, that as consumers, we can make a big difference in helping correct some of the problems in our environment. The days when we could blame major industrial

polluters for most of our problems are over—they still do their share, but *small consumers are now the major contributors to the pollution of our environment.* As an example, deforestation is driven by consumer demand for products. We panel and furnish our homes and offices with teak and mahogany from giant trees harvested by Japanese and Danish companies from deep within virgin rain forest lands. We eat more than 330 million pounds of beef purchased by U.S. companies from Central American countries alone—an amount that represents 90 percent of that region's beef exports.[9] As long as consumers keep buying this teak, mahogany, and beef, the trees continue to fall.

For another example of U.S. citizens' responsibility for the environmental problems of today, consider air pollution. People-generated pollution is continuous, concentrated, and in many cases growing more intense from year to year. People-generated pollutants come from four main sources: fuel burned to heat and cool homes, fuel burned to run appliances, wastes from industrial activity, and materials being burned for disposal. These add large amounts of pollutants to the air—among them, compounds that reduce its clarity (hampering photosynthesis) and compounds such as acids that render it toxic to plants (directly damaging them or making them vulnerable to disease).

Many avenues are open to us to help make positive changes in our lives to save our resources. Valuable suggestions for ways to accomplish this in each person's own life are offered by many inspired and creative

groups of thinkers.* We can also encourage our political leaders to work with other U.S. politicians to correct some of our country's environmental problems and with other world leaders to take global action. Finally, we need to renew our own earth consciousness and instill it in our children. Our Native American predecessors, the American Indians, have always known:

This we know. The Earth does not belong to man; man belongs to the Earth. This we know. All things are connected like the blood which unites one family. All things are connected. Whatever befalls the Earth befalls the sons of the Earth. Man did not weave the web of life, he is merely a strand in it. Whatever he does to the web, he does to himself.—Chief Seattle, 1854

Notes

1. National Academy of Sciences, *Resources and Man* (1969 report), as cited by L. J. Gordon, Popullution: The 1981 APHA presidential address, *American Journal of Public Health* 72 (1982): 341–346.
2. L. R. Brown, *The Changing World Food Prospect: The Nineties and Beyond,* Worldwatch paper 85 (Washington, D.C.: Worldwatch Institute, October 1988), available from the Worldwatch Institute, 1776 Massachusetts Ave. NW, Washington, DC 20036.
3. T. Peterson, Hunger and the environment, *Seeds,* October 1987, pp. 6–13.

*One book of excellent suggestions for meeting personal responsibilities to the world is produced under the auspices of the American Friends Service Committee: J. Bodner, ed., *Taking Charge of Our Lives: Living Responsibly in a Troubled World* (San Francisco: Harper and Row, 1984).

4. S. Begley, M. Miller, and M. Hager. The endless summer? *Newsweek,* 11 July 1988, pp. 18–20.

5. C. Uhl and G. Parker, Viewpoint: Our steak in the jungle, *Bioscience* 36 (1986): 642.

6. Letter (December 1988) from Conservation International, 1015 18th St. NW, Suite 1000, Washington, DC 20036.

7. J. D. Nations and D. I. Komer, Rainforests and the hamburger society, *Environment,* April 1983, pp. 12–20.

8. Letter from Conservation International, 1988.

9. Nations and Komer, 1983.

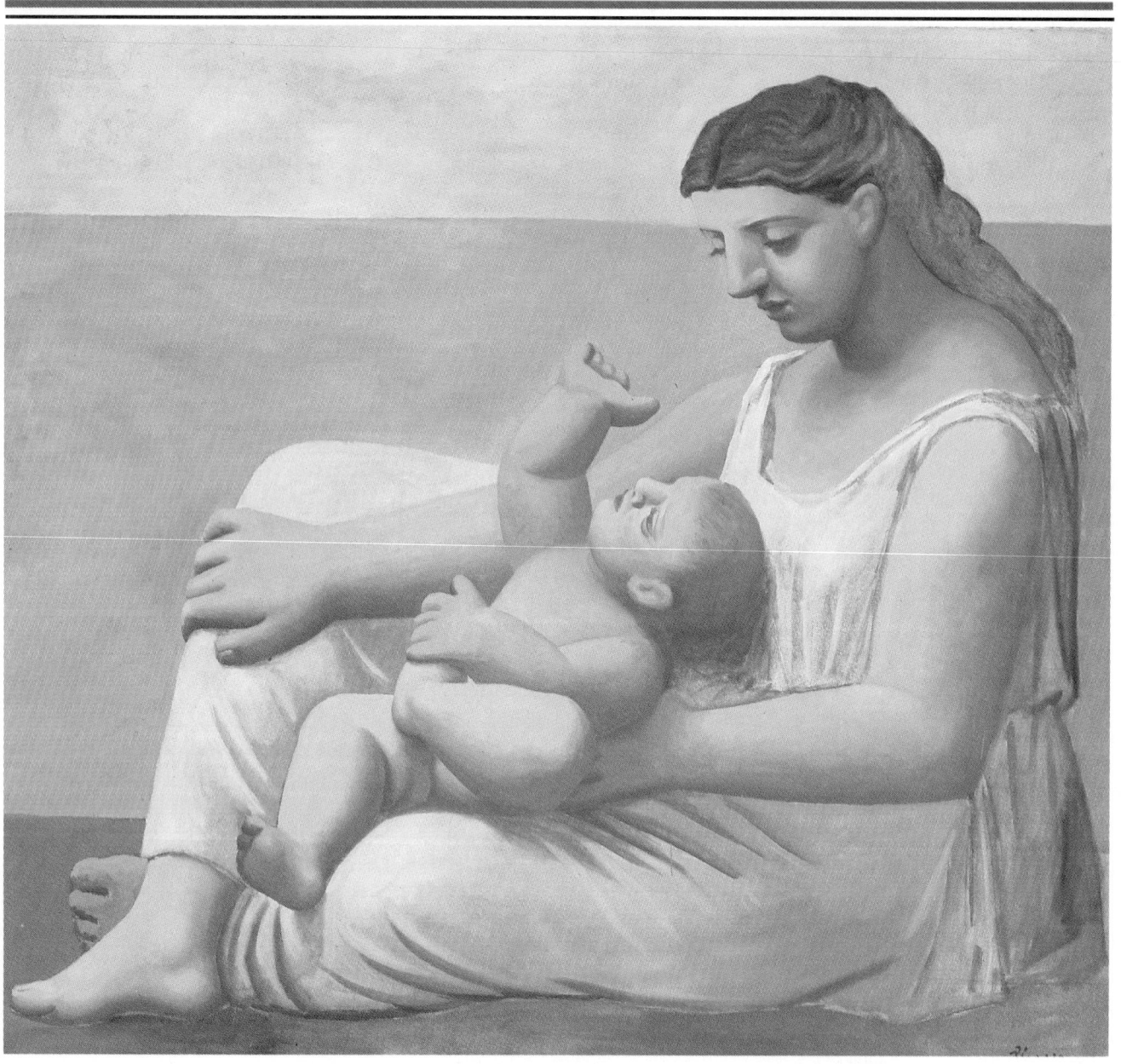

Pablo Picasso, Spanish, 1881–1973, Mother and Child, oil on canvas, 1921,
143.5 × 162.6 cm; Gift of Maymar Corporation, Mrs. Maurice L. Rothschild,
Mr. and Mrs. Chauncey McCormick; Mary and Leigh Block Charitable Fund;
Ada Turnbull Hertle Endowment; through prior gift of Mr. and Mrs Edwin E. Hokin,
1954. 270 © 1991 The Art Institute of Chicago, All Rights Reserved.

CHAPTER

11

Nutrition During Pregnancy and Infancy

CONTENTS

CHAPTER

11

The effects of nutrition extend over years. A woman's nutrition prior to and throughout pregnancy not only affects her own health but also is critical to the growth, development, and health of her child, even long after it has been born. The pregnant woman and the health professional advising her will be strongly motivated to attend to the woman's nutrition needs if they both understand how critical the nutrients are to the woman's health and her child's future. Similarly, sound nutrition during infancy promotes the rapid growth that characterizes this stage of life, and influences the child's future health. This chapter focuses on the special importance of nutrition during pregnancy and infancy.

Pregnancy: The Impact of Nutrition on the Future

The woman who enters pregnancy with full nutrient stores, sound eating habits, and a healthy body weight has done all she can nutritionally to ensure an optimal pregnancy outcome. Then, during the pregnancy itself, if she eats a variety of nutrient-dense foods, her own health and that of her developing child will benefit considerably.

Preparing for Pregnancy

Nutrition before conception is important. In the early weeks of pregnancy, before many women are even aware that they are pregnant, significant developmental changes occur that depend on a woman's nutrient intake and nutrient stores. A woman who has established sound eating habits already will optimally nourish the growing fetus and herself. If her habits are poor, and dietary changes do not correct deficiencies, nutrient supplementation may be warranted.

Appropriate weight for height prior to pregnancy also benefits pregnancy outcome. Women who enter pregnancy 10 percent or more below or 20 percent or more above standard weight for height and age face a greater risk than normal-weight women of impaired pregnancy outcome.[1] Underweight women are therefore advised to try to gain weight before becoming pregnant; overweight women are wise to lose excess weight to maximize the chances of having healthy babies, as well as to maintain their own good health.

A strong correlation exists between prepregnancy weight and infant birthweight. In turn, infant birthweight is the most potent single indicator of the infant's future health status. A low-birthweight baby, defined as one who weighs 5½ pounds (2,500 grams) or less, has a statistically greater chance than a normal-weight baby of contracting diseases and of dying early in life. In fact, low-birthweight babies are nearly 40 times as likely to die in the first month of life than normal-weight babies are.[2]

A major reason why the mother's prepregnancy nutrition is so crucial to a healthy pregnancy is that it determines whether she will be able to grow a healthy placenta during the first month of gestation. The only way nutrients can reach the developing fetus in the uterus is through the placenta.

low birthweight (LBW): a birthweight of 5½ lb (2,500 g) or less, used as a predictor of poor health in the newborn and as a probable indicator of poor nutrition status of the mother during and/or before pregnancy. Normal birthweight is 6½ lb (3,000 g) or more. Low-birthweight infants are of two different types. Some are **premature;** they are born early and are the right size for their gestational age. Others have suffered growth failure in the uterus; they may or may not be born early, but they are **small for gestational age (small for date).**

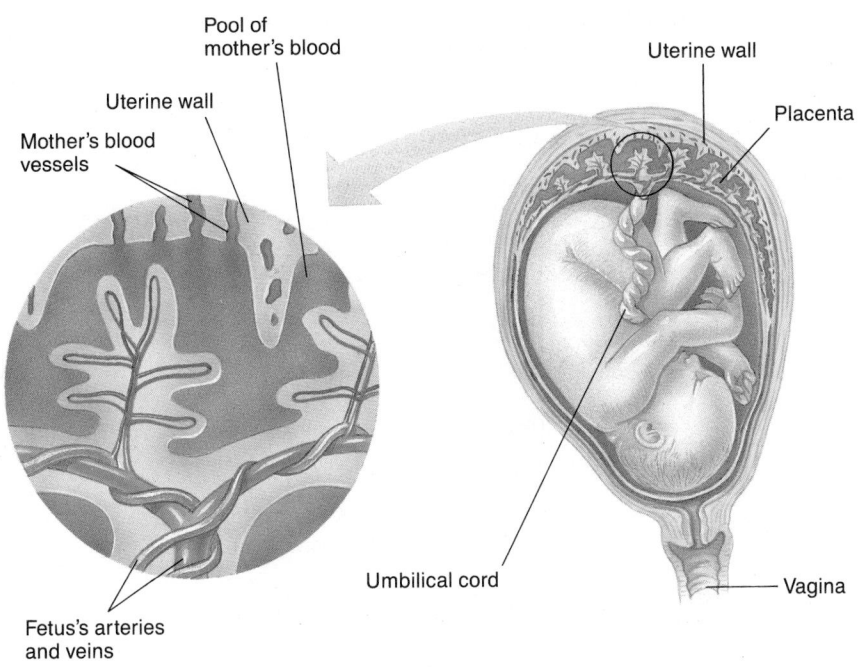

Pool of
mother's blood

Uterine wall

Mother's blood
vessels

Uterine wall

Placenta

Umbilical cord

Vagina

Fetus's arteries
and veins

FIGURE 11–1 **The Placenta**
In the placenta maternal blood vessels
lie side by side with fetal blood vessels
entering it through the umbilical cord.
This close association between the two
circulatory systems permits the mother's
bloodstream to deliver nutrients and
oxygen to the fetus and to carry away
fetal waste products.

The placenta is shown in Figure 11–1; it is a sort of cushion in which the mother's and baby's blood vessels intertwine and exchange materials— nutrients and oxygen going into the baby's system, and wastes leaving it to be excreted by the mother. The placenta must develop normally if the developing fetus is to attain full genetic potential.

If the mother's nutrient stores are inadequate during placental development, then no matter how well she eats later, the fetus will not receive optimum nourishment. The infant will be a low-birthweight baby, with all of the attendant health consequences.

Nutrient Needs during Pregnancy

Between the moment of conception and the moment of birth, innumerable events determine the course and outcome of fetal development and, ultimately, the health of the newborn infant. Each organ needs nutrients most during its own intensive growth period. A nutrient deficiency during one stage of development might affect the heart and during another stage, the developing limbs.

A woman's nutrient needs during pregnancy and lactation are higher than at any other time in her adult life and are greater for certain nutrients than for others. Figure 11–2 compares the nutrient needs of nonpregnant, pregnant, and lactating women. A study of the figure reveals some of the key needs.

ENERGY. During pregnancy, one of the smallest increases apparent is in food energy. An increase of only 15 percent (about 300 kcalories per day during

placenta (pla-SEN-tuh): an organ that develops inside the uterus early in pregnancy in which the mother's and fetus's circulatory systems intertwine, and in which exchange of materials between maternal and fetal blood takes place. The fetus receives nutrients and oxygen across the placenta; the mother's blood picks up carbon dioxide and other waste materials to be excreted via her lungs and kidneys.

gestation: the period from conception to birth; for human beings, the normal length of gestation is from 38 to 42 weeks.

fetus (FEET-us): the developing infant from eight weeks after conception until its birth.

uterus (Yoo-ter-us): the womb, the muscular organ within which the infant develops before birth.

A finite period occurs during development in which the events that take place will have irreversible, determining effects on later developmental stages. This is a **critical period,** usually a period of cell division in a body organ.

FIGURE 11-2 **Comparison of Nutrient Needs of Nonpregnant, Pregnant, and Lactating Women**

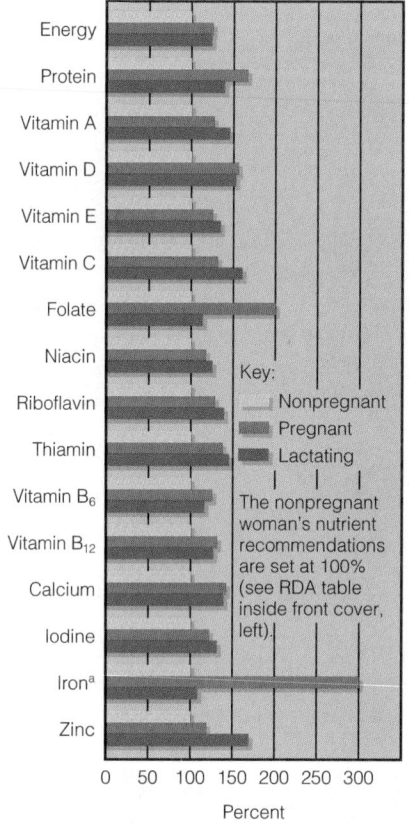

Key:
Nonpregnant
Pregnant
Lactating

The nonpregnant woman's nutrient recommendations are set at 100% (see RDA table inside front cover, left).

Energy
Protein
Vitamin A
Vitamin D
Vitamin E
Vitamin C
Folate
Niacin
Riboflavin
Thiamin
Vitamin B$_6$
Vitamin B$_{12}$
Calcium
Iodine
Iron[a]
Zinc

0 50 100 150 200 250 300

Percent

[a]The increased needs of pregnancy cannot be met by diet or by existing iron stores. Therefore, pregnant women need to take an iron supplement.

For a 120-lb woman, this represents at least 2,000 kcal/day, and preferably 2,200 kcal/day.

Recommended energy intake: 40 kcal/kg (18 kcal/lb).

Minimum energy intake: 36 kcal/kg (17 kcal/lb).

Recommended protein intake: 60 g/day.

Recommended carbohydrate intake: about 50% of energy intake. In a 2,000-kcal/day intake, this represents 1,000 kcal of carbohydrate, or about 250 g. Four cups of milk will contribute about 50 g carbohydrate. An apple provides 15 g carbohydrate, and a slice of bread provides 15 g, so generous intakes of fruit and bread are clearly beneficial.

the second and third trimesters) above the allowance for nonpregnant women is recommended. Pregnant teenagers, underweight women, or physically active women may need more. In each case, enough energy should be consumed to spare the protein needed for growth.

PROTEIN. The recommendation for protein allows an additional 10 grams per day throughout pregnancy. The results of food consumption surveys indicate that many women in the United States exceed the recommended protein intake each day.[3] Thus some women already receive the 10 grams of additional daily protein recommended during pregnancy. Adequate protein consumption during pregnancy is important, but excessive protein may have adverse effects, as Chapter 3 described.

Some people choose to exclude all foods of animal origin from their diets. For these individuals, the selection of protein-rich foods is limited, and the need for abundant high-quality protein during pregnancy demands careful attention. The inclusion of adequate food energy each day and several servings of plant-protein foods such as legumes, whole grains, nuts, and seeds in generous quantities is imperative.

TABLE 11–1   **Women at Nutritional Risk during Pregnancy**

- Women who ordinarily consume an inadequate diet (for example, those who avoid consumption of all animal-derived foods)
- Women who are lactose intolerant
- Women who are carrying multiple fetuses
- Women who smoke cigarettes or use alcohol or illicit drugs
- Women who are underweight or overweight at conception
- Women who gain insufficient or excessive weight during pregnancy
- Women who lack nutrition knowledge or who have insufficient financial resources to purchase adequate food
- Adolescents

Source: Compiled from information in National Academy of Sciences, Food and Nutrition Board, *Nutrition During Pregnancy* (Washington, D.C.: National Academy Press, 1990).

CARBOHYDRATE. Pregnant women need generous amounts of carbohydrate to spare the protein they eat. If added energy is needed, it is best obtained from carbohydrate.

VITAMINS. The vitamins required for blood production and rapid cell proliferation—folate and vitamin B_{12}—are needed in large amounts during pregnancy. New cells are laid down at a tremendous pace as the fetus grows and develops. At the same time, the mother's red blood cell mass expands. The RDA for folate more than doubles during pregnancy. It is possible to obtain the recommended folate amounts from foods, but some diets may be inadequate in this respect. Although routine folate supplementation of pregnant women is not recommended, if the folate adequacy of a pregnant woman's diet is in doubt, then folate supplementation of 300 micrograms per day is recommended.[4]

The pregnant woman has a slightly greater need for the vitamin that assists folate in the manufacture of red blood cells—vitamin B_{12}. (The vitamin B_{12} RDA for adults is 2 micrograms. During pregnancy, the RDA increases to 2.2 micrograms.) Generally, the body's stores of vitamin B_{12} can meet the needs of pregnancy, and because the vitamin is found almost exclusively in foods of animal origin, meat eaters and lacto-ovo vegetarians are protected from deficiency. For women who eat all-plant diets, a daily vitamin B_{12} supplement of 2.0 micrograms is recommended.[5]

Dietary improvements are always preferred as the means to improve nutrient inadequacies, but when such improvements are unlikely, then nutrient supplementation becomes necessary. The National Academy of Sciences subcommittee for the publication *Nutrition during Pregnancy* defines certain women as nutritionally at risk during pregnancy (see Table 11–1).[6] Unfortunately, the categories of "at risk" women undoubtedly include a majority of pregnant women in the United States.[7] The subcommittee recommends a multivitamin-mineral supplement containing the nutrient amounts shown in Table 11–2 for these women.

TABLE 11–2   **Nutrient Supplements during Pregnancy**[a]

NUTRIENT	AMOUNT
Folate	300 μg
Vitamin B_6	2 mg
Vitamin C	50 mg
Vitamin D	5 μg
Calcium	250 mg
Copper	2 mg
Iron	30 mg
Zinc	15 mg

[a]For pregnant women at nutritional risk (see Table 11–1).

Source: Reprinted with permission from *Nutrition During Pregnancy* c. 1990 by the National Academy of Sciences. Published by National Academy Press, Washington, D.C.

The RDA for folate more than doubles during pregnancy, increasing from 180 to 400 μg per day.

Foods containing folate:
Green leafy vegetables.
Legumes.
Liver.
Orange juice and cantaloupe.
Other vegetables.
Whole-wheat products.

MINERALS. Among the minerals, those involved in building the skeleton—calcium, phosphorus, and magnesium—are in great demand during pregnancy. Intestinal absorption of calcium doubles early in pregnancy; the mother's bones store the mineral. Later, as the fetal bones begin to calcify, there is a dramatic shift of calcium across the placenta, and the mother's bone stores are drawn upon. Recommendations for calcium and phosphorus are 1,200 milligrams per day. The recommendation for magnesium during pregnancy is slightly higher than for nonpregnant women based on its role in bone and tissue growth.

Mineralization of the baby's teeth begins in the fifth month after conception. For this and for the bones, fluoride may be needed. Fluoride does cross the placenta, but whether the placenta can defend against excess intakes is questionable. Therefore, fluoride supplements are not recommended for pregnant women who drink fluoridated water. For women who live in communities without fluoridated water, a fluoride supplement may protect fetal teeth.

The body conserves iron even more than usual during pregnancy: menstruation ceases, and absorption of iron increases up to threefold due to a rise in the blood concentration of the blood's iron-absorbing and iron-carrying protein, transferrin. However, iron stores dwindle during pregnancy. The developing fetus draws on the mother's iron stores to create stores of its own to last through the first three to six months of life. Iron losses also occur with the blood losses inevitable at the time of birth. These drains on the mother's supply may precipitate a deficiency.

Few women enter pregnancy with adequate iron stores, so a daily iron supplement containing 30 milligrams is recommended during the second and third trimesters for all pregnant women.[8] Meats and legumes top the list of iron-rich foods.

Zinc is another nutrient of vital importance in pregnancy; it is required for DNA and RNA synthesis and thus for protein synthesis. The results of a study of more than 400 pregnant women revealed that blood zinc concentration is a significant predictor of low birth weight.[9] The incidence of low-birthweight babies was 8 times higher among women with the lowest blood zinc concentrations as compared with women who had the highest blood zinc concentrations. Zinc is most abundant in foods of high protein content, such as shellfish, meat, and nuts, but the presence of other trace elements and fiber in foods may adversely affect zinc absorption. Zinc nutrition is the focus of intense study at the present time, and many questions remain to be answered regarding zinc metabolism and availability from foods. In the meantime, however, daily consumption of zinc-rich foods is no doubt beneficial to the pregnant woman and her fetus.

FOOD CHOICES. An adequate nutrient and energy intake throughout pregnancy will help to support the growth and health of both mother and baby. The dietary challenge during pregnancy is to meet nutrient needs without overconsuming kcalories. Because food energy needs increase less than nutrient needs, the pregnant woman must select foods of high nutrient density. For most women, appropriate choices include foods like nonfat milk, nonfat plain yogurt, lean meats, eggs, liver, dark green vegetables, vitamin C–rich fruits, and whole-grain breads and cereals. Table 11–3 provides a suggested food pattern.

Four cups of milk a day will supply 1,200 mg calcium. For other food sources, see Chapter 8.

In pregnancy, hemoglobin values of 12 g are not unusual, and 11 g is where the line defining "too low" is often drawn. It is usually desirable to use more sensitive measures than hemoglobin tests if questions about the woman's iron status arise.

Food sources of iron:
  Liver, oysters.
  Fish, red meat, other meat.
  Dried fruits.
  Legumes (dried beans, peas, lima beans).
  Dark green vegetables.

TABLE 11–3 Daily Food Choices for Pregnant and Lactating Women

| | Number of Servings | |
FOOD GROUP	ADULTS	PREGNANT OR LACTATING WOMEN
Meat/meat alternates	2	3
Milk/milk products	2	4
Vegetables	3 to 5	3 to 5
Fruits	2 to 4	2 to 4
Breads/cereals	6 to 11	6 to 11

Some women develop cravings for, or aversions to, some foods and beverages during pregnancy. Individual food cravings during pregnancy do not seem to reflect real physiological needs.[10] In other words, a woman who craves pickles does not necessarily need salt, nor does a chocolate craving indicate a need for caffeine or fat. The craving for ice cream is the most common craving in pregnancy, but does not signify a calcium deficiency. Food aversions and cravings that arise during pregnancy are probably due to changes in taste and smell sensitivities.

Craving of nonfood items such as clay, ice, and cornstarch is known as *pica*.

Weight Gain and Exercise

The pregnant woman must gain weight. Table 11–4 shows the components of an example weight gain of 31 pounds. A pregnancy weight gain of 25 to 35 pounds is recommended for women who begin pregnancy at a normal weight for height, carrying a single fetus.[11] For underweight women, a slightly higher weight gain (28 to 40 pounds) is recommended. The recommended weight gain for overweight women is lower—15 to 25 pounds. Some women should strive for gains at the upper end of the target range,

TABLE 11–4 Components of Weight Gain during Pregnancy

DEVELOPMENT	WEIGHT GAIN (lb)
Infant at birth	7½
Placenta	1
Increase in mother's blood volume to supply placenta	4
Increase in mother's fluid volume	4
Increase in size of mother's uterus and muscles to support it	2½
Increase in size of mother's breasts	3
Fluid to surround infant in amniotic sac	2
Mother's fat stores	7
Total	31

Weight-for-height categories for prepregnant women are based on body mass index (BMI) measures (see Appendix B). A BMI of 19.8 to 26.0 defines the normal range. A BMI less than 19.8 defines the low range. A BMI greater than 26.0 to 29.0 defines the high, or overweight, range. A BMI above 29.0 defines obesity.

notably adolescents, who are still growing themselves. Short women (5 feet 2 inches and under) should strive for gains at the lower end of the target range.

The ideal pattern is thought to be about 2 to 4 pounds during the first three months and a pound per week thereafter. Women lose some of the weight gained during pregnancy at delivery, and most of the remainder within a few weeks or months, as blood volume returns to normal and accumulated fluids are lost.

If a woman has gained more than the expected amount of weight early in pregnancy, she should not try to diet in the last weeks. A sudden large weight gain, however, is a danger signal that may indicate the onset of a complication known as pregnancy-induced hypertension (discussed later in the chapter).

Weight gain during pregnancy, like prepregnancy weight, directly relates to infant birthweight.[12] If the mother does not gain the full amount of weight recommended, she may give birth to an underweight baby.

Chapter 9 described another lifestyle component that promotes health and well-being: exercise. The active, physically fit woman experiencing a normal pregnancy can continue to enjoy the benefits of exercise throughout pregnancy, adjusting the duration and intensity as needed. One study found that women who participated in a balanced, 45-minute exercise session three days per week had fewer surgical births, shorter hospital stays, and infants who were in stronger physical condition at birth than women who did not.[13] Table 11–5 provides some guidelines for exercise during pregnancy.

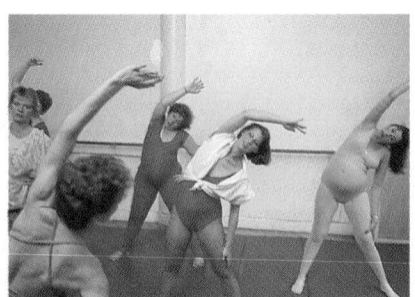

Pregnant women can enjoy the benefits of exercise.

Practices to Avoid

A general guideline can be offered to the pregnant woman: eat a normal, healthy diet, and practice moderation. A woman's daily choices, her lifestyle habits, may normally affect her only slightly, but during pregnancy, these same choices take on enormous importance. Forewarned, pregnant women can choose to abstain from or avoid potentially harmful practices. The following practices or substances may adversely affect dietary intake and nutritional status during pregnancy, as well as pregnancy outcome.

TABLE 11–5   **Exercise Guidelines for Pregnancy**

- Stop exercising if you feel overheated.
- Drink plenty of fluids before you exercise.
- Avoid exercising in hot, humid weather.
- Protect the abdomen from injury, especially in games like baseball or basketball, in which accidents are likely.
- Discontinue any exercise that causes discomfort.
- Do not exercise while lying on your back after about the fourth month.
- Do not allow your heart rate to exceed 140 beats per minute.

CIGARETTE SMOKING. Smoking restricts the blood supply to the growing fetus, and so limits the delivery of oxygen and nutrients and the removal of wastes. Cigarette smoking is by far the single most important modifiable risk factor responsible for fetal growth retardation in developed countries.[14] Smoking also causes these adverse effects: premature births, spontaneous abortions (fetal deaths), and increased risks of infants' dying early in life.[15] In addition, smoking adversely affects the pregnant woman's nutrition status, which in turn impairs fetal nutrition. Cigarette smoking increases iron needs and decreases the availability of vitamin B^{12}, vitamin C, folate, and zinc.[16] Smoking never conveys a health advantage, and pregnancy dramatically magnifies the disadvantages of smoking.

CAFFEINE. Caffeine consumption during pregnancy should be limited. Caffeine is a potentially harmful drug, and it does cross the placenta. So far, there is no convincing evidence that caffeine causes birth defects in human beings, but there is limited evidence that caffeine retards fetal growth.[17] The Food and Drug Administration recommends that pregnant women either avoid caffeine-containing products or use them sparingly. Pregnant women's caffeine consumption should be minimal (less than 150 milligrams per day, the amount contained in one cup of coffee or two 12-ounce colas).

A table of the caffeine amounts in beverages and medications is provided in Chapter 12.

DRUGS. Drugs taken during pregnancy can cause serious birth defects. The use of over-the-counter drugs is routine for many people, and drugs of abuse are a major problem. Research shows that marijuana or cocaine use during pregnancy adversely affects fetal growth and development.[18] Without prior physician consultation, the use of any drugs or even vitamin supplements is contraindicated.

DIETING. Dieting, even for short periods, is hazardous during pregnancy. Low-carbohydrate diets or fasts that cause ketosis deprive the growing brain of needed glucose and may impair its development. Energy restriction during pregnancy is dangerous for all women, regardless of their prepregnancy weights.

ALCOHOL CONSUMPTION. Alcohol consumption during pregnancy can cause irreversible brain damage and mental and physical retardation in the fetus—the abnormalities that define fetal alcohol syndrome (FAS). The potential for fetal damage arises when the mother's liver receives more alcohol than it can detoxify. Alcohol-laden blood then circulates to all parts of the mother's body and freely crosses the placenta to impair fetal development. Alcohol also interferes with placental transport of nutrients to the fetus.[19]

Of the leading causes of mental retardation, FAS is the only one that is totally preventable.[20] The surgeon general has issued a statement that pregnant women should drink absolutely no alcohol. All containers of beer, wine, and liquor now must carry the following warning: Women should not drink alcoholic beverages during pregnancy because of the risk of birth defects.

fetal alcohol syndrome: the cluster of symptoms seen in a person whose mother consumed excess alcohol during her pregnancy; includes mental and physical retardation with facial and other body deformities.

Medical Complications and Other Problems of Pregnancy

Some nutrition measures can help alleviate the most common problems encountered during pregnancy. Pregnancy precipitates the onset of diabetes in some women. This condition is known as gestational diabetes. Without proper management, gestational diabetes can lead to infant sickness and death. Health care professionals screen all pregnant women for diabetes at or before the sixth month. Women with gestational diabetes should not reduce their carbohydrate intakes but should choose foods rich in complex carbohydrates, such as vegetables and whole-grain breads, and should limit their intakes of concentrated sweets.

A certain degree of edema is to be expected in late pregnancy. This is due to the raised secretion of the hormone estrogen—which promotes water retention and helps to ready the uterus for delivery—toward the end of pregnancy. For some women, however, edema may be a part of a larger problem known as pregnancy-induced hypertension (PIH). Preexisting hypertension and PIH are the most common medical complications of pregnancy. They can cause maternal death, infant death, retarded growth, lung problems, and other birth defects. Prenatal care includes keeping track of maternal blood pressure throughout pregnancy and, if PIH is diagnosed, initiating treatment promptly.* Treatment requires medical attention; salt restriction is not a part of treatment until and unless the kidneys prove unable to handle a normal sodium load. A normal salt intake is necessary for health.

The nausea of "morning" (actually, anytime) sickness seems unavoidable, because it arises from the hormonal changes taking place early in pregnancy; however, it can often be alleviated. A strategy some expectant mothers have found effective in quelling nausea is to start the day with a few sips of water

gestational diabetes: the appearance of abnormal glucose tolerance during pregnancy, with subsequent return to normal postpartum.

The normal edema of pregnancy responds to gravity; blood pools in the ankles. The edema of PIH is a generalized edema. The distinction helps with diagnosis.

pregnancy-induced hypertension (PIH), formerly known as **toxemia** (tox-EEM-ee-uh): a cluster of symptoms seen in pregnancy, including edema, hypertension, and kidney complications. A variety of terms are associated with PIH. Most common is **eclampsia;** its symptoms include convulsions and coma, associated with hypertension, edema, and protein in the urine. Eclampsia may be preceded by **preeclampsia,** an abnormal condition of pregnancy characterized by edema, increasing hypertension, and protein in the urine.*

Hints for controlling nausea and vomiting:
  Eat soda crackers before getting out of bed.
  Eat frequent, small meals. Keep something in your stomach.
  Drink liquids before or after meals rather than during meals.
  Avoid fried foods, and limit the fat you use in foods.
  Avoid using foods with strong odors if the odors make you feel nauseated.
  Everybody is different. Keep track of what you eat and when you feel nauseated, and do what's best for you.
  Take prenatal vitamin and iron supplements on a full stomach or at a time of day when you are not nauseated.
  Allow for some quiet time after eating. Rushing around after meals increases nausea.

Don't be fooled into thinking that the nausea many pregnant women experience is always a minor complaint. True, occasional nausea does not threaten health. And true, nausea may not be a problem for the woman with a small touch of it that subsides after a short time. But for the woman who has nausea all day long (sometimes accompanied by vomiting), the problem can be depressing.

Comments like "Don't worry, nausea usually subsides after the first trimester" may actually make things worse. The woman may be thinking, "You mean I'm going to feel like this for *two more months?*" Think of how much worse the woman who is nauseated for a longer time may feel.

How can you help? For one thing, don't ignore the problem or treat it as unimportant. Let your client know that you understand what she is going through. Offer the suggestions given here for dealing with nausea. If appropriate (if the woman is happy about having a baby), it may help to focus her attention on the end result of her efforts—the beautiful baby she has been waiting for.

---

*Blood pressure of 140/90 millimeters of mercury during the second half of pregnancy in a woman who has not previously exhibited hypertension indicates PIH. So does a rise in systolic blood pressure of 30 millimeters or in diastolic blood pressure of 15 millimeters on at least two occasions more than six hours apart. R. J. Worley, Pathophysiology of pregnancy-induced hypertension, *Clinical Obstetrics and Gynecology* 27 (1984): 821–835.

and a few nibbles of a soda cracker or other bland carbohydrate food, to get something in their stomachs before getting out of bed. Carbonated beverages also may help. The margin note offers further suggestions to alleviate nausea.

As the hormones of pregnancy alter muscle tone and the thriving infant crowds intestinal organs, an expectant mother might complain of constipation. A high-fiber diet, exercise, and a plentiful fluid intake will help relieve this condition. Also, responding promptly to the urge to defecate can help. Laxatives should be used only as prescribed by the physician. Mineral oil should not be used, because it robs the body of fat-soluble vitamins.

Pregnancy for many women is a time of adjustment to major changes. The woman who is expecting a baby is a growing person in more ways than one. Her needs are changing, not only physically but also emotionally. If it is her first baby, she senses that her lifestyle will have to change as she takes on the new responsibility of caring for a child. Ideally, she will be encouraged to develop this sense of responsibility by caring for herself during pregnancy. The expectant mother needs support in thinking of herself as a thoroughly worthwhile and important person with a new and challenging task that she can and will perform well.

Breastfeeding

Adequate nutrition of the mother makes a highly significant contribution to successful lactation. Without it, lactation is likely to falter or fail.

The Mother's Nutrient Needs

By continuing to eat high-quality foods, not restricting weight gain unduly, and enjoying ample food and fluid at frequent intervals throughout lactation, the mother who chooses to breastfeed her infant will be nutritionally prepared to do so. An inadequate diet does not support the stamina, patience, and self-confidence that nursing an infant demands.

A nursing mother produces an average of 25 ounces of milk a day, with wide variations possible.[21] At 21 kcalories per ounce, this milk output amounts to about 525 kcalories per day. In addition, the woman's body requires extra energy to produce this milk. The energy allowance for a woman during the first six months of lactation is a generous 640 kcalories a day above her ordinary need. The Committee on RDA suggests that 500 kcalories come from added food, and the rest from the body stores of fat accumulated during pregnancy for that purpose. Some research suggests that for many women, energy needed for milk production may be less than current recommendations.[22] Severe energy restriction, however, hinders milk production.

The period of lactation is the natural time for a woman to lose the extra body fat that was accumulated to support lactation. If she chooses nutrient-dense foods, she will gradually lose weight, even though her energy intake may be greater than normal.[23]

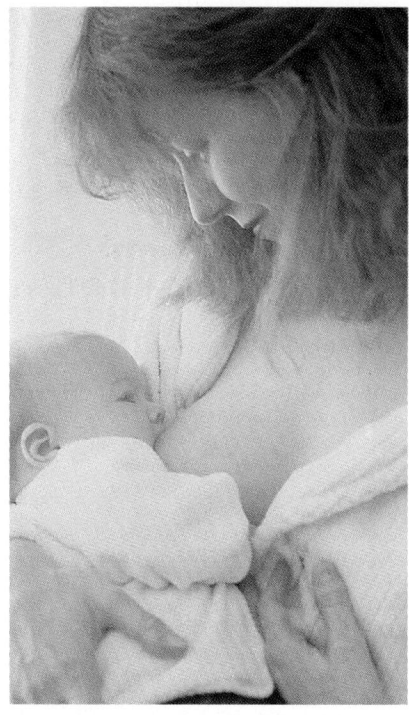

Breastfeeding is a natural extension of pregnancy—of the mother's body nourishing the infant.

In addition to providing energy, the foods consumed by the nursing mother should offer abundant nutrients—especially those needed to make milk, such as calcium, protein, magnesium, zinc, and plenty of fluid. Figure 11–2 shows the differences between a lactating woman's nutrient needs and those of a nonpregnant woman, and Table 11–3 shows a food pattern that meets those needs.

Despite previous misconceptions, increasing maternal fluid intake does not increase breast milk volume.[24] Nevertheless, a lactating woman will want to drink at least 2 quarts of liquids each day to protect herself from dehydration. A convenient way to ensure adequate fluid consumption is to drink a glass of milk, juice, or water each time the baby nurses, as well as at mealtimes.

The question is often raised whether a mother's milk may lack a nutrient if she fails to get enough in her diet. The answer differs from one nutrient to the next, but in general, the effect of nutritional deprivation of the mother is to reduce the *quantity,* not the *quality,* of her milk. For protein, carbohydrate, and most minerals, the milk of a healthy mother has a fairly constant composition. The taking of a vitamin-mineral supplement that contains nutrient levels close to 100 percent of the RDA seems not to raise nutrient concentrations in the breast milk of an otherwise well-nourished mother. The concentrations of most of the water-soluble vitamins reach saturation levels in well-nourished women; excesses are excreted. Vitamin B_6 is the exception; its concentration in breast milk continues to rise with increasing intakes.[25] The levels of fat-soluble vitamins in human milk can be altered, however, by excessive or deficient intakes of the mother. For example, large doses of vitamin A correspondingly raise the concentration of this vitamin in breast milk. Furthermore, vitamin supplementation of *undernourished* women appears to raise the vitamin concentration of their milk, and it may be beneficial.[26]

Foods with strong or spicy flavors may alter the taste of breast milk. A sudden change in the taste of the milk may annoy some infants. Infants who are sensitive to particular foods, such as cow's milk protein, may become uncomfortable when the mother's diet includes these foods. While this may be true of a few infants, it is not a basis for all nursing mothers to avoid cow's milk. The nutrients provided by milk products make a significant contribution to both the infant's and the mother's health.

Contraindications of Breastfeeding

Some substances impair maternal milk production or enter the breast milk and interfere with infant development. Alcohol easily enters breast milk. One study showed that the alcohol concentration of breast milk peaks within one hour after ingestion of even small amounts of alcohol (½ ounce).[27] In this study, alcohol consumption by lactating women significantly reduced the breast milk intake of their infants. The researchers suggest that the following three factors, acting separately or together, may explain the change in breast milk consumption:

■ The alcohol may have altered the flavor of the breast milk, which in turn influenced the infants' feeding behavior.

▬ Infants have a limited capacity to metabolize alcohol; even low doses may become potent enough to change infant feeding response.
▬ The alcohol reduced the women's milk production.

Regardless of the exact mechanism, alcohol consumption by lactating women led to decreased milk consumption by infants. In the past, alcohol has been recommended to lactating mothers to facilitate milk production, despite a lack of scientific support for such recommendations. The research discussed here supports the concept that alcohol actually impairs milk production. An occasional glass of wine or beer is considered within safe limits, but in general, alcohol consumption by lactating women should be discouraged.

Excessive caffeine consumption during lactation may cause irritability and wakefulness in the breastfed infant. As during pregnancy, caffeine consumption should be moderate.

Health care professionals should actively discourage smoking by lactating women. Smoking may reduce milk volume, and it also has numerous harmful effects on both mother and child.[28]

If a woman has an ordinary cold, she can go on nursing without worry. If susceptible, the infant will catch it from her anyway, and thanks to immunological protection, a breastfed baby may be less susceptible than a formula-fed baby would be. If a woman has a communicable disease such as tuberculosis or hepatitis, which could threaten the infant's health, then mother and baby have to be separated. Breastfeeding would be possible only by pumping the mother's breasts several times a day. The Centers for Disease Control recommend that women who test positive for the human immunodeficiency virus (HIV-1), the virus that causes acquired immune deficiency syndrome (AIDS), should not breastfeed their infants.[29]

Similarly, if a nursing mother must take medication that is secreted in breast milk and that is known to affect the infant, then breastfeeding is contraindicated. Drug addicts, including alcohol abusers, are capable of taking such high doses that their infants can become addicts by way of breast milk; in these cases, too, breastfeeding is contraindicated. Many prescription drugs do not reach nursing infants in sufficient quantities to affect them adversely. Some, however, do. As a precaution, a nursing mother should consult with the prescribing physician prior to ingesting any drug.

A lactating woman is wise to avoid oral contraceptives until after she has weaned her infant, and to use another method of contraception in the meantime. Standard oral contraceptives contain estrogen, which reduces milk volume and the protein content of breast milk.[30]

A woman sometimes hesitates to breastfeed because she has heard that environmental contaminants may enter breast milk and harm her infant. The decision whether to breastfeed on this basis might best be made after consultation with a physician or dietitian familiar with the local circumstances.

Nutrition of the Infant

For a while, the infant drinks only breast milk or formula, but later other foods become appropriate. All who are involved in caring for an infant need to understand the nutrient needs and proper feeding of infants. Early nutrition affects later development, and early feeding sets the stage for eating habits that will influence nutrition status for a lifetime.

Trends change, and experts argue about the fine points, but properly nourishing a baby is relatively simple, overall. Common sense in the selection of infant foods and a nurturing, relaxed environment go far to promote an infant's health and well-being.

Nutrient Needs

An infant grows faster during the first year than ever again, as Figure 11–3 shows. The growth of infants and children directly reflects their nutritional well-being and is an important parameter in assessing their nutrition status. The birthweight doubles around four months of age, and it triples by the age of one year. (Consider that if an adult, starting at 150 pounds, were to do this, the person's weight would increase to 450 pounds in a single year.) By the end of the first year, the growth rate slows considerably, so that between the first and second birthdays, the weight gained amounts to less than 10 pounds.

The rapid growth and metabolism of the infant demands an ample supply of *all* the nutrients. However, the energy nutrients and those vitamins and minerals critical to the growth process, such as vitamin A, vitamin D, calcium, and iron, have special importance during infancy.

Infants, because of their small size, need smaller total amounts of the nutrients than adults do; but as a percentage of body weight, infants need over twice as much as most nutrients. Figure 11–4 compares a three-month-old infant's needs per kilogram of body weight with those of an adult male; as you can see, some of the differences are extraordinary. After six months, energy needs increase less rapidly as the growth rate begins to slow down, but some of the energy saved by slower growth is spent in increased activity.

The most important nutrient of all, for infants as for everyone, is the one easiest to forget: water. The younger the infant, the greater the percentage of body weight is water. Proportionately more of the infant's body water than the adult's is between the cells and in the vascular space, so this water is easy to lose. Conditions that cause fluid loss, such as vomiting, diarrhea, sweating, or obligatory urinary loss without replacement, can rapidly propel an infant into life-threatening dehydration. In early infancy, breast milk or infant formula normally provides enough water for a healthy infant to replace water losses from the skin, lungs, feces, and urine.[31] An infant who is exposed to hot weather, has diarrhea, or vomits repeatedly, however, needs supplemental water to prevent dehydration. Infants cannot tell you what they are crying for; remember that they may need water, and let them drink it until they quench their thirst.

In developed, well-nourished countries, such as the United States and Canada, the dietary practices that influence infants' nutrition status the most center upon which type of milk the infant receives and the age at which solid foods are introduced. The remainder of this discussion is devoted to feeding the infant and identifying the nutrients most often deficient in infant diets.

Infant's metabolism
Heart rate: 120 to 140 beats per minute.
Respiration rate: 20 per minute.

Adult's metabolism
Heart rate: 70 to 80 beats per minute.
Respiration rate: 12 to 14 per minute.

FIGURE 11–3   Weight Gain of Human Infants in Their First Five Years of Life
The colored vertical bars show how the yearly increase in weight gain diminishes over the years.

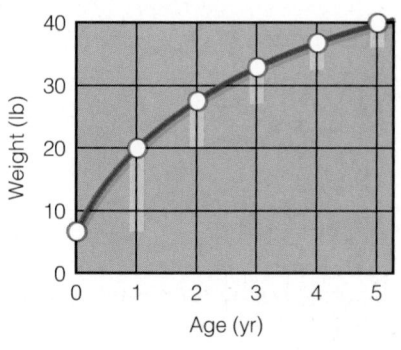

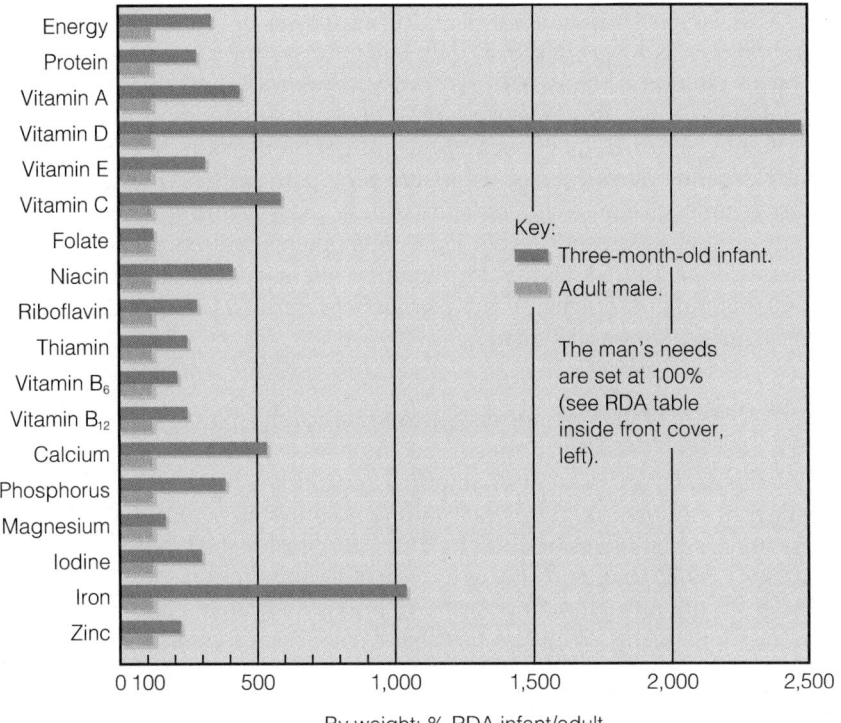

Under most circumstances, a woman can freely choose to feed breast milk or formula, knowing that either mode of feeding suits the infant. However, if the family is poor, or if other factors act to the baby's disadvantage, then breastfeeding becomes the preferred choice.

Breast Milk

With the possible exceptions of vitamin D and fluoride, breast milk provides all the nutrients needed by the healthy infant for the first four to six months of life. But the attributes of breast milk go beyond its nutrient content, as the later section on immunological protection describes.

ENERGY-YIELDING NUTRIENTS. Tailor-made to meet the nutrient needs of the human infant, breast milk offers its carbohydrate as lactose and its fat as a mixture with a generous proportion of the essential fatty acid linoleic acid. The unique composition of the fat in breast milk, in combination with the fat-digesting enzymes present, contributes to highly efficient fat absorption by the breastfed infant. The protein in breast milk is largely alpha-lactalbumin, a protein the human infant can easily digest.

VITAMINS. The vitamin content of breast milk is ample. Even vitamin C, for which cow's milk is a poor source, is supplied generously by breast milk

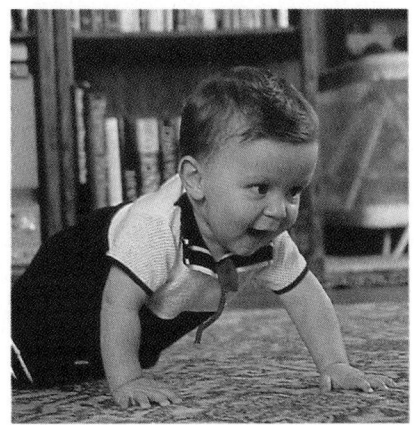

At six months, the energy saved by slower growth is spent on increased activity.

alpha-lactalbumin (lact-AL-byoo-min): the chief protein in human breast milk, as opposed to **casein** (CAY-seen), the chief protein in cow's milk.

from a well-nourished mother. The concentration of vitamin D in breast milk, however, is low. Vitamin D deficiency causes impaired bone mineralization in children. Manufacturers fortify cow's milk and infant formulas with vitamin D, but the concentration in breast milk falls short of adequacy. The vitamin is formed by the action of sunlight on the skin, but the amount formed depends on skin color, exposure time, atmospheric pollution, time of year (summer versus winter), and latitude (how far from the sun). Lack of daily sunlight exposure; prolonged, unsupplemented breastfeeding; and pigmented skin are risk factors for vitamin D deficiency in infants. For this reason, vitamin D supplements are routinely prescribed for breastfed infants in the United States and Canada.

MINERALS. As for minerals, the 2-to-1 calcium-to-phosphorus ratio of breast milk is ideal for the absorption of calcium; both of these minerals, along with magnesium, are present in amounts appropriate for the rate of growth expected in a human infant. Breast milk is also low in sodium. The iron in breast milk is highly absorbable. Its zinc, too, is absorbed better than zinc from cow's milk, thanks to the presence of a zinc-binding protein.[32] Normally, given the nutrient composition of breast milk, infants do not require nutrient supplements, with the possible exceptions of vitamin D and fluoride. After age four to six months, depending on food intake, infants may also require iron supplements, as Table 11–6 shows.

TABLE 11–6   **Supplements for Full-Term Infants**

	VITAMIN D[a]	IRON[b]	FLUORIDE[c]
Breastfed infants:			
Birth to six months of age	✓		✓
Six months to one year	✓	✓	✓
Formula-fed infants:			
Birth to six months of age			✓
Six months to one year		✓	✓

[a]Vitamin D supplements are recommended for breastfed infants for as long as breast milk is the major milk the infant consumes. Once infant formula or vitamin D–fortified cow's milk replaces breast milk in the infant's diet, vitamin D supplements are no longer needed.
[b]Iron-fortified infant cereal is a reliable source of iron for both breastfed and formula-fed infants during the second half of the first year. The Committee on Nutrition of the American Academy of Pediatrics recommends the use of iron-fortified infant formula for formula-fed infants. Most pediatricians recommend the use of iron-fortified formula from birth for formula-fed infants, although some infants are fed noniron-fortified formula for the first few months.
[c]The use of fluoride supplements for infants less than six months of age is controversial. The Committee on Nutrition of the American Academy of Pediatrics recommends initiating fluoride supplements for breastfed infants, formula-fed infants who receive ready-to-use formulas (these are prepared with water low in fluoride), or those who receive formula mixed with water that contains little or no fluoride (less than 0.3 ppm) shortly after birth. The committee acknowledges that fluoride supplementation could be initiated at six months of age, however.

Source: Adapted from American Academy of Pediatrics, Committee on Nutrition, Vitamin and mineral supplement needs of normal children in the United States, in *Pediatric Nutrition Handbook,* 2d ed., eds. G. B. Forbes and C. W. Woodruff (Elk Grove Village, Ill.: American Academy of Pediatrics, 1985), pp. 37–48.

IMMUNOLOGICAL PROTECTION. Breast milk offers the infant unsurpassed protection against infection. This barrier of protection includes antiviral agents, antibacterial agents, and other infection inhibitors.

During the first two or three days of lactation, the breasts produce colostrum, a premilk substance containing antibodies and white cells from the mother's blood. Colostrum is relatively sterile as it leaves the breast, and the baby cannot contract a bacterial infection from it even if the mother has one. Because it contains maternal immune factors, colostrum helps protect the newborn infant from those infections against which the mother has developed immunity. These diseases are the ones in her environment, and precisely those against which the infant needs protection. Entering the infant's body with the milk, maternal antibodies inactivate harmful bacteria within the digestive tract, where they would otherwise cause harm. Later, breast milk also delivers antibodies, although not as many as colostrum.

Other powerful agents against bacterial infection also are found in colostrum and breast milk. Certain factors known as bifidus factors favor the growth of the "friendly" bacteria *Lactobacillus bifidus* in the infant's digestive tract, so that other, harmful bacteria cannot grow there.

Another protein component of breast milk, lactoferrin, indirectly benefits the baby's iron nutrition and, at the same time, acts as an antibacterial agent. Lactoferrin is an iron-grabbing compound that keeps intestinal bacteria from getting the iron they need to grow on, helps absorb iron into the infant's bloodstream, and also works directly to kill some bacteria.[33]

Other factors in breast milk include several enzymes, several hormones (including thyroid hormone and prostaglandins), and lipids, all of which protect the infant against infection. Research suggests that breastfeeding offers better protection against wheezing during the first few months of life than formula feeding does.[34] It seems, too, that breastfed babies are less prone to develop stomach and intestinal disorders during the first few months of life, and so experience less vomiting and diarrhea than formula-fed infants do.[35] Much remains to be learned about the composition and characteristics of human milk, but clearly it is a very special substance. Nutrition in Practice 11 offers suggestions for successful breastfeeding.

colostrum (co-LAHS-strum): a milklike secretion from the breast, rich in protective factors, present during the first day or so after delivery, before milk appears.

bifidus (BIFF-id-us, by-FEED-us) **factors:** factors in colostrum and breast milk that favor the growth, in the infant's intestinal tract, of the "friendly" bacteria *Lactobacillus* (lack-toh-ba-SILL-us) *bifidus*, so that other, less desirable intestinal inhabitants will not flourish.

lactoferrin (lak-toe-FERR-in): a factor in breast milk that binds iron and keeps it from supporting the growth of the infant's intestinal bacteria.

Infant Formula

Because breastfeeding has so many advantages for both mother and infant, it should be encouraged whenever possible. However, the mother who has decided to feed her infant formula should be supported in her choice just as the breastfeeding mother should be. The mother who offers formula to her baby has valid reasons for making her choice, and she and her baby can benefit in many ways from the supportive approval of those around them.

Formulas can be prepared from cow's milk in such a way that they do not differ significantly from human milk in nutrient content. Although formulas do not contain protective antibodies for human babies, the high level of preventive medical care (vaccinations) and public health measures achieved in the developed countries make these considerations less important than they were in the past. Safety and sanitation can be achieved with either mode of feeding by the educated mother whose water supply is reliable.

The mother who feeds formula can offer the same closeness, warmth, and stimulation during feedings as the breastfeeding mother can. Furthermore, other family members can help with feedings and thus develop a warm relationship with the baby and allow the new mother additional time to rest. Formula feeding may enable a mother to contribute to the family's income by returning to work sooner.

Another advantage of formula feeding is that gained by the mother whose attempts at breastfeeding have met with frustration. If the mother truly doesn't want to breastfeed, or worse, if she earnestly does want to but can't, continuing to try is an agonizing course, as hard on the baby as on the mother. When the mother finally accepts the necessity of formula feeding and weans the baby to the bottle, a period of anguish for both may be followed by the onset of peace and the first real opportunity to develop the important mother-child love.

The attendant who is asked to advise a mother on breastfeeding versus formula-feeding should remember the advantages of both. In fact, when addressing any audience, you should remember that some members will be women who formula-fed their babies. To praise breastfeeding out of proportion or without qualification can only make these women feel guilty or angry.

Many mothers choose to breastfeed at first but wean their children within the first one to six months. Prior to six months of age, mothers must wean their infants onto *infant formula,* not onto plain milk of any kind—whole, low fat, or nonfat.

The American Academy of Pediatrics (AAP) recommends the use of iron-fortified formula for all formula-fed infants.[36] The AAP concludes that low-iron infant formulas have no role in infant feeding. The increasing use of iron-fortified formulas during the past few decades is credited as being the major factor in the declining prevalence of iron-deficiency anemia among infants in the United States.[37] Only iron-fortified formula, not plain milk, contains enough iron (to name but one of many factors) to support normal development in the infant's first months of life.

How to Feed Formula

National and international standards have been set for the nutrient contents of infant formulas. The Infant Formula Act of 1980 requires that formulas meet nutrient standards based on the American Academy of Pediatrics recommendations, and in 1982 the FDA adopted quality control procedures to ensure that formulas do. Formulas that meet the standards are nutritionally similar; small differences in nutrient content are sometimes confusing but not usually important.

Standard formulas are inappropriate for some infants (see Figure 11–5). For example, premature babies require special formulas. Special formulas based on soy protein are available for infants allergic to milk protein, and formulas with lactose replaced can be used for infants with lactose intolerance. For infants with other special needs, many other variations have been formulated.

The mother should be trained in formula preparation by an experienced person and should be observed and guided at least once as she goes through

Formula preparation:
  Liquid concentrate (moderately expensive, relatively easy)—mix with equal part water.
  Powdered formula (least expensive, lightest for travel)—read label directions.
  Ready-to-feed (easiest, most expensive)—pour directly into clean bottles.

FIGURE 11–5   **Choosing a Formula**

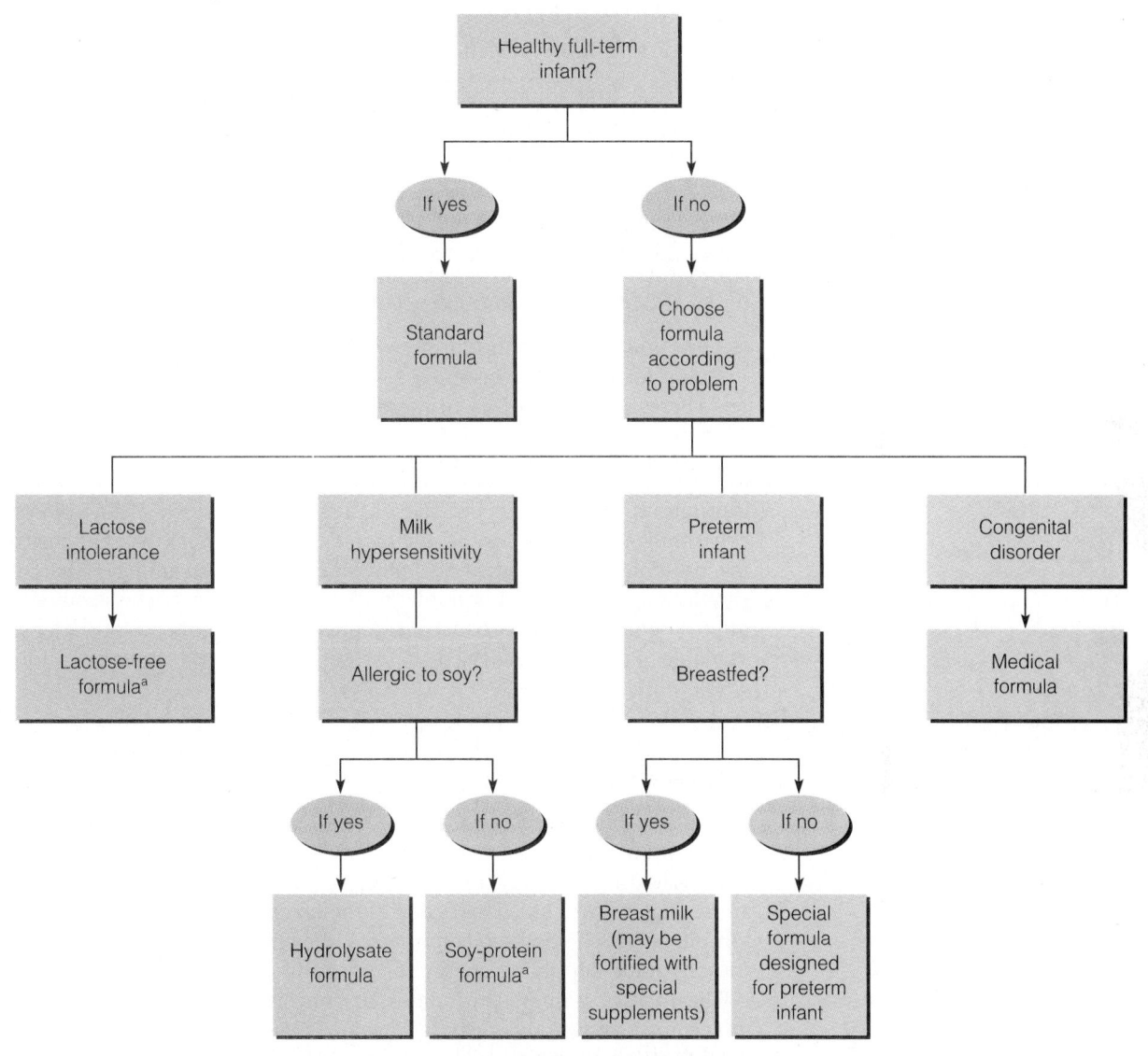

[a]Manufacturers design soy-based formulas for infants with milk sensitivities—whether lactose intolerance or milk allergy. These formulas use corn syrup or sucrose in place of lactose.

the steps herself. These safeguards are more important if the mother is inexperienced or not well educated, or if the baby is not strong and healthy. In poor areas, especially where a sanitary water supply is not dependable, these rules and training are crucial.

In an infant's first six months, the choice of formula is important, because whatever is chosen must supply the nutrients of human milk in similar forms and proportions. After the first year, the exact formulation of the milk selected is less critical, but the choice remains important—milk or its substitute occupies a place in the diet that no other type of food can fill.

Introducing Cow's Milk

During the first four to six months of life, when breast milk or infant formula is the baby's major food, ordinary milk is an inappropriate replacement—primarily because cow's milk provides insufficient vitamin C and iron. The AAP states that breast milk and formula continue to be optimal for the milk portion of infant diets during the second six months of life.[38] The AAP does acknowledge, however, that cow's milk could be substituted for breast milk or formula during the second six months of life under the following conditions:

- The energy contribution of cow's milk does not exceed 65 percent of total food energy consumed.
- The solid food portion of the diet replaces the iron and vitamins deficient in cow's milk.

Many pediatricians advise continued use of breast milk or infant formula throughout the first year because of the iron it provides. (Don't offer plain cow's milk before six months; the infant's digestive tract may be sensitive to the protein content and, if so, may bleed.) Children under a year of age should not drink low-fat or nonfat milk routinely; they need the fat of whole milk. Powdered milk is usually skimmed, but fat-containing varieties are available. Parents are advised to use vitamin A– and vitamin D–fortified whole milk.

Introducing First Foods

Changes in body organs during the first year affect the baby's readiness to accept solid foods. The immature stomach and intestines can digest milk sugar (lactose), but they don't develop the ability to digest starch until they are several months old. This is one of the many reasons why breast milk and formula are such good foods for babies; they provide simple, easily digested carbohydrate, supplying energy for the baby's growth and activity.

The infant's kidneys are unable to concentrate waste efficiently, so an infant must excrete relatively more water than an adult to carry off a comparable amount of waste. This means that the risk of dehydration is even greater once solid foods are introduced. Because infants can communicate their needs only by crying, it is important to remember that they may be crying for fluid. All infants require supplemental water once they receive solid foods in the diet. Foods with a high protein or electrolyte content, such as meat and eggs, in the absence of adequate water, can promote water loss to the point of dehydration. Water also provides fluid without additional food energy. Many adults would no doubt be healthier had they learned early to quench their thirst with water.

The timing for adding solid foods (beikost) to an infant's diet depends on several factors. As long as the infant receives formula or breast milk from a healthy, well-nourished mother, additions to the diet are not needed until the infant is four to six months old. Foods may be started gradually begin-

beikost (BYE-cost): a term used by many authorities to mean supplemental or weaning foods.

ning sometime between four and six months, depending on readiness. Indications of readiness include any one of the following:

- When the infant has doubled the birth weight.
- When the infant can consume 8 ounces of formula and still is hungry in less than four hours.
- When the infant can sit up.
- When the infant is consuming 32 ounces of formula a day and wanting more.
- When the infant is six months old.

Solids should not be introduced too early, because infants are most likely to develop allergies to them in the early months. But infants differ, and the program of additions depends on the individual baby's developmental readiness, not on any rigid schedule. Table 11–7 presents a suggested sequence for introducing new foods.

The addition of foods to an infant's diet should be governed by three considerations: the infant's nutrient needs, the infant's physical readiness to handle different forms of foods, and the need to detect and control allergic reactions. With respect to nutrient needs, the nutrient needed earliest is iron, then vitamin C.

Iron deficiency is a common nutrition problem, especially in young children, throughout the world. Iron deficiency is most prevalent in children between the ages of six months and three years due to their rapid growth rate and the significant place that milk, which is a poor source of iron, has in their diets. An infant's stored iron supply from before birth runs out after

TABLE 11–7 **First Foods for the Infant**

AGE (MONTHS)	ADDITION
4 to 6	Iron-fortified rice cereal, followed by other cereals (for iron; baby can swallow and can digest starch now)[a]
5 to 7	Strained vegetables and/or fruits and their juices,[b] one by one (perhaps vegetables before fruits, so the baby will learn to like their less sweet flavors)
6 to 8	Protein foods (cheese, yogurt, tofu, cooked beans, meat, fish, chicken, egg yolk)
9	Finely chopped meat (baby can chew now), toast, teething crackers (for emerging teeth)
10 to 12	Whole egg (allergies are less likely now), whole milk

[a]Later you can change cereals, but don't forget to keep on using the iron-fortified varieties. According to *Nutrition and the M.D.*, April 1981, the iron in cereal specially prepared for babies is so bioavailable that three level tablespoons a day is all they need.

[b]All baby juices are fortified with vitamin C. Orange juice causes allergies in some babies; apple juice is often recommended as the first juice to feed. Juices should be offered in a cup, not a bottle, to prevent nursing bottle syndrome.

Source: Adapted from *Recommendations for Infant Feeding Practices of the California Department of Health Services*, 1979, as presented in Current infant feeding practices, *Nutrition and the M.D.*, January 1980.

the birthweight doubles. One study showed that infants who were started on whole milk at six months of age had 33 percent lower serum ferritin concentrations than those who continued to drink iron-fortified formula until one year of age.[39] Iron ranks highest on the list of nutrients most needing attention in infant nutrition. Formula with iron, iron-fortified cereals, and later, meat or meat alternates such as legumes, are recommended to deliver iron to infants.

Vitamin C's best vehicles are fruits and vegetables. Some authorities suggest that the early introduction of sweet fruits to infants' diets might favor the development of a preference for sweets and lessen the liking for vegetables introduced later. To prevent this, the order can be reversed: vegetables first, fruits later. This practice now has a wide following. As for sweets of any other kind (including baby food "desserts"), they have no place in a baby's life. The added food energy they contribute can promote obesity, and they convey no nutrients to support growth.

Physical readiness to handle food develops in many small steps. For example, the ability to swallow solid food develops at around four to six months, and experience with the spoon and solid food at that time helps to develop swallowing ability by desensitizing the gag reflex. Later still, a baby can sit up, can handle finger foods, and begins to teethe. At that time, hard crackers and other hard finger foods may be introduced to promote the development of manual dexterity and control of the jaw muscles. These feedings must occur under the watchful eye of an adult, because the infant can also choke on such foods.

Some parents want to feed solids at an earlier age, on the theory that "stuffing the baby" at bedtime promotes sleeping through the night. There is no proof for this theory. On the average, babies start to sleep through the night at about the same age (three to four months) regardless of when solid foods are introduced.

New foods should be introduced singly and slowly, so that allergies can be detected. For example, when cereals are introduced, rice cereal is offered first for several days; it causes allergy least often. Wheat cereal is offered last; it is the most common offender. If a cereal causes an allergic reaction (irritability due to skin rash, digestive upset, or respiratory discomfort), its use should be discontinued before going on to the next food.

As for the choice of foods, baby foods commercially prepared in the United States and Canada are generally safe, nutritious, and of high quality. In response to consumer demand, baby food companies have removed all of the added salt and much of the sugar their products contained in the past, and baby foods also contain few or no additives. They generally have high nutrient density, except for mixed dinners and heavily sweetened desserts. An alternative for the parent who wants the baby to have family foods it to "blenderize" a small portion of the table food at each meal. This necessitates cooking without salt, though. Foods adults prepare for themselves often contain much more salt than commercial baby foods. Besides, when a person prepares a food without salting, deep-frying, or heavily seasoning, the flavor of the food itself comes through.

Some foods are best omitted from a baby's diet. Canned vegetables are inappropriate for infants; not only do they contain too much sodium, but those products packaged in lead-soldered cans present the risk of lead contamination. Honey should never be fed to infants because of the risk of botulism. Babies and even young children have difficulty swallowing foods such as popcorn, whole grapes, whole beans, hot dog slices, and nuts, and they can easily choke on these foods. It's not worth the risk. Also, an infant's caretaker must be on guard against food poisoning and take the precautions against it as described in Nutrition in Practice 14.

At a year of age, milk remains the obvious food to supply most of the nutrients the infant needs; 2 to 3½ cups a day meets those needs sufficiently. More milk than this displaces foods necessary to provide iron and can cause the iron-deficiency anemia known as milk anemia. Other foods—meat, iron-fortified cereal, enriched or whole-grain bread, fruits, and vegetables—should be supplied in variety and in amounts sufficient to round out total energy needs. Ideally, a one-year-old will sit at the table, eat many of the same foods everyone else eats, and drink liquids from a cup—not a bottle. Table 11–8 shows a meal plan that meets the requirements for the one-year-old.

milk anemia: iron-deficiency anemia caused by drinking so much milk that iron-rich foods are displaced from the diet.

Looking Ahead

The first year of life lays the foundation for future health. From the nutrition standpoint, the relevant problems most common in later years are obesity and dental disease. Prevention of obesity can also help prevent the development of the obesity-related diseases—atherosclerosis, diabetes, and cancer.

Infant obesity should be avoided. Probably the most important single measure to undertake during the first year is to encourage eating habits that will support continued normal weight as the child grows. Primarily, this means introducing a variety of nutritious foods in an inviting way; not forcing the baby to finish the bottle or the baby food jar; avoiding concentrated sweets and empty-kcalorie foods; and encouraging physical activity.

To discourage development of the behaviors and attitudes that plague obese people, parents should avoid teaching infants to seek food as a reward,

TABLE 11–8   **Meal Plan for a One-Year-Old**

BREAKFAST	SNACK
1 c milk 3 tbsp cereal 2 to 3 tbsp fruit Teething crackers	½ c milk Teething crackers 1 tbsp peanut butter
LUNCH	SUPPER
1 c milk 2 to 3 tbsp vegetables 2 tbsp chopped meat or well-cooked, mashed legumes	1 c milk 1 egg 2 tbsp cereal or potato 2 to 3 tbsp vegetables 2 to 3 tbsp fruit

to expect food as comfort for unhappiness, or to associate food deprivation with punishment. If infants cry for thirst, give them water, not milk or juice. Infants seem to have no internal "kcalorie counter," and they stop eating when their stomachs feel full. Nutrient-dense, low-kcalorie foods will satisfy as long as they provide bulk.

A "prudent diet," like that recommended for heart clients (restrict fat, increase the ratio of polyunsaturated to saturated fat, and reduce cholesterol intake), is inappropriate for infants. The AAP recommends against a fat-modified diet during infancy, stating that the evidence so far is insufficient and does not warrant dietary manipulation to lower serum cholesterol.

Normal dental development is promoted by the same strategies outlined above: supplying nutritious foods, avoiding sweets, and discouraging the association of food with reward or comfort. Dental health is the subject of Nutrition in Practice 2.

Mealtimes

The wise parent of a one-year-old offers nutrition and love together. Both promote growth. "Feeding with love" produces better growth in both weight and height of children than feeding the same foods in an emotionally negative climate.[40]

The person feeding a one-year-old has to be aware that this is a period in the child's life when exploring and experimenting are normal and desirable behaviors. The child is developing a sense of autonomy that, if allowed to flower, will provide the foundation for later confidence and effectiveness as an individual. The child's impulses, if consistently denied, can turn to shame and self-doubt. In light of the developmental and nutrient needs of one-year-olds, and in the face of their often contrary and willful behavior, a few feeding guidelines may be helpful:

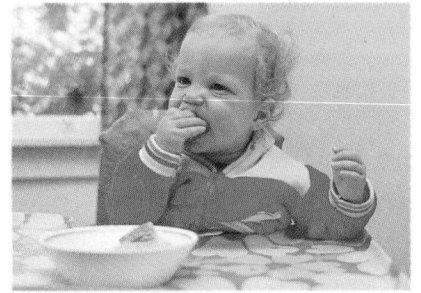

By the end of the first year, a baby can sit up and enjoy finger foods.

■ *Firmly discourage unacceptable behavior (such as standing at the table or throwing food) by removing the child from the table to wait until later to eat.* Be consistent and firm, not punitive. The child will soon learn to sit and eat.

■ *Let the child explore and enjoy food.* This may mean the child eats with fingers for a while. Use of the spoon will come in time.

■ *Don't force food on children.* Provide children with nutritious foods, and let them choose which ones and how much they will eat. Gradually they will acquire a taste for different foods. If children refuse milk, provide it in the form of cheese, cream soups, and yogurt.

■ *Limit sweets strictly.* Infants have no room in their 1,000-kcalorie allowance each day for empty-kcalorie sweets, except occasionally.

These recommendations reflect a spirit of tolerance that serves the best interest of the child emotionally as well as physically. The next chapter continues with the special nutrient needs of children and teenagers.

CASE STUDY

Overweight Pregnant Woman

Ellen is a 24-year-old housewife who is four months pregnant. It is her first pregnancy, and she is eager to know how to feed herself during pregnancy as well as her infant after birth. She is 5 feet 3 inches tall and currently weighs 150 pounds. Her prepregnancy weight was 148 pounds. Ellen is very concerned about her 2-pound weight gain.

1. Assess Ellen's weight. What would her ideal weight be if she were not pregnant? Should she be concerned about her 2-pound weight gain? Why? What advice should you give Ellen about her weight gain during pregnancy? What other dietary advice would you give her?
2. Discuss methods of infant feeding with Ellen. What advantages would breastfeeding offer her? What are the advantages of formula feeding? What advice will you give Ellen if she decides to breastfeed? What information should she have about formula-feeding?

Study Questions

1. What is the significance of infant birthweight in terms of the child's future health?
2. Describe the placenta and its function.
3. Which nutrients are needed in the greatest amounts during pregnancy? Why are they so important?
4. What is the recommended pattern of weight gain during pregnancy?
5. What practices should be avoided during pregnancy?
6. How do nutrient needs during lactation differ from nutrient needs during pregnancy?
7. Describe some of the nutrient and immunological attributes of breastmilk.
8. What are the advantages of formula-feeding?
9. What three considerations govern the addition of solid foods to an infant's diet?
10. Name some foods that are inappropriate for infants, and tell why they are inappropriate.

Notes

1. M. C. Mitchell and E. Lerner, Weight gain and pregnancy outcome in underweight and normal weight women, *Journal of the American Dietetic Association* 89 (1989): 634–638, 641.

2. National Academy of Sciences, Food and Nutrition Board, *Nutrition during Pregnancy* (Washington, D.C.: National Academy Press, 1990), pp. 176–211.

3. H. S. Wright and coauthors, The 1987–1988 Nationwide Food Consumption Survey: An update on the nutrient intake of respondents, *Nutrition Today,* May/June 1991, pp. 21–27.

4. National Academy of Sciences, Food and Nutrition Board, 1990, pp. 1–23.

5. National Academy of Sciences, Food and Nutrition Board, 1990 pp. 1–23.

6. National Academy of Sciences, Food and Nutrition Board, 1990 pp. 1–23.

7. J. E. Brown and M. Story, "Let them eat cake" or a prescription for improving the outcome of pregnancy? *Nutrition Today,* November/December 1990, pp. 18–23.

8. National Academy of Sciences, Food and Nutrition Board, 1990 1–23.

9. Y. H. Neggers and coauthors, A positive association between maternal serum zinc concentration and birth weight, *American Journal of Clinical Nutrition* 51 (1990): 678–684.

10. B. Worthington-Roberts and coauthors, Dietary cravings and aversions in the postpartum period, *Journal of the American Dietetic Association* 89 (1989): 647–651.

11. National Academy of Sciences, Food and Nutrition Board, 1990.

12. National Academy of Sciences, Food and Nutrition Board, 1990, pp. 176–211.

13. D. Hall and D. Kaufmann, Effects of aerobic and strength conditioning on pregnancy outcomes, *American Journal of Obstetrics and Gynecology* 157 (1987): 199–203.

14. National Academy of Sciences, Food and Nutrition Board, 1990, pp. 390–411.

15. M. J. Stjernfeldt and coauthors, Maternal smoking during pregnancy and risk of childhood cancer, *Lancet,* 14 June 1986, pp. 1350–1351; B. Haglund and S. Cnattingus, Cigarette smoking as a risk factor for sudden infant death syndrome, *American Journal of Public Health* 80 (1990): 29–32; J. Coste, N. Job-Spira, and H. Fernandez, Increased risk of ectopic pregnancy with maternal cigarette smoking, *American Journal of Public Health* 81 (1991): 199–200.

16. National Academy of Sciences, Food and Nutrition Board, 1990.

17. National Academy of Sciences, Food and Nutrition Board, 1990.

18. B. Zuckerman and coauthors, Effects of maternal marijuana and cocaine use on fetal growth, *New England Journal of Medicine* 320 (1989): 762–768.

19. S. Fisher and P. Karl, Maternal ethanol use and selective fetal malnutrition, *Alcoholism* (New York: Plenum Press, 1988), pp. 277–289.

20. K. R. Warren and R. J. Bast, Alcohol-related birth defects: An update, *Public Health Reports* 103 (1988): 638–642.

21. National Academy of Sciences, Food and Nutrition Board, Committee on Nutrition, *Recommended Dietary Allowances,* 10th ed. (Washington, D.C.: National Academy Press, 1989), pp. 24–38.

22. J. M. A. van Raaij and coauthors, Energy cost of lactation, and energy balances of well-nourished Dutch lactating women: Reappraisal of the extra energy requirements of lactation, *American Journal of Clinical Nutrition* 53 (1991): 612–619; A. Sadurskis and coauthors, Energy metabolism, body composition, and milk production in healthy Swedish women during lactation, *American Journal of Clinical Nutrition* 48 (1988): 44–49.

23. M. Brewer, M. R. Bates, and L. P. Vannoy, Postpartum changes in maternal weight and body fat depots in lactating vs nonlactating women, *American Journal of Clinical Nutrition* 49 (1989): 259–265.

24. Maternal nutrition during lactation, *Nutrition and the M.D.,* February 1987; L. B. Dusdieker and coauthors, Prolonged maternal fluid supplementation in breast-feeding, *Pediatrics* 86 (1990): 737–740.
25. Nutrition during lactation, *Nutrition Today,* May/June 1991, pp. 28–31.
26. Maternal nutrition during lactation, 1987.
27. J. A. Mennella and G. K. Beauchamp, The transfer of alcohol to human milk: Effects on flavor and the infant's behavior, *New England Journal of Medicine* 325 (1991): 981–985.
28. Nutrition during lactation, 1991, pp. 28–31.
29. B. Lonnerdal and M. F. Picciano, Mechanisms regulating lactation and infant nutrient utilization, *Nutrition Today,* May/June 1991, pp. 32–35.
30. American Academy of Pediatrics, Committee on Drugs, The transfer of drugs and other chemicals into human breast milk, *Pediatrics* 72 (1983): 375–381.
31. American Academy of Pediatrics, Committee on Nutrition, *Pediatric Nutrition Handbook,* 2d ed., eds. G. B. Forbes and C. W. Woodruff (Elk Grove Village, Ill.: American Academy of Pediatrics, 1985), p. 31.
32. C. Eckhert, Isolation of a protein from human milk that enhances zinc absorption in humans, *Biochemical and Biophysical Research Communications* 130 (1985): 264–269.
33. P. F. Hennart and coauthors, Lysozyme, lactoferrin, and secretory immunoglobulin A content in breast milk: Influence of duration of lactation, nutrition status, prolactin status, and parity of mother, *American Journal of Clinical Nutrition* 53 (1991): 32–39.
34. When deciding between feeding by breast or by bottle, *Tufts University Diet and Nutrition Letter,* December 1990, pp. 3–4.
35. When deciding between feeding by breast or by bottle, 1990, pp. 3–4.
36. American Academy of Pediatrics, Committee on Nutrition, Iron-fortified infant formulas, *Pediatrics* 84 (1989): 1114.
37. American Academy of Pediatrics, Committee on Nutrition, 1989.
38. American Academy of Pediatrics, Committee on Nutrition, Follow-up or weaning formulas, *Pediatrics* 83 (1989): 1067.
39. Ross Laboratories, Perspectives on nutrition in later infancy, *Public Health Currents* 28 (1988): 17–20.
40. E. M. Widdowson, Mental contentment and physical growth, *Lancet* 1 (1951): 1316–1318.

11

Encouraging Successful Breastfeeding

Breastfeeding offers benefits to both mother and infant. The American Academy of Pediatrics; the American Dietetic Association; the Special Food Supplemental Program for Women, Infants, and Children (WIC); and the U.S. Department of Health and Human Services advocate breastfeeding as the preferred means of infant feeding for the first six months of life.[1]

However, breastfeeding has been on the decline since the early 1980s, when it reached a high of about 60 percent.[2] Why has breastfeeding been declining? Many experts cite two major deterrents: public advertising of infant formula, and the medical community's failure to encourage breastfeeding. As an example of the medical lack of encouragement, in some hospitals, it is routine to separate mother and child soon after birth. The child's first feeding then comes from the bottle rather than the breast. Furthermore, many hospitals send new mothers home with free samples of infant formula. The World Health Organization opposes this practice because it sends a misleading message that medical authorities favor infant formula over breast milk for infants.

Even in hospitals where women are encouraged to breastfeed and are supported in doing so, little, if any, assistance is available after hospital discharge, and many breastfeeding women still need assistance. Of mothers who initially breastfeed their infants, up to half discontinue breastfeeding within a month—seemingly due to lack of knowledge.[3] Research shows that when women receive early and repeated breastfeeding information and support, they breastfeed their infants longer than other women do.[4] Health professionals can play a vital role in encouraging successful breastfeeding. That is why this Nutrition in Practice is devoted to ways to facilitate successful breastfeeding.

Should all women be encouraged to breastfeed?

No, not necessarily. Chapter 11 discussed some instances where breastfeeding is contraindicated, such as when a woman is addicted to drugs. Some women may simply not wish to breastfeed for their own personal reasons. Such women should not be pressured—the development of a relaxed, loving relationship between mother and child is as important to the child's well-being as optimal nourishment is. Women who do want to breastfeed their infants and those who are indecisive should be offered accurate information and instruction about breastfeeding.

I thought that breastfeeding was a natural process that didn't require any learning.

Although *lactation* is an automatic physiological process, *breastfeeding* requires some learning. This learning is most successful in a supportive environment. It begins with preparatory steps taken before the baby is born.

OK. What are the preparatory steps?

Toward the end of pregnancy and throughout lactation, a woman who intends to breastfeed should stop using soap and lotions on her breasts. The natural secretions of the breasts themselves lubricate the nipple area best. A few weeks before the baby is due, the woman should allow her breasts to rub against her outer clothing for a little while each day, to toughen them somewhat in preparation for the baby's sucking. Also, she should go without clothing at times, at home, to expose her breasts to air and light.

She can also condition her nipples for breastfeeding by doing a simple exercise called nipple rolling. This involves taking the nipple between her thumb and forefinger, pulling the nipple out slightly, and rolling it between the fingers several times.

A woman who plans to breastfeed should acquire at least two nursing bras before her baby is born. The bras should provide good support and have drop-flaps so that either breast can be freed for nursing.

How soon after birth should she start to breastfeed?

As soon as possible. Immediately after the delivery, for a short period, the baby is intensely alert and intent on suckling. This is the ideal time for the first breastfeeding and facilitates successful lactation.[5]

What does the new mother need to know in order to breastfeed her infant successfully?

She needs to learn how to relax and position herself so that she and the infant will be comfortable, and so that the infant can breathe freely while nursing. She also needs to understand that the infant has a rooting reflex that makes the infant turn toward any touch on the face. The mother shouldn't try to push the infant's face toward her nipple, because this tends to make the infant turn toward her hand instead, frustrating both her and the infant. Instead, she should touch the infant's cheek to her nipple so that the infant will automatically turn and start to nurse. The mother can then squeeze her areola, the colored ring around the nipple, between two fingers and slip enough of it into the infant's mouth so as to permit a good hold and strong pumping action (see Figure NP11–1). The nipple must rest well back on the infant's tongue, so that the infant's gums will squeeze on the glands that release the milk. Also, with the nipple far back in the mouth, as the infant's tongue and jaw suck milk from the breast, the swallow easily follows. To break the suction, if

necessary, the mother can slip a finger between the infant's mouth and her breast.

Doesn't it hurt to have the infant sucking so hard on the breast?

No, because the mother has a let-down reflex that forces milk to the front of her breast when the infant begins to nurse, virtually propelling the milk into the infant's mouth. Let-down has to occur for the infant to obtain milk easily, and the mother needs to relax for let-down to occur. The mother who assumes a comfortable position in a noninterrupting environment will find it easiest to relax.

How long should the baby be allowed to nurse at each feeding?

Although the infant sucks half the milk from the breast within the first 2 minutes, and 80 to 90 percent of it within 4 minutes, sucking on each breast for 10 to 15 minutes is encouraged. The sucking itself, as well as the complete removal of milk from the breast, stimulates the milk-producing glands to produce milk for the next nursing session. Sessions should start on alternate breasts to ensure that each breast is emptied regularly. This pattern maintains the same supply and demand for each breast, and thus prevents either breast from overfilling.

Infants should be fed "on demand" and not held to a rigid schedule. The breastfed baby may average 8 to 12

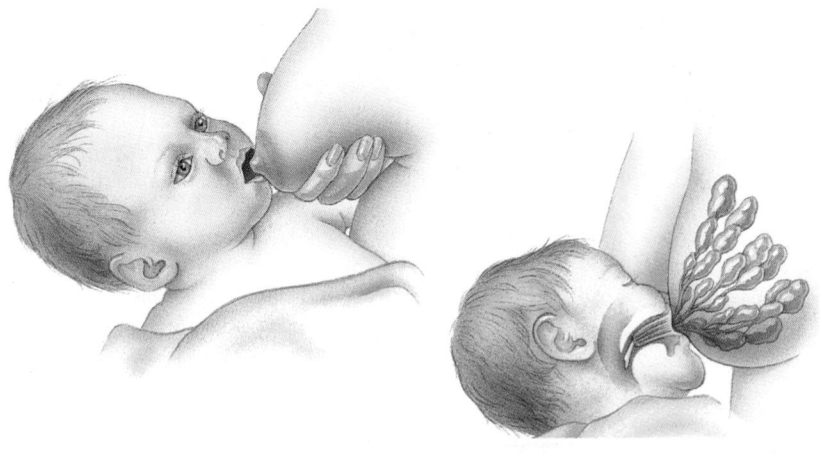

FIGURE NP11–1 **Infant's Grasp on Mother's Breast**
The mother squeezes the areola, slipping enough of it into the infant's mouth to promote good pumping action. The infant's lips and gums pump the areola, releasing milk from the mammary glands into the milk ducts that lie beneath the areola.

feedings per 24-hour period during the first month or so. Once the mother's milk supply is well established and the infant's capacity has increased, the intervals between feedings will become longer.

What if a mother wants to skip one or two feedings daily—for example, because she works outside the home?

A mother can substitute formula for those feedings and continue to breastfeed at other feedings. Or the mother can express breast milk into a bottle ahead of time, freeze the breast milk, and when needed, substitute the expressed breast milk for a nursing session. Breast milk can be kept refrigerated for 24 hours or frozen (at a freezer temperature below 0 degrees Fahrenheit) for several months.

The mother can hand express her breast milk, as shown in Figure NP11–2, or use one of several different breast pumps available. One type of manual breast pump is not recommended, however: the bicycle horn type. These pumps are difficult to keep clean; cylinder-type manual pumps or electric breast pumps are preferred and are more efficient.

What about problems associated with breastfeeding, such as sore nipples or infection of the breast?

Most problems associated with breastfeeding can be resolved. Many mothers experience sore nipples during the initial days of breastfeeding. Sore nipples need to be treated kindly, but nursing can continue. Improper feeding position is a frequent cause of sore nipples: the mother should make sure the infant is taking the entire nipple and part of the areola onto the tongue. She should nurse on the less sore breast first, to get let-down going while the infant is sucking hardest; then she can switch to the sore breast. Between times, she should expose her nipples to light and air to heal them.

Before lactation is well established, when the schedule changes, or when a feeding is missed, the breasts may become full and hard—an uncomfortable condition known as engorgement. The infant cannot grasp an engorged nipple and so cannot provide relief by nursing. A gentle massage or warming the breasts with a heating pad or in the shower helps to initiate let-down and to release some of the accumulated milk; then the mother can pump out some of her milk and allow the infant to nurse.

Infection of the breast, known as mastitis, is best managed by *continuing*

FIGURE NP11–2   **Milk Expression by Hand**

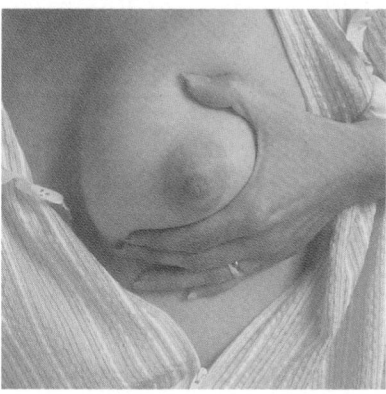

1. The hand is placed on the breast near the chest wall, with the thumb on top and the fingers cupped around and under the breast. The hands gently move toward the nipple.

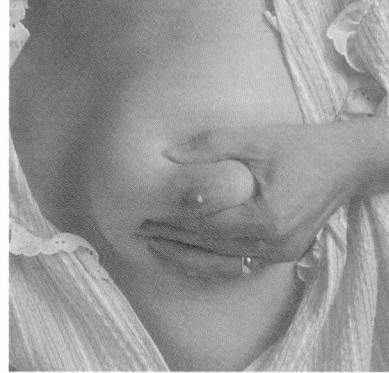

2. With the thumb and forefinger about an inch back from the nipple, the woman presses gently inward toward the chest wall and squeezes the thumb and fingers together. This "push back and squeeze" motion is continued until no more milk comes out. Then the fingers are rotated to another position, and the procedure is repeated.

to breastfeed. By drawing off the milk, the infant helps to relieve pressure in the infected area. The infant is safe, because the infection is between the milk-producing glands, not inside them.

Even if everything is going smoothly, the nursing mother should ideally have enough help and support so that she can rest in bed a few hours each day for the first week or so. Successful breastfeeding requires the support of all those who care. This, plus adequate nutrition, ample fluids, fresh air, and exercise will do much to enhance the well-being of mother and infant.

Notes

1. American Academy of Pediatrics, The promotion of breastfeeding: Policy statement based on task force report, *Pediatrics* 69 (1982): 654–661; Position of the American Dietetic Association: Promotion of breastfeeding, *Journal of the American Dietetic Association* 86 (1986): 1580; Position of National Association of WIC Directors on breastfeeding promotion in the WIC program, *Journal of the American Dietetic Association* 89 (1989): 1091; *Healthy People 2000: National Health Promotion/Disease Prevention Objectives,* conference ed. (Washington, D.C.: Government Printing Office, 1990), p. 377.

2. G. A. Martinez, Ross Laboratories mothers survey: Sample design and methodology, trends in infant milk feeding practices (Columbus, Ohio: Ross Laboratories, 1987), as cited in A. C. Gielen and coauthors, Maternal employment during the early postpartum period: Effects on initiation and continuation of breast-feeding, *Pediatrics* 87 (1991): 298–305.

3. S. E. Saunders and J. Carroll, Postpartum breast feeding support: Impact on duration, *Journal of the American Dietetic Association* 88 (1988): 213–215.

4. S. P. Barron and coauthors, Factors influencing duration of breast feeding among low-income women, *Journal of the American Dietetic Association* 88 (1988): 1557–1561.

5. M. Teitel, S. Delaney, and L. Fink, *Breastfeeding: The Art of Mothering* (Port Washington, N.Y.: Alive Productions, 1987).

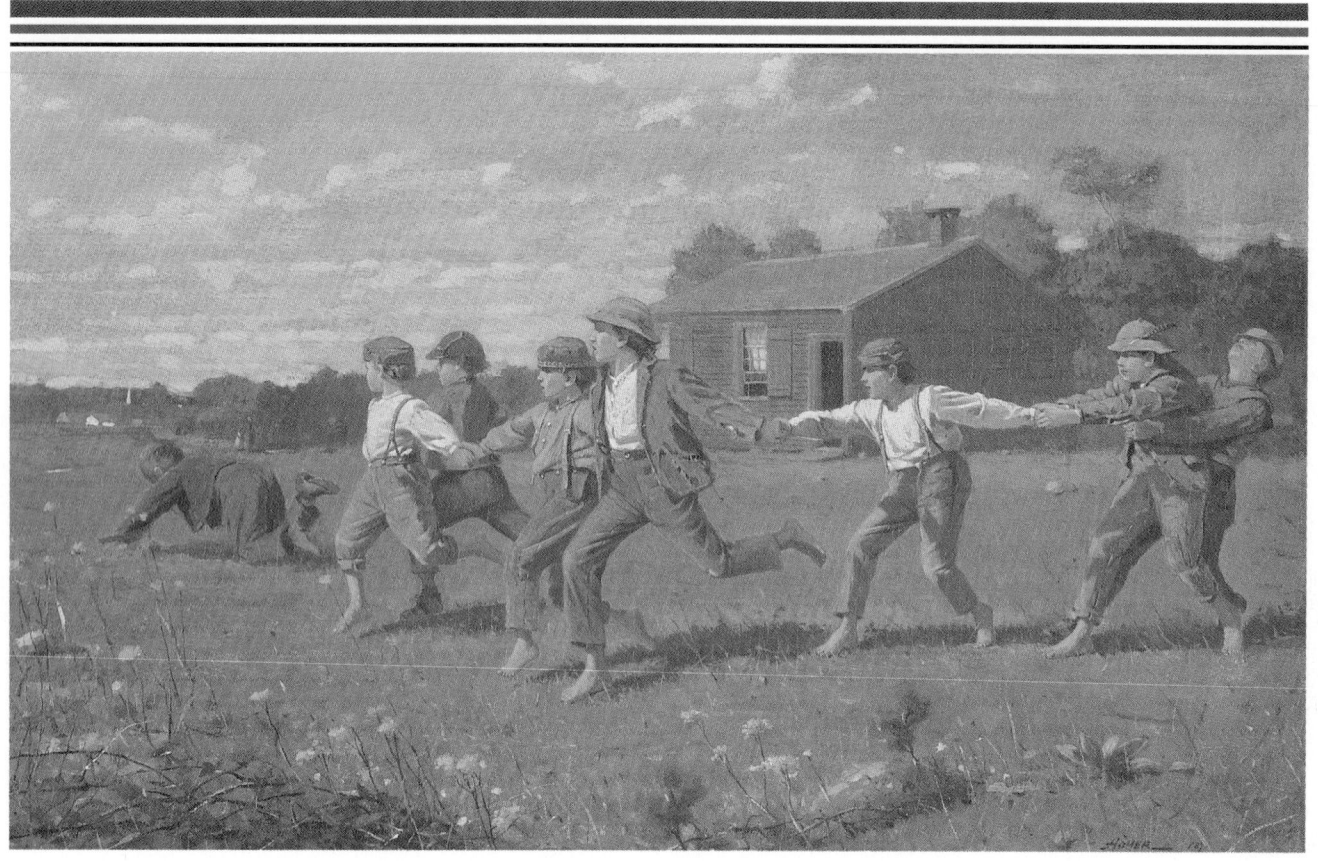

Winslow Homer, Snap the Whip; *The Metropolitan Museum of Art,*
Gift of Christian A. Zabriskie, 1950 (50.41).

CHAPTER

12

Nutrition for Children and Teenagers

CONTENTS

CHAPTER

12

Nutrient needs change steadily throughout life, depending on people's rates of growth, gender, activity level, and many other factors. Nutrient needs also vary from individual to individual, but generalizations are possible and useful. Sound nutrition throughout childhood promotes normal growth and development; facilitates academic and physical performance; and helps prevent obesity, heart disease, cancer, and other degenerative diseases in adulthood. As children enter the teen years, a nutrient foundation built on years of nutritious foods best prepares them to meet the demands of rapid growth that characterize this stage of life. This chapter begins with the nutrient needs of children. Later sections are devoted to the special concerns of teenagers.

Early and Middle Childhood

After the age of one, a child's growth rate slows, but the body continues to change dramatically. At one, infants have just learned to stand and toddle; by two, they can take long strides with solid confidence and are learning to run, jump, and climb. One of the internal changes that makes these new accomplishments possible is the accumulation of a larger mass and greater density of bone and muscle tissue. Thereafter, the same trend—a lengthening of the long bones and an increase in musculature—continues, unevenly and more slowly, until adolescence.

Growth and Nutrient Needs

An infant's appetite declines markedly around the first birthday, consistent with the reduction in growth rate. Thereafter, the appetite fluctuates; at times children seem to be insatiable, and at other times they seem to live on air and water. Parents need not worry about this—a child will need and demand much more food during periods of rapid growth than during slow periods. The perfection of appetite regulation in children of normal weight guarantees that their food energy intakes will be right for each stage of growth.

Many people mistakenly believe that they must control children's portion sizes; children's erratic eating patterns often reinforce this belief. However, research proves otherwise. Researchers studied preschool children's food intakes for six days. Each child's food energy intake was highly variable from meal to meal, but the total daily energy intake was remarkably constant.[1] The children adjusted their energy intakes at successive meals: if they ate less at one meal, they ate more at the next, and vice versa. (Overweight children may not adjust their energy intakes appropriately, however. They may eat in response to external cues, disregarding appetite-regulation signals.)

Steady growth during childhood is reflected in gradually increasing needs for all nutrients. The RDA table (inside front cover) lists average nutrient intakes recommended for each span of three years. Before adolescence, children accumulate stores of nutrients. Then, when they take off on the

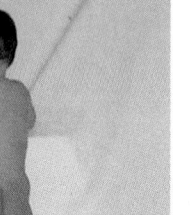

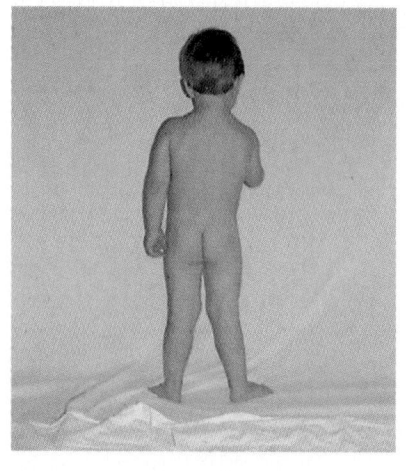

The body shape of a one-year-old (above) changes dramatically by age two (below). The two-year-old has lost much of the baby fat; the muscles (especially in the back, buttocks, and legs) have firmed and strengthened; and the leg bones have lengthened.

adolescent growth spurt, there comes a time during which their nutrient intakes cannot keep pace with the demands of rapid growth, and they draw on the nutrient stores accumulated earlier. This is especially true of calcium; the denser the bones are in childhood, the better prepared they will be to support teen growth, and still withstand the inevitable bone losses of later life. The way preteen children eat, then, influences their nutritional health both during their teen years and for the rest of their lives.

To provide all the needed nutrients, a variety of foods from each food group is recommended. Table 12–1 offers a daily food pattern for children. The portion sizes increase with the children's ages. A portion of meat, fruits, and vegetables for children is loosely defined as 1 tablespoon per year. Thus at four years of age, a serving of meat, fruit, or vegetable is about 4 tablespoons (¼ cup). Because the portion sizes adjust as children grow older, this rule of thumb is appropriate from age two to the teen years.

A parent or caretaker can do much to foster the development of healthy eating habits in a child. The challenge is to deliver nutrients in the form of meals and snacks that are nutritious and delicious to children, so as to accomplish the goal of teaching children to enjoy a variety of nutritious foods.

Every meal is important in a child's life. When a child skips a meal or when empty-kcalorie, sugary foods take the place of nourishing ones, it is virtually guaranteed that the child will fail to get enough of several nutrients. Experimentation with children's food patterns shows that candy, cola, and other concentrated sweets must be limited in a child's diet if the needed nutrients are to be supplied. If such foods are permitted in large quantities, the only possible outcomes are nutrient deficiencies, obesity, or both. The child can't be trusted to choose nutritious foods on the basis of taste alone; the preference for sweets is innate, and children naturally gravitate to them. They need help in sticking to nutrient-dense foods that will meet their nutrient needs within their energy intake allowances. However, under-

TABLE 12–1   **Children's Daily Food Patterns for Good Nutrition**

| FOOD GROUP | SERVINGS PER DAY | *Average Size of Serving* | | |
		1 TO 3 YEARS	4 TO 6 YEARS	7 TO 12 YEARS
Milk and milk products[a]	4	½ to ¾ c	¾ c	¾ to 1 c
Meat and meat alternates[b]	2 or more	1 to 2 oz	1 to 2 oz	2 to 3 oz
Fruits and vegetables[c]	4 or more	2 to 4 tbsp or ½ c juice	¼ to ½ c or ½ c juice	½ to ¾ c or ½ c juice
Bread and cereals (whole-grain or enriched)[d]	4 or more	½ slice	1 slice	1 to 2 slices

[a]½ c milk = ½ c cottage cheese, pudding, yogurt; ¾ oz cheese; 2 tbsp dried milk.
[b]1 oz meat, fish, poultry = 1 egg, 1 frankfurter, 2 tbsp peanut butter, ½ c legumes.
[c]Vitamin C source (citrus fruits, berries, tomatoes, broccoli, cabbage, cantaloupe) daily; vitamin A source (spinach, carrots, squash, tomatoes, cantaloupe) 3 to 4 times weekly.

[d]1 slice bread = ¾ c dry cereal; ½ c cooked cereal; ½ c potato, rice, or noodles.

Source: Adapted from P. M. Queen and R. R. Henry, Growth and nutrient requirements of children, in *Pediatric Nutrition: Theory and Practice,* eds. R. J. Grand, Jr., L. Sutphen, and W. H. Dietz, Jr. (Boston: Butterworths, 1987), p. 347.

weight children or children of normal weight who are very active can enjoy the higher-kcalorie nutritious foods in each category: ice cream or pudding in the milk group and pancakes or crackers (whole-grain or enriched only, however) in the bread group. These foods, made from milk and grain, carry valuable nutrients and encourage a child to learn appropriately that eating is fun.

In U.S. children and adolescents, iron-deficiency anemia is the most prevalent nutrient deficiency. This is also true for those in the latter half of infancy. Iron deficiency is especially common among children and teens from low-income families. However, the iron status of children in the United States is improving. Changing infant feeding practices, such as increased breastfeeding and increased use of iron-fortified formulas, may positively influence iron status in later childhood.[2] Among children from low-income families, the U.S. government's WIC program (Special Supplemental Food Program for Women, Infants, and Children) appears to have played a role in improving iron status. The WIC program provides supplemental iron-rich foods during infancy.

To avert iron-deficiency anemia, children's foods must deliver 10 milligrams of iron or more per day. To achieve this goal, milk intakes must be limited after infancy, because milk is a poor source of iron. Children should receive enough milk products to ensure adequate calcium and riboflavin intakes, but no more. That means 2 to 3 cups of milk per day up to age 3, grading on up to 3 to 4 cups per day from ages 6 to 12 (see Table 12–1). After age two, if low-fat milk is used instead of whole milk, saved kcalories can be invested in iron-rich foods such as lean meats, fish, poultry, eggs, and legumes. Whole-grain or enriched breads and cereals also contribute iron. The next section discusses the effects of nutrient deficiencies on behavior in children, with emphasis on iron deficiency.

Nutrient Deficiencies and Behavior

Earlier chapters emphasized the physical symptoms that nutrient deficiencies incur. Of particular interest to people involved in caring for children is that nutrient deficiencies might also have behavioral symptoms.

Iron deficiency presents the best-known and most widespread effects on behavior. Most people are familiar with the role of iron in carrying oxygen in the blood. Another important function of iron is transporting oxygen within cells, where it is used to help produce energy. A lack of iron not only causes an energy crisis but also directly affects behavior, mood, attention span, and learning ability. Iron is involved in the function of many molecules in the brain and nervous system. Iron deficiencies produced experimentally in animals cause abnormal synthesis and degradation of neurotransmitters—most notably those that regulate the ability to pay attention, which is crucial to learning.[3]

Iron deficiency is usually diagnosed by a deficit of iron in the *blood,* after the deficiency has progressed all the way to anemia. A child's *brain,* however, is sensitive to slightly lowered iron concentrations long before the blood effects appear. Iron's effects are hard to distinguish from the effects of other factors in children's lives, but it is likely that iron deficiency manifests itself in a lowering of "motivation to persist in intellectually challenging tasks," a shortening of the attention span, and a reduction of overall intellectual performance. Anemic children perform less well on tests and have more conduct disturbances than their nonanemic classmates.[4] The prevalence of iron deficiency among children in this country and throughout the world is a problem that has become the focus of major public health organizations. The Public Health Service of the U.S. Department of Health and Human Services identifies the goal of reducing iron deficiency among young children as one of the nation's foremost health priorities.[5] The World Health Organization is collaborating with a United Nations subcommittee on nutrition to develop a ten-year plan to eliminate iron deficiency.[6]

Iron is only one of several dozen nutrients that can be displaced in a diet high in nutrient-poor foods. Any of the other nutrients may be lacking as well, and the deficiencies of those nutrients may also cause behavioral, as well as physical, symptoms.

A child with behavioral symptoms of nutrient deficiencies might be irritable, aggressive, disagreeable, or sad and withdrawn. One might label such a child "hyperactive," "depressed," or "unlikable," when in fact these traits might arise from simple, albeit marginal, malnutrition. Should suspicion of dietary inadequacies be raised, *no matter what other causes may be implicated,* the people responsible for feeding the child should take steps to correct those inadequacies promptly.

Lead Poisoning and Behavior

The health impairment caused by malnutrition not only often involves multiple nutrient deficiencies but also is compounded by other factors. One example of a possible complicating factor is lead. Lead poisoning can cause iron-deficiency anemia, and iron deficiency impairs the body's defenses against lead absorption. In fact, the interactions between lead poisoning and iron deficiency are so strong that some researchers suggest it may be appropriate to consider lead poisoning an adverse consequence of iron deficiency.[7] A risk factor common to both iron deficiency and lead poisoning is a low socioeconomic background. The anemia brought on by lead poisoning may be mistaken for a simple iron deficiency. Like iron deficiency, mild lead toxicity has nonspecific effects, including diarrhea, irritability, reduced ability of the blood to carry oxygen, and fatigue. The symptoms may be reversible if exposure stops soon enough. With higher levels of lead, the signs become more pronounced, yet still difficult to pinpoint to a cause. Children lose their general cognitive, verbal, and perceptual abilities, developing learning disabilities and behavior problems. Still more severe lead toxicity can cause irreversible nerve damage, paralysis, mental retardation, and death. Only one year of exposure can permanently impair the brain, nervous system, and psychological functioning.[8] Furthermore, research shows that the effects occur with *lower* doses than has been thought in the past.[9] This research prompted the Centers for Disease Control to lower the lead poisoning guidelines—the amount of lead in the blood believed to cause lead poisoning. The new threshold is 10 micrograms per 100 milliliters of blood, a considerable drop from the previous 25 micrograms per 100 milliliters.[10] The U.S. Department of Health and Human Services has labeled lead poisoning "the most common and societally devastating environmental disease of young children."[11]

Lead toxicity symptoms are widespread among children under six years of age—as many as 3 to 4 million children may have blood lead concentrations high enough to cause mental and behavioral problems and other health problems.[12] Lead aggressively attacks fetuses, infants, and children, because the body absorbs lead most efficiently during times of rapid growth. Other factors also explain why infants and children are so vulnerable to lead poisoning. Children's behaviors and activities—putting their hands in their mouths, playing in dirt, and eating nonfood items—favor their chances of exposure to lead.[13] Blood concentrations of lead generally reach a peak in two-year-old children; age two is the typical time of exploring surroundings "hand to mouth" and ingesting lead-tainted dirt and debris.[14]

Reductions in the use of leaded products (such as leaded gasoline, lead-soldered food cans, and leaded house paint) mandated by federal law in recent years have helped to limit the amount of lead in the environment, but the problem of exposure to lead still pervades children's lives. Of all the sources of lead for children, paint remains the most important.[15] In the homes of 3 million young children, leaded surfaces are peeling and deteriorating. Each child in these homes is already poisoned, or at immediate risk of lead poisoning.

Recently, three major discoveries about lead toxicity have occurred simultaneously:

- Lead poisoning appears to have more *subtle* effects than previously appreciated.
- The effects of lead poisoning are more *permanent* than known earlier.
- The effects of lead poisoning occur at *lower levels of exposure* than realized before.

To prevent exposure is therefore more urgent than heretofore realized:

- In contaminated environments, prevent hand-to-mouth ingestion (keep small children from putting dirty or old painted objects in their mouths).
- Do not make baby formula from canned, evaporated milk.
- Once you have opened canned food, immediately remove it from the can, and keep it in a storage container to minimize lead migration into the food.
- Make sure children consume nutritious meals consistently.

Hunger and Behavior

Not only the content but also the timing of meals makes a difference in children's behavior and academic performance. A study of more than 1,000 elementary schoolchildren offers the latest evidence that children who eat a nutritious breakfast function better than their peers who do not.[16] Young children who participated in the School Breakfast Program, a child nutrition program that offers morning meals for children, improved their scores on achievement tests and were tardy or absent significantly less often than children who did not participate in the breakfast program. Common sense dictates that it is unreasonable to expect anyone to learn and perform work when no fuel has been provided. By the late morning, discomfort from hunger may become distracting even if a child *has* eaten breakfast.

The problem that arises for children who attempt morning schoolwork on an empty stomach appears to be at least partly due to hypoglycemia. The average child up to the age of ten or so needs to eat every four to six hours to maintain a blood glucose concentration high enough to support the activity of the brain and nervous system. A child's brain is as big as an adult's, and the brain is the body's chief glucose consumer. A child's liver is considerably smaller—and the liver is the organ responsible for storing glucose (as glycogen) and releasing it into the blood as needed. A child's liver can't store more than about four hours' worth of glycogen—hence the need to eat fairly often. Teachers aware of the late-morning slump in their classrooms wisely request that a midmorning snack be provided; it improves classroom performance all the way to lunchtime.

Food Allergies

Food allergies are frequently blamed for physical and behavioral abnormalities in children. The incidence of food allergies is highest in the first several years of life and tends to decline with age.[17] A true food allergy occurs when a whole food protein or other large molecule enters the system. (Recall that large molecules of food are normally dismantled in the digestive tract to smaller ones that are absorbed without problem.) The body's immune system reacts to a food protein or other large molecule as it does to an antigen—by producing antibodies, histamines, or other defensive agents.

Allergies may have one or two components. They always involve antibodies; they may or may not involve symptoms. A person may produce antibodies *without* having any symptoms (known as asymptomatic allergy) or may produce antibodies *and* have symptoms (known as symptomatic allergy). Symptoms without antibody production are *not* due to allergy. This means that allergies cannot be diagnosed from symptoms alone; they have to be diagnosed by testing for antibodies.

Even if a child's symptoms are exactly like those of an allergy, they may not be caused by one. A parent whose child has any kind of discomfort after eating—stomachache, headache, pain, rapid pulse rate, nausea, wheezing, hives, bronchial irritation, cough, or any other—may decide that an allergy is responsible, when in fact the cause is something else entirely. Only careful, skilled testing can distinguish the many possibilities, and such testing is seldom done.

Depending on the location of the allergic reaction in the body, a symptomatic allergy will exhibit different symptoms. In the digestive tract, it may cause nausea or vomiting; in the skin, it may cause rashes; and in the nasal passages and lungs, it can cause inflammation or asthma. A generalized, all-systems reaction is anaphylactic shock.

Allergic reactions to food can occur with different timings, simply classified as immediate and delayed. In both, the interaction of the antigen with the immune system is immediate, but the appearance of symptoms may come within minutes or after several (up to 24) hours.[18] Identifying the food that causes an immediate allergic reaction is easy, because symptoms correlate closely with the time of eating the food. Identifying the food that

antigen: a substance foreign to the body that elicits the formation of antibodies or an inflammation reaction from immune system cells. Food antigens are usually glycoproteins (large proteins with glucose molecules attached).

antibody: a large protein that is produced in response to an antigen, and that inactivates the antigen.

histamine: a substance produced by cells of the immune system as part of a local immune reaction to an antigen; participates in causing inflammation.

allergy: an immune reaction to a foreign substance (such as some components of food) in which antibodies are produced. (An immune reaction not involving antibody production is termed a **sensitivity** by some researchers.) Allergies may be **symptomatic** or **asymptomatic.**

anaphylactic (an-AFF-ill-LAC-tic) **shock:** a whole-body allergic reaction to an offending substance. Symptoms: abdominal pain, nausea, vomiting, diarrhea, inflamed nasal membranes, chest pain, hives, swelling, low blood pressure.

TABLE 12–2   **Foods That Most Often Cause Allergies**

Nuts	Peanuts
Eggs	Chicken
Milk	Fish
Soybeans	Shellfish
Wheat	Mollusks

Source: Adapted from D. D. Metcalfe, Diseases of food hypersensitivity, *New England Journal of Medicine* 321 (1989): 255–257; C. D. May. Food allergy: Perspective, Principles, practical management, *Nutrition Today,* November/December 1980, pp. 28–31.

may cause a delayed reaction is more difficult, because the symptoms may not appear until a day after the offending food is eaten; by this time, many other foods will have been eaten, too, complicating the picture.

The foods that most often cause immediate allergic reactions are listed in Table 12–2. According to the American Academy of Allergy and Immunology, most allergic reactions to foods are caused by cow's milk, egg white, peanuts, wheat, and soy. Shrimp, tomatoes, codfish, and crab also contain allergens to which some people are sensitive.[19] Allergic reactions to single foods are common. Reactions to multiple foods are the exception, not the rule.

A number of tests and food challenges are required to identify a true food allergy. Allergies are not always diagnosed by these time-consuming, laborious methods, however. In fact, the term *food allergy* is used loosely, even by many physicians, as a catchall term for any unexplained adverse reaction to foods. Among reactions to foods that are confused with true food allergies are:

- Allergic reactions to molds, antibiotics, and other contaminants of foods.
- Chinese restaurant syndrome, a reaction specific to the flavor enhancer monosodium glutamate, or MSG (trade name, Accent).
- Reactions to bacterial toxins, such as botulinal toxin, and other food poisoning.
- Reactions to chemicals in foods, such as the natural laxative in prunes.
- Symptoms of digestive diseases such as hernias and ulcers, aggravated by eating any food.
- Enzyme deficiencies, such as lactose intolerance, that cause symptoms superficially indistinguishable from those of food allergy.
- Psychological reactions based on the belief that certain foods cause certain symptoms.[20]

These reactions should be called *hypersensitivity reactions* or *adverse reactions,* not *allergies.*

Parents are advised to watch for signs of food dislikes and take them seriously: "Dislike of a food may be only a whim or fancy, but it should be regarded as significant until proven otherwise."[21] Children's food aversions may be the result of nature's efforts to protect them from allergic or other adverse reactions. Although many cases of suspected allergies turn out to be something else, real allergies do exist, as do other valid reasons to avoid certain foods. Don't prejudge, in any case.

Test, and then apply nutrition knowledge conscientiously in deciding how to alter the diet. Don't risk feeding the child an unbalanced diet, which could lead to nutrient deficiencies. Whenever a food is excluded from the diet, care must be taken to include other foods that offer the same nutrients as the omitted food contains. Remember that children with allergies need all their nutrients, just as other children do.

Hyperactivity and Diet

Because malnutrition and food allergies do impair children's functioning in many ways, people tend to look to food habits for explanations of hyperactivity. However, no behavior problems originate with diet other than the general misery caused by malnutrition, nor do food allergies cause hyperactivity. Misbehavior is seldom, if ever, attributable, or even linked, to dietary causes, although poor diet may be part of a cluster of factors seen in an unfortunate child's life.

Hyperactivity is a learning disability that occurs in 4 percent of young school-age children—that is, in 1 child in every classroom of 20 children.[22] It can lead to academic failure and major behavior problems. Parents and teachers need to deal effectively with it wherever it appears, to avert the grief that can otherwise result.

Physicians often diagnose hyperactivity by conducting a trial with stimulant drugs. Stimulants normally speed up people's activity, but they have a paradoxical effect with hyperactivity; they normalize it. (Perhaps they stimulate control centers in the brain.) If a child responds to stimulant drugs by calming down, it indicates that the drugs may be correcting a biochemical imbalance in the nervous system, and they can be used to help control the behavior. *In children who are responsive*, prescription medication should at least be considered as the treatment of choice.

Many parents fail to appreciate the utility of drug treatment for hyperactivity and resist its use, especially when they believe a solution may lie in manipulating the diet. Diet is one aspect of a child's life over which parents feel they can have some control. If problems can be solved by adding carrots or deleting cookies, then parents are eager to give diet advice a try. While it is true that nutrition should be considered whenever a person's physical or mental health is less than optimal, it is advised not to jump at appealing solutions that are unfounded.

Caffeine and Other Stimulants

One dietary excess that can irritate many children is that of caffeine, a matter of some concern to pediatricians. A 12-ounce cola beverage may contain as much as 50 milligrams caffeine; two or more such beverages are equivalent in the body of a 60-pound child to the caffeine in 8 cups of coffee for a 175-pound man. Chocolate bars also contribute caffeine. Children can be troubled by sleeplessness, restlessness, and irregular heartbeats due to excess caffeine consumption. A survey of over 1,000 children between the ages of 1 and 17 years found that 77 percent of them were caffeine consumers.[23] Table 12–3 lists caffeine contents of beverages, foods, and medications. As long as such undeniably attractive temptations as cola beverages and candy bars surround children, barriers against their abuse have to be provided by concerned adults until the children learn to control consumption themselves.

Common sense says that all children at times get wild and "hyper." There are many normal, everyday causes of such behavior:

- Desire for attention.
- Lack of sleep.
- Overstimulation.
- Too much TV.
- Lack of exercise.

hyperactivity syndrome in children: A cluster of symptoms in which the essential features are signs of developmentally inappropriate inattention, impulsivity, and high levels of motor activity. Other important features are onset before age seven, duration of six months or more, and proven absence of mental illness or mental retardation. Other names associated with hyperactivity: attention deficit disorder, hyperkinesis, minimal brain damage, minimal brain dysfunction, minor cerebral dysfunction.

learning disability: a defect in the ability to learn basic cognitive skills such as reading, writing, and mathematics; causes vary.

TABLE 12–3   **Caffeine Content of Beverages, Foods, and OTC Drugs**

	AVERAGE (mg)	RANGE (mg)
BEVERAGES AND FOOD		
Coffee (5-oz cup)		
Brewed, drip method	130	110–150
Brewed, percolator	94	64–124
Instant	74	40–108
Decaffeinated, brewed or instant	3	1–5
Tea (5-oz cup)		
Brewed, major U.S. brands	40	20–90
Brewed, imported brands	60	25–110
Instant	30	25–50
Iced (12-oz glass)	70	67–76
Soft drinks (12-oz can)		
Dr. Pepper		40
Colas and cherry cola		
Regular		30–46
Diet		2–58
Caffeine-free		0–trace
Jolt		72
Mountain Dew, Mello Yello		52
Fresca, Hires Root Beer, 7-Up, Sprite, Squirt, Sunkist Orange		0
Cocoa beverage (5-oz cup)	4	2–20
Chocolate milk beverage (8 oz)	5	2–7
Milk chocolate candy (1 oz)	6	1–15
Dark chocolate, semisweet (1 oz)	20	5–35
Baker's chocolate (1 oz)		26
Chocolate-flavored syrup (1 oz)		4
DRUGS[a]		
Cold remedies (standard dose)		
Dristan		0
Coryban-D, Triaminicin		30
Diuretics (standard dose)		
Aqua-ban, Permathene H_2Off		200
Pre-Mens Forte		100
Pain relievers (standard dose)		
Excedrin		130
Midol, Anacin		65
Aspirin, plain (any brand)		0
Stimulants		
Caffedrin, NoDoz, Vivarin		200
Weight-control aids (daily dose)		
Prolamine		280
Dexatrim, Dietac		200

[a]Because products change, contact the manufacturer for an update on products you use regularly.
Source: Data from C. Lecos, The latest caffeine scoreboard, *FDA Consumer,* March 1984, p. 14; Measuring your life with coffee spoons, *Tufts University Diet and Nutrition Letter,* April 1984, pp. 3–6; Institute of Food Technologists, Expert Panel on Food Safety and Nutrition, *Evaluation of Caffeine Safety,* a publication (1986) available from the Institute of Food Technologists, 221 N. LaSalle St., Chicago, IL 60601.

Together, these produce the tension-fatigue syndrome, which can be relieved by giving more consistent care to the child's welfare. It helps especially to insist on regular hours of sleep, regular mealtimes, and regular outdoor exercise.

tension-fatigue syndrome: apparent hyperactivity produced in a child by the combination of lack of sleep and overstimulation with anxiety.

Mealtimes with Children

The childhood years are a parent's last chance to influence food choices. By fostering healthy eating habits, parents help determine whether development will take place in a positive or negative direction for the rest of life. Food choices not only can promote healthy growth but, as mentioned earlier, also can help prevent the degenerative diseases of later life—cardiovascular disease, cancer, diabetes, and osteoporosis. Many experts agree that early childhood is the time to put into effect practices that, until recently, were recommended only for adults.

Most important is to avoid obesity. Train preschool children to eat slowly, to pause and enjoy their table companions, and to stop eating when they are full. Serve small portions of food that can be followed by additional servings, if needed. Discourage snacking on high-fat, high-sugar foods. Encourage frequent, adequate milk consumption. Follow recommendations like those of the *NRC Recommendations* (Table 1–3 in Chapter 1), emphasizing foods with high nutrient density. Encourage physical activity on a daily basis.

It is not surprising that problems over food often arise during the second or third year, when children are asserting their independence. Many of these problems stem from the conflict between children's developmental stages and capabilities and parents who, in attempting to do what they think is best for their children, try to control every aspect of eating. Such conflicts can disrupt children's abilities to regulate their own food intakes or to determine their own likes and dislikes. For example, many people share the misconception that children must be persuaded or coerced to try new foods. Research with children indicates the opposite. When children are forced to try new foods, even by way of rewards, they are less likely to try those foods again than are children who are left to decide for themselves.[24] One authority on childrens' eating behaviors makes a point relevant to the research just discussed: the parent is responsible for *what* the child is offered to eat, but the child is responsible for *how much* and even *whether* to eat.[25]

When introducing new foods at the table, parents are advised to offer them one at a time and only in small amounts at first. The more often a food is presented to a young child, the more likely the child will like that food. Whenever possible, the new food should be presented at the beginning of the meal, when the child is hungry. Offer the new food, and allow the child to make the decision to accept or reject it. Parents have inclinations and dislikes to which they feel entitled; children should be accorded the same privilege. Never make an issue of food acceptance. A power struggle almost invariably sets a firm pattern of resistance and permanently closes the child's mind.

It is desirable for children to learn to like a variety of nutritious foods within each of the food groups. With one exception, this liking usually develops naturally. The exception is vegetables, which young children frequently dislike and refuse. Even a tiny serving of spinach, cooked carrots, or squash may elicit an expression that registers the utmost in negative feelings. Since most youngsters need to eat more vegetables, the next few paragraphs are addressed to this problem.

Try to remember how you felt when first offered a cup of vegetable soup, a serving of runny spinach, or a pile of peas and carrots. If the soup burned your tongue, it may have been years before you were willing to try it again. As for the spinach, it was suspiciously murky looking. (Who could tell what might be lurking in that dark, stringy stuff?) The peas and carrots troubled your sense of order. Before you could eat them, you felt compelled to sort the peas onto one side of the plate and the carrots onto the other. Then you had to separate, into a reject pile, all those that got mashed in the process or contaminated with gravy from the mashed potatoes. Only then might you be willing to eat the intact, clean peas and carrots one by one—perhaps with your fingers, since the peas, especially, kept rolling off the fork.

Researchers attempting to explain children's food preferences are met with contradictions. Children describe liking colorful foods, yet most often reject vegetables while favoring brown peanut butter and white potatoes, apple wedges, and bread. They do, though, like raw vegetables better than cooked ones, so it is wise to offer vegetables that are raw or slightly undercooked and crunchy, and bright in color. They should be warm, not hot, because a child's mouth is much more sensitive than an adult's. The flavor should be mild (a child has more taste buds), and smooth foods, such as mashed potatoes or pea soup, should have no lumps (a child wonders, with some disgust, what the lumps might be). Vegetables should be served separately, and be easy to eat.

When feeding children, parents must always be alert to the dangers of choking. A choking child is a silent child—an adult should be present whenever a child is eating. Make sure the child sits when eating; choking is more likely when a child is running or falling. Round foods such as grapes, nuts, hard candies, and hot dog pieces are hard to control in a mouth with few teeth, and they can easily become lodged in the small opening of a child's trachea. Other potentially dangerous foods include tough meat, popcorn, and chips.

Small children like to eat at little tables and to be served little portions of food. They also love to eat with other children and have been observed to stay at the table longer and eat much more when in the company of their peers. Parents who serve the food in a relaxed and casual manner, without anxiety, provide the emotional climate in which a child's negative emotions will be minimized.

Ideally, each meal is preceded, not followed, by the activity the child looks forward to the most. In a number of schools, it has been discovered that children eat a much better lunch if recess occurs before, rather than after, the meal—otherwise they "hurry up and eat" so that they can go play. Before sitting down to eat, small children should be helped to clean themselves thoroughly, washing their hands and faces so that they can enjoy their meal with "that clean feeling."

Allowing children to help plan and prepare the family's meals provides enjoyable learning experiences and encourages children to eat the foods they have prepared. Vegetables are pretty, especially when fresh, and provide opportunities for children to learn about color, about growing things and

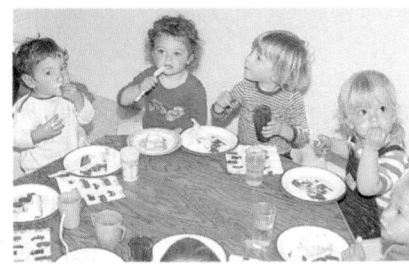

Eating is more fun when your friends are there.

their seeds, about shapes and textures — all of which are fascinating to young children. Measuring, stirring, decorating, cutting, and arranging vegetables are skills that even a very small child can practice with enjoyment and pride.

Parents may find that their children often snack so much that they aren't very hungry at mealtimes. Instead of teaching children *not* to snack, parents might be wise to teach them *how* to snack. Provide snacks that are as nutritious as the foods served at mealtimes. Snacks can even be mealtime foods that are served individually over time, instead of all at once on one plate. Snacks need to be easy to prepare and readily available to children. This is particularly important to children who return home after school without parental supervision.

Children sometimes lose their appetites when they are sick with colds or flu, and sometimes for no apparent reason at all. On a short-term basis, this is usually nothing to worry about. As children who are ill recover, so will their appetites. The child who is sick should be encouraged to drink plenty of fluids. Chapter 14 gives suggestions to improve the appetite of the hospitalized child.

Nutrition at School

While parents are doing what they can to establish favorable eating behavior in their children during the transition from infancy to childhood, other factors are entering the picture. During preschool or grade school, the child encounters foods prepared and served by outsiders. The U.S. government funds several programs to provide nutritious, high-quality meals for children at school. Under the National School Lunch Program, school lunches are designed to meet certain requirements and must include specified numbers of servings of milk, protein-rich food (meat, poultry, fish, cheese, eggs, legumes, or peanut butter), vegetables, fruits, and breads or other grain foods. The design of school lunches is intended to provide at least a third of the RDA for each of the nutrients. Table 12–4 shows different school lunch patterns for children of different ages.

Unlike the National School Lunch Program, which is available in nearly all schools, the School Breakfast Program is available in only about 40 percent of schools. As research results continue to emphasize the positive impact breakfast has on school performance and health, campaigns to expand school breakfast programs are under way.[26] The school breakfast must contain, at a minimum:

- One serving of fluid milk.
- One serving of fruit or vegetable or full-strength juice.
- Two servings of bread or bread alternate, two servings of meat or meat alternate, or one of each.

Surveys show that the majority of children who eat school breakfasts are from low-income families. In addition, survey results show that more students would participate in the School Breakfast Program if it were available in more schools.[27]

Both the National School Lunch Program and the School Breakfast Program provide meals at a reasonable cost to children from families with the

TABLE 12–4 **School Lunch Patterns for Different Ages**

FOOD GROUP	Preschool (Age)		Grade School through High School (Grade)		
	1 TO 2	3 TO 4	K TO 3	4 TO 6	7 TO 12
MEAT OR MEAT ALTERNATE					
1 serving:					
Lean meat, poultry, or fish	1 oz	1½ oz	1½ oz	2 oz	3 oz
Cheese	1 oz	1½ oz	1½ oz	2 oz	3 oz
Large egg(s)	1	1½	1½	2	3
Cooked dry beans or peas	½ c	¾ c	¾ c	1 c	1½ c
Peanut butter	2 tbsp	3 tbsp	3 tbsp	4 tbsp	6 tbsp
VEGETABLE AND/OR FRUIT					
2 or more servings, both to total	½ c	½ c	½ c	¾ c	¾ c
BREAD OR BREAD ALTERNATE					
Servings[a]	5 per week	8 per week	8 per week	8 per week	10 per week
MILK					
1 serving of fluid milk	¾ c	¾ c	1 c	1 c	1 c

[a]A serving is 1 slice of whole-grain or enriched bread; a whole-grain or enriched biscuit, roll, muffin, and so on; or ½ c cooked pasta or other cereal grain such as bulgur or grits.

Source: School lunch patterns: Ready, set, go! *School Food Service Journal,* August 1980, p. 31.

financial means to pay. Meals are available free or at reduced cost to children from low-income families.

Television and Vending Machines

For the most part, children learn nutrition from parents or teachers who know little about it. Meanwhile, they hear a great deal about foods from the television set. Many authorities are concerned that television commercials have a negative impact. Most of the concern centers on the issue of sugar. According to estimates, the average child sees more than 10,000 commercials a year, of which many more than half are for sugary foods. Hundreds of millions of dollars are spent in the effort to sell these foods to children. Not all the public disapproval of sugar is based on scientific findings, but there is widespread agreement on one point: sticky, sugary foods left on the teeth provide an ideal environment for the growth of mouth bacteria and for the formation of cavities (see Nutrition in Practice 2). Also, sugary foods may displace needed nutrients in the diet. No regulations to prevent the promotion of sticky, sugary foods are in force, however.

Television is not the only environmental force affecting children's food choices. Another is vending machines, especially those in schools. Children will choose more nutritious snacks, however, if offered to them side by side with sugary foods. When milk is made available, soft drink use drops.

The Teen Years

The teen years are a time of change—the child is becoming an adult. Changes are evident physically, emotionally, intellectually, and socially. Nutrient needs are high during this time of growth, and the challenge to make sure that nutrient needs are met continues.

A transition of importance is that teens make many more choices for themselves than they did as children. Teenagers are not fed; they eat. And they are not sent out to play; they choose whether to invest their energy in physical activity. Social pressures thrust choices at them: to drink or not to drink, to develop their bodies to meet sometimes extreme ideals of slimness or athletic prowess. The person concerned with the nutrition and health of teenagers cannot simply deliver food, but must instead deliver motivation. That means becoming knowledgeable about the subjects that teenagers are interested in and showing how nutrition relates to those subjects. The next few sections examine the nutrient needs of teenagers and how this unique time of life influences their food choices.

Growth and Nutrient Needs

The fairly steady rate of growth throughout childhood speeds up abruptly and dramatically with the onset of adolescence. Prior to adolescence, female and male growth patterns differ little; with the onset of puberty, they become distinct. A female's adolescent growth spurt begins at age 10 or 11 and reaches its peak at 12. A male's growth spurt begins at 12 or 13 and peaks at 14. The duration of the growth spurt is about two years, but of course, wide variations are seen for individuals.[28] Gender differences also become apparent in the skeletal system, lean body mass, and fat stores. In females, fat becomes a larger percentage of the total body weight, and in males, the lean body mass—muscle and bone—becomes much greater. This intensive growth period brings not only a dramatic increase in height and weight, but also hormonal changes that profoundly affect every organ of the body, including the brain, and culminate in the emergence of physically mature adults within two or three years.

Tremendous individual variations occur in teenagers' rates and patterns of growth. Growth charts used for children must be abandoned when the signs of puberty begin to appear. Age in years indicates little about development; one way to be sure a teenager is growing normally is to compare his or her height and weight with previous measures taken at intervals. Rating scales based on stages of adolescent development are available and widely used to record developmental changes during puberty.[29]

The energy needs of teenagers also vary to a great extent, depending on the intensity of the adolescent growth spurt, body size, and physical activity. The rapid growth of adolescence, especially if coupled with high activity, incurs high energy needs. The energy needs of teenage boys may be especially high. Boys experience a more intense growth spurt than girls do, and as mentioned, develop more lean body mass than girls do; both of these characteristics contribute to a greater energy need for teenage boys than teenage girls. In general, because girls enter their growth spurts earlier than boys, and because girls attain lower body weights than boys, their energy needs peak sooner and decline more quickly than those of their male peers.[30] Thus teenage girls need to pay special attention to selecting foods of high nutrient density in order to meet their nutrient needs without exceeding energy needs.

Total nutrient needs are greater during adolescence than at any time of life except for the times of pregnancy and lactation. Iron remains notable as a nutrient of concern. Iron needs increase in teen girls as they start to menstruate, and in boys as their lean body mass increases. Food intake surveys show that adolescent iron intakes often fail to keep pace with increasing needs, especially for females.[31] Female adolescents typically consume less meat and fewer total kcalories than males do. These dietary habits make it all the more difficult to obtain adequate iron. Chapter 9 offers a discussion of the iron needs of athletes, another group at risk for iron deficiency.

Another nutrient of concern during adolescence is calcium. Low calcium intakes during adolescence, especially during the adolescent growth spurt and especially if paired with physical inactivity, may compromise the development of peak bone mass. The attainment of maximal bone mass is considered the best protection against age-related bone loss and fractures.[32] Once again, teenage girls are at greatest risk, for their milk intakes begin to decline at the time when their calcium needs are greatest.[33] Calcium intakes among adolescents decline as milk consumption decreases. Research suggests that the low calcium intakes of teenagers are caused in part by their choice to replace milk with soft drinks.[34]

Other nutrients are also required in greater quantities during adolescence than in childhood. These nutrient requirements either level off or diminish slightly as the adolescent passes into adulthood.

The insidious problem of obesity becomes more apparent in adolescence and often continues into adulthood, especially in females. Young women who become interested in nutrition may make choices that will benefit their health, or they may become obsessed with weight control (see Nutrition in Practice 19).

Food Choices and Eating Habits of Teenagers

Teenagers come and go as they choose and eat what they want when they have time. With a multitude of after-school, social, and job activities, they almost inevitably fall into irregular eating habits. The adult becomes a gatekeeper, controlling the availability, but not the consumption, of food in the teenager's environment. The gatekeeper who wants to promote the desired choices effectively provides access to nutritious and economical energy foods that are low in sugar and fat at home and limits access to nonnutritious foods. The teenage snacker who finds only nutritious foods around the house is well provided for.

Snacks provide about a fourth of the average teenager's total daily food energy intake. Teens receive substantial amounts of protein, thiamin, riboflavin, vitamin B$_6$, magnesium, and zinc from snacks, and even calcium (if they snack on dairy products). The nutrients they most often fail to obtain are iron, vitamin A, and folate. Protein usually need not be stressed, but many teenagers need to be encouraged to recognize and consume more

gatekeeper: with respect to nutrition, a key person who controls other people's access to foods and thereby has a profound impact on their nutrition. Examples are the spouse who buys and cooks the food, the parent who feeds the children, and the caretaker in a day-care center.

dairy products (for calcium) and more vegetables (for vitamin A and folate). (Wherever vitamin A is lacking, folate is, too, because both are found in green vegetables.) Iron-rich snacks include hard-boiled eggs, bran muffins, and peanut butter and crackers.

Inevitably, teenagers do a lot of eating away from home. There, as well as at home, their nutritional welfare is favored or hindered by the choices they make. Nutrition in Practice 21 discusses the best choices for fast foods.

Teenagers are intensely involved in day-to-day life with their peers and in preparation for their future lives as adults. Adults need to remember that teenagers have the right to make their own decisions—even if they are in opposition to the adults' own views. The gatekeepers can set up the environment so that nutritious foods are available, and can stand by with reliable nutrition information and advice, but the rest is up to the teenagers. Ultimately, they make the choices.

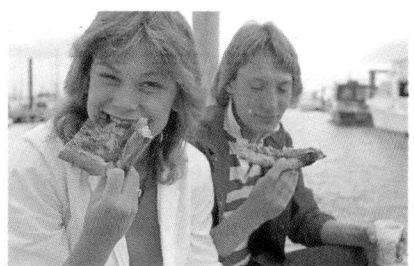

Teenagers are notorious snackers. Nutritious snacks play an important role in active teens' diets.

Drugs, Alcohol, Tobacco, and Nutrition

The teen years are a critical time in the development of problem behaviors such as drug, alcohol, and tobacco use. Three of every five high school seniors report that they have at least tried an illicit drug, most commonly marijuana.[35] One in 20 high school seniors reports having used cocaine at least once.[36]

Smoking a marijuana cigarette has several characteristic effects on the body, altering, among other things, the sense of taste. Among the apparent taste changes induced by marijuana is an enhanced enjoyment of eating, especially of sweets, commonly known as "the munchies." Why or how this effect occurs is not known. Some investigators speculate that the hunger induced by marijuana is actually a social effect caused by the suggestibility of the group in which it is smoked. Prolonged use of the drug does not seem to bring about a weight gain. Despite increased food intakes, marijuana abusers often consume fewer nutrients than do nonabusers. This is probably because the extra foods they choose are usually high-kcalorie, low-nutrient snack foods.

Marijuana users may think that because they usually smoke fewer marijuana cigarettes in a day than they would tobacco cigarettes, they will incur fewer harmful, long-term effects on their lungs. This is a myth. Research shows that one marijuana cigarette is as bad for the body as four or five tobacco cigarettes. People may smoke fewer marijuana cigarettes than tobacco cigarettes, but they inhale more smoke and hold it in their lungs longer. As a result, regular marijuana users may face the same risk of lung cancer as people who smoke a pack of tobacco cigarettes a day.[37]

Cocaine elicits effects such as intense euphoria, restlessness, heightened self-confidence, irritability, insomnia, and loss of appetite. Weight loss is a common side effect, and cocaine abusers often develop eating disorders.[38] Thus, unlike marijuana use, cocaine use brings major nutritional consequences. Notably, the craving for the drug replaces hunger; the stronger the craving for cocaine, the less a drug abuser wants food. Rats given unlimited cocaine will choose the drug over food until they die of starvation.[39]

Repeated cocaine use can cause rapid heart rate, irregular heartbeats, heart attacks, and even death. Cocaine use continues to escalate as cheaper and more dangerous forms of the drug become available. Cocaine in its smokable form, crack, is more addicting than any other drug.[40] The addictive power of cocaine is overwhelming. One former crack addict tells the story of holding a gun to his brother's head to steal money for his next crack purchase.

The effects of other addictive drugs vary in degree but are similar in kind to those of cocaine. Drug abusers face multiple nutrition problems:

- They spend money for drugs that could be spent on food.
- They lose interest in food during "high" times.
- Some drugs induce at least a temporary depression of appetite.
- Their lifestyles often lack the regularity and routine that promote good eating habits.
- They may contract hepatitis, a liver disease common in drug abusers, which causes taste changes and loss of appetite.
- They risk contracting AIDS.
- Their nutrition status may be altered by treatments and medicines.
- They often become ill with infectious diseases, which increase their need for nutrients.

During withdrawal from drugs, an important aspect of treatment is the identification and correction of nutrition problems.

The nutrition implications of alcohol use and the consequences of its abuse are described in Nutrition in Practice 6. To sum them all up, alcohol is an empty-kcalorie beverage that can displace needed nutrients from the diet while simultaneously altering absorption and metabolism of nutrients. Thus even if nutrient intake is adequate, imbalances result from altered nutrient absorption and metabolism. People who are unable to use alcohol with moderation must abstain completely from its use if they are to maintain good health.

Cigarette smoking is a pervasive health problem causing thousands of people to suffer from cancer and diseases of the cardiovascular, digestive, and respiratory systems. These effects are beyond the scope of nutrition, but smoking does influence hunger, body weight, and nutrient status. Links between smoking's nutrition effects and lung cancer are also known.

Beta-carotene, a precursor to vitamin A found in vegetables, has anticancer activity.[41] Specifically, the risk of lung cancer is greatest for smokers who have the lowest intakes of carotene. Of course, conclusions from such evidence should not be misinterpreted. Teenagers cannot be led to believe that as long as they eat their carrots they can safely smoke their cigarettes. Smokers are ten times more likely to get lung cancer than nonsmokers. People who do smoke, however, as well as those who do not, can lower their cancer risks by eating fruits and vegetables rich in carotene.

Smoking a cigarette eases feelings of hunger. A smoker who receives a hunger signal can quiet it with a cigarette instead of food. Such behavior ignores body signals and postpones energy and nutrient intake. Thus smokers tend to weigh less than nonsmokers and to gain weight upon cessation of smoking.[42] Weight gain is often a concern for people contemplating giving up cigarettes. The decision to quit weighs unhealthy smoking against unattractive (and potentially unhealthy) weight gain. The message to smokers wanting to quit is to adjust diet and exercise habits to maintain weight during and after cessation.

Nutrient intakes of smokers and nonsmokers differ. Smokers have lower intakes of dietary fiber, vitamin A, folate, and vitamin C.[43] The association between smoking and low vitamin intake may be noteworthy, considering the altered metabolism of vitamin C in smokers and the protective effect of vitamin A against lung cancer.

Research shows that the vitamin C requirement of smokers exceeds that of nonsmokers.[44] Smokers break down vitamin C faster, thus requiring more vitamin C to achieve steady body pools comparable to those of nonsmokers. It is estimated that the vitamin C requirement of smokers may be twice as high as that of nonsmokers. The evidence for this is so strong that it is reflected in the RDA for vitamin C—at least 100 milligrams per day for smokers compared with 60 milligrams for nonsmokers.[45]

In summary, the nutrition choices and other lifestyle choices people make as teenagers and young adults have immediate, as well as long-term, effects on their health. Few teenagers become interested in nutrition for its contribution to health. Lessons (and misinformation) in nutrition come to them by way of personal experiences—eating to improve athletic performance or dieting to lose unwanted pounds. The challenge for health professionals and other adults concerned with the well-being of teenagers is to motivate teens to make sound nutrition and health choices by showing them how such choices relate to their own interests.

CASE STUDY

Six-year-old Boy

Freddie is a 6-year-old boy who seldom sits still, often misbehaves, and is frequently sick. Freddie's eating habits are erratic and poor, as is his appetite. He often misses breakfast because he is too tired to get up in time to eat before school. By midmorning, Freddie is irritable and disruptive in the classroom. At lunchtime he trades the fruit his mother packed with his sandwich for a piece of cake. After school he hurries home to watch television while he eats his favorite snack—root beer and potato chips. At dinnertime, Freddie picks at his food because he isn't very hungry. Later on, when it's time for bed, Freddie complains that he's hungry. His parents let him stay up to have a bowl of cereal (the kind with marshmallows) before he finally falls asleep.

1. What factors in Freddie's daily routine might be contributing to his restless behavior?
2. Discuss some changes in diet that may improve Freddie's health and disposition.

Study Questions

1. What are the health consequences of allowing children to eat large quantities of nutrient-poor foods?
2. What is the most prevalent nutrient deficiency among children and adolescents in the United States? What dietary strategies can help prevent this deficiency?
3. Describe the relationship between iron deficiency and lead poisoning in children.
4. Explain why infants and children are so vulnerable to lead poisoning.
5. Explain what a true food allergy is. Which foods most often cause allergic reactions?
6. List some strategies for introducing new foods to young children.
7. Why are adolescent girls usually at greater risk of iron deficiency than adolescent boys?
8. What are some of the nutrition problems that drug abusers face?
9. How do nutrient intakes of smokers differ from nonsmokers? Why are those differences important?

Notes

1. L. L. Birch and coauthors, The variability of young children's energy intake, *New England Journal of Medicine* 324 (1991): 232–235.
2. R. Yip, The changing characteristics of childhood iron nutritional status in the United States, in *Dietary Iron: Birth to Two Years*, ed. L. J. Filer (New York, Raven Press, 1989), pp. 37–56.
3. B. Lozoff, Behavioral alterations in iron deficiency, *Advances in Pediatrics* 35 (1988): 331–360; N. S. Scrimshaw, Iron deficiency, *Scientific American*, October 1991, pp. 46–52.
4. J. D. Haas and M. W. Fairchild, Summary and conclusions of the International Conference on Iron Deficiency and Behavioral Development, October 10–12, 1988, *American Journal of Clinical Nutrition* 50 (1989): 703–705.
5. P. L. Splett and M. Story, Child nutrition: Objectives for the decade, *Journal of the American Dietetic Association* 91 (1991): 665–668.
6. Scrimshaw, 1991.
7. R. Yip, The interaction of lead and iron, in *Dietary Iron: Birth to Two Years*, ed. L. J. Filer (New York: Raven Press, 1989), pp. 179–181.
8. Getting the lead out, *Science News* 132 (1987): 269.
9. H. Needleman and coauthors, The long-term effects of exposure to low doses of lead in childhood: An 11-year follow-up report, *New England Journal of Medicine* 322 (1990): 83–88.
10. J. Murphy, Federal agencies gearing up for new efforts against lead, *Nation's Health*, May/June 1991, pp. 1, 23.
11. A. Greeley, Getting the lead out of just about everything, *FDA Consumer*, July/August 1991, pp. 27–31.
12. Murphy, 1991.
13. Greeley, 1991.

14. J. Raloff, Lead effects show in child's balance, *Science News* 135 (1989): 54.

15. Childhood lead poisoning: A disease for the history texts (editorial), *American Journal of Public Health* 81 (1991): 685.

16. Breakfast of little champions, *Tufts University Diet and Nutrition Letter,* May 1989, pp. 7–8.

17. S. A. Bock, The natural history of adverse reactions to food in young children. Address presented at the 70th Annual Meeting of the American Dietetic Association, Atlanta, Ga., 19 October 1987; Adverse reactions to food in young children, *Nutrition and the M.D.,* September 1988, p. 4.

18. A. Lake, Food allergy, in *Pediatric Nutrition: Theory and Practice,* eds. R. J. Grand, Jr., J. L. Sutphen, and W. H. Dietz, Jr., (Boston: Butterworths, 1987), pp. 615–625.

19. Questions readers ask, *Nutrition and the M.D.,* August 1987, pp. 5.

20. R. H. Buckley and D. D. Metcalfe, Food allergy, *Journal of the American Medical Association* 248 (1982): 2627–2631; D. D. Metcalfe, Diseases of food hypersensitivity, *New England Journal of Medicine* 321 (1989): 255–257.

21. Metcalfe, 1989.

22. Hyperactivity, latest news, *Health Gazette,* January 1991, p. 3.

23. M. L. Arbeit and coauthors, Caffeine intakes of children from a biracial population: The Bogalusa Heart Study, *Journal of the American Dietetic Association* 88 (1988): 466–471.

24. L. L. Birch, D. W. Marlin, and J. Rotter, Eating the "means" activity in contingency: Effects on young children's food preference, *Child Development* 55 (1984): 431–439.

25. E. Satter, *How to Get Your Kid to Eat . . . But Not Too Much* (Palo Alto, Calif.: Bull Publishing, 1987), 13–28.

26. P. E. McConnell, Good mornings begin with school breakfast, *Nutrition News* 52 (1989): 8.

27. McConnell, 1989.

28. L. E. Underwood, Normal adolescent growth and development, *Nutrition Today,* March/April 1991, pp. 11–16.

29. Underwood, 1991.

30. National Academy of Sciences, Food and Nutrition Board, Committee on Dietary Allowances, *Recommended Dietary Allowances,* 10th ed. (Washington, D.C.: National Academy Press, 1989), pp. 24–38.

31. J. B. Anderson, The status of adolescent nutrition, *Nutrition Today,* March/April 1991, pp. 7–10.

32. V. Matkovic, Diet, genetics, and peak bone mass of adolescent girls, *Nutrition Today,* March/April 1991, pp. 21–24.

33. Matkovic, 1991.

34. P. M. Guenther, Beverages in the diets of American teenagers, *Journal of the American Dietetic Association* 86 (1986): 493–499.

35. L. D. Johnston, P. M. O'Malley, and J. G. Bachman, Psychotherapeutic, licit, and illicit use of drugs among adolescents, *Journal of Adolescent Health Care* 8 (1987): 36–51.

36. American Council on Science and Health, *Cocaine: Facts and Dangers* (New York: American Council on Science and Health, 1990).

37. T. C. Wu and coauthors, Pulmonary hazards of smoking marijuana as compared with tobacco, *New England Journal of Medicine* 318 (1988): 347–351.

38. J. M. Jonas and M. S. Gold, Cocaine abuse and eating disorders, *Lancet* 1 (1986): 390–391.

39. M. A. Bozarth and R. A. Wise, Toxicity associated with long-term intravenous heroin and cocaine self-administration in the rat, *Journal of the American Medical Association* 254 (1985): 81–83.

40. American Council on Science and Health, 1990.

41. T. V. Ringer and coauthors, Beta-carotene's effects on serum lipoproteins and immunologic indices in humans, *American Journal of Clinical Nutrition* 53 (1991): 688–694.

42. M. E. Mohs, R. R. Watson, and T. Leonard-Green, Nutritional effects of marijuana, heroin, cocaine, and nicotine, *Journal of the American Dietetic Association* 90 (1990): 1261–1267.

43. A. F. Subar, L. C. Harlan, and M. E. Mattson, Food and nutrient intake differences between smokers and non-smokers in the US, *American Journal of Public Health* 80 (1990): 1323–1329.

44. G. Schectman, J. C. Byrd, and H. W. Gruchow, The influence of smoking on vitamin C status in adults, *American Journal of Public Health* 79 (1989): 158–162.

45. National Academy of Sciences, Food and Nutrition Board, Committee on Dietary Allowances, 1989, pp. 115–124.

12

Teenage Pregnancy

The nutrition implications of pregnancy are discussed in Chapter 11, where it is shown that the price a pregnant woman and her child pay for poor nutrition can be acute and long lasting. When the pregnant woman happens also to be a teenager, nutrient needs are greatly amplified, and malnutrition is more likely. Teenage pregnancy has been historically, and continues to be, a major public health problem in the United States. Pregnant teenagers have higher rates of miscarriages, premature births, stillbirths, and low-birthweight infants than do pregnant adult women.

Even when not pregnant, a teenage female is hard put to keep up with her own nutrient needs at this time of maximal growth. Nourishing a growing fetus adds to her burden. The teenager's own high nutrient requirements can compete with those of her fetus, especially if she is going through her most rapid growth phase. Adequate nutrition can substantially improve the course of events and the health of both mother and infant; it is an essential component of prenatal care.[1] This Nutrition in Practice discusses the special nutrient needs of pregnant teenagers.

Are there special recommendations for teenagers, then?

Yes. To support the needs of both mother and fetus, young teenagers (13 to 16 years old) are encouraged to strive for pregnancy weight gains at the upper end of the ranges recommended for pregnant women (see Chapter 11). For teens who enter pregnancy with a body mass index in the normal range, a pregnancy weight gain of about 35 pounds is recommended.[2] Those who gain between 30 and 35 pounds during pregnancy have significantly lower risks of delivering low-birthweight infants.[3] As discussed in Chapter 11, the smallest newborns are the ones most likely to sicken and die.

Is teenage pregnancy really a major public health concern? How common is it?

In 1985, more than 10,000 babies were born to girls under the age of 15. For young women between the ages of 15 and 19, there were more than 467,000 births.[4]

Do pregnant teenagers eat less well than other pregnant women?

Yes. The adequacy of many teen girls' diets is marginal anyway: they have irregular eating habits, often skipping meals or choosing foods of low nutrient density. As many as one-fifth of them skip breakfast, while many more eat nutrient-poor breakfasts.[5] As discussed in Chapter 11, many have iron deficiencies, and many have inadequate energy intakes.

When they become pregnant, their eating patterns do not change, according to research. One study showed the energy intakes of pregnant teenagers participating in the WIC program and receiving supplemental food to be substantially below the RDA.[6] Other research indicates that pregnant teens do make appropriate changes in dietary habits compared with nonpregnant teens, but that even so, their iron intakes lag behind recommended levels.[7]

What are the nutrient needs of pregnant teenagers?

Little information is available on their specific nutrient needs. For some nutrients, estimates are made by adding the increments of recommended nutrients of the pregnant adult woman to the RDA for nonpregnant females 15 to 18 years of age; for other nutrients, the RDA during pregnancy is set for all ages. Clearly, though, as Figure NP12-1 shows, their needs for many nutrients increase more than does their energy allowance.

If a young woman starts pregnancy already malnourished or lacks education, resources, and support, she

FIGURE NP12–1   **Nutrient Needs of Pregnant and Nonpregnant Teenage Girls Compared**

Most of the values derive from adding the increment of recommended nutrients for the pregnant adult woman to the RDA for females 15 to 18 years of age; the values for vitamin D, folate, calcium, phosphorus, and zinc are allowances for pregnant women of all ages. The nonpregnant teenager's nutrient recommendations are set at 100% RDA for females 15 to 18 years old.

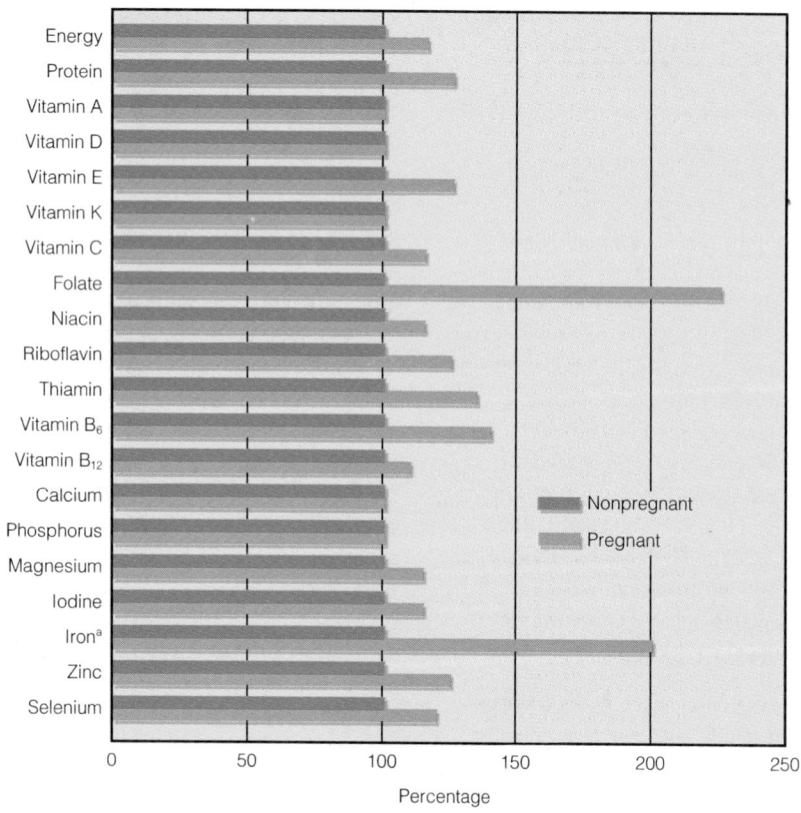

[a]Since the increased iron requirement cannot be met by typical diets or by iron stores, supplements are recommended.

TABLE NP12–1   **Nutrition-Related Risk Factors for Pregnant Adolescents**

- Low pregnancy weight gain.
- Low prepregnancy weight for height (or other evidence of malnutrition).
- Smoking.
- Young age at onset of pregnancy (less than 17 years of age).
- Excessive prepregnancy weight for height.
- Anemia.

Other Risk Factors Derived from History Information

- Unhealthy life-style (use of drugs or alcohol).
- Unfavorable reproductive history.
- Chronic diseases.
- History of eating disorders.

Source: Adapted from Nutrition management of adolescent pregnancy: Technical support paper, *Journal of the American Dietetic Association* 89 (1989): 104–109.

may encounter serious medical problems. Table NP12–1 lists nutrition-related risk factors for pregnant adolescents. Table NP12–2 provides a daily food guide for pregnant and lactating teenagers.

How can professionals persuade pregnant teens to eat better?

Counseling pregnant teenagers is a challenge. It is extremely important to establish rapport. Teenagers typically turn a deaf ear to lectures, but empathy and support can help them become willing to listen. Once the young woman feels comfortable enough to talk about herself, the counselor can use the information the client volunteers to employ nutrition counseling. For example, if she says she eats meals away from home, the counselor can provide tips on how to get the most nutrients for the money she spends. If she enjoys snacking, then she may welcome ideas for nutritious snacks. Whenever possible,

TABLE NP12-2   **Daily Food Guide for Pregnant and Lactating Teenagers**

	Number of Servings	
FOOD GROUP	TEENAGERS	PREGNANT OR LACTATING TEENAGERS
Meat and meat alternates	2 to 3	3
Milk and milk products	3	4
Vegetables	3 to 5	4 or more
Fruits	2 to 4	3 or ore
Breads and cereals	6 to 11	9 or more

she needs respect and support for whatever good judgment she is already exhibiting.

Among concrete items of advice acceptable to the teenager are these:

- Eat at least one serving every day of a vitamin C–rich food.
- Restrict soft drinks to one each day.
- Try a breakfast shake or snack made with milk, yogurt, and fruit.

Many different factors affect the outcome of adolescent pregnancy. Nutrition is a vital and modifiable factor that affects the health of mother and infant. The challenge for health professionals who counsel and monitor pregnant teenagers is to develop a rapport with their clients that encourages enthusiasm for nutrition and willingness to comply with sound diet advice.

Notes

1. Nutrition management of adolescent pregnancy (position of the American Dietetic Association), *Journal of the American Dietetic Association* 89 (1989): 104.
2. National Academy of Sciences, Food and Nutrition Board, *Nutrition during Pregnancy* (Washington, D.C.: National Academy Press, 1990), pp. 1–23.
3. M. L. Hediger and coauthors, Rate and amount of weight gain during adolescent pregnancy: Associations with maternal weight-for-height and birth weight, *American Journal of Clinical Nutrition* 52 (1990): 793–799.
4. National Center for Health Statistics: Advance report of final natality statistics, 1985, *Monthly Vital Statistics Report* 36, no. 4, July 17, 1987, as cited in Nutrition management of adolescent pregnancy: Technical support paper, *Journal of the American Dietetic Association* 89 (1989): 105–109.
5. Nutrition management of adolescent pregnancy: Technical support paper, *Journal of the American Dietetic Association* 89 (1989): 105–109.
6. J. Endres and coauthors, Older pregnant women and adolescents: Nutrition data after enrollment in WIC, *Journal of the American Dietetic Association* 87 (1987): 1011–1019.
7. J. D. Skinner and B. R. Carruth, Dietary quality of pregnant and nonpregnant adolescents, *Journal of the American Dietetic Association* 91 (1991): 718–720.

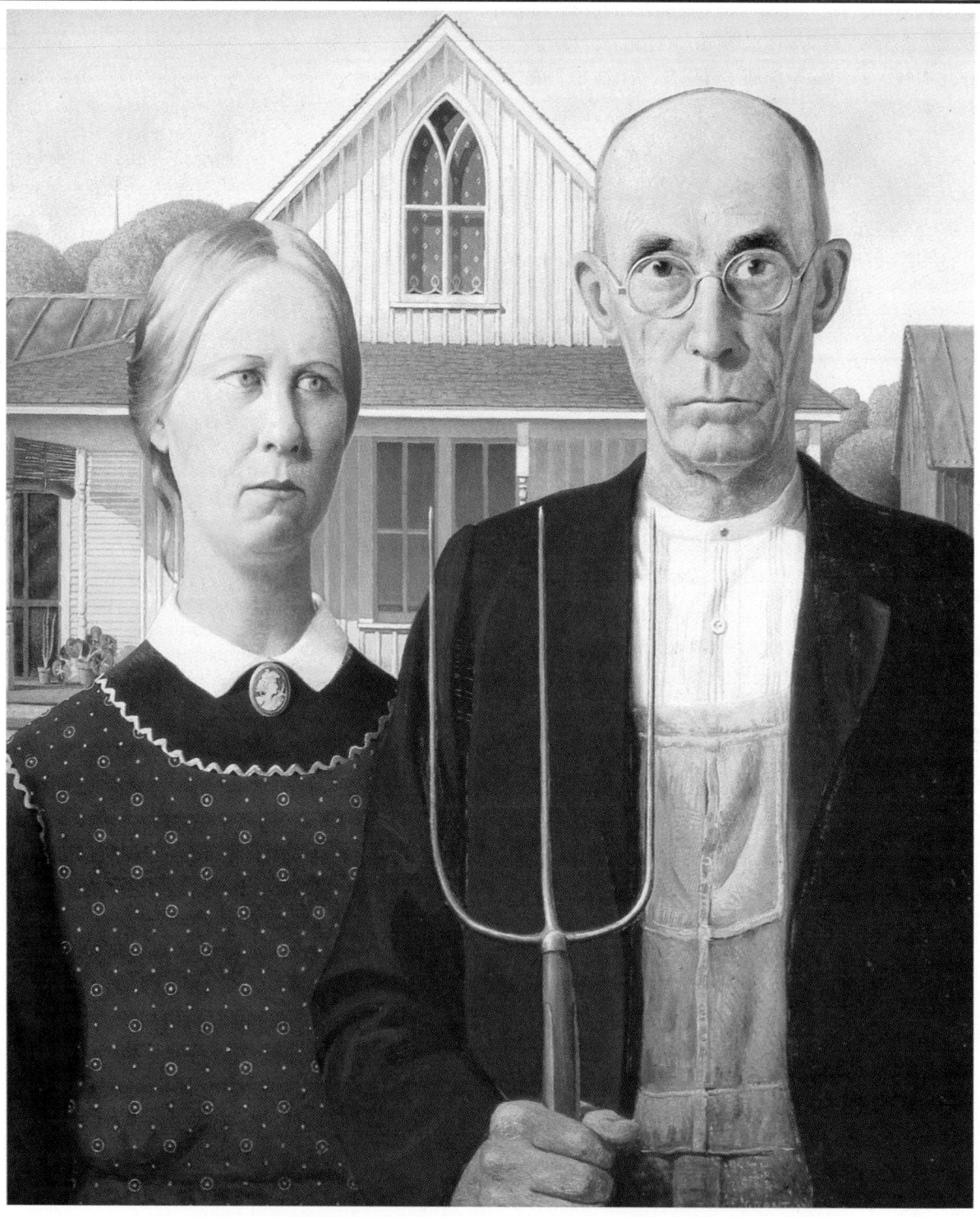

CHAPTER

13

Nutrition for Older Adults

CONTENTS

CHAPTER 13

After devoting ten chapters to adult nutrition, this book turned in the last two chapters to stages of the life cycle that require special nutrition attention: pregnancy, lactation, infancy, childhood, and adolescence. This chapter describes the special nutrition needs of the later adult years.

The most urgent nutrition need of older people, however, is to have made good food choices in the past! All of life's nutrition choices incur health consequences for the better or for the worse. A single day's intakes of nutrients may exert only a minute effect on body organs and their functions, but over years and decades their repeated effects accumulate to have major impacts. This being the case, it is of great importance for everyone, of every age, to pay close attention today to nutrition.

Aging and Nutrition

The majority of the U.S. population is now middle-aged, and the ratio of old people to young is growing steadily larger, as Figure 13–1 shows. The fastest-growing age group in the United States is people over 85.[1]

In 1983 in the United States, the life expectancy for women was 78 years and for men was 71 years, up from about 45 years in 1900. Advances in medical science—antibiotics and other treatments—are largely responsible for almost doubling the life expectancy in this century. Still, the biologic schedule that we call aging built into human beings cuts off life at a genetically fixed point in time. The life span (the maximum length of life possible for a species) of human beings— 115 years—has not changed over the years and is probably the upper limit of human longevity.

The study of the aging process in human beings is among the youngest of the scientific disciplines. It is only in this century that human beings have achieved a life expectancy worthy of a science devoted to studying it.[2] The idea that nutrition can influence the way human bodies age is particularly appealing, since it is one factor that people can control and change.

What has been learned so far about the effects of nutrition and environment on longevity provides incentive for researchers to keep asking questions about how and why human beings age. Among the questions they are asking are:

- To what extent is aging inevitable? Can aging be slowed through changes in lifestyle and environment?
- What roles does nutrition play in aging, and what roles can it play in retarding aging?

With respect to the first question, it seems that aging is an inevitable, natural process, programmed into the genes at conception, but that people can adopt lifestyle habits such as exercising and attention to work and recreational environments that will slow the process within the natural limits set by heredity. With respect to the second question, clearly, good nutrition can retard and ease the aging process in many significant ways.

One approach researchers use to gain insight into the prevention of aging has been to study other cultures in the hope of finding an extremely long-

life expectancy: the average number of years lived by people in a given society.

life span: the maximum number of years of life attainable by a member of a species.

longevity: long duration of life.

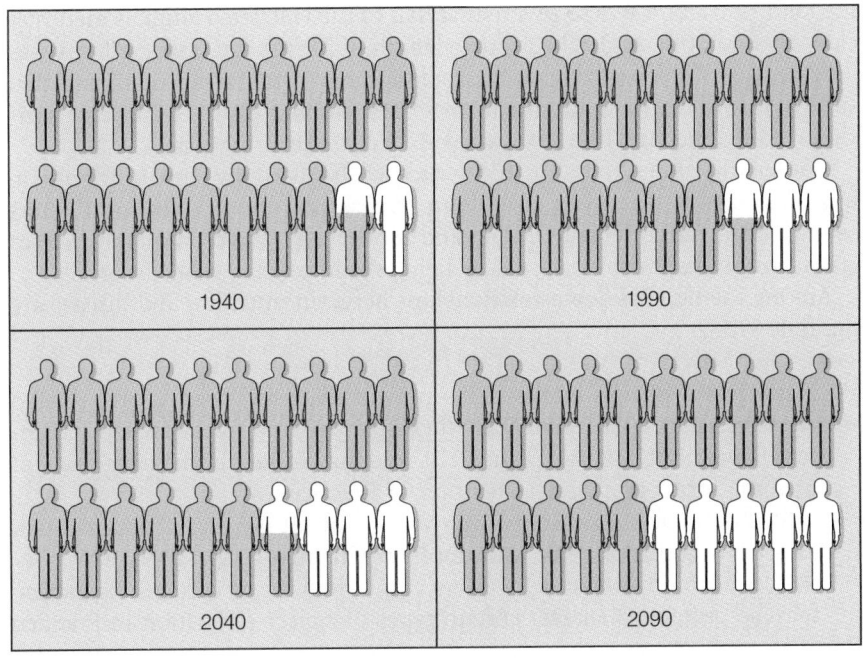

FIGURE 13–1   **The Aging of the U.S. Population (☖ = 65 Years or Older)** In 1940, 6.8% of the population was 65 or older. Today, 12.7% of us have reached age 65; by 2040, 21.7% will have reached age 65; and a century from now, nearly one out of four Americans will be 65 or older. An estimated 25,000 Americans now living are 100 years old or older.

Source: K. Flieger, Why do we age? *FDA Consumer*, October 1988, pp. 20–25.

lived race of people and then learning from them the secrets of long life. Scientists have found people who claimed to have lived over 100 years in two different geographical areas. Further study revealed, however, that some of these people only claimed to be 100 or older, because in their societies age was venerated. Still, some did prove to be not only remarkably old, but also remarkably healthy. The credit did not go to nutrition: these people did not eat according to any particular formula. The secret—the one thing they all seemed to have in common—was that they lived a physically active life, and they remained active into old age. Research on longevity bears this out in this society, too; vigorous exercise and long life seem to go together.[3] Even a moderate amount of physical activity—for example, a brisk 30-minute walk each day—is protective against early mortality.

Another approach to prevention of aging has been to try manipulating animals' diets and looking for effects on longevity. This has given rise to some interesting and suggestive findings.[4] For example, rats live longer when their food intake is restricted in the early weeks of their lives, or even when it is restricted after they are mature. Especially effective in lengthening rats' lives were drastic restrictions of their food intakes, and especially their fat intakes, during the growth period. In one experiment, animals allowed to eat freely lived to an average of 656 days, while those whose feed was restricted lived to an average of 949 days. In these experiments it was possible to study nutrition-induced growth retardation of various organ systems, and to speculate on the cause of the increased length of life of some of the animals—a delay in the onset of certain diseases, for example.

Experiments with food restriction and longevity in rats has *not* suggested any direct applications to human nutrition, though, and there have been distinct disadvantages to the animals given restricted feedings. For example, the food restriction was so severe that half of the restricted animals died *very* early (before 300 days). The average length of life for the restricted rats was long because the few survivors lived a long time. The restricted animals that survived were retarded and malformed in a number of ways. Extreme starvation to extend life, like any extreme, is not worth the price.

One of the ways that nutrition clearly affects aging and longevity in human beings is by way of its role in disease prevention. Nutrition alone, even if ideal, cannot ensure a long and robust life. However, many diseases are nutrition responsive, as well as being responsive to other factors.

Among the better-known relationships between nutrition and disease are the following:

- Appropriate energy intake helps prevent *diabetes, obesity,* and related *cardiovascular diseases* such as atherosclerosis and hypertension (Chapter 19 and Nutrition in Practice 22), and may influence the development of some forms of *cancer* (Nutrition in Practice 18).
- Adequate intakes of essential nutrients prevent *deficiency diseases* such as scurvy, goiter, anemia, and the like (Chapters 7 and 8).
- Variety in food intake, as well as ample intakes of certain vegetables, may be protective against certain types of *cancer* (Nutrition in Practice 18).
- Moderation in sugar intake helps prevent *dental caries* (Nutrition in Practice 2).
- Appropriate fiber intakes help prevent malfunctions of the digestive tract such as *constipation, diverticulosis,* and possibly *colon cancer* (Chapter 2).
- Moderate sodium and adequate intakes of potassium, calcium, and other minerals help prevent *hypertension,* at least in people who are genetically predisposed to it (Chapter 8 and Nutrition in Practice 22).
- Adequate calcium intake throughout life helps protect against *osteoporosis.*

Other, less well established links between nutrition and disease are being discovered each day. For example, research efforts to uncover clues about the relationship between nutrition and immunity become more and more urgent as AIDS takes its toll on human life.

The question whether nutrition is related to cataracts is under investigation. Cataracts are age-related changes in the lens of the eye, thickenings of the lenses that impair vision and can lead to blindness if not surgically removed. Cataracts occur even in well-nourished individuals due to injury, viral infections, toxic substances, and genetic disorders, but most cataracts are vaguely called senile cataracts—meaning "caused by aging." Close to 400,000 new cases of age-related cataracts occur in the United States each year.[5] Scientists have searched for possible roles of nutrient deficiencies, excesses, and imbalances in cataract causation. They have observed several possible (and, it should be emphasized, highly tentative) links: to sugar (galactose derived from lactose) excess; to excess food energy intake (in people with diabetes); and to deficiencies of the vitamins riboflavin, vitamin C, or vitamin E.

Arthritis, another disease that disables the elderly, is also suspected to have some relationships to nutrition. Arthritis is a painful swelling of the

arthritis: a usually painful inflammation of a joint caused by many conditions, including infections, metabolic disturbances, or injury; joint structure is usually altered, with loss of function.

joints that troubles many people as they grow older. During movement, the normal ends of bones are protected from wear by cartilage and by small sacs of fluid that act as a lubricant; but with age, bones sometimes disintegrate, and the joints become malformed and painful to move. The cause of arthritis is unknown, but it afflicts millions around the world and is a major problem of older adults.

Unfortunately, much nutrition quackery surrounds arthritis, making it difficult to ferret out whatever valid relationships to nutrition may exist. Many bizarre diets advertise themselves as arthritis cures. Two or three new popular books on diet for arthritis come out every year, urging people to eat no meat, or drink no milk, or eat all their foods raw, or eat only "natural" foods, or avoid all additives, or—who knows what will be next? Actually no known diet prevents, relieves, or cures arthritis, but as long as people keep buying the books that make these claims, the law of supply and demand dictates that such books will keep coming out.[6]

One possible link between arthritis and diet is through the immune system. Researchers believe that in one type of arthritis (rheumatoid arthritis), the immune system mistakenly attacks the tissues of the bone coverings as it normally would an invader.[7] The integrity of the immune system depends on adequate nutrition, and a poor diet probably worsens the condition. It is also possible that for some individuals, certain foods may stimulate the immune system to attack.[8] For example, milk and milk products seem to bring on symptoms of arthritis in some people.

Another nutrient link to arthritis is the now-famous fatty acid found in fish oil, EPA. Chapter 3 showed the links between EPA and heart health. Research shows, too, that the same diet recommended there—one low in saturated fat from red meats and dairy products and high in fish oil—can reduce the suffering of people with arthritis after three months of use.[9] The seemingly all-purpose low-fat diet with EPA added may prevent the inflammation in the joints that makes arthritis so painful. Researchers theorize that EPA probably interferes with the action of prostaglandins, chemicals involved in the inflammatory responses of body tissues.

A known connection between arthritis and nutrition exists in overweight persons. Weight loss is important for these people, because the joints affected are often weight-bearing joints that are stressed and irritated by having to carry excess poundage. Weight-loss diets alone often relieve the worst of the pain in arthritis clients. Interestingly, though, weight loss often helps relieve arthritis in the hands, which are not weight bearing; perhaps the drastic reduction in fat intake that accompanies the adoption of a kcalorie-restricted diet contributes to arthritis relief, with or without EPA added.

Still another nutrition connection with arthritis is through the drugs that are commonly used to relieve its symptoms. Some drugs may affect nutrient availability and require attention to nutrition status when used over long times.

These brief discussions of cataracts and arthritis could be multiplied manyfold, both to provide further details and to add other diseases, but they have sufficed to show that nutrition can provide at least some protection against certain diseases commonly associated with aging. In fact, in general, it is beginning to look as if nutrition through the prime years may play a greater role than has been realized in preventing many changes once thought to be inevitable consequences of growing older.

Not effective against arthritis:

- Alfalfa.
- Blackstrap molasses.
- Calcium.
- Cod liver oil.
- Fruit.
- Garlic.
- Honey.
- Lecithin.
- Vitamin megadoses.
- Wheat germ oil.
- Yeast.
- 100 other substances.

Nutrient Needs and Nutrition Status of Older Adults

Because old age is a relatively new phenomenon, and because the ranks of senior citizens have only recently been growing larger, scientists are only now working out the nutrient needs of the elderly. So far, there are no RDA for older age groups—everyone over 50 is grouped together, even though people's needs change as their bodies age. Clearly, the need for standards is becoming more and more urgent as the bulk of the population ages.

A problem attending the setting of standards for all groups, and especially for older people, is that their differences become more and more marked as they grow older. One person may tend to omit vegetables from his diet, and by the time he is old he will have an associated set of nutrition problems. Another may have omitted milk and milk products all her life—her nutrition problems will be different. Also, as people age, their individual health histories affect their nutrient needs: they will have suffered different diseases with different impacts. On top of all this, people start out with different genetic predispositions to faulty nutrient absorption, and the effects of these become magnified as the years go by. Still, some generalizations are valid, and until an improved version of the RDA exists, the present RDA for adults is useful. The next sections give special attention to a few nutrients of concern.

Water

Water recommendation for adults: 1 to 1½ oz/kg actual body weight.

A large percentage of nursing home operators note that one of the biggest problems with their elderly clients is getting them to drink more water and fruit juices. Dehydration is a risk for older adults, who may not notice or pay attention to their thirst, or who are unable to obtain water because of immobility. Research shows that older adults seem to have reduced thirst. In one study, despite fluid deprivation and obvious physiological need, older adults did not get thirsty or experience mouth dryness.[10] Another factor predisposing older adults to fluid imbalance is a decrease in total body water as people age. Even mild stress such as fever or hot climate can precipitate rapid dehydration in older adults.[11] Chapter 8 described the importance of water. An intake of six to eight glasses of water a day is recommended, enough to bring urine output to about 6 cups per day.

Energy and Energy-Yielding Nutrients

Energy needs decline with advancing age. For one thing, lean body mass diminishes as people age, resulting in a lower basal metabolic rate. For another, as people age, they usually reduce their physical activity (although they need not do so). The lower energy expenditures of older adults mean that they require less food energy to maintain their weight. Accordingly, the energy RDA for men and women decrease slightly starting at age 51.[12]

On such limited energy allowances, people must make sure that nearly all foods they eat are nutrient dense. There is little leeway for such low-nutrient-density foods as sugars, fats, oils, or alcohol. Because overweight is well recognized as a shortener of the life span, these seem to be life-

TABLE 13-1   **Daily Food Plan for Older Adults**

2 to 3 two-ounce servings of protein-rich food (lean meat, poultry, fish, eggs, dried
    beans and peas, nuts)

2 to 4 half-cup servings of milk, cheese, or yogurt[a]

6 or more servings of whole-grain breads or cereals

2 to 4 half-cup servings of fruits

3 to 5 half-cup servings of vegetables

[a]Women should aim for 4 servings of milk, cheese, or yogurt.
Source: Adapted from A. Greeley, Nutrition and the Elderly, *FDA Consumer*, October 1990, pp. 25–28.

sustaining recommendations. Table 13–1 offers a daily dietary framework
for older adults. Those who need additional food energy should choose
extra servings from the groups of listed foods.[13]

The many and remarkable benefits of regular physical activity are not
limited to the young. Activities of all kinds are recommended for older
adults to maintain and promote health. Ideally, exercise should be part of
each day's schedule, and should be intense enough to prevent muscle atrophy and to increase the heartbeat and respiration rate for at least 20 minutes.
Many older persons believe that they can't participate in strenuous exercise,
but studies show that they can do more than they think they can. Any
exercise—even a ten-minute walk a day—is better than none, and with
persistence, people can achieve great improvements at any age. Training not
only tones, firms, and strengthens muscles but also increases the blood flow
to the brain. Another reason to exercise: a person spending energy in physical activity can afford to eat more food, and with it, more nutrients.

PROTEIN. The protein needs of older adults appear to be about the same as,
or even greater than, those of younger people. Since energy needs decrease,
however, the protein has to be obtained from low-kcalorie sources of high-
quality protein. Foods such as lean meats, poultry, and fish; nonfat milk; and
low-fat cottage cheese are examples of protein-rich, low-kcalorie foods.

CARBOHYDRATE. Abundant carbohydrate is needed to protect protein from
being used as energy. Complex carbohydrate foods such as vegetables,
whole grains, and fruits are also rich in fiber and essential vitamins and
minerals.

High-fiber foods can alleviate constipation—a condition prevalent among
older adults, and especially among nursing home residents.[14] Some older
adults eat diets lacking in fiber, but one group of researchers has found that
the fiber intakes of the older adults they studied were not as low as they
expected.[15] The researchers compared independent-living older adults and
nursing home residents, and discovered that their fiber intakes were similar
(18 grams per day) and were comparable to the fiber contents of other
typical adult diets. Physical inactivity and medication use among nursing
home residents probably contributes to their high incidence of constipation,
but fiber lack probably does, too, in many cases. In fact, everyone's fiber

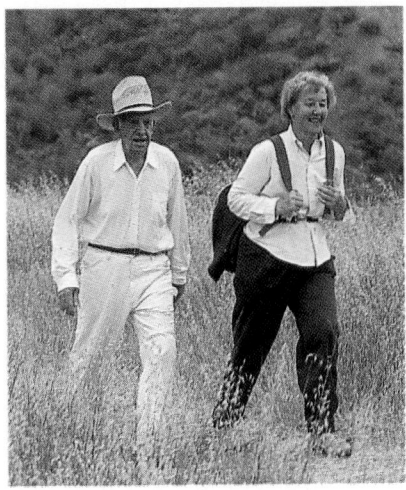

*Physical activity promotes health at any
age.*

Fiber is discussed in more detail in Chapter 2.

intakes are lower, on average, than current recommendations (20 to 35 grams).

A reminder for those who care for older adults in nursing homes is important here: notice who does, and who does not, need added fiber, for both extremes are always present. It has been estimated that as many as 50 percent of nursing home residents may be malnourished and underweight. For these people, a diet that emphasizes fiber-rich foods such as whole grains, fruits, and vegetables may be inappropriate because it is low in concentrated protein and energy.[16] Protein- and energy-dense snacks such as hard-boiled eggs, tuna fish and crackers, peanut butter on graham crackers, and homemade soups are valuable additions to the diets of underweight or malnourished older adults.

FAT. As is true for people of all ages, fat needs to be limited in the diet of most older adults, for many reasons. Cutting fat helps cut kcalories and may also help retard the development of cancer, atherosclerosis, and other degenerative diseases. It is a challenge for older adults to restrict their fat intakes to less than 30 percent of their total energy, when they are on limited energy intakes.

Vitamins

The roles of specific vitamins in disease prevention and development and the age-related physiological changes that affect vitamin metabolism are unclear. Until more is known, vitamin recommendations for older adults remain the same as for younger adults. Vitamins A and D illustrate why research focusing on the vitamin needs of older adults deserves attention.

Vitamin A stands alone in that there is an apparent *increase* in its absorption with aging.[17] When the vitamin A intake and plasma retinol concentrations of healthy older adults and young adults were compared, the older people had higher mean plasma vitamin A concentrations despite little difference in dietary intake between the two groups.[18] This research supports a proposal that has been advanced that the RDA for vitamin A should be lowered, but research into the role of the vitamin A precursor beta-carotene in preventing cancer should perhaps be considered before any final decisions are made.

Older adults face a greater risk of vitamin D deficiency than younger people do. Many older adults drink little or no milk.[19] Only vitamin D–fortified milk provides significant amounts of vitamin D. Many older adults have vitamin D intakes of less than half of the RDA.[20] Further compromising the vitamin D status of many older people is their limited exposure to sunlight, especially among those in nursing homes. Finally, the potential for vitamin D deficiency in older people is favored by age-related changes in vitamin D synthesis and metabolism.[21]

Adequate vitamin intakes can be ensured by including foods from all food groups. Studies have shown that older adults often omit vegetables and fruits.[22] About 18 percent of older people are reported to eat no vegetables at all, and up to one of every three older people reports never eating fruit. When almost 500 participants in a meal program were surveyed about their food likes and dislikes, nine of the top ten most-disliked foods were vegetables, which are often overcooked or canned in such programs.[23] Some older adults eat no whole-grain breads and cereals, a significant source of many B vitamins.

Minerals

Among the minerals, iron deserves first mention. Iron-deficiency anemia is not as common in older adults as it is in younger people, but it still occurs in some, especially those with low food energy intakes. Aside from diet, other factors in many older people's lives increase the likelihood of iron deficiency:

- Chronic blood loss from ulcers, hemorrhoids, or other disease conditions.
- Poor iron absorption due to reduced stomach acid secretion.
- Antacid use, which interferes with iron absorption.
- Use of medicines that cause blood loss, including anticoagulants, aspirin, and other arthritis medicines.

Anyone concerned with the nutrition status of an older person should not forget these possibilities.

Zinc deficiencies are common in older people. As many as 95 percent of older adults may not get the zinc they need, and many miss the mark by more than half.[24] It is possible that improved absorption compensates for low zinc intakes, but this has not been confirmed. Some research suggests that older adults absorb zinc less efficiently than younger people do.[25] A number of different factors can impair zinc absorption or enhance its excretion and thus lead to deficiency. Chronic malabsorption diseases such as Crohn's disease impair zinc absorption. Alcohol consumption and stresses such as surgery and burns increase zinc excretion. Many medications that older adults use, both prescription and over-the-counter, either impair zinc absorption or increase excretion.[26] Older adults who do not make special efforts to eat zinc-rich foods such as meats, fish, and poultry will no doubt fail to meet the RDA for this nutrient.

It is interesting to note that some symptoms of zinc deficiency resemble symptoms associated with aging—for example, a decline in taste acuity and dermatitis. However, it remains unclear whether the decline in taste acuity or the dermatitis associated with aging can be attributed to zinc deficiency.[27]

The importance of abundant dietary calcium throughout life, especially for women after menopause, to protect against osteoporosis was discussed in Chapter 8. Controversy surrounds the question of what the appropriate calcium intake for older adults is. Some researchers argue that current recommendations are too low for postmenopausal women.[28] The Committee on RDA contends that evidence is insufficient to warrant revising the calcium RDA upward for older women.[29]

While researchers attempt to reach agreement about the calcium requirements of older adults, especially those of women, one aspect of calcium nutrition is not controversial—calcium intakes of many people, especially women, in the United States are well below the RDA. If fresh milk causes stomach discomfort, as some older people report, then they should include some cheese in their diets. Dry nonfat milk can be incorporated into many foods.

The determination of mineral requirements for older adults poses many challenges for researchers. Food composition tables fail to include some of the trace minerals. The accuracy of dietary intake studies is hindered when the amounts of certain nutrients present in foods are unknown. Interactions of minerals with other nutrients and drugs affect the bioavailability of the minerals, complicating the process still further. When age-related metabolic changes and disease conditions are superimposed on these problems, the task of determining mineral requirements for older people becomes increasingly difficult, but it is not impossible. The ever-growing number of older people in the world creates an urgency to know more about how their nutrient needs differ from those of younger people, and how such knowledge can enhance their health. In the meantime, people judge for themselves how to manage their nutrition, and some turn to supplements.

Supplements for Older Adults

Advertisers target older people with their appeals to take supplements and eat "health foods," claiming that these products prevent disease and promote longevity. Despite this, and much to their credit, older adults are, for the most part, reasonable in their approaches to so-called health foods—most avoid health food stores, or buy less there than others do.

Older adults are not always so reasonable, however, in their approaches to supplement use. A study in a California retirement community showed that 72 percent of those surveyed were taking supplements—mostly vitamins C and E—but that these choices were not related to the users' dietary intakes.[30] The vitamins they were taking were not the ones they may have needed. Furthermore, some of the older people in this study consumed toxic levels of vitamin A (more than 25,000 IU per day) and more than ten times the RDA of vitamins C and E. One study found that supplement use correlated with medical problems and living alone.[31] Certain diseases or health problems may necessitate the taking of supplements, but in this study the vitamins taken had not been prescribed by a health care professional and were often inappropriate.

Can supplements meet the needs of older people? The answer is sometimes, depending on the nutrient being supplemented. For instance, calcium supplements for osteoporosis or iron for anemia, when recommended by a health care professional, may be beneficial. In most cases, though, the money people spend on supplements would be better spent on nutritious foods.

Older adults with food energy intakes less than about 1,500 kcalories should probably take vitamin-mineral supplements—not megavitamins, but just the once-daily type of supplements. Many older adults fall into this category and should take this precaution. Physically active older adults whose energy needs remain high are an exception.

A better choice than supplements for people with small energy allowances, however, would be to become more active and earn the right to eat more food. Food is the best source of nutrients for everybody. Supplements are just that—supplements to foods, not substitutes for them. For anyone who is motivated to obtain the best possible health, it is never too late to

TABLE 13-2   **Health Checklist for Older Adults**

- Drink water—6 to 8 glasses each day.
- Choose nutrient-dense foods—fresh fruits and vegetables; whole-grain breads and cereals; lean meats, poultry, fish, and legumes; and low-fat milk and milk products.
- Go outside for sunshine and fresh air as often as possible.
- Be physically active. Walk, run, dance, swim, bike, row, or climb for aerobic activity. Lift weights, do calisthenics, or pursue some other activity to tone, firm, and strengthen muscles.
- Limit or avoid alcohol and caffeine.
- Use drugs only as prescribed.
- Do not smoke. If you do smoke, quit.
- Be socially active—play bridge, join an exercise group, take a class, teach a class, invite friends to eat with you, or volunteer your time to help others.
- Stay interested in life—pursue a hobby, spend time with your grandchildren, take a trip, read, grow a garden, or go to the movies.
- Enjoy life.

learn to eat well, exercise regularly, and adopt other lifestyle changes to facilitate the achievement of that goal, such as quitting smoking, moderating alcohol use, and the like. Table 13–2 offers a health checklist for older adults.

The Effects of Drugs on Nutrients

As people grow older, illnesses tend to set in, and the use of medicines—from over-the-counter (OTC) types such as aspirin and laxatives to prescription drugs of all kinds—becomes commonplace. Most drugs interact with one or more nutrients in several ways, usually resulting in greater-than-normal needs for these nutrients.

The most common drug that can affect nutrition in older people is alcohol. A recent estimate sets the incidence of alcoholism in people over 60 in our society at 2 to 10 percent. The effects of alcohol on a person of any age are explained in Nutrition in Practice 6.

Over-the-counter (OTC) drugs are readily available and can be harmful to nutrition. These drugs are useful aids in the self-treatment of minor conditions, but they can easily be misused. For example, a person who uses laxatives daily for a long time may find that the intestines can no longer function without them. This dependence can lead to malnutrition. Laxatives cause foods to move rapidly through the intestine, so that many vitamins have too little time to be absorbed. The use of mineral oil as a laxative robs the person of the fat-soluble vitamins, including vitamin D. The vitamins dissolve in the indigestible oil and are excreted; calcium, too, is excreted. Antacids also have nutrition effects. A person who takes Alka-Seltzer may not realize it, but it is loaded with sodium—a single 2-tablet dose exceeds some people's safe sodium intakes for a whole day. Another antacid (Tums) makes claims to supplement calcium to the diet, but its action as a drug makes it unsuitable for this purpose. It neutralizes stomach acid, on which the absorption of many nutrients (possibly including calcium itself) depends. Taking Tums or any other antacid regularly will cause the body to excrete many nutrients as wastes, rather than absorb them.

Older people use more medications than any other age group. They often take multiple drugs simultaneously and need to be particularly aware of the nutrition consequences.

Food Choices and Eating Habits of Older Adults

Strategies and interventions to improve people's nutrition status must be based on knowledge of their food preferences and eating patterns to afford any benefit. Menus and feeding programs for older adults must take into consideration the food likes and dislikes, as well as the living conditions, economic status, and medical conditions, of this diverse group of people. It is essential to know what foods older adults prefer, in what settings they like to eat these foods, and whether they can buy and prepare meals, if nutrition intervention is to be successful.

Many factors affect food choices, eating habits, and the nutrition status of older adults. Information about specific subgroups of older people is lacking, making it difficult to interpret existing research. For instance, nutrition surveys do not always differentiate among older people living alone, those living with others, and those in institutions. Research shows that these factors make significant differences in the food practices of older adults.[32] In one study, work experience, education, housing (federally funded versus privately owned), and gender influenced food intake.[33] The results indicated that older adults most likely to be malnourished were women, those with the least education, those living alone in federally funded housing, and those who had recently experienced changes in lifestyle. In a different study, more men living alone ate poor-quality diets than those living with spouses.[34] In general, however, this same study showed more women than men to have poor-quality diets. The results indicate that older adults who live alone do not make poorer food choices than those who live with a companion, but rather that they consume fewer kcalories. Different subgroups of the aging population therefore appear to need programs designed to meet different specific nutrient deficiencies.

Results of national surveys give some indication of the food likes of older adults. It seems that older adults prefer low-fat milk and cheese from the milk group; grapefruit and melon among the fruits; potatoes and tomatoes from the vegetable group; bread, biscuits, and muffins from the grain group; and ground beef from the meats.[35]

Knowledge about the kinds of foods older people prefer and the reasons why they select or reject foods can be used to develop nutrition intervention programs and acceptable food products. Most older people are independent, productive, health-conscious consumers who know what they want from the foods they purchase. Older people spend more money per person on

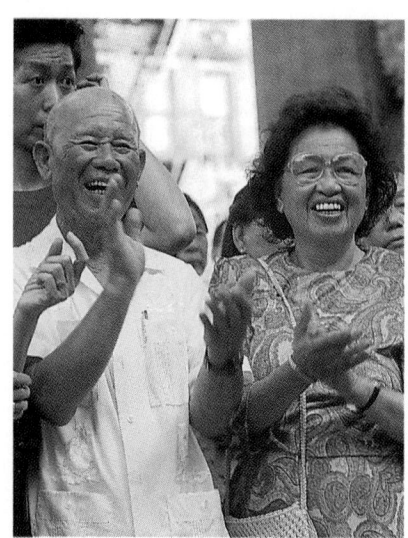

Spending time with friends adds enjoyment to life.

food they eat at home than other age groups and less money on food away from home. Manufacturers would be wise to cater to the preferences of older adults by providing good-tasting, nutritious foods in easy-to-open, single-serving packages with labels that are easy to read.

Researchers studying nutrition and aging are challenged by the physiological and psychosocial diversity of older adults. Many of the health problems older adults experience are presently attributed to normal, age-related processes, perhaps to the point of exaggeration.[36] Research that focuses on how nutrition and other life factors affect aging and disease processes is vital to ensuring that more and more people can look forward to long, healthy lives.

CASE STUDY

Elderly Man with a Poor Diet

Mr. Hawkins is a 75-year-old man who lives alone. He has been losing weight slowly since he lost his wife a year ago. At 5 feet 8 inches tall, he currently weighs 135 pounds. His previous weight was 150 pounds. In talking with Mr. Hawkins, you realize that he doesn't even like to talk about food, let alone eat it. "My wife always did the cooking before, and I ate well. Now I just don't feel like eating." You manage to find out that he skips breakfast, has soup and bread for lunch, and sometimes eats a cold-cut sandwich or a TV dinner for supper. He seldom sees friends or relatives. Mr. Hawkins has also lost several teeth and doesn't eat any raw fruits or vegetables, which he feels are hard to chew. He lives on a meager but adequate income.

1. What percent is Mr. Hawkins's weight in relationship to the ideal body weight of a 75-year-old man of his size (%IBW)? What is his percent usual body weight (%UBW)? Is his weight loss significant? What factors are contributing to his poor food intake? What nutrients are probably deficient in his diet?
2. Look at Mr. Hawkins as an individual. Suggest ways he can improve his diet that fit his lifestyle. What other aspects of Mr. Hawkins's physical and mental health should you consider in helping him to improve his food intake?

Study Questions

1. What roles does nutrition play in aging, and what roles can it play in retarding aging?
2. Name some factors that complicate the task of setting nutrient standards for older adults.
3. Why does the risk of dehydration increase as people age?
4. Why do energy needs usually decline with advancing age?
5. Why is the risk of vitamin D deficiency greater among older adults than younger adults?

Notes

1. R. Chernoff, Demographics of aging, in *Geriatric Nutrition: The Health Professional's Handbook,* ed. R. Chernoff (Gaithersburg, Md.: Aspen Publishers, 1991), pp. 1–9.
2. E. L. Schneider and J. D. Reed, Life extension, *New England Journal of Medicine* 312 (1985): 1159–1168.
3. R. S. Paffenbarger and coauthors, Physical activity, all-cause mortality, and longevity of college alumni, *New England Journal of Medicine* 314 (1986): 605–613; S. N. Blair and coauthors, Physical fitness and all-cause mortality, *Journal of the American Medical Association* 262 (1989): 2395–2401.
4. Curtailing calories may lengthen life, *FDA Consumer,* February 1989, pp. 3–4; E. J. Masoro, Food restriction in rodents: An evaluation of its role in the study of aging, *Journal of Gerontology* 43 (1988): B59–B64.
5. G. E. Burce and J. L. Hess, Cataract—What is the role of nutrition in lens health? *Nutrition Today,* December 1988, pp. 6–8.
6. P. G. Wolman, Management of patients using unproven regimens for arthritis, *Journal of the American Dietetic Association* 87 (1987): 1211–1214.
7. E. D. Harris, Rheumatoid arthritis: Pathophysiology and implications for therapy, *New England Journal of Medicine* 322 (1990): 1277–1289.
8. Rheumatoid arthritis and food, *Health Gazette,* February 1989, p. 3.
9. J. M. Kremer and coauthors, Fish-oil fatty acid supplementation in active rheumatoid arthritis: A double-blind, controlled crossover study, *Annals of Internal Medicine* 106 (1987): 497–503.
10. B. J. Rolls and P. A. Phillips, Aging and disturbances of thirst and fluid balance, *Nutrition Reviews* 48 (1990): 137–144.
11. R. Chernoff, Physiologic aging and nutritional status, *Nutrition in Clinical Practice,* February 1990, pp. 5–8.
12. National Academy of Sciences, Food and Nutrition Board, *Recommended Dietary Allowances,* 10th ed. (Washington, D.C.: National Academy of Sciences, 1989).
13. A. Greeley, Nutrition and the elderly, *FDA Consumer,* October 1990, pp. 25–28.
14. E. J. Johnson and coauthors, Dietary fiber intakes of nursing home residents and independent-living older adults, *American Journal of Clinical Nutrition* 48 (1988): 159–164.
15. Johnson and coauthors, 1988.
16. R. Andres and J. Hallfrisch, Nutrient intake recommendations for the older American, *Journal of the American Dietetic Association* 89 (1989): 1739–1741.
17. Processing of dietary retinoids is slowed in the elderly, *Nutrition Reviews* 49 (1991): 116–118.
18. P. J. Garry and coauthors, Vitamin A intake and plasma retinol levels in healthy elderly men and women, *American Journal of Clinical Nutrition* 46 (1987): 989–994.
19. Chernoff, 1990.
20. E. E. Delvin, A. Imbach, and M. Copti, Vitamin D nutritional status and related biochemical indices in an autonomous elderly population, *American Journal of Clinical Nutrition* 48 (1988): 373–378; H. Payette and K. Gray-Donald, Dietary intake and biochemical indices of nutritional status

in an elderly population with estimates of the precision of the 7-day food record, *American Journal of Clinical Nutrition* 54 (1991): 478–488.

21. Chernoff, 1990.

22. V. Holt, J. Nordstrom, and M. B. Kohrs, Food preferences of older adults (abstract), *Journal of the American Dietetic Association* 87 (1987): 1597.

23. Holt, Nordstrom, and Kohrs, 1987.

24. C. A. Swanson and coauthors, Zinc status of elderly adults: Response to supplement, *American Journal of Clinical Nutrition* 48 (1988): 343–349.

25. R. J. Cousins and J. M. Hempe, Zinc, in *Present Knowledge in Nutrition,* 6th ed., ed. M. L. Brown (Washington, D.C.: International Life Science Institute, 1990), pp. 251–260.

26. G. J. Fosmire, Trace mineral requirements, in *Geriatric Nutrition: The Health Professional's Handbook,* ed. R. Chernoff (Gaithersburg, Md.: Aspen Publishers, 1991), pp. 77–105.

27. Fosmire, 1991.

28. H. Spencer, Minerals and mineral interactions in human nutrition, *Journal of the American Dietetic Association* 86 (1986): 864–867.

29. National Academy of Sciences, Food and Nutrition Board, 1989, pp. 174–184.

30. G. E. Gray and coauthors, Vitamin supplement use in a Southern California retirement community, *Journal of the American Dietetic Association* 86 (1986): 800–802.

31. B. S. Ranno, G. M. Wardlaw, and C. J. Geiger, What characterizes elderly women who overuse vitamin and mineral supplements? *Journal of the American Dietetic Association* 88 (1988): 347–348.

32. J. V. White and coauthors, Consensus of the Nutrition Screening Initiative: Risk factors and indicators of poor nutritional status in older Americans, *Journal of the American Dietetic Association* 91 (1991): 783–787.

33. P. O'Hanlon and coauthors, Socioeconomic factors and dietary intake of elderly Missourians, *Journal of the American Dietetic Association* 82 (1983): 646–653.

34. M. A. Davis and coauthors, Living arrangements and dietary quality of older U.S. adults, *Journal of the American Dietetic Association* 90 (1990): 1667–1672.

35. A. Sorenson, N. Chapman, and D. N. Sundwall, Health promotion and disease prevention in the elderly, in *Geriatric Nutrition: The Health Professional's Handbook,* ed. R. Chernoff (Gaithersburg, Md.: Aspen Publishers, 1991), pp. 449–483.

36. J. W. Rowe and R. L. Kahn, Human aging: Usual and successful, *Science* 237 (1987): 143–149.

13

Food for Singles

Singles of all ages face problems concerning food purchasing, storage, and preparation. Large packages of meat and vegetables are often suitable for a family of four or more, and even a head of lettuce can spoil before one person can use it all. Many singles live in small dwellings, some without kitchens and freezers, and for them, purchasing and storage problems are compounded. Following is a collection of ideas to solve some of these problems.

My grandmother is on a fixed income and doesn't have much money for groceries once the rent, utilities, and other bills are paid. What advice can I give her?

First, make sure your grandmother knows about food assistance programs available to older adults who need help obtaining proper, nourishing meals because of financial or other difficulties. Table NP13–1 summarizes food assistance programs for the elderly.

For those who have the means to shop and cook for themselves, it is possible to lower a food bill just by being a wise shopper. The first decision a person with a tight grocery budget must make is where to shop. Large supermarkets are usually less expensive than independent stores, but the cost of transportation to the market is a consideration.

Once a person decides where to shop, a grocery list that includes specials and coupons will help reduce impulse buying. Specials and coupons are a bargain only when the items featured are those that the shopper needs and uses. Foods that are almost always a good buy include nonfat dry milk, which can be stored on a shelf for months at room temperature; whole pieces of cheese rather than sliced or shredded; fresh produce that is in season; variety meats such as chicken livers; cereals that require cooking instead of ready-to-serve cereals; and dried beans and peas.

All foods, whether featured as specials or not, are bargains only when they are available in quantities that can be used without waste or spoilage. For example, turkey may be on sale and is one of the most economical meats for nutrients it offers, but only a person with ample storage space for leftovers would benefit from buying a whole turkey.

That's a big problem for my grandmother. How can she buy small quantities when so many foods are packaged for families?

This is a problem for all singles. Packages of meat and fresh vegetables often come already wrapped in large servings. Even milk is often available only in gallons or half-gallons and can spoil before one person can use it all. Try these hints:

- *Milk and milk products.* Buy fresh milk in the size best suited for you. If your grocer doesn't carry pints or half-pints, try a nearby service station or convenience store. Pint-size and even cup-size boxes of heat-treated milk are also available and can be stored unopened on a shelf for up to three months without refrigeration. Dry powdered milk can be stored for months before it is reconstituted. You can use only the amount you need and store the rest.
- *Meats and meat alternates.* Buy only what you will use. Ask the grocer to break open a package of wrapped meat and rewrap the portion that you need. Buy eggs by the half dozen—break the carton of a dozen eggs in half. Eggs do keep for long periods, though, if stored in the refrigerator, and are such a good source of high-quality protein that you will probably use a dozen before they lose their freshness. Dried beans and peas offer high-quality protein, fiber, and many other nutrients for practically pennies and have a long shelf life.

If you have ample freezing space, you can buy large packages of meat, such as pork chops, ground beef, or chicken, when they are on sale. Then, immediately divide the package into individual servings. Wrap them in aluminum foil, not freezer paper: the foil can become the liner for the pan in which you bake or broil the meat, thus saving work over the sink. For those who want to microwave these items for quick defrosting, wrap in a microwaveable wrap. Don't label these individually; put them all in a brown bag marked "hamburger" or "chicken thighs" or whatever, along with the date. The bag is easy to locate in the freezer, and you'll know when your supply is running low.

■ *Fruits and vegetables.* Purchase fresh fruits and vegetables individually. Buy only three pieces of each kind of fresh fruit: a ripe one, a semiripe one, and a green one. Eat the first right away, eat the second soon after, and let the last one ripen on your windowsill. If vegetables are packaged in large quantities, ask the grocer to break open the package so that you can buy what you need. Buy small cans of fruits and vegetables even though they are more expensive per unit. Remember, it is expensive to buy a regular-size can and let the unused portion spoil in the refrigerator. If you have space in your freezing compartment, buy frozen vegetables in large bags rather than in small boxes. You can take out the exact amount you need and close the bag tightly with a rubber band. If you return the

TABLE NP13–1   **Food Assistance Programs for Older Adults**

TITLE IIIC NUTRITION PROGRAM FOR OLDER AMERICANS

Funding: U.S. Department of Health and Human Services.

Services: Congregate and home-delivered meals, therapeutic diets. Supportive services include transportation to congregate meal sites; shopping assistance; information and referral; and to some extent, nutrition counseling and education.

Impact: The Title IIIc program improves the nutrient content of high-risk older adults' diets and offers socialization and recreation. Many of the nutrition programs around the country go above and beyond federal requirements of congregate and home meals by offering lunch clubs, ethnic meals, acceptance of food stamps for meal payment, and meals for older homeless people.

FOOD STAMPS

Funding: U.S. Department of Agriculture.

Services: Income supplement to low-income households in the form of coupons to purchase food.

Impact: Some research results suggest that food stamps serve more as an income supplement to elderly participants than as a device to improve nutrition status.[a] Other research indicates that food stamp participants' nutrient intakes are higher than those of nonparticipants of similar incomes.[b]

MEALS ON WHEELS

Funding: Private funding to supplement the Title IIIc program; an example of private and public sector partnership responding to the needs of the growing numbers of older adults.

Services: Direct meal delivery to the homebound elderly, integrated into the meal delivery services provided by the Title IIIc program.

Impact: Meals on Wheels focuses on filling the need for weekend and holiday meals for homebound elderly people, a service that is limited in the Title IIIc program.

[a]J. S. Butler, J. C. Ohls, and B. M. Posner, The effect of the food stamp program on the nutrient intake of the eligible elderly, *Journal of Nutrition for the Elderly* 4 (1985): 25–51, as cited in M. B. Kohrs, Effectiveness of nutrition intervention programs for the elderly, in *Nutrition and Aging,* eds. M. L. Hutchinson and H. N. Munro (New York: Academic Press, 1986), pp. 139–167.

[b]J. S. Akin and coauthors, The impact of federal transfer programs on the nutrient intake of elderly individuals, *Journal of Human Resources* 20 (1985): 382–404, as cited in B. M. Posner and E. Levine, Nutrition services for older Americans, in *Geriatric Nutrition: The Health Professional's Handbook,* ed. R. Chernoff (Gaithersburg, Md.: Aspen Publishers, 1991), pp. 415–447.

Source: Adapted from B. M. Posner and E. Levine, Nutrition services for older Americans, in *Geriatric Nutrition: The Health Professional's Handbook,* ed. R. Chernoff.

package quickly to the freezer each time, the vegetables will stay fresh for a long time.

■ *Breads and cereals.* Breads and cereals usually must be purchased in larger quantities. When you buy bread, take out the amount you will use in a few days, and store the rest in the freezer (not the refrigerator, which will make it stale). Cereal grains (rice, barley, oatmeal) and pastas, like the dried beans mentioned earlier, generally have a long shelf life if you keep them sealed in jars.

Those are great suggestions! I know my grandmother can use them, and so can I. But sometimes you just have to buy more food than you can use. Do you have hints for what to do then?

One thing you can do is to make mixtures of leftovers that you have on hand. A thick stew prepared from leftover green beans, carrots, cauliflower, broccoli, and any meat with added onion, pepper, celery, and potatoes makes a complete and balanced meal—except for milk, but then you can add powdered milk to your stew.

You can also set aside a place in your kitchen for rows of glass jars containing shelf staple items that you can't buy in single-serving quantities—rice, tapioca, lentils or other dry beans, flour, cornmeal, nonfat dry milk, macaroni, cereal, or coconut, to name only a few possibilities. Freeze each filled jar for one night first, to kill any insect eggs that might be present. The jars will then keep bugs out of the food indefinitely. They make an attractive display and will remind you of different choices you can make to vary

your menus. Cut the directions-for-use labels from the package and store them in the jars.

Think up a variety of ways to use a vegetable when you must buy it in a quantity larger than you can use. For example, you can divide a head of cauliflower into thirds. Cook one third and eat it as a hot vegetable. Put the other two-thirds into a vinegar-and-oil marinade for use as an appetizer or in a salad. You can keep half a package of frozen vegetables with other vegetables to be used in soup or stew.

Also, when you cook a lot of food, invite someone to share it with you. Next thing you know, that person will invite you back, and you'll get to enjoy a meal you wouldn't have thought to cook for yourself.

Another problem is that sometimes my grandmother doesn't feel like cooking a meal for herself. I'm afraid that she may not be getting the nutrients she needs.

When your grandmother does feel like cooking, she can cook several meals at a time. For example, she can boil three potatoes with skins. She can eat one hot with margarine and chives. When the others have cooled, she can use one to make a potato-cheese casserole ready to be put into the oven for the next evening's meal. The third one she can slice into a covered bowl and pour the juice from pickles over it. The pickled potato will keep several days in the refrigerator and can be used in a salad.

Depending on her freezer space, she can make double or even six portions of a dish that takes time to prepare: a casserole, vegetable pie, or meatloaf. The little aluminum trays from frozen foods can be saved and used to freeze

the extra servings. Your grandmother needs to be sure to date them and use the oldest first. Somehow the work seems worthwhile when several meals are prepared at once.

An occasional frozen TV dinner can also be useful—although expensive—if it makes the difference between a person's eating and not eating. Many such dinners that are now available are low in kcalories and nutritious. Adding a fresh salad, a whole-wheat roll, and a glass of milk can make a nice meal.

But encourage her to socialize, too. Sometimes, the loneliness that results from a single person's isolation can impair the person's appetite and motivation to cook appetizing meals.

My grandmother never drinks milk. What can I suggest?

She can try using nonfat dry milk. It is the greatest convenience food there is. Dry milk can be used in just about everything: hamburgers; gravies; soups; casseroles; sauces; and beverages, such as iced coffee. The taste is negligible, but five heaping tablespoons would be the equivalent of a cup of fresh milk. Ask a friend who is a member of Weight Watchers to give you some recipes for delicious milk shakes and "ice cream" using nonfat dry milk. Their recipes are for single servings.

Your grandmother can also increase her calcium intake by making soup stock from pork and chicken bones soaked in vinegar. The bones release their calcium into the acid medium, and the vinegar boils off when the stock is boiled. One tablespoon of such stock may contain over 100 milligrams of calcium. Something can then be cooked in this stock every day: vegetables, rice, and stews. And of course, this stock can be used as soup base.

One more suggestion for those who are alone at mealtime is this: make it a special occasion. One way to do this is to set the table with a tablecloth, napkin, full set of utensils, and fresh flowers. Set a pot of stew or homemade soup with vegetables and fresh herbs on low heat to cook, and make a salad. Get comfortable in a stuffed chair, and enjoy a book or some soothing music until the rich aroma of your simmering dinner beckons. After serving your plate, light a candle, dim the lights, savor the food, and relish some of the best company you will ever have—your own.

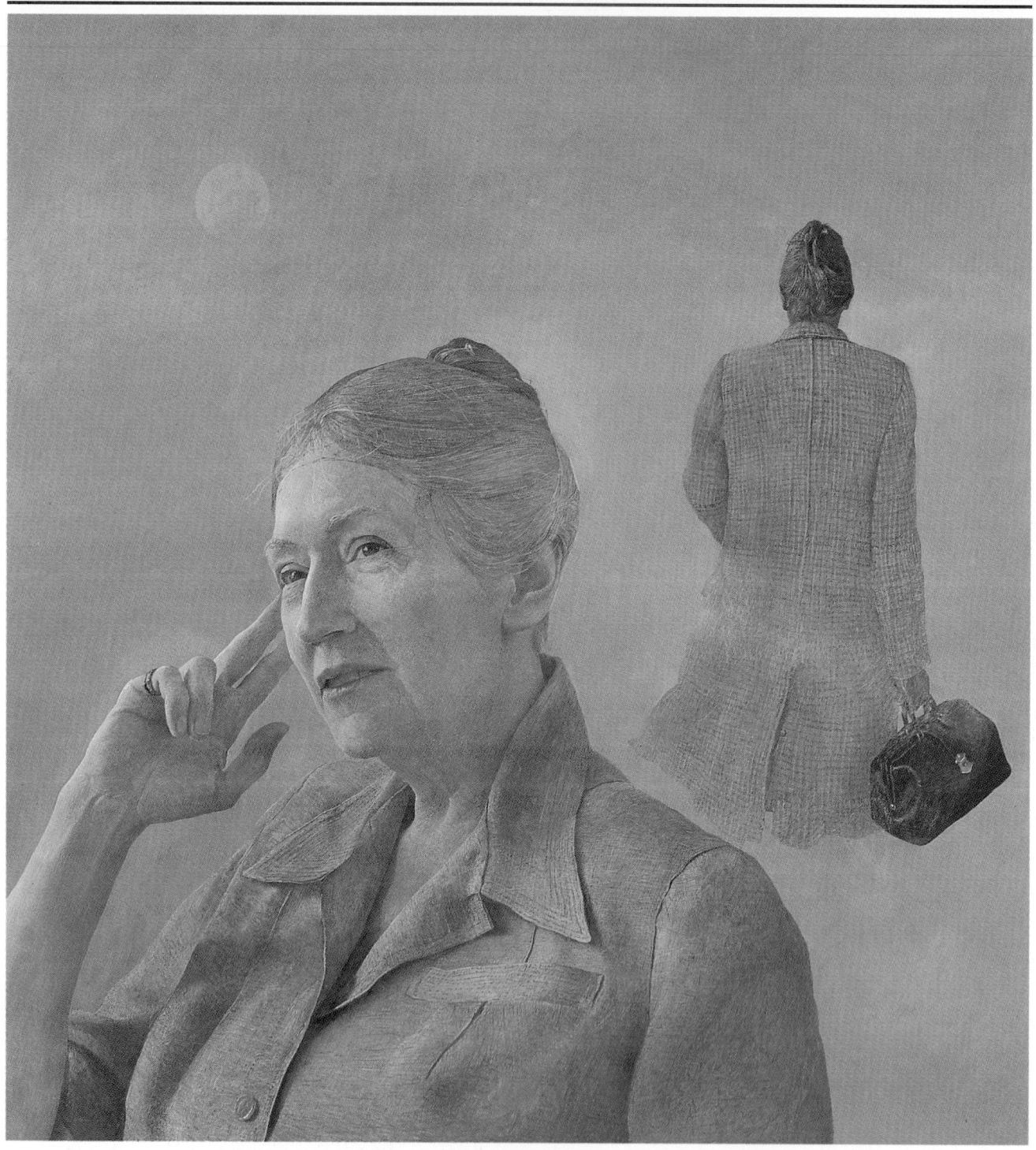

Andrew Wyeth, Children's Doctor, *1949, Tempera on panel, 26″ × 26″, Collection of the Brandywine River Museum.*

CHAPTER

14

Nutrition and Illness

CONTENTS

CHAPTER

14

It's tempting to take a simplistic view of nutrient needs, viewing them as fixed amounts determined using simple formulas. For example, because Ms. X is 22 years old, she needs Y amount of nutrient Z every day. In reality, though, nutrient needs are not fixed—they change in response to influences that change the body's internal environment. Aging is one such influence. As the last few chapters of this book demonstrate, nutrient needs throughout life fluctuate in response to the multitude of physical and physiological changes that accompany the aging process.

Illness is another influence that can significantly alter nutrient needs. Illnesses in general impose stresses on the body, and good nutrition status and attention to nutrient needs promote recovery from illness. This chapter first reviews general ways in which illness can affect nutrition status, then reviews the stress response and explores the relationships between nutrition and two types of defenses against illnesses—the immune system and drug therapy. Finally, the ways mental illnesses can affect nutrition status are described.

Interrelationships between Nutrition and Illness

While nutrient imbalances can predispose an individual to certain illnesses or interfere with recovery from illness, illness can also tax nutrient stores and lead to malnutrition. A malnourished person easily falls victim to illness, particularly infections, as the section on nutrition and immunity describes (see p. 346).

A particular illness inflicts damage on nutrition status to an extent that depends on the type, severity, and duration of the illness. An illness can:

▰ Alter food intake by causing a loss of appetite, changing the foods a person likes or dislikes, or by interfering with a person's ability to chew and/or swallow food.
▰ Alter the body's digestion of food or absorption of nutrients.
▰ Alter the body's metabolism of nutrients.
▰ Alter the body's excretion of nutrients.

Figure 14–1 summarizes and illustrates these interrelationships. Any or all of these effects can occur during illness. In addition, secondary effects of an illness, including immobility, emotional stress, diagnostic tests, medical procedures, and drug therapy can all further impair nutrition status.

Oftentimes when an ill person is weak or for other reasons is confined to bed, the resultant immobilization can affect nutrition status. First, the body loses nitrogen from muscle and calcium from bones when the muscle tension and weight bearing produced by normal activity do not occur. Then, in prolonged immobilization, blood and urine concentrations of calcium may rise, causing calcium stones to form in the bladder and kidney. Because physical activity is most effective at counteracting these losses, the bedridden or wheelchair-bound person should be encouraged to become active as soon as possible. Moderate exercise during a hospital stay appears to maintain the function of the vital organ systems necessary to recover from ill-

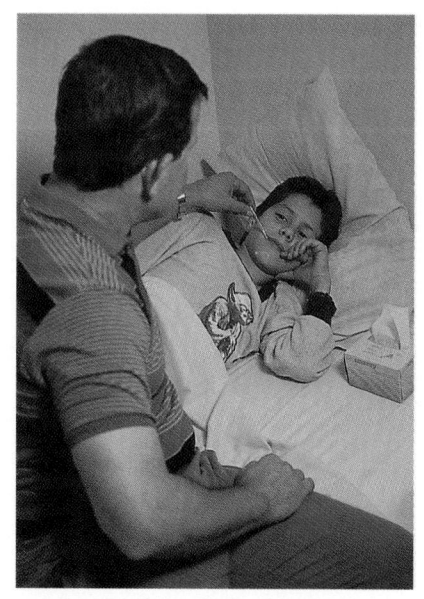

Although even the healthiest person sometimes gets sick, the person in poor nutrition status is an easier target.

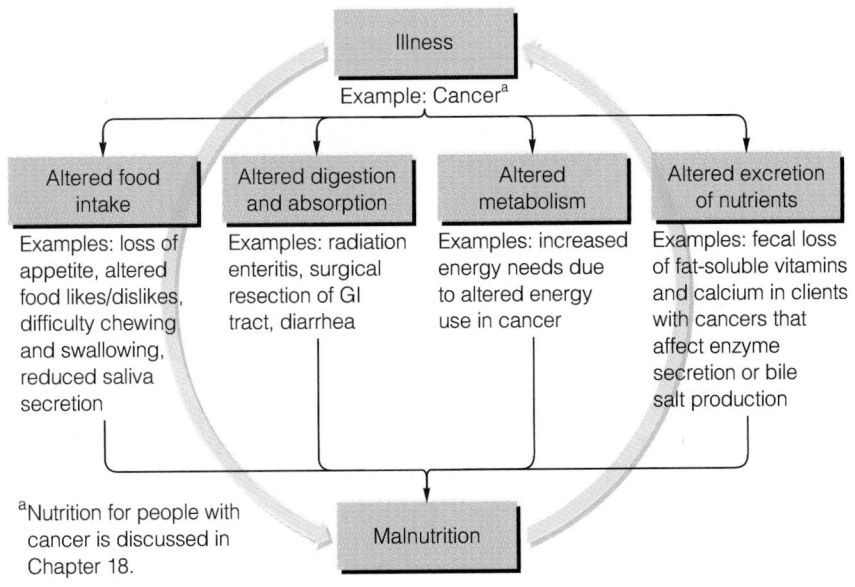

Illness
Example: Cancer[a]

Altered food intake
Examples: loss of appetite, altered food likes/dislikes, difficulty chewing and swallowing, reduced saliva secretion

Altered digestion and absorption
Examples: radiation enteritis, surgical resection of GI tract, diarrhea

Altered metabolism
Examples: increased energy needs due to altered energy use in cancer

Altered excretion of nutrients
Examples: fecal loss of fat-soluble vitamins and calcium in clients with cancers that affect enzyme secretion or bile salt production

[a]Nutrition for people with cancer is discussed in Chapter 18.

Malnutrition

FIGURE 14–1 **Interrelationships between Illness and Malnutrition**
Illness, and the treatment of illness, can contribute to malnutrition. Malnutrition enhances the chance of becoming ill. Thus a vicious cycle is set in motion.

ness.[1] However, it should be noted that people who are extremely ill or suffering from severe stress may be unable to tolerate much physical activity.

Bedsores are another problem associated with prolonged bed rest. Bedsores occur when the weight of the body exerts constant pressure on the skin, thus reducing blood flow to the area. Eventually, the skin breaks down and dies. The tissues and muscles under the skin, and even the bones, may also begin to break down. In addition to inadequate oxygen to the area, several nutrition risk factors have been associated with bedsores, including negative nitrogen balance, anemia, vitamin and mineral deficiencies, underweight, and overweight.

The best treatment for bedsores is to prevent their development by regularly turning and repositioning the bedridden person to relieve pressure. Those responsible for nutrition support should take special care to ensure that people with bedsores or those at risk for developing them receive diets that fully meet their nutrient needs.

In addition to the physical stresses of illness and immobilization, clients may be responding to the psychological stresses of fear and anxiety. They may be faced with life-threatening illnesses. They may be unfamiliar with their surroundings, the people who are caring for them, and the procedures they are being asked to undergo. These feelings stimulate stress hormone activity and suppress GI activity. Consequently, clients may lose their appetites. The best nutrition care that can be offered at such times is to alleviate fears and anxieties. Friendly words of assurance and explanations of procedures go a long way toward relaxing clients enough so that they can eat and digest their meals.

Diagnostic tests and medical procedures may require that a person not eat in order to obtain accurate test results. Thus, during the very time when an individual's nutrient needs are high due to illness, food intake declines. Little can be done to prevent this situation, except to ensure that restrictions

FIGURE 14–2   **Metabolic Responses to Starvation**

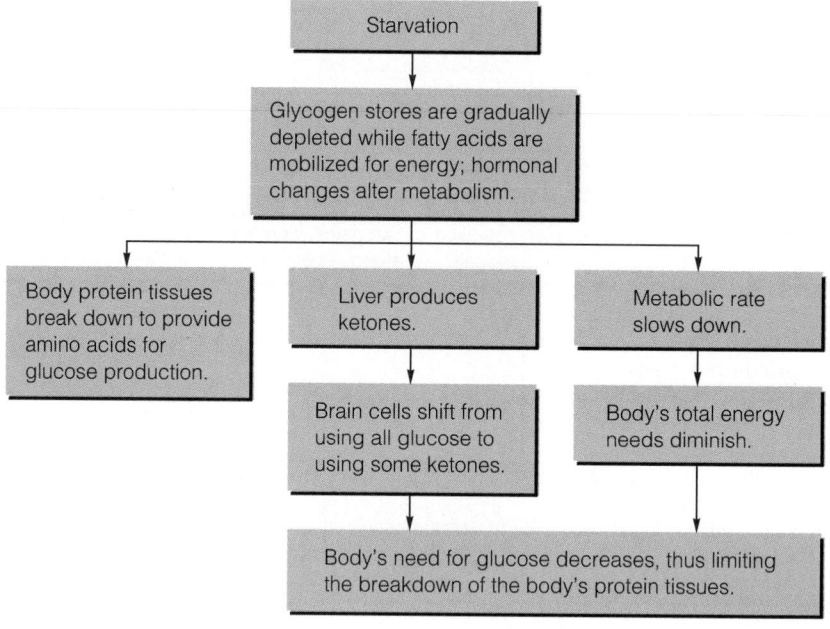

last no longer than absolutely necessary. Providing a nutrient-rich diet when the person is eating becomes imperative.

Disorders that markedly raise a person's metabolic rate over long periods of time tax nutrient stores and significantly raise the risk of nutrient deficiencies. These severe stresses and their effects are described in the next section.

The Stress Response

Stress is defined as any threat—physical or psychological—to a person's well-being. Surely, illnesses threaten a person's well-being, but even a healthy person visiting a physician for a regular checkup may feel anxious, triggering a mild stress response. It's all a matter of degree.

Under normal circumstances, the body efficiently maintains its internal balance, much like a finely tuned machine. Even small changes in the internal environment, such as the influx of nutrients entering the body following a meal, set in motion a series of metabolic events to restore homeostasis—that is, to bring the body back to a state of equilibrium. Occasionally, though, the body is confronted with a more severe change in the internal environment, such as a broken bone, an infection, or a burn. Because these conditions place greater stress on the body than normal, the body must employ more complicated mechanisms to reestablish balance.

The Response to Starvation and Severe Stress

The body's response to stress, then, depends on the type and severity of the insult. Understanding the initial metabolic changes that occur during star-

Some stress is part of the body's normal and healthy functioning; this type of stress is **physiological stress.** Additional stress imposed by disease or an abnormal bodily insult, such as surgery, burns, fever, or infection, can overwhelm the body; such stress is **pathological stress.** One type of pathological stress is **trauma**—physical injury to the body, such as a broken bone, a gunshot wound, or surgery.

homeostasis (HOME-ee-oh-STAY-sis): the maintenance of relatively constant internal conditions in the body.
  homeo = same
  stasis = staying

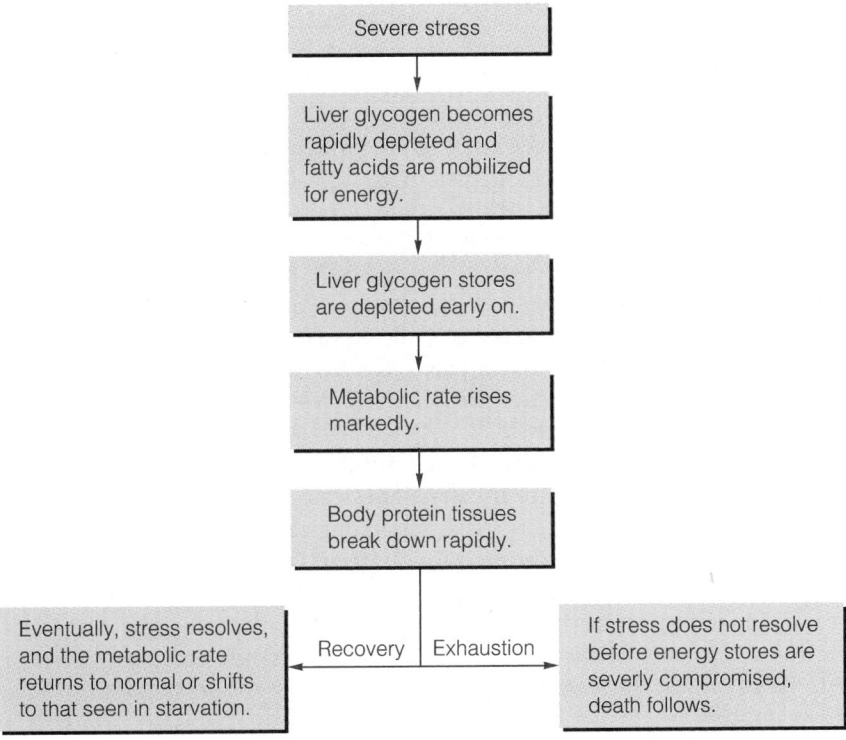

FIGURE 14–3 **Metabolic Response to Severe Stress**

vation, which is a relatively uncomplicated stress, lays the foundation for understanding the complex changes brought about by more complicated stresses. Chapter 6 provides this information (see pp. 101 to 103), and Figure 14–2 summarizes the metabolic changes that occur during starvation.

Severe stresses such as infection, and traumas such as surgery or fractures, generate a chain of metabolic events similar to those that occur in starvation, with some important differences. Most notably, the metabolic rate rises markedly (hypermetabolism) during severe stress, unlike the reduction in the metabolic rate that occurs during uncomplicated starvation (see Figure 14–3). In stress, changes in hormone levels result in an accelerated breakdown of body energy reserves (catabolism). Common hallmarks of the stress response during the period following injury include elevated blood glucose levels (hyperglycemia), negative nitrogen balance, exaggerated retention of fluid and sodium, and increased excretion of potassium.

While the general metabolic responses to all kinds of stress are similar, the body also responds uniquely to each type of stress. Consider that to mend a broken bone requires a different response than to heal a wound or to fight an infection. The body's response also depends on the severity of stress. For example, the response is less dramatic for a well-nourished person undergoing minor elective surgery (a moderate stress) than for a malnourished person with extensive burns (a severe stress). A severely malnourished person has few nutrient reserves with which to continue meeting the enhanced metabolic demands of a severe injury. The result is exhaustion, which may result in further complications such as infection or organ failure. This in turn compromises the person's physical state and makes recovery more difficult.

When several stresses occur at the same time, body tissues break down to a greater degree, amplifying the loss of vital protein. Multiple stresses can occur easily in one person—for example, a person may undergo surgery, receive no food following surgery, and then develop an infection with a fever.

As draining as the stress response may sound, medical researchers believe that the initial metabolic changes provide a positive service. These changes help to prevent further injury, repair damaged tissues, and maintain vital organ function. They facilitate the body's mobilization of its resources so that it can regain homeostasis.

The metabolic changes of stress constitute an adaptation that is sustained for as long as necessary or until exhaustion leads to death. In recovery, the rate of catabolism returns to normal, blood glucose levels fall, and nitrogen balance is slowly restored. The amount of time it takes for the body to return to normal depends on the degree of stress and the individual's state of health, including nutritional health. Figure 14–4 illustrates the phases of the stress response. Clearly, the better nourished people are at the onset of periods of stress, the better they are able to carry the metabolic burdens stress imposes.

The **acute,** or **flow, phase** of the stress response is the catabolic period immediately following the onset of stress. During the **adaptive phase,** the body adjusts to the stress to minimize losses. If adaptation succeeds, **recovery** follows. If adaptation fails, **exhaustion** follows.

Protein-Energy Malnutrition (PEM) and Severe Stress

Chapter 4 provides a description of protein-energy malnutrition (PEM) as a consequence of hunger throughout the world. This section explores the problem of PEM as it relates to illness. Such malnutrition knows no geographical, financial, age, or gender boundaries. It can strike a wealthy person in a hospital in an industrialized nation as readily as it can hit a poor person without access to any health care in a Third World country; it affects children and adults, men and women alike.

In fact, PEM associated with illness is a serious problem in the United States and throughout the world. Thus responsible health care professionals

Take a moment to imagine you are in a foreign country where you do not understand the language. As you walk down the street, you see signs that describe and direct. But the signs are meaningless to you, for you have yet to learn how to think, speak, or read this new language. Many health care professionals travel through hospitals looking at signs of malnutrition without recognizing them. They look at a person's pale complexion and lack of appetite, and see only that the person has a disease; they see a person's poor posture and lethargic attitude, and attribute these signs to old age. They have yet to learn to think "nutrition." Malnutrition is easy to miss if you are not looking for it. Caring for people requires that you at least consider the *possibility* that ill health may be due not just to a disease but perhaps to nutrient deficiencies. To overlook nutrition is to provide less than adequate care. The signs of malnutrition are there if you know where to look and how to read them.

FIGURE 14–4   **Phases of a Stress Response**
During the initial stress response, hypermetabolism sends nutrient reserves on a downhill course. As adaptation occurs, nutrient balances are gradually restored. If depleted of nutrients, the person will be unable to make the uphill trip and may not recover (exhaustion). A person who is carrying a heavier load (additional stress) will plunge downhill faster and have a more difficult climb.

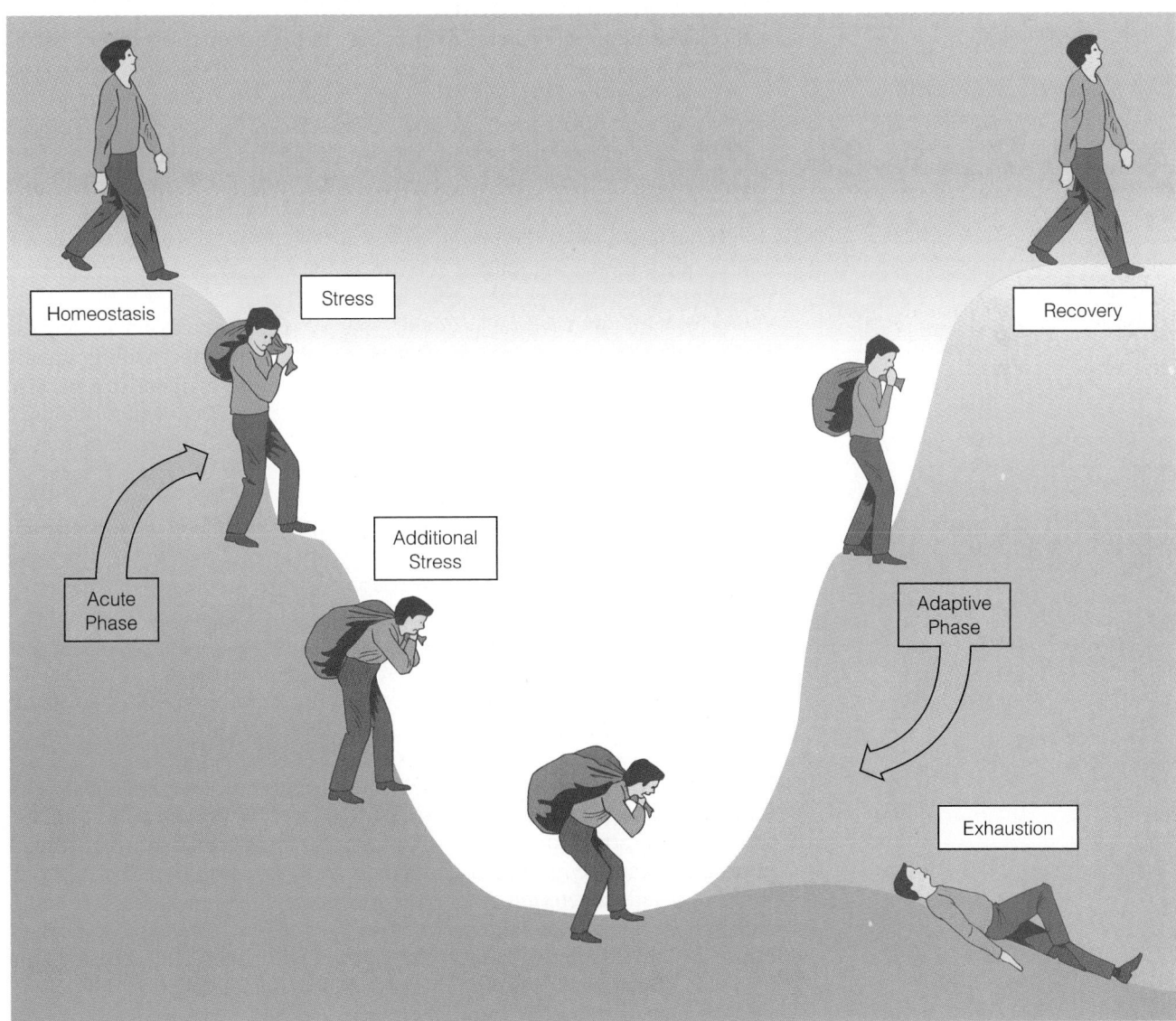

should learn to recognize the signs of PEM and the ways it interferes with a person's recovery. (Chapter 10 describes the nutrition assessment procedures used to detect PEM.)

While strong nutritional health supports a person in withstanding the stress of illness, poor nutritional health constitutes a stress that doubles the ill person's burden. Consider how the body must work to counteract the compound stresses of a serious illness combined with PEM. Because requirements for protein and energy rise remarkably during stress, the body's

It is technically incorrect to speak of body protein stores, because proteins (amino acids) are not stored in the body. All protein is functional; that is, it is being used in some capacity (as part of cell structure, as skeletal muscle, as enzymes or immune factors, or as other body protein components).

To understand the relationship of protein-energy malnutrition to serious illness, think of energy stores and protein status as money in the bank. Illness can be compared to a major expense that arises unexpectedly. The person who has saved enough money can pay off the expense without too much difficulty. However, if more and more expenses arise, the money may run out. The person with few or no savings is unable to pay even a small expense.

ability to respond depends, to a large extent, on available energy reserves and protein status. If the person is malnourished and hasn't received adequate protein or energy for a while, the body uses its protein tissues to meet its energy needs. As a result, the body loses functional protein from skeletal muscles, from organs, and from circulating pools of protein (such as albumin and immune factors).

For the well-nourished person, *some* loss of protein is acceptable, since sufficient protein will remain to support vital functions. However, for the person experiencing prolonged stress or malnutrition, the protein loss can be critical. Consider the consequences of protein loss to an accident victim who sustains multiple fractures and burns. Once other proteins have been used up, the demand for protein eats into lung cells and immune factors. The loss of a critical number of functioning lung cells combined with a reduced synthesis of immune factors can lead to deterioration of lung function and depression of the immune system. The result: pneumonia—on top of multiple fractures and burns. You can see how easily stresses can multiply if they are allowed to go unchecked.

Organs with rapid cell replacement—such as the GI tract—are among the first to suffer the consequences of PEM. The intestinal microvilli gradually shrink and become nonfunctional; up to 90 percent of them can be lost. Consequently, absorption fails and PEM worsens. Even when adequate nourishment is restored, the malnourished GI tract is so impaired that at first it has serious difficulty absorbing nutrients.

Within body cells, PEM hinders the synthesis of enzymes and other protein molecules that the body needs for proper metabolism and maintenance of the cells' structures. The rapid synthesis and degradation of these protein molecules help the body to adapt promptly to changes in the environment. Losing this ability to adapt leaves the body vulnerable and defenseless. PEM thus interferes with the body's ability to heal wounds, mount an immune response, and maintain the functions of vital organs and skeletal muscles. In addition, the person suffering from PEM often has other nutrient deficiencies as well, complicating the problems further.

Nutrition is only one of many factors that influence a person's ability to respond to illness, but it is an important one. Other important factors are the severity of the stress, the number of organ systems involved, other therapies in progress, and the responses of the individual to them. All of these factors working together determine whether a person will regain health. To summarize the role of nutrition described so far, adequate nutrition helps fight illness by providing the energy and nutrient reserves needed to fuel the metabolic changes associated with stress. But adequate nutrition does more. It also supports a healthy immune system.

The Immune System

The immune system alertly and silently defends the body against thousands of disease-causing microorganisms that bombard it every day. The immune system operates without a central organ of control; it depends on the interactions and secretions of various organs and white blood cells. The ac-

---

MINIGLOSSARY of Immunity Terms

acquired immunity: immunity directed at specific organisms (also called **specific immunity**). The lymphocytes mediate this type of immunity, which depends on prior exposure to, recognition of, and reaction to invading organisms. Two types of specific immunity are **cell-mediated immunity** and **humoral immunity**.

antibody: a protein of the type known as immunoglobulins, produced by the B-cells in response to invasion of the body by a foreign protein.

antigen: a substance that induces the formation of antibodies.

B-cells: a class of lymphocytes that secrete antibodies and are important in humoral immunity.

cell-mediated immunity: immunity conferred by the reaction of T-cells to an invading organism.

humoral immunity: immunity conferred by antibodies secreted by B-cells and carried to the invaded area by way of body fluids.

immune system: the body's natural defense system against foreign materials that have penetrated the skin or mucous membranes.

immunity: the body's ability to recognize and eliminate foreign materials.

immunoglobulin: a protein capable of acting as an antibody.

lymphocytes: white blood cells that participate in acquired immunity. Two classes of lymphocytes important in immunity are the T-cells and the B-cells.

phagocytes: cells that have the ability to ingest and destroy foreign substances.

phagocytosis (FAG-oh-sigh-TOE-sis): the process by which some cells (phagocytes) engulf and destroy foreign materials.
  phagein = to eat
  kytos = cell
  osis = intensive

T-cells: a class of lymphocytes that recognize antigens and stimulate other cells to join in the immune response. T-cells are important in cell-mediated immunity.

---

companying Miniglossary defines key terms related to the immune system and its components.

The immune system is called into play when a foreign substance penetrates the body's first lines of defense—the skin, the GI tract, and the mucous membranes. Normally, these formidable barriers successfully prevent entry of invaders into the body. The skin is thick and coated with protective waxes, and it is constantly shedding its outermost layers while its associated glands secrete sweat and oily secretions that are toxic to some types of bacteria.

The remarkably efficient cells of the GI tract rarely allow microorganisms to pass into the body, even though over 500 species of bacteria normally reside in the intestines.[2] Some harmless bacteria present in the intestines prevent other, harmful bacteria from entering the body.

Mucous membranes coat all of the body's openings—eyes, nose, mouth, lungs, GI tract, and genitourinary tract—and secrete protective mucus. The sticky mucus catches foreign materials and carries them along as it flows out

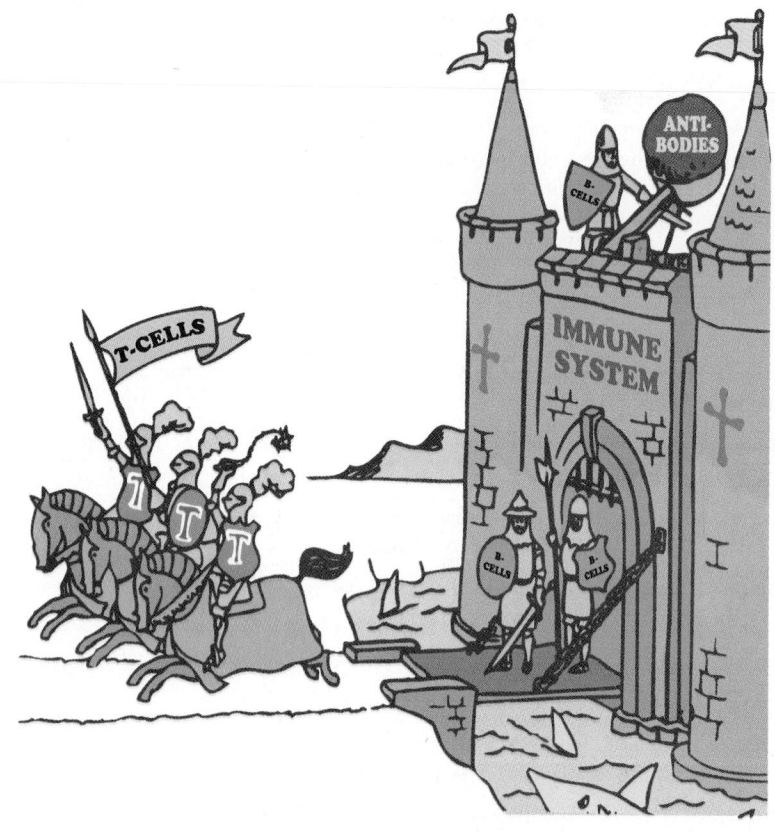

of the body. Moreover, mucus contains antimicrobial chemicals and enzymes that are lethal to invading organisms. If an invader does gain entry into the body (through a cut in the skin, for example), then the organs and cells of the immune system spring into action.

Three types of white blood cells—the phagocytes and two types of lymphocytes—are key players in the immune response (see Figure 14–5). Phagocytes engulf and digest some foreign substances. They also secrete proteins that activate some metabolic and immune responses to infection. In addition, phagocytes facilitate the action of the T-cells, one type of lymphocyte important in the immune system.

T-cells actively defend the body against fungi, viruses, parasites, and a few types of bacteria; they also destroy cancer cells. Unlike the phagocytes, which are capable of inactivating many types of invaders, each T-cell specifically attacks only one type of invader. T-cells participate in the rejection of newly transplanted tissues, which is why they must be inactivated by drugs when tissue transplantation is necessary.

The other lymphocytes important in immunity are the B-cells. B-cells respond to infection by rapidly dividing and then producing antibodies. Antibodies then travel to the site of infection, where they stick to the surfaces of the foreign particles and kill or otherwise inactivate them, making the foreign particles easy for the phagocytes to ingest. Antibodies react selectively to a specific foreign organism, just as T-cells do, and the B-cells retain a memory of how to make them. The next time the same foreign organism is encountered, the immune system can respond with greater speed.

The Role of Nutrition in the Immune Response

Nutrient imbalances impair a variety of immune system components and functions, including the skin and exterior barriers, as well as the activities of the cells of the immune system. For this reason, people who suffer from malnutrition develop more infections than well-nourished people. Infection, in turn, increases nutrient requirements, further taxing nutrition status. Figure 14–6 shows that malnutrition impairs immunity, that impaired immunity raises the risk of disease, and that disease further impairs nutrition status, creating a synergistic cycle that must be broken to recover from disease. In Third World countries, infection leads to mortality and morbidity in children with PEM. Table 14–1 shows how malnutrition affects immune system components.

Cell-mediated immunity, a function of the T-cells, appears to be markedly depressed by malnutrition. The areas of the lymphatic system that normally house the T-cells become depleted of lymphocytes. Because malnutrition impairs T-cell function, a depressed *lymphocyte count* and *antigen skin testing* indicate malnutrition, as Chapter 10 describes.

Severe Stress and Immunity

The immune system's response to the hormonal and metabolic changes that accompany stress is to temporarily suppress its disease-fighting activity. If malnutrition accompanies stress, the immune system is forced to work without adequate nutrient support, further impairing its activity. Indeed, malnutrition and infections present a serious threat to people who have severe medical problems, undergo complicated surgeries, suffer major trauma, or have advanced cancer.

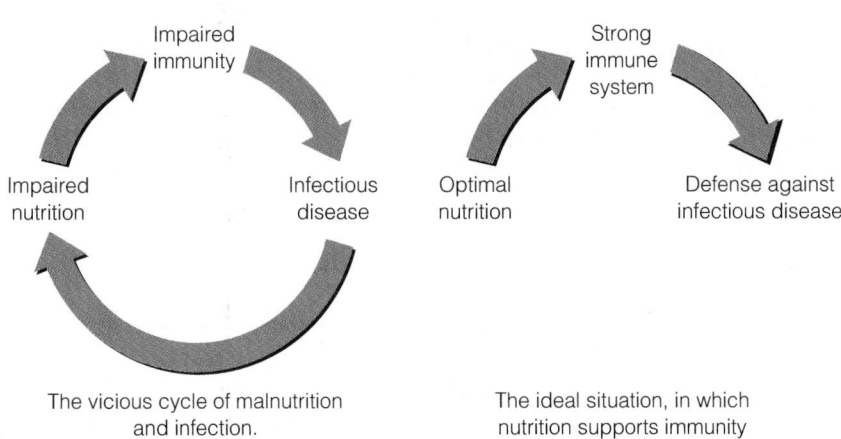

Impaired immunity

Impaired nutrition

Infectious disease

The vicious cycle of malnutrition and infection.

Strong immune system

Optimal nutrition

Defense against infectious disease

The ideal situation, in which nutrition supports immunity against diseases.

FIGURE 14–6 **Nutrition and Immunity**

TABLE 14–1   **Effects of General Malnutrition on Immune System Components**

IMMUNE SYSTEM COMPONENT	EFFECTS OF MALNUTRITION
Skin	Thinned, with less connective tissue
GI tract	Compounded likelihood of bacterial translocation when intestines are injured
Mucous membranes	Microvilli flattened; antibody secretions reduced
Lymph tissues	Thymus gland, lymph nodes, and spleen reduced in size; T-cell areas depleted of lymphocytes
Phagocytosis	Kill time delayed
Cell-medicated immunity	Circulating T-cells reduced
Humoral immunity	Circulating immunoglobulin levels normal; antibody response possibly impaired

translocation: the passage of microorganisms from the interior of the intestines to the inside of the body. Translocation of bacteria can occur from direct injury to the intestines or from indirect injuries such as reduced blood flow to the intestines, burn injuries, or certain drugs.

nucleotides: nitrogen-containing components of RNA and DNA. They can be synthesized in the body and therefore are not essential in the diets of healthy people. However, in severely stressed individuals, a dietary source of nucleotides may be helpful.

immunonutrition: nutrition support directed at maintaining or enhancing the function of the immune system.

Although it is clear that malnutrition diminishes immune function, it is less clear that nutrition therapy can help to restore it. When given nutrition therapy, severely stressed people show signs of weight gain and positive nitrogen balance, but benefits to the immune system are inconsistent.[3] Delivering nutrients into the GI tract appears to help the intestinal cells maintain a barrier that prevents bacteria from entering the body. Feeding the person by vein fails to confer this benefit. The translocation of bacteria into the body may trigger hypermetabolism and infection, which can ultimately lead to multiple organ failure.[4] The need for research to determine the most appropriate mixture of nutrients to restore immune function is indicated. Some preliminary studies point to arginine (a nonessential amino acid), dietary nucleotides, and omega-3 fatty acids as holding some promise in stimulating immune function.[5] Accordingly, a product containing arginine, nucleotides, and a balance of lipids, in addition to the other essential nutrients, is currently being marketed for maintaining immune function in severely stressed people. Whether this immunonutrition formula will be successful, though, remains to be seen.

The body's natural defenses against insults to its internal environment are vulnerable to poor nutrition. Thus poor nutrition impairs the individual's ability to mount both a stress response and an immune response when confronted with illness, trauma, and infection. In addition, nutrition affects the way the body responds to man-made weapons against disease, namely drugs.

Nutrition and Drug Therapy

Most people think of drugs as medicines that help them recover from illnesses, or as illegal substances that lead to addiction. Actually, both uses of the term *drug* are correct, because any substance taken into a living organism that modifies one or more of its functions is, technically, a drug. All drugs affect users physiologically, and their uses always involve side effects and risks. This discussion focuses on medical drugs, both nonprescription, or over-the-counter (OTC), drugs and prescription drugs.

To help explain the far-reaching chemical effects of nutrient-drug interactions on body systems, this discussion will begin with a look at a class of drugs called monoamine oxidase (MAO) inhibitors. Physicians sometimes prescribe MAO inhibitors to treat people with some forms of severe depression. MAO inhibitors block the action of the enzyme monoamine oxidase. Normally, monoamine oxidase converts tyramine, a substance found in some foods (see Table 14–2), into an inactive form. When people take MAO inhibitors, tyramine remains abnormally active and stimulates the release of norepinephrine. This action can lead to severe hypertension and headaches. If blood pressure rises high enough, it can be fatal.

Nicotine gum provides another example of how specific food items alter a drug's intended action. Physicians prescribe nicotine gum to help people quit smoking cigarettes. Recently, researchers discovered that acidic foods and beverages limit the effectiveness of nicotine gum. The acidity from these foods and beverages changes the chemical balance in the mouth, thus preventing the nicotine from being absorbed through the lining of the mouth into the blood.[6] The blocking action of acidic foods may help to explain why nicotine gum is successful in only about one-fourth of the people who use it to quit smoking. Other side effects of this food-drug interaction—nausea and hiccups—develop when the unabsorbed nicotine arrives in the stomach. In the end, then, the combination of acidic foods and nicotine gum both interferes with the drug's effectiveness and creates uncomfortable side effects.

Some acidic foods and beverages that may interfere with the effectiveness of nicotine gum:

- Apple juice.
- Beer.
- Catsup.
- Coffee.
- Colas.
- Grape juice.
- Lemon-lime soda.
- Mustard.
- Orange juice.
- Pineapple juice.
- Soy sauce.
- Tomato juice.

TABLE 14–2 **Foods Restricted from a Tyramine-Controlled Diet**

Beverages	Chianti; sherry; sauterne; champagne; imported beer; nonalcoholic beer; ale[a]
Cheeses	Aged cheeses, American, Camembert, cheddar, Gouda, Gruyère, mozzarella, Parmesan, provolone, Romano, Roquefort, Stilton;[b] cheese-filled breads, crackers, and desserts
Meats	Liver; dried, salted, smoked, or pickled fish; meat processed with tenderizers; sausage; pepperoni; dried meats; meat extracts
Vegetables	Fava beans; Italian broad beans; sauerkraut; fermented pickles and olives
Other	Brewer's yeast; monosodium glutamate; all aged and fermented products; caffeine and chocolate in large amounts

Note: The tyramine contents of foods vary from product to product according to the methods used to prepare, process, and store food. The amount of tyramine a person consumes depends on the quantity of the food eaten. In some cases, as little as 1 oz of cheese can cause a severe hypertensive reaction in people taking monoamine oxidase inhibitors. The items listed in this table contain significant enough quantities of tyramine that they are not allowed. In general, the following foods contain small enough quantities of tyramine that they can be consumed in small quantities: ripe avocados, bananas, yogurt, sour cream, acidophilus milk, buttermilk, raspberries, and peanuts.

[a]Most wine and domestic beer can be consumed in small quantities.

[b]Unfermented cheeses, such as ricotta, cottage cheese, and cream cheese, are allowed.

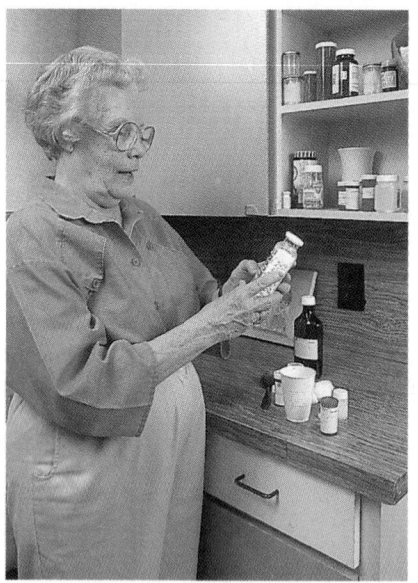

Taking several drugs over long periods of time intensifies the risk of nutrient-drug interactions.

Hundreds of medical drugs interact with nutrients, creating the possibility of imbalances whenever a person takes them. Drugs can profoundly affect nutrition status, and conversely, nutrients can profoundly affect the body's responses to drugs. Awareness of possible drug-nutrient interactions and the ways in which they can be prevented or controlled can help limit problems. Hospitals that have established a drug-nutrient interaction policy can limit drug-nutrient interactions significantly. In one study of a hospital with such a policy, researchers found clinically significant drug-nutrient interactions in only 2 of 493 cases that were reviewed.[7] The policy guided health care professionals in preventing, recognizing, and treating the most common and clinically significant interactions.

Adverse drug-nutrient interactions occur most commonly when drugs are taken over long periods, when several drugs are taken simultaneously, or when poor nutrition status is present or impending. Understandably, elderly people and people with serious illnesses that raise nutrient needs are most at risk, for they are most likely to be in poor nutrition status, to suffer chronic disorders, to use many drugs, and to take them over a long period.

Nutrients and drugs may interact in many ways:

- Drugs can alter food intake.
- Nutrients and foods can alter drug absorption.
- Drugs can alter nutrient absorption.
- Nutrients can alter the intended actions of drugs.
- Nutrients can alter the metabolism and excretion of drugs.
- Drugs can alter the metabolism and excretion of nutrients.

Table 14–3 summarizes the mechanisms by which these interactions occur and provides specific examples. The number of drug-nutrient actions that have been identified is mind-boggling, and it continues to grow. It would be difficult, if not impossible, to remember and apply all of this information in a clinical setting. Instead, health care professionals would serve their clients well to:

- Be aware of groups of people who are at high risk for developing drug-related nutrient deficiencies.
- Keep in mind that drug-nutrient interactions can and do occur.
- Be familiar with the nutrient interactions of drugs commonly used to treat the disorders of their clients.
- Be prepared to look up the nutrition effects of drugs their clients are taking.

Nutrient interactions and risks are not unique to prescription drugs. People may mistakenly believe that OTC drugs are harmless, but such drugs can be dangerous if they mask serious problems by covering up the symptoms. For example, a person who repeatedly takes antacids for stomach discomfort may be ignoring the signs of an ulcer. For another example, hidden ingredients in some OTC drugs can be undesirable—such as the significant amounts of sodium or calcium found in some antacids that aggravate certain medical conditions. The availability of OTC drugs allows people to treat themselves for minor ailments, but they should maintain an awareness of the potential dangers and seek professional care if symptoms persist.

TABLE 14–3 **Mechanisms and Examples of Food-Drug Interactions**

DRUGS CAN ALTER FOOD INTAKE BY:

- Altering the appetite (amphetamines suppress the appetite).
- Interfering with taste or smell (methotrexate changes taste sensations).
- Inducing nausea or vomiting (digitalis does both).

- Changing the oral environment (phenobarbital causes dry mouth).
- Irritating the GI tract (cyclophosphamide induces mucosal ulcers).
- Causing sores or inflammation of the mouth (methotrexate can cause painful mouth ulcers to form).

DRUGS CAN ALTER NUTRIENT ABSORPTION BY:

- Changing the acidity of the digestive tract (antacids can interfere with iron absorption).
- Altering digestive juices (cimetidine can improve fat absorption).
- Altering motility of the digestive tract (laxatives speed motility, causing the malabsorption of many nutrients).
- Inactivating enzyme systems (neomycin may reduce lipase activity).
- Damaging mucosal cells (chemotherapy can damage mucosal cells).
- Binding to nutrients (antacids bind phosphorus).

FOODS CAN ALTER DRUG ABSORPTION BY:

- Changing the acidity of the digestive tract (candy can change the acidity, thus dissolving slow-acting asthma medication too quickly).
- Stimulating secretion of digestive juices (griseofulvin is absorbed better when taken with foods that stimulate the release of digestive enzymes).
- Altering motility of the digestive tract (aspirin is absorbed more slowly when taken with food).
- Binding to drugs (tetracycline binds to calcium in dairy foods, limiting drug absorption).
- Competing for absorption sites in the intestines (dietary amino acids interfere with levodopa absorption this way).

DRUGS CAN ALTER NUTRIENT METABOLISM BY:

- Acting as structural analogues (as anticoagulants and vitamin K do).
- Interfering with metabolic enzyme systems (phenobarbital competes for folate coenzymes).

FOODS CAN ALTER DRUG METABOLISM BY:

- Interfering with a drug's action (phenobarbital action is limited by large amounts of folate in the diet).
- Contributing pharmacologically active substances (examples are tyramine from cheese and monoamine oxidase inhibitors).

DRUGS CAN ALTER NUTRIENT EXCRETION BY:

- Altering reabsorption in the kidneys (some diuretics increase the excretion of sodium and potassium).
- Displacing nutrients from their plasma protein carriers (aspirin displaces folate).

FOODS CAN ALTER DRUG EXCRETION BY:

- Changing the acidity of the urine (vitamin C can alter urinary pH and limit the excretion of aspirin).

For example, nurses working with people who have heart disease will want to become familiar with the drug-nutrient interactions that can occur with medications used to treat heart disease. Better yet, they might keep a reference handy, such as Table B–1B in appendix B, to check the possibility of drug-nutrient interactions.

As this chapter describes, physiological illnesses and their treatments interact in many ways with nutrition status. The next section explores the interactions of mental illness and nutrition status.

Nutrition and Mental Illness

Although it may be easy to visualize the effects of physiological illnesses on nutrient stores, it may be less apparent that mental illnesses, too, can affect nutrition status. Mental disorders characterized by depression, illogical thinking, dementia, paranoia, delusions, and inappropriate eating habits can alter food intake and thus interfere with nutrition status. These disorders include schizophrenia, Alzheimer's disease, mood disorders, substance abuse, and eating disorders (anorexia nervosa and bulimia). Nutrition in Practice 6 describes nutrition concerns associated with alcohol abuse—one type of substance abuse. Nutrition in Practice 19 explores eating disorders and their nutrition consequences. The accompanying Miniglossary defines terms related to mental illness.

Individuals suffering from depression, illogical thinking, or dementia may have little interest in food. Those who are paranoid may believe that foods are being used to poison them. People suffering from delusions may attribute magical powers to certain foods, and may therefore insist on eating only those foods.

In addition to the direct effects of some mental illnesses on food intake, drug therapy used in the treatment of mental illnesses can also have nutrition consequences. This chapter previously described the nutrition concerns associated with MAO inhibitors (see p. 351), which may be used in the treatment of depression. Other drugs used to treat mental illnesses may interfere with food intake, GI function, or nutrient absorption and metabolism.

Both physiological and mental illnesses can significantly alter nutrition needs. The attentive health care professional recognizes possible problems and takes corrective measures whenever possible.

CASE STUDY

Nutrition and Illness

Karen, a 20-year-old engineering student, went to the university clinic after developing a fever, sore throat, and nausea. From the clinical examination, the doctor suspected a streptococcal pharyngitis (strep throat), and a throat culture was taken. The results of the throat culture confirmed the diagnosis. A ten-day course of penicillin was prescribed, along with instructions to rest, drink plenty of fluids, use acetaminophen for pain, and complete the full dose of antibiotics.

Describe ways in which Karen's symptoms might interfere with her nutrition status. Why is it important for Karen to begin eating a well-balanced diet as quickly as possible?

Look up penicillin in Table B–1B in Appendix B. How should penicillin be given with respect to food intake? What side effects of penicillin might further impair Karen's nutrition status?

Study Questions

1. What effects do immobilization have on nutrient balances, and how can these effects be minimized?
2. What is a bedsore? How can bedsores be prevented and treated?
3. Describe the interrelationships between illness and nutrition.
4. What is the stress response, and what is its purpose?
5. How does the body's response to severe stress differ from the body's response to starvation?
6. Describe the effect of nutrition status on the body's ability to respond to stress.
7. How does the immune system defend the body against disease-causing microorganisms? What effect does nutrition have on this response?
8. Describe the conditions that increase the risk of drug-induced nutrient deficiencies. Based on your answer, which groups of people would most likely be at risk?
9. In what ways can drugs and foods interact? Give some examples of how drugs can interfere with food intake and of how nutrients can interfere with drug action.

Notes

1. J. A. Windsor and G. L. Hill, Weight loss with physiologic impairment: A basic indicator of surgical risk, *Annals of Surgery* 207 (1988): 290–296; J. D. Albert and coauthors, Preservation of functional aerobic capacity with daily submaximal exercise during intravenous feeding in hospitalized normal men, *World Journal of Surgery* 12 (1988): 123–131.
2. J. W. Alexander, Nutrition and translocation, *Journal of Parenteral and Enteral Nutrition* 14 (Supplement, 1990): 170–174.
3. M. D. Lieberman and coauthors, Effects of nutrient substrates on immune function, *Nutrition* 6 (Supplement, 1989): 88–91.
4. Alexander, 1990.
5. A. Barbul, Arginine and immune function, *Nutrition* 6 (Supplement, 1989): 53–58; F. B. Rudolph and coauthors, Role of RNA as a dietary source of pyrimidines and purines in immune function, *Nutrition* 6 (Supplement, 1989): 45–52; J. E. Kinsella and coauthors, Dietary polyunsaturated fatty acids and eicosanoids: Potential effects on the modulation of inflammatory and immune cells: An overview, *Nutrition* 6 (Supplement, 1989): 24–44.
6. J. E. Henningfield and coauthors, Drinking coffee and carbonated beverages blocks absorption of nicotine from nicotine polacrilex gum, *Journal of the American Medical Association* 264 (1990): 1560–1564.
7. V. L. Franse, N. Stark, and T. Powers, Drug-nutrient interactions in a Veterans Administration medical center teaching hospital, *Nutrition in Clinical Practice* 3 (1988): 145–147.

14

Food as a Source of Illness

Nutrition plays a pivotal role in the prevention of disease and the recovery from illness, but foods can also be a source of illness. Food hazards such as food-borne illness and food contaminants compel people to wonder about the safety of our food supply. Nutrition in Practice 14 discusses these concerns.

It seems that I've been hearing many reports about serious cases of food poisoning. What causes food poisoning?

Food poisoning is a real and frequent threat to people who consume food that has been contaminated by toxic microorganisms during processing, packaging, transport, storage, or preparation. Food poisoning can affect large numbers of people whenever batches of contaminated foods escape detection and are distributed and consumed. However, commercial processors are less frequently responsible for incidents of food poisoning than are individuals who prepare food in their home kitchens or restaurants, catering firms, and institutions where food is served to large groups.

All foods contain bacteria. Bacteria are widely distributed in nature but are usually harmless. For growth and reproduction, they require warmth, moisture, and a source of nutrients. When the conditions are right, such as in leftover foods improperly stored, bacteria will proliferate. The growth of harmful bacteria causes food-borne illness.

What are some types of harmful bacteria?

One type is *Salmonella*. *Salmonella* infection is rapidly spreading worldwide. Over the last decade, food poisoning cases linked to this infection have increased by 200 percent in the United States alone.[1] *Salmonella* organisms are frequently found on poultry and on egg shells. In one outbreak, *Salmonella* infected over 300 people attending a conference. *Staphylococcus aureus* microbes, found on human skin, are another common cause of food-borne illness in the United States. *Clostridium botulisum,* a bacteria producing a toxin, is found in foods that have been improperly canned. Botulism, the poisoning caused by ingesting this toxin, is rare, but it is so deadly that an amount as tiny as a single crystal of salt can kill several people within an hour.

Viruses, transmitted from sick people to well ones through seafood, can also cause food-borne illness. Certain types of seafood, such as oysters and clams that grow in water contaminated with human or animal waste products, can collect viruses from that waste—the hepatitis virus for example. If the clams or oysters have filtered the virus out of the water and have it in their bodies, there is a good possibility that a consumer of those shellfish will contract hepatitis. However, most seafood that is commercially harvested is safe, because it is harvested from water that is tested and known to be free of contamination.

How do you know if you have a food-borne illness?

Food-borne illnesses can be very painful. Symptoms vary depending on the type of toxin. However, diarrhea, abdominal cramps, fever, vomiting, headache, and gut pain are common complaints. Botulism, which is often fatal, causes nervous system symptoms including double vision, inability to swallow, speech difficulty, and progressive paralysis of the respiratory system. Infants and the elderly can be more seriously affected by food-borne diseases than others.

What steps can I take to prevent food-borne illness?

Harmful organisms cannot be kept out of foods. Every day, each of us ingests small numbers of microbes with no ill effects. The task at hand is not to eliminate, but to kill those organisms that are present or control their multiplication.

Three simple measures help prevent food-borne illnesses: keep hot foods hot; keep cold foods cold; and keep hands, utensils, and the kitchen clean. Table NP14–1 lists some specific food safety tips. The person who follows the suggestions provided in the table regarding the selection, storage, and preparation of food will greatly reduce the risk of food-borne illness.

If you suspect that you have a food-borne illness, these steps may be helpful:

1. Call your physician.
2. Wrap and label the remainder of the suspected food, along with its container, so that it can't be mistakenly used; place it in the refrigerator; and hold it for possible inspection by health authorities.
3. Notify the Health Hazard Evaluation Board of the FDA's Bureau of Foods,

a panel of scientists and health experts who assess how serious a threat to health a food may be.

Illnesses from foods also occur when nonnutrient substances find their way into the food supply. Such contaminants are of concern because they are increasingly present in the environment, from which they can migrate into foods.

TABLE NP14–1 **Suggestions for the Prevention of Food-Borne Illnesses**

To Keep Hot Foods Hot
- When cooking meats or poultry, use a thermometer to test the internal temperature. Insert the thermometer between the thigh and the body of the turkey, or in the thickest part of other meats, making sure the tip of the thermometer is not in contact with bone or the pan. Cook to the temperature indicated for that particular meat; cook hamburgers to at least medium well-done.
- Cook stuffing separately, or stuff poultry just prior to cooking.
- Do not cook large cuts of meats or turkey in a microwave oven.
- Cook eggs before eating them (boiled for 7 min, poached for 5 min, and fried for 3 min on each side).
- When serving foods, maintain temperatures above 140° F.
- Heat leftovers thoroughly.

To Keep Cold Foods Cold
- When running errands, stop at the grocery store last. When you get home, refrigerate the perishable groceries (such as meats and dairy products) immediately. Do not leave perishables in the car any longer than it takes for ice cream to melt.
- Buy only those foods that are solidly frozen and stored below the frost line in store freezers.
- Keep cold foods at 40° F or less.
- Refrigerate leftovers promptly; use shallow containers to help foods cool faster.
- Thaw meats or poultry in the refrigerator, not at room temperature. If you must hasten thawing, use cool running water or a microwave oven.

To Keep a Clean Kitchen
- Use hot, soapy water to wash hands, utensils, dishes, nonporous cutting boards, and countertops. Use a bleach solution to clean wooden cutting boards.
- Avoid cross-contamination by washing all surfaces that have been in contact with raw meats, poultry, or eggs.
- Mix foods with utensils, not hands; keep hands and utensils away from mouth, nose, and hair.
- Anyone may be a carrier of bacteria and should avoid coughing or sneezing over food. A person with a skin infection or infectious disease should not prepare food.

(continued)

What are contaminants?

A food contaminant is anything that doesn't belong there. Used broadly, the term includes the microbes already discussed, harmful substances from industry, pesticide residues, bits of packaging, and ordinary dirt. As used here, the term applies only to harmful substances from industry; it includes pesticides only when they are accidentally spilled in large quantities into food. Nutrition in Practice 8 describes lead, a contaminant of grave concern today. The number of contaminants and the amount of information available about them is far beyond the scope of this book. However, examples of metal contaminants are presented in Table NP14–2.

How do you know whether or not a contaminant will be harmful?

The potential harmfulness of a contaminant depends in part on its persistence—the extent to which it lingers in the environment or in the body. If the environment can break the contaminant down before it enters the food chain, then there may be no cause for concern; but when a substance resists breakdown, and furthermore when it accumulates from one species to the next, it builds up in

---

TABLE NP14–1   **Suggestions for the Prevention of Food-Borne Illnesses** (*continued*)

■ Wash or replace sponges and towels regularly. (Cook wet sponges and cloths on "high" in a microwave oven until they are steamy and hot, or launder them with bleach; sponge a bleach solution over the cutting board, to sterilize two kitchen items at once.)

■ Clean up food spills and crumb-filled crevices.

In General

■ Throw out foods with danger-signaling odors. Be aware, though, that most food poisoning bacteria are odorless, colorless, and tasteless.

■ Do not even taste food that is suspect.

■ Do not buy or use items that appear to have been opened.

■ Follow label instructions for storing and preparing packaged and frozen foods.

For Specific Food Items

■ *Canned goods.* Discard food from cans that leak or bulge in a manner that will protect other people and animals from its accidental ingestion; before canning, seek professional advice from the USDA Extension Service (check your phone book under United States government listings, or ask directory assistance).

■ *Cheeses.* Aged cheeses, such as Cheddar and Swiss, do well for an hour or two without refrigeration, but should be refrigerated or stored in an ice chest for longer periods.

■ *Eggs.* Use clean eggs with intact shells.

■ *Honey.* Honey may contain dormant bacterial spores, which can awaken in the human body to produce botulism. In adults, this poses little hazard, but infants under one year of age should never be fed honey. Honey can accumulate enough toxin to kill an infant; it has been implicated in several cases of sudden infant death. (Honey can also be contaminated with environmental pollutants picked up by the bees.)

■ *Mayonnaise.* Commercially prepared mayonnaise may actually help a food to resist spoilage because of its acid content. Still, keep mayonnaise cold after opening.

■ *Mixed salads.* Mixed salads of chopped ingredients spoil easily, because they have extensive surface area for bacteria to invade, and they have been in contact with cutting boards, hands, and kitchen utensils that easily transmit bacteria to food (regardless of their mayonnaise content). Chill them well before, during, and after serving.

■ *Picnic foods.* Choose foods that last without refrigeration, such as fresh fruits and vegetables, breads and crackers, and canned spreads and cheeses that can be opened and used immediately.

the food chain. Figure NP14–1 shows how this happens. Similarly, if the body can rapidly excrete the contaminant or metabolize it to a harmless compound, then its ingestion may not be cause for concern; the body may be able to survive a brief exposure time. But if the contaminant enters and interacts with the body's systems, without being metabolized or excreted, then it presents a danger.

Additional doses may accumulate and cause significant harm.

This brings us to another factor. The *amount* of contamination makes a difference; if the dose is low enough, then it can be tolerated without ill effects.

Doesn't the government guarantee our food supply to be safe?

Contaminants can be difficult to regulate. Sometimes they are hard to identify, and sometimes their presence is not even known. However, for the most part, the hazards appear to be small, because the FDA regulates the presence of contaminants in foods and removes foods with unsafe contamination.[2] But in the event of an accidental spill, the risk of toxicity can suddenly become great.

TABLE NP14–2 **Examples of Metal Contaminants**

METAL	COMMON SOURCES	TOXIC EFFECTS
Aluminum	Used to manufacture or process foods, cosmetics, and medicines; to purify water	Spinal cord and brain disease, skeletal pain
Cadmium[a]	Used in industrial processes, including electroplating, plastics, batteries, vapor lamps, alloys, pigments, and as a substitute for tin in solder; present in cigarette smoke	Emphysema, fatigue, headache, vomiting, anemia, loss of smell, kidney failure
Chromium	Used in car manufacturing	Lung cancer, kidney damage
Cobalt	Used as a superalloy for jet engines	Nausea, vomiting, anorexia, ear ringing, nerve damage, respiratory diseases, goiter, heart and kidney damage
Lead[b]	Added to gasoline, newspaper ink, batteries, shotgun ammunition, and some nonresidential paints (see Chapter 12)	Damage to the nervous system, the blood-forming system, the kidneys, the reproductive system, the endocrine system (see Chapter 12)
Mercury[c]	Widely dispersed in gases from the earth's crust; local high concentrations from industry, electrical equipment, paints, and agriculture	Damage to the nervous system causing emotional disturbances, including excitability and quick-tempered behavior, lack of concentration, loss of memory, depression, fatigue, weakness, headache, stomach and intestinal disorders

[a]The World Health Organization suggests not more than 400 to 500 μg per individual per week.
[b]The World Health Organization suggests not more than 3 mg per individual per week for adults.
[c]The World Health Organization notes adverse health effects at 200 μg/l blood.
Source: Adapted from R. W. Miller, The metal in our mettle, *FDA Consumer,* December 1988/January 1989, pp. 24–27.

FIGURE NP14–1 **How a Food Chain Works**

A person whose principal animal-protein source is fish may consume about 100 lb of fish in a year. These fish will, in turn, have consumed a few tons of plant-eating fish in the course of their lifetimes. The plant eaters, in their lifetimes, will have consumed several tons of photosynthetic producer organisms. The concern about persistent contaminants is implicit in this pyramid. Assuming 100% retention of the contaminant at each level (an oversimplification), a person, being at the top of the food chain, could ingest in a year the amount of contaminant that had accumulated in several tons of producer organisms.

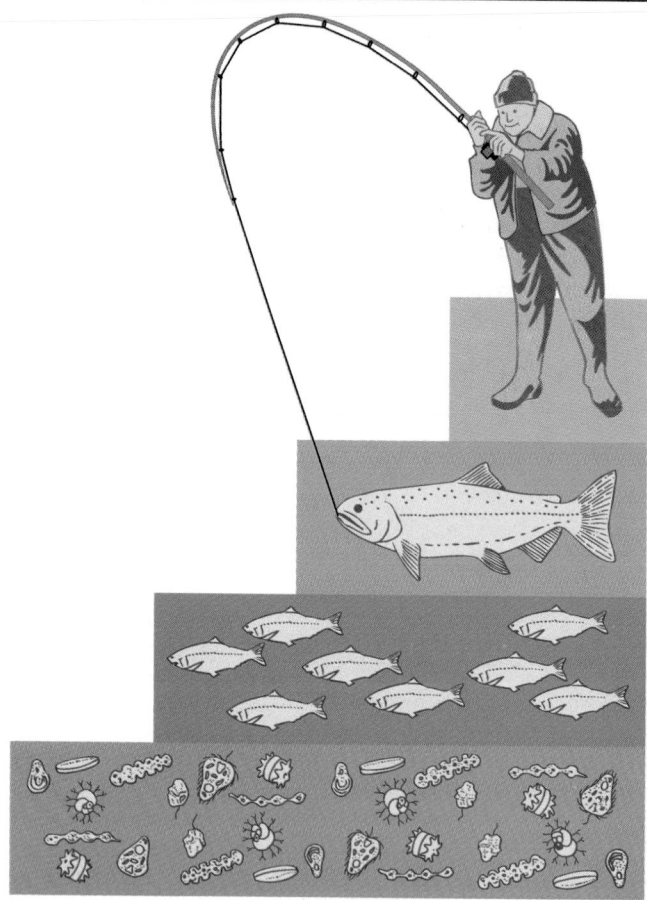

Level 1
A 150-lb person

Level 2
100 lb of fish

Level 3
A few tons of plant-eating fish

Level 4
Several tons of producer organisms

Has an accidental spill ever occurred?

Yes, more than once. One example occurred in Michigan in 1973, when half a ton of polybrominated biphenyl (PBB), a toxic chemical, was accidentally mixed into some livestock feed that was distributed throughout the state. The chemical found its way into millions of animals and then into people who ate their meat. By 1982, it was estimated that 97 percent of Michigan's residents had become contaminated with PBB. Nervous system aberrations and alterations in the liver and immune system were among the effects in exposed farm residents.[3]

When you consider the incredible challenge of supplying food safely to over 250 million people in the U.S., the job that has been done has been remarkably efficient. Although accidents do occur, and rigorous monitoring of the food supply must be continued, our efforts at keeping food safe have been successful.

Notes

1. Centers for Disease Control, as cited in *Atlanta Constitution,* 23 October 1990, p. E3.
2. D. Farley, Chemicals we'd rather dine without, *FDA Consumer,* September 1988, pp. 10–15.
3. 97% of Michigan population contaminated by 1973 spills, *Tallahassee Democrat,* 16 April 1982.

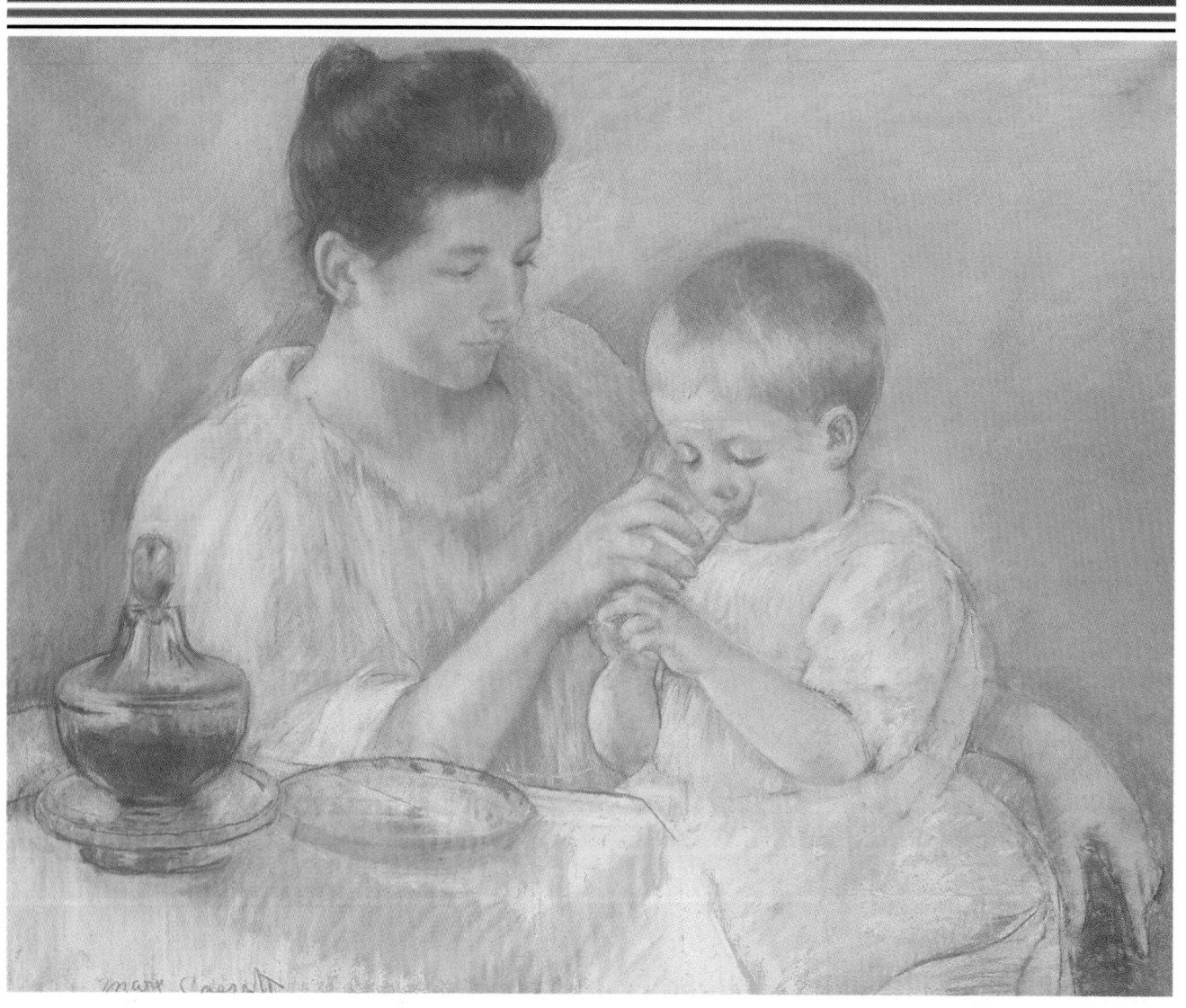

Mary Cassatt, Mother Feeding Child; *The Metropolitan Museum of Art, from the Collection of James Stillman, Gift of Dr. Ernest G. Stillman, 1922 (22.16.22).*

CHAPTER

15

Nutrition Intervention

CONTENTS

CHAPTER
15

Chapter 10 presented the first two steps in providing effective nutrition intervention: it showed how to assess a client's nutrition status and how to analyze the assessment data to determine a client's nutrient needs. Chapters 11 through 14 showed how a client's nutrient needs can be altered by pregnancy, growth, development, aging, and illness. This chapter begins by describing how to develop, implement, and evaluate nutrition care; then how to effectively communicate nutrition needs. Finally, because nutrition care includes the provision of nutrients through foods, this chapter ends by describing how foodservice is orchestrated to meet the varied needs of individuals in health care facilities.

The Nutrition Care Process

Effective nutrition intervention successfully meets the unique nutrient needs of each individual. Because these needs can be varied and complicated, applying a systematic and logical approach helps ensure success. The nutrition care process is such an approach. To identify and solve nutrition problems, follow these five steps:

nutrition care process: an organized approach to problem solving that consists of five steps (assessing, analyzing, planning, implementing, and evaluating).

nutrition care plan: a strategy for translating nutrition assessment data into a plan for meeting clients' nutrient and nutrition education needs.

1. Assess nutrition status.
2. Analyze assessment data to determine nutrient requirements.
3. Develop a plan of action, including client education, for meeting nutrition needs.
4. Implement the nutrition care plan.
5. Evaluate the effectiveness of the nutrition care plan through ongoing assessment, and make appropriate changes as needed.

As mentioned earlier, Chapter 10 described the first two steps in the nutrition care process. The focus here is on the development, implementation, and evaluation of nutrition care plans.

Nutrition Care Plans

Health care professionals use nutrition care plans to translate assessment data into strategies for meeting peoples' nutrient and nutrition education needs. Nutrition care plans define the goals of nutrition intervention and clearly describe the strategies to achieve these goals.

Developing Nutrition Care Plans

The first step in developing a nutrition care plan is to study the information gleaned from analyzing the nutrition assessment data. Does the diet history show inadequacies? Is body weight appropriate? Are lab values out of line? From this information the health care professional (usually the dietitian) generates a nutrition problem list that forms the basis of the care plan.

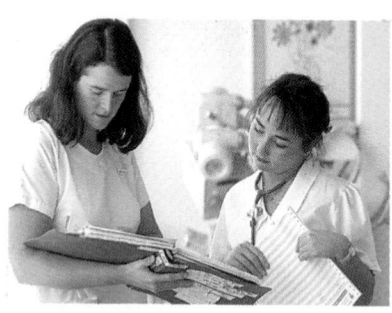

Successful nutrition intervention requires logical and systematic planning.

FORM 15-1 Sample Nutrition Assessment and Care Plan Summary

After analyzing the assessment data as described in Chapter 10, the health care provider summarizes the findings and develops a care plan using this form.

Client: _____ Diet Order: _____

ASSESSMENT SUMMARY

Anthropometric Data: _____
_____

Biochemical Data: _____
_____

Health Data: _____
_____

Socioeconomic Data: _____
_____

Drug-Nutrient Interactions: _____
_____

Dietary Intake Data: _____
_____

Recommend Additional Screening: Yes/No _____

NUTRITION CARE PLAN SUMMARY

Problem List: 1. _____
2. _____
3. _____
4. _____
5. _____

Proposed Nutrition Care: _____
_____

Other Therapy: _____
_____

Education: _____
_____

Compliance/Understanding: _____
_____

Follow-up: _____
_____

Date: _____ Dietitian: _____

Among the problems assessors list are current and past conditions that impair nutrition status, as well as areas that may present future problems. Form 15-1 provides a sample nutrition assessment and care plan summary.

Working together, health care professionals can help one another to assess clients' situations accurately. For example, a nurse may notice that the socioeconomic history section on the assessment form says that an elderly client lives with his son's family. That statement might bring to mind the image of family members gathered around a dining table, enjoying nutritious meals and one another's company. Yet the client has mentioned to the nurse that the family is always so busy coming and going that they never eat a meal together. Sure, there's always dinner for him at 6:00 each evening, but he usually eats alone. This could explain his lack of appetite and recent weight loss. By providing the dietitian with this bit of information, the nurse adds to the dietitian's understanding of the client's nutrition problems, and possibly leads to enhancement of the nutrition care the client receives.

With a problem list in hand, a dietitian can develop a plan that specifies the objectives of the diet, the content of counseling sessions, and a tentative time frame for accomplishing each objective. If, for example, a client needs to lose weight (the objective), the dietitian might set a goal of 1 pound a week for three months (the time frame). That specific goal helps the dietitian to design the weight-loss program. It determines that the diet will provide 500 kcalories less than the client's energy expenditure each day; that the diet will be low in fat and high in carbohydrate; and that exercise activity should be aerobic (the areas of content).

For each nutrition problem, the dietitian specifies the strategies needed to tackle it. The strategies provide detailed plans for reaching specific goals, and are tailored to deal with each nutrition problem's cause. For example, the problem of diarrhea requires an understanding of its cause before the dietitian can develop a successful strategy. If the diarrhea has developed in response to drug therapy, an appropriate strategy might be to request that the physician prescribe a different drug, or to provide the client with ample fluids and electrolytes to prevent dehydration. If the diarrhea is caused by a milk allergy, then eliminating milk and milk products from the diet is a critical problem-solving strategy.

In addition to strategies for meeting the client's nutrient needs, the nutrition care plan also provides for nutrition education. For example, the client needs instructions and suggestions for following a diet that eliminates milk and milk products.

Implementing Nutrition Care Plans

Once care plan strategies have been developed, the next step is to implement them. This step includes providing the appropriate diet and education. Again, thanks to frequent daily contact with clients, nurses can provide clients and dietitians with information that can improve nutrition care. It is not unusual for a client to have questions after a nutrition education session—quite often hours after the dietitian has left. And so, the client asks the next person who walks into the room—quite likely, the nurse. The nurse who is confident of the answers should provide them. Otherwise, the nurse should express honest uncertainty as to the answer and agree to check with the dietitian. The nurse may decide to inform the dietitian that the client needs a follow-up visit to clarify a few points.

As the care process continues, the plan may change. For example, a person admitted to the hospital for a diagnostic workup may later become a candidate for surgery. Adjustments in the care plan need to parallel the client's changing needs. Caretakers must be on the alert for changes in medical status so that nutrition needs will not be neglected, and should suggest new plans if original plans fall short.

Evaluating Nutrition Care Plans

As the planned strategies are implemented, the dietitian must begin to carefully evaluate the care plan. Are the strategies meeting the needs of the client? (If not, change strategies.) Have events occurred in the client's life that have changed nutrition status or altered nutrient needs? (If so, assess again.) Is the client able to make the suggested dietary changes? (If not, identify the obstacles and find solutions.)

The nutrition care process allows dietitians to identify nutrition needs and solve nutrition problems. But the plan is only as good as the information obtained to develop it. The contributions of nurses, dietetic technicians, and other care team members can add quality information to the plan. Therefore, effective communication plays a critical role in the nutrition care process.

Professional Communication Networks

One way professionals communicate is through the medical record. The medical record compiles the history, the diagnosis, the therapy, and the prognosis for each client. By reading the medical record and adding information to it, the health care team shares information about clients' conditions and their responses to therapy. This information helps determine how to proceed with the best possible care.

Medical records can be organized in many ways. Health care professionals today commonly use the problem-oriented medical record (POMR) approach. In this approach, health care team members start by generating a list of each problem the client has. Following each problem in the record are the actions being taken to deal with it. As new problems arise, they are added to the list. As problems resolve, they are deleted from the list with an explanation of how the problem was corrected.

Progress notes describe new information gleaned from the client, laboratory tests, or other objective measurements. Progress notes then provide a written assessment of the data and describe the actions to be taken based on the assessment.

Learn how to use the record effectively in the facility where you work. Regardless of the type of medical record approach used, be sure the client's medical record includes important nutrition-related information. Examples of important information include:

- Evaluation of the client's current diet.
- Nutrition assessment data.
- Recommended nutrition therapy.
- The client's acceptance and tolerance of the diet.
- Problems with the client's food intake.
- Documentation of diet counseling.
- Any planned follow-up or referral to another person or agency.
- The client's response to nutrition care.
- The client's response to diet counseling.

In addition to the formal medical record, various health care providers generally keep records of their own. For example, nurses keep nursing care

medical record: a continuous written account of a client's health, history, diagnosis, therapy, and prognosis.

diagnosis: the disease a person has or is thought to have.
  dia = through
  gnosis = knowing

prognosis: the predicted course and outcome of a disease.
  pro = ahead of time, before

An entry made in a POMR is generally written in the form of a **SOAP note.** SOAP stands for:

Subjective—Describes the client's perception of a problem or the client's feelings about a problem.

Objective—Lists new data from laboratory reports, physical exams, diagnostic tests, nutrition assessments, and other objective data.

Assessment—Evaluates the information from the subjective and objective data.

Plan—Describes actions to be taken based on the assessment.

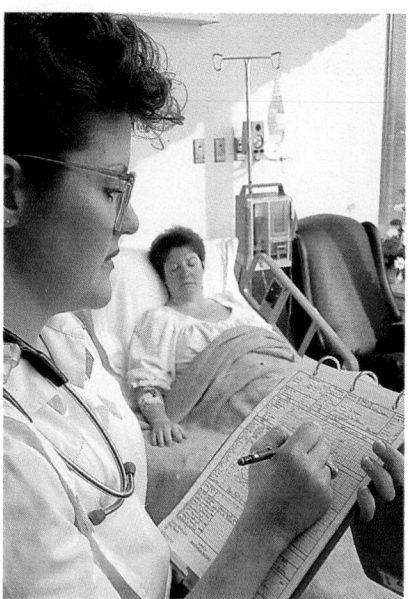

Take time to record important nutrition information in the client's medical record.

plans, and dietitians keep nutrition care plans (as described earlier). These records contain some of the same information contained in the formal medical record. However, they also include more detailed plans and notes specifically pertinent to the individual health care team member. For example, a nutrition care plan may include the details of a client's reaction to a diet, which the dietitian will later use in preparation for diet counseling. Nursing care plans may also contain information regarding a client's nutrition needs. The direct and frequent interactions nurses have with their clients generate valuable additions to the care plan.

In addition to the medical records, health team members can share other avenues of communication. Team members within a health care facility phone or page one another when they identify problems. Outside the health care facility, health care team members may be reached in their offices or through their answering services.

Bedside rounds provide an ideal opportunity for professional communication. During rounds, teams of professionals visit, examine, and discuss selected clients. Use discussion periods to talk over nutrition problems and to exchange information about clients' concerns and attitudes.

Nurses also report to one another at the end of each shift. You can use this time to pass along information regarding clients' special nutrition needs or requests. Often these requests deal with the foods the person receives while hospitalized. Because part of the nutrition care plan specifies how clients will receive the nutrients they need, it is important for health care providers to understand how foods are prepared and delivered to clients in the hospital.

Food Service in Health Care Facilities

This discussion uses the hospital as an example of a health care facility because of its familiarity to most health care providers. Other long-term care

Bedside rounds provide an excellent opportunity to discuss your concerns regarding a person's nutrition status.

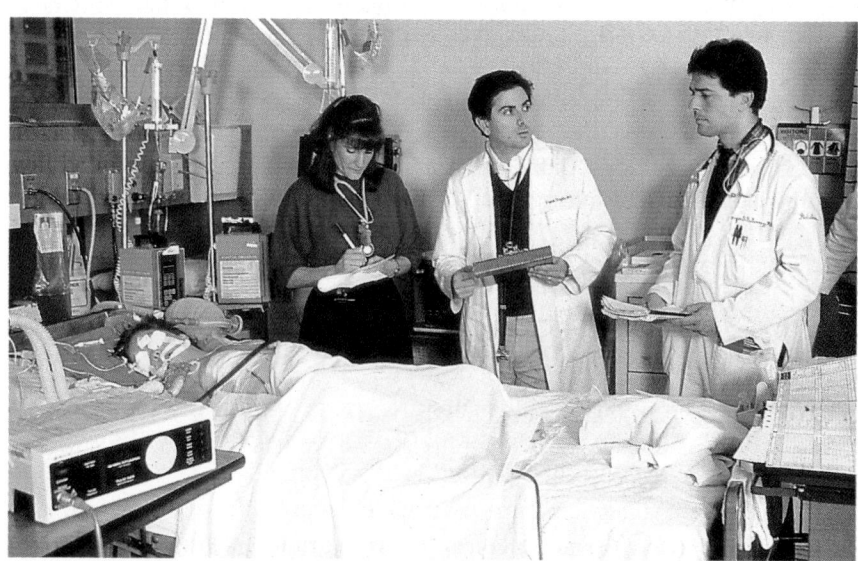

MINIGLOSSARY of Dietitian Terms

ADA: the American Dietetic Association, the professional organization of dietitians in the United States. The Canadian equivalent is the Canadian Dietetic Association, which operates similarly.

administrative dietitian: a dietitian who is primarily concerned with the management of a food service system that provides optimal nutrition and quality food. Administrative dietitians sometimes assume some clinical duties as well.

clinical dietitian: a dietitian responsible for direct client care—assessing nutrition needs, developing and implementing nutrition care plans, and evaluating and reporting the results.

dietetic technician: a technically skilled person with an associate's degree who meets the ADA's educational standards, and who works under the guidance of an RD (registered dietitian).

food service manager: a manager skilled in operating a food service system who generally is not a dietitian.

registered dietitian (RD): a trained professional with at least a bachelor's degree in nutrition and food science, a year's internship at an ADA-approved facility or the equivalent, and a passing score on the national registration exam (a four-hour qualifying exam administered over six competency areas by the ADA).

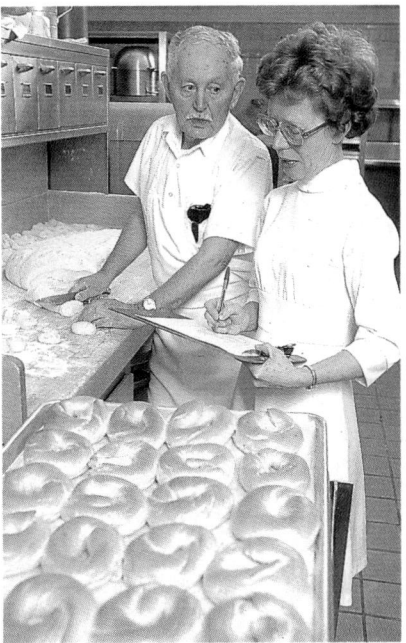

Coordination of food service in a health care facility requires the expertise of a specialist.

facilities such as nursing homes and mental institutions use similar food service systems, so the information presented applies to those settings as well. However, additional concerns arise in long-term care facilities. A person in a short-term care facility may eat poorly while hospitalized, but may make up for nutrient deficits by eating well at home. The resident in a long-term care facility continuously depends on the food service department to provide nutritious foods, and also to make them acceptable. It benefits no one, after all, to provide nutritious foods to a person who cannot or will not eat; the food service department of a long-term care facility must ensure that clients on special diets not only receive, but also eat, the appropriate foods.

The responsibility of preparing and serving food in a health care setting rests with either a chief administrative dietitian or a food service manager. (The accompanying Miniglossary defines these and related terms.) These professionals direct all aspects of food service—from purchasing foods to delivering meals to clients.

The clinical dietitian works directly with clients to assess their nutrition status, to plan appropriate diets, and to provide nutrition education. In some facilities, dietetic technicians assist dietitians in both administrative and clinical responsibilities. Other dietary employees include clerks, aides, cooks, porters, and other assistants. Keep in mind that only dietitians have extensive formal education in nutrition. Other dietary employees do not have such education, and their ability to interpret diet orders or provide accurate information may be limited.

Many hospitals provide menus from which clients can select their meals. Clients who must follow a special diet receive menus that list only appropriate food selections. This system helps to ensure that clients will receive foods they enjoy and will eat. It also gives clients the feeling of having control over something in the hospital environment.

Some facilities do not offer selective menus; their dietary departments serve a standard house diet, adjusting the basic, balanced diet according to dietary orders as necessary. Generally, even these menus provide some flexibility, though. For example, a client can find out what foods will be served at dinner and can request simple changes, such as the substitution of one vegetable for another.

You can help your clients greatly, as well as save yourself needless aggravation and time, by learning about the food service system in the health care facility where you work. Some of the things you will want to know include:

- The phone number to call and the procedure to follow to request a physician-ordered diet, make diet changes, or report problems with a client's tray.
- The phone number to reach the clinical dietitian in case a client needs special nutrition advice.
- The times when the dietary department serves meals, so that you can call in any requests before these times.
- The location of the diet manual—usually available at each nursing station—and its contents.

Once you understand how the dietary department operates, you will know where to turn for help when your clients have problems with meals or nutrition.

Hospital Foods: The Professional Perspective

Diet therapy strives to provide, for clients with specific diseases or disorders, the appropriate amounts of energy, protein, carbohydrate, fat, vitamins, major minerals, trace elements, and water in whatever form the clients can best use. For example, a person who cannot chew needs soft foods; a person whose GI tract is dysfunctional needs a formula delivered directly to the bloodstream.

Each prescribed diet has its own purpose and rationale. The purpose of a weight reduction diet may be to improve self-image in one case, or to improve blood glucose regulation in another. Its rationale is to provide limited food energy so that the person will use stored energy and lose body fat.

A person whose nutrition needs have been correctly identified and for whom an appropriate nutrition care plan has been designed benefits maximally from diet therapy. It is usually up to the physician and dietitian to select the diet therapy most appropriate to meet specific nutrition needs and to complement other medical therapies. As an example of how a diet must complement other therapies, a diet plan for an individual with insulin-dependent diabetes mellitus must coordinate meals with the times of delivery of insulin to the body.

Standard and Modified Diets

Regular or standard diets provide the recommended daily allowances of nutrients and include all foods. If such diets fail to meet specific needs of a client, modifications are made. Modifying the regular diet is much like tailoring a suit. A tailored suit is the same suit after alterations—only it fits better. So it is with the modified diet. A modified diet is a basic nutritious diet that emphasizes a variety of foods but that is tailored to meet a particular individual's needs. The tailoring may involve adjusting the consistency; adjusting the amounts of individual nutrients, energy, or fluid; altering the number of meals; or eliminating certain foods. Table 15–1 gives examples of modified diets used to treat diseases involving different organ systems. These diets are described further in Chapters 17 through 23.

It is helpful to think about modified diets in terms of the symptoms or conditions they relieve rather than in terms of the diseases they are used to treat. People differ, and so do the diets they need. Two people with the same disease may need different diets. Conversely, people in two completely different states of health may benefit from the same diet. Consider two people with cancer and a third who is pregnant. One person with cancer may be nauseated and needs dietary suggestions for controlling nausea. The other person with cancer may be overweight and not experiencing any nausea. The dietary suggestions you make to each cancer client will differ. However, a pregnant woman with nausea may benefit from some of the same recommendations as those for the nauseated person with cancer.

> In the chapters on modified diets that follow, different diets are introduced, along with the rationales for their uses. Also provided are examples of situations for which each diet may be used. As you read, keep in mind the advice you were given previously: diets should be used to treat people rather than diseases. If you know when a diet can help, you can apply your knowledge to help any individual regardless of the actual diagnosis.

Diet Manuals and Diet Orders

The exact foods excluded or included on a specific modified diet differ among hospitals, generally in minor ways. These variations reflect different schools of thought regarding diet. You can familiarize yourself with a particular institution's diets by reading the institution's diet manual.

In large hospitals, the staff of dietitians compiles a diet manual, subject to approval by the hospital administrator, several physicians, and representatives of the nursing service. A small hospital may adopt the diet manual of another hospital or of an organization such as the state dietetic association. The diet manual describes the foods allowed and not allowed on each diet, the rationale and indications for use of the diets, sample menus, and information regarding the nutritional adequacy of the diets. The dietary department then uses the manual to design menus for clients.

Diets are selected for clients in several ways. Commonly, the physician prescribes the client's diet and writes the diet order in the medical record. Alternatively, the dietitian or another health care team member may suggest

regular or **standard diet:** a diet that provides the recommended daily allowances of nutrients and includes all foods.

modified or **therapeutic diet:** a regular diet that is adjusted to meet special nutrition needs. Such diets can be adjusted in consistency, in level of energy and nutrients, in amount of fluid, in number of meals, or by the elimination of certain foods.

diet manual: a book that describes the foods allowed and restricted on a diet, the rationale and indications for use of the diet, and sample menus.

diet order: a physician's written statement in the medical record of what diet a client should receive.

TABLE 15–1   **Summary of Modified Diets by Organ System**

CONDITIONS AFFECTING OR INVOLVING THE GI TRACT, LIVER, AND EXOCRINE PANCREAS[a]	POSSIBLE DIET MODIFICATIONS
Blind loop syndrome	Low-fat
Broken jaw	Mechanical soft
Celiac disease	Gluten-restricted
Cirrhosis	Protein-restricted, sodium-restricted, fluid-restricted
Constipation	High-fiber, increased fluids
Cystic fibrosis	Low-fat, high-kcalorie, high-protein
Dental caries	Mechanical soft
Diarrhea	Liquid, low-fiber, regular, fluid and electrolyte replacement
Difficulty swallowing (dysphagia)	Mechanical soft, tube feeding, total parenteral nutrition (TPN)
Diverticulitis	Low-fiber
Diverticulosis	High-fiber
Dry mouth	Mechanical soft
Dumping syndrome	Carbohydrate-restricted; no concentrated sugars; small, frequent feedings; fluid and electrolyte replacement
Gastritis	Low-fiber, bland
Hepatic coma	Protein-restricted, sodium-restricted, fluid-restricted
Hepatitis	Regular, high-kcalorie, high-protein
Hiatal hernia	Small, frequent feedings; low-fat; bland; kcalorie-restricted
Ill-fitting dentures	Mechanical soft
Indigestion (dyspepsia)	Low-fiber; bland; small, frequent feedings
Inflammatory bowel disease	Low-fiber, low-fat, high-kcalorie, high-protein, fluid and electrolyte replacement, lactose-restricted, tube feeding, TPN
Irritable bowel syndrome	Low-fiber
Lactose intolerance	Lactose-restricted
Malabsorption	Low-fat, high-kcalorie, high-protein, fluid and electrolyte replacement
Missing teeth	Mechanical soft
Nausea	Low-fiber; bland; small, frequent feedings; no liquids with meals
Oral surgery	Mechanical soft
Pancreatitis	Low-fat; regular; small, frequent feedings; tube feeding; TPN
Peptic ulcer	Bland
Periodontal disease	Mechanical soft
Plastic surgery of head or neck	Mechanical soft, tube feeding, TPN
Reflux esophagitis	Small, frequent feedings; low-fat; bland; kcalorie-restricted
Short bowel syndrome	Low-fat, high-kcalorie, high-protein, fluid and electrolyte replacement
Ulcers of mouth or gums	Mechanical soft, bland
Vomiting	Fluid and electrolyte replacement
CONDITIONS AFFECTING THE ENDOCRINE PANCREAS[a]	**POSSIBLE DIET MODIFICATIONS**
Diabetes mellitus	Carbohydrate-controlled, kcalorie-restricted, fat-controlled, high-fiber
Hypoglycemia	No concentrated sweets; small, frequent feedings

[a]The pancreas produces both external (exocrine) and internal (endocrine) secretions. The external secretions (enzymes) play an important role in the digestion of food; the internal secretions (insulin and other hormones) play a primary role in the regulation of glucose metabolism.

TABLE 15-1 (*continued*)

CONDITIONS AFFECTING THE BLOOD VESSELS, HEART, AND LUNGS	POSSIBLE DIET MODIFICATIONS
Atherosclerosis	Fat-controlled, kcalorie-restricted, sodium-restricted, high-fiber
Congestive heart failure	Sodium-restricted; kcalorie-restricted; low-fiber; bland; small, frequent feedings; fluid-restricted
Coronary heart disease	(See *Atherosclerosis* above)
Hyperlipidemias	Fat-controlled, kcalorie-restricted, carbohydrate-controlled
Hypertension	Low-sodium, kcalorie-restricted, high-potassium, fat-controlled
Myocardial infarction	Low-sodium; kcalorie-restricted; low-fiber; bland; small, frequent feedings; moderate-temperature; fat-controlled
Pulmonary disease	High-kcalorie, high-protein

CONDITIONS AFFECTING THE KIDNEYS	POSSIBLE DIET MODIFICATIONS
Acute renal disease	Protein-restricted, high-kcalorie, fluid-controlled, sodium-controlled, potassium-controlled, fat-controlled, carbohydrate-controlled
Chronic renal disease	Protein-restricted, low-sodium, fluid-restricted, potassium-restricted, phosphorus-restricted
Kidney stones	Increased fluid intake, calcium-controlled, low-oxalate
Nephrotic syndrome	Sodium-restricted, high-kcalorie, high-protein, potassium-restricted

CONDITIONS AFFECTING MANY ORGAN SYSTEMS	POSSIBLE DIET MODIFICATIONS
Acquired immune deficiency syndrome (AIDS)	High-kcalorie, high-protein, low-fat, low-residue, low-fiber, fluid and electrolyte replacement, lactose-restricted, mechanical soft, tube feeding, TPN
Burns	High-kcalorie, high-protein, increased fluid intake
Cancer	High-kcalorie, high-protein (see also specific related conditions: *Dry mouth, Indigestion (dyspepsia), Malabsorption, Nausea, Plastic surgery of head or neck, Ulcers of mouth or gums, Vomiting,* and so on)
Food sensitivities	Elimination of offending substance
Galactosemia	Galactose-restricted
Obesity, overweight	kCalorie-restricted, high-fiber
Phenylketonuria (PKU)	Phenylalanine-restricted
Stroke	Mechanical soft, regular, tube feeding
Surgery	Regular, high-kcalorie, high-protein, increased fluids
Underweight	High-kcalorie, high-protein

a diet prescription to the physician or make recommendations when changes or clarity in the diet orders appears warranted. Whenever possible, the health care team should jointly recommend the most appropriate diet.

To avoid confusion, physicians order diets by the names given in the diet manual and describe exact modifications, when appropriate. For example, a physician should specify a 1200-kcalorie weight-loss diet rather than just a low-kcalorie diet. A "low-sodium diet" request should specify the amount of sodium; otherwise, it could be interpreted as containing any amount from 500 to 4000 milligrams of sodium.

When a physician is not available to clarify a vague order, the dietitian may determine the exact modification and record it in the medical record. If a dietitian is not available and the dietary department receives an unclear order from the nursing station, a house diet (usually specified in the diet manual) is sent.

Because the physician is ultimately responsible for a client's diet order, it is easy for others to follow the order without further consideration. But all health care providers share responsibility for the client's care.

Ideally, a dietitian or dietetic technician visits all clients and reviews the charts of every person admitted to the hospital. But often the dietitian is assigned to so many people that this is virtually impossible; therefore, most clinical dietitians see only people on modified diets or people they have been asked to see. Some smaller hospitals may not even employ full-time clinical dietitians.

Mistakes occur daily because of inappropriate diet orders. Consider, for example, the following:

- A grossly overweight individual is described as "well-nourished" and placed on a regular diet. Because the person is not on a modified diet, the dietitian does not see him, and he receives an inappropriate diet and no nutrition advice.
- A physician orders that a person be kept NPO after midnight for a lab test to be run in the morning. Because of a miscommunication, the physician thinks that the order is changed after the test, but it isn't. The individual is needlessly "starved" for several days.
- A person routinely enjoys foods low in sugar and salt. Foods served on the regular diet are too salty for her, so she eats very little food. Furthermore, she feels the hospital has totally neglected its responsibility to provide nutritious foods to its clients.

Why isn't the diet ordered correctly in the first place? In cases where many physicians, interns, and residents are seeing a client, miscommunication can easily occur. The individual may communicate needs more clearly and more often to the nurse or other health care provider than to the physician. Furthermore, the client's physician may not consider nutrition to be a significant part of the client's care. Whatever the reason, be aware that written diet orders are not always appropriate. When they are not, contact the dietitian or alert the physician.

Hospital Foods: The Client's Perspective

What do you think of when you see or hear the words *hospital food?* What are your own experiences with hospital food, or the experiences of someone close to you? Viewing hospital food from a client's perspective will add to your understanding of nutrition care.

Most people generally look forward to eating, and in the hospital, eating may become even more enjoyable than usual, for it offers clients familiarity in an otherwise strange environment. It also offers one of the few experiences in the hospital in which clients have a choice. Consider that clients usually cannot choose when they will receive tests, how much blood they will have drawn, what nurse will care for them, or what time they will have surgery. But for the most part, they can enjoy the opportunity to select their meals, and they can exercise some control: they can eat them or refuse to eat them!

Of course, clients may complain about hospital food. Complaining may have little to do with the food itself, but serves instead to vent fear, frustration, anger, and physical pain. Clients need opportunities to express their feelings, and often you may find that simply listening helps to resolve some problems without the need to make any diet changes. Actual food problems need to be corrected by the dietary department, of course.

Problems with food service unrelated to the client's physical or mental state can interfere with appetite. For one, the hospital does not cook food the same way as a client does at home—a considerable problem when the client must eat three meals a day for many days in the hospital. Unfortunately, the food may also be cold by the time it arrives in the room. In addition, the client receives meals at specified times, regardless of hunger, and often must eat alone in bed, which can be more of a chore than a pleasurable experience. Meals can also be unwelcome if they follow painful treatments. Food is so important to most people that a bad experience with it in the hospital can make them and those who work with them agitated and angry.

All this is not to say that every person in the hospital has problems with meals. The majority of people will eat adequate amounts of food, even if they complain about it. If their intakes decrease somewhat, the deficit will be easy to correct once they are at home eating familiar foods.

The loss of appetite can have a serious effect on the health or recovery of some people, however. These individuals lose their appetites at times when they can least afford nutrient deficits. By using the steps discussed in Chapter 10 (p. 248) to identify clients at risk for poor nutrition status, health care professionals can work to improve appetite and otherwise ensure that clients receive adequate nutrients.

Helping the Client Eat

Nurses and nursing assistants most often shoulder the responsibility for delivering food to the client's room. They prepare the client to eat, observe problems the client may be having with food, and communicate the client's needs to the appropriate person or department.

If a client has a poor appetite or constantly complains about food, try to get to the root of the problem. If the client is frightened, angry, or confused, simply showing that you care may help improve the situation. Be sure the client understands how important nutrition is in the recovery process. When it is permissible and possible, a friend or family member can bring

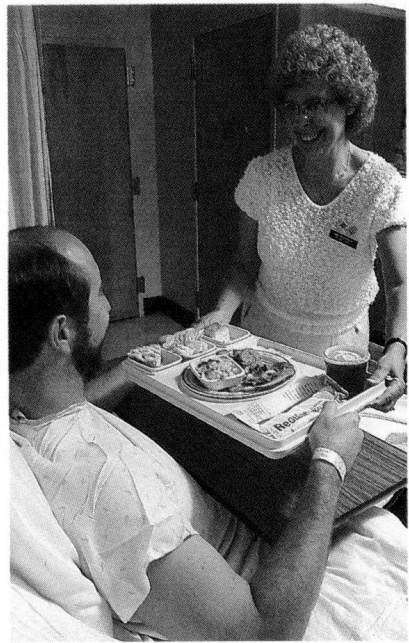

People enjoy eating when they feel comfortable and cared for.

vorite foods from outside the hospital, if these foods will improve food ʹake. This may be especially useful if the client is a child.

To help improve your client's food intake, ask yourself these questions:

- Does the client understand the importance of nutrition to the recovery process?
- Does the client understand how a modified diet supports the recovery process?
- Does the client know which foods are allowed on the diet and which are restricted?
- Does the client understand how to mark the menu correctly?

If clients need help in any of these areas, give the advice they need. Call a dietitian if the problem is one you cannot handle. Dietitians or dietetic technicians can work closely with clients to find acceptable foods.

Your own attitudes about the hospital's food can influence your client. Try to be positive; never say something like, "I couldn't eat this stuff either." Instead, say, "The dietary department really tries to make foods the way you like them. Let me call the dietitian. I'm sure we can find a solution." When a dietitian, dietetic technician, or food service manager is unavailable, look for the dietary department's list of alternative foods generally located at each nursing station.

Clients can also take a few steps to make mealtimes more enjoyable for themselves. Encourage them to wash their hands and faces and to brush their teeth or rinse their mouths before eating. Help your clients get comfortable, either in bed or sitting in a chair. Adjust the extension table to a comfortable height and distance, and make sure it is clean. Making sure that the room is clean and odor-free also helps. Take these steps before the tray arrives so that the client can enjoy the meal at the right temperature.

When the food cart arrives on the floor, check each tray:

- Verify that the name on the tray is the client's name. A client's room number may have been incorrectly recorded, or a new client may have been admitted to a room.
- Check to see that the client receives the right diet.
- Compare the tray with the selective menu that the client has filled out to make sure the client has received the foods that were ordered. Order a new tray if foods are not appropriate.
- Scan the tray for overall appearance. The client will eat better if the food is served attractively.

Once you have checked the trays, serve them immediately—while warm foods are still warm and cold foods are still cold. Help clients who need assistance in opening containers such as milk cartons. Your efforts can mean a lot to clients whose illnesses, fears, and frustrations significantly interfere with the desire to eat.

People appreciate receiving the right meal served attractively.

The Sick Child

A sick child often requires special care. Those who care for children must be sensitive to their needs and feelings. Many of the hints given in Chapter 12 for helping well children to eat are useful for working with ill children as well. Additional pointers from people experienced in working with children include:

- Notice the child's posture. Body language will tell you if a child feels fear, pain, or discomfort.
- Touch the child often and lovingly. Your touch communicates more than your words.
- As with adults, let the child choose what to eat as much as possible. Foods brought from outside the hospital can help, if permissible.
- Notice whether the child eats the food. Putting a tray of food in front of the child is not enough.
- Stay with the child during the meal, or make sure a loved person is there. The child will eat and assimilate food better if a caring person soothes away anxiety and loneliness.
- Encourage the child to eat the most nutritious foods first before he becomes too full to complete the meal.
- Let the child eat with other children, if possible. She'll enjoy mealtimes more, accept more food, and eat for longer periods.
- Avoid painful procedures near mealtimes. The stress of pain or fear shuts down digestion and turns off interest in food.

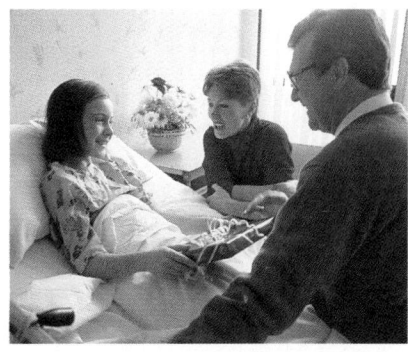

Foods taste better when you're not alone and scared.

Nutrition care contributes importantly to a child's recovery, even though its effects may not be immediately obvious.

Nutrition care means more than providing clients with food; it also means giving them attention. This chapter has described the techniques for both. The next chapter offers alternatives to feeding clients when standard oral diets cannot meet nutrient needs.

CASE STUDY

The Nutrition Care Process

Sam is a nine-year-old boy who was admitted to the hospital after an episode in which he passed out while playing with friends. Tests confirmed a diagnosis of juvenile-onset diabetes mellitus. Sam will be in the hospital for several days while his blood glucose levels are regulated. He and his family will also be learning about the special diet he will have to follow, how to use insulin, and how to coordinate diet, insulin, and exercise.

Relate the information you have been given with the nutrition care process. What steps will be necessary to develop a nutrition care plan? What are some general things you know from the description above that will be part of the nutrition care plan?

Different health care professionals will be working with Sam to help him deal with diabetes. For example, nurses will be teaching him how to give insulin injections, and dietitians will be helping him understand his diet. Describe ways these professionals can communicate with one another to ensure that Sam receives the best possible care.

Sam has been depressed about his diagnosis. He is worried about insulin injections and doesn't like the idea of limiting sweets. His appetite in the hospital has been very poor. Suggest ways for improving Sam's appetite.

Study Questions

1. What are the steps in the nutrition care process that can be used to identify nutrition problems and take corrective measures?
2. What is a nutrition care plan, and what does it include?
3. Why is continuous updating of a nutrition care plan important?
4. Describe several ways through which health care professionals can communicate.
5. What are some things you should learn about the food service system in the health care facility where you work?
6. What are modified diets, and how do they differ from standard diets?
7. What factors influence a client's response to food in the hospital?
8. Suggest ways to improve the appetites of adults and children who are having problems eating enough food in the hospital.

15

Cost Containment and Specialized Nutrition Support

Skyrocketing health care costs have become a crisis in health care today. Urgent action is needed to ensure the availability of quality health care for many lower- and middle-class families. This health care crisis troubles everyone—health care facilities, their employees, their clients, government agencies, and taxpayers. The costs of medical care have risen higher than the costs of any other service industry. It is beyond the scope of this section to discuss the reasons why health care costs continue to rise or to explore all of the implications of these rising costs. Rather, this Nutrition in Practice focuses on how spiraling costs have prompted changes in health care delivery, and how they may affect nutrition care. The accompanying Miniglossary defines some terms related to cost containment issues.

I was shocked at the cost of my physical exam to get into college, and I'm concerned about what to expect in the future. What steps are being taken to contain health care costs?

The introduction of the prospective payment system for paying the medical bills of people on Medicare represents a major step by the government to control health care costs. Before the prospective payment system was enacted in September 1983, Medicare reimbursed hospitals for a portion of the costs incurred during the

treatment of an eligible client. Using this system, hospitals had little incentive to control costs, since they received payment for any expenses incurred.

Prospective payment is quite different. Under this system, hospitals receive a fixed payment for the care of a client with a particular diagnosis. In effect, the hospital is given a budget for each case: it receives specified amounts for delivering care for specified disorders—so much for gallbladder surgery, so much for treating a broken arm, and so on. The diagnoses that qualify for a given amount of money are grouped together; hence the term diagnosis-related group, or DRG, for the categories of care funded by the system.

The DRG system motivates hospitals to cut costs, for each client's

---

MINIGLOSSARY

comorbidity: a condition that exists at the time a person is hospitalized that usually adds at least one extra day of hospitalization.

complication: a condition that develops during hospitalization that usually adds at least one extra day of hospitalization.

cost containment: measures that reduce costs.

cost effective: promoting quality care at the least cost.

diagnosis-related groups (DRG): classification of disorders that provides a basis for reimbursement under Medicare's prospective payment system.

Medicare: health insurance for eligible recipients that is administered from the Social Security Administration.

outliers: unusual cases in which the person develops severe complications or must be hospitalized much longer than expected for a particular DRG.

prospective payment system: a system for reimbursing medical costs for eligible recipients that is based on the person's diagnosis rather than actual costs.

DRG determines how much money the hospital will receive when that client leaves the hospital. The payment made to the hospital is independent of actual costs the hospital incurred. If, for example, the hospital can care for the client in fewer days with fewer tests than provided for under the DRG system, the hospital makes money. If, on the other hand, a client must remain in the hospital longer, or if physicians request too many tests, the hospital may lose money.

I can see how this affects people on Medicare, but what about people with private insurance?

Good question. Currently, unlike the prospective payment system, private insurance companies operate on a fee-for-service basis. Clients with private insurance bolster hospital revenues when they have extended hospital stays or when they receive additional services or tests. These clients help limit the losses a hospital might incur under the DRG system, but they also contribute to rising health care costs. Between 1982 and 1988, Medicare expenditures under the DRG system fell steadily so that by 1987 and 1988 the increase averaged less than one percent per year. During this same period, non-Medicare expenditures rose to almost 9 percent.[1] Private insurers are carrying a higher cost burden, which the consumer eventually pays for. For these reasons, private carriers may switch to prospective payment systems in the future if the DRG system proves effective.

The prospective payment system sounds good in a way, but it scares me, too. What about a person with a particular

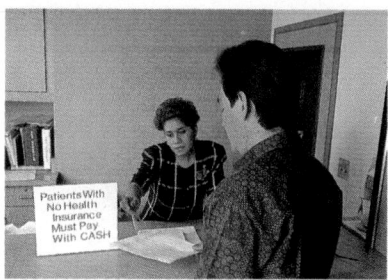

Soaring health care costs threaten the availability of health care for many individuals.

illness who gets unusually sick or needs extra care? How can you be sure that the client will not be shortchanged in an effort to reduce costs?

Your concern is a concern shared by others. However, hospitals and their staffs exist to treat disease and to relieve suffering and pain. This commitment to quality care, coupled with the competition among hospitals for clients as well as the threat of malpractice suits, balances the situation. The Prospective Payment Assessment Commission, created by Congress to oversee the DRG system, has found no evidence of reduced quality of care created by the system.[2]

In addition, some safeguards built into the program help prevent this problem to some extent. If a client must be hospitalized for much longer than normal, or incurs much higher hospital costs for a particular DRG, the hospital may receive additional support for the case. Still, in most of these cases, called outliers, the hospital's costs exceed what it receives in reimbursement; the hospital loses money. This is of concern for people who need special nutrition support, because these individuals are

frequently more ill and require longer hospital stays.

What is special nutrition support?

Chapter 16 discusses special nutrition support in detail. For now, what you need to know is that special nutrition support includes feeding clients by tube and by vein. These techniques provide an alternative source of nutrients for people who cannot meet their nutrient needs from a conventional diet.

For our purposes here, feeding by tube is also called enteral nutrition, and feeding by vein is total parenteral nutrition (TPN). These terms will be clarified further in Chapter 16.

I'm confused. In Chapter 14 we learned that attention to good nutrition would result in lower mortality rates, fewer complications, and reduced length of hospital stay. Now it sounds as if the opposite is true. Please explain.

First of all, it's important to note that studies *suggest* that appropriate nutrition support lowers mortality rates, results in fewer complications, and reduces length of hospital stays. Common sense dictates that no disease process benefits from starvation. However, the degree to which nutrition support alleviates disease is difficult to quantify. Malnourished people who need specialized nutrition support are usually quite ill. Their diseases may lead to complications or death regardless of their nutrition status. Furthermore, the severity of a given disease and the degree of malnutrition differ from case to case. Therefore, health care professionals cannot prove, when one person recovers faster than another, that one factor, such as nutrition, was directly responsible for the difference.

Studies have clearly shown that aggressive nutrition support can improve nutrition status, but few studies have documented that nutrition support speeds up recovery from disease. The effects simply have not been dramatic.[3] This does not mean that nutrition support does not help clients, but it may help in ways that are difficult to justify directly in terms of costs. Unfortunately, subjective improvements, like energy level and quality of life, do not come with price tags attached. Although it might be cheaper to keep someone in the hospital for an extra day than to give several days of nutrition support, what price do you put on the individual's comfort and desire to go home? Nutrition support can also affect the individual's risk of becoming ill again. All of these factors are difficult to justify in a context where cost containment is a high priority.

How much do enteral nutrition and total parenteral nutrition (TPN) really cost? How much do they affect the hospital's revenues?

Providing nutrition support, particularly TPN, is expensive. The average cost of parenteral nutrition runs about $365 per day.[4] Since the average person placed on parenteral nutrition needs the therapy for about 21 days, the cost of parenteral nutrition alone during an average hospitalization exceeds $7,500. The total cost of providing parenteral nutrition solutions in hospitals in 1984 was estimated at $3 billion.[5]

By comparison, enteral nutrition is a far less expensive therapy. On the average, enteral nutrition costs about $30 per day and requires about 19 days.[6] Using these figures, the average cost of enteral nutrition during a typical hospitalization is about $570.

The combination of high costs for parenteral nutrition and extended hospital stays for clients who require any type of special nutrition support puts a serious financial burden on hospitals. The Prospective Payment Assessment Committee estimated that in 1987 hospitals were reimbursed 62 cents for every dollar spent on people receiving TPN.[7] Financial pressures may force hospitals to discontinue the use of specialized nutrition support or to discourage its use.[8] Either of these measures could impair the nutrition status and support of hospital clients.

What can be done to ease the problem?

While some practitioners are pessimistic about the future of specialized nutrition support under the DRG system, others are more optimistic. It is hoped that the government will provide additional money under the DRG system to cover the costs of specialized nutrition support. Meanwhile, health care professionals need to work within the system to reduce costs associated with specialized nutrition support, as well as to justify its use.

Nutrition support teams can help control the costs of specialized nutrition support.[9] Among the steps health care professionals can take to keep nutrition care costs down are these:

■ Identify people with malnutrition at entry into the system, so that mal-

nutrition can be documented as a diagnosis and, in some cases, hospital reimbursement can be increased for the malnourished individual.[10]

■ Recommend the most cost-efficient method of feeding (enteral versus parenteral), as well as the most suitable feeding solution.

■ Evaluate and purchase nutrition support supplies that will provide the needed service at minimum cost.

■ Monitor clients who are receiving nutrition support, so as to avoid or promptly correct metabolic, mechanical, and other problems that can lead to costly complications.

■ Document the positive effects of specialized nutrition support to show that costs would be higher had nutrition support not been provided.

■ Continuously evaluate new methods of delivering nutrition support that could save money.

One study compared the costs of nutrition support recommended by a nutrition support team versus the costs of nutrition support initiated by attending physicians.[11] In 14 cases, the team had recommended enteral nutrition but the physician initiated parenteral nutrition. Had the team's advice been followed, the potential savings to clients would have amounted to $5,000 per client, or over $70,000 in all.

Teams limit the cost of nutrition support by following procedures that reduce the likelihood of complications. One group of authors reports an estimated cost savings of $400,000 a year to their hospital due to the low rate of total parenteral nutrition catheter sepsis (a complication associated with TPN) in their hospital.[12] The authors credit their nutrition support nurse with the much-lowered sepsis rate (1 percent per client catheter) compared with the rate observed in hospitals without a nutrition support nurse (33 percent per client catheter). Such documentation justifies the nurse's position and increases the probability that clients will continue to receive needed special nutrition support.

These examples illustrate how health care professionals can help ensure that specialized nutrition support will continue to be safely and readily available for people who need it. Professionals must understand the problems associated with reimbursement under the DRG system and take the necessary steps to ensure that clients will have access to optimal nutrition care.

Notes

1. W. B. Schwartz and D. N. Mendelson, Hospital cost containment in the 1980s, *New England Journal of Medicine* 324 (1991): 1037–1042.
2. American Society for Parenteral and Enteral Nutrition, *PENline* (newsletter discussing the DRG system), February 1987.
3. J. A. Sargent, Assessing the utility and improving the effectiveness of nutritional support, *Nutrition in Clinical Practice* 1 (1986): 29–39.
4. M. Regenstein, Reimbursement for nutrition support, *Nutrition in Clinical Practice* 4 (1989): 194–202.
5. G. F. Anderson and E. P. Steinberg, *Prospective payment and nutritional support: The need for reform,* Journal of Parenteral and Enteral Nutrition 10 (1986): 47–52.
6. Regenstein, 1989.
7. Regenstein, 1989.
8. J. M. Mirtallo and coauthors, Cost-effective nutrition support, *Nutrition in Clinical Practice* 2 (1987): 142–151.
9. K. S. Christensen, Hospitalwide screening increases revenue under prospective payment system, *Journal of the American Dietetic Association* 89 (1989): 1234–1235.
10. D. M. Delhey, E. J. Anderson, and S. H. Laramee, Implications of malnutrition and diagnosis-related groups (DRGs), *Journal of the American Dietetic Association* 89 (1989): 1444–1451.
11. D. D. O'Brien and coauthors, Recommendations of nutrition support team promote cost containment, *Journal of Parenteral and Enteral Nutrition* 10 (1986): 300–302.
12. M. V. Kaminiski and coauthors, Confusion of cost containment and cost effectiveness in nutritional support therapy, *Nutritional Support Services* 8 (April 1988): 27–28.

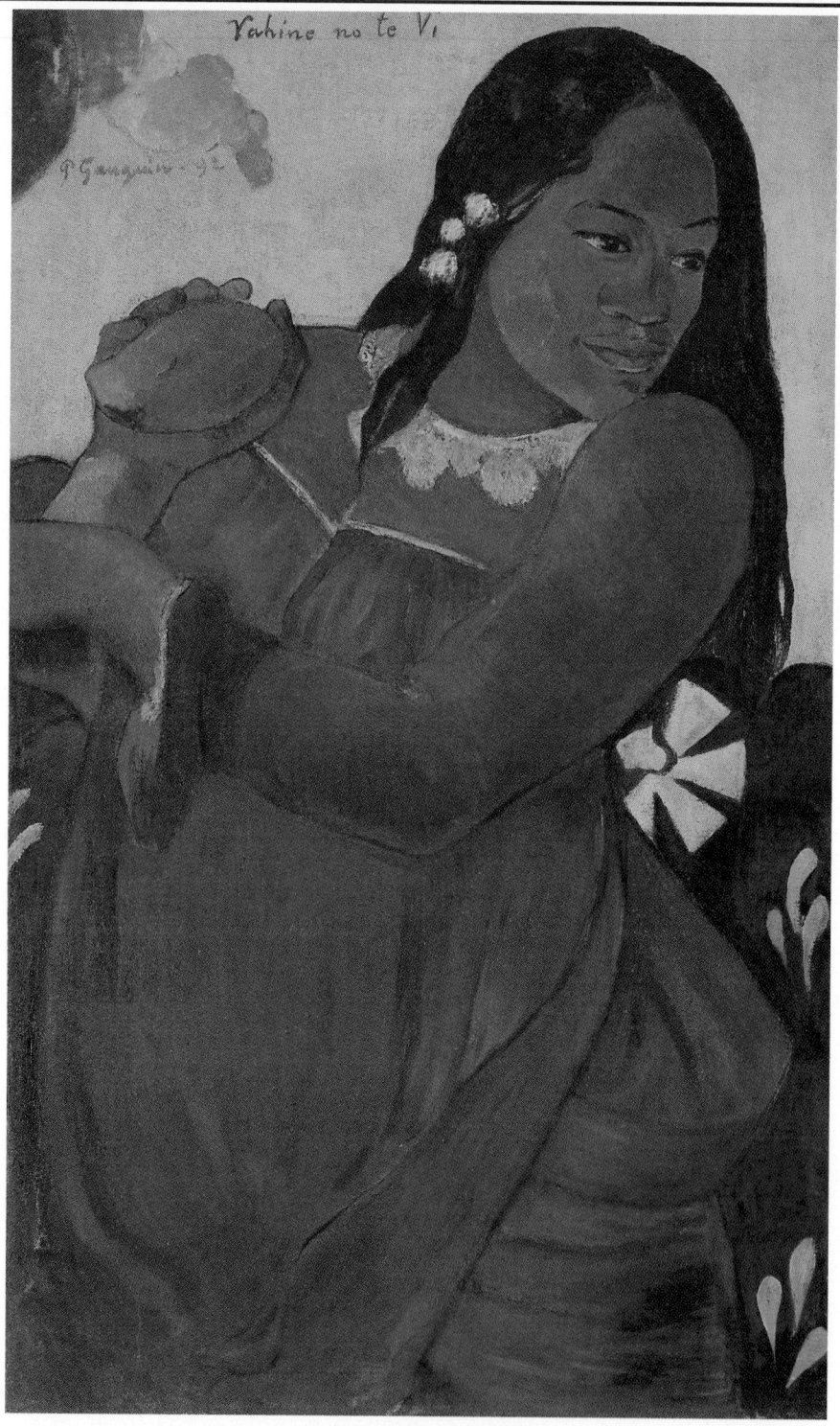

Paul Gauguin, Woman of the Mango, *1892, The Baltimore Museum of Art; the Cone Collection, formed by Dr. Claribel Cone and Miss Etta Cone of Baltimore, Maryland, BMA 1950, 213.*

Specialized Nutrition Support

CONTENTS

CHAPTER

16

As Chapter 14 describes, illness can alter nutrient needs in a variety of ways. Chapter 15 shows how foodservice departments translate these nutrient needs (by way of diet orders) into conventional foods for people who can eat them. However, conventional foods fail to meet some people's nutrient needs. This chapter looks at the ways these people are fed: by way of supplemental feedings, tube feedings, and intravenous nutrition. Figure 16–1 summarizes some of the factors involved in deciding the most appropriate way to feed a client.

Supplemental Nutrition

The term **supplements** often just means *food*—snacks or drinks between meals, for example.

When a person can't eat enough food from regular meals, the first step is to supplement the diet with extra foods between meals. To encourage intake, try to give nutritious snacks that the person truly enjoys. Many clients do well with such snacks, and for people who find it easier to drink than to eat, liquid snacks are useful. Psychologically, liquids seem less filling, and they are easy for debilitated, weak, or tired people to handle.

Liquid supplements can be common drinks like milk, milk shakes, or instant breakfast drinks. Commercially prepared liquid formulas also are available (some of these formulas are listed in Appendix D). Adding powdered milk to these liquids makes them high in protein, and adding a source of carbohydrate such as corn syrup or sugar can boost energy intakes. Commercial products (also listed in Appendix D) can be used to raise the protein, fat, or carbohydrate content of any liquid supplement.

Even when a person enjoys a liquid supplement, palatability becomes a problem after long-term use. Help relieve boredom by using more than one type of supplemental feeding. Try adding flavorings such as chocolate, decaffeinated instant coffee, or strawberry or other fruit flavorings to the supplement. A wide variety of commercially prepared flavor packets are available; these packets can be kept at the bedside for use as desired.

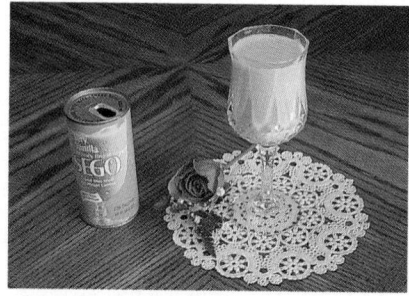

Both contain the same formula. Which would you rather drink?

complete formula: a liquid formula that, when given in sufficient volume, supplies all the nutrients a person needs.

Serve liquid feedings attractively. Liquids served in a glass are far more appealing than those served from a can. Remember to serve formula cold, and provide an ice bath to keep the formula cold so that it can be sipped as desired.

A liquid formula that supplies all the nutrients a client needs is called a complete formula. Such a formula should always be used when it is to be the sole source of nutrients. However, complete formulas can be (and often are) used as supplemental feedings. When used in this way, they boost the amounts of nutrients delivered by the diet even though they may not be given in quantities large enough to meet all nutrient needs by themselves.

Tube Feedings

An individual who has a functioning GI tract but who is unable to ingest enough nutrients orally to meet present needs is a candidate for a tube

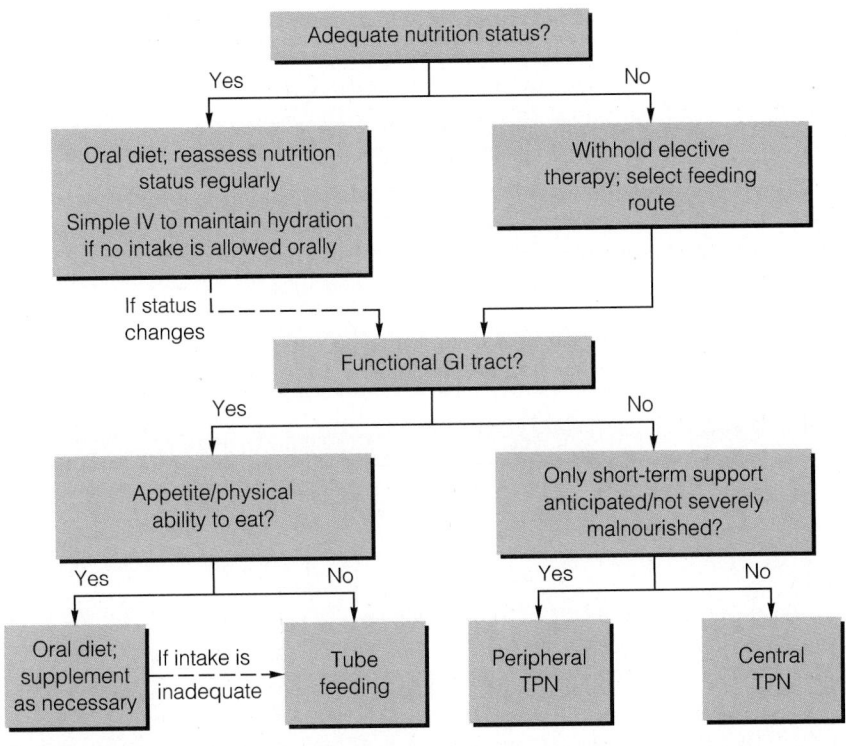

FIGURE 16–1   **Selection of the Feeding Method**

feeding. Such a person may have physical problems that make chewing and swallowing difficult, may have no appetite, may be in a coma, or may have very high nutrient requirements. Table 16–1 (p. 388) lists indications and contraindications for feeding people by tube.

For people who cannot eat oral diets, tube feedings are preferred to feedings by vein whenever possible, because enteral nutrition helps maintain normal gut function. When the GI tract is not used for a long time, the cellular structures of the intestine (the villi) shrink, and their enzyme activity slows. In addition, enteral feedings in those who are critically ill may prevent the translocation of intestinal bacteria from the gut to the portal vein and lymphatic system, a recognized source of sepsis in individuals who are critically ill.[1] Enteral nutrition is also associated with fewer complications and is less costly than feeding by vein (see Nutrition in Practice 15). The Miniglossary of Tube Feeding Terms (p. 391) defines some words you may encounter while working with clients who are fed by tube.

Feeding tubes are most commonly inserted through the nose and passed into the stomach or intestine. Feeding tubes can also be inserted through surgically made openings in the esophagus, stomach, or jejunum. Figure 16–2 (p. 389) illustrates the locations of various feeding tube placement sites. Table 16–2 (p. 390) compares some of the features of each.

Feeding tubes in wide use today are soft, flexible, and small in diameter. They are more comfortable and safer to use than older types of feeding tubes. The client on a tube feeding often becomes unaware of the tube's presence within only a few hours of its insertion.

tube feeding: delivery of a nutrient solution via a tube into the stomach or intestine.

enteral nutrition: delivering nutrients into the GI tract. Oral diets and tube feedings are types of enteral nutrition. However, *enteral nutrition* is frequently used interchangeably with *tube feeding*.

A typical feeding tube has an outer diameter of about 2.0 mm and an inner diameter of about 1.3 mm, as shown here.

TABLE 16–1 **Indications and Contraindications for the Use of Tube Feedings**

SITUATIONS IN WHICH TUBE FEEDINGS SHOULD BE RECOMMENDED

Protein-energy malnutrition with inadequate oral nutrient intake for 5 or more days
Less than 50% of required nutrient intake orally for 7 to 10 days
Severe dysphagia (difficulty swallowing)
Major burns
Major bowel resections when used along with TPN
Low-output enterocutaneous fistulas (abnormal openings between an internal organ and the skin)

SITUATIONS IN WHICH TUBE FEEDINGS MAY BE USEFUL

Inflammatory bowel disease
Major trauma
Radiation therapy
Mild chemotherapy
Liver failure
Kidney dysfunction

SITUATIONS IN WHICH TUBE FEEDINGS ARE OF LIMITED OR UNDETERMINED VALUE

Intensive chemotherapy
Immediate postoperative or poststress period if adequate oral intake is anticipated in 5 to 7 days
Enteritis (inflammation of the intestine due to radiation therapy or infection)
Major small bowel resections without the use of TPN

SITUATIONS IN WHICH TUBE FEEDINGS ARE GENERALLY NOT RECOMMENDED

Intestinal obstruction
Ileus (paralysis of the intestine)
Hypomotility of the intestine (lack of normal intestinal contractions)
Severe diarrhea
High-output enterocutaneous fistulas
Severe acute pancreatitis (inflammation of the pancreas)
Shock
Client or legal guardian does not desire aggressive nutrition support
Prognosis does not warrant aggressive nutrition support

Source: Adapted from A.S.P.E.N. Board of Directors, Guidelines for the use of eternal nutrition in the adult patient, *Journal of Parenteral and Enteral Nutrition* 11 (1987): 435, 439.

Feeding tubes come in a variety of diameters and lengths, and many have special characteristics that make them desirable for specific uses. Selection of the appropriate feeding tube depends on where the tube will be placed (stomach or intestine), as well as the inner diameter of the tube. Once the appropriate length is selected, the smallest tube through which the feeding will flow readily is best, but it is important that the tube not be so small that it becomes clogged from formula. Unclogging a tube is difficult, and attempts are frequently unsuccessful.[2] Insertion of a new tube can cause stress and anxiety.

The inner open space of a tube or hollow organ is called the **lumen.**

FIGURE 16–2   **Feeding Tube Placement Sites**

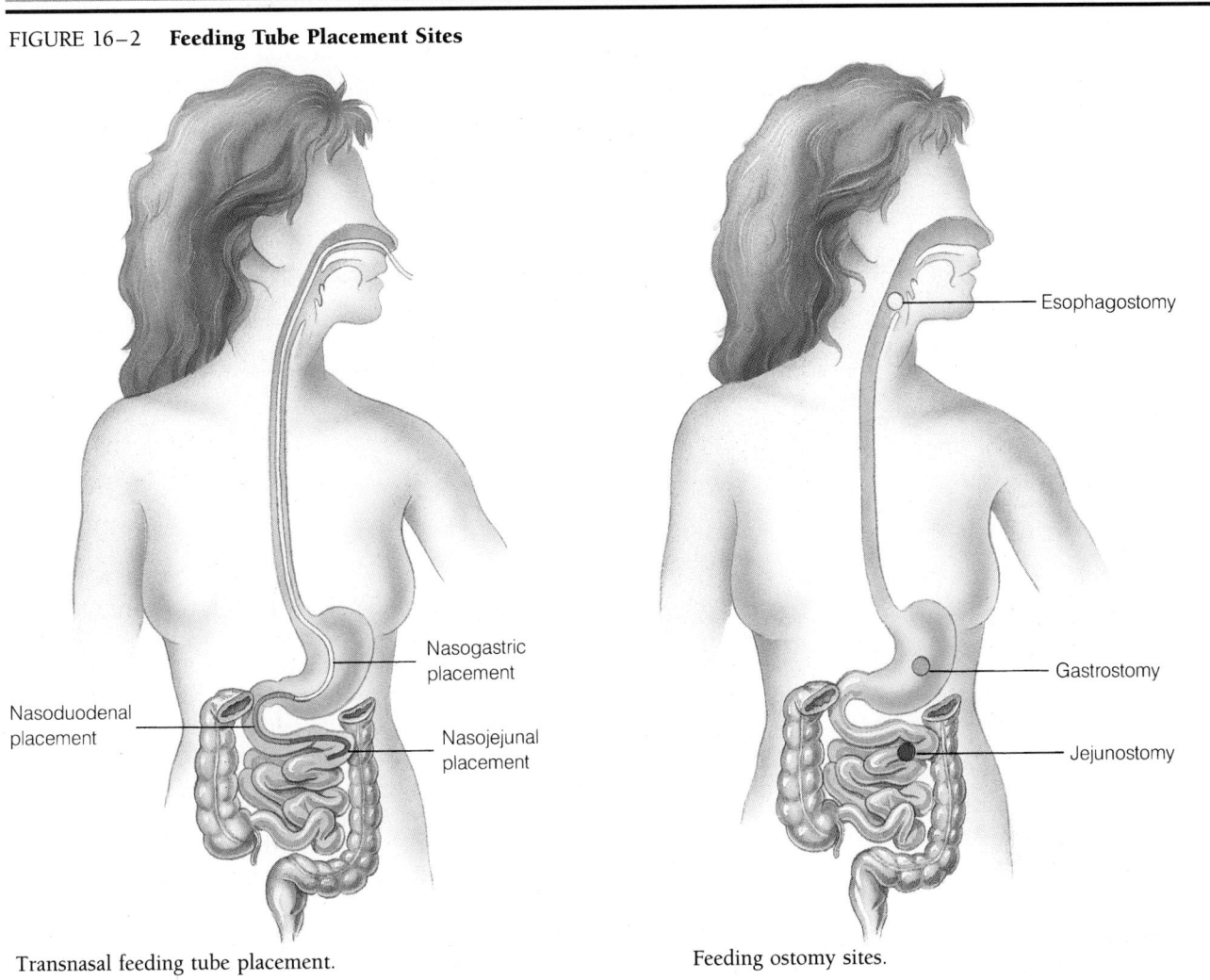

Transnasal feeding tube placement.

Feeding ostomy sites.

Although the newer tubes have greatly enhanced client comfort during tube feeding, some complications have been associated with their use. The most common complications result from inadvertent placement of the tube in the lungs and from obstruction of the tube itself. Complications can be serious and even life threatening.

Formula Characteristics

The number of formulas available to feed people either orally or by tube is staggering (some are listed in Appendix D). Formulas designed to meet a variety of medical and nutrition needs can be used alone or modified using other supplements to meet an even wider range of needs.

TABLE 16-2   **Features of Feeding Tube Placement Sites**

SITE	INSERTION	POTENTIAL IRRITATIONS	RISK OF REGURGITATION[a]	LONG-TERM TOLERANCE	CHANCE OF REMOVAL BY UNCOOPERATIVE CLIENT
Nasogastric	Nonsurgical	Nasal passages, esophagus	High	Fair[b]	Likely
Nasoduodenal	Nonsurgical	Nasal passages, esophagus	Low	Fair[b]	Likely
Nasojejunal	Nonsurgical	Nasal passages, esophagus	Low	Fair[b]	Likely
Esophagostomy	Surgery required	—	High	Good	Unlikely
Gastrostomy	Surgery required	Skin irritation	Moderate	Good	Unlikely
Jejunostomy	Surgery required	Skin irritation	Low	Good	Unlikely

[a]Relative to the other feeding sites. The absolute risk of regurgitation is small.
[b]When the appropriate type and size of tube are used.

Types of Formulas

The client's specific nutrition needs, identified through a careful nutrition assessment, determine the most appropriate formula. To simplify the classification of formulas, it is reasonable to think of formulas as belonging to one of two types. Those that contain proteins, carbohydrates, and fats of high molecular weights are called *intact formulas*. Those that contain smaller molecules of proteins, fats, and carbohydrates are called *hydrolyzed formulas*.

Intact formulas are appropriate for people who are able to digest and absorb nutrients without difficulty; they come in the form of either protein isolate formulas or blenderized formulas. A protein isolate formula contains a purified protein. A blenderized formula can be made in a blender or purchased commercially, and it usually contains pureed meats, vegetables, fruit, milk, and starches with vitamins and minerals added as necessary.

Hydrolyzed formulas are, in a sense, "predigested," and therefore only minimal further digestion is needed. People who lack digestive capabilities or who have a smaller than normal area for absorbing nutrients may benefit from these formulas.

Commercial formulas come in ready-to-use liquid form, as liquid concentrates, or in powdered form. Standard formulas provide about 1 kcalorie per milliliter. Formulas containing 1.5 and 2.0 kcalories per milliliter and higher protein contents than standard formulas meet energy and protein needs in a smaller volume. Other special formulas meet the needs of people with disorders (such as liver, kidney, and lung disorders) who require different proportions or types of protein, amino acids, carbohydrate, fat, and electrolytes.

A small number of formulas are termed *modular formulas*. Modules contain different forms of individual nutrients (see Appendix D). A module can be added to another formula to alter the composition of that formula (for example, to add protein to that formula) or can be used with other modules to construct totally individualized formulas. Modular formulas can be con-

intact formula: a liquid diet that contains complete molecules of proteins, carbohydrates, and fats; also called **polymeric formulas.**

hydrolyzed formula: a liquid diet that contains broken-down molecules of proteins, carbohydrates, and fats, such as amino acids or short peptide chains; also called **monomeric formulas.**

protein isolate: a protein of high biological value that has been separated from a source containing a variety of proteins. Examples include casein and albumin.

modular formulas: formulas that contain specific nutrients for use as supplements.

MINIGLOSSARY of Tube Feeding Terms

transnasal: through the nose. A **transnasal feeding tube** is one that is passed through the nose.

nasogastric (NG): from the nose to the stomach.

nasoenteric: from the nose to the intestine. **Nasoenteric feedings** include both nasoduodenal and nasojejunal feedings.

nasoduodenal (ND): from the nose to the duodenum.
 naso = nose

nasojejunal (NJ): from the nose to the jejunum.

feeding ostomy: surgical opening in the esophagus, stomach, or intestine through which a feeding tube can be passed.

esophagostomy: (ee-soff-uh-GOSS-toe-mee): a surgically made opening in the esophagus through which a feeding tube can be passed.
 ostomy = a surgically formed opening

gastrostomy: (gas-TROSS-toe-mee): a surgically made opening in the stomach through which a feeding tube can be passed.

jejunostomy: (JEE-ju-NOSS-toe-mee): a surgically made opening in the jejunum through which a feeding tube can be passed. A **duodenostomy** (DEW-odd-eh-NOSS-toe-mee) is not used as a feeding ostomy site because the duodenum swings toward the back of the body and is not easily accessible.

structed to meet specific nutrient requirements more closely than regular commercial formulas and can also be less expensive in some cases. However, the person formulating a modular feeding must have in-depth nutrition knowledge to carefully design a formula that will meet all of a client's nutrient needs.

Formula Osmolality

Osmolality is a measurement of the concentration of molecular and ionic particles in a solution. The greater the number of particles in a solution, the greater the osmolality. The osmolality of normal blood serum is about 300 milliosmoles (mOsm) per liter. The osmolality of formulas ranges from about 250 to over 800 milliosmoles. A formula that approximates the osmolality of the serum is referred to as an isotonic formula. A hypertonic formula has a higher osmolality than serum.

A hypertonic formula in the intestine can cause water to be drawn from in and around the body cells into the intestine. If an individual's body has had time to adapt to the hypertonic solution, this is usually not a problem. However, if adaptation has not occurred, diarrhea, vomiting, cramps, or nausea can result. Because people placed on tube feedings often have been unable to eat for some time, the most desirable formulas are often those as near isotonic as possible.

osmolality: the number of molecular and ionic particles (measured in osmoles) per liter of water in a solution.

isotonic formula: a formula with an osmolality similar to that of blood serum (300 mOsm/l).
 iso = the same
 ton = tension

hypertonic formula: a formula with an osmolality higher than that of blood serum.
 hyper = greater, more

Residue and Fiber

Dietary fibers are the structural parts of plant foods that cannot be digested by enzymes in the human digestive tract. Residue includes fiber, together with intestinal secretions, bacteria, and shed intestinal cells in the colon. The residue content of the diet is largely responsible for fecal bulk. As you will see in later chapters, people with certain GI disorders need low-residue diets.

Higher-fiber diets benefit people who can tolerate them, because they help maintain gut integrity.[3] Research has not yet defined which people on tube feedings benefit from fiber-enriched formulas.[4] However, some research suggests that fiber may benefit those with diarrhea or constipation and those who must have tube feedings for long periods of time.[5] Furthermore, certain fibers (pectins) may be digested by bacteria in the intestine to short-chain fatty acids. These fatty acids provide fuel to support growth, maintenance, and repair of the lining of the intestine, enabling it to adapt more readily after large portions of the small bowel have been resected (see Chapter 21).[6]

Other Characteristics of Formulas

Formulas can be made from many different ingredients. For example, some contain lactose, while others are lactose-free. One formula may derive its protein from a source of higher biological value (see pp. 64–65) than other formulas. Health care professionals must keep these characteristics in mind when choosing formulas for a client.

Another characteristic important in comparing different formulas is their cost. Costs vary widely for individual products in different parts of the country and for different hospitals. However, as a general rule, hydrolyzed formulas are more costly than intact formulas, because they require more commercial modification. Nutrition in Practice 15 describes the importance of cost considerations in health care today.

Formula Selection

No formula is perfect. In general, the more digestible the formula, the higher its osmolality, the lower its palatability, and the higher its cost. Because hydrolyzed formulas are more costly and more likely than other formulas to cause complications, they should be used only for people who can't digest and absorb nutrients adequately. As a rule of thumb, the formula that meets the client's nutrient needs with the least risk of complications and at the least cost is the best choice. If a formula does not meet all nutrient needs, it should be supplemented with the appropriate nutrients. Figure 16–3 shows some of the considerations required to select the appropriate formula.

A formula given orally also needs to taste good. As a general guide, the more hydrolyzed a formula and the lower its fat content, the less tasty it will be. However, remember that people's likes and dislikes vary greatly, and what is unpalatable to one person might be perfectly acceptable to another.

Some additional factors in formula selection include:

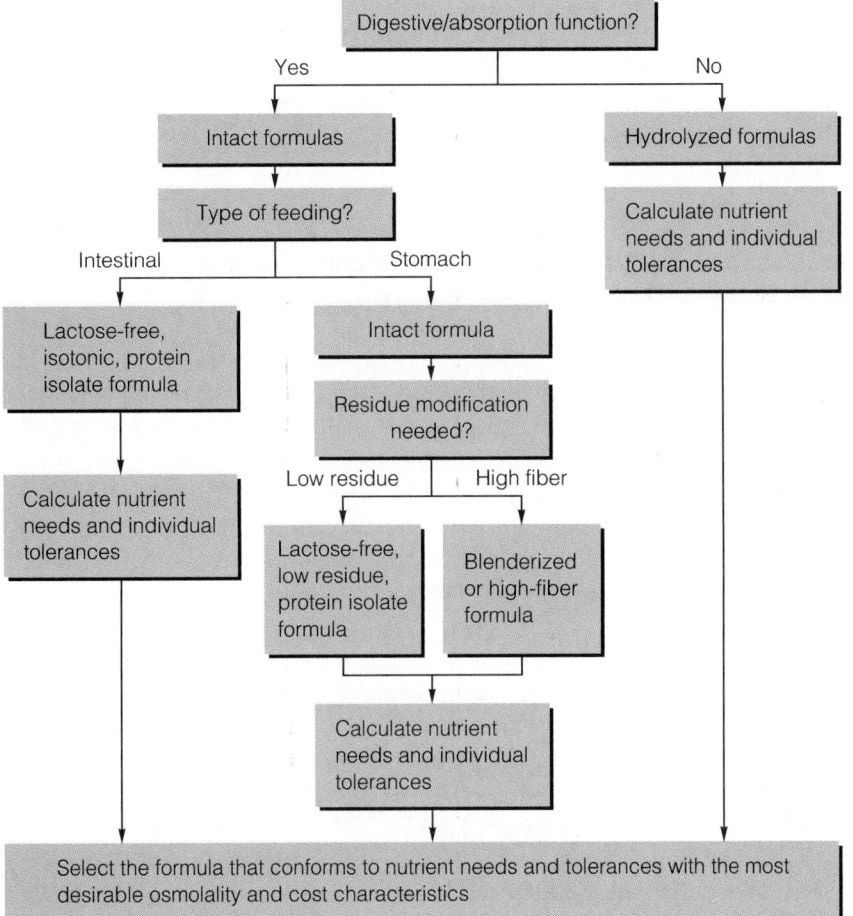

FIGURE 16–3 **Selection of Formulas**

■ *The client's digestive and absorptive function.* A person who doesn't have a functioning GI tract is not a candidate for an oral or tube feeding. However, people with minimal GI function may be able to benefit from hydrolyzed formulas.

■ *The placement of the feeding tube (stomach versus intestine).* Feedings delivered directly into the intestine must be easily digested, but if the GI tract is functional, they do not have to be hydrolyzed. Isotonic formulas are preferred for intestinal feedings, because the intestine is more sensitive than the stomach to hypertonic formulas.

■ *Nutrient requirements.* Nutrient requirements are estimated based on careful nutrition assessment. The client's medical condition, nutrition status, and metabolic rate are all important considerations in estimating nutrient requirements.

■ *Individual preferences and tolerances (food allergies and sensitivities).* Lactose-free formulas are frequently selected, because temporary and permanent lactose intolerances are common problems.

In the final analysis, the health care provider can, at best, make only an educated or informed guess about the best formula for an individual. After the selection is made, monitor each person's nutrition status and tolerance to the formula, and be prepared to make or recommend a change to help ensure that individual needs are being met. As a later section in this chapter describes, the procedure for monitoring people on tube feedings includes daily weighings and weekly assessments to make sure nutrition status is satisfactory or improving.

Administration of Tube Feedings

Attention to formula preparation and administration helps ensure the successful use of tube feedings. The formula container should be labeled with the client's name, the client's room number, and the date and time that the formula was prepared. Bacterial contamination of formulas can lead to food-borne illness. Mounting evidence suggests that people with suppressed immune systems may be particularly vulnerable to infection from food-borne illness.[7] These steps reduce the risk of contaminating formula with bacteria during preparation and administration:

- Prepare formula in a clean environment with clean equipment and clean hands.
- Store opened or mixed formulas in the refrigerator.
- Discard unlabeled or improperly labeled containers and all opened containers of formula not used within 24 hours.
- Deliver formula in a fresh container daily. Never add fresh formula to formula still in the container.
- Before adding formula to the feeding bag or bottle, rinse the feeding container, the tubing attached to it, and the feeding tube itself with water.
- Change the feeding bag or bottle and the tubing attached to it (except the feeding tube itself) every 12 to 24 hours.

Tube feeding formulas sometimes come prepackaged in containers that can be used to dispense formula without being added to another feeding bag; such systems may significantly reduce the risk of bacterial contamination.[8]

Many people can receive undiluted formulas at the start of a tube feeding, particularly when the selected formula is isotonic or slightly hypertonic. However, people with severe stress or those who have not eaten for several weeks may not be able to tolerate large volumes or highly concentrated formulas. As a rule of thumb, people who have low serum albumin levels (less than 3.5 grams per 100 milliliters) are more likely to have problems tolerating concentrated formulas. For these individuals, formulas may at first need to be diluted to one-half or one-third strength (see Figure 16–4). Initially, give the formula slowly, 30 to 50 milliliters per hour. If the person tolerates the formula, increase the rate of feeding by 25 milliliters per hour every 8 to 12 hours. Once the final desired rate is reached, the strength is increased. If the client cannot tolerate a new rate or strength, back up and proceed more slowly, giving the person more time to adapt.

Water is important for the individual who is fed by tube. Supplemental water is often needed to meet the client's daily fluid requirements. As a

Formulas themselves contain considerable amounts of water. A standard formula (1 kcal/ml) contains about 850 ml of water per liter of formula. Higher-kcalorie formulas contain less water: formulas that contain 1.5 kcal/ml and 2.0 kcal/ml provide about 775 ml and 600 ml of water per liter of formula, respectively.

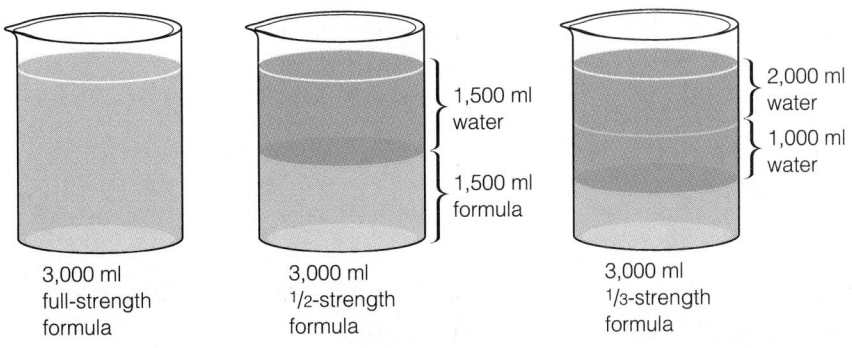

3,000 ml
full-strength
formula

1,500 ml
water

1,500 ml
formula

3,000 ml
1/2-strength
formula

2,000 ml
water

1,000 ml
water

3,000 ml
1/3-strength
formula

FIGURE 16-4   **Formula Dilution**

guideline, adults require from 1500 to 2000 milliliters of water daily. A person with a high fever may require an additional 500 to 1500 or more milliliters. Other conditions such as excessive sweating, severe vomiting, diarrhea, blood loss, and some types of kidney disease also raise water requirements. In other types of kidney, liver, and heart diseases, total water intake may need to be restricted.

Attention to indicators of body water balance can help determine individual water requirements. Thirst, in alert adults, is a good regulator of water needs; a person complaining of thirst generally needs water. Body weight changes can also help determine if fluid needs are being met. An unexplained body weight change of 2.2 pounds (1 kilogram) can represent a fluid loss or gain of about 1 liter.[9] Serum electrolytes, hematocrit, and blood pressure should also be monitored regularly; high values suggest dehydration.

Water used to flush the feeding tube before and after a feeding or when the feeding apparatus is being changed not only helps prevent the feeding tube from becoming clogged but also helps keep the client hydrated. Water can also be given orally if the person can drink it.

A day's volume of a formula can be given in many ways. For example, a person can be fed four to six times daily. In such a case, the total volume of formula needed for the day is divided by 4 or 6, respectively. The client given intermittent feedings can move about more freely between feeding times than the client being fed continuously.

Optimal tolerance to intermittent delivery of feedings occurs when a feeding volume of no more than 250 milliliters is infused over 30 minutes. Larger volumes of formulas or formulas delivered too quickly often lead to complaints of abdominal discomfort, nausea, fullness, and cramping. This makes sense. After all, you do not gobble down a meal in just a few minutes, especially when you are not feeling well.

Feedings delivered slowly over a 16- to 24-hour period—continuous drip feedings—benefit people intolerant of larger formula volumes. People being fed by tube who have not received any food through the GI tract for long periods of time or those receiving jejunal feedings often benefit from continuous drip feedings. Infusion pumps (similar to those used for delivering intravenous solutions) help ensure accurate and constant flow rates (see Figure 16-5 on p. 396), although continuous drip feedings can be delivered without

intermittent feedings: delivery of a 4- to 6-hour volume of feeding solution over 20 to 30 minutes.

continuous drip administration: delivery of a feeding solution continuously over a 16- to 24-hour period.

FIGURE 16–5   **Tube Feeding Administration**

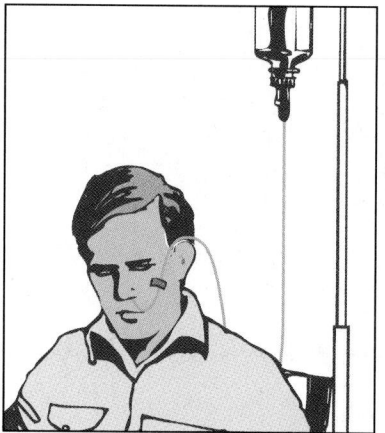

A person being fed by tube. This feeding is being delivered by gravity drip.

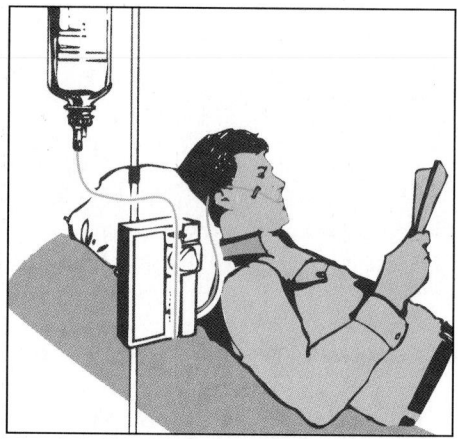

A tube feeding delivered by pump. A typical setup is shown here.

Source: Illustrations Courtesy of Ross Laboratories.

them. The accompanying box, "How to Administer a Tube Feeding," provides examples of different tube feeding delivery schedules.

Regardless of the method used to deliver a formula, elevate the client's head to at least a 30-degree angle during the feeding and for 30 minutes following an intermittent feeding to minimize the possibility of regurgitation.

Prevention of Tube Feeding Complications

People receiving the proper formula, prepared and administered correctly, seldom have major problems with tube feedings. Tube feedings can go smoothly if a few simple measures are taken to eliminate problems, but faithful and frequent monitoring of each person is crucial to success. Table 16–3 (p. 398) provides a schedule for monitoring that helps ensure early detection of problems.

Complications can be related to the tube itself (such as inappropriate placement, clogging of the lumen of the tube, and skin irritation around a feeding ostomy site) or can be related to the formula or its administration. Table 16–4 (pp. 400–401) identifies many complications associated with tube feedings and suggests ways to prevent or correct them.

Feeding Tubes Used to Administer Drugs

Advances in the understanding of nutrition, as well as the availability of many new products for feeding people by tube, have resulted in a dramatic growth in the use of the tube feeding method. The method is widely used for people who are seriously ill, and such people are also likely to be receiving numerous medications. Often these medicines are delivered through the feeding tube, and in some cases, undesirable interactions can occur.

How to Administer a Tube Feeding

To determine a tube feeding schedule, the planner needs to know how much formula a person needs in a day to meet nutrient needs. This amount will be the final goal for the person once she is able to tolerate the full volume of feeding. For example, let's take a client who needs 3000 milliliters of formula per day to meet his nutrient requirements. If the client is to receive the formula intermittently six times a day, then at each feeding he will need:

3000 milliliters ÷ 6 feedings = 500 milliliters per feeding.

If he is to receive the same volume of formula intermittently four times a day, at each feeding he needs:

3000 milliliters ÷ 4 feedings = 750 milliliters per feeding.

He would probably tolerate this volume of formula poorly if it were given to him within a few minutes at each feeding.

If the client is to receive the formula continuously over 16 hours, he needs 187.5 milliliters of formula each hour during the administration period:

3000 milliliters ÷ 16 hours = 187.5 milliliters per hour.

If the total volume of solution is to be given by continuous drip over 24 hours, he will receive 125 milliliters of formula each hour:

3000 milliliters ÷ 24 hours = 125 milliliters per hour.

Regardless of the delivery rate, the feeding is started at small volumes and gradually increased. A sample administration schedule for a person who is eventually to receive 125 milliliters of continuous drip feedings per hour for 24 hours might go like this:

- Start the feeding at 50 milliliters per hour at full strength.
- Administer the formula at 75 milliliters per hour at full strength after 8 hours.
- Administer the formula at 100 milliliters per hour at full strength after 16 hours.
- Administer the formula at 125 milliliters per hour at full strength after 24 hours.

Of course, the rate is not increased if the person is not tolerating the tube feeding. It may be necessary to back up and increase the rate more gradually in some cases.

Crushing tablets and mixing them with water so that they will flow through the feeding tube is a common practice, but it should be avoided if possible. If the particles are too large for the lumen of the feeding tube, the tube becomes clogged and may need to be reinserted at the cost of considerable discomfort to the client. Also, some types of tablets and capsules are intended to release their contents slowly; they should not be crushed, or the

TABLE 16–3   **Checklist for Monitoring Clients on Tube Feedings**

Before starting a new or intermittent feeding:	Complete a nutrition assessment. Check tube placement. Check residual formula in stomach (if 150 ml or more, consider possible reasons for delayed gastric emptying.)
Every half hour:	Check gravity drip rate, when applicable.
Every hour:	Check pump drip rate, when applicable.
Every two to four hours of continuous feeding:	Check gastric residual.
Every four hours:	Check vital signs, including blood pressure, temperature, pulse, and respiration. Check glucose and acetone in urine; monitoring glucose and acetone can be discontinued after 48 hours if test results are consistently negative in a nondiabetic client. Refill feeding container.
Every eight hours:	Check intake and output. Check specific gravity of urine. Chart client's total intake of, acceptance of, and tolerance to, tube feeding.
Every day:	Weigh client. Change feeding bag and tubing. Check electrolytes, blood urea nitrogen, and blood glucose daily until stabilized.
Every seven to ten days:	Check all laboratory findings. Reassess nutrition status.
As needed:	Observe client for any undesirable responses to tube feeding (for example, nausea, vomiting, or diarrhea). Check tube placement (for nasogastric placement only). Check nitrogen balance. Check laboratory data. Clean feeding equipment. Chart significant details.

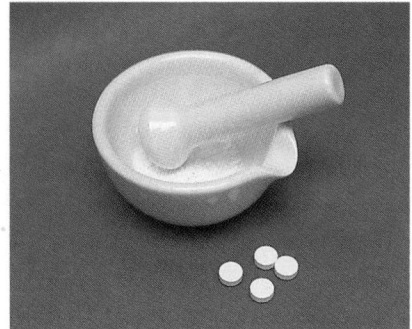

Use liquid medicines for delivery through feeding tubes whenever they are available; if not, finely crush the tablets and mix them with water.

person might be exposed to an excessive dose of the drug at one time. When administering drugs through feeding tubes, follow these guidelines:

■ Give medications orally whenever possible.
■ If a client cannot take medication by mouth, deliver a liquid form of the medication through the tube, using a syringe whenever it is available.
■ Consider giving the drug by injection or intravenously if available.

■ If tablets are the only form in which a medicine is available, crush them *finely* and mix them with water before administering them.

■ Flush the feeding tube with at least 30 milliliters of warm water or saline before and after giving any form of medicine.[10]

The location of the feeding (whether gastric or intestinal) is also of considerable importance. Some drugs are designed to dissolve in the acidic environment of the stomach. Delivered directly to the duodenum or jejunum, such drugs may not be as readily absorbed. Similarly, a drug that is absorbed optimally in the duodenum may be poorly absorbed in the jejunum. In such cases, oral, intravenous, or injectable forms of the drug should be used.

Some drugs are not compatible with feeding solutions. A common example is drugs that are highly acidic; these can thicken and clump formulas, which in turn clog feeding tubes. Some drugs that are known to be incompatible with formulas are listed in Table 16–5 (p. 402). Medications should never be added directly to formulas, because too little is known about the interactions of drugs with formulas. Instead, deliver medication through the tube using a syringe.

In some cases, drugs added to formulas are incompatible because the drug effects are hindered. One example is phenytoin (a drug used to control seizures). Absorption of phenytoin may be markedly reduced if a person is on continuous drip tube feedings. To help remedy the problem, stop tube feeding for two hours before and two hours after giving phenytoin whenever possible.

An important consideration in delivering a medication through a feeding tube is the medication's osmolality. Hyperosmolar medications given too rapidly cause the same undesirable side effects as hyperosmolar formulas. If a medication is compatible with the tube feeding formula, it can be added directly to the formula and given slowly over a long time. To avoid problems with hyperosmolality:

■ Mix incompatible drugs with water, and administer them slowly; then resume the feeding.

■ Consider using injectable forms of the drugs.

■ Do not mix drugs together and give them all at once; give each drug individually, and flush the feeding tube with water after each one. This measure also reduces the likelihood of drug-drug interactions.

Drugs can trigger GI side effects similar to those associated with tube-feedings. Nausea, vomiting, diarrhea, and electrolyte disturbances are a few of these possible complications. When tube feedings are being given, side effects of drugs should be considered as a possible source of problems. In some cases, a substitute drug with similar pharmaceutical action, but without the side effects, can be used to reduce GI problems. Finally, keep in mind that tube feeding formulas can interact with drugs in the same ways that everyday foods can (see Appendix B).

Psychological Implications of Tube Feedings

Chapter 1 discusses many reasons why people choose the foods they eat. The person fed by tube is denied the right to select food for any reason, even

Some drugs that may clog feeding tubes include:

■ Dyazide.
■ Ibuprofen.
■ Magnesium oxide.
■ Metamucil.
■ Micro K.
■ Theo-Dur Sprinkles*

*Source: M. L. Gora, M. M. Tschampel, and J. A. Visconti, Considerations of drug therapy in patients receiving enteral nutrition, *Nutrition in Clinical Practice* 4 (1989): 105–110.

TABLE 16-4   **Causes and Prevention or Correction of Tube Complications**

COMPLICATION	POSSIBLE CAUSES	PREVENTIVE/CORRECTIVE MEASURES
Aspiration pneumonia	Regurgitation of formula, which is subsequently inhaled into lungs	Use nasoenteric, gastrostomy, or jejunostomy feedings in high-risk clients; use small-diameter transnasal tube; elevate head of bed during feeding; use continuous drip method of delivery; check gastric residual.
Clogged feeding tube	Formula too thick for tube	Select appropriate tube size; dilute formula with water; flush tubing with water before and after giving formula.
	Medications given through tube inadequately crushed or incompatible with formula	Use liquid medications whenever possible; crush tablets finely and mix with water; flush tubing with water before and after medicines are given; give medicine individually; do not mix medication with formula.
Constipation	Low-fiber formula	Provide additional fluids; use high-fiber formula; give laxatives or enemas if necessary.
	Lack of exercise	Encourage walking and other activities, if appropriate.
	Drug therapy	Change drug therapy if possible; use laxatives if indicated.
Dehydration and electrolyte imbalance[a]	Excessive diarrhea	See items under "Diarrhea."
	Inadequate fluid intake	Provide additional fluid.
	Carbohydrate intolerance	Use continuous drip administration of formula; monitor glucose levels in blood and urine; consider administering insulin; change amount or type of carbohydrate.
Diarrhea, cramps, distention	Excessive protein intake	Monitor blood electrolyte levels; reduce protein intake.
	Bacterial contamination	Use fresh formula every 24 hours; store opened or mixed formula in a refrigerator; rinse feeding bag and tube before adding fresh formula; change feeding bag every 24 hours; prepare formula with clean hands using clean equipment in a clean environment.

TABLE 16–4 (*continued*)

COMPLICATION	POSSIBLE CAUSES	PREVENTIVE/CORRECTIVE MEASURES
	Lactose intolerance	Use lactose-free formula in lactose-intolerant and high-risk clients.
	Hypertonic formula	Dilute formula and increase concentration gradually; use isotonic formula.
	Rapid formula administration	Use continuous drip administration of formula.
	Malnutrition/low serum albumin	Dilute formula and increase concentration gradually; supplement enteral with parenteral nutrition.
	Drug therapy	Use antidiarrheal agents; change drug therapy if possible.
	Low-fiber formula	Provide high-fiber formula.
	Fat intolerance	Use low-fat formula or formulas containing MCT (medium-chain triglycerides).
Hyperglycemia	Diabetes, hypermetabolism, drug therapy	Check glucose in blood and urine; slow administration rate; provide adequate fluids; limit type or amount of carbohydrate; consider hypoglycemic drug therapy.
Nausea and vomiting	Obstruction	Discontinue tube feeding.
	Delayed gastric emptying	Check gastric residual; use continuous drip method of administration.
	Intolerance to concentration or volume of formula	Dilute formula, increasing strength gradually; use continuous drip method of administration.
	Drug therapy	Change drug therapy if possible; use antinausea and antiemetic drugs.
	Psychological reaction to tube feeding	Address clients' concerns.
Skin irritation around feeding ostomy site	Leakage of GI secretions and friction caused by tube	Keep site clean; inspect area for redness, tenderness, and drainage.

Note: Many of the complications presented here can be caused by the client's primary disorder rather than the tube feeding itself. In such a case, the corrective measure would include treatment of the disorder.

[a]This cluster of symptoms is sometimes called the tube feeding syndrome. Imbalances of any electrolytes are possible, and corrective measures would vary.

TABLE 16–5   Selected Drugs That Are Incompatible with Some Formulas

Chlorpromazine concentrate	Mellaril concentrate
Cibalith-S syrup	Mellaril oral solution
Dimetane elixir	Neo-Calglucon syrup
Dimetapp elixir	Paragoric elixir
Feosol elixir	Potassium chloride
Fleet's Phospho-Soda	Reglan syrup
Gevrabon liquid	Robitussin expectorant
Klorvess syrup	Sudafed syrup
Mandelamine Forte suspension	Thorazine concentrate
MCT oil	Zinc sulfate capsules

Note: These substances may be compatible with some formulas and not others.
Sources: P. E. Burns, L. McCall, and R. Wirsching, Physical compatibility of enteral formulas with various common medications, *Journal of the American Dietetic Association* 88 (1988): 1094–1096; A. J. Cutie, E. Altman, and L. Lenkel, Compatibility of enteral products with commonly employed drug additives, *Journal of Parenteral and Enteral Nutrition* 7 (1983): 186–191.

for its nutrition benefits. Feeding becomes merely nourishment, not an expression of personal preference, social pressure, or cultural tradition. To compound the problem, the person may experience physical and emotional discomforts from the tube, the tube feeding formula, the illness itself, or hospitalization.

Help allay the client's fears as much as possible. Explain the procedure for inserting the tube and administering the formula. Answer all questions, and try to gain the client's cooperation. Be sure the client and the client's family understand the objective of the tube feeding and how it will aid in recovery.

The person may also feel self-conscious about how the tube looks and may feel tied down by the feeding equipment. Show the client how to manipulate the equipment so that he can get out of bed. Encourage him to walk about and socialize whenever possible. Walking around will help the client realize that movement is not impossible and that exercise feels good. Socializing may help the individual to forget about the tube.

You can take other steps to make the tube feeding experience more tolerable. The person who is allowed to eat or drink other foods should be given the foods she prefers. Sometimes a person can "drink" a favorite beverage or food (blenderized) through a tube for psychological satisfaction.

> The more complex the procedure that a health care provider is responsible for, the more likely she is to focus on the procedure and forget the client's feelings. Remember, no matter how many technicalities you have to keep in mind, you must never forget the person who is the object of your care.

What to Chart

An earlier discussion emphasized the importance of the medical record as a communication tool. Document this information about tube feedings:

- Type of feeding tube.
- Tube placement.
- Client's response to tube insertion.
- Nutrients being delivered by formula (energy, protein, carbohydrate, fat, and water).
- Administration schedule (concentration and rate).
- Method of delivery (intermittent or continuous).
- Client's tolerance to tube feeding (note any complications and any corrective actions taken).
- Client's response to tube feeding.
- Reasons that a tube feeding was interrupted or could not be delivered (if applicable).
- Drugs and forms of drugs delivered through the feeding tube.
- Education given to the client about tube feeding.

If a person on a tube feeding does not seem to be responding adequately, investigate to see if the tube feeding has been delivered as intended. In one study of 35 people on tube feedings, researchers found that only 16 received 100 percent of their estimated energy needs on *any* day during the period they were tube fed. Intakes averaged only 61 percent of estimated energy needs. Furthermore, it was found that physicians typically ordered only 75 percent of clients' actual (calculated) energy needs.[11] If these problems are prevented or corrected early, clients can benefit maximally from tube feeding programs. Some guidelines include:

- Be alert to signs that the tube feeding is not being delivered as ordered.
- When changing the feeding bag or adding fresh formula to a bag that has been rinsed with water, check and record the amount of formula left from a previous feeding. Is the client receiving the amount of formula that has been ordered? If not, why not?
- Is the formula correctly labeled? Is it the right one?
- Has the formula been stored properly?

Be sure to correct any problems early. Appropriate charting helps all members of the health care team to maintain optimal care.

In many situations, tube feedings provide a practical solution to feeding the person who is unable to consume adequate nutrients by mouth. However, a person without a functional GI tract cannot benefit from a tube feeding. In such a case, intravenous nutrition can be a lifesaving treatment option.

Intravenous Nutrition

A variety of nutrient solutions can be administered by vein to people unable to eat or drink. These intravenous (IV), or parenteral, solutions may consist of some or all of the essential nutrients: water, amino acids, dextrose, lipids, electrolytes (minerals), vitamins, and trace elements.

In contrast to complete parenteral solutions containing all of the nutrients, simple IV solutions generally provide water, dextrose, and electrolytes.

intravenous (IV): through a vein.
Parenteral nutrition refers to the delivery of nutrients directly through a vein, bypassing the intestines.
intra = within
vena = vein
para = opposite
enteron = intestine

dextrose: a form of glucose that is especially soluble in water and is therefore used in IV solutions. Dextrose contains some water, so it provides only 3.4 kcal/g, whereas glucose provides 4 kcal/g.

Simple IV solutions are far from complete nutritionally, but they help to maintain fluid and electrolyte, as well as acid-base, balances. For the well-nourished person who is expected to eat within a few days following surgery, simple IV solutions are adequate.

Generally, an adult with normally functioning kidneys receives from 2½ to 3½ liters of a 5 percent dextrose solution per day following a major trauma or surgery (see the accompanying box "How to Read IV Solution Abbreviations."). Three liters of a 5 percent dextrose solution contributes about 510 kcalories per day (see the box "How to Calculate the Nutrient Content of IV Solutions"). Electrolytes are replaced as needed.

People who can't eat for long periods of time, those who are malnourished, and those who have high nutrient requirements need more complete solutions than a simple IV solution offers. The next section describes how to meet their needs.

Intravenous (IV) Fat Emulsions and Peripheral Total Parenteral Nutrition

Simple glucose solutions or solutions containing only amino acids present a major drawback—they fall far short of meeting total nutrient needs. The problem with the infusion of highly concentrated nutrient solutions is that the small-diameter peripheral veins become irritated and eventually collapse. If less-concentrated solutions were used, though, it would take 12 to 15 liters of solution a day to deliver all the needed nutrients, a fluid volume far greater than the body can safely handle.

peripheral veins: the smaller-diameter veins that bring blood to the extremities (arms and legs).

Intravenous fat emulsions make it possible to deliver needed nutrients by peripheral vein for two reasons. First, they provide a concentrated source of kcalories. Ten percent fat emulsions provide 1.1 kcalories per milliliter, and 20 percent fat emulsions provide 2.0 kcalories per milliliter. Second, IV fat is isotonic to blood and does not irritate the veins the way hypertonic glucose and amino acid solutions do.

How to Read IV Solution Abbreviations

Several abbreviations are used to name IV solutions, including:

D: dextrose.
NS: normal saline (0.9 percent sodium chloride solution).
W: water.

These abbreviations are combined to specify IV solutions as follows:

D_5W: Read as: 5 percent dextrose in water (the subscript following the D tells you the percentage of dextrose required).
$D_{10}W$: Read as: 10 percent dextrose in water.
D_5½ **normal saline:** Read as: 5 percent dextrose in a ½ normal saline solution (0.45 percent sodium chloride).

How would you read $D_{50}W$?

<hr>

How to Calculate the Nutrient Content of IV Solutions

You will have confidence in IV solutions if you know what is in them. The basic thing to remember is that the percentage of a substance in a solution tells you how many grams of that substance are present in 100 milliliters. For example, in a 5 percent dextrose solution, there are 5 grams of dextrose per 100 milliliters. A 3.5 percent amino acid solution contains 3.5 grams of amino acids (protein equivalents) per 100 milliliters. A 0.9 percent normal saline solution contains 0.9 gram of sodium chloride per 100 milliliters.

A person receiving 1500 milliliters of 50 percent dextrose and 1500 milliliters of 7 percent amino acid solution would get:

$$\frac{50 \text{ g dextrose}}{100 \text{ ml}} \text{ as } \frac{X \text{ g glucose}}{1500 \text{ ml}}$$
$$(50 \text{ g} \times 1500 \text{ ml}) \div 100 \text{ ml} = 150 \text{ g dextrose.}$$

And for amino acids:

$$\frac{7 \text{ g amino acids}}{100 \text{ ml}} \text{ as } \frac{X \text{ g amino acids}}{1500 \text{ ml}}$$
$$(7 \text{ g} \times 1500 \text{ ml}) \div 100 \text{ ml} = 105 \text{ g amino acids.}$$

To calculate the total kcalories in the mixture, simply multiply by kcalories per gram:

$$750 \text{ g dextrose} \times 3.4 \text{ kcal/g} = 2550 \text{ kcal.}$$
$$105 \text{ g amino acids} \times 4.0 \text{ kcal/g} = 420 \text{ kcal.}$$
$$\text{Total} = 2970 \text{ kcal.}$$

<hr>

Intravenous fat emulsions are also valuable because they provides essential fatty acids, thus preventing deficiencies. Intravenous fat can safely provide about 50 percent of the total daily energy requirement for the unstressed client.[12] For clients under stress, further studies are needed to define optimal fat intakes, but restricting fat kcalories to 30 percent of the total daily energy need is widely practiced.[13]

Current research suggests that the source of lipid may also be important.[14] The IV fat emulsions presently available are rich sources of long-chain omega-6 fatty acids. These fatty acids may exert a negative impact on immune function and, therefore, may be less than desirable for critically ill clients. Alternate lipid sources such as fish oils (a rich source of omega-3 fatty acids) and triglycerides chemically modified to contain both long- and medium-chain fatty acids are currently under investigation.

The use of IV fat, amino acids, and dextrose given by peripheral vein to meet all energy needs is called *peripheral total parenteral nutrition (peripheral TPN)*. Vitamins, minerals, and trace elements can also be given intravenously so that all nutrient needs can be met. Peripheral TPN works well for many clients but cannot deliver quite enough nutrients for people with very high energy needs. Peripheral TPN best suits people who need only short-term nutrition support (about 7 to 14 days), people with normal renal function who do not have excessive energy requirements, people in whom inserting an IV catheter into a central vein might be difficult, and people on oral or tube feedings who may need additional nutrients temporarily.

IV fat emulsions are made from egg phospholipids and plant-derived (safflower and soybean) oils. Omega-6 and omega-3 fatty acids are described on p. 48.

peripheral total parenteral nutrition (peripheral TPN): the provision of a nutrient solution that meets nutrient needs by peripheral vein.

A typical peripheral TPN solution provides about 2500 kcal and 90 g of amino acids per day.

bilirubin: a pigment in bile whose concentration becomes elevated in the blood as a result of some disorders.

Hyperlipidemias and atherosclerosis are discussed in Chapter 22 and liver disease, in Chapter 23.

palpitations: rapid fluttering or throbbing of the heart.

cyanosis: a bluish or grayish color of the skin.

total parenteral nutrition (TPN): a method of meeting all nutrient needs by infusing formulas into large-diameter central veins; also called **intravenous hyperalimentation.** *Hyperalimentation* means feeding higher-than-normal amounts of nutrients either enterally or parenterally.

    hyper = greater than normal
    alimentation = the process of providing nutrients to the body.

IV catheter: the thin tube inserted into a vein through which nutrient solutions or medications can be given directly.

central veins: the large-diameter veins located close to the heart (see Figure 16–6).

One liter of a traditional central TPN formula contains 25% dextrose and 3.5% amino acids. Often, 3 l of the solution is given daily and provides 3,000 kcal and 105 g protein.

respiratory acidosis: a condition of too much acid in the blood caused by failure of the lungs to ventilate properly. Excess acids are normally released from the lungs during exhalation; compromised lungs, however, are unable to perform this function adequately.

Intravenous fat emulsions are contraindicated in newborns with markedly elevated bilirubin levels and in people with some types of hyperlipidemias, severe liver disease, and severe egg allergies. Cautious use of IV fats is recommended for people with atherosclerosis, moderate liver disease, blood coagulation disorders, pancreatitis, and some types of lung problems.

Although infrequent, adverse reactions to IV fat emulsions occur in some people, particularly when IV fats are given in excessive doses or administered too rapidly. Immediate reactions can include fever, warmth, chills, backache, chest pain, allergic reactions, palpitations, rapid breathing, wheezing, cyanosis, nausea, and an unpleasant taste in the mouth. Irritation and inflammation of the vein are also possible. After long-term administration, the most commonly observed adverse effect is the deposition of a brown pigment in certain liver cells. These pigments disappear after parenteral therapy is stopped, and their effects on liver function, if any, are unknown. Other effects of long-term administration may include an enlarged liver and spleen, as well as a reduced number of blood platelets and white blood cells.

TPN by Central Vein

Another method used to meet all nutrient needs by vein is TPN by central vein. This may be called *central total parenteral nutrition,* but it is abbreviated simply *TPN.* In TPN, the IV catheter is surgically placed in a large-diameter central vein (see Figure 16–6). Almost a gallon of blood rushes through one such vein, the superior vena cava, each minute. Here, highly concentrated solutions can be quickly diluted. By the time these solutions reach the peripheral veins, they are not irritating.

Enteral nutrition is always preferred to parenteral nutrition, but TPN offers the advantage that concentrated solutions of nutrients can be delivered to people who cannot or should not be fed through the GI tract. TPN is indicated whenever long-term parenteral nutrition will be required, when nutrient requirements are high, or when people are severely malnourished. Some specific conditions that may necessitate its use are listed in Table 16–6 (p. 408). The actual need for TPN must be determined by the individual's medical and nutrition needs. Ideally, the person should not reach a severely depleted state before TPN is initiated. It is much easier to maintain nutrition status than to try to replenish lost nutrient stores with TPN.

The actual concentrations of amino acids and dextrose that compose the final TPN formula are determined by each person's unique nutrient needs. Traditionally, TPN solutions provide energy needs primarily from dextrose. Intravenous fat is given periodically (two 500-milliliter bottles per week) to meet essential fatty acid requirements. However, the current practice is to use IV fat emulsions more frequently as a kcalorie source. People with severe stress may become intolerant of high glucose loads. Providing fat allows glucose to be reduced, thus helping to alleviate this problem. Providing more energy as lipid is also beneficial for people in respiratory failure, because oxidation of glucose in the body results in an increased output of carbon dioxide and can lead to respiratory acidosis.

Electrolytes, vitamins, and trace elements are added to the TPN solution in addition to dextrose, amino acids, and fat. Without the addition of these

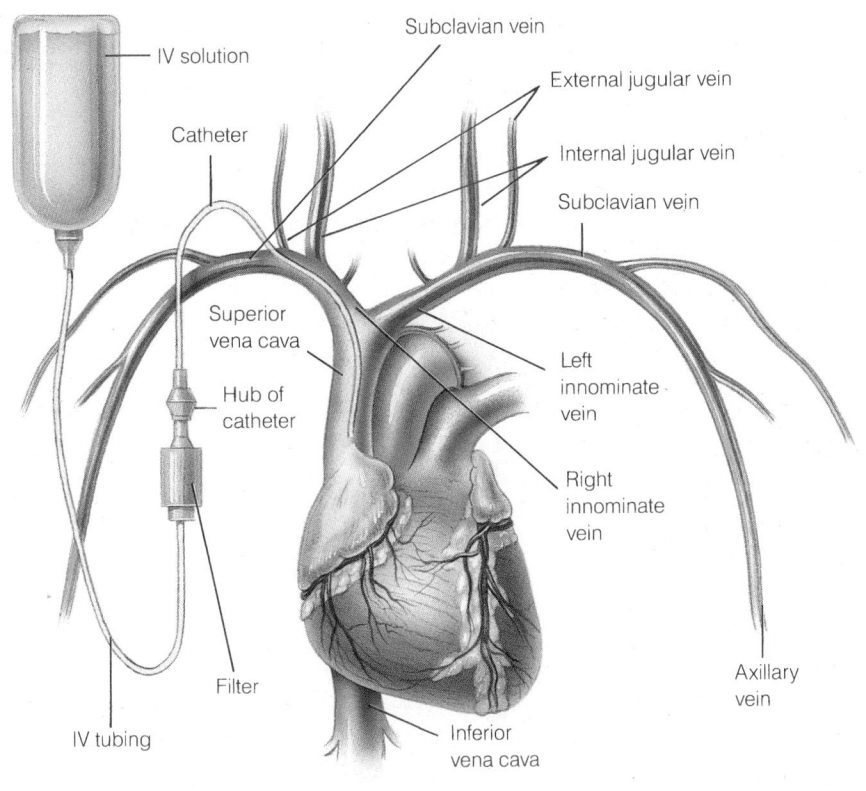

IV solution

Catheter

Subclavian vein

External jugular vein

Internal jugular vein

Subclavian vein

Superior vena cava

Hub of catheter

Left innominate vein

Right innominate vein

Filter

IV tubing

Inferior vena cava

Axillary vein

FIGURE 16–6 **The Central Veins Used for TPN**
The superior vena cava is one of the largest-diameter veins and is usually used for giving TPN solutions. When it cannot be used, the internal jugular vein is the next choice, followed by the external jugular vein. Can you see why?

utrients, deficiencies can occur. Essential fatty acid requirements are met giving IV fat. Other possible additions to the TPN formula include:

- Albumin, to raise serum albumin concentration.
- Heparin, to prevent clots from forming on the IV catheter that might obstruct the flow of the TPN formula.
- Insulin, to help regulate blood glucose levels.

Adding albumin, heparin, and insulin directly to the TPN solution is a controversial practice. Not all institutions consider these substances TPN additives. Where they are used, only those additives needed by each individual are given.

An exciting new area of research in the area of TPN involves the amino acid glutamine. Glutamine appears to be an important fuel source for the gut. It is often depleted from tissues during severe stress. At the same time, parenteral formulas are currently glutamine-free. Early animal investigations suggest that providing glutamine helps maintain gut integrity during total parenteral nutrition.[15] If further research verifies early findings and shows glutamine to be a safe addition to TPN formulas, it may help make it easier to begin enterally refeeding a client who has been on TPN.

Like a tube feeding, a TPN feeding is started slowly to give the client time to adapt to the high glucose concentration and osmolality of the TPN formula. Health team members monitor the client regularly to ensure that the formula is appropriate for the person's needs and that the person is toler-

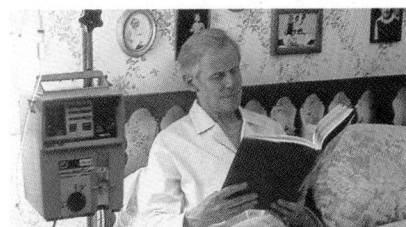

Infusion pumps ensure a controlled delivery rate of the TPN formula.

TABLE 16-6   **Possible Indications for TPN by Central Vein**

Major small bowel resections
Radiation enteritis (inflammation of intestine caused by radiation)
Severe diarrhea
Intractable vomiting
Intensive chemotherapy
Bone marrow transplants
Inflammatory bowel diseases
Moderate to severe acute pancreatitis
Severe malnutrition when GI tract is nonfunctional
Hypermetabolic disorders or major surgery (when it is anticipated that the GI tract will be unusable for 5 to 7 days)
Moderate stress if adequate nutrient intake cannot be achieved for more than 7 to 10 days
Enterocutaneous fistulas
Severe nausea and vomiting associated with pregnancy (hyperemesis gravidarum) when it lasts more than 5 to 7 days
Moderate malnutrition if surgical or intensive medical intervention is necessary
When adequate enteral nutrition cannot be established within 7 to 10 days of hospitalization

Source: Adapted from A.S.P.E.N. Board of Directors, Guidelines for the use of total parenteral nutrition in the hospitalized adult patient, *Journal of Parenteral and Enteral Nutrition* 10 (1986): 441–445.

ating the formula. Guidelines for monitoring the person on TPN are given in Table 16-7.

Transitional/Combination Feedings

Once the problem causing the need for tube feedings or IV nutrition has resolved, the client can gradually shift onto an oral diet while the volume of the special feeding is tapered. Dietitians work with the health care team to ensure that the individual's nutrient needs will continue to be met. For example, a person on a tube feeding should be eating adequate amounts of food by mouth before the tube feeding is discontinued. The person can eat orally with the tube in place as the volume of the tube feeding is gradually tapered off. In many cases, the person can drink the same formula that was earlier given by tube.

The transition from IV feeding to an oral diet can be accomplished in different ways. One way is to start by placing the client on a tube feeding. Then reduce the volume of the IV nutrition solution while offering an increased volume of tube feeding, as tolerated. The person who cannot tolerate the tube feeding can still rely on TPN to meet nutrient needs. A person can also be weaned from a TPN solution while increasing oral intake, bypassing the use of the tube. Parenteral nutrition can be discontinued when

TABLE 16-7 **Checklist for Monitoring People on TPN**

Every four to six hours:	Check urinary glucose. Monitor vital signs (respiration, pulse, temperature).
Daily:	Monitor weight changes. Record intake and output carefully. Check urine specific gravity.
Daily until stable, and then two or three times weekly:	Monitor serum glucose. Monitor serum electrolytes. Monitor blood urea nitrogen.
Weekly:	Conduct a nutrition assessment. Monitor serum protein. Monitor serum calcium. Monitor serum phosphorus. Monitor serum ammonia. Monitor complete blood count.

60 percent of estimated energy needs are being met by oral intake, tube feeding, or a combination of the two.[16]

The transition to enteral nutrition after a person has been on intravenous feedings for long periods of time demands careful attention. Following long periods of disuse, the intestinal villi shrink and lose some of their function. The return to enteral nutrition must be gradual to avoid problems of malabsorption and other GI discomforts. The appropriate introduction of nutrients to the GI tract stimulates the progressive return of the villi to normal structure and function.

The return of oral intake for the person who has been fed either intravenously or by tube can have a variety of psychological effects. Some people may be extremely eager to eat again, and food can be an important morale booster. Others may be apprehensive about eating, particularly if they have had extensive GI problems. Appetite may be slow to return for some. In such circumstances, all members of the health care team can play important roles in the successful reintroduction of food. Throughout the process, recognize the person's concerns, and reassure the person that you will be there to help for as long as necessary.

Specialized Nutrition Support at Home

Occasionally clients must continue to receive specialized nutrition support (tube feedings or parenteral nutrition) after their primary medical conditions have stabilized. In such cases, hospitalization often remains necessary primarily to support nutrition status rather than to provide intensive medical care. An option in such cases is continuance of nutrition support at home.

The main objective of home parenteral and enteral nutrition, as with TPN and tube feedings in the hospital, is to maintain or achieve adequate nutrition status. However, nutrition support at home has an added dimension: it permits a person to get the needed nutrition care in familiar surroundings. If you have ever been in a hospital yourself—or taken a long trip, for that matter—you probably remember what comfort and relaxation you experienced when you returned to your own bed, could get things when you needed them, and knew where things were. In some cases, people who require nutrition support at home can resume many activities, such as going to work, driving, and playing sports. In general, home parenteral and enteral nutrition allow people the opportunity to lead more normal lives.

An additional benefit of nutrition support at home is cost savings. Considerable savings result when the responsibilities formerly performed by hospital staff are assumed by the client or the family. One institution reports a cost savings of $1.5 million a year for ten clients maintained on home TPN versus TPN in the hospital.[17]

Since the first report of a person sent home successfully on home TPN in 1969,[18] the use of nutrition support at home has expanded rapidly. The number of people benefitting from home programs continues to grow, and health care professionals who work with these programs are gaining valuable experience in improving the quality of specialized nutrition support at home. Although the exact number of people on home nutrition support programs is unknown, a 1986 survey estimated that about 14,300 people were on home TPN and as many as 52,000 people were on home tube feedings at that time.[19] Many medical supply companies provide the equipment, formulations, and service necessary to support home nutrition care.

While one person may require home nutrition support for a relatively short time (for example, a few months), another may need it permanently. Medical considerations must be analyzed. In addition, the candidate for home nutrition support and those who care for that person must have rational, stable personalities so that problems can be successfully handled as they arise. The person or those who care for the person must be capable of learning the techniques of nutrition support and of dealing with complications. Additionally, the person must have financial resources to support the program, as well as access to the equipment, supplies, and professional support that are integral components of a successful home program. The members of the nutrition support team are usually the ones who must decide if a client is a candidate for home parenteral or enteral nutrition.

Once a home nutrition program is initiated, a nurse visits the client at home, and the person also sees a physician at regular intervals. In some programs, dietitians make home visits also. A qualified nurse, dietitian, or physician must be available to answer questions and handle problems as they arise.

Home Parenteral Nutrition

People on home TPN most commonly have cancer, Crohn's disease, or ischemic bowel disease (death of a portion of the intestine). Different types of home TPN programs are in current use. Ideally, clients are given as much responsibility for their own care as they can handle. For example, a client who is capable of mixing the solutions and changing the catheter dressings is trained to do so. Typically, family members also learn the techniques so that they can assist in the procedures whenever necessary.

Special types of catheters often are inserted for home TPN. One type makes it possible for the client to see the catheter site and to inspect it for changes, as well as to perform dressing changes (see Figure 16–7). Another type of catheter is implanted under the skin; this allows the client more freedom of movement and is associated with a lower risk of infection.

Most commonly, the client is instructed to use an infusion pump set to deliver the total volume of solution needed for the day within 8 to 12 hours. The total volume of solution can be placed in large-capacity IV bags so that the client can infuse the solution while sleeping or at any other convenient time. This method of delivery allows freedom of movement during much of the day.

For people who cannot tolerate an 8- to 12-hour infusion rate, nutrients are infused over 24 hours. Those who are ambulatory can benefit from a lightweight carrying case that holds a small pump and IV bags. This system allows the client to move around freely with little inconvenience.

Some people prepare their own home TPN solutions from bottles of IV dextrose and amino acids. Others receive their bottles premixed. Premixed solutions are more convenient and are essential when the client's (or family members') ability to correctly mix the solution is questionable.

Home Enteral Nutrition

People on home enteral nutrition programs most commonly have cancer or swallowing disorders. Enteral nutrition is the preferred feeding method for people at home, as well as those in the hospital. Home enteral nutrition programs are similar to home TPN programs in many ways.

Feeding ostomies often are placed for long-term tube feedings. Some people learn to use a transnasal tube, which they insert at each feeding. When possible, an intermittent feeding schedule is arranged so that the person is free to move around between meals. Infusion pumps are used only if necessary; they are expensive to purchase or rent. People who must receive a continuous drip feeding are trained to use small pumps that are easy to transport and allow the client freedom of movement.

The person on a home enteral program can make tube feedings from blenderized table foods or purchase a commercially prepared, premixed formula. Most clients prefer to purchase formula. A premixed formula should be used whenever the person's (or family members') ability to mix the formula is questionable.

How Do People on HPEN Cope?

The person on home enteral or parenteral nutrition has succeeded in working out a way of obtaining nutrients daily via tube feeding or through a vein. At its best, this represents a remarkably courageous adaptation to a challenging way of life.

People in home nutrition programs adapt to their programs with time and appear to enjoy a reasonable quality of life.[20] Home programs allow people to resume many activities, including employment, sexual activity, recreation, swimming, social activity, and travel. Women on home TPN successfully carry and deliver babies. Students return to college.

FIGURE 16–7 **Placement of a Home TPN Catheter**
In this case, the catheter is tunneled under the skin before going into the subclavian vein; in other cases, the catheter may enter the subclavian directly.

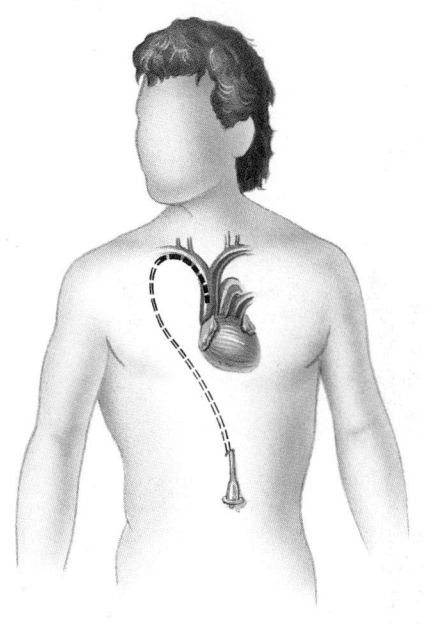

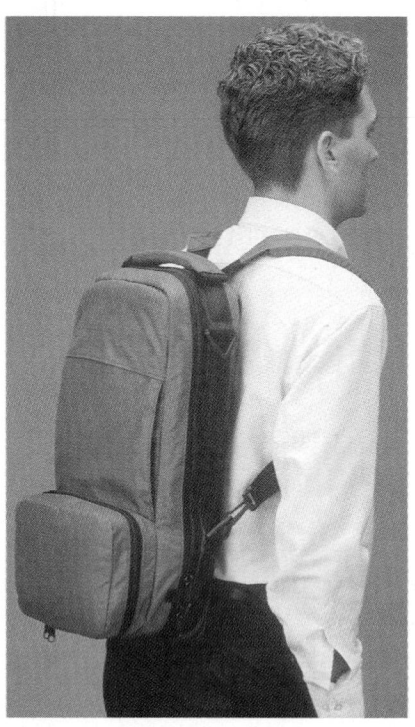

A 3-liter bag of solution allow people on home TPN to lead normal lives, free from a pole-mounted apparatus.

Even so, people on home nutrition programs do have unique problems. In a 1987 survey of people on home nutrition support programs, participants were asked to rank their psychosocial concerns.[21] Depression, lack of control over their lives, and loss of independence were cited most frequently, followed by restricted food intakes, impaired relationships with spouses or significant others, unfavorable body image, and sexual concerns. To deal with emotional problems, clients might benefit from support groups or psychological counseling.

Clients also worry about the substantial costs associated with long-term nutrition support. Although techniques of home support have become safer and simpler, these changes have come at a financial cost. Financial problems can be major for the individual on expensive therapy who often cannot continue to work full time. Social workers might be able to find ways to handle some of the financial problems.

No doubt, enteral and parenteral nutrition provide lifesaving alternatives for nourishing people with special problems. The remaining chapters provide many examples of specific instances in which these therapies are useful.

Enteral and Parenteral Nutrition

Mr. Small has been admitted to the hospital for a diagnostic workup. He has been steadily losing weight. He appears emaciated and states that he can't swallow and has lost his appetite. He was afraid to come to the hospital and has waited a long time before checking in. After a thorough examination, Mr. Small has been found to have an obstruction in his esophagus. The nutrition assessment reveals severe PCM. Surgery will be required as soon as possible. Mr. Small is placed on TPN before surgery. He progresses well, gains weight, and undergoes surgery about two weeks after admission. During surgery, a feeding jejunostomy is made.

What factors in Mr. Small's history indicate the need for TPN? How would you explain the need for TPN to Mr. Small?

About two days after surgery, Mr. Small begins to receive feedings through the jejunostomy. His digestive and absorptive capacity are intact. Was the placement of a feeding jejunostomy during surgery a good idea? Why or why not? What general type of formula would you recommend for Mr. Small's tube feedings? How does the feeding route influence this selection?

After the formula has been selected, a plan for administering the formula is necessary. How would you begin the tube feeding? How would you have it progress? What method of delivery would you use? How would you monitor its effectiveness?

Mr. Small is now ready to begin jejunal feedings at low concentrations. When should Mr. Small be taken off TPN? How should this be accomplished?

After several weeks, Mr. Small is ready to take some food by mouth. How does this affect his tube feeding? If Mr. Small's medical condition stabilized but he was unable to consume enough food by mouth to go off tube feedings, he might be a candidate for a home enteral nutrition program. What are some of the advantages of such a program?

Study Questions

1. What are tube feedings? How are feeding tubes placed?
2. What are the two major types of formulas, and how do they differ from each other?
3. What factors are considered in selecting a formula?
4. Describe different ways that formulas can be administered to clients.
5. Describe the problems that can occur when drugs are delivered through feeding tubes. What guidelines can be used to help prevent these problems?
6. Define the differences between routine IV formulas, peripheral TPN formulas, and central TPN formulas. When would each type be used?
7. How many kcalories are in 1 liter of a TPN solution containing 25 percent dextrose and 5 percent amino acids?
8. How have IV fat emulsions made it possible to deliver energy requirements by peripheral vein?
9. Describe some ways in which a person on tube feedings or parenteral nutrition can be weaned to ordinary table foods.
10. What are the advantages of home enteral and parenteral nutrition programs?

Notes

1. J. W. Alexander, Nutrition and translocation, *Journal of Parenteral and Enteral Nutrition* 14 (Supplement, 1990): 170–174; E. A. Deitch, J. Winterton, and M. Li, The gut as a portal of entry for bacteremia: Role of protein nutrition, *Annals of Surgery* 205 (1987): 681–884.
2. S. P. Marcuard, K. L. Stegall, and S. Trogdon, Clearing obstructed feeding tubes, *Journal of Parenteral and Enteral Nutrition* 13 (1989): 81–83.
3. D. C. Frankenfield and P. L. Beyer, Dietary fiber and bowel function in tube-fed patients, *Journal of the American Dietetic Association* 91 (1991): 590–596.
4. J. Slavin, Commercially available enteral formulas with fiber and bowel function measures, *Nutrition in Clinical Practice* 5 (1990): 247–250.
5. J. C. Palacio and J. L. Rombeau, Dietary fiber: A brief review and potential application to enteral nutrition, *Nutrition in Clinical Practice* 5 (1990): 99–106; K. Shankardass and coauthors, Bowel function of long-term tube-fed patients consuming formulae with or without dietary fiber, *Journal of Parenteral and Enteral Nutrition* 14 (1990): 508–512.
6. Palacio and Rombeau, 1990.
7. G. Moe, Enteral feeding and infection in the immunocompromised patient, *Nutrition in Clinical Practice* 6 (1991): 55–64.
8. L. Vaughan, M. Manore, and D. Wilson, Bacterial safety of a closed-administration system for enteral nutrition solutions, *Journal of the American Dietetic Association* 88 (1988): 35–37.
9. C. Austin, Water: Guidelines for nutritional support, *Nutritional Support Services,* September 1986, pp. 27–29.

10. M. L. Gora, M. M. Tschampel, and J. A. Visconti, Considerations of drug therapy in patients receiving enteral nutrition, *Nutrition in Clinical Practice* 4 (1989): 105–110.

11. G. B. Abernathy and coauthors, Efficacy of tube feeding in supplying energy requirements of hospitalized patients, *Journal of Parenteral and Enteral Nutrition* 13 (1989): 387–391.

12. M. Roesner and J. P. Grant, Intravenous lipid emulsions, *Nutrition in Clinical Practice* 2 (1987): 96–107.

13. R. H. Bower, Nutritional and metabolic support of critically ill patients, *Journal of Parenteral and Enteral Nutrition* 14 (Supplement, 1990): 257–259; G. L. Blackburn, In search of the "preferred fuel," *Nutrition in Clinical Practice* 4 (1989): 3–5.

14. S. J. Bell and coauthors, Alternative lipid sources for enteral and parenteral nutrition: Long- and medium-chain triglycerides, structured triglycerides, and fish oils, *Journal of the American Dietetic Association* 91 (1991): 74–78.

15. D. Jacobs and coauthors, Trophic effects of glutamine-enriched parenteral nutrition on colonic mucosa, 12th Clinical Congress Abstracts, *Journal of Parenteral and Enteral Nutrition* 12 (Supplement, 1988): 6; S. T. O'Dwyer and coauthors, Maintenance of small bowel mucosa with glutamine-enriched parenteral nutrition, *Journal of Parenteral and Enteral Nutrition* 13 (1989): 579–585.

16. M. F. Winkler and coauthors, Transitional feeding: The relationship between nutritional intake and plasma protein components, *Journal of the American Dietetic Association* 89 (1989): 969–970.

17. E. T. Herfindal and coauthors, Survey of home nutritional support patients, *Journal of Parenteral and Enteral Nutrition* 13 (1989): 255–261.

18. M. E. Shils and coauthors, Long-term parenteral nutrition through an external arteriovenous shunt, *New England Journal of Medicine* 283 (1970): 341–344.

19. The Oley Foundation of A.S.P.E.N., *OASIS Home Nutritional Support Patient Registry: Annual Report* (Albany, N.Y.: Oley Foundation for Home Parenteral and Enteral Nutrition, 1986).

20. Herfindal and coauthors, 1989.

21. As cited in K. C. Hoffman, Psychosocial concerns of home nutrition therapy consumers, *Nutrition in Clinical Practice* 4 (1989): 51–56.

16

Ethical Issues in Clinical Nutrition

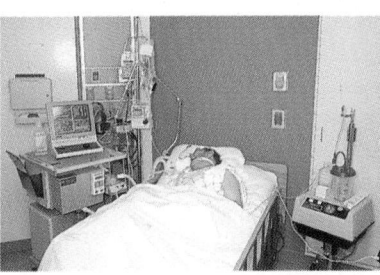

When is it morally and legally appropriate to use special nutrition support techniques?

Chapter 16 described in some detail the techniques of parenteral and enteral nutrition. The capability of providing nourishment to people unable to eat by mouth has only become available in recent years. The technical advances made in the areas of parenteral and enteral nutrition have been lifesaving for many people. However, as is true with many new technologies, the availability of special nutrition support forces health care professionals and society to face ethical issues—specifically, when it is morally and legally appropriate to use special nutrition support techniques. We must ask ourselves when such treatments prolong life and when they merely delay death.

The highly publicized Nancy Cruzan case called the public's attention to just this dilemma. This Nutrition in Practice reviews some of the ethical questions that surround the use of special nutrition support. Its intent is not to draw conclusions or solve problems; rather, it seeks to present the issues for your consideration. The Miniglossary defines many of the terms used in this section.

What ethical problems face health care professionals with respect to nutrition support?

To put the problem into perspective, consider for a moment the circumstances under which health care professionals make their decisions to feed clients. Most often, they readily provide whatever form of nutrition is necessary to support all clients who have any chance of recovering from a disease and sustaining an acceptable quality of life. Clearly, health care professionals cannot rightfully withhold nutrition support because of poor judgment or negligence. If a client were to die because nourishment was withheld, the staff and facility would be held responsible, and in all likelihood, a malpractice lawsuit would result.

The decision of whether to feed a client becomes less clear, however, when the client is not expected to recover. How aggressively do we support the person who is terminally ill or in a persistent vegetative state? How do we respond to elderly or physically disabled people who refuse special nutrition support because they feel the quality of their lives is so poor that they do not wish to be sustained? Do we (as a society) allow them such choices? Are health care professionals morally and legally obligated to comply with, or to deny, requests to discontinue feedings? Furthermore, when clients are incompetent and unable to speak for themselves, who, if anyone, should be allowed to make such life-and-death decisions? These questions are but a few those that have evolved along with the technology of nutrition support.

What was the Nancy Cruzan case? Why did it go to court?

Nancy Cruzan was a young woman who suffered permanent and irreversible brain damage in a car accident in 1983. After that, she was in a persistent vegetative state—awake but unaware. Her physicians and parents held no hope for recovery, yet given food and water, she might have lived for another 30 years. Her parents' requested permission to discontinue tube feeding, but their request was rejected by the Missouri Supreme Court in 1987. The Court held that Nancy Cruzan had never definitively stated her "right-to-die" wishes, and that the parents had no legal right to make such a request for her. The Court stated that preserving life, no matter what its quality, took precedence over all other considerations.

Unsatisfied with the Missouri Supreme Court decision, the Cruzan parents took further legal action. In 1989 the U.S. Supreme Court agreed to hear the case. Several professional organizations—including the American Medical Association, the American Academy of Family Physicians, the American Association of Neurological Surgeons, the American College of Surgeons, the American College of Physicians, and the American Society for Parenteral and Enteral Nutrition—filed briefs with the Supreme Court in support of the parents.

The U.S. Supreme Court recognized that competent people have the right to decide whether to accept or refuse medical treatment, including lifesaving hydration and nutrition. However, the question before the Supreme Court was not what the best decision would be in the Nancy Cruzan case, but rather, whether the U.S. Constitution prohibited Missouri from making the decision it made in the Cruzan case. The answer was no.[1] Missouri did not violate the Constitution.[2] The U.S. Supreme Court entrusted state legislatures with the task of establishing laws to address the issue of whether families (or other third parties) could authorize the withdrawal of life-sustaining treatment on behalf of incompetent persons in the absence of exacting evidence on incompetent persons' wishes.

The Cruzan case did not end with the U.S. Supreme Court decision. Newly discovered evidence presented to a trial judge in Missouri led thecourt to conclude that, clearly and convincingly, Nancy Cruzan would not want the tube feeding continued in her condition. The feeding tube was removed on December 14, 1990, and she died two weeks later of dehydration.

That's quite a bit to think about. It sounds like the best bet is for people to be sure their wishes about life-sustaining measures are known.

You're right; it is very important for people to make their wishes about life-sustaining measures known. The emerging ethical, medical, and legal consensus seems to support the opinion that state interests do not outweigh those of individual rights. Individuals have a legal right to refuse medical treatments—including artificial feedings—even when medical experts consider those treatments necessary to sustain life.[3] That is, even when treatment is lifesaving and its refusal may bring an earlier death, clients' rights remain paramount.

Many people will agree that competent adults have the right to accept or refuse medical treatment. However, the controversy grows louder when the person is comatose, incompetent, or otherwise unable to refuse or accept medical treatment—especially when the person's wishes are not known.

Without knowledge of an incompetent person's wishes, the court decides in the client's "best interest." For many families, it becomes their burden to convince the court that discontinuing feeding is in the client's "best interest." Such was the case in the Cruzans' situation.

What can people do to make sure their wishes are known?

Health care professionals should encourage their competent clients to express ahead of time their preferences for medical treatments, including artificial feedings, should terminal illness or coma develop.[4] These preferences should be noted in medical records. Any health care professional who is unwilling to abide by these stated preferences should arrange for continuing care by an equally qualified professional and then withdraw from that client's care.[5] Clients should expect that physicians and facilities will comply with their preferences and not merely tolerate them grudgingly.[6]

In addition, clients can state their preferences in legal documents known as living wills (see Form NP16–1 on p. 418). Many states have enacted laws that authorize the use of living wills. A living will stands as a clear expression of a competent adult's wishes.[7] It may specify that no extraordinary treatments be administered in the event that the person is unable to make the necessary decisions at that time. Alternatively, a living will may declare a person's wish to have every effort made to maintain life in the event of terminal illness or irreversible loss of consciousness. Each individual's preference should be known to the attending physicians and family.

In some states, the durable power of attorney offers clients the protection of having their wishes carried out. A durable power of attorney allows a competent adult to designate another competent adult as agent to make decisions in the event of incapacitation. Some states have enacted statutes authorizing the use of durable powers of attorney specifically for health care.[8]

An added advantage of planning ahead for future care in the case of a terminal illness or irreversible state of unconsciousness is that others are freed from the guilt and anxiety of having to make decisions. Imagine the anxiety a family member goes through in directing the health care team to stop nutrition support, knowing that it will hasten death. That decision would be far easier if the family member knew that was what the individual would want or, better yet, if a legal document took the decision out of the family's hands altogether.

Health care professionals, particularly physicians, can find themselves in awkward and difficult positions regarding aggressive nutrition support. On the one hand, they are obligated to provide optimal care. Negligence could result in a malpractice suit. On the other hand, health care professionals are client advocates. In this role, they must respect the wishes of the people in their care. Again, there is no easy answer to this dilemma. Each case must be carefully decided individually.

Most hospitals have established ethics committees to deal with ethical problems such as those presented here. Health care professionals should ensure that their disciplines are represented on such committees and become familiar with their profession's ethics guidelines.[9]

Notes

1. Supreme Court of the United States Syllabus, *Cruzan, by her parents and co-guardians,* Cruzan it ux. v. Director, Missouri Department of Health, et al., no. 88-1503. Argued December 6, 1989 — Decided June 25, 1990.
2. A. M. Capron, The implications of the *Cruzan* decision for clinical nutrition teams, *Nutrition in Clinical Practice* 6 (1991): 89–94.
3. S. H. Miles, P. A. Singer, and M. Siegler, Conflicts between patients' wishes to forgo treatment and the policies of health care facilities, *New England Journal of Medicine* 321 (1989): 48–50; R. Steinbrook and B. Lo, Artificial feeding—Solid ground, not a slippery slope, *New England Journal of Medicine* 318 (1988): 286–290.
4. Capron, 1991.
5. C. R. Gallagher-Allred, Managing ethical issues in nutrition support of terminally ill patients, *Nutrition in Clinical Practice* 6 (1991): 113–116.
6. Miles, Singer, and Siegler, 1989.
7. J. E. Ruark, T. A. Raffin, and the Stanford University Medical Center Committee on Ethics, Initiating and withdrawing life support—Principles and practice in adult medicine, *New England Journal of Medicine* 318 (1988): 25–30.
8. Capron, 1991.
9. American Dietetic Association, Position of the American Dietetic Association: Issues in feeding the terminally ill adult, *Journal of the American Dietetic Association* 87 (1987): 78–85.

FORM NP16–1   **A Living Will**

To My Family, My Physician, My Lawyer
And All Others Whom It May Concern

Death is as much a reality as birth, growth, and aging—it is the one certainty of life. In anticipation of decisions that may have to be made about my own dying and as an expression of my right to refuse treatment,
I _____ ,

(print name)

being of sound mind, make this statement of my wishes and instructions concerning treatment.

By means of this document, which I intend to be legally binding, I direct my physician and other care providers, my family, and any surrogate designated by me or appointed by a court, to carry out my wishes. If I become unable, by reason of physical or mental incapacity, to make decisions about my medical care, let this document provide the guidance and authority needed to make any and all such decisions.

If I am permanently unconscious or there is no reasonable expectation of my recovery from a seriously incapacitating or lethal illness or condition, I do not wish to be kept alive by artificial means. I request that I be given all care necessary to keep me comfortable and free of pain, even if pain-relieving medications may hasten my death, and I direct that no life-sustaining treatment be provided except as I or my surrogate specifically authorize.

This request may appear to place a heavy responsibility upon you, but by making this decision according to my strong convictions, I intend to ease that burden. I am acting after careful consideration and with understanding of the consequences of your carrying out my wishes. *List optional specific provisions in the space below.*[a]

I sign this document knowingly, voluntarily, and after careful deliberation, this _____ day of _____ ,19 _____ .

_____
(signature)
Address _____

I do hereby certify that the within document was executed and acknowledged before me by the principal this _____ day of _____ , 19 _____ .

_____
Notary Public

Witness _____
Printed Name _____
Address _____

Witness _____
Printed Name _____
Address _____

Copies of this document have been given to:
_____
_____
_____
_____
_____

[a]The Living Will should clearly state your preference about life-sustaining treatment. You may wish to add specific statements that concern cardiopulmonary resuscitation, artificial or invasive measures for providing nutrition and hydration, kidney dialysis, mechanical or artificial respiration, blood transfusion, surgery (such as amputation), and antibiotics. You may also wish to indicate any preferences you have about such matters as dying at home.

Source: Reprinted by permission of Concern for Dying/Society for the Right to Die, 250 West 57th Street, New York, NY 10107. For a copy of "A Living Will" and other information write or call (212) 246-6973.

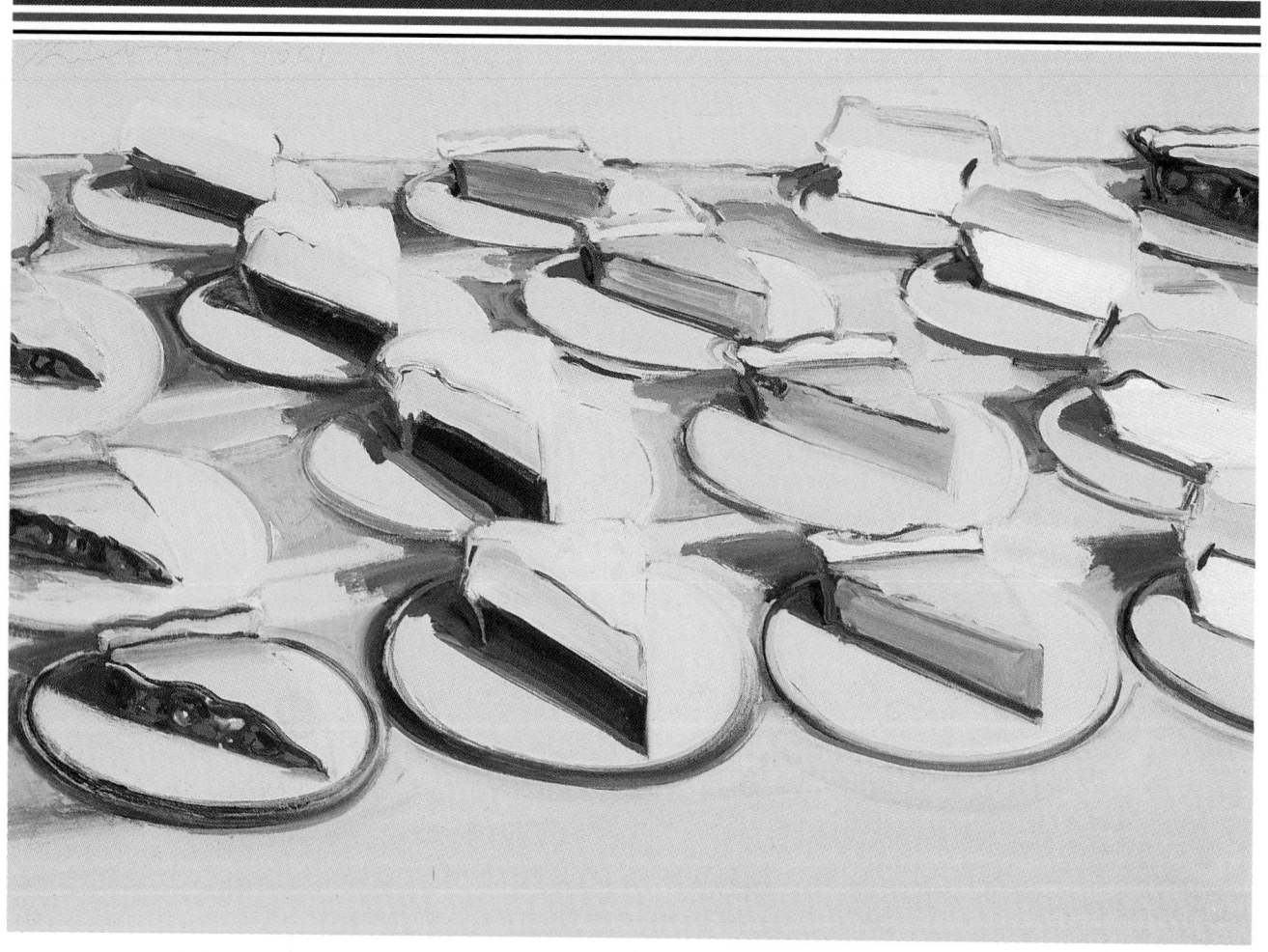

Wayne Thiebaud, Sixteen Pies, 1961, Oil on canvas, 20″ × 30″, Private Collection.

Diets Modified in Consistency, Texture, and Number of Meals

CONTENTS

CHAPTER

17

Modified diets complement other medical therapies in the prevention or treatment of many disorders. In some instances, diet therapy is crucial. In others, modified diets comprise a small part of the total treatment plan. Sometimes the only diet required is a well-balanced one. The remaining chapters of this book describe modified diets and the reasons for their uses in different disorders.

This chapter begins the study of modified diets by explaining diets that differ from the regular diet in consistency, texture, and frequency of feedings. Table 17–1 summarizes these diets and lists conditions for which they are indicated. Diets modified in consistency, texture, and frequency of feedings often aid in the treatment of GI disorders or conditions that affect the GI tract (surgery, for example). If you think about it, this makes sense. The consistency or texture of a food makes a difference only in the GI tract. Once digested and absorbed, the cells use the basic units of foods regardless of which foods provided these units.

residue: bulk in the colon that includes undigested food, intestinal secretions, bacteria, and the turnover of intestinal cells.

Liquid Diets

There are two types of liquid diets—clear-liquid diets and full-liquid diets. Table 17–2 (p. 425) shows foods allowed on these diets. Clear-liquid diets serve the primary function of providing fluids and electrolytes to prevent dehydration. As you might expect, they consist of foods that are relatively transparent to light, such as gelatin, tea, broth, and the like. They are liquid at body temperature, although they may be semisolid when cool (as gelatin is). The body digests and absorbs these liquids easily, and they contribute little or no residue in the GI tract. The sample menu shows an example of a day's meals.

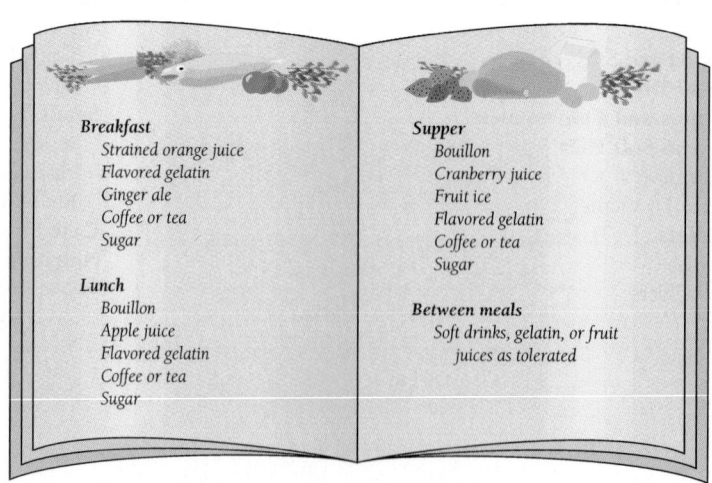

Breakfast
Strained orange juice
Flavored gelatin
Ginger ale
Coffee or tea
Sugar

Lunch
Bouillon
Apple juice
Flavored gelatin
Coffee or tea
Sugar

Supper
Bouillon
Cranberry juice
Fruit ice
Flavored gelatin
Coffee or tea
Sugar

Between meals
Soft drinks, gelatin, or fruit
*   juices as tolerated*

Sample Clear-Liquid Diet Menu

TABLE 17–1   **Indications for the Use of Diets Modified in Consistency, Texture, and Number of Meals**

CLEAR-LIQUID DIET

Postsurgical diet
Bowel preparation for surgery or diagnostic test
Diarrhea
Early refeeding after complete bowel rest
Early feeding in protein-energy malnutrition

FULL-LIQUID DIET

Postsurgical diet
Diarrhea
Dysphagia
(See also *Mechanical Soft Diet*)

LOW-FIBER OR SOFT DIET

Postsurgical diet
Indigestion
Nausea
Esophageal varices (cirrhosis)
Gastritis
Diarrhea
Diverticulitis
Inflammatory bowel disease
Myocardial infarction (heart attack)
Congestive heart failure

MECHANICAL SOFT DIET

Severe dental caries
Missing or no teeth
Ill-fitting dentures
Dry mouth
Periodontal disease
Ulceration of mouth or gums
Oral surgery
Broken jaw
Plastic surgery of the head or neck
Dysphagia
Stroke
Acquired immune deficiency syndrome (AIDS)

BLAND DIET

Ulcers of the mouth or gums
Nausea
Reflux esophagitis
Hiatal hernia

(continued)

TABLE 17–1 *(continued)*

BLAND DIET *(continued)*
Gastritis Peptic ulcers Myocardial infarction Congestive heart failure

HIGH-FIBER DIET
Constipation Irritable bowel syndrome Diverticulosis Weight loss Obesity Diabetes mellitus Heart disease

SMALL, FREQUENT MEALS
Indigestion Nausea Reflux esophagitis Hiatal hernia Dumping syndrome Hypoglycemia Pancreatitis Myocardial infarction

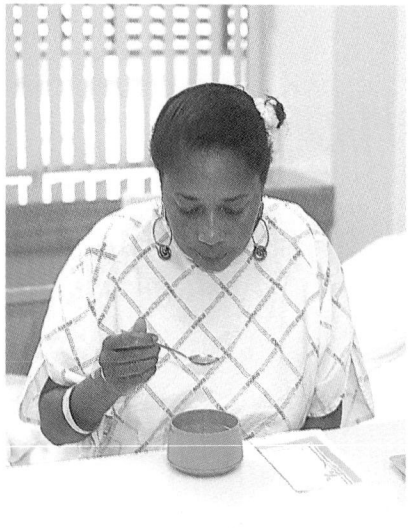

Liquid diets help to prevent dehydration.

If you take a close look at the foods allowed on a clear-liquid diet, you will see why many people find these foods unappetizing and boring. Even more disturbing, consider the nutritional quality of the diet—it is deficient in energy and most nutrients. Then consider the nutrient requirements of a stressed person. No one should stay on a standard clear-liquid diet for more than a day or two, and the aware health care provider will make sure that regular foods are offered as soon as possible.

Clear-liquid diets may be used to prepare the intestine for surgery or diagnostic tests or as a first diet after surgery. They can also be used as an initial diet to treat diarrhea, or to feed a malnourished person, or to feed a person who has not had any oral intake for some time. The diet is usually temporary; as the client can tolerate other foods, the diet is progressed.

The full-liquid diet includes both clear and opaque liquid foods and those that liquefy at body temperature. Table 17–2 lists the foods allowed on full-liquid diets, and the sample menu shows an example of a day's meals. Full-liquid diets may be used as a second diet (after clear liquids) following surgery or for a person who is unable to chew or swallow (see "Mechanical Soft Diet" later in the chapter). As with clear-liquid diets, it can be difficult to meet nutrient needs with a full-liquid diet.

To meet the energy and nutrient needs of people on liquid diets, health care professionals use nutrition formulas or fortified nutrition supplements.

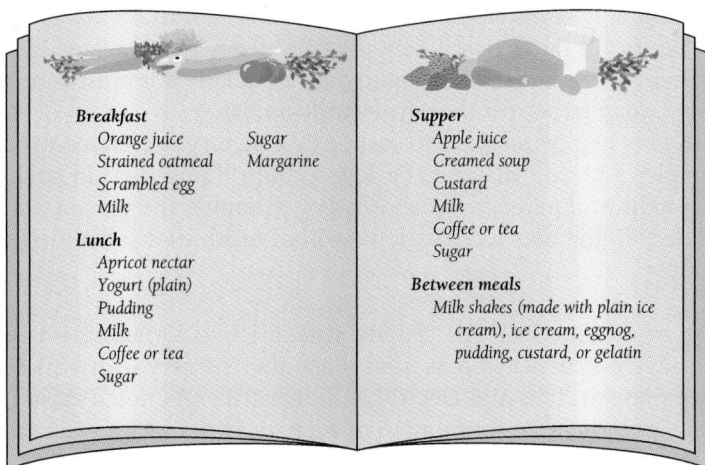

Breakfast
Orange juice   Sugar
Strained oatmeal   Margarine
Scrambled egg
Milk

Lunch
Apricot nectar
Yogurt (plain)
Pudding
Milk
Coffee or tea
Sugar

Supper
Apple juice
Creamed soup
Custard
Milk
Coffee or tea
Sugar

Between meals
Milk shakes (made with plain ice
    cream), ice cream, eggnog,
    pudding, custard, or gelatin

Sample Full-Liquid Diet Menu

Some of these supplements include special gelatins and puddings fortified with nutrients. Some hospitals routinely use these formulas and supplements to prevent energy and protein deficits incurred by standard liquid

TABLE 17–2   **Foods Included on Liquid Diets**

CLEAR-LIQUID DIETS	FULL-LIQUID DIETS
Bouillon	All clear liquids
Broth, clear	Butter
Carbonated beverages	Cheese, cottage[a]
Coffee, regular and decaffeinated	Commercially prepared liquid
Commercially prepared clear liquid	formulas (all)
formulas	Cooked cereals, strained
Fruit drinks	Cream
Fruit ices	Custard
Fruit juices, strained	Eggs, soft cooked or scrambled[a]
Gelatin	Flavorings
Hard candy	Ice cream, plain
Honey	Instant breakfast drinks
Lemonade	Margarine
Popsicles	Milk, all types
Salt	Potatoes, mashed and diluted in cream
Salt substitutes	soups
Sugar	Pudding
Sugar substitutes	Sherbet
Tea	Soups, strained vegetable, meat, or
	cream
	Sour cream
	Vegetable juices, strained
	Vegetable purees, diluted in cream soups
	Yogurt

[a]As tolerated.

diets. Additionally, formulas of specific osmolalities or those that are lactose-free can be useful for people likely to suffer from GI problems. For these reasons, individuals who need a liquid diet, especially if it must continue for more than a day or so, can benefit from formulas.

Liquid diets can be adapted to meet other dietary requirements as well. For example, a person may need a low-sodium liquid diet. In such cases, only low-sodium liquids are provided. For example, the person on a low-sodium clear-liquid diet receives low-sodium broth as a substitute for regular broth.

The next two sections of this chapter describe two situations—as a treatment for severe diarrhea and as a first diet after surgery—for which liquid diets help prevent fluid and electrolyte imbalances. As noted earlier, when these diets must be used for more than a day or two, nutritionally complete liquid formulas are the appropriate choice.

Diarrhea

Diarrhea that results from unabsorbed water and electrolytes, increasing the osmolarity of the intestinal contents, is called **osmotic diarrhea.** Diarrhea that results from an accelerated movement of fluids and electrolytes from the intestinal capillaries into the lumen of the intestine is called **secretory diarrhea.** Severe, chronic diarrhea is often called **intractable diarrhea.**

Diarrhea occurs either when fluids are not absorbed as the intestinal contents move quickly through the GI tract or when water is drawn from cells lining the intestinal tract and added to the food residue. The result is frequent, watery bowel movements.

Mild diarrhea that remits in 24 to 48 hours is seldom a cause for concern unless it is very severe or the individual is already dehydrated. A person with severe, persistent diarrhea may rapidly develop dehydration, weight loss, and multiple nutrient deficiencies. It is urgent to prevent or correct these problems by starting nutrition support before severe depletion occurs.

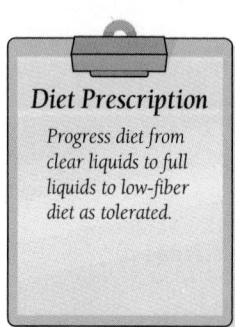

Diet Prescription

Progress diet from clear liquids to full liquids to low-fiber diet as tolerated.

Diarrhea can have many causes. Emotional and physiological stress, nervous tension, food allergies, overeating, food contaminated with infectious bacteria (see Nutrition in Practice 14), bacterial overgrowth in the gut (see Chapter 21), and malnutrition can trigger diarrhea, as can some drugs that irritate the GI tract. Many people on tube feedings develop diarrhea (as you may recall from Chapter 16). Infants and children frequently develop diarrhea when they are ill or given formulas that their immature GI tracts cannot tolerate.

A variety of foods and spices can cause diarrhea in different individuals and at different times. Food sensitivities, such as lactose intolerance, are a frequent cause. Aspartame and sorbitol used in large doses have been known to cause diarrhea in some people. Generally, adults who have food sensitivities that result in diarrhea are aware of the offending foods. For those who don't know the cause of their diarrhea, keeping a food diary and a record of bowel movements can help pinpoint offending foods.

Mild diarrhea does not require medical treatment. Health care professionals can recommend eliminating food irritants and drinking clear liquids to help alleviate mild diarrhea.

Severe diarrhea, on the other hand, can quickly lead to serious dehydration. An average-sized adult producing a large volume of watery stools can lose more than 1 liter of fluid and electrolytes per hour—a fluid loss that can be fatal in six hours or less.[1] Severe or persistent diarrhea in infants and children is of particular concern, because a greater percentage of body weight in infants and children is water—and it can be depleted even more quickly.

Chronic diarrhea is also a cause for concern. Chronic diarrhea can result from other disorders such as malabsorption or protein-energy malnutrition (PEM) or from medical treatments such as radiation therapy or drugs. The person with chronic diarrhea can gradually become dehydrated as large amounts of water and electrolytes are lost over a long period of time.

Oral rehydration therapy formulas may successfully prevent dehydration in some cases of severe diarrhea. Oftentimes, however, especially in seriously ill individuals, it becomes necessary to stop placing demands on the GI tract and let it rest while investigating the cause of the diarrhea. The diagnostician may order all foods and beverages withheld for 24 to 48 hours, during which time treatment primarily focuses on maintaining fluid and electrolyte balance intravenously. After a day or so of intravenous fluids, the person tries a clear-liquid diet, and then progresses to a full-liquid diet, a low-fiber diet (described later in this chapter), and finally a regular diet as tolerated. Once a person receives an oral diet, applesauce or scraped raw apples may be given every two to four hours. These foods contain pectin, a carbohydrate that attracts water and improves the consistency of the stools. Of course, if a food is known to have irritated the intestine, it is eliminated. The exact treatment plan depends on the cause of the diarrhea.

If the diarrhea worsens as the diet progresses, then alternate feeding programs are appropriate. Enteral nutrition is always preferred to parenteral nutrition, so a first choice is to try hydrolyzed formulas, either orally or by tube. However, some people with chronic diarrhea are unable to tolerate any type of enteral feeding. For these people, parenteral nutrition is indicated, and nothing is given by mouth.

Drug therapy also plays an important role in the treatment of diarrhea. Table 17–3 lists antidiarrheal agents and their nutrition consequences.

oral rehydration therapy formulas: formulas containing glucose and a combination of sodium and potassium salts used to prevent or treat dehydration associated with diarrhea.

TABLE 17–3 **Antidiarrheal Agents**

DRUG NAME	TIMING WITH MEALS	COMMON SIDE EFFECTS THAT MAY INFLUENCE NUTRITION STATUS
Diphenoxylate hydrochloride	May give with food.	Nausea, vomiting, bloating, anorexia, dry mouth, sore or swollen gums.
Kaolin, pectin	Mix at room temperature with milk or juice.	Constipation, dry mouth, altered taste perception.
Loperamide hydrochloride		Abdominal pain, constipation, bloating, dry mouth, vomiting, nausea.
Opium, belladonna, paregoric	May give with food.	Nausea, vomiting, constipation. Sedation.

Source: Adapted from D. E. Powers and A. O. Moore, *Food Medication Interactions* (Phoenix: Food Medication Interactions, 1991), and *Nursing 91 Drug Handbook* (Springhouse, Pa.: Springhouse Corp., 1991).

Nutrition and Surgery

Ideally, all clients enter surgery at appropriate weight, with full nutrient reserves. However, such optimal status may be difficult to achieve. The illness that necessitates the surgery, or the psychological stress associated with it, may interfere with a person's food intake or the body's use of nutrients. Additionally, the person may have to fast or follow a nutritionally inadequate liquid diet before undergoing diagnostic and laboratory tests in preparation for surgery.

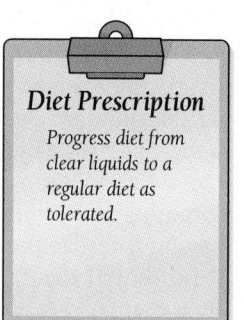

Diet Prescription

Progress diet from clear liquids to a regular diet as tolerated.

Before surgery, a well-nourished client who is expected to have an uncomplicated recovery usually receives a regular diet. Regular hospital diets provide ample food energy and protein. Given such a diet, a well-nourished person can withstand short-term starvation and some degree of protein catabolism without serious consequences.

Malnourished people require diets high in energy and protein prior to surgery (see Chapter 18). Most hospitals provide malnourished clients with high-kcalorie, high-protein supplements and snacks between meals. For people with functioning GI tracts who cannot eat enough food orally, tube feedings may be indicated. TPN may be initiated before surgery to supply nutrients when use of the GI tract is contraindicated. Studies suggest that preoperative TPN may be useful in preventing some types of postoperative complications in severely malnourished clients.[2] Health care professionals offer a valuable service when they explain to clients the highly supportive role that nutrition plays in immunity and recovery from stress; such explanations encourage clients to eat or to accept tube feedings or intravenous nutrition cooperatively.

Physicians generally order all foods and fluids withheld for at least eight hours before surgery. This measure helps to prevent regurgitation and aspiration, which can occur during anesthesia or recovery. People undergoing GI surgery receive liquids or foods low in residue for two or three days before surgery to minimize the amount of fecal material in the gut and to help prevent distention after surgery. People restricted to liquid diets may receive low-residue and residue-free liquid supplements either orally or by tube to meet nutrient needs.

The immediate nutrition-related task for the health care team following surgery is to maintain fluid and electrolyte balance. Clients lose blood, fluid, and electrolytes during surgery, and they may lose additional fluids following surgery from fever, draining wounds, vomiting, and diarrhea. Excessive losses without replacement can lead to dehydration and shock. To replace lost fluids and electrolytes, clients receive IV infusions after surgery. The intravenous, rather than gastrointestinal, route is used because peristalsis in the GI tract is inactive in the immediate postoperative period; until peristalsis returns, food and fluids are generally not given orally. The physician determines the client's fluid needs based on the person's blood pressure, pulse rate, urinary output, level of consciousness, breathing patterns, and body temperature, among other factors.

Some studies suggest that feeding immediately after surgery, even before peristalsis returns, may have some benefits. However, more research is

A diet high in energy and protein provides about 1000 kcal more than a person needs to maintain weight and about 1.5 g protein per kilogram of body weight daily.

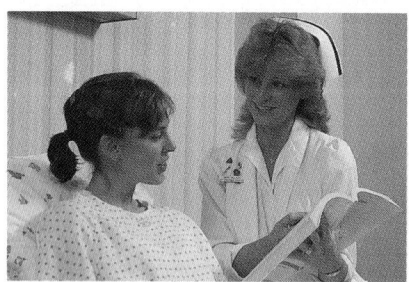

Health care professionals relieve clients' anxieties when they explain procedures to them.

Some types of GI surgeries described later in this book include ileostomies and colostomies (later in this chapter), gastrectomies (Chapter 20), and intestinal resections (Chapter 21).

shock: a sudden drop in the blood volume that disrupts the supply of oxygen to the tissues and the return of blood to the heart. Many events can lead to shock; some include severe bleeding from trauma or surgery, or severe dehydration.

needed to determine if the benefits of early feeding outweigh the risks. The risks of feeding in the absence of peristalsis include abdominal distention with possible perforation of the bowel and consequent infection.

Although fluids and electrolytes are of primary concern, other nutrients cannot be ignored. If you think about the roles nutrients play, you'll see why. Consider protein: it is the material of antibodies needed to fight infection, of collagen to form scars, of all cells to rebuild damaged tissue, of plasma proteins that maintain fluid and electrolyte balance, of the matrix on which bones are rebuilt after fractures, and of many crucial tissue constituents. In addition, some amino acids provide glucose when the body's glucose needs exceed its glycogen stores. Deficiencies of other nutrients hinders recovery in similar ways. Depending on the type of surgery and the quality of the diet, supplements of some nutrients may be necessary.

When GI tract activity returns, the postoperative client may be ready to eat. After uncomplicated surgery, a well-nourished person who can tolerate solid foods is ready for a standard hospital diet adequate in all nutrients.

People with depleted nutrient stores and people with postsurgical complications need high-kcalorie, high-protein diets. This is true even for overweight people, for they, too, have high postsurgical nutrient needs and risk nutrient depletion. They may have surplus fat stores, but they may also have lost vital proteins.

The need for many of the B vitamins increases when energy and protein intakes increase. However, diets high in food energy and protein usually contain large amounts of B vitamins as well; thus the person who consumes a variety of foods in adequate amounts needs no supplements. However, vitamin C deserves special attention; it helps form collagen, which plays an important role in wound healing. Similarly, zinc also participates in wound healing. Vitamin K serves an important function in helping blood to clot after surgery. Keep an eye open for signs of deficiencies and the possible need for supplements.

The risk of malnutrition after surgery may be further complicated by anorexia and immobilization. Individualizing the diet is very important. Exercise is important, too: encourage clients to get out of bed and to begin minimal exercise, such as walking, as soon as medically safe.

People on tube feedings or parenteral nutrition before surgery usually stay on specialized nutrition support until they are able to meet most of their nutrient needs with oral diets. The surgeon who anticipates that a person may have difficulties in resuming oral intake after surgery may construct a feeding gastrostomy or jejunostomy during surgery. Tube feedings can then be continued until oral intake is adequate.

Depending on the type of surgery, additional nutrition consequences are possible (see Table 17–4, p. 430). People who develop complications following surgery are even more likely to become malnourished due to the additional stress placed on the body.

In summary, postsurgical nutrition support aims to minimize the loss of vital body tissue and the depletion of nutrients. Generally, the diets of people who are not receiving special nutrition support progress from clear liquids or full liquids on to low-fiber foods (discussed next) and regular foods as tolerated.

Chapter 14 describes how anorexia and immobilization interfere with nutrition status.

The general progression of diets after surgery from clear liquids to full liquids to a low-fiber diet to a regular diet is collectively called a **progressive diet.**

TABLE 17–4   **Possible Effects of Surgery on Nutrition Status**

HEAD AND NECK RESECTION	
Difficulty in chewing/swallowing	Inability to chew/swallow

ESOPHAGEAL RESECTION	
Reduced gastric motility	Steatorrhea (fat malabsorption)
Reduced gastric acid production	Fistula formation (Chapter 21)
Diarrhea	Stenosis (constriction)

STOMACH RESECTION	
Dumping syndrome	Vitamin B_{12} malabsorption
Hypoglycemia	General malabsorption
Lack of gastric acid	

INTESTINAL RESECTION	
General malabsorption	Hyperoxaluria (Chapter 21)
Steatorrhea	Fluid and electrolyte imbalance
Diarrhea	Blind loop syndrome (Chapter 21)

PANCREATIC RESECTION	
General malabsorption	Diabetes mellitus

Often the postsurgical diet order simply says "diet as tolerated." Nursing personnel consult with the client and use their discretion in advancing the diet from a liquid to a regular diet. Many times someone forgets to advance the diet and the client is provided an inadequate diet for no reason. Other times a person truly cannot tolerate foods except for clear liquids; in such cases, alert the dietitian or suggest to the physician that a supplemental formula be considered. Occasionally, tube feedings or total or supplemental intravenous nutrition may be necessary. If you work with people after surgery, remember to check their diets.

Low-Fiber Diets

Low-fiber diet, **soft** diet, and **low-residue** diet all describe the same diet. Traditional **low-residue** diets inappropriately restrict milk and milk products.[3]

Low-fiber diets supply foods that are least likely to form an obstruction when the intestinal tract is narrowed by inflammation or scarring or when GI motility is slowed. Low-fiber diets often serve as intermediate diets after intestinal or rectal surgery as a person progresses from a liquid to a regular diet. People with inflammatory bowel diseases, ileostomies, colostomies, or partial obstructions of the intestine may benefit from low-fiber diets. Table 17–5 on p. 432 lists foods included in and eliminated from a low-fiber diet, and the sample menu shows how a low-fiber diet translates into a meal plan.

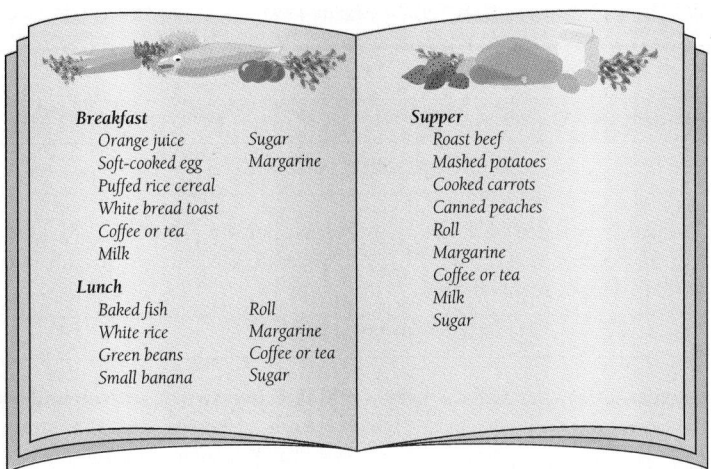

Sample Low-Fiber/Low-Residue Diet Menu

Two terms, *fiber* and *residue,* describe components of the diet that affect the contents of the colon. People often use these terms interchangeably, although it is incorrect to do so. *Fiber* describes the portion of food that is found in the colon because people don't have the enzymes to digest it. *Residue* refers to the total amount of material in the colon (see margin, p. 392).

Earlier in this chapter, the use of low-fiber diets as transitional diets following surgery was discussed. For people who undergo ileostomies or colostomies—two types of intestinal surgery—the low-fiber diet may be required for a longer period of time, as described below.

Ileostomies and Colostomies

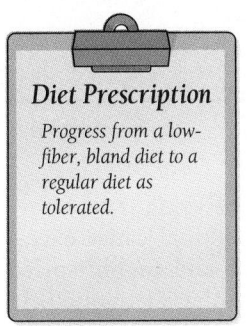

Diet Prescription

Progress from a low-fiber, bland diet to a regular diet as tolerated.

In some clients, certain intestinal obstructions or lesions necessitate the removal of all or a portion of the large intestine. An ileostomy involves the removal of the entire colon, rectum, and anus; a stoma, or opening, made from the ileum is brought out through the abdomen to allow for defecation (see Figure 17–1, p. 433). A colostomy involves removal of only the rectum and anus, with the stoma formed from the remaining part of the colon. Watery stools result from ileostomies, while more formed stools result from colostomies.

stoma (STOH-ma): a surgically formed opening; after an ileostomy or colostomy, a stoma is formed from the cut-off end of the intestine through the abdominal wall, rerouting the excretion of wastes.
stoma = window

After oral intake is initiated following surgery, people who have undergone ileostomies or colostomies generally receive low-fiber, bland diets to help promote healing of the stoma and to prevent irritation. However, encourage clients to resume normal diets as soon as possible. Add foods individually and in small amounts so that their effects can be assessed. If a new food causes problems, encourage clients to try it again a few months later.

TABLE 17-5   **Low-Fiber Diet**

FOODS ALLOWED	FOODS AVOIDED
MEAT AND MEAT ALTERNATES	
Baked, broiled, or roasted beef, fish, lamb, liver, poultry, veal, crisp bacon; hard- or soft-cooked eggs	Fried poultry or meats, cold cuts, sardines, fried eggs, peanut butter
MILK AND MILK PRODUCTS	
Whole, nonfat, or low-fat milk; yogurt; mild cheeses	Milk drinks or yogurt containing whole fruits or berries, seeds, or skins; strongly flavored cheeses
FRUITS AND VEGETABLES	
Cooked or canned fruits without seeds and skins; ripe bananas, orange sections, grapefruit sections; all fruit juices; cooked asparagus tips, beets, broccoli, carrots, green beans, tomato juice, wax beans, winter squash; strained peas, spinach, summer squash, or potatoes	Berries; avocados; prune juice; raw fruits except those listed; legumes, raw vegetables, and all other vegetables except those listed
GRAINS	
Refined, enriched white-bread; plain muffins or rolls; white-flour crackers (saltines, melba toast, zwieback); refined, ready-to-eat, or cooked cereals; noodles; macaroni; spaghetti; strained oatmeal	Whole-grain breads and cereals or those containing nuts, bran, or seeds; fried breads such as doughnuts
MISCELLANEOUS	
Tea, coffee, fruit drinks, carbonated beverages, butter, cream, margarine, mayonnaise	Any dishes made with foods to be avoided; coconut

ostomate (OSS-toe-mate): a person who has a surgically formed opening from the bowel to the outside of the body, bypassing the anus. An *ileostomate* (ILL-ee-OSS-toe-mate) has had an *ileostomy;* a *colostomate* (ko-LOSS-toe-mate) has had a *colostomy.*

Ostomates are often concerned about gas, odor, and loose and watery stools. Each person individually must identify the foods that cause excessively watery stools. Certain raw fruits and vegetables and highly spiced foods cause problems for some ileostomates. Beer and other alcoholic beverages may cause diarrhea and gas. Gas and odors can also arise from such foods as beans, onions, green peppers, cabbage, turnips, and beets.

Ostomates may restrict their fluid intakes for fear of aggravating diarrhea. Explain to them the importance of drinking plenty of fluids, and reassure them that excess fluid taken above and beyond the amount lost through the ostomy will be absorbed and excreted by the kidneys and will not aggravate diarrhea.

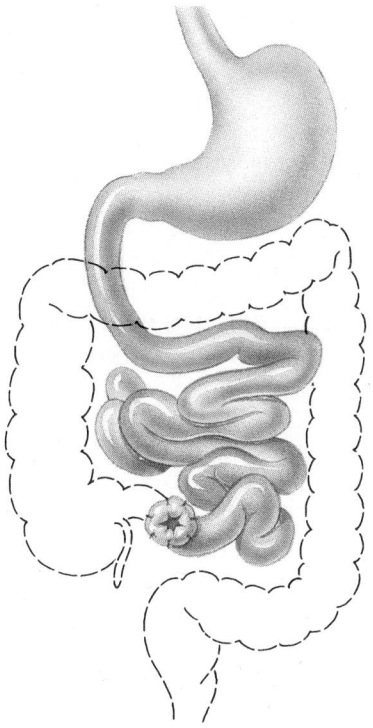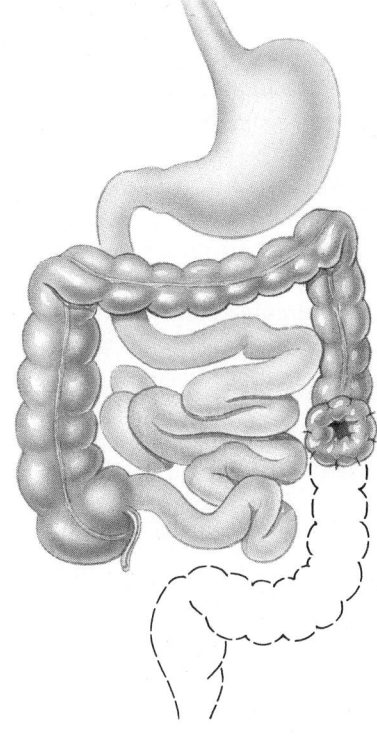

FIGURE 17–1   **Ileostomy and Colostomy**

A. Ileostomy. The entire colon, rectum, and anus are removed, and the stoma is formed from the ileum.

B. Colostomy. The rectum and anus are removed, and the stoma is formed from the remaining colon.

New ostomates face many adjustments after surgery. They may feel loss of control over a basic and private function. The retraining required to care for the ostomy and maintain bowel function may be difficult. Ostomates may also worry that loved ones, particularly spouses, may find them unattractive. The health care team must work closely with each person and that person's family to help everyone make the necessary adjustments and resume normal activities.

A health care professional specially educated to assist ostomates in learning the proper methods of caring for ostomy sites and adjusting to the ostomy is the **enterostomal** (en-ter-oh-STOME-al) **therapist (E.T.).**

Mechanical Soft Diet

A variety of dental, medical, and surgical conditions can temporarily or permanently interfere with chewing or swallowing (see Table 17–6, p. 435). Without the appropriate adjustments in diet, people with these conditions might eat too little, lose too much weight, and suffer the consequences of a deteriorating nutrition status.

To ease the task of chewing and swallowing, the mechanical soft diet eliminates those foods the person cannot easily chew or swallow. All foods and seasonings are permitted on mechanical soft diets; liquid, chopped, pureed, or regular foods with a soft consistency are best tolerated. Any

mechanical soft diet: a diet that excludes all foods that are difficult to chew or swallow; also called a **dental soft diet.**

person who cannot eat enough foods or drink enough liquids to meet nutrient needs should be fed by tube.

People's tolerances of food consistency vary greatly. Health care professionals should work closely with individuals to identify those tolerances and to make needed adjustments. For example, a person with a newly broken jaw may be able to consume only liquids; a person without teeth, however, may be able to eat baked chicken or fish, ground beef, casseroles, canned fruits, and soft-cooked vegetables. Encourage the client to eat a variety of foods that are as similar as possible to those of a regular diet to enhance the client's acceptance of them and to lessen the likelihood of nutrient deficiencies. Provide plenty of fluids with meals to ease chewing and swallowing of foods. Sucking fluids through a straw may be easier than drinking them from a cup or glass.

All seasonings and types of foods are allowed on a mechanical soft diet. However, people with mouth ulcers may experience pain from eating highly seasoned or acidic foods (such as citrus fruits and tomatoes). In addition, foods that contain nuts or seeds (such as breads with sesame or poppy seeds) can easily become trapped in the ulcer and cause discomfort. Clients with mouth sores often find foods served at cooler temperatures soothing.

Clients who have difficulty chewing and swallowing foods due to a reduced flow of saliva often can increase salivary flow by sucking on sour candy or gum. Encourage such clients to practice good oral and dental hygiene and to avoid concentrated sweets to prevent dental caries.

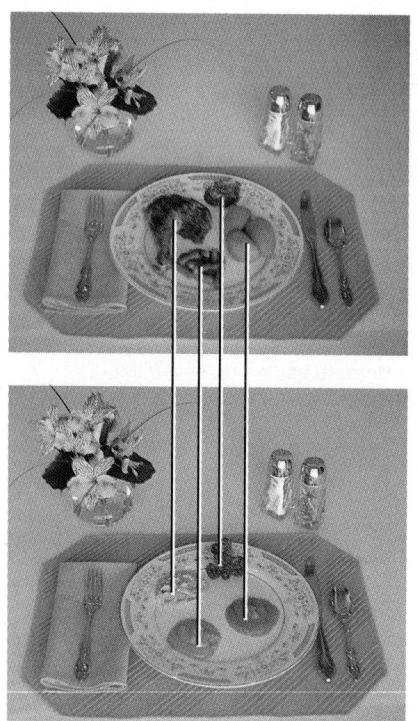

Serve colorful pureed meals at the appropriate temperature, seasoned to taste.

Take a moment to think about a pureed diet. A typical dinner of baked chicken, boiled potatoes, and green beans is now white mush, more white mush, and a green blob. However, creative and caring people in the kitchen can make a difference. By arranging and shaping foods attractively on a plate, and adding garnishes for color, they can enhance the eye appeal of a meal.

In many hospitals, baby foods routinely replace pureed foods. While baby foods offer nutrients, they often taste bland, since manufacturers prepare them without salt or spices. Regardless of whether the client receives pureed food or baby food, the consistency creates a psychological block to eating, and malnutrition can result.

Can you improve the situation? The answer is yes. First, determine whether the client truly needs pureed rather than chopped or soft foods. Second, help the client select well-balanced, colorful meals. For example, substitute mashed sweet potatoes for mashed white potatoes. Such a change adds appetizing color to the meal. Serve the food attractively and at the right temperature. Lastly, unless the physician has ordered otherwise, suggest spices that will enliven the flavor of foods. Many people think that because they must follow a special diet, the foods must not be spicy.

If pureed foods consistently present a problem for a client, talk to the administrative dietitian or food service manager. Pureed foods should be smooth and thick—not watery or thin. Whenever possible, regular foods that have been pureed should be served instead of baby foods. The use of blenders, food processors, and grinders simplifies the process of making pureed foods.

TABLE 17–6   **Conditions That May Interfere with Chewing or Swallowing**

Achalasia	No teeth
Acquired immune deficiency syndrome (AIDS)	Oral surgery
	Periodontal disease
Broken jaw	Radiation therapy of the head and neck
Cancer or chemotherapy	Sensitivity to hot or cold
Dental caries	Strokes (sometimes)
Dryness of the mouth	Surgery of the head and neck
Dysphagia	Ulceration of the mouth or gums
Ill-fitting dentures	
Missing teeth	

People with dysphagia and those who have suffered from strokes often benefit from mechanical soft diets. The next sections describe these disorders.

Dysphagia

Dysphagia results from any disorder that impairs the ability to swallow. A person may be unable to initiate swallowing, to chew foods and mix them with saliva, or to push foods to the back of the throat and into the esophagus. Other disorders specifically interfere with the muscular contraction of the esophagus.

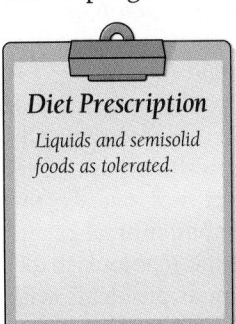

Diet Prescription

Liquids and semisolid foods as tolerated.

Diets for swallowing disorders are highly individualized based on each client's unique needs. Often, the client can handle only liquids and semisolid foods. Many prefer thickened liquids and pureed foods, because these flow slowly enough to allow time to coordinate oral movements. Naturally thick liquids include fruit nectars, milk shakes, eggnog, and vegetable juices. Liquids thickened with commercially available thickeners or baby cereal, as well as soft, smooth solids such as puddings, custards, and smooth yogurts, are frequently well tolerated. Recommend that clients experiment with tilting the head forward and backward to see if swallowing can be made easier with the head positioned differently.

Another cause of dysphagia is achalasia. In achalasia, nerves that control the esophageal movement fail to function properly; the muscles of the esophagus cannot propel the food bolus downward toward the stomach, and the cardiac sphincter remains closed, thus preventing food from passing out of the esophagus into the stomach. Foods and fluids accumulate in the esophagus, which explains the sensation of food sticking in the throat. Eventually, either the pressure of the food causes the cardiac sphincter to open or the person regurgitates the food.

At first, the person with achalasia may experience only temporary and mild dysphagia. As the condition worsens, the esophagus widens, and the

dysphagia (dis-FAY-gee-ah): difficulty in swallowing.
dys = bad
phagein = to eat

Conditions sometimes associated with dysphagia include strokes (described later), brain tumors, surgery for cancer of the head and neck, congenital defects, reflux esophagitis, Lou Gehrig's disease, Guillain-Barré syndrome, multiple sclerosis, polio, head injury, myasthenia gravis, Alzheimer's disease, and Parkinson's disease.

achalasia (ack-ah-LAY-zee-ah): dysfunction of the esophagus; sometimes called **esophageal dyssynergia** (ee-SOF-ah-GEE-al dis-sin-ER-gee-ah) or **cardiospasm.**
a = not
chalasis = relaxation
dys = bad
synergia = cooperation

The **cardiac sphincter** is often called the **lower esophageal sphincter (LES)** or the **gastroesophageal sphincter.** (The passage of food through the GI tract is described on p. 76.)

The fear of eating is called **sitophobia** (SIGH-toe-FOE-bee-ah).

sitos = food

phobos = fear

symptoms become painful. The person becomes fearful of eating and begins to eat less food. By the time the person seeks medical attention, weight loss and signs of nutrient deficiencies are frequently evident. A further danger exists—the person may aspirate into the lung food that has been stagnating in the esophagus. This can lead to a serious lung infection.

The person with achalasia may be able to tolerate liquid or semiliquid foods in small servings. Suggest liquid supplements to meet nutrient needs. Tube feedings and parenteral nutrition may be beneficial for people with any type of dysphagia, particularly if they are severely malnourished or unable to consume adequate nutrients orally. However, nasogastric or gastrostomy feedings may be contraindicated; a high risk of complications, particularly aspiration pneumonia (see p. 400), is associated with their use in some clients with dysphagia.[4]

The Stroke Victim

When blood flow to the brain is insufficient or when blood vessels burst and blood flows into the brain, a stroke, or cerebrovascular accident (CVA), results. Recovery for some stroke victims is unremarkable. The optimal diet in such a case is based on the underlying medical condition (for example, hyperlipidemia, hypertension, or obesity or a combination of these).

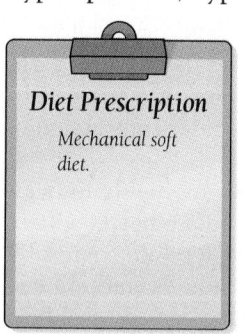

Diet Prescription

Mechanical soft diet.

Many stroke victims, however, require many months of rehabilitative therapy to recover. They may suffer from temporary or permanent problems that interfere with the ability to communicate. Inability to communicate effectively makes it difficult for these clients to tell health care professionals what foods they would like to eat or about problems they may be having with foods or meals.

Food energy in the diet of a stroke victim may need to be limited due to the client's inactivity. Clients who must relearn how to walk or use other muscle groups will be better able to do so if they are not overweight. However, underweight can be a problem for physical rehabilitation also, and care should be taken to ensure that clients do not become malnourished.

Many stroke victims have either temporary or permanent problems with chewing, swallowing, and the physical process of eating. Tube feedings often are indicated initially. Later, a mechanical soft diet may be useful. Those people who have problems with the physical aspects of eating often benefit from special feeding devices, several of which are shown in Figure 17–2.

Bland Diets

Bland diets eliminate foods that stimulate gastric acid secretion or those that are irritating to the gastric mucosa, such as the ones described in Table 17–7. Health care professionals individualize the diet based on each person's tolerances. Most practitioners recommend that alcohol and both reg-

TABLE 17-7 **Liberal Bland Diet**

A liberal bland diet provides three meals a day and includes all foods except those that irritate the gastric mucosa. Substances generally contraindicated on a liberal bland diet include:
- Any foods an individual identifies as irritating to the GI tract.
- Alcohol.
- Caffeine and caffeine-containing beverages (including cola beverages, cocoa, coffee, and tea).
- Decaffeinated coffee.
- Pepper and spicy foods (except as tolerated).

Note: Read Nutrition in Practice 17 for a more complete discussion of the liberal bland diet and its development over the years.

ular and decaffeinated coffee be avoided. There is less agreement about pepper and beverages other than coffee that contain caffeine.

Practitioners frequently prescribe bland diets for gastritis, ulcers, and reflux esophagitis (all discussed later in this chapter). People who suffer heart attacks or people with congestive heart failure (see Chapter 22) may benefit from temporary bland diets. Bland foods are thought to be less likely to form gas than regular diets—important, because gas can distend the stomach, causing the diaphragm to be pushed upward toward the heart, adding to the heart's work load.

The bland diet has changed so dramatically over the years that it is virtually a different diet from the bland diet of the past. Nutrition in Practice 17 describes these changes. The next two sections discuss uses of the bland diet.

Gastritis

Gastritis is a common disorder characterized by inflammation of the mucosal lining of the stomach. The person with gastritis may complain of anorexia, nausea, vomiting, belching, a feeling of fullness, and stomach pain.

gastritis: inflammation of the lining of the stomach.

Diet Prescription
Bland diet as tolerated.

Acute gastritis most often follows ingestion of aspirin or other drugs that irritate the gastric mucosa. Alcohol abuse, food irritants, food allergies, food poisoning, radiation, stress, and infections can also cause gastritis. The dietary management of acute gastritis rests on two principles:

- Eliminate irritating foods.
- Reduce gastric acidity.

For the person with gastritis who cannot eat because of nausea or vomiting, food is generally withheld for one or two days. Then the diet progresses from liquids to liberal bland as tolerated. Antacids may also be given.

FIGURE 17–2   **Special Feeding Devices**
Utensils

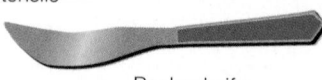

Rocker knife

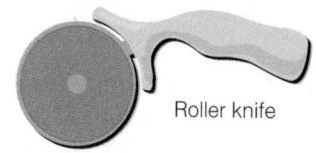

Roller knife

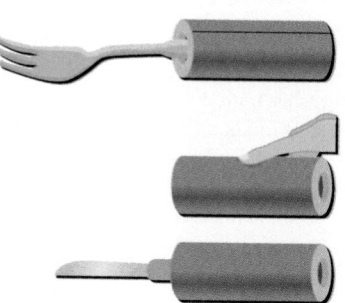

A. People with only one arm or hand may have difficulty cutting foods and may appreciate using a *rocker knife* or a *roller knife*.

B. People with a limited range of motion can feed themselves better when they use *flatware with built-up handles*.

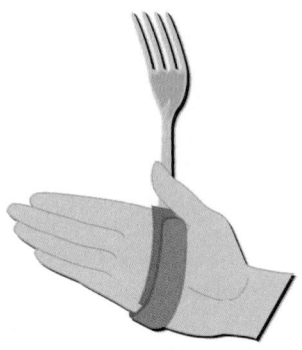

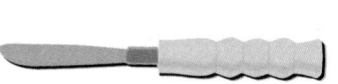

C. People with extreme muscle weakness may be able to eat with a *utensil holder*.

D. For people with tremors, spasticity, and uneven jerky movements, *weighted utensils* can aid the feeding process.

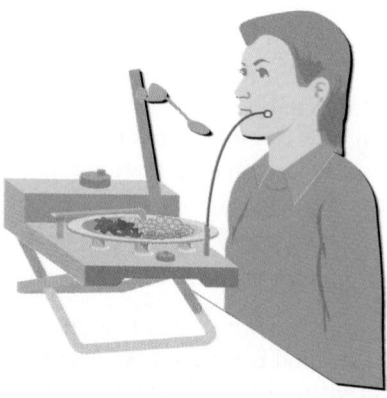

E. For people with severe limitations, *battery-powered feeding machines* require less feeding assistance from others.

FIGURE 17–2   (*continued*)

Plates

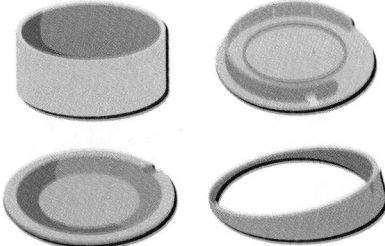

F. People who have limited dexterity and difficulty maneuvering food find *scoop dishes* or *food guards* useful.

G. People with uncontrolled or excessive movements might move dishes around while eating and may benefit from using *unbreakable dishes with suction cups.*

Cups

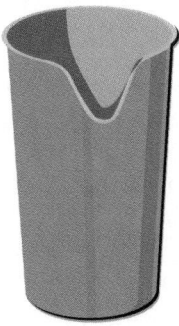

H. People with limited neck motion can use a *cut-out plastic cup.*

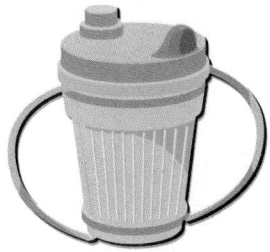

I. *Two-handled cups* enable people with moderate muscle weakness to lift a cup with two hands.

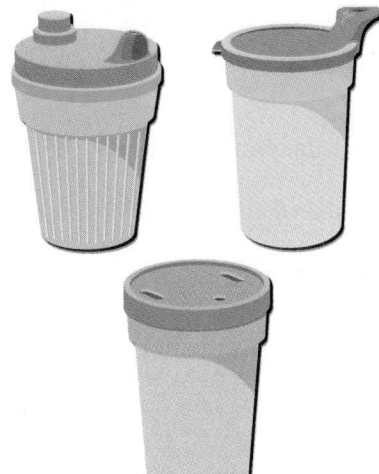

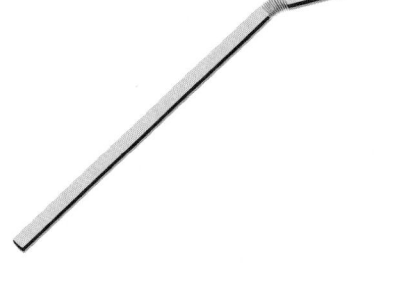

J. People with uncontrolled or excessive movements might prefer to drink liquids from a *covered cup* or glass with a *slotted opening* or *spout*.
K. A soft, flexible, long plastic straw may also ease the task of drinking.

Chronic gastritis has the same symptoms as acute gastritis but persists for a longer time. As gastritis progresses, the gastric cells atrophy, and gastric secretions decline. Unlike acute gastritis, chronic gastritis has no known cause. Because so little is known about chronic gastritis, finding the appropriate diet may be a matter of trial and error. A bland diet seems to relieve GI symptoms in some cases.

Peptic Ulcers

peptic ulcer: an eroded lesion of the stomach (gastric ulcer) or duodenum (duodenal ulcer). Ulcers that develop following a severe physiological stress (surgery, burns, shock, or infection) are called *stress ulcers*.

Recall that **pepsin** is a gastric enzyme that digests protein.

peritonitis: infection of the lining of the abdominal cavity.

Ulcers can develop both inside and outside the body, but the term *ulcer* used alone generally refers to a *peptic ulcer*. A peptic ulcer is an erosion of the top layer of cells from the mucosa of the stomach or duodenum (occasionally peptic ulcers may develop in the esophagus). This erosion leaves the underlying layers of cells exposed to gastric juices, and to erosion by hydrochloric acid and the enzyme pepsin. The erosion may proceed until it eats into the capillaries and the nerves surrounding the area, leading to bleeding and pain. If the erosion penetrates all the way through the mucosal lining, a major and sometimes fatal infection known as peritonitis can rapidly develop.

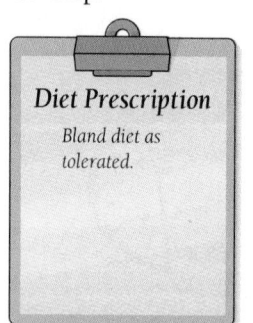

Diet Prescription

Bland diet as tolerated.

A person with an ulcer may experience a gnawing, burning pain that lasts up to several weeks. Although symptoms generally disappear for periods of time, they usually recur. People with gastric ulcers almost always have chronic gastritis.

Currently there is no cure for ulcers. Instead, treatment aims at relieving pain, healing the ulcer, and minimizing the likelihood of recurrence. Both gastric and duodenal ulcers share the same treatment regimen.

Peptic ulcer therapy attempts to neutralize gastric acidity and to reduce gastric acid secretion. These measures help protect the stomach and duodenum wall from the eroding effect of gastric acid. Thanks to the development of drugs that prevent ulcer formation, drug therapy has become the primary therapy for ulcers, with diet playing a minor role. The client with ulcers may be instructed to:

- Follow prescribed drug therapy, which may include any of the drugs listed in Table 17–8.
- Use antacids, taken one hour after meals, when gastric acid secretion is high.
- Eliminate any food that routinely causes indigestion or pain. Avoid caffeine- and alcohol-containing beverages.
- Reduce stress, which stimulates gastric acid secretion.
- Learn how to handle stress without overreacting or becoming upset; learn how to relax, get enough sleep, and enjoy life. Engage in regular physical activity, which effectively reduces stress.
- Eliminate drugs that irritate the stomach (for example, aspirin).
- Reduce or eliminate cigarette smoking, which also stimulates gastric acid secretion.

TABLE 17-8 **Antacids and Other Antiulcer Medications**

DRUG NAME	TIMING WITH MEALS	COMMON SIDE EFFECTS THAT MAY INFLUENCE NUTRITION STATUS
Aluminum hydroxide	Give 1 to 3 hr after meals.	Constipation, cramps, bloating, nausea, vomiting, anorexia, chalky taste. Inactivates thiamin; decreases absorption of vitamin A, phosphorus, and calcium.
Calcium carbonate	Give 1 to 3 hr after meals. Give iron supplements 1 to 2 hr before or after use. Do not take with large amounts of dairy products.	Belching, nausea, constipation, steatorrhea, chalky taste. May decrease iron absorption.
Cimetidine	Give with meals; caffeine and alcohol reduce effectiveness.	Diarrhea, reduced gastric secretion. May induce hyperglycemia.
Dihydroxyaluminum sodium carbonate	Give 1 to 3 hr after meals.	Constipation, diarrhea, anorexia, weight loss.
Magaldrate	Give on empty stomach.	Chalky taste. May decrease absorption of fat-soluble vitamins, especially vitamin A.
Magnesium hydroxide	Give 1 hr after meals.	Constipation. May decrease absorption of vitamin A, phosphorus, and calcium; inactivates thiamin.
Ranitidine		Constipation, nausea, abdominal discomfort. (Fewer reported side effects and interactions than with cimetidine.)
Sodium bicarbonate	Give 1 to 3 hr after meals.	Belching, gas, bloating, weight gain. Decreases iron absorption.
Sucralfate	Give on empty stomach 1 hr before meals and at bedtime.	Constipation, diarrhea, nausea, cramps, dry mouth. Interferes with absorption of fat-soluable vitamins.

Source: Adapted from D. E. Powers and A. O. Moore, *Food Medication Interactions* (Phoenix: Food Medication Interactions, 1991), and *Nursing 91 Drug Handbook* (Springhouse, Pa.: Springhouse Corp., 1991).

Ulcers are painful, but the pain is intermittent. The person with an ulcer who is bothered by particular foods has one great advantage over the person with a "silent" disease or one that causes chronic pain. The pain of an ulcer promptly follows the commission of a dietary indiscretion, and the client can quickly learn which foods and beverages hurt and which do not. Use this information to help clients tailor their dietary routines to their own tolerances.

High-Fiber Diets

Health care professionals frequently advise clients to adopt high-fiber diets by increasing the consumption of whole-grain breads and cereals, fruits and vegetables, dried beans and peas, and nuts. As Chapter 2 described, foods contain many types of fibers; the effects that fiber has in the body depend on the type of fiber.

The addition of high-fiber foods is often recommended to reduce the risk of cancer (Nutrition in Practice 18), to help in weight loss efforts (Chapter 19), to help regulate blood glucose in people with diabetes mellitus (Chapter 20), and to help control blood cholesterol in people with heart disease (Chapter 22).

The major impact of dietary fiber is on the colon, and the most clearly defined and least controversial use of high-fiber diets is in the treatment of constipation and diverticular disease. High-fiber diets work by adding volume and weight to the stool, speeding the transit of undigested materials through the intestine, and minimizing pressure within the colon. Table 2–3 (p. 37) lists foods useful for adding fiber to the diet, and a sample menu is shown here. High-fiber diets provide about 20 to 25 grams of dietary fiber daily. Bran sprinkled on cereals, salads, applesauce, and other food items, or added to beverages, significantly increases the fiber content of the diet.

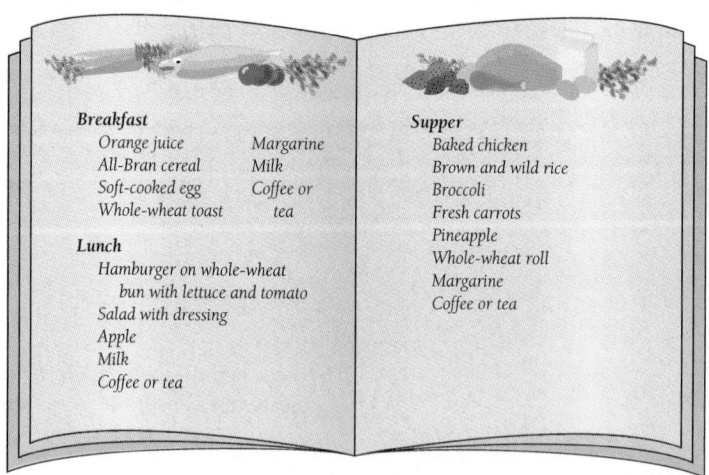

Breakfast
Orange juice   Margarine
All-Bran cereal   Milk
Soft-cooked egg   Coffee or
Whole-wheat toast   tea

Lunch
Hamburger on whole-wheat
    bun with lettuce and tomato
Salad with dressing
Apple
Milk
Coffee or tea

Supper
Baked chicken
Brown and wild rice
Broccoli
Fresh carrots
Pineapple
Whole-wheat roll
Margarine
Coffee or tea

Sample High-Fiber Diet Menu

Clients adjust best to high-fiber diets when fiber is gradually added to the diet. During the first few weeks on the diet, the person may feel bloated, pass gas frequently, or experience heartburn. Forewarn the person about these symptoms to dispel unnecessary fears and to foster compliance. Reassure the client that it won't be a problem for long.

The cautious use of certain high-fiber foods is recommended for people prone to form phytobezoars.[5] At risk are people with disorders that delay gastric emptying or reduce gastric acidity. Some high-fiber foods may con-

Some of the different types of fibers in foods are **cellulose, hemicellulose, gums, pectins,** and **lignins.** See pp. 30 for a review of fiber.

phytobezoar (FIGH-toh-BEE-zor): a collection of plant matter (fibers, leaves, skins) that forms a ball in the stomach or intestine.

tribute to phytobezoar formation, which, in turn, can interfere with normal GI tract function or lead to ulcers or abdominal infections. Foods to avoid include oranges, persimmons, coconut, berries, green beans, figs, apples, sauerkraut, brussels sprouts, and potato skins.

Disorders for which high-fiber diets play a primary role are described below. Other disorders for which high-fiber intakes are encouraged in addition to other dietary recommendations are discussed in later chapters.

Some types of gastric surgery and a condition of reduced gastric motility that affects some people with diabetes mellitus (Chapter 20) are associated with an increased risk of phytobezoar formation.

Constipation

Each person's GI tract responds to food in its own way, with its own rhythm, the fecal matter arriving at the rectal area in a fairly constant number of hours. Each GI tract thus has its own cycle, which depends on its owner's physical makeup and such environmental considerations as the type of food eaten, when it was eaten, and when the person's schedule allows time to defecate. If several days pass between movements, but these movements take place without discomfort, then the person is not constipated. Bowel movements that are hard and passed with difficulty, discomfort, or pain, however, indicate constipation, regardless of the amount of time that has elapsed since the previous bowel movement.

constipation: difficult or painful bowel movements; elapsed time between movements is irrelevant.

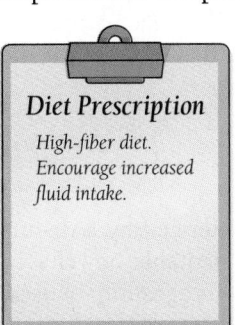

Diet Prescription

High-fiber diet. Encourage increased fluid intake.

Constipation occurs when the muscles of the colon fail to push the intestinal contents along. Hospitalized or institutionalized individuals often suffer from constipation. Certain disorders, stress, nervous tension, inactivity, failure to respond to signals to defecate, laxative abuse, and some drugs can lead to constipation. Constipation can also occur as a result of irregular and excessive contractions of the colon. This disorder—the irritable bowel syndrome—is discussed in the following section.

Disorders associated with constipation include intestinal obstructions, tumors, and diverticular disease (described later in this chapter).

When constipation is not the result of a disorder, careful review of daily habits may reveal its causes. Being too busy to respond to the signal to defecate is a common complaint. A person's daily regimen may need to be reexamined with the idea of instituting regular eating and sleeping times that will allow time in the day's schedule to have a bowel movement at the dictate of the person's body. Regular physical activity can also help. Recommend these dietary measures to help relieve constipation:

- Follow a high-fiber diet. Several types of fibers can aid in the treatment of constipation.
- Drink more fluids. Apparently, increased bulk physically stimulates the upper intestine, promoting peristalsis throughout.
- Eat prunes and drink prune juice; prunes contain a substance that acts as a laxative.

Adding fat to the diet relieves constipation in some cases. Fat in the intestine stimulates the release of bile, which has a high salt content. The salt in bile draws water from the intestinal wall equalizing the high osmolality in the intestine, which in turn stimulates peristalsis and softens the fecal matter.

TABLE 17–9 **Laxatives**

DRUG NAME	TIMING WITH MEALS	COMMON SIDE EFFECTS THAT MAY INFLUENCE NUTRITION STATUS
Bisacodyl	Do not give with milk or antacids.	Nausea, vomiting, abdominal cramps.
Castor oil	Give with juice or carbonated beverages to mask taste.	Nausea, abdominal cramps. May reduce absorption of fat-soluble vitamins.
Lactulose		Nausea, constipation, abdominal cramps.
Mineral oil	Give with juice or carbonated beverages to mask taste; do not give with meals.	Nausea, abdominal cramps. May reduce absorption of fat-soluble vitamins.

Source: Adapted from D. E. Powers and A. O. Moore, *Food Medication Interactions* (Phoenix: Food-Medication Interactions, 1991), and *Nursing 91 Drug Handbook* (Springbook, Pa.: Springhouse Corp. 1991).

If diet and lifestyle changes fail to correct the constipation, a physician should be consulted. The physician examines the client for underlying disorders that may result in constipation and prescribes laxatives (see Table 17–9), if indicated. Chronic constipation is associated with other problems; the constant pressure of straining to defecate may cause hemorrhoids or the formation of diverticula (discussed later).

Irritable Bowel Syndrome

Irritable bowel syndrome is a common disorder characterized by a disturbance in the motility of the GI tract. The person with irritable bowel syndrome may experience a variety of symptoms including indigestion, nausea,

People troubled by gas benefit from avoiding foods such as beans, broccoli, cabbage, and onions.

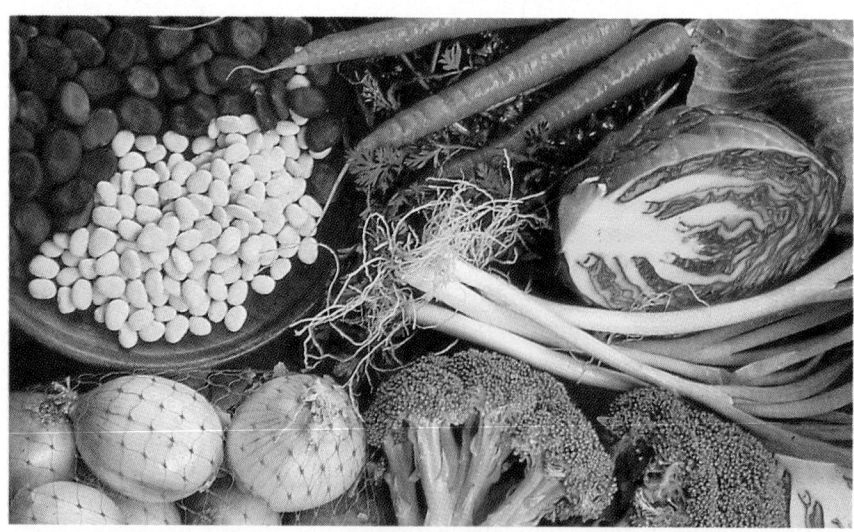

TABLE 17–10   **Foods That May Produce Gas**

Apples	Honey
Artichokes, Chinese	Kohlrabi
Barley	Melons
Beans	Milk
Bran	Molasses
Broccoli	Mulberries
Brussels sprouts	Nuts
Cabbage	Onions
Celery	Radishes
Cherries	Rye seeds
Coconut	Soybeans
Eggplant	Wheat
Figs	Yeast

abdominal pain, flatulence, diarrhea, constipation, or constipation alternating with diarrhea.

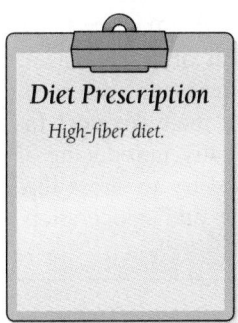

Diet Prescription

High-fiber diet.

When the primary symptom of the disorder is alternating constipation and diarrhea, adding fruits and vegetables to the diet may help.[6] People with irritable bowel syndrome who complain of gas and abdominal pain might benefit from avoiding foods that contain raffinose and stacchyose, complex carbohydrates that the body cannot digest or absorb. (Instead, bacteria in the colon metabolize these complex carbohydrates and produce gas in the process.) Table 17–10 lists some foods containing these complex carbohydrates. Excessive gas production often subsides if the person avoids gas-producing foods for about four to six weeks. Many people with irritable bowel syndrome find that adding bran to their diets or taking hydrophilic colloids will return bowel function to normal. If they also have gas, though, they should use the colloids only; they should avoid the foods listed in Table 17–10, including bran, because bran can also produce gas.

hydrophilic colloids: a type of laxative that attracts water into the intestine to form a bulky stool, which then stimulates peristalsis. (Metamucil and Fiberall are examples of hydrophilic colloids.)

Diverticular Disease

Sometimes pouches, or diverticula, form along the intestine in areas where the intestinal muscles are weak—often at points where blood vessels enter the muscles. Evidence suggests that the pouches result from high pressure in the intestinal lumen, combined with weakness of the supporting muscles in the intestinal wall. Strong intestinal contractions pinch off segments of the intestine; pressure then builds in these segments and forces parts of the membrane of the intestine to balloon outward through the weakened intestinal muscle layer. Diverticulosis is the condition in which diverticula have formed in the intestine.

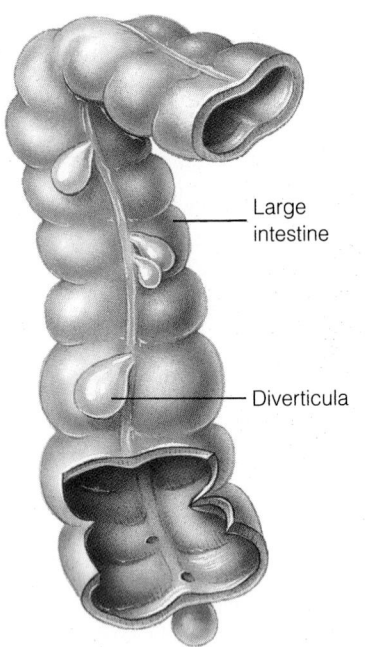

The outpocketings of the intestinal wall that balloon through the weakened muscles of the intestine are known as **diverticula.**

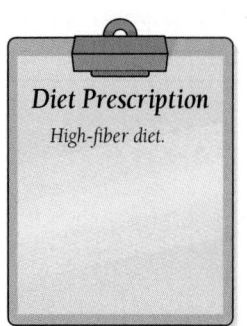

Diet Prescription
High-fiber diet.

People with diverticulosis are frequently symptom-free and unaware of the disorder. However, in some people, fecal material gets trapped in the diverticula, causing inflammation and infection, a condition called diverticulitis. People with diverticulitis may complain of cramps, alternating periods of diarrhea and constipation, dyspepsia, gas, and abdominal distention. Occasionally, a diverticulum ruptures, creating a life-threatening infection.

For many years, health care professionals advised people with diverticulosis to adopt low-fiber diets, believing that fiber would become trapped in the diverticula and cause irritation. However, this advice has changed dramatically. Now health care professionals believe a high-fiber diet may actually reduce the incidence of diverticulosis. Furthermore, many people with established diverticular disease remain symptom-free while following a high-fiber diet. However, foods with seeds, such as okra and strawberries, may need to be avoided; the seeds may get trapped in the diverticula and cause irritation.

People with diverticulosis, particularly older people, often have been following a low-fiber diet for many years. They may be apprehensive about switching to a high-fiber diet. After all, they had been told that the low-fiber diet would prevent symptoms, and they may be fearful of trying once-forbidden foods. They may be skeptical about any diet after having received such contradictory advice. What can you do to relieve their anxiety? In addition to following the advice given earlier for gradually introducing a high-fiber diet, you can acknowledge their concerns and try to stress the value of the diet. Also, try gaining their involvement and cooperation during the teaching process.

Small, Frequent Feedings

Any regular or modified diet can be given in small, frequent feedings. Small feedings are useful whenever distention of the stomach causes pain or discomfort. Thus people suffering from indigestion or nausea may benefit from small, frequent feedings—for example, six a day, each half the size of a regular meal. People who lack the energy to eat regular meals or who have problems with chewing or swallowing may also benefit from this modification. Small, frequent feedings also aid in the treatment of reflux esophagitis and hiatal hernia.

Indigestion

Indigestion or dyspepsia describes vague discomfort in the GI tract. It is not a specific disease, but rather a common problem associated with a variety of disorders. Emotional tension, underlying medical conditions, eating too much, eating too rapidly, or chewing poorly frequently result in indigestion.

dyspepsia: vague abdominal discomfort. Remember, dyspepsia is a symptom, not a disease.
 dys = bad
 peptein = to digest

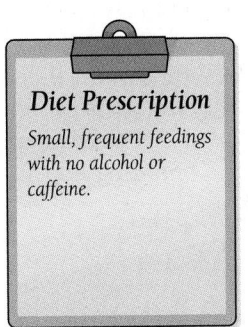

Diet Prescription

Small, frequent feedings with no alcohol or caffeine.

A temporary bout of indigestion requires no dietary intervention. Persistent indigestion, however, suggests underlying medical problems, such as gastritis and peptic ulcers (described earlier in this chapter), that should be identified. Persistent indigestion may lead to a depressed appetite and malnutrition. Dietary advice that may help control indigestion includes eating small servings; eating slowly, at regular times, and in a relaxed atmosphere; avoiding gas-forming foods; and avoiding excessive amounts of alcohol and caffeine-containing beverages. Of course, people should avoid any foods that they know give them indigestion. Antacids may also provide relief in some cases.

All drugs, even over-the-counter drugs such as antacids, should be used cautiously. A serious problem can be masked by covering up symptoms. A person who repeatedly takes antacids for stomach discomfort may be ignoring the signs of an ulcer.

Antacids also contain ingredients that may be undesirable. Some antacids contribute significant amounts of sodium or calcium to these mineral intakes. Although these ingredients may not be a problem for healthy individuals, they can aggravate some medical conditions. Aluminum-containing antacids can lead to phosphorus depletion and bone disease. Table B-1B in Appendix B lists many other nutrition-related side effects of antacids. All drugs—prescription and nonprescription alike—should be taken with caution.

Nausea and Vomiting

Nausea describes a feeling that one is about to vomit. Many medical conditions, certain smells, or even disturbing sights can trigger nausea. Generally, a nauseated person does not want to eat, which is fine when nausea is temporary. When nausea is persistent, as it may be in people with cancer or during pregnancy, the individual must eat, or malnutrition will result.

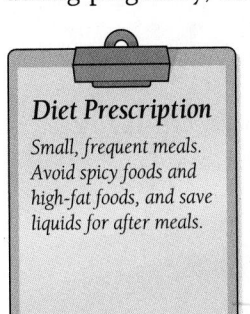

Diet Prescription

Small, frequent meals. Avoid spicy foods and high-fat foods, and save liquids for after meals.

You can make several suggestions that may help: eat smaller meals, avoid spicy and high-fat foods, save liquids for between meals, avoid foods with odors that cause nausea, sip clear liquids slowly, or suck popsicles or ice cubes made from a favorite liquid. Loosening the clothing and getting fresh air can help relieve nausea.

If nausea leads to vomiting, other concerns may arise. Simple vomiting is certainly unpleasant and wearying for the nauseated person but is no cause for alarm. It is merely one of the body's adaptive mechanisms to rid itself of something irritating.

Prolonged vomiting, however, can be serious and dangerous enough to require professional medical care, because fluid is lost from the body's cells. Leaving the cells with the fluid are electrolytes—particularly sodium, po-

Chapter 8 (pp. 153–156) describes fluid and electrolyte balance in more detail.

tassium, chloride, and bicarbonate—that are absolutely essential to the life of the cells. Dehydration and electrolyte imbalances can occur. Electrolytes and fluids may be difficult to replace if vomiting continues. If possible, fluids and electrolytes are replaced orally using clear liquids. If oral liquids cannot be tolerated, IV feedings of saline and glucose with added electrolytes are necessary until the physician diagnoses the cause of the vomiting and institutes corrective therapy.

Reflux Esophagitis and Hiatal Hernia

In reflux esophagitis, the cardiac sphincter fails to close tightly, and so allows the highly acidic gastric contents to splash backward into the esophagus and irritate the esophageal mucosa. People with hiatal hernias often develop reflux esophagitis, and the goals of nutrition care of people with either condition are the same. Figure 17–3 shows the relationship of the upper GI tract to the diaphragm and the changes that occur in the presence of a hernia.

hiatal hernia (high-A-tal HER-knee-uh): a protrusion of a portion of the stomach through the esophageal hiatus of the diaphragm. In a *sliding hiatal hernia* (the most common type), the portion of the stomach that contains the cardiac sphincter protrudes through the esophageal hiatus. In a *rolling hernia*, the cardiac sphincter remains below the diaphragm while a portion of the stomach protrudes through the esophageal hiatus.

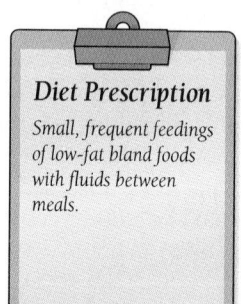

Diet Prescription

Small, frequent feedings of low-fat bland foods with fluids between meals.

A burning pain called heartburn occurs when the gastric juices reflux into the esophagus. At times, the pain may be so severe as to awaken a sleeping person. Heartburn usually hurts behind the sternum (see Figure 17–4), often spreading into the neck and back of the throat in waves. Because heartburn occurs when pressure in the stomach exceeds pressure in the esophagus, it most frequently flares up when a person lies down or bends over.

The best treatment of reflux esophagitis is prevention. Encourage clients to avoid substances or activities that lower cardiac sphincter pressure or raise pressure in the stomach (see Table 17–11). Treatment for active reflux esophagitis aims at reducing gastric acidity and limiting irritation of an already inflamed esophagus.

FIGURE 17–3   **Relationship of the Upper GI Tract to the Diaphragm**

(*near right*)
Normally the stomach lies below the diaphragm, and the esophagus passes through the esophageal hiatus (opening in the diaphragm).

(*far right*)
A *sliding hiatal hernia* results when the part of the stomach that contains the cardiac sphincter slips through the diaphragm. This type of hiatal hernia is the most common.

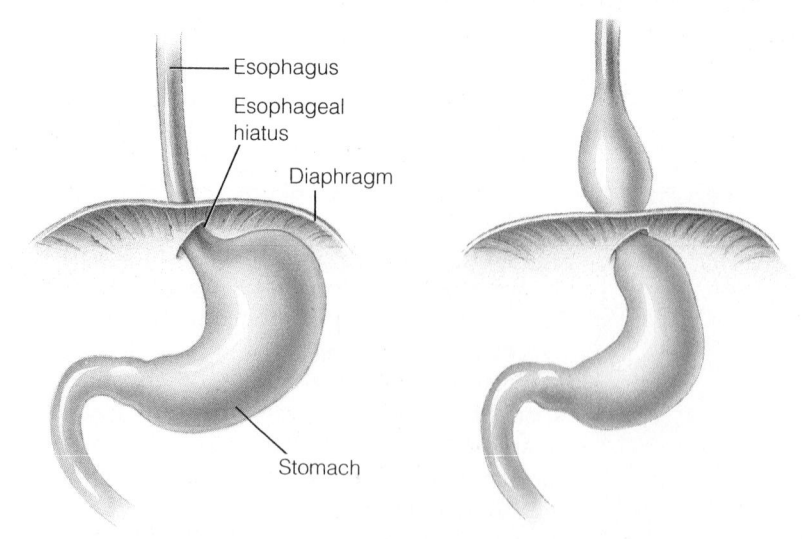

Esophagus
Esophageal hiatus
Diaphragm
Stomach

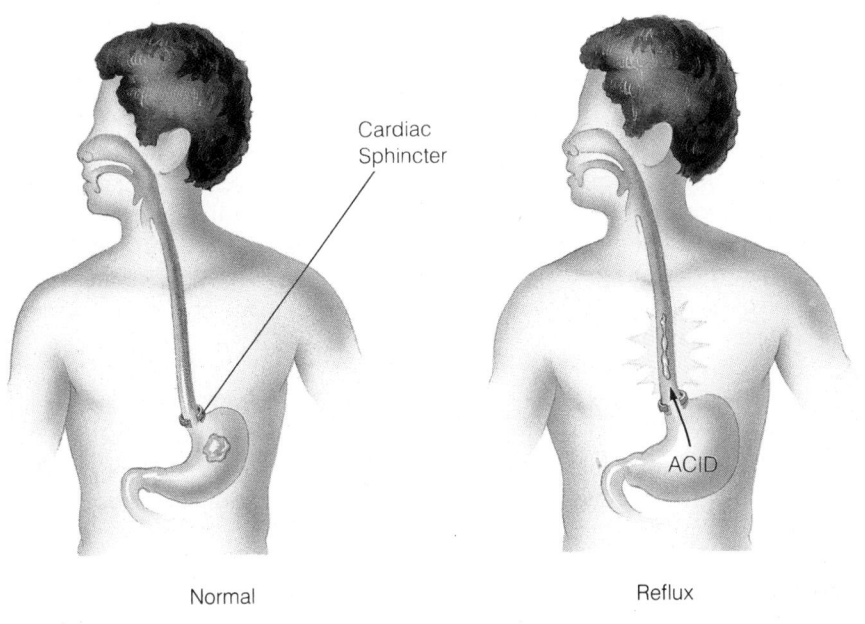

Cardiac Sphincter

ACID

Normal

Reflux

FIGURE 17-4 Effects of Gastric Pressure on Reflux
Overeating and overdrinking can increase the pressure in the stomach. Whenever the pressure in the stomach exceeds the pressure in the esophagus, the chance of reflux increases.

Diet plays an important role in the prevention and treatment of reflux esophagitis. Instruct clients to:

- Eat small, frequent meals and drink liquids one hour before or after meals to avoid distending the stomach.
- Refrain from lying down or bending over, and from wearing tight-fitting garments, particularly after eating, to avoid elevating pressure in the stomach.
- Lose weight, if necessary.
- Limit fat, alcohol, and peppermint and spearmint oil intakes to avoid lowering cardiac sphincter pressure.
- Limit decaffeinated coffee, caffeine-containing foods and beverages, and red pepper to avoid stimulating gastric acid secretion.

TABLE 17-11 **Substances That Affect Cardiac Sphincter Pressure**

ELEVATES PRESSURE	LOWERS PRESSURE
Bethanechol chloride	Alcohol
Metoclopramide hydrochloride	Anticholinergic agents
Protein	Atropine
	Caffeine-containing beverages
	Chocolate
	Cigarette smoking
	Fat
	Peppermint and spearmint oils

■ Avoid acidic juices such as orange, grapefruit, and tomato juice when experiencing symptoms of reflux esophagitis to minimize irritation to the esophagus.

Other measures also help. Advise clients not to smoke cigarettes, since cigarette smoking can reduce cardiac sphincter pressure. In addition, physicians may prescribe antacids or other drugs to neutralize gastric acidity. Advise clients to sleep with the head of the bed elevated; keeping the chest higher than the stomach helps to prevent reflux. Generally, these measures can control esophagitis. However, in some cases, if medical management fails, surgery may be indicated.

This chapter presents an overview of diets that differ from a regular diet in consistency, texture, and number of meals. In addition, you have seen how each diet is used in at least one condition or disorder. The following chapters look at different types of modified diets—those modified in nutrients.

CASE STUDY

Businessman with a Peptic Ulcer

Mr. Kelly is a busy executive living a high-stress life. He entertains many clients, so he eats many meals out and drinks alcoholic beverages regularly. He smokes and gets little sleep. Mr. Kelly visited his physician after he began experiencing severe, gnawing stomach pain; the physician diagnosed a peptic ulcer.

Having assessed Mr. Kelly's medical situation, you are ready to counsel him. What changes in lifestyle would you suggest to help Mr. Kelly treat his ulcer? What diet do you recommend he follow? From the limited information you have about his eating habits, what practical suggestions can you offer Mr. Kelly? What questions could you ask Mr. Kelly to help him design an acceptable diet? How could you help him identify foods that irritate his ulcer?

Study Questions

1. Identify the two major types of liquid diets, and distinguish between the two. What are the uses of liquid diets? Are standard liquid diets nutritionally complete?

2. What are some causes of diarrhea? When is diarrhea a cause for concern? How can diet be used to treat diarrhea?

3. Name some factors that can lead to poor nutrition status prior to surgery? What type of diet should be eaten in the days before and after surgery, and why?

4. What are low-fiber diets, and how are they used?

5. Describe the differences between an ileostomy and a colostomy. What diet, if any, can benefit the person who has undergone one of these procedures?

6. How are diets adjusted for people who have difficulties with chewing and swallowing? What special concerns arise for the person with mouth ulcers or with a reduced flow of saliva?

7. Consider the numerous medical and dental problems that can interfere with a person's ability to chew and swallow foods. What is the most important step health care professionals must take in planning a diet for these clients?

8. Reflect upon ways in which a person's nutrition needs can be affected by a stroke. How can nutrition affect a person's response to physical therapy?

9. Discuss the liberal bland diet and its role in the treatment of peptic ulcers.

10. Review some of the suggested uses for high-fiber diets. What foods add fiber to the diet? What precautions should the person trying a high-fiber diet for the first time take? Under what circumstances might high-fiber diets be contraindicated?

11. What is constipation? What suggestions can be made to clients to help them alleviate constipation?

12. Discuss irritable bowel syndrome, and describe the dietary modifications that are helpful in alleviating symptoms of the disorder.

13. What theory explains the development of diverticula in the intestine? What dangers are associated with diverticular disease? What diet is useful for treating diverticular disease?

14. When would a diet of small, frequent feedings be desirable?

15. Under what conditions do indigestion and nausea become causes for concern? What dietary suggestions can be offered to help treat and prevent indigestion and nausea?

16. What is reflux esophagitis? What is a hiatal hernia? What advice can you give the person with reflux esophagitis to prevent and treat the symptoms?

Notes

1. W. E. Woodward and T. E. Woodward, Management of dehydrating diarrhea, *Hospital Practice,* 30 March 1986, pp. 60–70.

2. Veterans Affairs Total Parenteral Nutrition Cooperative Study Group, Perioperative total parenteral nutrition in surgical patients, *New England Journal of Medicine* 325 (1991): 525–532.

3. G. M. Christian and coauthors, Milk and milk products in low-residue diets: Current hospital practices do not match dietitians' beliefs, *Journal of the American Dietetic Association* 91 (1991): 341–342.

4. J. V. Sizmann, Nutritional support of the dysphagic patient: Methods, risks, and complications of therapy, *Journal of Parenteral and Enteral Nutrition* 14 (1990): 60–63.

5. A. P. Emerson, Foods high in fiber and phytobezoar formation, *Journal of the American Dietetic Association* 87 (1987): 1675–1677.

6. A. D. Schwabe, Dietary management of the irritable bowel syndrome, *Nutrition and the M.D.,* July 1987, pp. 1–2.

17

The Seasoning of the Bland Diet

At its best, diet therapy applies valid findings from nutrition science so that they benefit clients. In other words, diet therapy puts the facts to work to help people. Often, however, gaps exist in the knowledge base from which these facts are derived. Logic and educated guesses fill these gaps until further study generates more information that either validates the original presumptions or invalidates them. If necessary, diet therapy eventually changes to accommodate the newly acquired information. This Nutrition in Practice provides a dramatic example of such evolution; it presents a historical look at changes in ulcer treatment over the years.

How has diet therapy for ulcers changed?

First of all, diet has lost importance in therapy for ulcers now that effective drugs are available. Secondly, the diets recommended today are much more liberal than the old traditional bland diets. Traditional bland diets were developed during a time when few drugs were available to alter gastric acid secretion. Diet was therefore the cornerstone of therapy. The rationale for the bland diet, as it was originally designed, was to provide foods that did not irritate the gastric mucosa. The theory was that certain foods could neutralize or reduce gastric acid secretion, and thus help relieve the pain and damage of ulcers.

The actual diet consisted of a series of diets that progressed through stages. As shown in Table NP17–1, the first stage generally provided only milk and cream, given frequently throughout the day, with the belief that milk would coat the stomach and intestine and buffer stomach acids. Even as the diet progressed to the final stage, many foods were restricted. Basically, only foods mild in flavor and low in fiber were included to minimize the possibility of irritating the stomach and intestinal linings. Small meals were provided several times a day, for that way, the stomach would never be empty and exposed to undiluted acid. Caffeine and alcohol were excluded, to avoid stimulating acid secretion.

All that makes sense to me. What was the problem?

All of the recommendations did seem to make sense. They were based on logical assumptions about how diet affects the GI tract. However, health care practitioners held widely varying beliefs about which foods irritated the GI tract. In the 1970s the disagreements prompted the American

Dietetic Association (ADA) to review the literature and issue a position paper on bland diets.[1] The ADA concluded that the traditional bland diet was mostly supported by tradition and folklore, not by scientific research. Well-controlled research studies failed to demonstrate that most of the restrictions on foods in traditional bland diets helped ulcers to heal. The ADA questioned the recommendation to include milk frequently and found no support for eliminating high-fiber foods. *Logic* in this case was not supported by *facts*.

What foods were found to irritate an ulcer?

The ADA found that a few of the substances commonly eliminated in bland diets were, indeed, irritating to the gastric mucosa. True irritants included black pepper, chili powder, caffeine, tea, cocoa, alcohol, and a few drugs—most notably, aspirin. The ADA did conclude, though, that small, frequent meals were beneficial (but wait; that item changed later). The ADA recommended individualizing the diet based on specific food intolerances.

What other information about bland diets has since come to light?

Since publication of the ADA position paper, further changes in bland diets have been made. For one thing, *decaffeinated* coffee was found to stimulate gastric acid secretion to the same degree as caffeinated coffee; therefore, all coffee should be restricted. For another, advice to eat small, frequent meals, as mentioned earlier, has changed. Since food stimulates gastric acid secretion, frequent eating is contraindicated; instead, three regular meals are preferred.

With respect to spices, individuals who do not regularly eat spicy foods may experience discomfort when they do eat such foods. However, contrary to popular belief, spicy foods do not damage the GI tract lining.[2] Individuals who regularly eat spicy foods are probably not at a higher risk of developing ulcers or of having ulcers recur.[3]

Although only minimal information is available, some research has shown that milk may actually impair recovery from ulcers. In one study of people with ulcers who were taking the drug cimetidine, the ulcers healed in 78 percent of the people who ate a normal diet but in only 53 percent of those whose main food was milk.[4]

If you look closely at the traditional bland diet, you will notice that some of its recommendations oppose dietary recommendations for a healthy diet. Milk and cream—mainstays of the traditional bland diet—are high in saturated fats and cholesterol, which may aggravate the risk of cardiovascular disease. Similarly, eliminating high-fiber foods may do more harm than good. Health care professionals recommend high-fiber foods to maintain optimal function of the GI tract, for weight control, for blood glucose regulation, and for blood lipid control. Unless fiber restrictions confer a greater advantage on the person with ulcers than the risks they pose, they are unwarranted and possibly harmful.

Scientific facts thus seem to contradict the rationale for the traditional bland diet, which was based on theory without much research. Table NP17-2 on p. 454 summarizes the differences between the traditional and liberal bland diets.

It is important to note that current research is not substantial, and the liberal bland diet of today may change further as new information becomes available. To stay knowledgeable about diet therapies that really work, keep up with research. Learning about what's new in research will enhance client care.

Notes

1. American Dietetic Association, Position paper on bland diets in the treat-

TABLE NP17-1   **Traditional Bland Diet**

STAGE I
3 to 4 oz milk and cream (half-and-half) every one to two hours.

STAGE II
Add to the Stage I diet small feedings of low-fiber foods at frequent and regular intervals throughout the waking hours (seven to eight feedings per 24 hours). *Foods allowed* include milk; white bread; soft-cooked or poached eggs; cream of wheat; farina; boiled rice, oatmeal; strained creamed soup; white crackers; butter; margarine; small servings of tender boiled, broiled, baked, roasted, creamed, or stewed beef, chicken, fish, lamb, liver, pork, sweetbreads, turkey, or veal; plain cake; cookies; ice cream; bread; cornstarch; rice; or tapioca pudding. *Foods not allowed* include all others.

STAGE III
Add to the Stage II diet small feedings given six times a day, as well as decaffeinated coffee. *Foods allowed* include all foods except those listed below. *Foods not allowed* include fried foods; most raw fruits and vegetables; dried peas and beans; broccoli; brussels sprouts; cabbage; onions; cauliflower; cucumbers; green peppers; rutabagas; turnips; sauerkraut; berries; figs; highly seasoned or cured meats, poultry, or fish; salad dressings; caffeine; alcohol; high-fiber breads and cereals; highly seasoned foods; catsup; pepper; barbecue sauce; chili pepper; horseradish; garlic; mustard; vinegar; olives; pickles; popcorn; nuts; coconut.

TABLE NP17–2   Traditional and Liberal Bland Diets Compared

DIET MODIFICATION	TRADITIONAL BLAND	LIBERAL BLAND
Frequency of feedings	Six small feedings	Three feedings
Milk	Use liberally	Use in moderation
Alcohol	Restricted	Restricted
Caffeine and caffeine-containing beverages	Restricted	Restricted
Decaffeinated coffee	Not restricted	Restricted
Pepper and spicy foods	Restricted	As tolerated
High-fiber foods	Restricted	Not restricted

ment of chronic duodenal ulcer disease, *Journal of the American Dietetic Association* 59 (1971): 244–245.

2. D. Y. Graham, J. L. Smith, and A. R. Opekun, Spicy food and the stomach, *Journal of the American Medical Association* 260 (1988): 3473–3475.

3. K. Holt and D. Hollander, Gastric mucosal injury, *Annual Review of Medicine* 37 (1986): 107.

4. N. Kumar and coauthors, Effect of milk on patients with duodenal ulcers, *British Medical Journal* 293 (1986): 666.

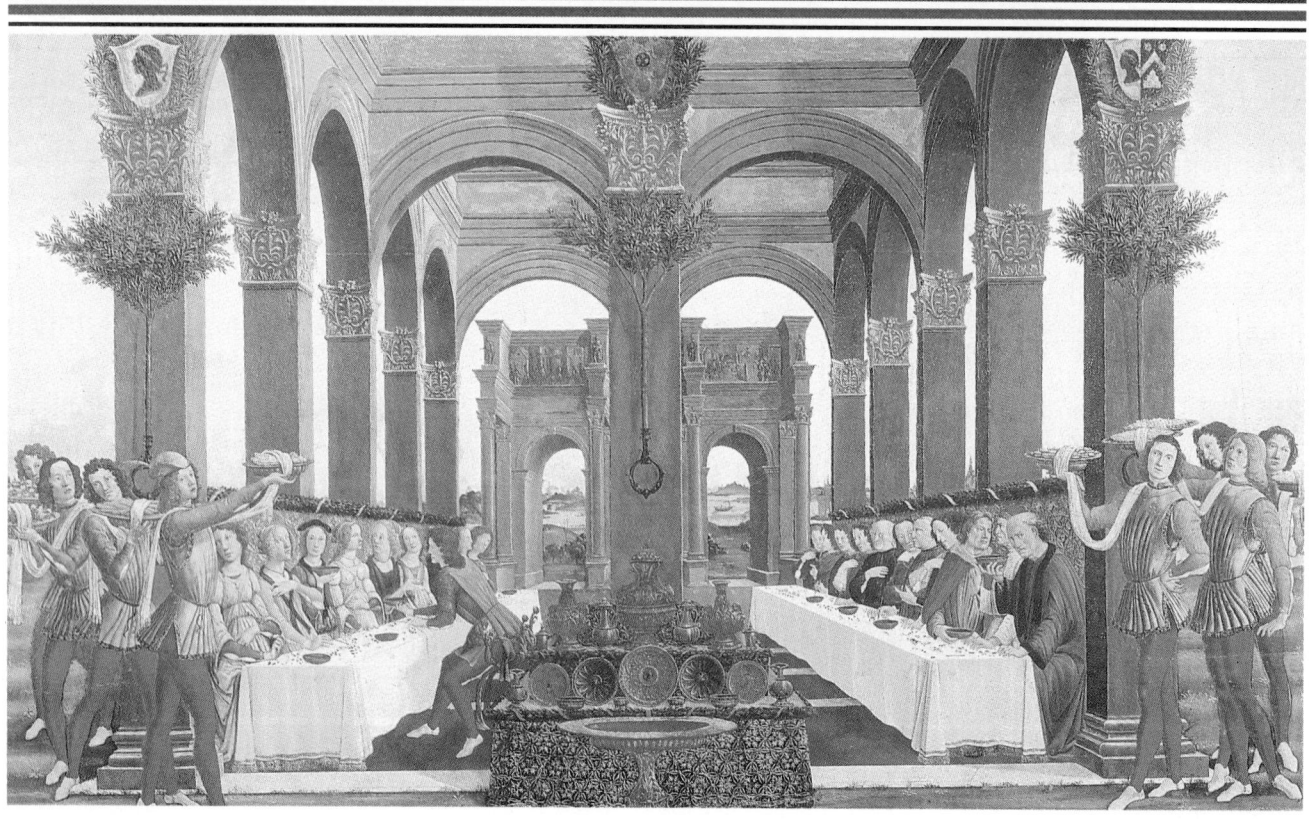

Sandro Botticelli, The Wedding Feast, *Bridgeman Art Library/Art Resource, N.Y.*

CHAPTER

18

Diets Modified in kCalories: I. High-kCalorie Diets

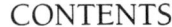

CONTENTS

CHAPTER

18

High-kcalorie diets are often used to rehabilitate people who are malnourished or underweight and to prevent malnutrition and weight loss in conditions that greatly raise energy needs. Such conditions include severe stress and burns, cancer cachexia, acquired immune deficiency syndrome (AIDS), chronic obstructive pulmonary diseases (COPD), and respiratory failure.

High-kCalorie Diets

High-kcalorie diets are also high-protein diets, because the purpose of such diets is to build or maintain lean body mass. To prevent the use of protein for energy, adequate energy must be provided. A typical high-kcalorie diet provides an extra 1000 kcalories above those the person normally needs to maintain weight. One and one-half grams of protein per kilogram of body weight is provided, as opposed to the 0.8 gram per kilogram normally considered adequate. Table 18–1 lists indications for the use of high-kcalorie, high-protein diets, and the accompanying sample menu provides an example of one such diet.

TABLE 18–1 **Indications for the Use of High-kCalorie, High-Protein Diets**

Acquired immune deficiency
    syndrome (AIDS)
Burns
Cancer cachexia
Chronic obstructive pulmonary
    diseases
Cystic fibrosis
Fractured bones
Hepatitis
Infections
Inflammatory bowel diseases
Malabsorption syndromes
Nephrotic syndrome
Protein-kcalorie malnutrition
Short bowel syndrome
Surgery
Underweight

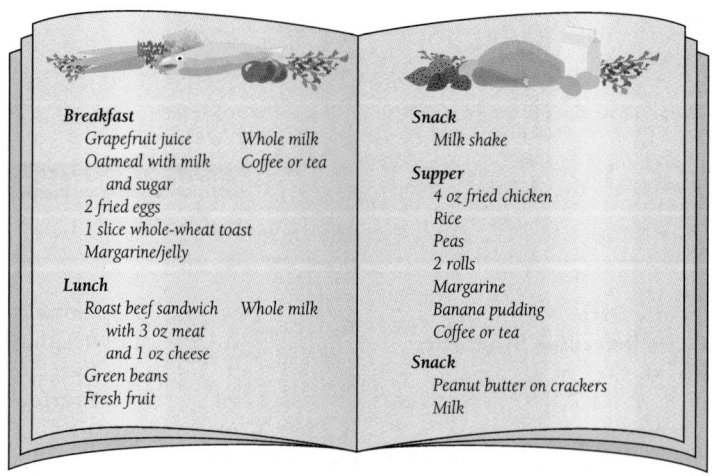

Sample High-kCalorie, High-Protein Diet Menu

Energy-dense foods, meaning those that provide the greatest number of kcalories in the smallest possible volume, hold the key to successful weight gain. Using such foods, clients can eat many kcalories without feeling uncomfortably full. To help clients gain weight, health care professionals can make these suggestions:

■ Select the highest-kcalorie items from each food group (see Figure 1–3 on p. 11). For example, use milk shakes instead of milk, peanut butter instead of lean meat, avocados instead of cucumbers, and whole-wheat muffins instead of whole-wheat bread.

■ Add fats to foods whenever possible, because fats add kcalories without adding much bulk to the diet. For example, eat margarine on cooked vegetables and mayonnaise on sandwiches; use cream with coffee, creamy dressings with salads, whipped cream with fruit, and sour cream on potatoes.

■ Add nuts and dried fruits such as raisins to desserts or cereals.

■ Add sugar to foods, and eat high-kcalorie desserts. For example, add sugar to coffee, tea, cereal, or strawberries.

■ Snack systematically between meals. Milk shakes, instant breakfast drinks, commercially prepared formulas (see Appendix D), and sandwiches make good snacks.

■ Preplan your meals. Many people who are underweight have simply been too busy to eat. In addition to preplanning meals, spend more time eating each meal; learn to eat more food within the first 20 minutes of a meal; eat higher-kcalorie foods first in the meal.

Consumption of high-fat foods is not healthy for most people, but it may be essential for the underweight person who needs to gain weight.

Underweight clients accustomed to eating small quantities of food can expect to feel full when they begin eating high-kcalorie diets. This is normal, and it passes with time. Additionally, the person attempting weight gain should anticipate a plateau—a period without weight gain even with the added food intake.

Although exercise costs kcalories, it can help the underweight person build lean body mass—the main goal of weight gain. A person who is not dangerously underweight can adopt an exercise program designed to increase lean body mass.

For people who are underweight due to illness, commercially prepared liquid formulas, tube feedings, or parenteral nutrition may be required. Chapter 16 provided the details of these feeding methods.

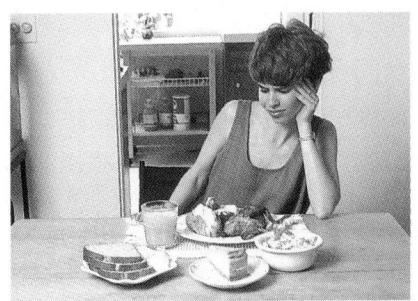

The thought of eating large quantities of food may overwhelm the person presented with a high-kcalorie diet.

Although the advice given to help someone gain weight might sound like a dream come true for the person who is overweight, eating all this extra food can be a nightmare for the person who needs the diet—especially for the person who is very ill.

Imagine feeling almost too sick to move or too tired to sit up. To someone in this state, the effort of eating even normal amounts of food three times a day seems monumental. It is even harder to eat extra foods.

You can help in several ways. As with other diets, be sure the person knows why the extra food is important. Work closely with individuals to find the high-kcalorie foods they enjoy most and are most likely to eat. Encourage people to select foods that require little effort to eat. For example, eating a roast beef sandwich requires less effort than cooking, cutting, and eating a steak. Drinking a high-kcalorie creamed soup is easier than eating it with a spoon. Finally, let the person know that you understand the difficulty involved.

PEM and the Refeeding Syndrome

No serious health hazards accompany mild degrees of underweight, unless it is accompanied by undernutrition. An inadequate supply of nutrients leaves the body unprepared to handle its many metabolic and physical tasks, particularly if a condition develops that greatly increases nutrient needs.

> *Diet Prescription*
>
> *Gradually progress diet from lactose-free liquids to a high-kcalorie, high-protein diet.*

Whenever a person is extremely underweight, is chronically underweight, or develops a clinical condition that greatly increases nutrient needs, PEM can develop. The problems associated with PEM are discussed in Chapters 4 and 14. The object of diet therapy is to enable the client to consume a high-kcalorie, high-protein diet, but this may not be possible right away. The PEM may have incurred such severe physiological and metabolic consequences that only a gradual approach will succeed in reversing the client's debilitated state. After such an approach, the person with PEM can safely assimilate nutrients, but if the reintroduction of adequate nutrition occurs too rapidly, severe complications, including malabsorption, cardiac insufficiency, respiratory distress, congestive heart failure, convulsions, coma, and even death, can result. These complications have collectively been termed the refeeding syndrome.

It may seem difficult to believe that simply feeding a malnourished individual can have such dire consequences. However, a review of the body's response to starvation helps clarify why this is so. During the course of chronic or severe PEM, the body loses protein from skeletal muscle and vital organs to support its energy needs. The organs most affected include those of the GI tract, the lungs, and the heart. In the GI tract, the loss of protein results in reduced GI motility, atrophy of the intestinal villi, and markedly reduced concentrations of digestive enzymes. Thus the person with PEM often experiences nausea, vomiting, diarrhea, and malabsorption, until the cells of the GI tract regenerate. This adaptation normally occurs fairly quickly after initiating enteral nutrition.

During starvation, the body attempts to conserve lean body mass by lowering its metabolic rate (to reduce the demand for energy) and sparing glucose by producing ketone bodies (to reduce the demand for glucose). As nutrients are reintroduced, the basal metabolic rate speeds up, thereby accelerating the production of oxygen and carbon dioxide. The lung and heart muscles, already weakened by malnutrition, must therefore work harder to keep the body's gases in balance. Overfeeding during this period markedly raises the metabolic rate and can raise the production of carbon dioxide so far as to overstress the lungs and heart.

Metabolic imbalances may also occur as the body shifts from a fasting state to a fed state. As the metabolic rate speeds up and glucose becomes available, glucose again becomes the body's primary energy source. The body immediately begins rebuilding lost tissue. As glucose and amino acids move into cells for this rebuilding process, intracellular electrolytes (potassium, phosphorus, magnesium, and calcium) move into the cells as well. As

refeeding syndrome: the physiological and metabolic complications associated with reintroducing adequate nutrition too rapidly for a person with severe PEM; these complications can include malabsorption, cardiac insufficiency, respiratory distress, congestive heart failure, convulsions, coma, and possibly death.

atrophy (ATT-ro-fee)**:** to waste away.
a = without
trophy = growth

these electrolytes shift into the intracellular fluid, circulating levels can plummet rapidly, resulting in life-threatening complications.

To avoid the refeeding syndrome, the reintroduction of nutrients to the severely malnourished individual must proceed slowly, with vigilant monitoring of medical and metabolic status. Although the reason is unclear, a high-carbohydrate intake seems to result in sodium and fluid retention; and sodium itself can increase fluid retention as well. Early feedings are therefore low in kcalories, moderate in carbohydrate, and low in sodium.[1] Fluid status and electrolyte balances are carefully monitored and maintained. Vitamin supplements are routinely provided.

Early feedings are also lactose-free. When enteral nutrition begins after a long period of GI tract disuse, diarrhea should be expected; it generally resolves within a few days. Enteral feeding rapidly stimulates intestinal enzyme activity, although lactose intolerance may persist. Hydrolyzed formulas are not necessary; animal studies suggest that intact formulas stimulate intestinal enzymes to a greater extent than hydrolyzed formulas.

Any disorder that leads to chronic malnutrition places people at risk for the refeeding syndrome. Many such disorders are described in this chapter, and one other such condition is covered later: anorexia nervosa, the self-starvation eating disorder, which results in chronic malnutrition. (Anorexia nervosa and the related disorder, bulimia, are discussed in Nutrition in Practice 19.)

Severe Stress

As described in Chapter 14 (see pp. 342), severe stress creates a state of hypermetabolism that results in a marked increase in energy expenditure and a rapid loss of lean body mass. The type of stress and its severity, as well as the person's nutrition status prior to the stress, determine the amount of time it will take the body to regain its normal balance. Figure 18–1 summarizes the metabolic response to stress.

While the goal of nutrition support in the malnourished person who is not stressed is to restore lean body mass and to promote weight gain, this goal is not realistic for the severely stressed individual. Instead, the goal is to minimize nutrient losses and to preserve organ structure and function. Generally, weight gain and positive nitrogen balance are not possible during the hypermetabolic period of severe stress.

Overzealous nutrition support during the hypermetabolic period can be detrimental. Supplying too little energy compromises the ability to recover from stress, heal wounds, and fight infection; but supplying too much energy can overwork the heart and lungs and lead to metabolic complications as in the refeeding syndrome, already described. The accurate determination of the stressed client's energy needs is therefore crucial to providing appropriate therapy.

Indirect calorimetry provides the most accurate assessment of energy expenditure and, thus, of energy needs in critically ill people. Using a portable machine that measures oxygen consumption and carbon dioxide production, a skilled clinician can determine an individual's resting energy

indirect calorimetry: a method of estimating energy needs from the measurement of oxygen consumption and carbon dioxide production.

FIGURE 18–1 **Metabolic Response to Stress**

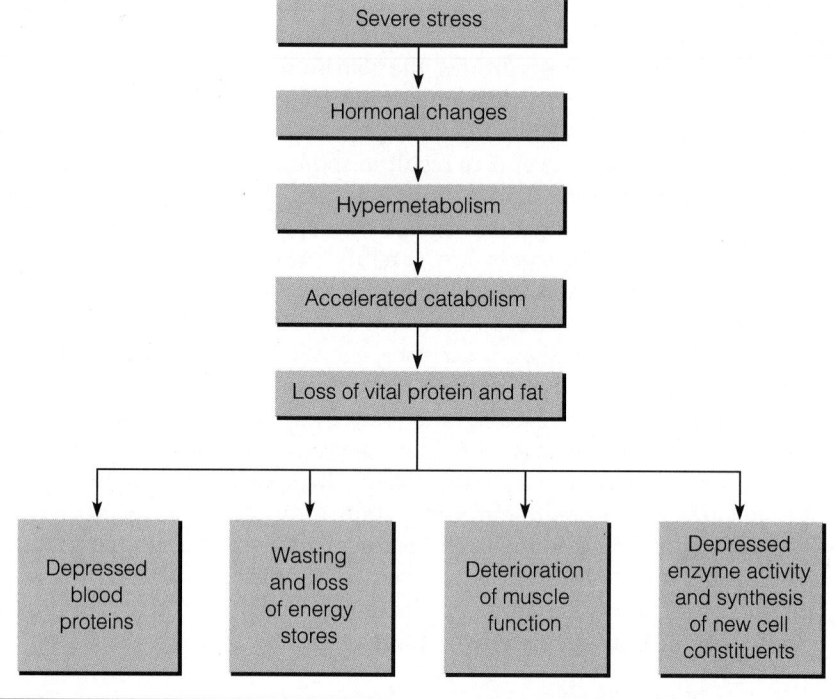

Severe stress → Hormonal changes → Hypermetabolism → Accelerated catabolism → Loss of vital protein and fat → Depressed blood proteins | Wasting and loss of energy stores | Deterioration of muscle function | Depressed enzyme activity and synthesis of new cell constituents

Although the Harris-Benedict equation is commonly used for estimating energy needs, many researchers have found wide variations in energy needs in severely stressed individuals. Although no consensus has been reached on the best formula, it is important to remember that energy needs determined from equations are estimates only. Clinical judgment and consistent monitoring of weight changes are always necessary.

expenditure. However, many facilities lack the equipment necessary to perform this measurement. In these cases, formulas provide estimates of energy needs. Table 18–2 shows the Harris-Benedict equation for calculating the basal energy expenditure (BEE) and determining total energy needs. Alternatively, some clinicians simply provide 25 to 30 nonprotein kcalories per kilogram of body weight per day. Protein is then provided at 1.5 grams per kilogram of body weight per day, adding more kcalories. The accompanying box shows an example of how these formulas are used.

Energy sources for severely stressed people have received increasing attention in recent years. Although the best mix of glucose and lipids to provide nonprotein kcalories is unknown, studies suggest that a mixture of 70 to 75 percent glucose and 25 to 30 percent lipids may be beneficial.[2] This ratio changes for some conditions (see the discussions of burns and respiratory failure later in this chapter). A person with a functional GI tract receives nutrients enterally; however, often the severely stressed person needs parenteral nutrition.

Vitamin and mineral needs in stress are highly variable, and specific requirements are unknown. The need for many B vitamins increase when energy and protein intakes increase. Vitamins and minerals act as important cofactors in the metabolic reactions that are occurring, and at the same time their levels are being drained. Therefore, vitamins and minerals are frequently supplemented at levels above the RDA. As stated earlier, serum electrolyte levels are closely monitored, and electrolytes are replaced as necessary.

TABLE 18–2   **The Harris-Benedict Equation for Estimating Energy Needs**

Basal energy expenditure (BEE)[a]:

Women:

BEE = 655 + (9.6 × weight in kg[b]) + (1.7 × height in cm[b]) − (4.7 × age in years).

Men:

BEE = 66 + (13.7 × weight in kg) + (5 × height in cm) − (6.8 × age in years).

Add to BEE for activity:

20%, sedentary.

35%, moderately active.

50%, active.

Add to BEE for stress:

10 to 15%, uncomplicated elective surgery.

20 to 40%, complicated surgery or fractures.

50 to 100%, major burn.

Add to BEE for fever (if present):

13% per degree centigrade over normal body temperature (37° C).[b]

Add to BEE for growth (if necessary):

5%, moderate weight loss.

10 to 15%, severe weight loss.

For people with a %IBW greater than 125, adjust the weight used in the BEE equation by following this equation:[c]

(Actual body weight − IBW) × 25%[d] + IBW = adjusted body weight.

[a]The equation used to determine basal energy expenditure (BEE) is the Harris-Benedict equation. Basal metabolic rate (BMR, described on p. 105) and BEE express the same thing: basal energy need. The equation for BMR is traditionally used in physiology and fitness laboratories; that for BEE, in hospitals. The two equations yield slightly different results, each suitable for the purposes intended. The increments for activity used in the hospital differ from those on p. 106 for similar reasons. All are approximations; all require judgment in their application.
[b]See Appendix for equations to convert kilograms, centimeters, and degrees centigrade.
[c]Source: J. M. Karkeck, Adjustment for obesity, *American Dietetic Association Renal Practice Group Newsletter,* Winter 1984.
[d]Approximately 25% of body fat tissue is metabolically active.

Severe stresses such as burns, infections, surgery, and broken bones, demand attention to nutrition to enhance recovery. The dietary treatments of these stresses are, in general, similar to that already described. However, some unique nutrition concerns are also associated with each specific stress, as the next sections reveal.

Burns

The person with extensive burns represents an extreme case of severe stress. The metabolic response to a burn includes major shifts in fluid and elec-

A burn is sometimes called a **thermal injury.**

How to Estimate Energy and Protein Needs

Mrs. Kelvin is a 50-year-old woman who is 5 ft 4 inches tall and weighs 118 lb. She has been in a car accident that has left her with several broken bones.

Before using the Harris-Benedict equation for BEE, convert weight in pounds to weight in kilograms:

$$\frac{118 \text{ lb}}{2.2 \text{ lb/kg}} = 54 \text{ kg}.$$

Then convert height in inches to height in centimeters:

$$64 \text{ inches} \times 2.54 \text{ cm/inch} = 163 \text{ cm}.$$

Then place the weight, height, and age factors into the equation for women:

$$\text{BEE} = 655 + (9.6 \times 54 \text{ kg}) + (1.7 \times 163 \text{ cm}) - (4.7 \times 50).$$

$$\text{BEE} = 655 + 518 + 277 - 235 = 1215 \text{ kcal}.$$

Thus Mrs. Kelvin needs 1215 kcal to meet her basal energy needs. Next, to account for stress, multiply the BEE by 30%:

$$1215 \text{ kcal} \times 0.30 = 364.5.$$

Add the BEE and the stress factor to determine total energy needs:

$$1215 \text{ kcal} + 365 = 1579 \text{ kcal}.$$

Mrs. Kelvin's nonprotein energy needs would be about 1600 kcal.

For comparison, the alternate approach to calculating energy requirements for stress (25 to 30 kcal/kg body weight) yields a similar estimate:

$$25 \text{ kcal/kg} \times 54 \text{ kg} = 1350 \text{ kcal}.$$

$$30 \text{ kcal/kg} \times 54 \text{ kg} = 1620 \text{ kcal}.$$

Thus a kcalorie range of 1350 to 1620 kcal would be appropriate. Keep in mind that these approximations would change (and probably increase) once the hypermetabolic phase of stress ended, and lean body mass and weight could be restored.

To estimate protein needs at 1.5 g protein/kg body weight:

$$54 \text{ kg} \times \frac{1.5 \text{ g}}{\text{kg}} = 81 \text{ g protein}.$$

$$81 \text{ g protein} \times 4 \text{ kcal/g protein} = 324 \text{ kcal}.$$

Note that the 324 kcal available from protein is given in addition to the 1600 kcalories determined from the Harris-Benedict equation.

trolyte balance, rapid tissue catabolism, and a rapid loss of body mass. The body of a person with extensive burns rapidly uses up its energy reserves and vital protein in the effort to survive. Therefore, these individuals have exceptionally high nutrient needs. Moreover, most people with burns experience anorexia and depression, leading to poor food intake and further deterioration of nutrition status. Further aggravating the situation, the burn injury itself may make eating difficult because of the associated pain or because of the injury's physical location (for example, the hands). Immobilization and lack of exercise further intensify the catabolic decline.

Immediately after a person is burned, dramatic changes take place in the circulatory system. Blood proteins (mainly albumin) and electrolytes leak

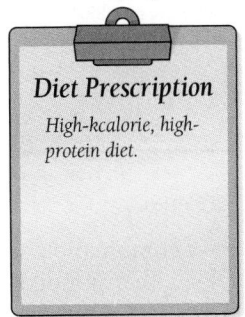

Diet Prescription

High-kcalorie, high-protein diet.

through the capillaries into the interstial space (the space between the blood vessels and the cells) and into the burned area. This leakage causes considerable edema and can reduce blood volume by half or more of its normal volume in people with extensive burns.

The primary goal of therapy at first is therefore to provide enough fluid, electrolytes, and albumin to maintain blood volume and prevent shock. When the burn is greater than 20 percent of the body surface area, isotonic fluids are given intravenously, because the person generally cannot take enough fluids by mouth. On average, a burned person requires 3 to 5 liters of fluid daily to replace losses; however, some clients may require over 10 liters per day.

The hypermetabolic state triggered by a severe burn greatly increases nutrient needs. The typical person will need about 4000 kcalories (two times the basal energy expenditure) and 200 grams of protein (1.5 to 3 grams of protein per kilogram of body weight) daily.

Tube feedings or parenteral nutrition should be initiated without delay for clients who cannot or will not eat adequate amounts of food by mouth. Enteral nutrition is preferred; it is less expensive, it helps to maintain the normal size and function of the intestinal cells, and it is associated with a lower risk of infection in burned clients.[3] Studies of animal suggest that providing enteral nutrition in the immediate postburn period may modulate the hypermetabolic response and limit weight loss.[4]

The proportions of nutrients supplying energy for the person with burns may also be important. Current recommendations advocate restricting fat to about 15 percent of the nonprotein kcalories.[5] Furthermore, the type of fat may be important. Providing a portion of the lipid kcalories as omega-3 fatty acids (see p. 48) is associated with improved immune function and tolerance to tube feeding.[6]

Specific vitamin and mineral requirements for people with burns have not been established. Researchers reviewing the micronutrient needs of burned people suggest that only vitamin C and vitamin A need to be supplemented above the RDA amounts.[7] Other supplements are provided as appropriate to the individual.

To encourage the person with a burn to eat, remember to offer emotional support. Understandably, food may seem unappealing to the person who faces a lengthy hospital stay, a great deal of pain, and fear of permanent disfigurement. Burn therapy, which generally includes whirlpool baths and the cutting away of dead skin and tissue, is extremely painful. If possible, schedule these treatments so as not to interfere with mealtimes. Give pain medications prior to meals so that mealtimes can be enjoyed.

A client may feel awkward about eating when the location of a burn interferes with self-feeding. An occupational therapist may be able to adapt

shock: a sudden drop in blood volume that disrupts the supply of oxygen to the tissues and the return of blood to the heart. Many events can lead to shock; some include major blood loss, trauma, and dehydration.

Whirlpool baths are known as **hydrotherapy.** They are used to cleanse the burn wound and help loosen the dead, burned skin, which is called **eschar** (es-CAR). As the eschar becomes loose, its removal reduces the risk of infection and allows the burn wound to heal as quickly as possible.

feeding utensils to assist the client. Encourage the client to get up, walk around, and begin physical therapy as soon as possible. This measure helps to prevent further tissue breakdown associated with injury, improves morale, and may also help to stimulate the appetite.

The person with a severe burn provides a dramatic example of how energy and protein needs can increase greatly as a result of hypermetabolism. Energy and protein needs can also increase for many other reasons, as described in the following sections.

Cancer Cachexia

cancer cachexia (ka-KEKS-ee-ah): anorexia with inadequate food intake, speeded-up metabolism and wasting, and general ill health associated with cancer.
  kakos = bad, poor
  hexis = condition

About two-thirds of people with cancer develop cachexia—a combination of loss of appetite with accelerated and abnormal metabolism that simultaneously reduces the supply of energy and nutrients and increases the demand for them. People with cachexia swiftly fall into a downward spiral. Their poor nutrient intakes lead to muscle wasting and poor health, and those conditions further contribute to inadequate intakes of nutrients. Malnutrition interferes with the quality of life, and contributes to the morbidity and mortality associated with the disease process. Loss of appetite, weight loss, and depletion of lean body mass and serum proteins typify the cancer cachexia syndrome. Factors that contribute to cancer cachexia are summarized in Figure 18–2.

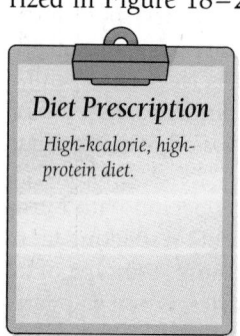

Diet Prescription

High-kcalorie, high-protein diet.

Cancer cachexia is a multifactorial problem. It begins early in tumor development, even before weight loss occurs. Cachexia appears to be tumor induced; that is, the tumor itself causes the changes that lead to cachexia, and removal of the tumor can reverse the cachexia.[8] Investigators continue to search for clues as to what tumor-related factors might be involved. Anorexia, accelerated nutrient losses, and altered metabolism all contribute to cancer cachexia; however, anorexia is widely recognized as the major precipitating factor.

Factors contributing to anorexia in the person with cancer include:

■ Psychological stress.
■ Cancer itself. Often anorexia and weight loss are the complaints that bring the person to visit the doctor in the first place.
■ A premature feeling of fullness after eating small amounts of food.
■ Lack of energy to prepare and eat food.
■ Tumor obstructing some portion of the GI tract, which, depending on the tumor's location, can interfere with the ability to chew or swallow or cause nausea and vomiting.
■ Cancer therapies. Treatments for cancer include surgery, chemotherapy, radiation therapy, and bone marrow transplants. Cancer therapies can contribute to anorexia by causing nausea; vomiting; altered taste perceptions; damage to the teeth and jawbones; altered taste perceptions;

chemotherapy: the use of drugs to arrest or destroy cancer cells. Drugs used for chemotherapy are sometimes called **antineoplastic agents.**
  chemo = chemical

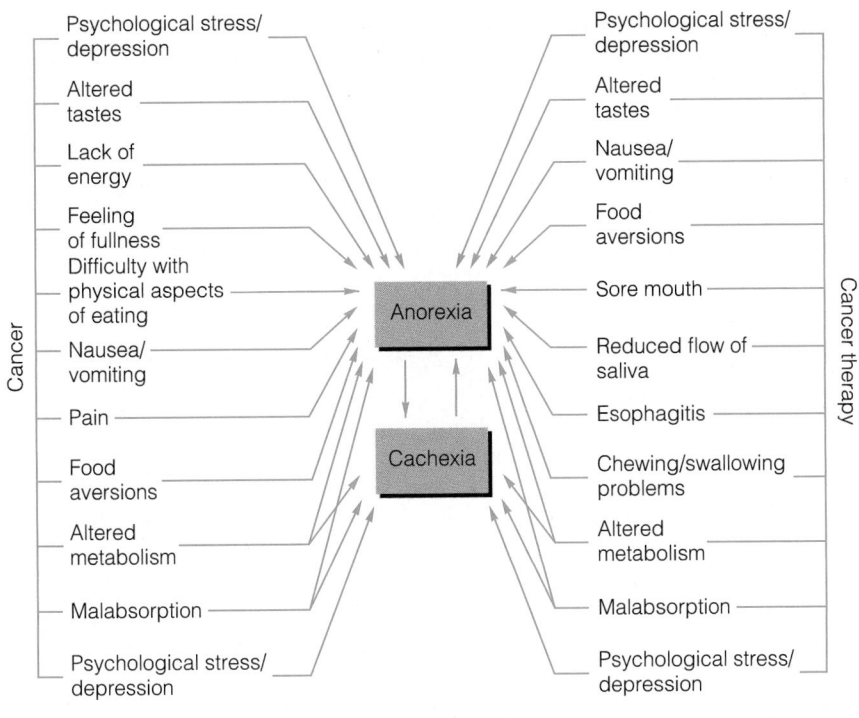

FIGURE 18–2 **Causes of the Cancer Cachexia Syndrome**
Anorexia and cachexia contribute to each other. Cancer itself and the available treatments for it make both problems worse.

reduced flow of saliva or thick saliva; inflammation of the tongue, mouth, or esophagus; mouth ulcers; food aversions; and depression.

Like anorexia, cancer and cancer therapies can accelerate nutrient losses by causing vomiting, diarrhea, and malabsorption. People treated with either radiation or chemotherapy may develop strong dislikes for certain foods, tastes, and odors that are associated too closely in time with unpleasant side effects of therapy, such as nausea and vomiting.

The problems caused by reduced nutrient intakes and excessive nutrient losses are compounded by changes in metabolism that further tax nutrition status. Studies suggest that some people with cancer are hypermetabolic, while others are not.[9] It may be that metabolic changes vary with different types of tumors or their locations in the body. However, even in the absence of hypermetabolism, metabolic pathways are altered, and nutrients are cycled in less efficient ways. The end result is that these metabolic changes raise energy needs. Other factors, such as the need for surgery or the development of an infection, can further raise nutrient needs. Drugs used for chemotherapy can interfere with normal metabolic pathways and create nutrient deficiencies as well. Table 17–4 in Chapter 17 described how different types of surgery can alter nutrition status. Table 18–3 describes the nutrition-related side effects of some drugs used in the treatment of cancer. Table 18–4 shows how radiation therapy can affect nutrition status. The nutrition consequences of bone marrow transplants are those caused by chemotherapy, radiation, and infections.

radiation therapy: the use of radiation to arrest or destroy cancer cells.

bone marrow transplants: the transfer of healthy bone marrow from a donor to a recipient, used as a treatment for leukemia (cancer of the white blood cells) and other blood disorders. The bone marrow recipient is prepared for the procedure with high doses of chemotherapy and sometimes whole body radiation to kill the cancerous cells before providing healthy cells. However, because healthy white blood cells are killed as well, the individual becomes very susceptible to infection.

TABLE 18–3   **Drugs Used in the Treatment of Cancer**

DRUG NAME	TIMING WITH MEALS	COMMON SIDE EFFECTS THAT MAY INFLUENCE NUTRITION STATUS
Adrenocorticosteroids	Give with food	Increased appetite, GI upset, glucose intolerance, negative nitrogen and calcium balance
Asparaginase	Give parenterally	Anorexia, nausea, vomiting, pancreatitis, hepatitis, glucose intolerance
Bleomycin	Give parenterally, intramuscularly, or subcutaneously	Anorexia, nausea, vomiting, mouth ulcers, stomatitis, weight loss, altered taste perceptions
Busulfan	Give with food	Nausea, vomiting, diarrhea, cracking at corners of mouth, inflammation of the tongue, anemias, weight loss, dry mouth
Carmustine	Give parenterally	Anorexia, nausea, vomiting, esophagitis, diarrhea, impaired liver function
Mithramycin	Give parenterally; slow infusion reduces nausea	Anorexia, nausea, vomiting, diarrhea, inflammation of the tongue, metallic taste
Procarbazine	Give with food; avoid foods containing tyramine (see Table 14–2)	Anorexia, nausea, vomiting, diarrhea, constipation, anemia, sore throat, dry mouth, difficulty swallowing
Vinblastine	Give parenterally	Anorexia, nausea, vomiting, diarrhea, constipation, stomatitis, sore throat, reduced bowel activity, abdominal pain, bowel inflammation
Vincristine	Give parenterally	Anorexia, nausea, vomiting, diarrhea, constipation, abdominal pain, mouth ulcers, anemia, thirst, weight loss, altered taste perceptions

Source: Adapted from D. E. Powers and A. O. Moore, *Food Medication Interactions,* (Phoenix: Food Medication Interactions, 1991), *Nursing 91 Handbook* (Springhouse, Pa.: Springhouse Corporation, 1991).

For many years, the deteriorating nutrition status that accompanies cancer was largely ignored. Many practitioners believed that emaciation and physical debilitation were an inevitable result of cancer. Others believed that if you fed the client, you also fed the tumor, so to "starve" the tumor, they would almost starve the client.

Today, experts recognize that attention to the diet in cancer treatment can prevent or reverse poor nutrition status. The malnourished person is less active and becomes weak, eats less, becomes weaker, and goes into a downward spiral. The person in good nutrition status:

- Enjoys a better quality of life.
- Is less susceptible to infections (see Chapter 14).
- Probably tolerates cancer therapies better.

Although it makes sense to prevent PEM in the person with cancer, actual research into ways of restoring and maintaining lean body mass has been disappointing. Despite seemingly adequate nutrition support, people with cancer cachexia often fail to replete their lean body masses. They may gain

TABLE 18–4 **Effects of Radiation on Nutrition Status**

EFFECTS LEADING TO REDUCED NUTRIENT INTAKE

Anorexia
Damage to teeth and jawbones
Depression
Esophagitis
Food aversions
Inflammation of mouth or tongue
Nausea
Reduced salivary secretions
Taste alterations
Thick salivary secretions
Vomiting

EFFECTS LEADING TO ACCELERATED NUTRIENT LOSSES

Chronic blood loss from intestine and bladder
Diarrhea
Fistula formation
Intestinal obstructions
Malabsorption
Vomiting

EFFECTS LEADING TO ALTERED METABOLISM

Altered metabolism occurs secondary to malnutrition

weight, but this weight often represents fat and water weight rather than lean body mass. Research continues to identify individual nutrients and other substances that might aid in repleting lean body mass.

People with cancer, particularly those who feel they cannot be helped by therapy, are easy targets for peddlers of cancer ''cures.'' Such people may take massive doses of vitamins and/or minerals, some of which may be toxic, or they may be following other programs that can impair nutrition status. Generally, people will not volunteer such information. Health care professionals should try to find out what supplements, products, or procedures the client may be using, for stopping these treatments may be as important to nutrition therapy's success as the design of the therapy.

People with cancer often benefit from a high-kcalorie, high-protein diet. One method of estimating the energy and protein needs for people with cancer is shown in the box. Table 18–5 shows diet modifications that may be necessary for different types of cancer.

Recognizing the many obstacles affecting the appetite of the person with cancer, health care professionals are faced with an enormous challenge in

TABLE 18–5   **Dietary Considerations for Various Cancers**

LOCATION OF CANCER	DIETARY CONSIDERATIONS
Brain	Physical feeding disabilities; chewing and swallowing problems.
Head/neck	Chewing and swallowing problems.
Mouth/esophagus	Chewing and swallowing problems; if obstructed, tube feeding below the obstruction may be necessary.
Stomach	Nausea, vomiting; if obstructed, tube feeding below the obstruction may be necessary; if resection is performed, a postgastrectomy diet (see Chapter 20) may be needed; nutrient deficiencies due to blind loop syndrome (Chapter 21) may occur.
Intestine	If obstructed, tube feeding or TPN may be necessary; resections or inflammation may cause multiple nutrition problems (see Chapter 21); low-fat, lactose-restricted diet may be useful.
Liver	Protein-, sodium-, and fluid-restricted diet may be necessary (see Chapter 23).
Pancreas	Low-fat diet and enzyme replacements may be necessary (see Chapter 21); diabetic diet may be necessary if insulin production is affected (see Chapter 20).
Kidneys	Protein-, electrolyte-, and fluid-controlled diet may be necessary (see Chapter 23).

Note: The considerations listed here are specific to the type of cancer; they do not include the effects of treatment. Other factors described for all cancers, such as anorexia, nausea, and vomiting, are considered in addition to the interventions discussed here.

How to Determine Energy and Protein Needs for Cancer

Energy: Calculate the basal energy expenditure (BEE) using the Harris-Benedict equation provided in Table 18–2 on p. 463. Energy needs range from 1.5 to 2.0 times the BEE.

Calculate protein at 1.5 to 2.0 grams protein per kilogram ideal body weight.

---

helping these individuals maintain their nutrition status. Every bit of interpersonal skill and nutrition knowledge can help, beginning with the professional's awareness of the client's predicament. Point out the proven benefits of aggressive nutrition therapy in cancer treatment, and offer all the practical pointers you can to help clients help themselves. Table 18–6 (pp. 472–473) describes specific problems a client may have and offers suggestions for alleviating them. Persistent anorexia and the inability to eat an adequate diet orally indicate the need for tube feedings or parenteral nutrition, particularly during and immediately after treatments.

The person receiving a bone marrow transplant often receives parenteral nutrition support because the GI tract is severely compromised by the preparation procedure. As GI function returns, the person begins to receive food orally, and parenteral nutrition is tapered off as oral intake improves. Early oral feedings start with lactose-free, low-residue, low-fat liquids to maximize absorption and minimize the risk of nausea, vomiting, and malabsorption. Gradually, solids are introduced. As individual tolerances allow, fiber, lactose, and fat can be added back to the diet.

Any discussion of nutrition and cancer pales in relation to actual experience in working with the person with cancer. Because this is so important to understand, and to show just how varied these effects can be, we would like to share with you an example from personal experience. Kathy was a 36-year-old, vibrant, intelligent woman who developed a malignant brain tumor that progressively affected her speech center and the right side of her body. Because this type of tumor progresses rapidly, the prognosis was poor, with an expected survival time of six months.

As her ability to communicate declined, Kathy found it more and more difficult to express her desires and needs regarding foods she would like to eat. Simultaneously, she became less able to prepare and physically eat foods herself because she was losing control of the right side of her body. Learning to use her left hand, particularly to handle feeding utensils, was hard for her. One solution to this problem was to service foods that she could eat with her fingers. She was an intelligent adult who did not want to be treated like a child, so the types of foods served this way had to be consistent with her need to preserve her dignity. She found that breads, cheeses, fruits, and luncheon meats were easy to handle, but the depression and frustration that resulted from her inability to communicate made it even more difficult for her to eat.

Another problem arose when foods were too small. Kathy lost the ability to move her tongue back and forth, and when small foods lodged in the right side of her mouth, she could not feel them and could choke.

Kathy was taking a steroid medication to reduce swelling in the brain, as well as narcotics to deal with the severe headaches associated with the tumor. Both the tumor itself and the steroids caused nausea, although in Kathy's case, she ate more rather than less to alleviate the nausea. She stated that she felt much more nauseated when she had an empty stomach. The tumor itself and the narcotics also made Kathy sleepy, which compounded the difficulty she had with physical aspects of eating.

As you can see, many factors affect food intake in the person with cancer. Consider also that nutrition is only one part of many treatments in the care of the person with cancer. In Kathy's case, the prognosis was poor, so the effects on long-term nutrition status were not as critical as helping Kathy preserve her feelings of self-esteem, dignity, comfort, and independence. These considerations are particularly important for the person whose disease is terminal. When time is short, you want the person to enjoy, rather than be burdened by, the routine experiences of everyday life.

TABLE 18–6   **Suggestions for Improving Food Intake**

TO IMPROVE THE APPETITE

- Explain why eating is important.
- Encourage clients to eat the most when they feel the best.
- Suggest that clients eat nutrient-dense foods first.
- Recommend indulging in favorite foods throughout the day.
- Suggest foods that are easy to prepare and eat.
- Let others prepare foods.
- Encourage clients to eat with family and friends.
- Recommend smaller, more frequent meals.
- Advise clients not to drink liquids with meals.
- Recommend the use of time-saving food preparation appliances.
- Give pain or antinausea medications when they will work best (usually before meals).
- Provide a pleasant and relaxed environment.
- Reassess clients regularly to solve feeding problems as they may arise.

TO COMBAT BITTER OR METALLIC TASTE PERCEPTIONS

- Encourage the use of eggs, fish, poultry, and dairy products instead of meats.
- Recommend adding sauces and seasonings to meats.
- Suggest that meats be served cold or at room temperature.
- Advise clients to brush teeth or use a mouthwash before eating.
- Encourage clients to try new foods and experiment with herbs and spices.

TO CONTROL NAUSEA AND VOMITING

- Recommend small meals.
- Advise clients to avoid spicy and high-fat foods.
- Suggest that clients avoid odors that cause nausea.
- Encourage clients to save liquids for after meals. Clear liquids or Popsicles after meals help prevent dehydration.
- Suggest that clients get fresh air, loosen clothing, or rest after meals.
- Advise clients to avoid eating their favorite foods during the times of the day when they frequently experience nausea or vomiting.
- Give antinausea drugs before mealtimes.
- Recommend that others prepare meals, if possible.

TO AVOID FOOD AVERSIONS

- Advise clients to avoid favorite foods when nauseated.
- Suggest to clients that they do not eat for one or two hours before or after treatments that cause nausea or vomiting.

TO ALLEVIATE PROBLEMS WITH CHEWING AND SWALLOWING

- Work with clients to find the consistency of food that will be easiest to handle. Thin liquids, true solids, and sticky foods are often difficult to swallow.
- Provide fluids with meals to ease chewing and swallowing.

(continued)

TABLE 18–6 *(continued)*

TO ALLEVIATE PROBLEMS WITH CHEWING AND SWALLOWING *(continued)*

- Advise the client with mouth sores to try foods at cooler temperatures. They are often soothing.
- Recommend that clients with mouth ulcers avoid foods that are spicy, acidic, or coarse or that contain seeds that can be trapped in an ulcer.
- Recommend that clients experiment with tilting the head forward and backward to see if swallowing can be made easier with the head positioned differently.
- Suggest a straw for drinking.
- Encourage clients who suffer from a reduced flow of saliva to rinse the mouth frequently and to avoid concentrated sweets. Artificial saliva from the pharmacy can also help. Sour candy or gum can stimulate the flow of saliva.
- Encourage good oral and dental hygiene.

TO ADD kCALORIES AND PROTEIN

- Add 2 tbsp milk powder to liquid milk, recipes, soups, puddings, and cereals.
- Add ground meats, chicken, fish, or grated cheeses to sauces, soups, casseroles, or vegetables.
- Use extra butter, margarine, or cream cheese on breads.
- Eat peanut butter on fruit, celery, or crackers.
- Use butter or margarine whenever possible (on breads, potatoes, vegetables, pasta, and rice).
- Use yogurt, sour cream, or a sour cream dip with vegetables.
- Use mayonnaise as a salad dressing and on sandwiches.
- Add whipping cream to desserts and hot chocolate, or use it to lighten coffee.
- Have snacks available at all times.
- Add nuts and dried fruits such as raisins to desserts or cereals.
- Use cream instead of milk with cereal.
- Try commercially available liquid supplements or instant breakfast mixes for meals or between-meal snacks.

Human Immunodeficiency Virus (HIV) Infection and Acquired Immune Deficiency Syndrome (AIDS)

Infection by the human immunodeficiency virus (HIV) eventually causes AIDS, the devastating disorder that affects young and old, rich and poor, urban and rural dwellers, men and women. An estimated 50 million people worldwide have been infected with the virus, and virtually all of these people will likely develop the disorder.[10] As its incidence rises sharply, prevention and treatment of HIV infection become critical concerns of health care professionals around the world.

HIV infection attacks the immune system and leaves its victims defenseless against opportunistic infections and other disorders from which most people are protected. The disorder begins with infection by the human

human immunodeficiency virus (HIV): a virus transmitted from one person to another by direct contact of their body fluids. The result of infection is a progressive immune system disorder that leaves its victims defenseless against numerous infections. In the early, symptomless stages, the person is said to have an HIV infection. The term **acquired immune deficiency syndrome (AIDS)** refers to the end stage of the infection, when the severe complications are manifested. HIV infections are most often transmitted through sexual intercourse, through contaminated needles or blood products, or from mother to infant during pregnancy or lactation.

opportunistic infections: infections caused by microorganisms that normally do not cause disease in the general population but can infect people once their immune systems are compromised (as in AIDS).

The cluster of signs and symptoms that are not life threatening and precede the development of AIDS is referred to as **AIDS-related complex (ARC).**

thrush: a fungal infection of the mouth caused by *Candida albicans;* the technical term for this infection is *candidiasis.*

The type of cancer, which is rare in the general population but common in people with AIDS, is **Kaposi's sarcoma.**

immunodeficiency virus (HIV) and progresses in stages. At first, the HIV-infected individual is symptom-free. Later, as the infection progresses, the person develops symptoms that may include fatigue, skin rashes, fevers, diarrhea, muscle pain, night sweats, weight loss, thrush, oral lesions, and other opportunistic infections that are not life threatening. In the final stages, serious infections of the lungs, central nervous system, GI tract, and skin, as well as pneumonia, a type of cancer, and severe diarrhea, are frequent and often fatal complications.

Currently an HIV infection has no cure. Treatment focuses on slowing its course and controlling its symptoms to improve the individual's comfort and quality of life. However, researchers and clinicians remain optimistic that they will be able to develop effective therapies and, possibly, an AIDS vaccine. AIDS research has spurred tremendous growth in our understanding of the immune system. This knowledge has unraveled some of the mysteries of AIDS and other immune system disorders as well.

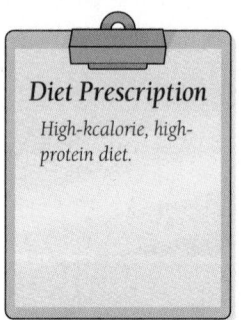

Diet Prescription

High-kcalorie, high-protein diet.

The severe PEM and wasting associated with HIV infections, much as in cancer, are multifactorial: they are caused by inadequate food intake, excessive nutrient losses, hypermetabolism, and drug-nutrient interactions as shown in Table 18–7. The exact causes of wasting depend on the particular complications the individual develops. Repeated infections and cancer accelerate wasting dramatically. Weight loss typically begins in the early stages of HIV infection and becomes more severe as the disease progresses. Table 18–8 lists the nutrition-related side effects of drugs used in the treatment of HIV infections and their complications.

Although attention to nutrition cannot change the ultimate outcome of AIDS, it is possible that good nutrition status can slow its progression and

TABLE 18–7   **Causes of Malnutrition in HIV Infections**

REDUCED FOOD INTAKE	ACCELERATED NUTRIENT LOSSES
Drug therapy	Diarrhea
Lack of energy to eat	Malabsorption
Pain associated with eating	Low serum albumin levels
Fever/infection	PEM
Nausea and vomiting	Drug therapy
Psychological factors such as fear, depression, and dementia	**ALTERED METABOLISM**
Oral lesions	Infections
Dry mouth	Cancer
Altered taste perceptions	Drug therapy
Difficulty chewing/swallowing	
Esophageal lesions and obstructions	
Use of oxygen masks	

TABLE 18–8 **Drugs Used in the Treatment of HIV Infections**

DRUG NAME	TIMING WITH MEALS	COMMON SIDE EFFECTS THAT MAY INFLUENCE NUTRITION STATUS
Acyclovir	Give parenterally or orally with food	Nausea, diarrhea, vomiting, anorexia
Amphotericin B	Give parenterally	Nausea, vomiting, fever, anemia, kidney dysfunction
Ampicillin	Give with water 1 hr before or 2 hr after meals; do not give with fruit juice, beer, or wine	Nausea, vomiting, diarrhea, steatorrhea, anemia, inflammation of the mouth and tongue, stomatitis, altered taste perceptions, hypokalemia
Azidothymidine (AZT)		Anorexia, nausea, vomiting, diarrhea, constipation, altered taste perceptions, mouth ulcers, edema of tongue and lips, abdominal pain, anemia
Bleomycin	(See Table 18–3)	
Cisplatin	Give parenterally	Anorexia, nausea, vomiting, altered taste perceptions
Clotrimazole	Dissolve slowly in mouth and swallow saliva	Nausea, vomiting
Cyclophosphamide	Give during or after meals	Anorexia, nausea, vomiting, mouth ulcers, inflammation of the colon, anemia
Dactinomycin	Give parenterally	Anorexia, nausea, vomiting, mouth ulcers, heartburn, anemia
Doxorubicin	Give parenterally	Anorexia, nausea, vomiting, diarrhea, stomach pain, sore throat, mouth ulcers, mouth blindness, esophagitis
Erythromycin	Give on empty stomach 1 hr before or 2 hr after meals; if GI distress, give with meals, not milk, fruit juice, beer, or wine	Nausea, vomiting, cramps, abdominal pain, diarrhea, inflammation of the mouth
Estrogens	Give with food at same time each day	Anorexia, nausea, vomiting, edema, weight change altering glucose tolerance
Ethambutol hydrochloride		Anorexia, nausea, vomiting, abdominal pain
Fluconazole	Give orally or parenterally	Nausea, vomiting, diarrhea, intestinal inflammation
Fluorouracil	Give parenterally; if given orally, give with water, not acidic beverages	Anorexia, nausea, vomiting, stomatitis, diarrhea, heartburn, sore mouth, altered taste perceptions, GI bleeding, esophagitis
Ganciclovir	Give parenterally	Anorexia, nausea, vomiting
Hydroxyurea	Give with food	Anorexia, nausea, vomiting, mouth ulcers
Isoniazid	Give 1 hr before or 2 hr after meals; may give with food to relieve GI distress	Anorexia, nausea, vomiting, dry mouth, diarrhea, anemia, cracked lips
Ketoconazole	Give with food to reduce nausea and vomiting	Nausea, vomiting, abdominal pain, diarrhea, anemia
Mercaptopurine	Give with food	Anorexia, nausea, vomiting, stomatitis, stomach pain, diarrhea, anemia, vitamin B_6 depletion
Methotrexate	Give on an empty stomach; give with food to reduce gastric distress; do not give with milk	Anorexia, nausea, vomiting, diarrhea, GI ulcers, GI inflammation, anemia, stomatitis, steatorrhea, mouth ulcers
Metronidazole	Give with food	Anorexia, nausea, vomiting, diarrhea, altered taste perceptions, dry mouth, constipation, stomatitis, abnormal discomfort
Nystatin	Give orally as directed; retain drug in mouth as long as possible	Diarrhea, nausea, vomiting, GI pain (occasionally)

(continued)

TABLE 18–8   *(continued)*

DRUG NAME	TIMING WITH MEALS	COMMON SIDE EFFECTS THAT MAY INFLUENCE NUTRITION STATUS
Pentamidine isethionate	Give parenterally or as an inhalant	Nausea, vomiting, taste alternations, kidney dysfunction, hypoglycemia or hyperglycemia, diabetes
Pyrimethamine	Give with food	Anorexia, nausea, vomiting, diarrhea, anemia
Rifampin	Give with water on empty stomach	Anorexia, nausea, vomiting, cramps, diarrhea, altered taste perceptions, abdfominal distress
Sulfadiazide	Give with water	Anorexia, nausea, vomiting, diarrhea
Trimethoprim	Give with water on empty stomach	Nausea, vomiting, anorexia, anemia, diarrhea, stomatitis, GI distress
Vinblastine	(See Table 18–3)	
Vincristine	(See Table 18–3)	

Source: Adapted from D. E. Powers and A. O. Moore, *Food Medication Interactions,* (Phoenix: Food Medication Interactions, 1991; *Nursing 91 Drug Handbook* (Springhouse, Pa.: Springhouse Corporation, 1991).

meanwhile improve the quality of life. Good nutrition status supports optimal immune function, possibly reducing susceptibility to HIV infections. Good nutrition status may also improve clients' responses to drug therapy. Maintaining nutrition status may make the difference between an individual's being able to stay at home or having to move to a nursing home.[11]

A positive test for HIV infection in an individual alerts the health care professional to the need for aggressive nutrition intervention right away.[12] Although the person may still have no symptoms, early intervention may detect and correct subclinical deficiencies in preparation for the stresses ahead; it also establishes baseline assessment parameters to assist in monitoring changes in nutrition status. Researchers suggest that weight loss, reduced percent body fat, and reduced body mass index are early signs of nutrition status deterioration in people with AIDS.[13]

Presently, controlled studies documenting specific nutrient needs of people with HIV infections are lacking. However, practitioners have begun to make recommendations for care based on clinical experiences. For people with AIDS, as for all individuals, oral diets are appropriate as long as they are possible. Nutrient needs depend on the complications experienced in each case. The Harris-Benedict equation on p. 463 for estimating energy needs can be used for people with AIDS. Although the exact vitamin and mineral needs of people with AIDS have not been determined, at least 100 percent of the RDA for these nutrients should be provided daily. People who are unable to consume sufficient foods to make up an adequate diet might benefit from a multivitamin-mineral supplement containing at least 100 percent of the RDA of these nutrients. Many clinicians prescribe a daily prenatal vitamin supplement for people with HIV infections.[14]

The tips that help people with cancer are also useful for people with HIV infections. Suggestions for alleviating the problems of anorexia, altered taste sensations, nausea and vomiting, food aversions, and difficulty with chewing and swallowing were presented in Table 18–6 (on pp. 472–473).

TABLE 18–9 **Dietary Modifications for Managing Diarrhea and Malabsorption in HIV-Related GI Infections**

AREA OF INTESTINE AFFECTED	DIET MODIFICATIONS
Total small intestine	Low fat (less than 20% of total energy), low fiber, low residue, no lactose, no caffeine; parenteral nutrition is often necessary.
Partial small intestine	Low fat (less than 20% of total energy), low residue, low lactose, no caffeine.
Large intestine	Low fat, medium-chain triglycerides (MCT), low fiber, low residue, low lactose, no caffeine.
Nonspecific involvement	Bulking agent (pectin), low lactose, fat as tolerated.

Source: Adapted from Task Force on Nutrition Support in AIDS, Guidelines for nutrition support in AIDS, *Nutrition* 5 (1989): 39–46.

Nutrition therapy in the person with AIDS is frequently complicated by malabsorption and severe diarrhea. From 50 to 90 percent of people with AIDS experience chronic or recurrent diarrhea. In many cases, diarrhea is severe—the person may lose from 10 to 15 liters of diarrheal fluids daily. Treatment of diarrhea and malabsorption varies, depending on the cause and the extent to which the intestine is affected. Appropriate drug therapy and the provision of adequate fluids and electrolytes set the cornerstones of treatment. Salty broths and high-potassium juices can help replace fluids and electrolytes. Table 18–9 shows the dietary modifications recommended for the treatment of diarrhea and malabsorption based on the part of the intestine involved.

Among the infections against which clients with AIDS are relatively defenseless are food-borne illnesses. Susceptibility to these infections requires that the people with AIDS be given written and oral instructions on the safe handling of foods. Table NP14–1 in Nutrition in Practice 14 describes such precautions.

Individuals unable to consume enough food to prevent nutrition complications and unintentional weight loss need aggressive nutrition support. As a guideline, aggressive nutrition support should be considered when:

■ A person loses 5 percent of body weight within a month.
■ A person has lost more than 10 percent of body weight over the last six months.[15]

As always, enteral feeding is preferred to parenteral feeding. Sometimes liquid formulas given with or between regular meals can help maintain or restore nutrition status; otherwise, tube feedings can be used. Tube feedings given at night can supplement oral diets during the day, especially for people at home. If pain or obstructions in the upper GI tract make it difficult or painful for a client to tolerate a nasogastric feeding tube, gastrostomy or jejunostomy feedings are indicated.

Caretakers must take special precautions to keep tube feeding from causing diarrhea unrelated to the HIV infection. Table 16–4 on pp. 400–401 describes the causes and prevention of diarrhea associated with tube feeding. Preventing bacterial contamination of the formula is particularly important because of the susceptibility of HIV-infected individuals to GI infections.

The use of TPN in people with AIDS is controversial, especially in the final stages of the disorder. Generally, it is used only when people are expected to benefit from other therapy and need to maintain their nutrition status while undergoing that therapy. TPN may be more useful in repleting the body mass of people whose primary problems are reduced food intake or malabsorption, rather than those who have complications affecting the whole body (rather than one organ system).[16] People with GI tract obstructions, severe vomiting, or GI infections affecting the entire small bowel may benefit from TPN. The Case Study at the end of this chapter describes a person with an HIV infection.

Up to now, this chapter has shown how high-kcalorie diets are used to treat people with burns, cancer, and HIV infections. Another use of the high-kcalorie diet is in the treatment of pulmonary diseases, as described below.

Chronic Obstructive Pulmonary Diseases

chronic obstructive pulmonary diseases (COPD): disorders that cause blockage of the lungs' air passages and thus interfere with the exchange of gases between the air and the body.

emphysema (EM-fe-SEE-ma)**:** a type of COPD in which the lungs lose their elasticity and the victim has difficulty breathing.

bronchitis (bron-KYE-tis)**:** inflammation of the lungs' air passages.
  bronchos = windpipe
  itis = inflammation

alveoli (al-VEE-oh-lie)**:** air sacs in the lungs; one sac is an *alveolus.*

elastin: a structural protein in the lung.

bronchioles (BRON-key-ohls)**:** the small air passages from the trachea to the lungs.
  bronchos = windpipe

Chronic obstructive pulmonary diseases (COPD) are conditions characterized by persistent obstruction of airflow through the lungs. The two major types of COPD are emphysema and chronic bronchitis. Smoking is a primary risk factor for COPD. Heredity also plays a role: a family history of respiratory disorders predicts susceptibility. Other risk factors are exposure to environmental pollution (including exposure of nonsmokers to cigarette smoke); alcohol consumption; and possibly, repeated respiratory tract infections in young children.

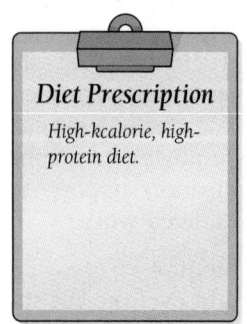

Diet Prescription

High-kcalorie, high-protein diet.

In emphysema, the small passages and air sacs (alveoli) within the lungs lose their elasticity. The victim can breathe air in but has trouble exhaling it. Stale air containing an excess of carbon dioxide becomes trapped in the rigid pockets in the lung, and the lung enlarges to accommodate the increased air volume. As the lung tissue expands, it thins out, and its small air passages then tend to collapse during exhalation. Emphysema is believed to be caused by the destruction of elastin, the major structural protein in the normal lung.

The individual with chronic bronchitis suffers from a different problem. In chronic bronchitis, excessive mucus is produced and clogs the air passages (bronchioles). These passages also become inflamed, obstructing the airways further.

Regardless of the type of COPD, it gradually becomes more difficult for the lungs to deliver oxygen to the tissues and to remove carbon dioxide (a waste product of metabolism). No cure for COPD is available; treatment is aimed at relieving the symptoms.

People with COPD frequently experience weight loss, PEM, and infection. People with pulmonary diseases account for many cases of malnutrition in hospitals. The extent of malnutrition appears to correlate with the severity of pulmonary disease.

As COPD advances, the lungs lose mass and strength, and body weight decreases. Lung function is compromised, and pulmonary infections become more and more likely. Heart failure and mortality rates are highest in people with COPD who lose weight.

Possible explanations as to why many individuals with COPD are at risk for poor nutrition status include:

- Anorexia and poor food intake.
- Increased energy expenditure associated with labored breathing.
- Steroid drug therapy that raises nutrient requirements and compromises nutrition status.
- Use of mechanical ventilators (people who require them are in a hypermetabolic state). Also, people requiring mechanical ventilation often experience weakness and discomfort, which can interfere with nutrient intake.
- Repeated infections, which raise nutrient needs and cause nutrient deficiencies. These deficiencies, in turn, increase the likelihood of infection, a vicious cycle.

mechanical ventilator: a machine that "breathes" for the person who can't, by forcing air into the person's lungs at intervals.

Weight loss in COPD may result from these factors, and also from high resting energy expenditure, which may be more greatly accelerated in malnourished people with stable COPD than in adequately nourished people with stable COPD.[17] In one study, clients with stable COPD who weighed less than 75 percent of standard body weight reported higher energy and protein intakes than COPD clients with body weights closer to standard.[18] The authors of the study concluded that energy needs rise as the disease progresses, and that it was increased needs, not poor intakes, that explained the weight loss in their subjects. Actually, though, both may contribute. A person with COPD may be unable to verbalize feelings of hunger and may not be able to take adequate nourishment. When on a mechanical ventilator, the person may feel weak, uncomfortable, and overwhelmed.

Repleting and maintaining nutrient stores for the person with COPD help to maintain lung function and to prevent lung infections. However, overfeeding can be just as harmful as underfeeding people with COPD (see the discussion of the refeeding syndrome on p. 460). Clients replete their nutrient stores best when refed gradually.

Respiratory Failure

In today's intensive care units, respiratory failure is a frequent cause of illness and death. Respiratory failure can result from advanced COPD, severe stress, and many other disorders. In respiratory failure, a person's lungs are unable to exchange gases, and the person requires mechanical ventilation until able to breathe again.

respiratory failure: failure of the lungs to perform.

People in respiratory failure spend much energy breathing, eating, and moving in any way, especially during attempts to wean them from mechanical ventilation. The types of nutrients used to supply this energy make a difference. During metabolism, glucose generates more carbon dioxide per kcalorie delivered than does fat. Therefore, carbohydrate in excess of the body's needs taxes the lungs to rid the body of excess carbon dioxide. For this reason, authorities currently recommend that for clients in respiratory failure, lipids supply from 50 to 60 percent of the total daily energy needs.[19]

People in respiratory failure are often candidates for TPN. TPN solutions that contain less glucose than standard solutions, and that are given with IV lipid instead to augment energy intake, are appropriate. Enteral formulas (see Appendix D) designed to meet the needs of people in respiratory failure have also been developed, but little information is available regarding the use of tube feedings for nutrition support of these individuals.

This chapter has described high-kcalorie diets and disorders for which such diets are used to help prevent severe consequences for nutrition status. Chapter 19 looks at low-kcalorie diets and the risks that excess weight can have on the body.

CASE STUDY

Nutrition and HIV Infections

Kevin sought medical help at age 34 when he began feeling run-down and developed a painful white coating over his mouth and tongue. The diagnosis of anemia and thrush alerted Kevin's physician to the possibility of an HIV infection. When Kevin tested positive for an HIV infection, the news was devastating both to him and to his family and friends. Fortunately, those closest to him have supported him through this difficult time, and he has a strong desire to live out his life as independently as possible. Four months after the diagnosis of HIV infection, Kevin developed a serious, continuous diarrhea that required hospitalization to classify and control. Since the diagnosis of HIV infection was made, Kevin has lost 10 pounds. At 6 feet tall, he currently weighs 158 pounds.

Describe how AIDS can lead to reduced food intake, nutrient losses, and hypermetabolism. From the limited information given here, what factors could have contributed to Kevin's weight loss?

Discuss nutrition strategies for dealing with thrush and diarrhea. Why is nutrition an important consideration early in the course of an HIV infection? Is Kevin's weight loss significant? What is his %IBW? What steps could be effective in preventing further weight loss?

Study Questions

1. Describe the uses of a high-kcalorie, high-protein diet. What are some specific suggestions that can help the person who needs to eat a high-kcalorie diet?
2. What is the refeeding syndrome? Describe why it is important to gradually reintroduce nutrients to the person who is nutritionally depleted.
3. Describe the changes in body fluids that occur immediately after a person suffers an extensive burn. What is the primary concern during this period? How are these needs met?
4. What metabolic events occur during a burn injury, and how do they affect nutrient needs?
5. What is cancer cachexia? What factors contribute to the development of cancer cachexia? Can nutrition intervention help prevent this problem?
6. What are the possible advantages of good nutrition status for the person with cancer? In the person with cancer, what strategies can combat anorexia? A bitter or metallic taste in the mouth? Nausea and vomiting? Problems with chewing and swallowing? Mouth ulcers? Reduced flow of saliva?
7. What is AIDS? What factors contribute to the wasting associated with AIDS?
8. In what ways can good nutrition status possibly alter the course of AIDS?
9. What is COPD? What factors play a role in the weight loss frequently seen in people with COPD?
10. What is respiratory failure? Describe how the nutrient needs of the person with respiratory failure should be met.

Notes

1. S. M. Solomon and D. F. Kirby, The refeeding syndrome: A review, *Journal of Parenteral and Enteral Nutrition* 14 (1990): 90–97; T. Havala and E. Shronts, Managing the complications associated with refeeding, *Nutrition in Clinical Practice* 5 (1990): 23–29.
2. F. Negro and F. Cerra, Nutritional monitoring in the ICU: Rational and practical application, *Critical Care Clinics* 4 (1988): 34–47.
3. C. S. Ireton-Jones and C. R. Baxter, Nutrition for adult burn patients: A review, *Nutrition in Clinical Practice* 6 (1991): 3–7.
4. S. Inque and coauthors, Prevention of yeast translocation across the gut by a single enteral feeding after burn injury, *Journal of Parenteral and Enteral Nutrition* 13 (1989): 565–571; H. Saito and coauthors, The effect of route of nutrient administration on nutritional state, catabolic hormone secretion, and gut mucosal injury after burn injury, *Journal of Parenteral and Enteral Nutrition* 11 (1987): 1–7.
5. Ireton-Jones and Baxter, 1991.
6. M. M. Gottschlich and coauthors, Differential effects of three enteral dietary regimens on selected outcome variables in burn patients, *Journal of Parenteral and Enteral Nutrition* 14 (1990): 225–236.

7. M. M. Gottschlich and G. D. Warden, Vitamin supplementation in the patient with burns, *Journal of Burn Care Rehabilitation* 11 (1990): 275–279.

8. K. A. Kern and J. A. Norton, Cancer cachexia, *Journal of Parenteral and Enteral Nutrition* 12 (1988): 286–298.

9. W. W. Souba and E. M. Copeland, Parenteral nutrition and metabolic observations in cancer, *Nutrition in Clinical Practice* 3 (1988): 183–190.

10. D. P. Kotler, Protein-energy malnutrition in AIDS, *Nutrition in Clinical Practice* 5 (1990): 41–42.

11. P. A. Cuff, Acquired immunodeficiency syndrome and malnutrition: Role of gastrointestinal pathology, *Nutrition in Clinical Practice* 5 (1990): 43–53; Department of Continuing Education in Health Sciences, UCLA Extension, *Nutritional Aspects of the AIDS Patient* (Los Angeles: 1989).

12. Federation of American Societies for Experimental Biology, Life Sciences Research Office, Nutrition and HIV infection: A review and evaluation of the extant knowledge of the relationship between nutrition and HIV infection, *Nutrition in Clinical Practice* 6 (Supplement, 1990): 1–94.

13. C. McCorkindale and coauthors, Nutritional status of HIV-infected patients during the early disease stages, *Journal of the American Dietetic Association* 90 (1990): 1236–1241.

14. Department of Continuing Education in Health Sciences, UCLA Extension, 1989.

15. Department of Continuing Education in Health Sciences, UCLA Extension, 1989.

16. D. B. Kotler and coauthors, Effect of home total parenteral nutrition on body composition in patients with acquired immunodeficiency syndrome, *Journal of Parenteral and Enteral Nutrition* 14 (1990): 454–458.

17. S. Goldstein and coauthors, Energy expenditure in patients with chronic obstructive pulmonary disease, *Chest* 91 (1987): 222–224; D. O. Wilson and coauthors, Metabolic rate and weight loss in chronic obstructive lung disease, *Journal of Parenteral and Enteral Nutrition* 14 (1990): 7–11.

18. N. L. Keim and coauthors, Dietary evaluation of outpatients with chronic obstructive pulmonary disease, *Journal of the American Dietetic Association* 86 (1986): 902–906.

19. M. M. Rothkopf and coauthors, Nutritional support in respiratory failure, *Nutrition in Clinical Practice* 4 (1989): 166–172.

18

Nutrition and Cancer Prevention

Chapter 18 shows how nutrition therapy supports the person being treated for cancer. Cancer is a concern for all of us; one out of every four people now alive will eventually contract cancer. We know that factors beyond our control, such as genetic predisposition, and factors within our control, such as cigarette smoking, have a strong influence on the development of cancer. Research suggests that the way we eat, another factor within our control, may make us more or less susceptible to certain kinds of cancer. Constituents in foods may be cancer causing, cancer promoting, or protective against cancer. This Nutrition in Practice looks at the role of diet in preventing cancer, and its Miniglossary explains the terms used.

What does research reveal about the relationships between diet and cancer?

Researchers have been attempting to discover what dietary differences exist between people who do and don't get cancer. Seventh-Day Adventists are one group of people with a remarkably lower death rate from cancers of all kinds than that of the rest of the population. This religious group has rules against smoking and using alcohol, discourages the use of hot condiments and spices, and encourages a lacto-ovo vegetarian diet. After cancers linked to smoking and alcohol

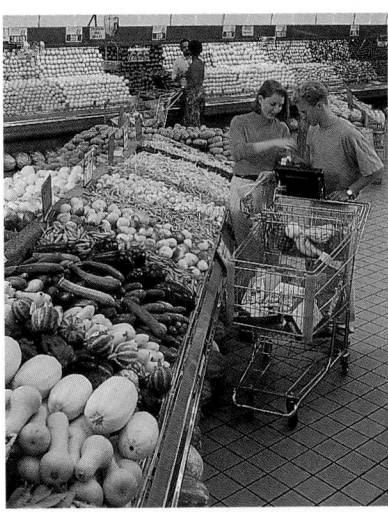

Concerned consumers carefully select foods that may help reduce the risk of cancer.

are discounted, Seventh-Day Adventists still have a cancer mortality rate about one-half to two-thirds that of the rest of the population. This may be due to their low meat and fat intakes, their high intakes of vegetables and cereal grains, or both—or to other lifestyle factors.

Studies of closely matched groups of people in which researchers study dietary factors in a context relatively free of interference by nondiet variables also implicate diet in cancer causation. In various studies, for example, people with colon cancer have been observed to eat more meat, less fiber, and more saturated fat than others without cancer.[1]

Studies have shown that the incidence of certain cancers varies both by geographic area and by racial group. For example, Japanese people living in Japan develop more stomach cancers and fewer colon cancers than people in the United States. However, when Japanese people come to the United States, their children develop both stomach and colon cancers at a rate similar to that of U.S. citizens. Japan and the United States are both industrial countries, and their environmental pollution rates are similar. However, something in the environment must account for the changed cancer pattern in immigrants, and an obvious candidate is diet.

Laboratory studies using animals confirm suspicions that fat, of all dietary components, is uniquely correlated with cancer. Fat does not initiate the cancers, however; to get the tumors started, an experimenter has to expose the animals to a known carcinogen. After that exposure, a high-fat diet makes more cancers develop and makes them develop earlier than they would with a low-fat diet. Thus fat appears to be a cancer promoter, rather than an initiator.

Is anything known about how fat exerts this effect?

Not all is known but a high-fat diet is thought to promote cancer in any of a number of ways:

- By causing the body to secrete more of certain hormones (for example, estrogen), thus creating a climate favorable to the development of certain cancers (for example, breast cancer).
- By promoting the secretion of bile into the intestine; bile may then be converted by organisms in the colon into compounds that cause cancer.
- By causing fat to be incorporated into cell membranes and changing them so that they become permeable to cancer-causing invaders.

It may not be fat in general that has these effects, but rather certain forms of fat. The finding that linoleic acid, the polyunsaturated fatty acid of vegetable oils, is particularly implicated in cancer causation is especially noteworthy. (On the other hand, omega-3 fatty acids and monounsaturated fatty acids do not promote cancer.)

What does this mean people should do about the fat in their diets?

The person wishing to apply this information should reduce consumption of all forms of fat, at least to the point where it contributes no more than 30 percent of total kcalories. Some cancer researchers suggest an even stricter limit: 20

"average American" to accomplish this degree of fat restriction in practice means drastically reducing the amount of fat used in food preparation, and excluding many traditional foods almost entirely: butter, margarine,

---

MINIGLOSSARY

carcinogen (car-SIN-oh-jen): a cancer-causing substance. A carcinogen is one kind of initiator; another is radiation.
> *carcin* = cancer
> *gen* = gives rise to

cruciferous vegetables: a group of vegetables named for their cross-shaped blossoms. They have been shown to protect against cancer in laboratory animals. Examples are cauliflower, cabbage, brussels sprouts, broccoli, turnips, and rutabagas.

dithiolthiones: a class of compounds important in connection with diet and cancer because some are found in plant foods and seem to exhibit anticancer activity.

indoles: a family of compounds with a structure resembling that of the amino acid tryptophan, mentioned here because some of those found in cruciferous vegetables have anticancer activity.

initiating event: an event caused by radiation of chemical reaction that can give rise to cancer.

promoter: a substance that does not initiate cancer, but that favors its development once the initiating event has taken place.

---

mayonnaise, and salad dressings. Of the fats used, olive oil and fish oils would seem to be the most desirable.

Besides fat, what other dietary factors that have a connection with cancer?

Fibers and certain plant foods may act as cancer antipromoters. Fibers may help protect against some cancers—by promoting the excretion of bile from the body, or by speeding up the transit time of all materials through the colon so that the colon walls are not exposed for long to cancer-causing substances. That fiber does have an independent protective effect of some kind is supported by evidence from Finland. The Finns eat a high-fat diet, but unlike other such diets, theirs is high in fiber as well. Their colon cancer rate is low, suggesting that fiber has a protective effect even in the presence of a high-fat diet.

A number of studies have supported special roles for plant foods in cancer resistance. One study found less frequent use of vegetables in people with colon cancer; another found, specifically, less use of cabbage, broccoli, and brussels sprouts in colon cancer victims. Stomach cancer, too, correlates with low vegetable intakes—in one study, with vegetables in general; in another, with fresh vegetables; in others, with lettuce and other fresh greens, or with vegetables containing vitamin C.

Cancers of the head and neck seem to correlate best not with diet but with the combination of alcohol and tobacco consumption. However, some dietary factors are implicated as protective, particularly fruits and raw vegetables, and specifically the fruits and vegetables that contribute carotene (the vitamin A precursor) and the B vitamin riboflavin. Carotene and its relatives, the retinoids, are also important in preventing cancers of epithelial origin, including skin cancer.

Vitamin A regulates cellular differentiation, which goes awry in cancer. This vitamin also helps maintain the immune system. Immunity can work against cancer even after a tumor has begun to form. Lung cancer incidence can be as much as 60 to 80 percent lower in people with high vitamin A intakes than in those with low intakes. In Japan, a study of 280,000 people showed lung cancer rates to be 20 to 30 percent lower in smokers who ate yellow or green vegetables daily than in those who did not. In ex-smokers who ingested yellow or green vegetables daily, the reduction was much greater, as if the *repair* of damage done by smoking after the initiation of cancer was enhanced by something in the vegetables.

Could people take vitamin A, carotene, vitamin C, and fiber to obtain this anticancer effect?

No. Green vegetables appear to have an additional protective effect beyond that supplied by these vitamins and fiber. Among other nutrients cited as possible antipromoters are vitamin B_6, folate, pantothenic acid, vitamin B_{12}, vitamin E, iron, zinc, selenium—and more. And not only nutrients but also some nonnutrient substances in vegetables may act as antipromoters.

What nonnutrient compounds have been identified as protective?

Some nonnutrient compounds, known as indoles, dithiolthiones, and other chemicals, occur in vegetables of the cabbage family—the so-called cruciferous vegetables. These compounds activate enzymes that destroy carcinogens. Another class of possible anticancer compounds, protease inhibitors, occurs in beans and plant seeds. These are thought to inhibit enzymes associated with the spreading of tumors.

Other vegetables and fruits contain other constituents that may activate the enzyme system that degrades carcinogens. These constituents are so widespread among plants that the single most valuable application of the information obtained to date is *not* to eat cabbages, for example, but to eat lots of of vegetables and fruits of all kinds in generous quantities.

How would you sum up the best ways to eat to prevent cancer?

Although we clearly still have much to learn, many researchers believe that we know enough to take the first preventive steps. The Committee on Diet, Nutrition, and Cancer of the National Research Council has published these provisional guidelines:

- Control total food energy intake.
- Reduce consumption of both saturated and unsaturated fats.
- Include fruits (especially citrus fruits), vegetables (particularly carotene-rich and cruciferous vegetables), and whole-grain products in the daily diet.
- Avoid possible carcinogens by limiting consumption of foods preserved by salt curing, salt packing, or smoking.
- Minimize contamination of foods with carcinogens from any source.
- Reduce the concentration of mutagens in foods when feasible.

- Consume only moderate amounts of alcohol, if any.
- Monitor drinking water with an eye out for toxic substances.

The committee also recommended to evaluate food additives for carcinogenic activity specifically stated that additives now legally permitted in foods were not implicated in cancer causation.

To the recommendations made in these guidelines, we would add one other: vary your choices. Don't let your diet become monotonous. This last suggestion is based on an important concept that is specific to the prevention of cancer initiation—dilution. Whenever you switch from food to food, you are diluting whatever is in one food with what is in the others. For example, it is safe to eat some salt-cured or smoked meats, but don't eat them all the time. Eat many green, yellow, and orange vegetables and fruits; they are all needed in the diet for many good reasons. If you include high-fiber foods and reduce your fat intake as well, you have every reason to feel confident that you are providing your body with the best nutrition at the lowest possible risk.

Notes

1. M. B. Grosvenor, Diet and colon cancer, *Nutrition and the M.D.,* April 1989; S. A. Bingham, Meat, starch, and nonstarch polysaccharides and large bowel cancer, *American Journal of Clinical Nutrition* 48 (1988): 762–776; B. S. Reddy and coauthors, Nutrition and its relationship to cancer, *Advances in Cancer Research* 32 (1980): 238–245.

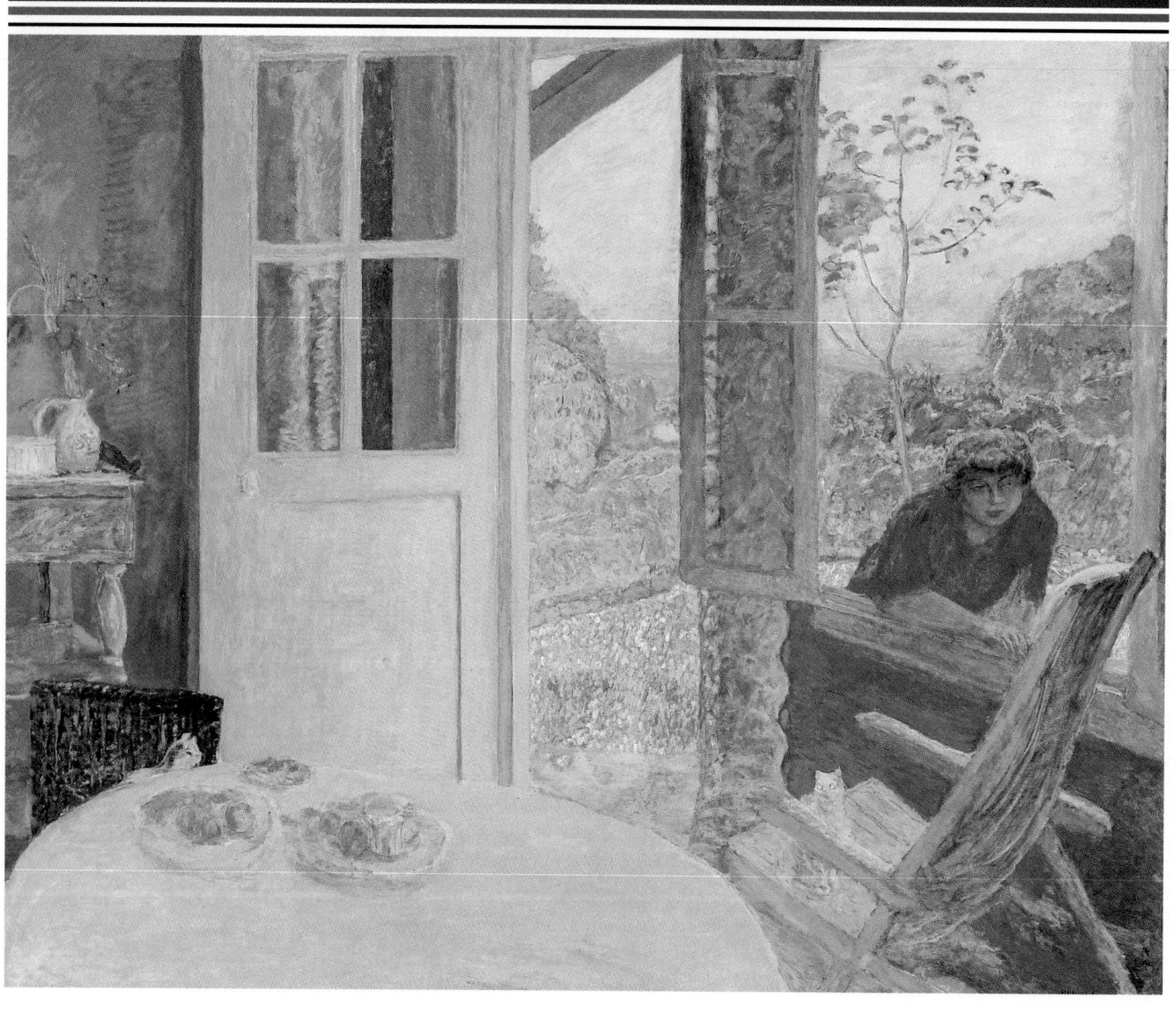

Pierre Bonnard, Dining Room in the Country, *1913, The John R. Van Derlip Fund, The Minneapolis Institute of Arts.*

CHAPTER

19

Diets Modified in kCalories: II. Maintenance and Low-kCalorie Diets

CONTENTS

CHAPTER
19
Obesity occurs to an alarming extent and is on the rise in developed countries. In the United States 10 to 25 percent of all teenagers and 25 to 50 percent of all adults are obese. This chapter discusses the problems of overweight and obesity and introduces the most widely used exchange system for diet planning, the one employed to plan diets for weight control, diabetes, and other conditions requiring regulation of kcalories and energy nutrients.

Diet Planning Using Exchange Lists

Unlike a food group system that sorts foods by protein, vitamin, and mineral contents only, the exchange system pays special attention to energy; proportions of carbohydrate, fat, and protein; and portion sizes. The U.S. exchange system described here consists of six lists of foods. Each list has a typical member—with portion size specified—that you can remember it by. All the food portions on a list contain approximately the same amount of energy and the same amounts of protein, fat, and carbohydrate. Figure 19–1 on pp. 492–493 shows the six lists and their typical representatives. Table 19–1 provides the energy, protein, fat, and carbohydrate values that pertain to each list. Appendix E provides detailed exchange lists.

The exchange system encourages the user to think of nonfat milk as milk and of whole milk as milk with added fat. A glass of whole milk is described, in fact, as "one milk plus two fats," and a glass of low-fat milk as "one milk

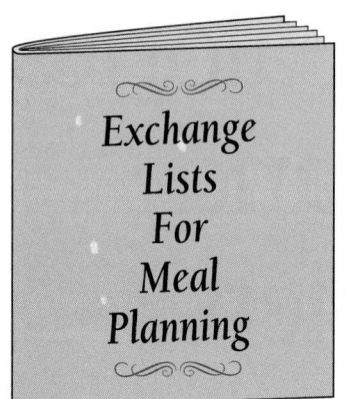

*Exchange
Lists
For
Meal
Planning*

The exchange lists were originally developed for people with diabetes. They proved so useful, however, that they are now in general use for diet planning. Weight Watchers, a well-known organization that helps people control their weight while eating a nutritious diet, bases its eating plans on the exchange system. Other kinds of exchange systems also exist—for example, those based on the sodium content of foods.

TABLE 19–1   **The Six Exchange Lists**

LIST	PORTION SIZE	CARBOHYDRATE (g)	PROTEIN (g)	FAT (g)	ENERGY (kcal)
Starches/breads[a]	1 slice	15	3	Trace	80
Meats[b]	1 oz				
Lean		—	7	3	55
Medium-fat		—	7	5	75
High-fat		—	7	8	100
Vegetables[c]	½ c	5	2	—	25
Fruits	1 portion	15	—	—	60
Milks	1 c				
Nonfat		12	8	Trace	90
Low-fat		12	8	5	120
Whole		12	8	8	150
Fats	1 tsp	—	—	5	45

Note: This is the U.S. exchange system. The complete lists are provided in Appendix E.

[a]This list includes starchy vegetables such as lima beans and corn, as well as cereal, bread, pasta, and other grain products. For portion sizes, see Appendix E.
[b]This list includes cheese and peanut butter, as well as meat.
[c]This list includes low-kcalorie vegetables only.

plus one fat." The vegetable list includes only low-kcalorie vegetables, so that a half-cup of any vegetable on the list will provide about 25 kcalories. The fruit list specifies "no added sugar or sugar syrup." Portion sizes are adjusted so that fruit portions are equal in kcalories. One small banana counts as "two fruits." A piece of cherry pie, however, is *not* "a fruit." It *includes* a fruit if it contains 12 large cherries, but it also includes bread and fat exchanges and added sugar. Thus a piece of cherry pie might be counted as "one fruit, two breads, and three fats with 3 teaspoons of sugar." The bread list also specifies portion sizes and makes clear which grain products contain added fat. Corn, lima beans, and other starchy vegetables are listed with the breads, not the vegetables, because they are similar to breads in energy and carbohydrate content.

Meats and cheeses are separated into three categories—lean, medium fat, and high fat. By including such items as bacon and olives, the fat list alerts the user to foods that are unexpectedly high in fat kcalories.

Most often, the dietitian assumes the responsibility of planning an exchange list diet. However, those interested in intelligently managing their own diets find the exchange system a useful and versatile tool for many purposes. The system works equally well for planning a weight-loss diet, an ordinary nutritious diet, a fat-controlled diet (see Chapter 22), or any other diet, including a diabetic diet. The accompanying box, "How to Plan a Diet Using Exchange Lists," shows how to use this diet plan effectively.

How to Plan a Diet Using Exchange Lists

The dietitian usually assumes the responsibility of planning the diabetic diet. A careful look at the individual's diet history helps to plan a diet that will meet both the person's needs and the needs imposed by the disease.

At first, using exchange lists to plan diets may take hours. However, with practice, dietitians learn to prepare complete diet plans in a matter of minutes by using a few shortcuts. This diet plan follows the shortcut steps.

1. *Estimate desirable body weight.*
   Males: Allow 106 lb for the first 5 ft; then add 6 lb for each inch over 5 ft.
   Females: Allow 100 lb for the first 5 ft; then add 5 lb for each inch over 5 ft.
   Adjustment: Add 10% for large-framed individuals; subtract 10% for small-framed individuals.
   Children: Refer to the growth charts in Appendix B.

   This example uses a woman of medium-frame who is 5 ft 8 inches tall and weighs 160 lb. IBW is:

$$100 \text{ lb} + (5 \text{ lb} \times 8 \text{ inches}) = 140 \text{ lb}.$$

   By comparing the person's actual weight to her desirable weight, you can determine whether or not she needs a weight-loss or weight-maintenance diet. For the person in our example, a weight-loss diet is in order.

(continued)

2. *Calculate energy needs in kcalories.* Multiply desirable body weight by 15 for men and active women; by 13 for most women, sedentary men, and adults over age 55; and by 10 for sedentary women, obese people, and sedentary adults over age 55.[1]

Children require about 1000 kcal for the first year of life plus 100 kcal per year, up to 2000 kcal at age 11. From age 12 to 15, add 100 kcal per year for girls and 200 kcal per year for boys. Remember, this is an estimate, and children's needs depend more on size than on age.

In this example, the woman is sedentary and needs the following number of kcalories:

$$140 \text{ lb} \times 10 \text{ kcal/lb} = 1{,}400 \text{ kcal.}$$

Note: The Harris-Benedict equation shown in Table 18–2 on p. 463 can also be used to determine energy requirements.

3. *Determine the grams of carbohydrate, fat, and protein.*

- 55 to 60% of the kcalories from carbohydrate.
- 25 to 30% of the kcalories from fat.
- 12 to 20% of the kcalories from protein.

For 1400 kcal, this division of kcalories translates into nutrients as follows:
Carbohydrate:

$$55\% \times 1400 \text{ kcal} = 770 \text{ kcal.} \qquad 770 \text{ kcal} \div 4 \text{ kcal/g} = 193 \text{ g.}$$
$$60\% \times 1400 \text{ kcal} = 840 \text{ kcal.} \qquad 840 \text{ kcal} \div 4 \text{ kcal/g} = 210 \text{ g.}$$

(The woman needs between 193 and 210 g carbohydrate.)
Fat:

$$25\% \times 1400 \text{ kcal} = 350 \text{ kcal.} \qquad 350 \text{ kcal} \div 9 \text{ kcal/g} = 39 \text{ g.}$$
$$30\% \times 1400 \text{ kcal} = 420 \text{ kcal.} \qquad 420 \text{ kcal} \div 9 \text{ kcal/g} = 47 \text{ g.}$$

(The woman needs between 39 and 47 g fat.)

TABLE 19–2   **Diet Patterns for Different Energy Intakes**

EXCHANGE	Energy Level (kcal)[a]						
	1200	1500	1800	2000	2200	2600	3000
Starches/breads	4	6	8	9	11	13	15
Meats	5	5	5	6	6	7	8
Vegetables	3	3	4	5	5	6	6
Fruits	3	3	4	4	4	5	6
Milks	2	3	3	3	3	3	3
Fats	4	5	6	7	8	10	12

[a]These patterns of exchanges supply about 30% of the kcalories as fat, in accordance with the view that a moderate fat intake is desirable.

TABLE 19–3   **A Day's Exchanges for a Sample 1400-kCalorie**

EXCHANGE ITEM	NUMBER OF EXCHANGES	CARBOHYDRATE (g)	PROTEIN (g)	FAT (g)	kCALORIES
Starches/breads	6	90	18	—	480
Meats (lean)	4	—	28	12	220
Vegetables	4	20	8	—	100
Fruits	4	60	—	—	240
Milks (nonfat)	2	24	16	—	180
Fats	4	—	—	20	180
		194	70	32	1400

ªThis diet supplies 55% of the energy as carbohydrate, 20% as protein, and 21% as fat. The percentages do not add up to 100% because the kcalorie values used in the exchange system are approximations, and percentages are rounded off.

Protein:

   $12\% \times 1400 \text{ kcal} = 168 \text{ kcal.}$ $168 \text{ kcal} \div 4 \text{ kcal/g} = 42 \text{ g.}$

   $20\% \times 1400 \text{ kcal} = 280 \text{ kcal.}$ $280 \text{ kcal} \div 4 \text{ kcal/g} = 70 \text{ g.}$

(The woman needs between 42 to 70 g protein.)

4. *Translate the diet prescription into a meal plan.* Table 19–2 provides examples of diet patterns for different energy intakes. Using that table as a guide, a dietitian might select the pattern of exchanges shown in Table 19–3, columns 1 and 2. The dietitian could then calculate the grams of energy nutrients by referring to Table 19–1 on p. 488 and come up with the next three columns in Table 19–3. Total energy and percentages of kcalories contributed by each nutrient are shown at the bottom of the table. As you can see, the diet delivers 55 percent of its energy from carbohydrate, 20 percent from protein, and 21 percent from fat, a balance that meets recommended standards.

With this information in hand, the dietitian and client can begin to fill in the plan with real foods to create a menu (see Figure 19–1 on pp. 492–493 and Appendix E). Developing menus takes time and patience; it is a matter of trial and error until the actual plan comes "close enough" to the goals.

Exchange lists ease the task of tailoring a diet to an individual's preferences. For example, the planner can substitute one bread exchange (80 kcalories, 15 grams carbohydrate) for one and a half fruit exchanges (90 kcalories, 15 grams carbohydrate). If the client doesn't drink milk (90 kcalories, 12 grams carbohydrate), the planner can substitute a half serving of bread and 1 ounce of lean meat (95 kcalories, 8 grams carbohydrate). Adjusting the diet to the client's preferences helps to ensure compliance with it.

FIGURE 19–1   **The Exchange System**

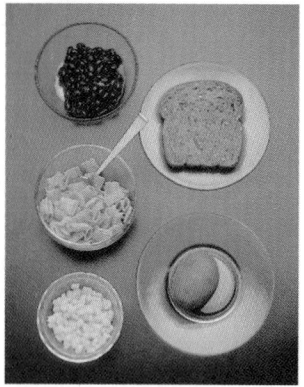

1. Starch/Breads

1 slice bread is like:

   ¾ c ready-to-eat cereal.

   ⅓ c cooked beans.

   ½ c corn.

   1 small (3-oz) potato.

(1 bread = 15 g carbohydrate, 3 g protein, trace of fat, and 80 kcal.)

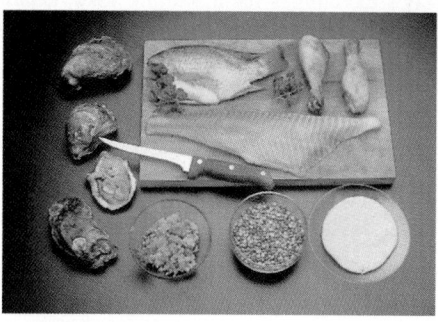

2a. Meats (Lean)

1 oz lean meat is like:

   1 oz chicken meat without the skin.

   1 oz any fish.

   ¼ c canned tuna.

   1 oz low-fat cheese.[a]

(1 lean meat = 7 g protein, 3 g fat, and 55 kcal.)

(One 3-oz portion of meat [such as a hamburger patty] = 3 meat exchanges.

One meat exchange = ⅓ of a 3-oz hamburger patty.)

[a]Cheeses are grouped with milk in food group plans because of their calcium content but with meats in this system because, like meat, they contribute kcalories from protein and fat and have negligible carbohydrate content.

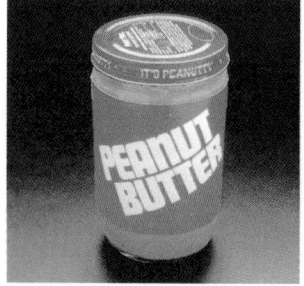

2e. Peanut Butter

Peanut butter is like a meat in terms of its protein content. It is estimated as:

   1 tbsp peanut butter = 1 high-fat meat.

(1 tbsp peanut butter = 7 g protein, 8 g fat, and 100 kcal.)

(Don't stop reading now, and don't swear off peanut butter, necessarily. You'll need to read about the polyunsaturated character of its fat in Chapter 3, and the B vitamin contributions it makes in Chapter 7, before deciding how much of a place it should have in your diet.)

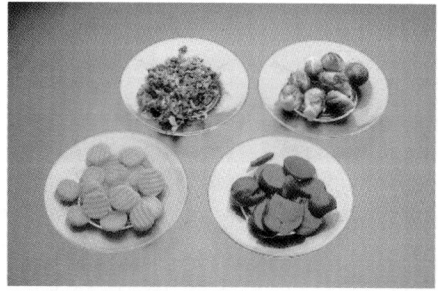

3. Vegetables

½ c carrots is like:

   ½ c greens.

   ½ c brussels sprouts.

   ½ c beets.

(1 vegetable = 5 g carbohydrate, 2 g protein, and 25 kcal.)

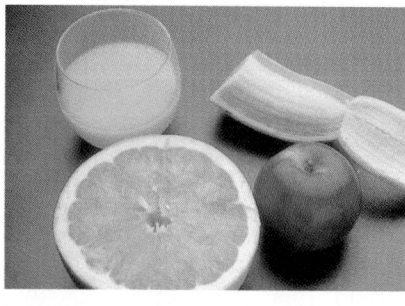

4. Fruits

½ small banana is like:

   1 small apple.

   ½ grapefruit.

   ½ c orange juice.

(1 fruit = 15 g carbohydrate and 60 kcal.)

FIGURE 19–1 (*continued*)

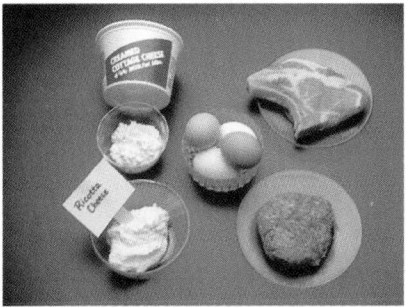

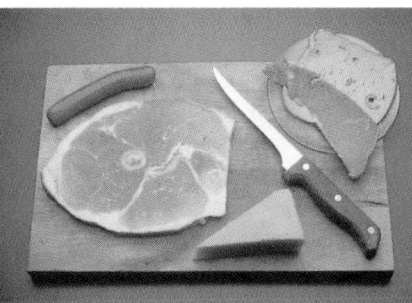

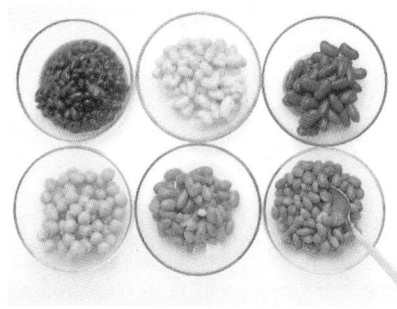

2b. Meats Medium-Fat

1 oz medium-fat meat is like 1 oz lean meat in protein content, but has 5 g fat (2 g more fat than lean meat).
Examples:

   1 oz pork loin.

   1 egg.

   ¼ c creamed cottage cheese.[a]

(1 medium-fat meat = 7 g protein, 5 g fat, and about 75 kcal.)

2c. Meats High-Fat

1 oz high-fat meat is like 1 oz lean meat in protein content but is estimated to have an **extra "1 fat"**—that is, to have the 3 g fat of a lean meat and 5 g additional fat.
Examples:

   1 oz country-style ham.

   1 oz Cheddar cheese.[a]

   1 small hot dog (frankfurter).[b]

(1 high-fat meat = 7 g protein, 8 g fat, and 100 kcal.)

[b]The frankfurter counts as 1 high-fat meat exchange plus 1 fat exchange.

2d. Legumes

Legumes are an odd kind of plant food. They are like meats because they are rich in protein and iron, but many are lower in fat than meat. Besides, they contain a lot of starch. They can be treated as follows:

   1 c legumes = 1 lean meat + 2 starch.

(1 c legumes = 30 g carbohydrate, 13 g protein, 3 + g fat, and 215 kcal.) Legumes can also be considered similar to breads in being rich in complex carbohydrate, and the additional protein can be ignored. However, this treatment underestimates their kcalorie value, especially that of the higher-fat legumes such as peanuts.

   Whatever you do with legumes on paper, however, use them often in cooking. You will learn many more reasons why they are an inexpensive, nutritious, high-quality, and health-promoting food.

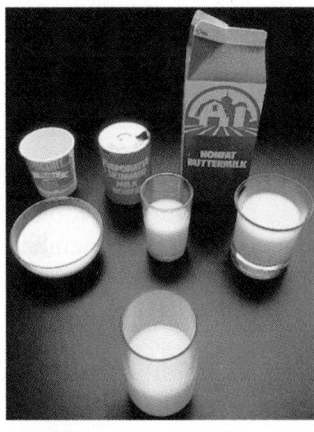

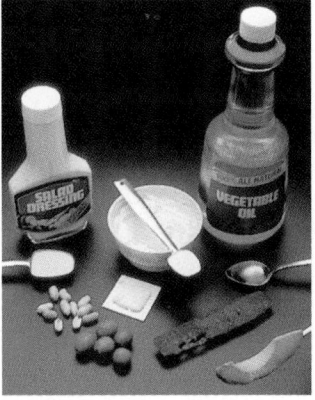

5. Milks

1 c nonfat milk is like:

   1 c nonfat yogurt, plain.

   1 c nonfat buttermilk.

   ½ c evaporated nonfat milk.

(1 milk = 12 g carbohydrate, 8 g protein, trace of fat, and 90 kcal.)

6. Fats

1 tsp butter is like:

   1 tsp margarine.

   1 tsp any oil.

   1 tbsp salad dressing.

   1 strip crisp bacon.

   5 large olives.

   10 whole Virginia peanuts.

(1 fat = 5 g fat and 45 kcal.)

The accompanying sample menu shows one possible way to approximate the goals of a 1400-kcalorie diet. You might see ways to improve it, or you might want to try planning another day's meals to see how close you get to distributing energy and carbohydrate as recommended.

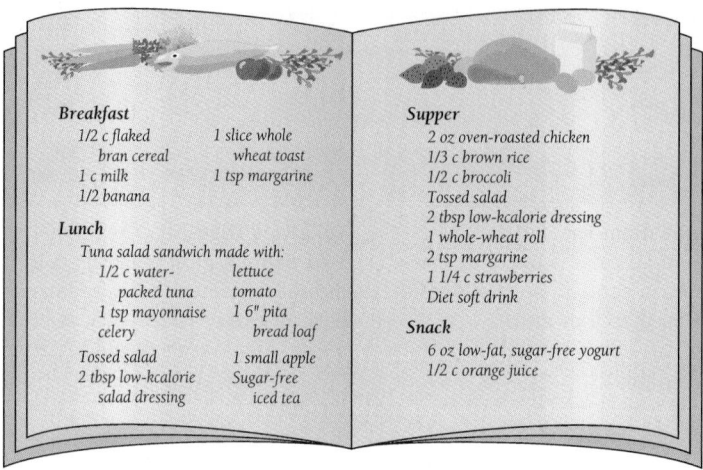

Breakfast
1/2 c flaked
  bran cereal
1 c milk
1/2 banana
1 slice whole
  wheat toast
1 tsp margarine

Lunch
Tuna salad sandwich made with:
1/2 c water-
  packed tuna
1 tsp mayonnaise
celery
Tossed salad
2 tbsp low-kcalorie
  salad dressing
lettuce
tomato
1 6" pita
  bread loaf
1 small apple
Sugar-free
  iced tea

Supper
2 oz oven-roasted chicken
1/3 c brown rice
1/2 c broccoli
Tossed salad
2 tbsp low-kcalorie dressing
1 whole-wheat roll
2 tsp margarine
1 1/4 c strawberries
Diet soft drink

Snack
6 oz low-fat, sugar-free yogurt
1/2 c orange juice

Sample 1400 kCalorie Diet Menu

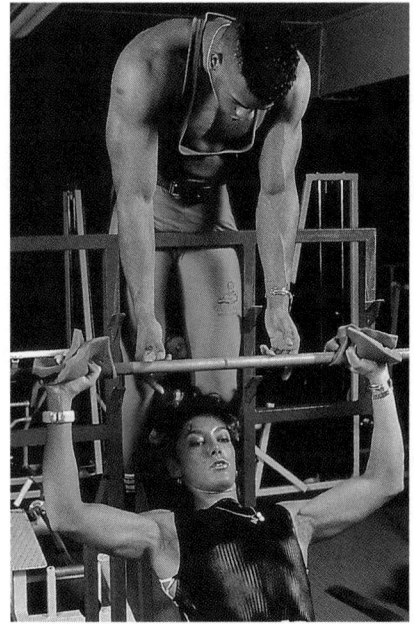

It is not body weight but the proportion of the weight contributed by lean body mass that makes a difference.

overweight: body weight 10% above the average table weight.

obesity: excessive body fatness; often loosely defined as a condition of being overweight by 20% or more.

Weight: How Much Is Too Much?

It isn't always possible to tell from the bathroom scale if a person is overweight, because body weight says little about body fat. A person who doesn't seem to weigh too much may be too fat; a person who seems to weigh too much may not be too fat. An athlete, whose muscles are well developed and whose bones have become well mineralized by responding to constant stress, may weigh the same as a sedentary person of the same height, yet the athlete may be at the right weight, and the sedentary person may be too fat. Chapter 9 provided a thorough discussion of body weight and included shortcut tips for assessing body fat. Chapter 10 and Appendix B describe clinical methods for assessing body fat, including fatfold tests, bioelectrical impedance, and underwater weighing.

Granted that weight poorly measures body fatness, it is still the measure people most commonly use as an index of body composition. Ideal weights are estimated from formulas such as the one on p. 236 or from tables (see p. 235 and the inside back cover). The person whose weight is 10 percent above the table weight is considered overweight. A person weighing 20 percent or more above the table weight is considered obese. Obviously, many problems exist with defining ideal weight, and any calculation of ideal weight must be interpreted less cautiously.

Weight Reduction: The Need

Obesity is a major nutrition problem in developed countries. Obesity brings many health hazards with it, as Table 19–4 demonstrates. Insurance companies report that overweight people die younger from a host of causes, including heart attacks, strokes, and complications of diabetes. The greater the degree of overweight, the higher the excess death rate, especially in the young. Even after the effects of diagnosed diseases are discounted, the risk of death remains twice as great for obese people, especially for those with lifelong weight problems.

The location of fat on the body may be as critical as (or even more critical than) the total amount. Fat around the abdomen may represent a greater risk to health than fat elsewhere on the body. Abdominal fat (most common in males), even in the absence of obesity, is associated with heart disease, diabetes, and hypertension. In contrast, fat around the hips and thighs (most common in females) seems relatively harmless. If weight loss is to benefit health, then it should reduce upper-body fat. A simple comparison of the waist and hip measurements better assesses abdominal fat than other methods and is quickly becoming a standard part of the assessment of body fatness.

Beyond all these hazards is the risk incurred by millions of obese people throughout much of their lives—the risk of ill-advised, misguided dieting.

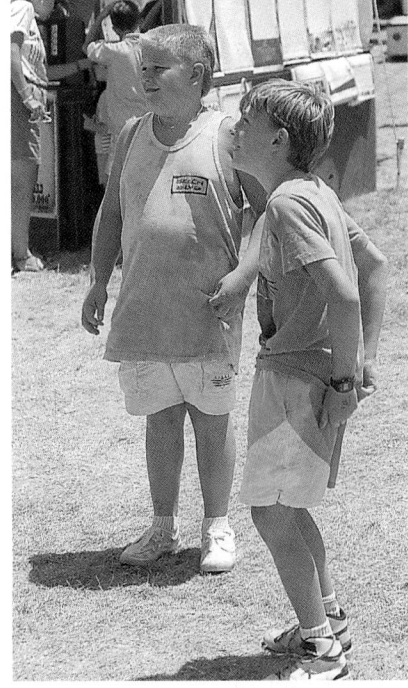

The overweight child who becomes obese invites a host of health risks and social disadvantages to follow in adult life.

TABLE 19–4   **Health Hazards Associated with Obesity**

IN GENERAL:

- Abdominal hernias
- Accidents
- Arthritis—especially in the knees, hips, and lower spine
- Complications after surgery
- Gout
- High blood cholesterol concentrations (a risk factor for coronary heart disease)
- Hypertension
- Respiratory problems
- Varicose veins

FOR MEN:

- Risk of cancers of the colon, rectum, and prostate gland

FOR WOMEN:

- Gynecological irregularities
- Pregnancy-induced hypertension
- Risk of cancers of the breast, uterus, ovaries, gallbladder, and bile ducts

Some fad diets are more hazardous to health than obesity itself. Research suggests that some very-low-kcalorie diets, when used without medical supervision, can lead to many side effects, including anemia, constipation, diarrhea, menstrual irregularities, gallbladder disease, and heart malfunctions.[2] Psychological problems associated with struggling to lose weight and self-blame for relapses are significant and negative effects of dieting.[3]

Social and economic disadvantages also plague the overweight person. Obese people are less often sought after for marriage, pay higher insurance premiums, meet discrimination when applying for college admissions and jobs, can't find attractive clothes easily, and are limited in their choice of sports.

Causes of Obesity

Excess body fat accumulates when people take in more food energy than they need to provide for the day's metabolic, muscular, and digestive activities. Why do they do this? Is it genetic? Metabolic? Psychological? Behavioral? Biological? All of these? Perhaps obesity has many causes; some experts in the field speak of many different *obesities*.

One way to approach the question of what causes obesity is to ask whether it is hereditary. One way to study this question in human beings is to study twins who have been raised by different families. If genes determine fatness, both twins will be equally fat or thin. But if the environment is responsible, then each twin will resemble the family he or she grows up in. Another approach is to study adopted children to see whether they resemble their natural or adoptive parents. Studies of both types suggest that the tendency to obesity is inherited but that the environment is influential in the sense that it can prevent or permit the development of obesity when the potential is there.

That obesity runs in families, though, does not support a hereditary cause alone, for clearly, learning plays a role. Habits learned in childhood tend to persist throughout life. Food-centered families encourage such behaviors as overeating at mealtimes, rapid eating, excessive snacking, and eating to meet needs other than hunger. Children readily imitate overeating parents, and their behaviors at the table tend to persist outside the home.

Still another approach to the question of what causes obesity is to study people from childhood on, asking the question, Do fat babies become fat adults? Several studies show that most fat babies don't become fat adults; they grow out of their obesity in childhood. However, most overweight *children* (80 percent) remain overweight into adulthood.

Research on fat cells suggests a possible reason why childhood-onset obesity persists. Simply stated, early overfeeding is thought by some researchers to stimulate fat cells so that they increase abnormally in *number*. The number of fat cells is thought to become fixed by adulthood; if it is, then a gain or loss in weight thereafter can take place only through an increase or decrease in the *size* of the fat cells. People with the greatest number of fat cells are least likely to lose weight successfully.

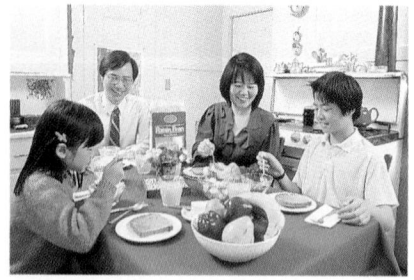

Family eating habits, as well as hereditary factors, influence the risk of obesity.

However, fat is always hard to lose, even if it is due to an increase in cell size. One possible explanation involves the hormone insulin. Enlarged fat cells become sluggish in their responses to insulin (the hormone that allows glucose to enter cells and promotes the making and storage of fat), even though insulin concentrations are high.[4] The delayed response allows excess glucose to remain in the bloodstream longer than normal, which, in turn, stimulates the insulin-producing cells of the pancreas to secrete more insulin. When the fat cells finally respond, they store more fat than normal in response to the raised insulin level. As if this were not enough, enlarged fat cells tend also to be insensitive to hormones that promote fat breakdown. Weight loss restores insulin levels to normal, but it first has to be achieved against great odds.

Another popular explanation as to what causes obesity is the set-point theory. Subscribers to the set-point theory hold that the body sends out signals to establish, regulate, and maintain a set body weight. These signals do more than maintain a constant body weight; they *defend* that body weight when it is challenged. People who have lost 25 percent of their body weight by restricting their dietary intake return to their normal weight when allowed to eat as they please. Similarly, people who increase their food energy intake and gain 15 to 25 percent of their body weight return to their normal weights when allowed to eat as usual. This tenacious defense of body weight deters obese people from losing weight and promotes the regain of any weight that is successfully lost.

Still another point of view is that obesity is environmentally determined. Proponents of this view hold that people overeat because they are pushed to do so by factors in their surroundings—foremost among them, the availability of a multitude of delectable foods.

Psychological stimuli also trigger inappropriate eating behavior in some people. Appropriate eating behavior is a response to hunger. However, eating behavior easily becomes conditioned to occur automatically in response to a wide variety of inappropriate stimuli, because food itself rewards the eater with its good taste and calming effects. Inappropriate eating becomes a routine in the brain's response to stressors such as pain, anxiety, arousal, excitement, and even the presence of food. On experiencing these stimuli, the brain responds by producing endogenous opiates. They soothe pain and lessen arousal, and they have two effects on energy balance. They enhance appetite for palatable foods, and they reduce physical activity. Combine these effects with a tendency to be supersensitive to particular stressors anyway, and one is likely to overeat and gain weight in response to any kind of stress, positive or negative. (What do I do when I'm depressed? Eat. What do I do when I'm excited? Eat!) Some people do respond to anxiety, or in fact to any kind of arousal short of severe stress, by eating.

Food behavior is also intimately connected to deep emotional needs such as the primitive fear of starvation and the infant's association of food with mother love. Yearnings, cravings, and addictions with profound psychological significance can express themselves in people's food behavior. An emotionally insecure person might eat rather than call a friend and risk rejection. Another person might use eating to relieve boredom or to ward off depression.

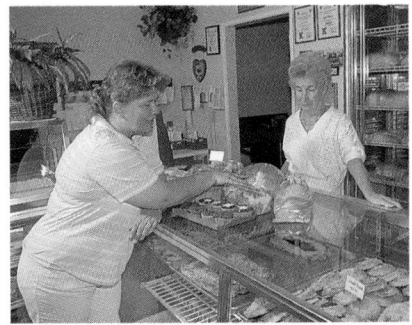

The environment sometimes motivates inappropriate eating behaviors.

Several terms related to eating include *hunger, appetite,* and *satiety.* The distinctions among these terms are as follows:

hunger: the physiological need to eat; a negative, unpleasant sensation.

appetite: the desire to eat, which normally accompanies hunger; by itself a pleasant sensation.

satiety (sat-EYE-uh-tee): the feeling of fullness or satisfaction at the end of a meal that prompts a person to stop eating.

The possible causes of obesity mentioned so far all relate to the input side of the energy equation. What about output? People may be obese because they eat too much, but another possibility is that they spend too little energy. The control of hunger/appetite actually works quite well in active people and only fails when activity falls below a certain minimum level. Obese people under close observation are often seen to eat less than lean people, but they are sometimes so extraordinarily inactive or efficient in their way of moving that they still manage to have an energy surplus.

No two people are alike either physically or psychologically, and the causes of obesity may be as varied as the people who are obese. Many factors may contribute to the problem in each person. Given this complexity, it is obvious that there is no panacea. The top priority should be prevention, but where prevention has failed, the treatment of obesity must involve a simultaneous attack on many fronts.

Strategies for Weight Loss

The only realistic and sensible way for the obese person to achieve and maintain a healthy body weight is to cut kcalories, to increase activity, and to maintain this changed lifestyle for life. This is a tall order. Only 5 to 10 percent of people who try meet with long-term success.[5] To succeed means modifying all the attitudes and behaviors that have contributed to the problem in the first place, sometimes against forces that can't be changed. Still, it can be, and has been, done successfully. A multiple approach works best, involving changes in diet, exercise, behavior, and attitude.

The way a person loses weight is a highly individual matter. Two weight-loss plans may both be successful and yet have little or nothing in common. Dietitians often recommend weight-reduction diets based on the exchange list system. However, many other weight-reduction diets are in use. Some are adequate; others are not. Table 19–5 describes a system to evaluate weight-loss diets. Inappropriate ways of treating obesity are listed in the Miniglossary of Poor Treatment Choices for Obesity on p. 500.

To heighten the sense of individuality, the following sections are written in terms of advice to "you." This is not intended to put "you" under pressure to take it personally, but to give you the illusion of listening in on a conversation in which an obese person (with, say, 50 pounds to lose) is being competently counseled by someone familiar with the techniques known to be effective. Margin notes at intervals highlight the principles involved.

Diet

No particular diet is magical, and no particular food must either be included or avoided. You are the one who will have to live with the diet, so you had better be involved in its planning. Don't think of it as a diet you are going "on"—because then you may be tempted to go "off." The diet can be called successful only if the pounds do not return. Think of it as an eating plan that

■ Be involved in planning your own diet.

TABLE 19–5   **How to Evaluate Weight-Loss Diets**

With a balanced perspective on foods and a sense of what is important in diet planning and what is not, you can evaluate the many different diets people consume. Here's a summary of the questions you might ask. Start with 100 points, and subtract if any of these criteria are not met:

1.   Does the diet provide a reasonable number of kcalories (about 10 kcal per pound of current weight and not fewer than 1200 kcal for the average-sized person)? If not, give it a **minus 10.**

2.   Does it provide enough, but not too much, protein (at least the recommended intake of RDA, but not more than twice that much)? If not, **minus 10.**

3.   Does it provide enough fat for balance and satiety, but not so much fat as to go against current recommendations (say, between 20 and 30% of the kcalories from fat)? If not, **minus 10.**

4.   Does it provide enough carbohydrate to spare protein and prevent ketosis (100 g carbohydrate for the average-sized person or at least 55% of total kcalories)? Is it mostly complex carbohydrate (not more than 10% of the kcalories as concentrated sugar)? If no to either or both, **minus 10.**

5.   Does it offer a balanced assortment of vitamins and minerals from meats, vegetables (especially dark green and yellow ones), fruits (especially citrus fruits), breads, cereals, legumes, and low-fat milk products? If a food group is omitted (for example, meats), is a suitable substitute provided? For *each* food group omitted and not adequately substituted for, **minus 10.**

6.   Does it offer variety, in the sense that different foods can be selected each day? If you'd class it as "monotonous," **minus 10.**

7.   Does it consist of ordinary foods that are available locally (for example, in the main grocery stores) at the prices people normally pay? Or does the dieter have to buy special, expensive, or unusual foods to adhere to the diet? If you'd class it as "bizarre" or "requiring unusual foods," **minus 10.**

you will adopt for life. It must consist of foods that you like, that are available to you, and that are within your means.

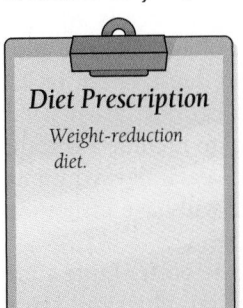

Diet Prescription

Weight-reduction diet.

To be successful, people have to first lose weight; then, maintain the weight loss. If you adopt an "eating plan" rather than a "diet," you can be practicing maintenance behaviors all the time you are losing weight. You will be ready to succeed for the rest of your life, once you arrive at your goal weight.

Choose an energy level you can live with. Nutritional adequacy is difficult for most people to achieve on fewer than 1,200 kcalories a day—1,000 at the very least. A rule of thumb is that you need at least 10 kcalories per pound of current weight. You will experience a healthier and more successful weight loss with a small kcalorie deficit that provides an adequate intake than with a larger kcalorie deficit that creates feelings of starvation and deprivation, which can lead to an irresistible urge to binge. Table 19–2 shows samples of balanced weight-

▮ Keep in mind that you will want to maintain your lost weight. Practice the needed behaviors as you go.

▮ Adopt a realistic plan.

MINIGLOSSARY of Poor Treatment Choices for Obesity

diet pills: pills that depress the appetite temporarily; often, physician-prescribed amphetamines (speed). It is generally agreed that these drugs are of little value for weight loss and that their use can cause a dangerous dependency; over-the-counter diet pills containing phenylpropanolamine hydrochloride carry the risk of stroke.

diuretics: pills that promote water excretion; dieters sometimes take these pills because they believe their weight excesses are due to water accumulation.

fad diets: diets designed to bring about quick weight loss that are usually unbalanced nutritionally and are sometimes dangerous.

HCG or **human chorionic gonadotropin** (core-ee-ON-ic go-nad-o-TROPE-in): a hormone excreted in the urine of pregnant women believed to enhance weight loss and reduce hunger. It does neither.

intestinal bypass surgery: surgery that involves removing or disconnecting a portion of the small intestine to reduce absorption of energy nutrients. Such surgery has severe side effects, including liver failure and deranged fluid and electrolyte balance.

very-low-kcalorie diets (VLCD): diets that provide from 400 to 800 kcal per day to promote weight loss; they may be appropriate for carefully selected and supervised clients, but in general are often nutritionally inadequate, and clients on these diets frequently meet with failure.

---

loss diets using the exchange system. (Dietitians frequently recommend the exchange system for weight-loss diets.)

This recommendation probably doesn't apply to people who are morbidly obese (twice their ideal body weights). Such individuals may need to lose weight more quickly, because they are at high risk for serious medical problems or may already have serious medical problems.

Put diet adequacy high on your list of priorities. This is a way of putting yourself first. "I like me, and I'm going to take good care of me" is the attitude to adopt. This means including low-kcalorie foods that are rich in valuable nutrients; tasty vegetables and fruits; whole-grain breads and cereals; modest portions of lean, protein-rich foods like poultry, fish, and veal; nutritious meat alternates like dried beans and peas; and low-fat milk products such as nonfat milk and yogurt. Within these categories, learn what foods you like, and use them often. If you plan resolutely to include a certain number of servings of food from each of these categories each day, you may be so busy making sure you get what you need that you will have little time or appetite left for high-kcalorie or empty-kcalorie foods.

Measure your dietary fat with extra caution. A slip of the butter knife adds even more kcalories than a slip of the sugar spoon. Even given the same number of kcalories, less fat in the diet means less fat in the body. Dietary fat correlates positively with body fat, whereas dietary carbohydrate and fiber correlate negatively with body fat.[6]

Learn to use water, not food, to satisfy thirst. A generous water intake will fill your stomach between meals and keep you busy. It will dilute the met-

■ Make the diet adequate by emphasizing nutrient-dense foods that you like.

■ Make tasty vegetables and fruits central to your weight-control plan.

■ Emphasize complex carbohydrate–rich foods high in bulk.

■ Use fats cautiously.

■ Drink plenty of water.

abolic wastes you generate from breaking down fat so that you can excrete them easily. Drinking water is a kcalorie-free oral pleasure; cultivate it enthusiastically.

Keep a food diary (see p. 231), and take well-spaced weighings so you can see your progress. If you see a weight gain and your diary shows you have strictly followed your diet, this probably represents a shift in water weight. Many dieters experience a temporary plateau after about three weeks—not because they are slipping, but because they have gained water weight temporarily while they are still losing body fat. If you faithfully follow your plan, one day the plateau will break. You can tell from your frequent urination.

A dieter who undertakes an exercise program may arrive at a plateau for another reason: gain in muscle mass at the expense of body fat. Chapter 9 (pp. 206–208) discusses the role of exercise in a weight-control program.

Finally, plan to put as much effort into the maintenance of goal weight as you did into achieving it. No doubt you've heard someone say, "I've lost 200 pounds, but I was never more than 20 pounds overweight." What this person means is that frequent dieting alternating with weight gain is an expected pattern of life. With each bout of dieting, this person is trading a small amount of healthy lean body tissue for a slightly higher body fat content. This weight-cycling pattern, known as the ratchet or "yo-yo" effect of dieting, was illustrated in Figure 9–5 on p. 208.

Researchers studying this repeated pattern of weight loss and weight gain propose that the body adapts by increasing the efficiency with which it stores food energy, thus creating a "dieting-induced obesity."[7] This increased efficiency shows itself in a way familiar to dieters who have lost and gained—and lost and gained again. With each attempt, it becomes harder and takes longer to lose weight, and it becomes easier and quicker to gain it back. The body's metabolic rate has declined so that the same body weight can be maintained on a lower food energy intake than was required prior to the dieting cycle.

■ Anticipate a plateau (have realistic expectations from the start).

■ Learn, practice, and eat right for the rest of your life.

weight cycling: the effect that repeated cycles of weight loss and gain, without exercise, have on body composition. The body fat content increases and kcaloric needs fall after each round, making the next round of weight loss harder; popularly called the **ratchet** or **yo-yo effect**.

Exercise

The importance of physical activity in a weight-loss program was thoroughly discussed in Chapter 9. The health advantages of regular physical activity are well documented. Physical activity can help speed weight loss and can help you look, feel, and be healthier.

Behavior Modification

People who overeat often need to change their eating behavior—a part of our lives that most of us are only faintly aware of. How often do you put down your fork (if at all)? How often do you interrupt your eating to converse with a friend? How fast do you chew your food? Do you always clean your plate?

Behavioral psychologists view human behavior as regulated by environmental conditions, those that precede a behavior and those that follow it. A behavior occurs in response to cues or stimuli; the more intense these cues, the more likely the behavior is to occur. The behavior leads to consequences,

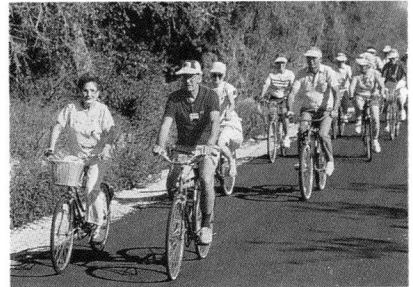

Enjoy exercise as a part of your weight-loss strategy.

stimulus: anything that triggers a certain behavior.

A conversation overheard in the cafeteria went like this:

Ms. A: I'm jogging half an hour every day to lose weight.

Ms. B: That's an awfully hard way to lose weight. Half an hour of jogging for someone your size would spend only 150 kcalories. I'd rather leave off a glass of milk every day, myself.

Ms. B is right, but she doesn't know the *other* advantages of jogging and the disadvantages of leaving off milk. If Ms. A keeps up her routine, her body will gradually change. She'll develop more lean tissue so that even her basal metabolic rate *at rest* will be faster. That means she'll burn more kcalories all day and night, not just during exercise. She'll have a higher kcalorie need, so she'll be able to drink that glass of milk and more besides, obtaining all the nutrients it offers. Also, her muscles will become conditioned, so that she'll be able to jog longer or faster and spend *more* energy. Meanwhile, Ms. B will be losing lean body mass as she sits around getting into poorer and poorer shape and, possibly, nutrition status. Let's hope Ms. A knows enough to defend her choice to Ms. B and perhaps even to persuade Ms. B to join her on her daily run.

and the more intense these are, the more or less likely the behavior is to occur again. Behavior modification involves manipulating these environmental conditions so as to favor the repeated occurrence of desired behaviors and extinguish the occurrence of unwanted behaviors.

Behavior modification can be used to change the behaviors of overeating and underexercising that lead to, and perpetuate, obesity. Books and pamphlets on behavior modification techniques abound, but it is beyond the scope of this book to list the techniques in detail. However, some suggestions include:

- *Control the stimuli that prompt you to eat inappropriately.* This involves purchasing appropriate foods, planning meals and activity times, and altering food-related activities.
- *Strengthen the cues to appropriate eating and physical activity.* Keep appropriate foods in the front of the refrigerator, and make exercise equipment easily available.
- *Alter eating behaviors.* By chewing food thoroughly and putting the fork down between bites, you will eat more slowly (overeaters eat faster than others).
- *Make sure that positive consequences follow your display of the desired behaviors.* Material rewards, such as buying a new dress when you reach a goal, or verbal rewards, such as praise from family and friends, are examples of positive consequences.
- *Monitor yourself.* Keep a record of your eating and activity behaviors against which to monitor future progress.
- *Learn about nutrition.* Be able to identify problem foods in your diet and make appropriate substitutions.
- *Increase your physical activity.* Park the car at the far end of the parking lot; use the stairs instead of the elevator; do a deep knee bend each time you get up from your chair. If you also incorporate regular aerobic

exercise into your schedule (see Chapter 9), your heart and lungs, as well as your muscles, will be fit.

■ *Change your outlook about weight reduction.* Set realistic goals, and think positively about reaching them.

From all the behavior changes available to you, you can choose the ones to begin with. Don't try to master them all at once. No one who attempts too many changes at one time is successful. Set your own priorities. Pick one trouble area that you think you can handle, start with that, and practice your strategy until it is habitual and automatic. Then you can select another trouble area to work on. Throughout the process, enjoy your new emerging self.

Keep in mind that it can be harder to maintain weight loss than to lose weight. On arriving at the goal weight after months of self-discipline and new habit formation, the victorious weight loser must at all cost avoid "celebrating" by resuming old eating habits. They are gone forever—remember? Membership in an ongoing weight-control organization and continued physical activity can provide indispensable support for the formerly overweight person who wants to remain trim.

Personal Attitude

When behavioral therapists view overeating and underexercising as maladaptive behaviors that people can change, they ignore the positive contribution that overeating plays in a person's life. They also miss that being overweight may have become a part of a person's identity. For many people, overeating and being overweight have become integral parts of activities, work, health, self-concept, and emotional states. To change diet and exercise behaviors without attention to the person's self-concept is to meet failure.

Many people overeat to cope with the stresses of life. To break out of that pattern, they must first identify the particular stressors that trigger their urges to overeat. Then, when faced with these situations, they must learn to practice problem-solving skills. When the problems that trigger the urge to overeat are dealt with in alternative ways, people may find that they eat less and that their eating behavior begins to occur appropriately in response to internal cues of hunger rather than inappropriately to external signals of stress. The message is that sound emotional health supports your ability to take care of your health in all ways—including nutrition, weight control, and fitness.

A surefire remedy for obesity has yet to be found, although most people find a combination of the approaches just described to be most effective. Diet and exercise shift energy balance so that more kcalories are being spent than taken in; the exercise maintains or even builds the lean body so that fat is preferentially lost and metabolic energy needs remain high; the behavior modification retrains habits so that once the weight is lost, it will not return; and improvement in inner self helps a person to manage life without a dependency on food. This treatment package requires time, individualization, and skilled health care providers.

CASE STUDY

Obesity

Allison is a 24-year-old woman of medium frame who weighs 185 pounds and is 5 feet 4 inches. She has been obese since her early teen years and has tried dieting unsuccessfully many times. Allison works as a telephone operator. She enjoys needlework and is an avid moviegoer. Although Allison has a few friends, she is frequently lonely. She wants to get out and socialize more frequently, but she feels awkward about her weight problem. Allison states that she has tried "every diet in the book." Now she has come to you for help.

Using the tables on the inside back cover or the formula shown on p. 236, estimate Allison's appropriate body weight. What is her percent ideal body weight?

Plan a diet for Allison at her current weight using the exchange list system. (In real life, you would be helping her plan this diet.) How many kcalories and how much carbohydrate, protein, and fat will you recommend? What tips can you give Allison to help her with her diet?

What things other than diet can help Allison reach and maintain a safer body weight? What important concept must Allison understand if she is to maintain her weight?

Study Questions

1. Describe how an exchange system works. Why is it well suited to a variety of dietary needs?
2. Discuss the limitations for the definition of ideal or desirable weight.
3. What are the dangers of excess weight? List factors that tend to increase the risk of obesity.
4. What considerations are essential to any successful weight-loss program?
5. What is weight cycling, and what are its risks?
6. What are the benefits of increased physical activity in a weight-loss program?
7. Describe the behavior modification techniques recommended for changing an individual's dietary habits.

Notes

1. M. J. Franz, Diabetes and nutrition: State of the science and the art, *Topics in Clinical Nutrition* 3 (1988): 1–16.
2. T. A. Wadden, T. B. Van Itallie, and G. L. Blackburn, Responsible and irresponsible use of very-low-calorie diets in the treatment of obesity, *Journal of the American Medical Association* 263 (1990): 83–85.

3. S. C. Wooley and D. M. Garner, Obesity treatment: The high cost of false hope, *Journal of the American Dietetic Association* 91 (1991): 1248–1251.

4. D. R. Krieger and L. Landsberg, Role of hormones in the etiology and pathogenesis of obesity, in *Obesity and Weight Control: The Health Professional's Guide to Understanding and Treatment,* eds. R. T. Frankle and M. Yang (Rockville, Md.: Aspen, 1988), pp. 35–54.

5. G. K. Goodrick and J. P. Foreyt, Why treatments for obesity don't last, *Journal of the American Dietetic Association* 91 (1991): 1243–1247.

6. D. M. Dreon and coauthors, Dietary fat: Carbohydrate ratio and obesity in middle-aged men, *American Journal of Clinical Nutrition* 47 (1988): 995–1000.

7. L. Buckmaster and K. D. Brownell, Behavior modification: The state of the art, in *Obesity and Weight Control: The Health Professional's Guide to Understanding and Treatment,* eds. R. T. Frankle and M. U. Yang (Rockville, Md.: Aspen, 1988), pp. 225–240.

19

Eating Disorders

When and how does dieting to lose weight progress to the point that it is dangerous and obsessive? The specific causes of eating disorders baffle clinicians. Some speculate that society's excessive pressure to be thin is to blame; others point to neurological links with depression and impulsive behaviors or other biological malfunctions; and still others believe the cause to be an inability to cope. Their point of agreement is that the disorders, like obesity itself, are most likely multifactorial—sociocultural, neurochemical, and psychological—and the treatment requires a multidisciplinary approach.

What are eating disorders?

The two major types of eating disorders of concern today are anorexia nervosa and bulimia. In the last decade a dramatic rise in the incidence of these disorders challenges health care professionals to prevent and treat them.

People with anorexia nervosa suffer from an extreme preoccupation with weight loss that seriously endangers their health and even lives. People with bulimia engage in episodes of binge eating alternating with periods of severe dieting or self-starvation. Some bulimics also follow binge eating with self-induced vomiting, laxative abuse, or diuretic abuse to "undo the damage."

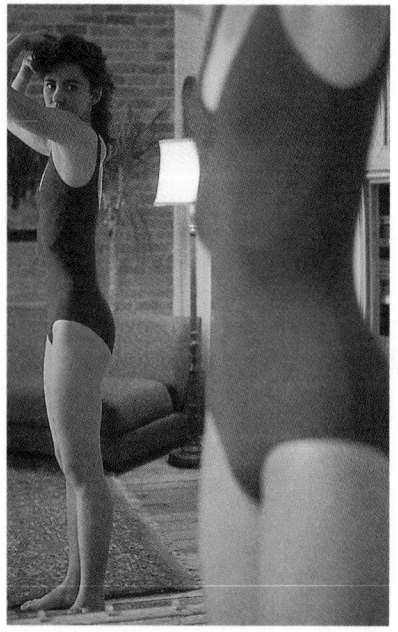

Women with anorexia nervosa see themselves as fat, even when they are dangerously underweight.

I remember a high school friend who had anorexia nervosa. She was a very bright girl and seemed to have it all. Is that uncommon for a girl with anorexia nervosa?

Not at all. The person with anorexia is almost always female and in her teens. She comes from an educated, middle- or upper-class family. A typical psychological profile includes depression, early developmental failure, and a characteristic cluster of family circumstances. Such families are usually mother dominated, with absentee or distant fathers. These families value achievement and outward appearances more than an inner sense of self-worth and self-actualization.

The person with anorexia nervosa is often a perfectionist who works hard to please her parents. She may identify so strongly with her parents' ideals and goals for her that she sometimes feels she has no identity of her own. She earnestly desires to control her own destiny, but she feels controlled by others. When she does not eat, she gains control.

Anorexia nervosa frequently develops shortly after a girl begins her menstrual periods. Distressed by the physical signs of womanhood, she may view thinness as an escape from physical and psychological maturity.

So many teenagers go on diets. How do you know when a diet is going too far?

Many young women diet to lose weight. However, take the person who loses weight to well below the average for her height and is no longer slim, but too slim, and still doesn't stop—she has gone too far. Regardless of how thin she is, she looks in the mirror and sees herself as fat. Anorexia nervosa resembles an addiction. The characteristic behavior is obsessive and compulsive. She is afraid of losing control, and she allows her self-imposed regimen to rule her life.

The anorexic controls her food intake with tremendous discipline. She avoids carbohydrates and fats as if they were poison and eats strictly limited amounts of lean meat and low-kcalorie vegetables. She knows the number of kcalories of dozens of different foods, and thinks and talks about foods constantly. She may cook elaborate meals for others, but she never partakes of them herself. If she feels that she has gained an ounce of weight, she exercises to work if off. Once in a while she eats more than she intends to, and when she has done that, she takes laxatives to hasten the exit of the food from her system. She is unaware that this doesn't work, because her other ways of staying thin are so effective. Her preoccupation with foods reveals that she is starving and is desperately hungry; the reason she doesn't eat is because of her fierce determination to achieve self-control, not because she isn't hungry.

Anorexia nervosa is hard to diagnose, because nearly everyone in our society is engaged in the "pursuit of thinness." It takes a skilled clinician to make the actual diagnosis. Denial runs high among people with anorexia, and they deceive their families effectively.

What are the consequences of anorexia nervosa?

The physical consequences of anorexia are those of PEM. Table NP19–1 lists some of these consequences. The malnutrition of anorexia nervosa can be so severe as to throw a person into severe electrolyte imbalance, create

---

TABLE NP19–1 Consequences of Protein-Energy Malnutrition in Anorexia Nervosa

GI TRACT

Reduced GI motility
Delayed gastric emptying
Atrophy of the cells of the digestive tract
Limited availability of digestive enzymes

CIRCULATORY SYSTEM

Weakened heart muscle with less efficient pumping action
Reduced blood pressure
Anemia
Altered serum lipid levels
Elevated concentrations of vitamin A and carotene
Reduced blood proteins

SKIN

Increased amount of fine body hair
Skin dryness
Decreased skin temperature

NERVOUS SYSTEM

Decreased core body temperature
Abnormal electrical brain activity
Disturbed sleep patterns and bad dreams

REPRODUCTIVE SYSTEM

Amenorrhea
Infertility
Loss of sex drive
Impotency

IMMUNE SYSTEM

Many abnormalities are possible (see Chapter 14)

tremendous metabolic stress by way of infection, cause depression to the point of suicide, and even stop the heart. Women with the disorder always have amenorrhea. Young men with the disorder lose their sex drive and become impotent. To resume normal menstrual cycles, a female must gain body fat to 17 to 22 percent of body weight before periods will resume. Some never restart, even after they have gained the weight.

What treatments help people with anorexia nervosa?

Successful treatment combines the expertise of various health care professionals to educate and motivate the individual with anorexia to initiate and sustain weight gain. Teams of physicians, nurses, psychiatrists, family psychologists, and dietitians work together to treat clients with anorexia.

Appropriate nutrition treatment is crucial and tailored to the needs of the individual. People with anorexia nervosa are usually younger than people with other medical conditions and are usually not ill with other diseases, so they are under less physical stress. Seldom are they willing to feed themselves, but if they are, chances are they can recover without other interventions.

It is suggested that clients be classed as being at low, intermediate, or high risk, depending on how they score on several indicators of PEM. Low-risk people need nutrition counseling by a dietitian and psychological counseling simultaneously. Intermediate-risk people may need nutritional supplements such as high-kcalorie, high-protein formulas besides regular meals but may not have to be hospitalized. The initial goal is to provide 250 to 500 kcalories above the daily energy requirement—about the maximum that most people will accept. Additionally, refeeding should proceed gradually to prevent complications (see pp. 462). Drugs may be used to improve gastric motility and help people become able to tolerate larger meals. If the risk is high, then hospitalization is indicated, and daily energy supplementation may be greater. The hope is that the person will gain about 2 to 4 pounds (1 to 2 kilograms) a month. For a person who refuses to eat, tube feedings or TPN may be necessary to forestall death.

Three-quarters of those in treatment may regain weight up to within 25 percent of the desired weight. Half to three-quarters may resume normal menstrual cycles. About two-thirds fail to eat normally on follow-up, but they may eat better than they did before. About 6 percent die, 1 percent by suicide. Social and family relationships may remain impaired. It seems that anorexia nervosa can adversely affect a person's social, psychological, and family functioning for life.

Well, that sounds good and bad. At least the majority of people with anorexia nervosa are helped, but quite a few aren't helped or have permanent effects from the disorder. Do people with bulimia also have permanent effects?

At this time, the answer to that question remains unclear. Long-term follow-up studies on people with bulimia remain to be undertaken. It may be possible to separate people with bulimia into roughly three categories: college students who engage in the disorder briefly and then recover; bingers/vomiters who also begin during college and who require more intensive therapy and hospitalization; and older people who have chronic and stable bulimia and whose binge eating and self-starving or vomiting patterns are regular and established.

How is bulimia similar to anorexia nervosa?

Bulimia is a distinct eating disorder that shares some characteristics with anorexia nervosa. It is more common than anorexia nervosa. Like anorexia nervosa, bulimia is more common in females than in males, although the proportion of males with bulimia is higher than that of males with anorexia nervosa.

The typical person with bulimia is well educated, in her early twenties, and close to ideal body weight. She is a high achiever, with a strong feeling of dependence on her parents. She experiences considerable social anxiety and has difficulty establishing personal relationships. She is sometimes depressed and often exhibits impulsive behavior.

Like the person with anorexia nervosa, the person with bulimia spends much time thinking about her body weight and food. Her preoccupation with food manifests itself in secretive binge-eating episodes followed by self-induced vomiting, fasting, or the use of laxatives or diuretics. Such behaviors typically begin in late adolescence after a long series of various unsuccessful weight-reduction diets. People with bulimia commonly follow a pattern of restrictive dieting interspersed with bulimic behaviors and experience weight fluctuations of more than 10 pounds up and down over short periods of time.

Unlike the person with anorexia

nervosa, the person with bulimia is aware of the consequences of her behavior, feels that it is abnormal, and is deeply ashamed of it. She feels inadequate, unable to control her eating; and so she tends to be passive and to look to men for confirmation of her sense of worth. When rejected, either in reality or in her imagination, her bulimia becomes worse. If she gets carried away by bulimia, she may not only experience a deepening of her depression, but may move on to drug or alcohol abuse.

What exactly is binge eating?

Binge eating is not like normal eating. It is not primarily a response to hunger, and the food is not consumed for its nutritional value. It is a compulsion to eat. A typical binge occurs periodically and is done in secret, usually at night, and lasts an hour or more. A binge frequently follows a period of rigid dieting, so that binge eating is accelerated by hunger. During a binge the person with bulimia may consume between one thousand and many thousands of kcalories of food containing little fiber or water, smooth in texture, and high in sugar and fat, so that it is easy to consume vast amounts rapidly, with little chewing.

What are the consequences of this behavior?

After a binge, the person develops swollen hands and feet, bloating, fatigue, headache, nausea, and pain. Repeated binges result in more serious consequences. A fluid and electrolyte imbalance caused by vomiting can lead to abnormal heart rhythms and injury to the kidneys, which have to cope with the altered balance. Infections of

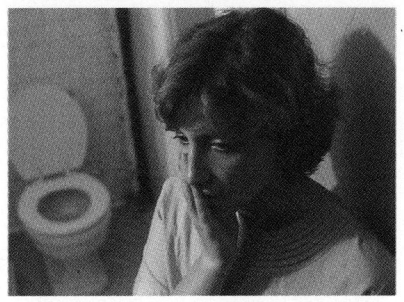

For many people with bulimia, guilt, depression, and self-condemnation follow a binge-eating episode.

the bladder and kidneys can lead to kidney failure. Vomiting causes irritation and infection of the pharynx, esophagus, and salivary glands; erosion of the teeth; and dental caries. The esophagus may rupture or tear, as may the stomach. Sometimes the eyes become red from pressure on vomiting. The hands may be bruised and lacerated from scraping on the teeth while inducing vomiting.

Some people use cathartics—violent laxatives that can injure the lower intestinal tract. Others use emetics, drugs that induce vomiting. Repeated use can lead to heart failure due to poisoning; it was emetic abuse that caused the death of popular singer Karen Carpenter in 1983.

What is the treatment for bulimia?

A team approach, as for people with anorexia nervosa, provides the most effective treatment for people with bulimia. Bulimia is in many respects easier to treat than anorexia nervosa, because it seems to be more of a chosen behavior. People with bulimia know that their behavior is abnormal, and many are willing to try to cooperate.

The goal of the dietary plan to treat bulimia is to help clients gain control,

establish regular eating patterns, and restore nutritional health.[1] The person needs to learn to eat a quantity of nutritious food sufficient to nourish her body and leave her satisfied without bringing on the feared and detested weight gain. Energy intake should not be severely restricted.

A mental health professional should be on the treatment team. Almost 90 percent of people with bulimia are clinically depressed, and the rates of alcohol, marijuana, and cigarette abuse are high.

At so tender an age as 12 years, beautifully growing, normal-weight female youngsters are already worried that they are too fat. Most are "on diets." Magazines, newspapers, and television all present the message that to be beautiful and happy is to be thin. Anorexia nervosa and bulimia are not a form of rebellion against these unreasonable expectations, but rather the exaggerated acceptance of them. Perhaps a person's best defense against these disorders is to learn to appreciate her own uniqueness. The author Eda LeShan beautifully described her recovery from overeating: "Deep inside there had always been a small child begging for my attention. . . . All I gave her was food. Now I give her love."[2] To respect and value oneself may be lifesaving.

Notes

1. S. H. Krey, Eating disorders: The clinical dietitian's changing role, *Journal of the American Dietetic Association* 89 (1989): 41–43.
2. E. LeShan, *Winning the Losing Battle: Why I Will Never Be Fat Again* (New York: Crowell, 1979).

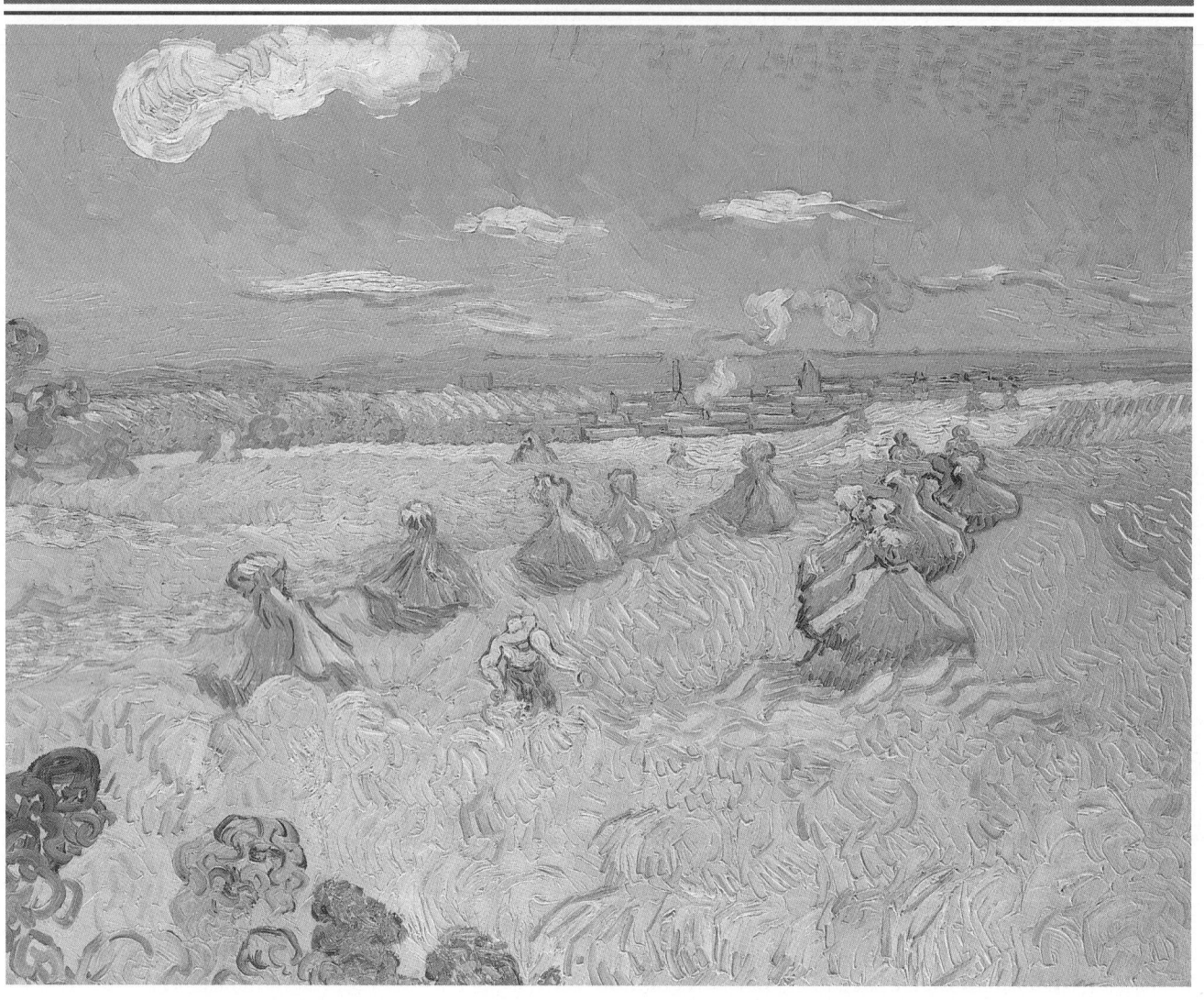

*Vincent Van Gogh, Wheat Fields with Reaper, Auvers, 1890, Oil on canvas, 29 ×
36⅝," The Toledo Museum of Art, Toledo, Ohio; Purchased with funds from the Libbey
Endowment, Gift of Edward Drummond Libbey.*

Most clinicians recommend that carbohydrate-controlled diets planned for people with diabetes, hypoglycemia, or dumping syndrome should limit concentrated sweets, because they may cause blood glucose levels to rise rapidly. In fact, different types of either complex or simple carbohydrates may affect blood glucose levels differently. The effect that food has on a person's blood glucose level and insulin response—how fast and how high the blood glucose rises, and how quickly the body responds by bringing it back to normal—is called the glycemic effect. Many practitioners have the impression that simple sugars produce a major surge in blood glucose, whereas complex carbohydrates produce a flatter response curve. However, the case is not so simple. The effects of different foods on blood glucose apparently depend on many factors:

- The digestibility of the starch in the food.
- Interactions of the starch with the protein in the food.
- The amounts and kinds of fat, sugar, and fiber in the food.
- The presence of other constituents, such as molecules that bind starch.
- The form of the food (dry, paste, or liquid; coarsely or finely ground; how thoroughly cooked; and so forth).
- The *combination* of foods consumed at a given time.

All these factors work together to produce a food's glycemic effect, and the effect is not always what is expected.[1] Ice cream, for example, produces less of a response than potatoes. More importantly, a food's glycemic effect differs when it is eaten alone or as part of a mixed meal. This one factor is actually quite significant, considering that most people eat a variety of foods in a meal.

Although the glycemic effect of foods may be important to people with disorders of blood glucose regulation, developing a ranking of how foods affect blood glucose levels has been difficult. Food combinations fail to yield predictable results. Therefore, the glycemic effects of food combinations are currently of little value in planning carbohydrate-controlled diets.

Diabetes Mellitus

Diabetes mellitus is a metabolic disorder characterized by either an absolute or a relative deficiency of insulin and by elevated blood glucose concentrations.

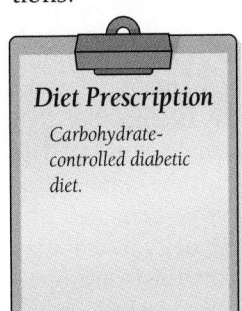

Diet Prescription

Carbohydrate-controlled diabetic diet.

Diabetes is not a single disease. Rather, it is a group of disorders with different causes, clinical features, and outcomes. Table 20–2 on p. 513 summarizes the distinguishing features of the two main forms of diabetes. In the first, less common type, known as Type I, the pancreas becomes unable to synthesize the hormone insulin, so after each meal the blood glucose rises and remains elevated even though the body's cells are simultaneously starved for glucose. The person must inject insulin at intervals to assist the cells in taking up the needed glucose; therefore, Type I diabetes is also called insulin-dependent diabetes mellitus (IDDM).

diabetes mellitus (DYE-uh-BEET-eez MELL-ih-tus or mell-EYE-tus): a disorder of blood glucose regulation caused by insufficiency or relative ineffectiveness of insulin. When the word *diabetes* is used alone, it refers to diabetes mellitus.

mellitus = honey sweet (from sugar in the urine)

Another type of diabetes, caused by inadequate secretion of antidiuretic hormone, is called **diabetes insipidus** (in-SIP-id-us). It is treated by giving the hormone.

insipid = without taste (no sugar in the urine)

Type I diabetes or **insulin-dependent diabetes mellitus (IDDM):** the less common type of diabetes, caused by an insufficiency of insulin; also called **juvenile-onset diabetes,** because it frequently develops in childhood.

TABLE 20–2   **Features of IDDM and NIDDM**

	IDDM	NIDDM
Other names	Type I diabetes	Type II diabetes
	Juvenile-onset diabetes	Adult-onset diabetes
	Ketosis-prone diabetes	Ketosis-resistant diabetes
	Brittle diabetes	Lipoplethoric diabetes
		Stable diabetes
Age of onset	<40 (mean age, 12)	>40
Associated conditions	Viral infection	Obesity
Insulin required?	Yes	Sometimes
Insulin receptors	Normal	Low or normal
Symptoms	Relatively severe	Relatively moderate
Prevalence in diabetic population	5 to 10%	85 to 90%

Type II diabetes or **non-insulin-dependent diabetes mellitus (NIDDM):** the more common form of diabetes, caused by a resistance to insulin; also called **adult-onset diabetes,** because it usually develops later in life. A type of NIDDM that develops during the teen years has been termed **maturity-onset diabetes in the young (MODY).**

The symptoms of diabetes:
Hyperglycemia.
Glycosuria (GLIGH-cose-YOUR-ee-uh).
Dehydration.
Polyuria (PAUL-ee-YOUR-ee-uh).
Polydipsia (PAUL-ee-DIP-see-uh).
Weight loss.
Polyphagia (PAUL-ee-FAY-gee-uh).
Acetone breath.
Ketosis.
Ketonuria.
Diabetic coma.
Hyperglycemic nonketotic coma.

Why the pancreas fails to produce insulin in IDDM is the subject of much research. Researchers theorize that perhaps in individuals with a genetic tendency for diabetes, immune cells mistakenly attack and destroy insulin-producing pancreatic cells. Evidence also suggests that environmental factors influence the development of diabetes; if this is true, then some cases may be preventable.

In the second, more predominant type of diabetes, known as Type II, the person's cells become resistant to insulin. The pancreas does produce insulin, but the cells respond to it less sensitively. Blood glucose first rises too high, as in IDDM, but then, because some insulin is available and the cells are sluggishly responding to it, some glucose finally moves slowly into the cells. This type of diabetes is therefore called non-insulin-dependent diabetes mellitus (NIDDM).

NIDDM tends to develop later in life than IDDM, and it has a strong familial component. People with the disorder often become quite obese. Obesity can also precipitate diabetes, and in most people with NIDDM, precedes it.[2] The incidence of diabetes also rises with increasing age, for in all people, pancreatic cells progressively lose their function with time.[3] In some people, this age-related decline in cell function is more rapid or more severe than in others, and these are the ones who need to beware especially of weight gain.

Whatever the type of diabetes, glucose fails to gain entry into cells, builds up in the blood, and leads to hyperglycemia. As the blood glucose concentration rises, water moves from the cells into the blood. (Remember that water moves from a less concentrated to a more concentrated solution.) The kidneys then begin excreting the excess glucose, along with the water. Thus both the intracellular fluid and the extracellular fluid become depleted. The person produces excessive urine (polyuria) and, becoming dehydrated, may become excessively thirsty (polydipsia). Polyuria and polydipsia are often early symptoms of diabetes. Figure 20–1 summarizes these events.

Normally, insulin signals the body that it has been fed and directs cellular activities that favor the uptake of amino acids, carbohydrate, and fat. The net

FIGURE 20–1   **Overview of Diabetes**
As you can see, when glucose cannot enter the cells, a cascade of changes follows. The symptoms of diabetes are highlighted in white.

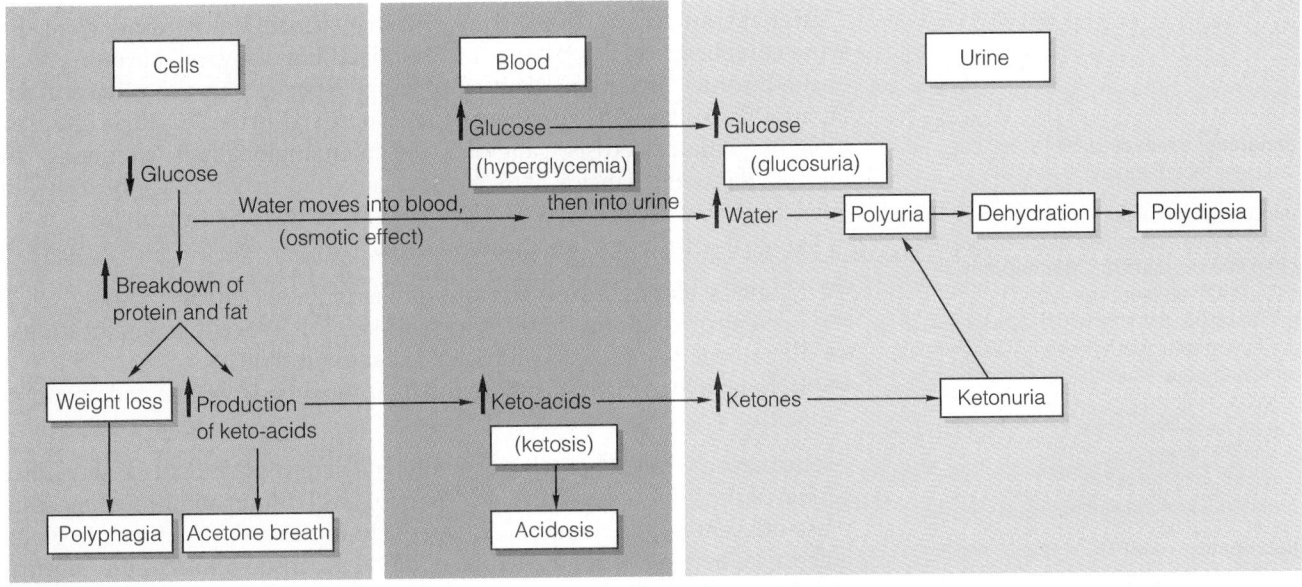

effect is to reduce blood glucose levels. Then between meals during fasting, the continued presence of some insulin prevents the body's energy stores from being mobilized excessively.

When not enough insulin is produced or when the cells cannot respond to insulin, the cells are deprived of the substrates they need for energy. Amino acids and glucose may abound in the cells' fluid environment, but the cells have limited access to them and therefore must mobilize their own proteins and fats as energy sources. Because of the large amounts of fat being broken down, the liver begins making ketone bodies, which also accumulate in the blood. The losses of both glucose and ketone bodies (both energy substrates) in the urine and the breakdown of protein lead to weight loss. This is why the insulin-dependent diabetic person is likely to be thin. It is also why the person may eat excessively (polyphagia).

People with Type II diabetes, as mentioned earlier, tend to be obese rather than thin. They overeat because their cells, lacking energy fuels, are hungry. Then the insulin they do have slowly takes effect, and the body ends up storing fat from the excess energy they have consumed.

If Type I diabetes goes uncontrolled, excessive levels of ketones persist in the blood (ketosis). The presence of one type of ketone (acetone) can be detected by a fruity odor on the breath. The ketones are acidic and lower the blood pH (acidosis). Ketones begin to appear in the urine (ketonuria); sodium and potassium are excreted along with them by a mechanism that worsens the acidosis. When acidosis becomes severe enough, the person can lapse into a fatal coma.

People with Type II diabetes generally are not prone to ketosis, because they have enough insulin to prevent the excessive buildup of ketones. They can develop another kind of coma, however, caused by extremely high blood glucose levels without acidosis. Logically, this kind of coma is termed hyperglycemic nonketotic coma.

Over the long term, the person with diabetes suffers not only from the acute complications of diabetes just described but also from chronic effects of the disorder. Infections tend to develop, especially in the urinary tract, because bacteria thrive on glucose-rich blood and urine. Vascular diseases, including atherosclerosis, gangrene, and microangiopathies, commonly afflict people with diabetes. Atherosclerosis is the major cause of death in NIDDM. Nerve tissues also may deteriorate, causing neuropathy.

The goals of therapy for diabetes are to:

■ Maintain blood glucose concentrations in an acceptable range.
■ Prevent or delay the onset or progression of associated complications.
■ Encourage people to resume normal activities.
■ Help people to achieve and maintain optimal body weight and nutrition status.

The person with diabetes has the same nutrient requirements as any other person of the same age, stature, and activity level. But in addition to meeting those nutrient requirements, food must help minimize fluctuations in blood glucose. Whether the maintenance of blood glucose within a fairly normal range can prevent the complications of diabetes remains uncertain; however, mounting evidence suggests that control of blood glucose does confer this benefit. (Methods of monitoring blood glucose control as well as testing for the presence of diabetes are described in the box entitled "Biochemical Tests for Diabetes Mellitus.")

gangrene: death of tissue, usually due to deficient blood supply.

microangiopathies (MY-crow-ANN-gee-OP-ah-thees): disorders of the capillaries, often seen in diabetes. **Retinopathy** (RET-in-OP-ah-thee) is a type of microangiopathy affecting the capillaries of the eye; **nephropathy** (nee-FROP-ah-thee) affects the capillaries of the kidney.
  micro = tiny
  angio = blood vessel
  pathy = disease
  retino = of the retina
  nephro = of the kidney

neuropathy (new-ROP-ah-thee): any disease of the nerves.

Biochemical Tests for Diabetes Mellitus

Urine tests often provide the first clue that a person may have diabetes. The person performing the test dips indicator paper into the urine sample. The paper changes color, and the person then compares it with a color chart to determine the approximate concentration of glucose. The results appear as percentages, indicating how much glucose is present in the urine, thus providing an indirect measure of glucose in the blood. Health care providers often perform urine tests for glucose and ketones as part of routine examinations. High concentrations of both ketones and glucose indicate diabetes. Positive test results for ketones alone, however, do not always mean diabetes (for example, ketones may be present in people who are following low-carbohydrate diets or fasting). Nor does the presence of glucose alone clinch a diagnosis of diabetes, but it does suggest the need for a follow-up blood test—usually, a glucose tolerance test.

A glucose tolerance test works like this. First, the health care professional performing the test draws blood from the client (who has fasted overnight) to obtain the fasting glucose level. The client then drinks a measured amount of glucose in the form of a flavored beverage. Blood is

(continued)

drawn again at regular intervals of 30 to 60 minutes (different clinics use different intervals). Table 20–3 lists the upper limits considered normal and the values suggestive of diabetes for each time interval. At least two of the glucose readings should be in the range characteristic of diabetes to confirm a diagnosis. A person whose glucose levels fall above the upper limits of normal but below the range suggestive of diabetes is diagnosed as having impaired glucose tolerance.

Once diabetes has been diagnosed, part of the treatment regimen includes monitoring glucose concentrations at regular intervals. Clients can check their urine or blood at home using the methods taught by professionals at the hospital or clinic. This enables them to be sure their insulin and diet are appropriate. Health care members will want to review records of test results at medical appointments.

In one home method of urine testing, the client drops a tablet into the urine sample and then compares the color that develops with a color chart. In another method, the client dips a piece of indicator paper briefly into the urine sample and compares the color of the paper with a color chart. Clients are instructed to check their urine at least twice a day, generally before meals and at bedtime.

Direct monitoring of blood glucose at home is more sensitive and more accurate than urine testing and is preferable to urine testing, because it helps individuals maintain control of their own glucose levels. More and more people with diabetes are using monitoring systems. Blood glucose must exceed 180 milligrams per 100 milliliters before glucose spills into the urine. When used properly, home monitoring of blood glucose can help maintain blood glucose between 60 and 140 milligrams per 100 milliliters.

To perform a home test of blood glucose, the client pricks a finger to get a blood sample (the same method used to determine hematocrit) and touches the blood to a paper strip. As with urine samples, the color indicates the blood glucose concentration. Meters that provide a more accurate readout of the actual glucose concentration are also available, although they are more expensive as well.

Ideally, until blood glucose control has been reliably established, the client performs blood tests seven times during the day: before each meal, two hours after each meal, and at bedtime. However, realizing the strain

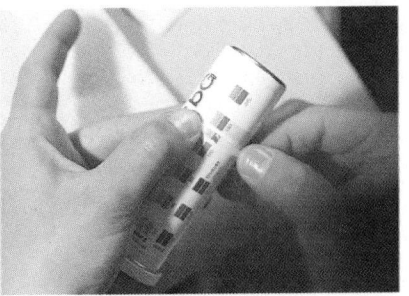

Diabetes care includes regular monitoring of glucose in the blood and urine.

TABLE 20–3   **Interpretation of Glucose Tolerance Test Results**

TIME (minutes)	UPPER LIMITS OF NORMAL (mg/100 ml)	VALUES SUGGESTIVE OF DIABETES (mg/100 ml)
0	115	140
60	200	>200
120	140	200

Note: This is one of many variations of the glucose tolerance test.

(continued)

this may place on a client, many practitioners instead recommend four tests daily. The person can test at any of the seven times listed above; the times of the tests should vary daily. Once the client has established blood glucose control, one or two tests a day are sufficient for further monitoring.

Physicians will want to see clients at regular intervals to determine whether they are controlling their blood glucose adequately. One test physicians use to monitor control of blood glucose levels is the measurement of *glycosylated hemoglobin* (or hemoglobin A_{1c}). As the blood glucose concentration rises, small glucose molecules spontaneously attach to an amino acid on each hemoglobin. The altered hemoglobin remains in circulation for the life of the red blood cell (approximately 120 days), and no longer releases oxygen properly. Normally, only 4 to 8 percent of a person's hemoglobin is glycosylated, but in diabetes, because blood glucose remains high for periods of time, the percentage can go up to 16 percent.

Measurement of glycosylated hemoglobin allows the physician to determine how successful diabetes control has been over the past two to four months. The test has another advantage. Urine and blood glucose tests permit ''cheating'' because they reflect diabetes control only just prior to the test. A person who has managed control poorly can produce normal urine or blood test results just by starving or using extra insulin the day before going to the doctor. But glycosylated hemoglobin reflects control over several months, so the client can't easily outfox the test.

Treatment of the Person with Insulin-Dependent Diabetes

A diagnosis of IDDM can be devastating to anyone. The parents of a young child with IDDM may feel overwhelmed, angry, anxious, and even guilty. To an adolescent, it may seem like the end of the world. In fact, to a person of any age, the prospect of daily insulin injections and possible complications may bring fear. In addition to insulin therapy, the person must carefully follow a new diet. Finally, successful control of blood glucose requires that the person master the impressive task of coordinating diet, insulin, and physical activity. Overwhelming as these assignments may seem at first, a person can manage them and lead an active and full life. The next sections provide details.

Insulin

As mentioned, the treatment plan for the person with IDDM involves coordinating insulin, diet, and physical activity. Because people with IDDM can't make insulin, they must receive it from another source. Although the availability of insulin has been lifesaving, insulin therapy cannot achieve the same degree of blood glucose control as a body that functions normally.

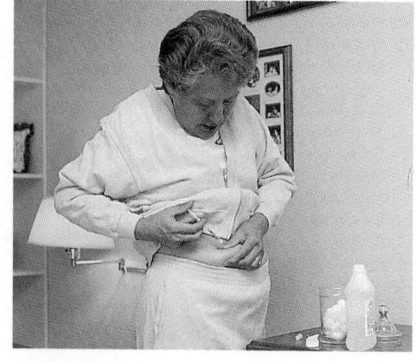

When the pancreas fails to produce insulin, the person with IDDM turns to commercially available injections of the lifesaving hormone.

TABLE 20–4   **Actions of Some Types of Insulin**[a]

TYPE	DURATION OF ACTIVITY	PEAK OF ACTION
Rapid acting		
Regular crystalline	5 to 7 hours	2 to 4 hours
Semilente	12 to 16 hours	2 to 8 hours
Intermediate acting		
Globin	12 to 18 hours	6 to 8 hours
NPH/lente	18 to 24 hours	8 to 14 hours
Long acting		
Protamine zinc	24 to 30 hours	16 to 24 hours
Ultralente	30 to 36 hours	18 to 29 hours

[a]Human insulins can be either rapid acting, intermediate acting, or long acting.

Commercially made insulin is commonly extracted from the pancreas of cattle. Insulins made from porcine pancreatic extracts and, more recently, human insulins are also available. The many types of insulin are described as rapid acting, intermediate acting, or long acting, depending on how quickly they begin to work and on how long they remain active. Table 20–4 lists examples of the various types of insulin and their actions. Because insulin is a protein, it would be digested if taken by mouth; therefore, it must be injected.

Normally, the body secretes a constant, baseline amount of insulin at all times. After a meal, insulin secretion surges to help store energy nutrients when they are plentiful. The person with IDDM needs insulin both to meet baseline needs and to process energy nutrients. The physician prescribes the exact type, dosage, and administration schedule of insulin based on the individual's stage of growth, activity patterns, eating habits, and individual responses. The accompanying box provides an example of one way insulin might be administered. Generally, individuals receive a mixture of two or more types of insulin several times a day to approximate the normal level of insulin in the body.

An Example of Insulin Administration

- 30 to 45 minutes before breakfast—an injection of a mixture of rapid-acting and long-acting insulin.
- 30 minutes before lunch—an injection of rapid-acting insulin.
- 30 minutes before supper—an injection of a mixture of rapid-acting and long-acting insulin.

The person who gets too little insulin or doesn't get insulin when glucose from foods is available risks hyperglycemia and diabetic ketoacidosis. The person who gets too much insulin or has too little glucose available when insulin is high risks severe hypoglycemia.

Symptoms of hyperglycemia:

- Dizziness.
- Double vision.
- Nervousness.
- Shallow breathing.
- Sweating.
- Weakness.

Symptoms of hypoglycemia:

- Acetone breath.
- Confusion.
- Glucosuria.
- Intense thirst.
- Labored breathing.
- Nausea.
- Vomiting.

Insulin needs rise as body weight increases. Stresses such as pregnancy, surgery, infection, and some illnesses also increase insulin needs. In contrast, activity reduces insulin needs, for physical activity acts like insulin in lowering blood glucose concentrations.

To ensure the coordination of insulin schedule, diet, and exercise regimen, the client must learn to monitor urine or blood glucose levels at home. Home monitoring of blood glucose is gradually replacing urine testing, because it is more accurate.

Researchers continue to search for ways to improve methods of delivering insulin. Implantable pumps that automatically deliver scheduled doses of insulin may soon be available to the majority of people with IDDM. These pumps, approximately the size of hockey pucks, hold a three-months' supply of insulin; they allow the client to release extra doses of insulin if needed, by sending a signal with a radio-sized transmitter. Clients return to their physicians to have the pumps refilled at the end of three months.

Diet in IDDM

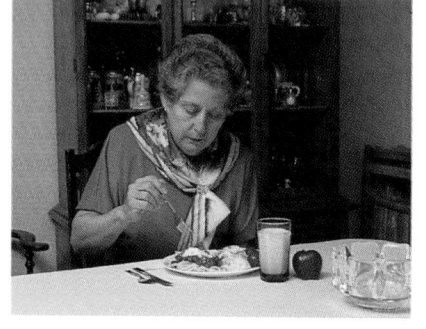

The person with IDDM coordinates food intake with her insulin schedule.

To control IDDM requires a lifelong commitment to a carefully orchestrated diet, insulin, and physical activity program. Therefore, the plan must honor the person's lifestyle habits and food preferences. Most frequently, diet planners use the exchange patterns described in Chapter 19 (pp. 488–494).

The diet for the person with IDDM first focuses on providing adequate food energy to achieve or maintain a healthy body weight, or, in children, to support growth. Of the total kcalories, carbohydrate should contribute 55 to 60 percent, fat should provide 25 to 30 percent, and protein intake should fall between 12 and 20 percent.[4] The diet planner divides these energy nutrients into meals that, in turn, coordinate with the insulin schedule.

In IDDM, consistency in the timing and composition of meals and snacks from day to day improves glucose control. In general, a plan of small meals

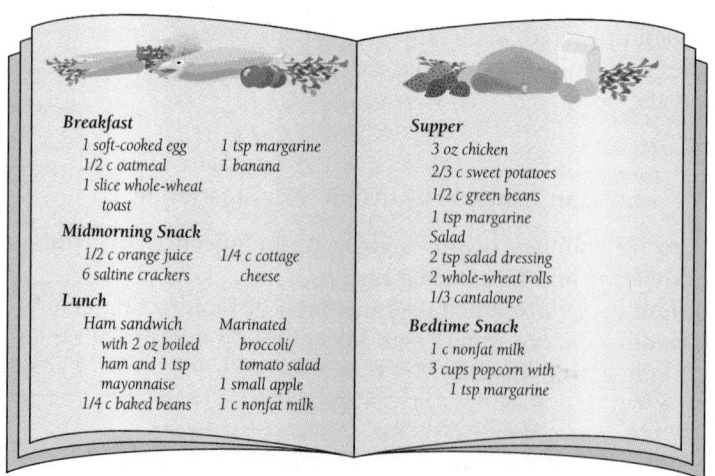

Breakfast
1 soft-cooked egg   1 tsp margarine
1/2 c oatmeal   1 banana
1 slice whole-wheat
    toast

Midmorning Snack
1/2 c orange juice   1/4 c cottage
6 saltine crackers   cheese

Lunch
Ham sandwich   Marinated
    with 2 oz boiled   broccoli/
    ham and 1 tsp   tomato salad
    mayonnaise   1 small apple
1/4 c baked beans   1 c nonfat milk

Supper
3 oz chicken
2/3 c sweet potatoes
1/2 c green beans
1 tsp margarine
Salad
2 tsp salad dressing
2 whole-wheat rolls
1/3 cantaloupe

Bedtime Snack
1 c nonfat milk
3 cups popcorn with
    1 tsp margarine

Sample 2200 kCalorie Diabetic Diet Menu

TABLE 20–5　**Distribution of Energy and Carbohydrate in a Sample Diabetic Diet**

	BREAKFAST (2/10)	MIDMORNING SNACK (1/10)	LUNCH (3/10)	SUPPER (3/10)	BEDTIME SNACK (1/10)	TOTAL
Energy (kcal)	440	220	660	660	220	2200
Carbohydrate (g)	60	30	91	91	30	302

Note: These figures are approximations. Chances are that you will not be able to divide meals so that the kcalories and carbohydrate are distributed exactly as you would wish. (See the sample 2200-kcal diabetic diet menu.)

with snacks between them maintains blood glucose control best. Carbohydrate is included in every meal and snack. Each meal usually contains from 20 to 40 percent of the day's total kcalories and carbohydrate, and each snack contains about 10 percent. The distribution often consists of three meals, a bedtime snack, and sometimes a midafternoon or midmorning snack, depending on the individual's blood glucose levels and insulin schedule. Table 20–5 shows how this distribution works for a sample 2200-kcalorie diabetic diet. The sample menu shows how this distribution is translated into foods.

Notice that although the carbohydrate-controlled diet for IDDM does restrict carbohydrate, its carbohydrate content is actually fairly high. In providing advice on a diet like this, encourage the liberal use of complex carbohydrates that provide fiber to fill the prescribed carbohydrate allowance. Whole-grain breads and cereals, dried beans and peas, fruits, and vegetables are excellent choices.

In most cases, the diabetic diet excludes concentrated sweets. However, because the "absolutely no sugar" rule would be difficult to follow, many health care professionals allow clients (particularly children) to consume modest amounts of concentrated sweets with meals (not to exceed 5 percent of the total kcalories). Additionally, people with IDDM may need concentrated sweets before vigorous exercise or during illness.

Because people with diabetes have a high risk of developing cardiovascular disease and hypertension, their diet plans should follow dietary guidelines to help protect against those conditions. Encourage the use of low-fat and nonfat milks, moderate use of lean meats, and small amounts of polyunsaturated fats in place of saturated fats. Restrict sodium intake to less than 3000 milligrams per day.[5] Chapter 22 provides more details on nutrition and disorders of the heart and blood vessels.

The person whose blood glucose is well controlled can usually include some alcoholic beverages with the consent of the physician. However, alcohol can cause hypoglycemia in any normal person, and the person with diabetes, who is susceptible to hypoglycemia anyway, should be especially careful in using it. Recommend that the person use alcohol not more than once or twice a week; only in moderate amounts (less than 6 percent of the total kcalories); and with, or shortly before or after, meals. Furthermore, of course, everyone should limit alcohol because of its low nutrient density.

People with IDDM should carry sugar cubes or hard candy at all times. Why? If they mistakenly take too much insulin, engage in excessive physical activity, skip meals, or eat too little food, they may develop hypoglycemia, which can be fatal. As soon as the earliest symptoms appear, they should ingest some form of readily absorbable glucose, such as fruit juice, hard candy, sugar, or glucose solutions.

Unrecognized hypoglycemia can result in tragedy. The person suffering from hypoglycemia may appear to be intoxicated and can die. To prevent such a mistake, the person is advised to wear identification in the form of a bracelet or necklace. A card in the wallet may not serve the purpose, because onlookers might not think to check a wallet immediately.

People with diabetes often wonder about replacing sweet foods in the diet. In general, they do not need special dietetic foods. People often misinterpret *dietetic* to mean *no kcalories,* but this is not the case. Some dietetic foods may be low in sodium instead of sugar, or they may contain reduced but still significant numbers of kcalories.

Some dietetic foods may be helpful, however. They include artificially sweetened soft drinks, artificial sweeteners, and water-packed canned fruits. kCalorie-free soft drinks and beverages, such as artificially sweetened tea, can be used freely and are often well liked. Artificial sweeteners that do not contain significant kcalories can help make low-kcalorie foods more acceptable. Nutrition in Practice 20 provides more information about these sweeteners.

Like most people, people with IDDM occasionally miss a meal. When this happens, they need to eat some carbohydrate to protect against hypoglycemia. Usually 15 to 30 grams of complex carbohydrate will forestall hypoglycemia for one to two hours on such occasions.

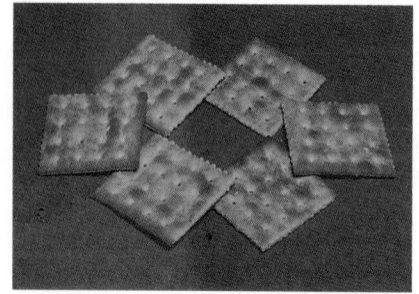

Six saltine crackers = 15 g carbohydrate.

In the hospital, the person with IDDM may miss meals in preparation for diagnostic tests, following surgery, of if GI problems prevent food intake. Procedures for dealing with this problem vary with each hospital. One procedure is to replace at least half the prescribed carbohydrate and kcalories within three hours after the missed meal. If this cannot be done, the physician may decide to take some other measure, such as changing the insulin schedule or giving IV dextrose. Sometimes the physician will add more simple carbohydrates to the diet prescription.

During an illness or other stress, blood glucose levels may rise, thus raising insulin requirements. This precarious time requires clients with diabetes to follow insulin and dietary instructions especially carefully. Physicians may advise clients to reduce total energy and carbohydrate intakes somewhat to limit the need for extra insulin. If appetite is poor, people with diabetes can use juice, flavored gelatin, soft drinks, or frozen fruit juice bars to meet their needs for energy and carbohydrates. The prevention of starvation, dehydration, and vomiting become main concerns.

Sugar is sometimes found in certain drugs. People with diabetes need to be aware that some liquid and chewable over-the-counter and prescription drugs may contain sugar. Members of the health care team, too, must be alert to this possibility and take appropriate measures.

People with diabetes may require central TPN or commercial tube feedings that contain considerable amounts of simple sugars. Health care professionals must take extra care in monitoring these people and adjust insulin dosages to meet higher carbohydrate loads. Even with added insulin, some people may be unable to tolerate the high carbohydrate in TPN. For these people, the concentration of glucose may have to be reduced and some of its energy delivered by IV fat emulsions instead (see Chapter 16). People who cannot tolerate any simple carbohydrates from tube feedings may require specially designed blenderized feedings or commercial formulas that contain no simple sugars.

Physical Activity

In addition to insulin therapy and diet, the management of diabetes requires attention to physical activity, partly because, as mentioned, physical activity produces an insulin-like effect and so can improve diabetes control. Activity programs can also help significantly to strengthen the heart, control blood pressure, and provide many other benefits to the cardiovascular system that people with diabetes especially need (see Chapter 9 for more on the benefits of exercise). For the person with IDDM, regular physical activity may lower insulin requirements. For those with NIDDM, physical activity can improve glucose tolerance.[6]

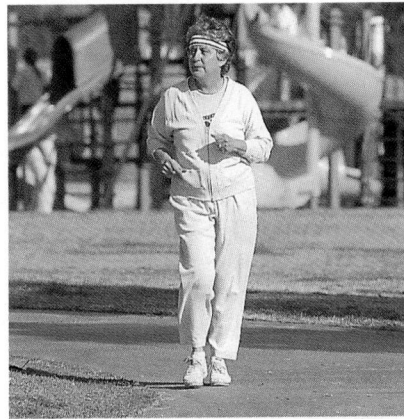

Exercise plays an important role in the management of diabetes.

For nondiabetic people, blood glucose levels generally vary little during physical activity. In contrast, blood glucose levels can vary markedly when people with IDDM engage in physical activity. Those with mild hyperglycemia may experience a fall in blood glucose during activity, whereas those with marked hyperglycemia may experience a still greater rise. For this reason, physicians generally advise people with IDDM to refrain from physical activity until blood glucose falls below 300 milligrams per 100 milliliters. When blood glucose stabilizes, the physician will prescribe the type, intensity, duration, and frequency of physical activity.

The person with IDDM may need to eat before, during, and after physical activity. Especially important is carbohydrate, which should come from fruits, fruit juices, yogurt, crackers, and other starches.[7] As a general guideline, the active person should take about 10 to 15 grams of additional carbohydrate before moderate activity, or about 20 to 30 grams of carbohydrate before vigorous activity. People with IDDM must coordinate the dose and timing of insulin injections with exercise. Vigorous exercise and warm temperatures increase blood flow, thus increasing the rate of insulin absorption and setting the stage for a hypoglycemic reaction. Reducing the insulin dosage can help to prevent this sequence of events. The best way to determine the appropriate course of action is to monitor blood glucose 30 minutes before and 1 hour after exercise. Table 20–6 on p. 524 provides some general guidelines.

Children with Diabetes

Diet planning for the child with diabetes involves some special problems. Growth is sporadic, and it is difficult to predict how many kcalories a child

Table 20–6   **Guidelines for Providing Additional Carbohydrate for Activity in IDDM**

EXERCISE INTENSITY	BLOOD GLUCOSE LEVEL (mg/ml)	ADDITIONAL CARBOHYDRATE TO PROVIDE (g)
Low intensity	<100	10 to 15
	>100	None
Moderate intensity	<100	15 to 20
	100 to 180	10 to 15
	180 to 300	None
Strenuous	<100	35 to 40
	100 to 180	25 to 50
	180 to 300	10 to 15

Source: Adapted from M. J. Franz, Exercise and the management of diabetes mellitus, *Journal of the American Dietetic Association* 87 (1987): 872–880.
Note: These values are estimates only. The individual should monitor blood glucose levels to more accurately determine specific needs.

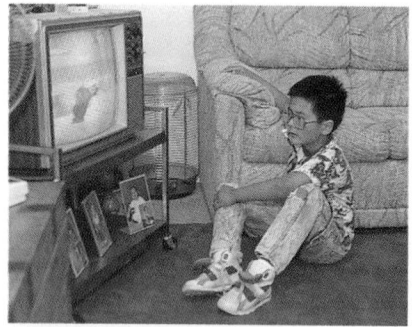

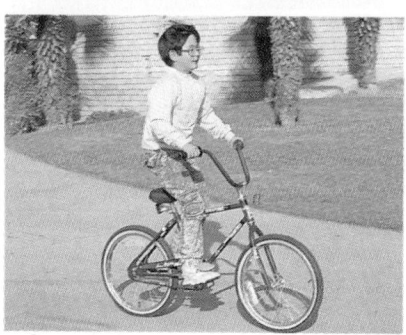

A flexible diet can help meet a child's needs, which vary from day to day.

Hypoglycemia that develops during the night is called **nocturnal hypoglycemia.** It is particularly dangerous, because it can go unrecognized in the sleeping person, who may go into shock. Adults as well as children can develop nocturnal hypoglycemia, but children are particularly susceptible.

will need during any one period of time. Appetite and activity vary widely from day to day. One day a child may eat like a horse, and the next like a mouse. Children may run and play after school on a sunny day, but sit quietly in front of the television on a rainy day. Growth, appetite, and activity levels can change the need for food or insulin.

To support growth and development, provide balanced meals that offer a wide variety of foods from the six exchange lists. Calculate energy needs based on age, gender, activity level, and growth status, and adjust them as necessary. Allow concentrated sweets only at times of vigorous physical activity or to treat hypoglycemia. Do not force children to finish meals, but encourage them not to skip meals either, since hypoglycemia can result. Plan meals for approximately the same times each day, and serve children the same foods as the rest of the family. Successful diet management incorporates prescribed meals into existing family lifestyles and eating patterns. Depending on insulin administration and personal preferences, children generally receive three meals with two to three snacks a day.[8] Vary snacks to prevent boredom. Providing extra snacks to share with friends helps to prevent the feeling of being different. Avoid identifying foods as "good" or "bad." Such connotations create unrealistic expectations or fears, and invite the development of manipulative eating behaviors. (The case study at the end of this chapter discusses a child with IDDM.)

Parents of a child with diabetes may fear that their child will develop hypoglycemia during the night, when the symptoms will go unrecognized. Snacks before bedtime may be helpful in preventing this, especially if the child engages in strenuous activity late in the day. Additionally, the child or parents can monitor blood glucose levels before bedtime (especially in the child newly diagnosed with diabetes) to help parents know when to make special efforts to protect against hypoglycemia during the night.

Treatment of the Person with Non-Insulin-Dependent Diabetes

In some ways, treatment for NIDDM parallels that of IDDM. In both, the primary goal of therapy is to maintain glucose homeostasis. However, because NIDDM develops from resistance to insulin rather than from lack of insulin, the approaches to attaining this goal differ. People with NIDDM can frequently control their blood glucose levels by diet alone. In other cases, drugs, in addition to diet, can maintain acceptable blood glucose levels.

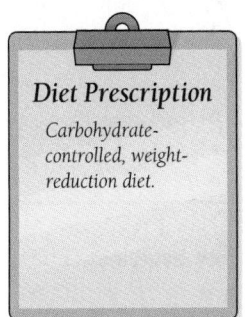

Diet Prescription

Carbohydrate-controlled, weight-reduction diet.

Diet therapy in NIDDM focuses on weight control. The majority of people with NIDDM are obese, and obesity aggravates insulin resistance. Weight loss in these people can lower blood glucose levels, ameliorate hypertension, and reduce blood lipid levels. Table 20–7 compares the key components of diet therapy in IDDM and NIDDM.

Obese people with diabetes and severe hyperglycemia are occasionally placed on medically supervised fasts temporarily or on diets very low in kcalories (600 kcalories per day) until blood glucose levels are under control. They can then follow less restrictive weight reduction diets until they reach their desired weights. Although such programs can be successful, oftentimes people who lose weight on fasts or very-low-

TABLE 20–7 **Comparison of IDDM and NIDDM Diet Therapies**

DIET APPROACH	IDDM	NIDDM
Reduce food energy intake	Usually not necessary	Almost invariably necessary
Keep ratio of carbohydrate, protein, and fat consistent for each feeding	Yes	No
Eat meals at regular times	Yes	Not necessary
Eat more frequent meals	Yes	No
Use food to treat or prevent hypoglycemia	Yes	No[a]
Replace carbohydrate when appetite is poor or meals are missed	Yes	No
Eat extra food for intense exercise	Yes	No
Restrict sodium to 3000 mg/day	Yes	Yes
Follow dietary pattern of 30% kcal fat, 55% kcal carbohydrate, and 15% kcal protein	Yes	Yes
Use exchange system	Yes	Yes

Note: Philosophies vary. Not every diet therapist would follow these guidelines in every case.
[a]Food may be needed to treat or prevent hypoglycemia when oral hypoglycemic agents are given.

TABLE 20-8   Foods Avoided on Diets That Exclude Concentrated Sweets

Cakes	Gelatin, sweetened	Puddings
Candy	Granola	Sherbet
Cereals, sweetened	Honey	Soft drinks
Cookies	Ice cream	Sugar
Cranberry sauce	Jam	Sweet rolls
Doughnuts	Jelly	Syrup
Frappés	Marmalade	Vegetables, glazed
Frosting	Milk, chocolate or	Yogurt, fruit flavored (if
Fruit drinks	condensed	sweetened with sugar)
Fruit ices	Milk shakes	
Fruit juices, sweetened	Molasses	
Fruits, canned, glazed,	Pastries	
frozen or cooked with	Pies	
sugar	Popsicles	

kcalorie diets quickly regain some or all of the weight they have lost. These diets, therefore, are not generally recommended.

Diets moderately restricted in kcalories that promote a 1- to 2-pound weight loss per week are recommended. Such diets permit clients to eat enough food to obtain the nutrients they need, if they make the proper selections, and thus can be followed until the desired weight is reached. The diet is then easily adapted for weight maintenance.

While the timing and distribution of meals for people with NIDDM is not critical, they should limit concentrated sweets as well as their energy intakes. A plan of three meals a day with no snacks helps prevent weight gain. The exchange list system frequently provides the basis for the diet. If the person is already at a healthy weight, an ordinary balanced diet that excludes concentrated sweets may be recommended. Table 20-8 lists foods to avoid on such a diet.

A program of moderate physical activity offers many benefits. Physical activity helps improve blood glucose control, glucose tolerance, and insulin action in NIDDM.[9] Many clinicians believe that 80 to 90 percent of all people with NIDDM who are overweight can achieve metabolic control if they follow a low-kcalorie diet combined with regular moderate physical activity.[10] While physical activity helps to lower blood glucose and improve insulin resistance in NIDDM, its greatest value is in contributing to weight loss.[11]

In some people with NIDDM, diet alone fails to adequately control hyperglycemia. These people may need to take insulin or other drugs. Remind clients that drugs do not replace their diets; advise them to continue their diets as instructed.

The drugs used in NIDDM include **oral hypoglycemic agents** (drugs taken by mouth that lower blood glucose levels) or insulin. Unlike insulin injections that actually replace the missing hormone, oral agents work, in part, by stimulating the release of insulin from the pancreas, and therefore are effective only in NIDDM.

Treatment of Diabetes during Pregnancy

Diabetes during pregnancy poses special problems for both mother and infant. Without management of maternal diabetes, women may experience episodes of severe hypoglycemia or hyperglycemia. Hypoglycemia can occur early in pregnancy because of placental transfer of glucose to the fetus, vomiting, or limited food intake resulting from nausea. Therefore, for the woman with IDDM, reduced insulin dosage early in pregnancy may be necessary. Insulin requirements rise in the latter half of pregnancy, however, because the placenta begins secreting hormones that oppose insulin's actions. The pregnant woman with IDDM must monitor her blood glucose and adjust her insulin dosages accordingly.

For the pregnant woman with NIDDM, diet is central to therapy. Physicians may prescribe oral hypoglycemic agents occasionally, or insulin in some cases. Oral agents must be discontinued late in pregnancy and be replaced with insulin if needed; hypoglycemic agents promote hypoglycemia in the newborn infant.

The risk of developing NIDDM or glucose intolerance later in life increases with each pregnancy.[12] This association may not appear until many years after childbearing and cannot be explained fully by age, obesity, or family history.

Gestational diabetes is a type of diabetes that develops during pregnancy, usually late in gestation. Gestational diabetes requires dietary management, just as NIDDM does. An important aspect of nutrition management is prevention of excessive weight gain, but weight-reduction diets are not normally recommended during pregnancy. Women with gestational diabetes should not reduce their carbohydrate intakes but should choose foods rich in complex carbohydrates, such as vegetables and whole-grain breads, and should limit their intakes of concentrated sweets. Optimal protein intakes are also important. Dietary recommendations encourage three meals a day plus two snacks, each containing protein, carbohydrate, and moderate fat.

Almost one-third of women who have gestational diabetes develop NIDDM within five years. Research indicates that the incidence of NIDDM in women with previous gestational diabetes is twice as high in those who are 20 percent or more overweight as in those who are not overweight.

Obstetricians recommend blood glucose monitoring for all pregnant women with any type of diabetes. Establishing blood glucose control is important to the health of both mother and infant. In addition to monitoring their blood glucose, pregnant women may also monitor their urine for ketones. Ketosis in early pregnancy can lead to congenital malformations, central nervous system disorders, and low IQs in infants.

Education for People with Diabetes

After physicians resolve the immediate crisis and restore glucose homeostasis in newly diagnosed cases of diabetes, clients and their caretakers must begin making adjustments to living with the disorder. These adjustments require establishing new attitudes and behaviors that will provide for a healthy life. Clients with diabetes, especially those with IDDM, have a lot to deal with at first, and all the new information can be overwhelming. They may find the diagnosis of diabetes hard to accept, and all it entails difficult to grasp. To ensure that clients and their caretakers receive the education and support they need to meet the many demands of diabetes care, health care professionals provide the following:

- Instruction on blood and urine testing (how to administer the tests, interpret results, and record the findings).
- Instruction on diet (how to use the exchange lists, time meals, and choose foods to include and exclude).
- Descriptions of the complications associated with diabetes and instructions on how to prevent or treat their development.
- Suggestions on ways to cope with fears and guilt feelings.
- Encouragement to have confidence in their own abilities to manage the disorder.
- Individualized programs for care, education, and support.

The person with IDDM and their caretakers must be given additional information:

- Instruction on insulin (the appropriate dose and schedule, how to draw insulin and administer an injection, and how to rotate injection sites).
- Instruction on changes in insulin and diet to accommodate physical activity or illness.
- Instruction on preventing hypoglycemia.

All oral instructions should be reinforced with printed information that clients and their caretakers can review whenever necessary.

To meet all the goals of diabetes education requires support from the diabetes care team—physicians, nurses, dietitians, counselors, and physical therapists. Each member of the team covers a specific area of instruction and reinforces instructions given by others.

Diabetes, a metabolic disorder of glucose metabolism, is characterized by elevated blood glucose concentrations. Another disorder of glucose metabolism, hypoglycemia, is characterized by low blood glucose. Ironically, a similar diet may help correct both of these disorders.

Hypoglycemia

Strictly speaking, the term *hypoglycemia* simply means low blood glucose. It refers to a symptom, not a disease. It may or may not be accompanied by other symptoms, some of which may be uncomfortable. The symptoms most people associate with hypoglycemia are similar to those of an anxiety attack: weakness, rapid heartbeat, sweating, agitation, hunger, and trembling. These symptoms are not surprising, since they are triggered by the "emergency hormone," epinephrine, but they do not arise in most people after meals. Most people, after eating, experience a gradual rise in blood glucose, followed by a gradual decline. During the decline, the cells are beginning to take up glucose to use as fuel—the physiological activity characteristic of the "fed state." When glucose stops entering the body from the small intestine, metabolism shifts gently into the reverse condition—the "fasting state," in which the liver cells start to release glucose from stored glycogen for the body's use. Throughout, blood glucose remains in the normal range, and the transition occurs without notice.

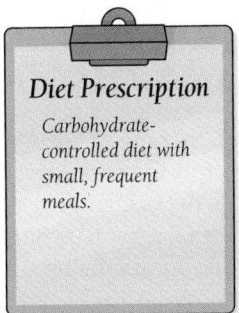

Diet Prescription

Carbohydrate-controlled diet with small, frequent meals.

In some people, however, the transition from the fed to the fasting state causes stress because of the associated effects of epinephrine. When hypoglycemia, with the symptoms of anxiety, arises several hours after a meal and causes distress, the condition is called reactive hypoglycemia. This type of hypoglycemia has attracted a lot of attention, is often misdiagnosed, and has been the subject of much misguided advice. To establish a valid diagnosis requires physicians' taking blood glucose measurements during the symptomatic episodes.[13]

A different kind of hypoglycemia exists in a person who has symptoms while well advanced into the fasting state (for example, overnight). The symptoms of fasting hypoglycemia differ from those of reactive hypoglycemia: headache, mental dullness, fatigue, confusion, amnesia, and even seizures and unconsciousness. These symptoms arise from medically diverse causes that interfere with normal blood glucose regulation, such as tumors of the pancreas or liver. Table 20–9 lists the major distinguishing characteristics of fasting and reactive hypoglycemia.

Because hypoglycemias vary and can arise from a multitude of causes, no one treatment is appropriate for all of them. Many dishonest or ill-informed practitioners "diagnose" hypoglycemia on the basis of their clients' verbal reports alone, and prescribe all sorts of "remedies" for it with transparently thin rationale. People also "diagnose" themselves so commonly that physicians have identified a special category for their condition: *non*hypoglycemia.

The finding that a person has reactive hypoglycemia requires three simultaneous observations: (1) a low blood glucose concentration, (2) the

reactive hypoglycemia: hypoglycemia experienced simultaneously with epinephrine-release symptoms two to five hours after a meal; also called **postprandial hypoglycemia.**

fasting hypoglycemia: hypoglycemia that occurs after 8 to 14 hours of fasting.

nonhypoglycemia: a term used when people think they have hypoglycemia but don't.

TABLE 20–9 **Characteristics of Fasting and Reactive Hypoglycemia**

	FASTING TYPE	**REACTIVE TYPE**
Onset of symptoms	Gradual; occurs after fasting	Sudden; occurs two to five hours after meals
Type of symptoms	Headache, mental dullness, fatigue, confusion, amnesia, seizures, unconsciousness	Anxiety, weakness, sweating, rapid heartbeat, hunger, trembling
Duration of symptoms	Persistent	Transient
Possible causes	Hormonal imbalance, drugs, tumors	Early NIDDM, gastric surgery, TPN
Clinical course	Can be serious; treat underlying problems	Less serious; treat with diet
Other names	—	Alimentary, postprandial, idiopathic, functional

simultaneous presence of symptoms, and (3) the occurrence of these after the passage of four to six hours after a meal or after a dose of glucose. Even people *not* prone to reactive hypoglycemia can wreak havoc with glucose regulation by depriving the body of carbohydrate and then dumping in a large dose all at once. The remedy, then, requires people to eat regularly, to eat balanced meals, and to avoid sugary snacks.

In true, fasting hypoglycemia, diet is a key part of therapy. The diet planner develops a diet similar to the diabetic diet, which is appropriate to achieve or maintain a healthy body weight, and often uses the exchange lists for instruction. To prevent episodes of hypoglycemia, the person avoids concentrated sweets, eats four to six small meals a day, and limits the use of alcohol.

Hypoglycemia may also develop as a complication of another medical problem—for example, when central TPN solutions are discontinued too quickly, in some inborn metabolic disorders, and sometimes in early NIDDM. The next section describes how hypoglycemia can occur as a result of gastric surgery.

Dumping Syndrome

Surgery in which part or all of the stomach has been removed is called a **gastrectomy** or **gastric resection.** The management of gastric cancer or of damage to the stomach during trauma (gunshot wound or auto accident) may include gastric surgery.

dumping syndrome: the symptoms that result from the rapid emptying of undigested food into the jejunum: sweating, weakness, and diarrhea shortly after eating and hypoglycemia later.

The type of hypoglycemia that occurs following gastric surgery is called **alimentary** (AL-ee-MEN-tah-ree) or **postgastrectomy hypoglycemia.**

A person who has had surgery to remove a significant portion of the stomach may experience complications that include hypoglycemia. A typical scenario goes something like this: Mr. Fremont had a fairly extensive gastric resection about a week ago and has just begun eating solid foods. He swallows the food; then, about 15 minutes later, he begins to feel weak and dizzy. He looks pale, his heartbeat is rapid, and he breaks out into a sweat. Shortly thereafter, he develops diarrhea. What causes this sequence of events?

Diet Prescription

Carbohydrate-controlled, postgastrectomy diet.

Mr. Fremont has lost an important function of his stomach. Food no longer empties at a controlled rate into the intestine. Instead, it gets "dumped" rapidly into the jejunum. (Even if the duodenum was not bypassed during surgery, it is so short that food passes quickly into the jejunum.) As the food is digested, the intestinal contents become concentrated. Water from the body moves into the intestinal lumen to dilute the concentration. The volume of circulating blood diminishes rapidly, causing weakness, dizziness, and rapid heartbeat. The large fluid load in the jejunum causes pain and hyperperistalsis, and diarrhea results. Figure 20–2 outlines the sequence of events that occur in dumping syndrome.

After about two to three hours, Mr. Fremont develops many of the same symptoms again: dizziness, fainting, nausea, and sweating. This time the cause is different. Carbohydrates from the meal were rapidly digested and then absorbed, causing blood glucose levels to rise quickly. The pancreas responded by overproducing insulin, making blood glucose levels fall sharply. The symptoms this time are resulting from hypoglycemia.

Not all people who have had gastrectomies experience the diarrhea of dumping syndrome; even fewer develop hypoglycemia. Many people who

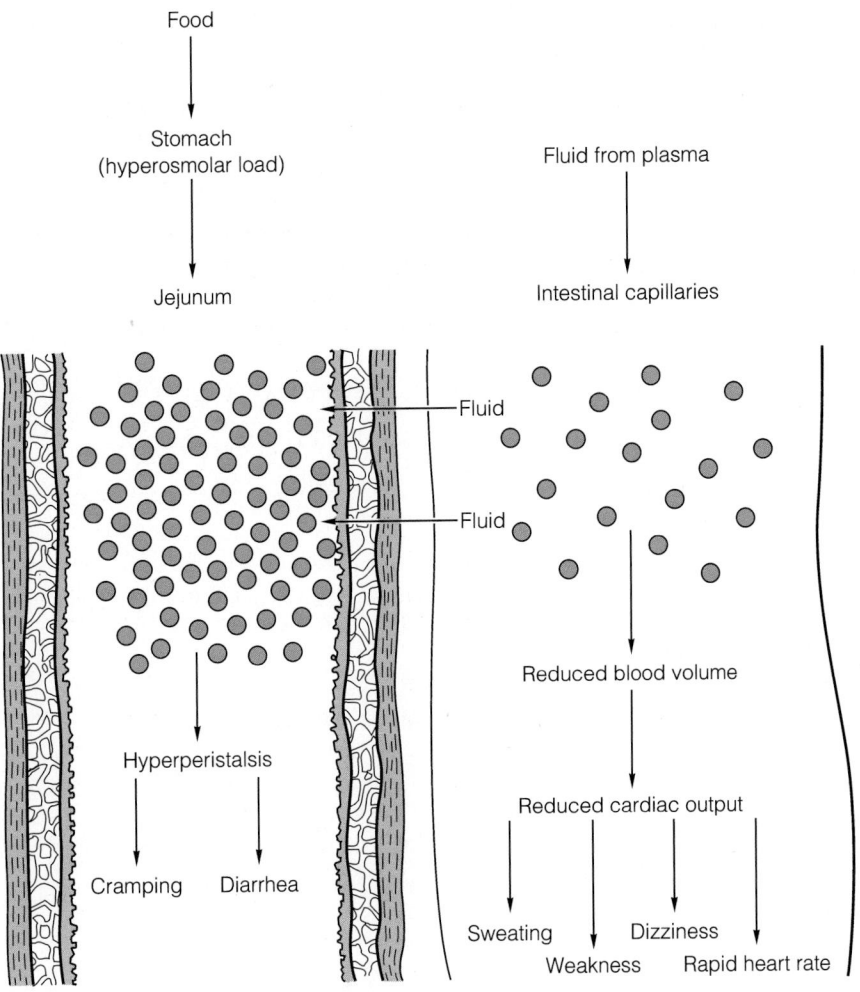

FIGURE 20-2 **Dumping Syndrome** When partially digested food rapidly enters the jejunum, it creates a hyperosmolar load. Fluid from the intestinal capillaries enters the jejunum, diminishing blood volume and stimulating peristalsis. The result: low blood pressure and diarrhea.

initially experience dumping syndrome gradually adapt to a fairly normal diet. However, a special diet benefits people during the immediate postsurgical period and in prolonged or severe cases.

The postgastrectomy diet is a carbohydrate-controlled diet designed to alleviate the symptoms of dumping syndrome. Health care professionals monitor fluid and electrolyte balances carefully, correcting any imbalances that occur. The diet emphasizes foods containing protein and fat. Because proteins and fats are digested more slowly than carbohydrates, they do not attract fluids as rapidly as do carbohydrates.

Advise the client not to eat concentrated sweets (sugar, cookies, cakes, pies, or soft drinks), because the body digests these carbohydrates most rapidly. Recommend small, frequent meals to fit the reduced storage capacity of the stomach. Suggest that clients wait about 45 minutes after each meal before drinking liquids. This precaution helps slow the rate of food's passage from the stomach to the intestine. Encourage clients to lie down immediately after eating to help slow the transit of food to the intestine. Pectin, a type of dietary fiber, can be added to the diet to help prevent

postgastrectomy diet: a diet given to prevent the symptoms of dumping syndrome and hypoglycemia that sometimes follow gastric surgery.

TABLE 20–10   **Postgastrectomy Diet**

FOOD ITEM	ALLOWED	EXCLUDED	COMMENTS
MEATS/MEAT ALTERNATES	X		Any type
GRAINS/STARCHY VEGETABLES			
Plain breads, crackers, rolls, unsweetened cereals, rice, pasta, corn, lima beans, parsnips, peas, white potatoes, sweet potatoes, pumpkin, yams, winter squash	X		Limit to 5 servings daily
Sweetened cereals; cereals containing dates, raisins, or brown sugar		X	
NONSTARCHY VEGETABLES			
Chicory, Chinese cabbage, endive, escarole, lettuce, parsley, radishes, watercress	X		As desired
Asparagus, bean sprouts, beets, broccoli, brussels sprouts, cabbage, carrots, cauliflower, celery, cucumbers, eggplant, green pepper, greens, mushrooms, okra, onions, rhubarb, sauerkraut, string beans, summer squash, tomatoes, turnips, zucchini	X		Limit to two ½-c servings daily; individual tolerances will vary
Vegetables prepared with sugar		X	
FRUITS			
Unsweetened fruits and fruit juices	X		Limit to 3 servings daily
Sweetened fruits and fruit juices		X	
FATS	X		Any type
BEVERAGES			
Milk (whole milk, nonfat milk, or buttermilk)	X		If tolerated
Coffee, tea, dietetic carbonated beverages	X		
Alcohol, carbonated beverages, sweetened milk, cocoa, fruit drinks		X	
DESSERTS			
Cakes, cookies, ice cream, sherbet		X	
OTHER			
Honey, jam, jelly, syrup, sugar		X	

dumping syndrome. Table 20–10 lists foods included on, and excluded from, the postgastrectomy diet. A sample postgastrectomy diet menu is also provided.

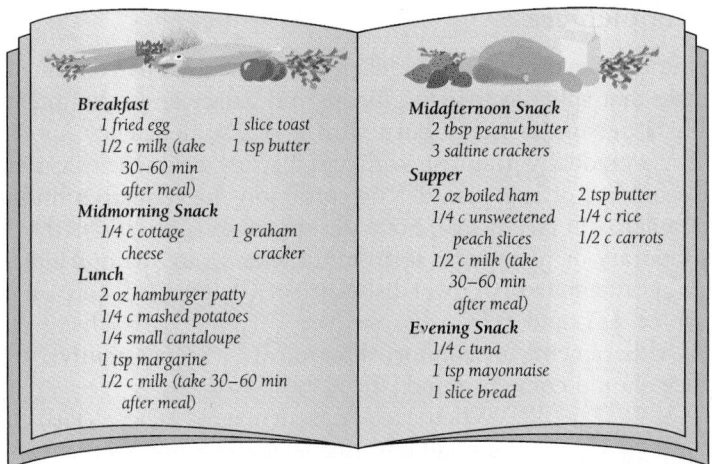

Sample Postgastrectomy Diet Menu

Breakfast
1 fried egg   1 slice toast
1/2 c milk (take   1 tsp butter
    30–60 min
    after meal)
Midmorning Snack
1/4 c cottage   1 graham
    cheese   cracker
Lunch
2 oz hamburger patty
1/4 c mashed potatoes
1/4 small cantaloupe
1 tsp margarine
1/2 c milk (take 30–60 min
    after meal)

Midafternoon Snack
2 tbsp peanut butter
3 saltine crackers
Supper
2 oz boiled ham   2 tsp butter
1/4 c unsweetened   1/4 c rice
    peach slices   1/2 c carrots
1/2 c milk (take
    30–60 min
    after meal)
Evening Snack
1/4 c tuna
1 tsp mayonnaise
1 slice bread

Dietitians carefully tailor the diet to meet the client's needs. Initially, visits to the client after each meal uncover food intolerances. For example, some people may be unable to tolerate any milk at all because they have developed lactose intolerance (see the next section).

Gradually, many people with dumping syndrome become able to tolerate small amounts of concentrated sweets, larger quantities of food, and some liquids with meals. Unfortunately, however, diet does not correct the symptoms of dumping syndrome for everyone. When all dietary measures fail, additional surgery may be necessary to resolve the problem.

Other nutrition concerns arise in people with gastrectomies. For example, clients may develop iron-deficiency anemia. Blood loss from surgery, accompanied by inadequate nutrition and poor iron absorption, contributes to the problem. An iron supplement helps to correct the deficiency. Anemia also can be caused by deficiency of vitamin B_{12} or folate. Recall that vitamin B_{12} cannot be absorbed without the intrinsic factor, which is synthesized in the stomach. Depending on the location and extent of the gastric resection, intrinsic factor production may be minimal or absent, and vitamin B_{12} absorption correspondingly impaired. To correct the deficiency, clients receive vitamin B_{12} by injection (to bypass the need for absorption) and supplemental folate orally.

Malabsorption of fat and many nutrients can also occur as a consequence of surgery in which a portion of the stomach has been removed. Chapter 21 discusses malabsorption.

Diets Restricted in Simple Carbohydrate

In some conditions requiring carbohydrate-controlled diets, certain types of simple sugars must be avoided. The most common diet of this kind is the one used to treat lactose intolerance.

Lactose Intolerance

A person born with little or no lactase activity has **primary lactose intolerance.** Lactase deficiency caused by another disease or condition is **secondary lactose intolerance.** A lactase deficiency that develops as a person ages is **developmental lactose intolerance.**

Lactose intolerance results from a deficiency of the digestive enzyme lactase, the enzyme that splits lactose to glucose and galactose in the intestine. In rare cases, a person is simply born with a lactase deficiency; more often, lactase levels gradually diminish with age. Lactase deficiencies can develop as a consequence of any disorder or condition that damages the delicate intestinal microvilli (see p. 86). Some disorders and conditions that lead to either temporary or permanent lactose intolerance are malnutrition, radiation therapy, inflammatory bowel diseases (see Chapter 21), GI tract surgery (see Chapter 21), and celiac disease (see Chapter 23). Whenever an ill person is experiencing discomfort after meals, the possibility of lactose intolerance should come to mind.

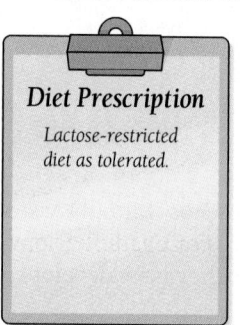

Diet Prescription

Lactose-restricted diet as tolerated.

When lactase is deficient, lactose absorption in the small intestine is blocked, and the intestinal contents become hyperosmolar. Large volumes of water are drawn into the gut to equalize the osmolarity, causing cramps, distention, and diarrhea. Bacteria in the intestine metabolize the undigested sugars to irritating acids and gases, further contributing to cramping and diarrhea.

An appropriately individualized lactose-restricted diet alleviates lactose intolerance. Because people vary widely in the amounts of lactose they can tolerate, lactose-restricted diets must be individualized. People sensitive to the smallest amounts of lactose must follow a lactose-free diet as shown in Table 20–11 and the accompanying sample menu. As you can see, hidden lactose makes this diet difficult to follow. People on lactose-free diets must read labels and avoid foods that include milk, milk solids, lactose, whey, and casein. They also need to check all drugs with the pharmacist, because some drugs contain lactose.

Be alert to the presence of lactose in a food whenever the label lists any of these ingredients:

- Milk.
- Milk solids.
- Lactose.
- Whey.
- Casein.

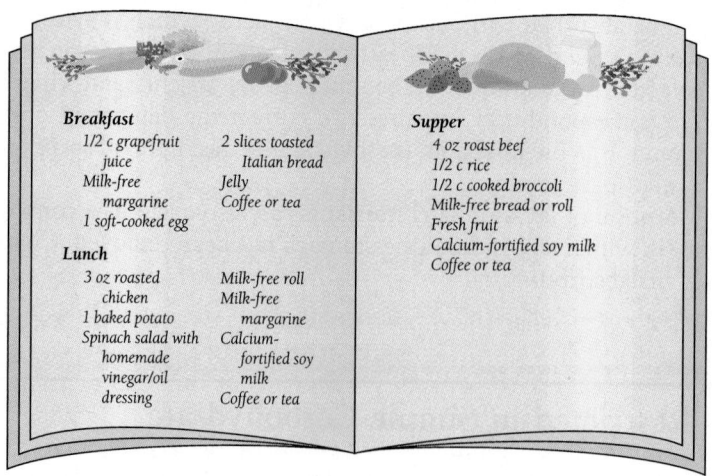

Breakfast
1/2 c grapefruit juice
Milk-free margarine
1 soft-cooked egg
2 slices toasted Italian bread
Jelly
Coffee or tea

Lunch
3 oz roasted chicken
1 baked potato
Spinach salad with homemade vinegar/oil dressing
Milk-free roll
Milk-free margarine
Calcium-fortified soy milk
Coffee or tea

Supper
4 oz roast beef
1/2 c rice
1/2 c cooked broccoli
Milk-free bread or roll
Fresh fruit
Calcium-fortified soy milk
Coffee or tea

Sample Lactose-Free Diet Menu

TABLE 20–11   **Foods to Avoid on a Lactose-Free Diet**

MEAT AND MEAT ALTERNATES
Breaded or creamed meats, fish, or poultry; sausage or cold cuts containing nonfat-milk solids; omelets or soufflés made with milk; some peanut butter
MILK AND MILK PRODUCTS
Whole, nonfat, evaporated, condensed, or dried milk; yogurt; cheese; ice cream; sherbet; whey and casein milk treated with lactobacillus/acidophilus culture; custard; pudding
FRUITS AND VEGETABLES
Any canned or frozen fruit or vegetable processed with lactose; creamed, breaded, or buttered vegetables
GRAINS
Breads and rolls made with milk; prepared muffin, biscuit, waffle, pancake, cake, or cookie mixes; some dry cereals; French toast; pie crusts made with butter or margarine
OTHER
Some cocoas, instant coffees, margarines, and dressings; butter; cream; creamed soups; chewing gum; chocolate; toffee; peppermint; butterscotch; caramels; some drugs and vitamin-mineral supplements; monosodium glutamate; sugar substitutes containing lactose

Fortunately, not all people with lactose intolerance must avoid lactose completely. Individual tolerances determine the amounts of lactose that clients can consume. Many times people need to eliminate only milk, milk beverages, creamed foods, and ice cream from their diets. Often people with mild lactose intolerance can eat cheeses, particularly aged cheeses, and drink buttermilk, because these items contain less lactose. They generally tolerate yogurt well, some brands better than others.[14] If a client cannot tolerate one brand of yogurt, suggest trying a different brand.

Many people can use commercially prepared products containing lactose without difficulty. Some may even be able to use milk or ice cream in limited quantities. Others can add an enzyme preparation (Lact-Aid) to milk before they drink it or take enzyme tablets (Dairy Ease) whenever they eat lactose-containing foods. The enzyme splits much of the lactose in milk to glucose and galactose. Alternatively, commercially prepared milk products that have been enzyme treated are also available.

A word of caution: people who consume little or no milk and milk products often have calcium-deficient diets. Encourage the use of milk and milk products whenever people can tolerate them; in some cases, a calcium

Lactose-restricted diets may be deficient in calcium.

supplement may be indicated. Other food sources of calcium (see Chapter 8, p. 159) can be used frequently.

Galactosemia

galactosemia (ga-lac-toe-SEE-mee-uh): an inherited disorder characterized by a deficiency of one of several enzymes necessary to convert galactose to glucose in the body.

Another type of diet restricted in simple carbohydrate is the galactose-free diet, which plays an important role in the treatment of galactosemia. Galactosemia is an inherited disorder of carbohydrate metabolism in which the body cannot use the monosaccharide galactose. When given milk-based formulas (which contain a galactose unit in each molecule of lactose), infants with galactosemia vomit and have diarrhea. The unmetabolized galactose follows an alternative metabolic pathway to form an abnormal product that causes growth failure, liver enlargement, and other neurological abnormalities that lead to coma and death. Early introduction of a galactose-restricted diet prevents or minimizes most of these symptoms. However, it may not prevent ovarian damage, some visual and speech problems, or other neurological abnormalities. Breastfeeding the infant with galactosemia is contraindicated, because breast milk contains galactose. Instead, infants receive soy-based formulas to replace standard (lactose-containing) infant formulas.

Diet Prescription

Galactose-restricted diet.

All foods omitted from a lactose-free diet must be strictly excluded from a galactose-free diet. (Recall from Chapter 2 that galactose is a part of the lactose molecule.) In addition, peas, organ meats such as liver and brain, and monosodium glutamate must be avoided.

Peas contain galactose, and organ meats and monosodium glutamate can be metabolized to galactose.

Carbohydrate-modified diets help control symptoms and prevent complications of several metabolic disorders. Chapter 22 shows how fat-modified diets help correct metabolic abnormalities of blood lipid levels. Other fat-modified diets, low-fat diets, are valuable in treating disorders of the GI tract. Chapter 21 describes these diets.

CASE STUDY

Insulin-Dependent Diabetes Mellitus

One year ago, Sam, a 10-year-old boy, was diagnosed with IDDM. He is 5 feet tall and weighs 80 pounds. The initial diagnosis was made after Sam's parents became concerned when Sam began to lose weight, to urinate excessively, and to complain of thirst. Aware of a family history of diabetes, Sam's parents quickly sought medical help. Since that time Sam's diabetes had been well-controlled. Recently, however, Sam was admitted to the emergency room, complaining of nausea, vomiting, and intense thirst. The physician noted that Sam was confused and was breathing with difficulty, and further noted the smell of acetone on his breath. Urine tests were positive for glucosuria and ketonuria, and his blood glucose level was 400 milligrams per 100 milliliters. The diagnosis was diabetic ketoacidosis.

  Describe the metabolic events that lead to the symptoms associated with diabetes (before diagnosis), as well as those associated with diabetic ketoacidosis. Were Sam's physical symptoms and laboratory tests consistent with this diagnosis? How can you distinguish between diabetic ketoacidosis and insulin shock?

  When Sam recovers, what advice can you offer him in order to prevent future incidents of ketoacidosis? Assume that Sam had never had a diabetic diet instruction. What dietary modifications would you advise him to follow?

  Think about and discuss the influence of Sam's age on his outlook and ability to cope with diabetes. What problems does his age pose? Consider some ways you might help him deal with these problems. Regarding his future, describe the possible role of diet in preventing the vascular complications of diabetes.

Study Questions

1. Name the two major types of diabetes. Which type is more common? Identify some differences between the two types.
2. Describe the basic problem in diabetes, and tell how it leads to these symptoms: hyperglycemia, glucosuria, dehydration, polyuria, polydipsia, weight loss, polyphagia, acetone breath, ketosis, and ketonuria.
3. What types of complications can arise from diabetes?
4. What are the goals of therapy for all people with diabetes? Describe the three components of lifestyle that must be coordinated for the person with IDDM.
5. What biochemical tests are used to diagnose diabetes? What methods can the person with diabetes use to monitor glucose levels? What is glycosylated hemoglobin, and what advantage is there in measuring it in the blood?

6. Why is insulin not taken orally? How do insulin needs change with body weight?

7. What is the recommended distribution of nutrients for the diet in the treatment of IDDM? What types of carbohydrates are recommended? What type of fat is recommended?

8. Why are the timing and composition of meals important considerations in planning a diet for a person with IDDM? How is the diet adjusted if a person misses meals? How is the carbohydrate content of the diet adjusted for physical activity?

9. What is the primary goal of diet therapy in the person with NIDDM? How does diet therapy for IDDM differ from that for NIDDM?

10. How is the pregnant woman with IDDM managed? How is the pregnant woman with NIDDM managed?

11. What is hypoglycemia? What type of hypoglycemia is treated with diet? For this type of hypoglycemia, what diet is recommended?

12. Describe the events associated with the dumping syndrome. What diet helps prevent these symptoms?

13. Discuss lactose intolerance. What types of foods are avoided on a lactose-restricted diet? Describe the variability of lactose-restricted diets for people with lactose intolerance.

14. What is galactosemia? Discuss the ways in which the lactose-restricted diet differs in the treatment of lactose intolerance and galactosemia.

Notes

1. G. M. Reaven, Parma Symposium: Current controversies in nutrition, *American Journal of Clinical Nutrition* 47 (1988): 1078–1082.

2. S. Lillioja and coauthors, Impaired glucose tolerance as a disorder of insulin action, *New England Journal of Medicine* 318 (1988): 1217–1225.

3. G. F. Cahill, Beta-cell deficiency, insulin resistance, or both? *New England Journal of Medicine* 318 (1988): 1268–1270.

4. M. J. Franz, Diabetes and nutrition: State of the science and the art, *Topics in Clinical Nutrition* 3 (1988): 1–16.

5. Franz, 1988.

6. M. J. Franz, Exercise and the management of diabetes mellitus, *Journal of the American Dietetic Association* 87 (1987): 28–34.

7. Franz, 1987.

8. K. H. Gabbay, Treatment of diabetes mellitus, in *Pediatric Nutrition,* eds. R. J. Grand, J. L. Stutphen, and W. H. Dietz (Boston: Butterworths, 1987), pp. 539–547.

9. M. L. Wheeler, L. Delahanty, and J. Wylie-Rosett, Diet and exercise in noninsulin-dependent diabetes mellitus: Implications for dietitians from the NIH Consensus Development Conference, *Journal of the American Dietetic Association* 87 (1987): 480–485.

10. M. Berger, Oral agents in the treatment of diabetes mellitus, in *Clinical Diabetes Mellitus: A Problem Oriented Approach,* ed. J. K. Davison (New York: Thieme, 1986), pp. 262–273.

11. Wheeler, Delahanty, and Wylie-Rosett, 1987.

12. D. K. Silverstein, E. B. Connor, and D. L. Wingard, The effect of parity on the later development of non-insulin-dependent diabetes mellitus or impaired glucose tolerance, *New England Journal of Medicine* 321 (1989): 1214–1219.

13. J. Palardy and coauthors, Blood glucose measurements during symptomatic episodes in patients with suspected postprandial hypoglycemia, *New England Journal of Medicine* 321 (1989): 1421–1425.

14. D. H. Whytock and J. A. DiPalma, All yogurts are not created equal, *American Journal of Clinical Nutrition* 47 (1988): 454–457.

20

Sugar Alternatives

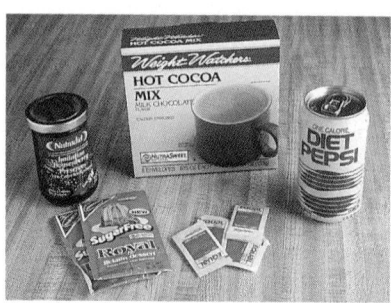

Many commonly used products contain sugar alternatives.

People who wish to avoid sugar or cut down on their use of it often look for substitutes to satisfy their taste for sweets. Nutrition in Practice 20 discusses several sugar alternatives and addresses many concerns regarding their safety.

I'm mixed up about kcalories in sugar alternatives. In some sugar-free things I use, like soft drinks, the products are also low in kcalories. But when I buy sugar-free gum, the label says that the gum isn't low in kcalories. Why?

The two sugar-free products you mentioned, soft drinks and chewing gum, contain two different kinds of sugar alternatives. Artificial sweeteners (saccharin, aspartame, cyclamate, and acesulfame potassium) do not contain appreciable kcalories in the amounts typically used.

On the other hand, the sugar alternatives are sugar alcohols (mannitol, sorbitol, xylitol, and maltitol), and they do contain kcalories. The body either absorbs these carbohydrates more slowly or metabolizes them to glucose more slowly than most other sugars, but it does absorb and metabolize them. These sugars were once widely used by people with diabetes who could not handle large amounts of glucose, but their associated side effects and their energy contribution make them less attractive than the artificial sweeteners. The accompanying Miniglossary describes the sugar alternatives further.

I am not diabetic or overweight, but I try to limit the amount of sugar I eat and drink. I have read that saccharin causes cancer and that it was almost banned. Is it safe for me to use?

That's a hard question to answer. Questions concerning the safety of saccharin have not been fully answered. One large-scale population study, involving 9000 people, showed a distinctly *greater risk* of cancers in some groups, such as women who drank two or more diet sodas a day and people who both smoked heavily and used artificial sweeteners heavily. Another study, involving over 1000 people, showed little or no excess risk of bladder cancers, but could not conclude that there was no risk at all.

As of now, two alternative conclusions are possible:

1. Saccharin causes tumors, possibly cancerous, in rats but not in people.
2. Saccharin is a weak carcinogen in people, and its effects will take more years of exposure to become apparent.

What about aspartame? I have also heard that it isn't safe to use.

First of all, before you can understand some of the concerns that have been raised about aspartame, it is important to know what aspartame is. Aspartame is the active ingredient in NutraSweet and is composed of two amino acids, phenylalanine and aspartic acid, connected by a single carbon.

One concern regarding aspartame centers around people who cannot metabolize phenylalanine normally. In the extreme case, phenylketonuria (PKU), there is an inherited inability to dispose of excess phenylalanine. An infant with PKU must have some phenylalanine to grow (phenylalanine is an essential amino acid), but too much can lead to severe mental retardation (see Chapter 23). For children with PKU, products containing aspartame should be avoided altogether.

Another objection to aspartame relates to its molecular size and the fact that it is rapidly digested and absorbed. Concern arises over the idea that a sudden rise in phenylalanine

FIGURE NP20-1 **Structure of Aspartame**

Aspartic Acid | Phenylalanine | Methyl Group

could affect the brain's chemical balance, and thus alter behavior and produce functional changes in certain individuals.

Still another concern about aspartame's safety has to do with its chemical structure (see Figure NP20-1). During metabolism, the methyl group becomes methyl alcohol (methanol) momentarily—a toxic compound. Then it is converted to formaldehyde, another toxic compound, and finally, to carbon dioxide. The quantities generated from normal use of aspartame are below the threshold at which these compounds cause harm, but in the testing of aspartame, that threshold had to be determined and its acceptability evaluated.

Still another concern is about the product that aspartame breaks down to—diketopiperazine, or DKP for short. Long-term studies using animals have directly tested this product and eliminated it as a source of concern. Another concern was over the effect aspartame use might have on the brain. Experiments with rats, monkeys, and human beings were performed,

and none showed any cause for concern. Some 500 individual complaints received after its approval were reviewed by the Centers for Disease Control, which concluded that some individuals may exhibit vague, but not dangerous, symptoms due to unusual sensitivity to aspartame, but that the product is generally safe.

So far, then, there is no concrete evidence that aspartame is harmful, although there are some concerns about its use. Is that why I am seeing so many new products that are sweetened with NutraSweet?

The FDA has approved aspartame based on the assumption that no one will consume more than 50 milligrams per kilogram of body weight in a day. This maximum daily intake is indeed a lot: for a 132-pound person, this adds up to 80 packets of Equal or about 15 soft drinks sweetened with aspartame only. The company that produces aspartame estimates that only if all the sugar and saccharin in the U.S. diet were replaced with aspartame, would even 1 percent of the population be consuming the FDA maximum. Some people actually do consume this amount, however. A child who drinks a quart of Kool-Aid sweetened with aspartame on a hot day, and who also has pudding, chewing gum, cereal, and other products sweetened with aspartame that day, packs in more than the FDA maximum level.

From what you've said, I gather that saccharin and aspartame are probably safe, but they could pose some risks. Until more is known, should I use these artificial sweeteners?

To decide whether or not to use artificial sweeteners in your diet, you must decide if the benefits you will

receive are worth any risks you may be taking. We have just discussed the possible risks. What are the benefits? One is better dental health, because artificial sweeteners that replace sugar don't cause tooth decay, while sugar does. Another may be weight loss,

Miniglossary

acesulfame (AY-see-sul-fame) **potassium:** a low-kcalorie sweetener recently approved by the FDA.

aspartame: a compound of phenylalanine and aspartic acid that tastes like the sugar sucrose but is much sweeter. It provides 4 kcal/g, as does protein, but because so little is used, it is virtually kcalorie-free. In powdered form it is mixed with lactose, however, so a 1-g packet contains 4 kcal. It is used in both the United States and Canada.

cyclamate: a 0-kcal sweetener banned in the United States and used restrictively in Canada.

diketopiperazine (dye-KEY-toe-pie-PER-a-zeen), or **DKP:** a product to which aspartame breaks down during metabolism.

maltitol, mannitol, sorbitol, xylitol: sugar alcohols, which can be derived from fruits or commercially produced from dextrose; absorbed more slowly and metabolized differently than other sugars in the human body, and not readily utilized by ordinary mouth bacteria.

saccharin: a 0-kcal sweetener used in the United States but banned in Canada.

because aspartame certainly lowers the kcalorie contents of foods in which it replaces sugar. If you want to lose weight, however, you may or may not find artificial sweeteners helpful. They are useful only if they replace sugar, not if they are simply added to the diet. An additional benefit for people with diabetes or hypoglycemia is taste: they can enjoy the sweet taste of sugar without changing their blood glucose levels.

The most important consideration when using artificial sweeteners is to remember to use them in moderation. Almost every substance, including water, can be harmful if the dose is high enough.

And don't forget: when you want something sweet, your choice is not just between sugar and artificial sweeteners. You can reach for natural foods such as fruit to satisfy your sweet tooth.

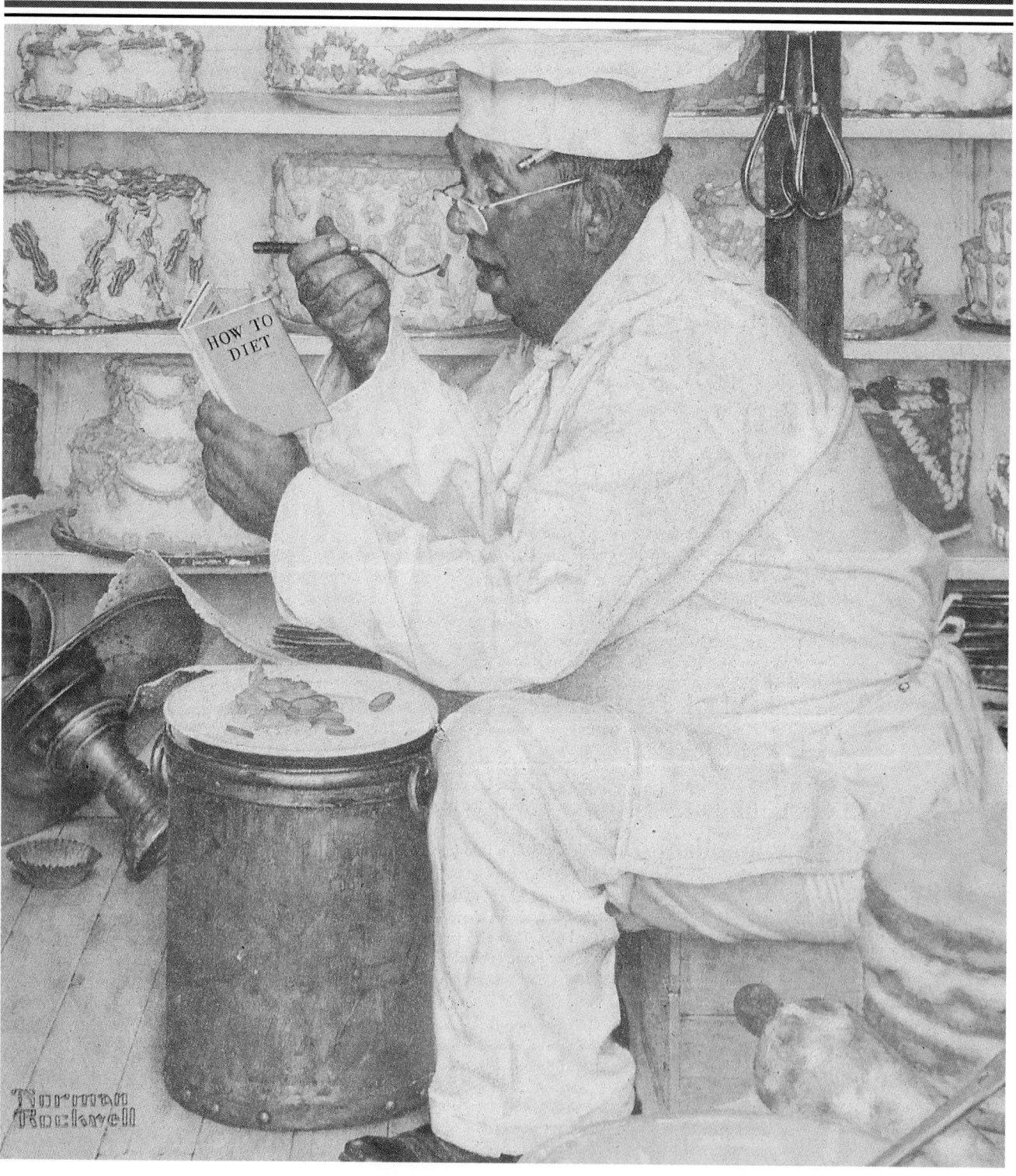

Diets Modified in Fat:
I. Fat-Restricted Diets

CONTENTS

fat-restricted diet: a diet in which the total amount of fat is limited.

fat-controlled diet: a diet in which both the amount of fat *and* the type of fat are controlled.

CHAPTER

21

Diets modified in fat are of two basic types. People on fat-restricted diets limit the total amount of fat in their diets. People on fat-controlled diets watch not only how much fat they eat but also the type of fat—polyunsaturated versus saturated. These two types of diets are frequently confused in the clinical setting, even though there is a considerable difference between them. This chapter discusses fat-restricted diets and Table 21–1 lists indications for their use. Chapter 22 discusses fat-controlled diets and Table 22–2 shows disorders for which they are used.

TABLE 21–1   Indications for the Use of Fat-Restricted Diets

Acquired immune deficiency
    syndrome (AIDS)
Blind loop syndrome
Cystic fibrosis
Fat malabsorption (steatorrhea)
Hiatal hernia
Inflammatory bowel diseases
Liver disease
Pancreatitis
Reflux esophagitis
Short bowel syndrome

Fat-Restricted Diets

Any condition in which fat malabsorption occurs can benefit from use of a fat-restricted diet. These diets prevent many of the problems associated with the malabsorption of fat. Fat-restricted diets limit the total amount of fat to 15 to 35 percent of the total kcalories. Table 21–2 details a typical fat-restricted diet. Fat-restricted diets can also be planned using the exchange list system presented in Chapter 19. To use this system, the client is instructed to select low-fat milk and meat exchanges and to limit the total number of fat and meat exchange servings. The exact number of servings allowed depends on the specific diet; for example, on a 30-gram fat-restricted diet, the client would be allowed 5 lean meat exchanges (15 grams of fat) and 3 fat exchanges (15 grams of fat). A sample menu is shown in the text.

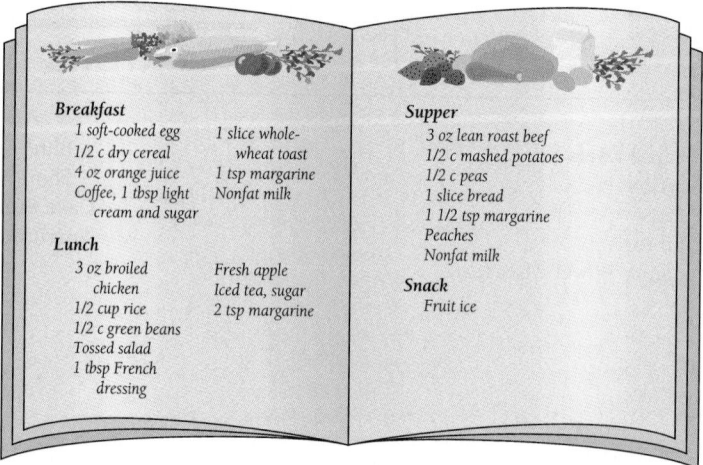

Sample Fat-Restricted Diet Menu

A fat-restricted diet can be difficult to follow. Fats give flavors to foods—flavors that some people may miss. Tips to reduce fat intake include:

■ Read labels and purchase low-fat foods. Nutrition labels state the fat contents of a product in grams per serving.

TABLE 21–2   **Fat-Restricted Diet**

USE:

1. Nonfat milk, nonfat-milk cheeses, yogurt made from nonfat milk, sherbet, and fruit ices.
2. Low-fat egg substitutes and up to three regular eggs per week.
3. Up to 6 oz of lean meats and poultry without skin daily.
4. Up to 6 servings of fat daily. One serving is any one of the following:
    1 tsp butter, margarine, shortening, oil, or mayonnaise.
    1 strip crisp bacon.
    1 tbsp heavy cream or Italian or French dressing.
    ⅛ avocado.
    2 tbsp light cream.
    6 small nuts.
    5 small olives.
    If fat is used to cook or season food, it must be taken from this allowance.
5. All vegetables prepared without fat.
6. All fruits prepared without fat.
7. Plain white or whole-grain bread; nonfat cereals, pasta, rice, noodles, and macaroni.
8. Clear soups and cream soups made with nonfat milk.
9. Angel food cake and fruit whips made with gelatin, sugar, and egg-white meringues.
10. Jelly, jam, honey, gumdrops, jelly beans, and marshmallows.

DO NOT USE:

1. Whole milk, chocolate milk, whole milk cheeses, and ice cream.
2. Pastries, cakes, pies, sweet rolls, or breads made with fat.
3. More than one egg a day, fried or fatty meats (sausage, luncheon meats, spareribs, frankfurters), duck, goose, or tuna packed in oil (unless well drained).
4. More than 6 servings of fat.
5. Desserts, candy, or anything made with chocolate or nuts.
6. Creamed soups made with whole milk.

SUGGESTIONS:

1. To make the diet still lower in fat, reduce the fat and meat (and egg) servings.
2. To raise the fat content, give additional fat or meat servings.
3. To improve acceptance of the diet, check the fat content of a well-liked food and allow that food if possible. Use the exchange system fat list for alternate suggestions for fat servings.

- Purchase low-fat meats. Fish, poultry, and veal are lower in fat than red meats. For ground meat without too much fat, buy a lean piece of beef or pork and have the butcher remove any excess fat from the meat and grind it. Ground turkey or chicken can be an excellent substitute for ground beef or pork.
- Tempt the taste buds by cooking meats in mixtures of vegetables such as tomatoes, green peppers, carrots, mushrooms, and onions.

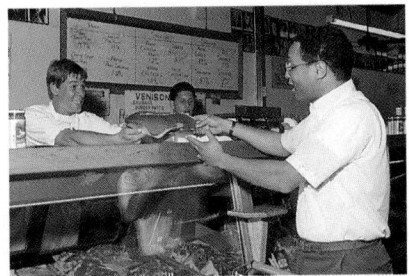

Grocers can trim excess fat from meats before you purchase them.

- Remember to use herbs and spices. Unless otherwise indicated, salt is not limited on a fat-restricted diet.
- Make gravy from bouillon or broth seasoned with wine and herbs and thickened with cornstarch or flour.
- Blenderize low-fat cottage cheese or yogurt made from nonfat milk with herbs for a zesty salad dressing.
- Substitute reduced-kcalorie margarine for regular margarine, because it has half the fat.
- Use butter salt or imitation butter flavoring to season food.
- Broil, bake, or steam foods instead of frying. If you pan fry on occasion, use vegetable cooking sprays and no-stick pans instead of fat.
- Make homemade stews and soups, and refrigerate them overnight. Skim off the excess fat that forms on top before using them the next day.

Both low-kcalorie and low-fat cookbooks feature recipes low in fat. Nutrition in Practice 21 offers guidelines for limiting fat when eating at fast food restaurants.

People on very-low-fat diets may find it difficult to get enough food energy. In such cases, products made from medium-chain triglycerides (MCT) can supplement the diet. MCT provides as many kcalories as regular fats, but the body digests and absorbs MCT differently than it does long-chain triglycerides. MCT oil can replace regular oil in salad dressings and can be used in beverages, desserts, and other dishes. However, MCT does not provide essential fatty acids, so the diet must include a source of long-chain fats. Clients can obtain MCT through the dietary department or pharmacy; they are expensive, but their delivery of needed energy often justifies their cost.

Malabsorption

Conditions that involve or affect the digestive organs often result in the malabsorption of nutrients either by hindering the digestion of food or the absorption of nutrients. Many disorders can lead to malabsorption; several are discussed throughout the remainder of this chapter. Table 21–3 highlights the reasons why malnutrition is especially likely in malabsorption syndromes.

Malabsorption of fat, carbohydrate, protein, vitamins, and minerals, or any combination of these nutrients, is possible. Most commonly, it is fat that is malabsorbed, because fat is digested and absorbed in a different, more involved way than either carbohydrate or protein (see Chapter 5). Unabsorbed fat is excreted from the body in the stools, causing the type of diarrhea known as steatorrhea.

The effects of fat malabsorption can be quite severe (see Figure 21–1). Fat lost in the stools carries with it valuable food energy and fat-soluble vitamins. Calcium and magnesium form soaps with unabsorbed fatty acids, so they, too, are lost in the stools. Vitamin D loss further adds to calcium depletion.

The loss of calcium with fatty acids can cause another problem, enteric hyperoxaluria. Oxalate, present in some foods, normally binds with calcium

steatorrhea (STEE-at-oh-REE-uh): fatty diarrhea characterized by stools that are foamy, greasy, and malodorous.

enteric hyperoxaluria (en-TER-ick HIGH-per-oxa-LOO-ree-ah): a condition of excess oxalate absorption that comes about because calcium is unable to bind oxalate in the gut; it leads to kidney stone formation.

Table 21–3   **Causes of Poor Nutrition Status in Malabsorption Syndromes**

REDUCED INTAKE	EXCESSIVE NUTRIENT LOSSES	RAISED NUTRIENT NEEDS
Abdominal pain	Blind loop syndrome	Drug therapy
Anorexia	Diarrhea	Surgery
Bowel rest	General malabsorption	
Emotional stress	Short bowel syndrome	
Food intolerance	Steatorrhea	
Indigestion		
Nausea		
Obstructions		

in the gut, and the body excretes both of them together. But when calcium binds instead to fatty acids, the oxalate remains unbound and available for absorption. The body does not metabolize oxalate, so this increased absorption leads to increased excretion of oxalate in the urine. High urinary oxalate favors the formation of kidney stones. (Nutrition in Practice 23 discusses kidney stones and presents a list of foods high in oxalate.)

The primary treatment of steatorrhea is to treat the underlying disorder. Along with this treatment, dietary fat is restricted, and fat-soluble vitamins are supplemented in a water-miscible form that facilitates their absorption. Often, the person with malabsorption initially receives a diet containing about 50 grams of fat per day. Gradually, the person may add fat if in need of additional energy and if the client is able to tolerate it. The client who cannot tolerate additional fat can use medium-chain triglycerides to increase energy intake.

water-miscible (MISS-i-bull) **vitamins:** fat-soluble vitamins that readily mix with water and can be absorbed without fat.

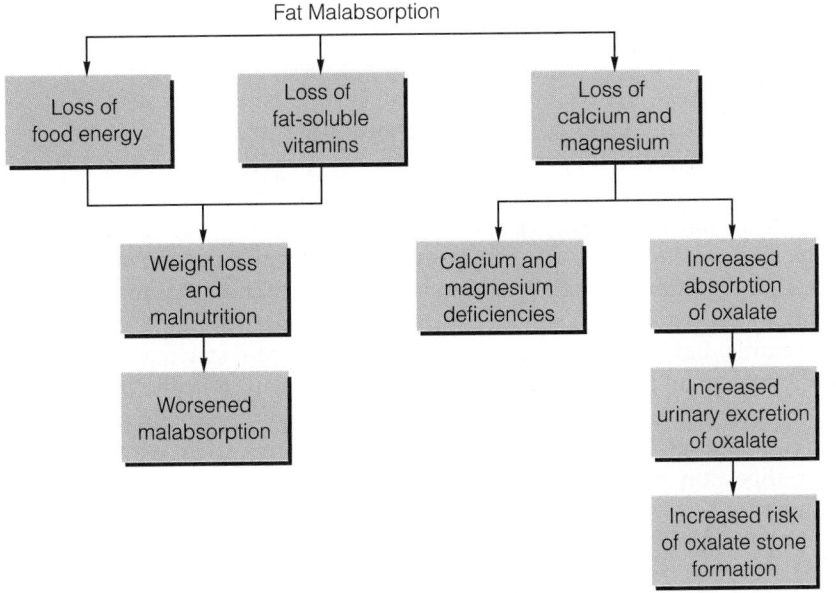

FIGURE 21–1   **The Effects of Fat Malabsorption**

Pancreatitis

pancreatitis (PAN-cree-uh-TIE-tis): inflammation of the pancreas.

amylase: a starch-digesting enzyme secreted by the pancreas.

lipase: a lipid-digesting enzyme secreted by the pancreas.

One disorder that can cause malabsorption is pancreatitis. Biliary tract disease, surgery (often of the stomach or biliary tract), and alcoholism most often precipitate pancreatitis. The damaged pancreas retains pancreatic secretions, including digestive enzymes, which begin to destroy the pancreas itself. The blood picks up some of these enzymes, raising serum amylase and lipase levels. These elevated enzyme levels serve as indicators of pancreatitis. Typical symptoms of pancreatitis include severe abdominal pain, nausea, and vomiting.

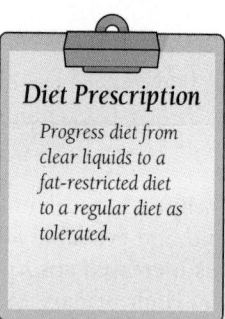

Diet Prescription

Progress diet from clear liquids to a fat-restricted diet to a regular diet as tolerated.

The goal of therapy in pancreatitis is to reduce pancreatic secretions. Food is withheld, since food stimulates bicarbonate and enzyme secretions from the pancreas. A nasogastric tube is inserted, not for feeding but rather to serve as a straw to suction out the stomach's secretions, so as to further reduce stimulation of the pancreas.

Clients receive intravenous fluids to maintain fluid and electrolyte balance. Edema, losses through nasogastric suction, and lack of oral intake can disrupt this balance. If pancreatitis is severe, or if the person is malnourished, TPN may be indicated. Some studies suggest that TPN does not stimulate pancreatic secretions to the degree an enteral diet would, but results of experiments in this area are unclear. Some people with pancreatitis may benefit from tube feedings of hydrolyzed formulas, delivered into the jejunum.[1]

When abdominal pain subsides, active bowel sounds resume, and serum amylase levels return to normal or near-normal, the client with pancreatitis can begin an oral diet. The diet progresses from a clear-liquid diet to a fat-restricted diet and, finally, to a regular diet as tolerated. At the first sign of pain, or if serum amylase levels rise, food is withheld; when these signs and symptoms subside, the person can eat again. Clients may tolerate six small meals better than large, less frequent meals.

If an acute attack of pancreatitis doesn't subside or if episodes occur at frequent intervals, the pancreatic cells can be permanently destroyed, leading to chronic pancreatitis. Chronic alcohol abuse is the most frequent cause of chronic pancreatitis.

The pancreas normally excretes enzymes far in excess of needs, so even after considerable damage has occurred, digestion may still proceed normally. However, with chronic pancreatitis and extensive degeneration of the pancreas, digestion, especially of fat, becomes permanently impaired.

Diet therapy during active attacks of pancreatitis is the same as for acute pancreatitis. Between attacks, the client follows a fat-restricted, bland diet. Small meals may be easiest to digest. The person with chronic pancreatitis usually tolerates about 50 to 70 grams of fat per day; restricting fat to less than this amount is unnecessary. Enzyme replacements taken with meals aid in the digestion and absorption of fat and protein. Absolutely no alcohol is permitted.

If steatorrhea persists, physicians prescribe fat-soluble vitamins in an easily absorbed, water-miscible, form. Vitamin B_{12} absorption may be reduced, so injections of vitamin B_{12} may be necessary.

acute: developing rapidly and lasting for only a short time.

chronic: developing slowly and lasting for long periods of time.

Goals of diet therapy in chronic pancreatitis:

- Maintain optimal nutrition status.
- Reduce steatorrhea, if present.
- Minimize pain.
- Avoid subsequent attacks of active pancreatitis.

A bland diet eliminates foods that stimulate gastric acid secretion, which in turn stimulate the secretions of the pancreas.

Sometimes pancreatitis damages the cells that produce insulin. In these cases, the individual becomes glucose intolerant, as in diabetes (Chapter 20), and must follow a diabetic diet in addition to the restrictions already mentioned.

Enzyme replacements are extracts of hog or beef pancreatic enzymes that help with digestion.

Cystic Fibrosis

Cystic fibrosis (CF) is a hereditary disease that affects many organs, including the pancreas, lungs, liver, heart, gallbladder, and small intestine. People with CF often have three major symptoms: chronic lung disease, pancreatic insufficiency (malabsorption), and abnormal electrolyte levels in the sweat. Cystic fibrosis is characterized by the production of thick mucus by glands throughout the body. The airways of the lungs become plugged with mucus, making it hard to breathe. Lung infections become likely and are the usual cause of death in people with CF.

cystic fibrosis (CF): a hereditary disorder characterized by the production of thick mucus that affects many organs, including the pancreas, lungs, liver, heart, gallbladder, and small intestine.

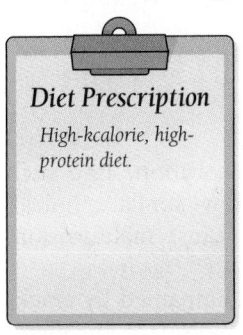

Diet Prescription

High-kcalorie, high-protein diet.

Cystic fibrosis affects the pancreas in 80 to 85 percent of cases. The thick mucus obstructs the small pancreatic ducts and interferes with the secretion of digestive enzymes and pancreatic juices. Malabsorption of many nutrients (including fat, protein, vitamins, and minerals) results, often leading to malnutrition. Although malabsorption is usually treated with a fat-restricted diet, malabsorption associated with cystic fibrosis is an exception to the rule. The extremely high energy needs and poor growth in most children and young people with CF make it necessary to treat malabsorption with enzyme replacements.

Energy needs of people with CF reach 150 percent of the RDA for sex and age; protein needs may be greater than 200 percent of the RDA. Energy and nutrient needs rise due to nutrient losses through malabsorption, frequent infections, higher than normal turnover of protein and essential fatty acids, and higher than normal protein catabolism and energy expenditure.[2] Extra energy is required simply to breathe. The combination of these factors and their effects on energy expenditure explain why growth failure is common.

For the infant with cystic fibrosis, breastfeeding is recommended, as it is for any infant; breast milk is optimally digestible. Infants who are not breastfed often tolerate regular infant formulas if they receive enzyme replacements with them. Infants intolerant to regular formulas need fat-restricted formulas. Energy can be added to any formula by adding carbohydrate and fat supplements, including MCT oil (see Appendix D).

After being weaned from breast milk or infant formula, a child with cystic fibrosis receives a high-kcalorie, high-protein, nutritionally balanced diet carefully tailored to individual tolerances. In the past, diets for people with CF were severely restricted in fat. However, growth failure and essential fatty acid deficiencies commonly occur in children with CF. Since fat is an important energy source and provides essential fatty acids, current recommendations do not restrict fat. Instead, clients use enzyme replacements to control steatorrhea, as mentioned earlier.

Enyzme replacements lessen malabsorption but do not fully correct it. People who have persistent steatorrhea, gas, and abdominal distention often benefit more from higher doses of enzyme replacements than from reduced fat intakes.

Abnormally high levels of electrolytes (sodium and chloride) in sweat are characteristic of CF. Fever, high environmental temperature, or diarrhea can rapidly precipitate electrolyte depletion in people with CF. When these conditions exist, extra salt is needed.

Vitamin supplements are prescribed; people with CF need their fat-soluble vitamins in a water-miscible form. They may also need zinc supplements. Regular nutrition assessments help to ensure that nutrient needs are being met. Height and weight measurements are particularly relevant. Despite the widespread use of unrestricted-fat diets, fat intakes in those with CF are often too low to meet their high needs.[3]

Maintaining adequate nutrition status is extremely important; it appears to be related to the severity of pulmonary disease. Home parenteral and enteral nutrition programs may help clients meet their high nutrient needs. Children might benefit from having both regular diets during waking hours and tube feedings or parenteral nutrition at night.

Inflammatory Bowel Diseases

Several conditions inflame the bowel and cause malabsorption. Two such disorders, Crohn's disease and ulcerative colitis, show similar clinical, pathologic, and biologic features, and both frequently cause malnutrition. Their cause or causes remain unknown.

In Crohn's disease, inflammation of the bowel is accompanied by crack-like ulcers and many granulomas. Symptoms most often occur in the ileum and colon, but can arise anywhere in the GI tract. The disease may be self-limited and eventually may be cured, but it often recurs. Inflammation and scarring may narrow the intestinal lumen, sometimes causing obstruction. The intestine may rupture and cause a severe, and sometimes fatal, infection (peritonitis). Bleeding from the ulcers can lead to anemia.

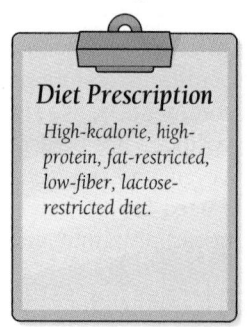

Diet Prescription

High-kcalorie, high-protein, fat-restricted, low-fiber, lactose-restricted diet.

The person with Crohn's disease often experiences anorexia, weight loss, fever, diarrhea, malabsorption, cramping abdominal pain, and anemia, and thus is at high risk for developing nutrient deficiencies. In addition, oral intake may be withheld so that the bowel can rest, particularly when the person develops an obstruction or when a fistula forms. Furthermore, drug therapy for Crohn's disease, which includes steroids and antibiotics, can also impair nutrition status (see Table 21–4). If the client requires surgery, nutrient needs become even greater.

To restore and maintain nutrition status for the person with Crohn's disease can be a challenging task. PEM and deficiencies of calcium, magnesium, zinc, iron, vitamin B_{12}, folate, vitamin C, and fat-soluble vitamins are commonly reported. Low serum albumin due to malnutrition and GI losses is common. Multiple nutrient deficiencies may reduce the effectiveness of drug therapy and threaten immune function.

Traditionally, enteral nutrition is withheld during the acute stage of Crohn's disease. However, hydrolyzed formulas (given by tube) have suc-

---

Crohn's disease: inflammation and ulceration along the length of the GI tract, often with granulomas.

granulomas (gran-you-LOH-mahz): a granular tumor or growth.
  granulum = little grain
  oma = tumor

fistula (FIS-too-lah): an abnormal opening between two organs or from an organ to the skin.
  fistula = pipe

TABLE 21–4   **Drugs Used in the Treatment of Crohn's Disease**

Drug Name	Timing with Meals	Common Side Effects That May Influence Nutrition Status
Prednisone	Give with food.	Fluid retention, stomach upset, peptic ulcers, blood glucose abnormalities, growth inhibition in children, decreased resistance to infection, weight gain. May decrease effects of insulin or antidiabetic medicine. May induce edema. Alters protein and carbohydrate metabolism. Decreases absorption of calcium and phosphorous.
Sulfasalazine	Give with food or milk.	May cause anorexia, nausea, and GI distress.

Source: Adapted from D. E. Powers and A. O. Moore, *Food Medication Interactions*, (City: Phoenix, 1991); *Nursing 91 Drug Handbook* (Springhouse, Pa.: Springhouse Corp., 1991).

cessfully resolved active Crohn's disease without the need for TPN or steroids.[4] The upper small intestine easily absorbs these formulas, allowing the remaining bowel to rest. Although hydrolyzed formulas are hypertonic and may contribute to diarrhea in some people, many people with Crohn's disease can tolerate hydrolyzed formulas given at full strength and so can receive all needed nutrients quickly.

In some cases, however, the bowel may need complete rest. When enteral nutrition significantly aggravates diarrhea, when the bowel is obstructed, or when rest might help a fistula to close, TPN can successfully deliver needed nutrients (see Chapter 16).

As the acute stage of Crohn's disease resolves, the client is gradually progressed to an oral diet as tolerated. A high-kcalorie, high-protein, fat-restricted, low-fiber diet is often recommended. Lactose intolerance frequently develops, and the person is then advised to eliminate milk and milk products. Supplemental vitamin and mineral preparations are frequently prescribed. Encourage clients to eat a nutrient-rich, well-balanced diet, and reassess nutrition status frequently to ensure that nutrient needs are being met.

Low-fiber diets may benefit people with Crohn's disease by reducing the risk of obstructions forming in the intestinal tract.

The incidence of Crohn's disease is highest in teenagers, so the individual who has it is typically young and depressed. The disease is highly unpredictable; just when a person feels well, a relapse may occur, necessitating another round of hospitalization or surgery. The person may feel that food itself causes the disease and may react by eating very little. The person with Crohn's disease therefore often needs a lot of emotional support.

Unlike Crohn's disease, which can occur anywhere along the GI tract, ulcerative colitis develops only in the large intestine. Ulcerative colitis is characterized by severe diarrhea, rectal bleeding, cramping, abdominal pain, anorexia, and weight loss. Diarrhea can be almost continuous, resulting in poor absorption of nutrients and great losses of fluids and electrolytes. Anemia may develop because of blood loss from rectal bleeding.

ulcerative colitis (ko-LYE-tis):
inflammation and ulceration of the colon.

Many of the dietary principles outlined for Crohn's disease apply to the person with ulcerative colitis. A primary concern is to ensure adequate intake of fluid and electrolytes. Clients need to avoid high-fiber foods, because these foods can irritate the colon. The diet includes high-kcalorie, high-protein foods and restricts fat if the client has symptoms of fat malabsorption. Milk and milk products may need to be eliminated if lactose intolerance is present. Supplemental vitamins or minerals may be necessary.

Blind Loop Syndrome

blind loop syndrome: the problems of fat malabsorption and folate and vitamin B$_{12}$ deficiencies that result from the overgrowth of bacteria in a bypassed segment of the intestine.

The blind loop syndrome represents another cause of fat malabsorption. The blind loop syndrome results from some types of gastric resections in which a portion of the small intestine is bypassed, making that portion nonfunctional. The bypassed portion is called a blind loop. Figure 21–2 illustrates a blind loop.

FIGURE 21–2   **A Blind Loop Resulting from a Gastric Resection**
Note that the segment of the intestine bypassed is no longer flushed by the steady flow of secretions that would normally go through it.

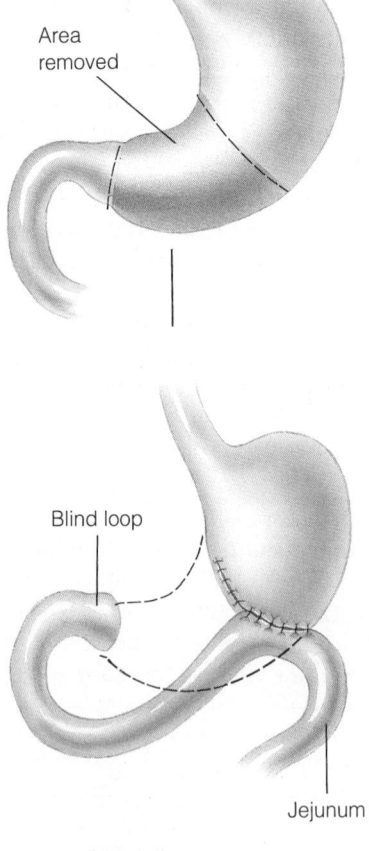

Area removed

Blind loop

Jejunum

Billroth II
(gastrojejunostomy)

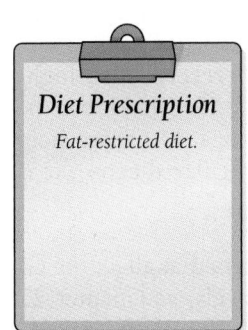

Diet Prescription

Fat-restricted diet.

Stasis occurs in the blind loop, and bacteria normally not present in that part of the intestine may begin to flourish there. The bacteria compete with the body for vitamin B_{12} and folate, limiting the available supply. The bacteria also partly dismantle bile salts, hampering fat digestion and absorption. The bacterial overgrowth that occurs in a blind loop leads to fat malabsorption, and to vitamin B_{12} and folate deficiencies. To correct these problems, the client receives a fat-restricted diet, parenteral vitamin B_{12}, and/or oral folate supplements. Physicians also prescribe antibiotics to inhibit bacterial growth. Sometimes the blind loop must be removed surgically.

stasis (STAY-sis): standing still. Normal actions of the intestines keep a steady stream of secretions flowing through them. Stasis in a blind loop allows bacteria to flourish.

Parenteral vitamin B_{12} must be provided because intrinsic factor, necessary for vitamin B_{12} absorption, is produced in the portion of the stomach which has been removed.

Short Bowel Syndrome

Pancreatitis, cystic fibrosis, and blind loop syndrome cause malabsorption because they interfere with the digestion of nutrients. Short bowel syndrome causes malabsorption by reducing the surface area of the intestine normally available for nutrient absorption.

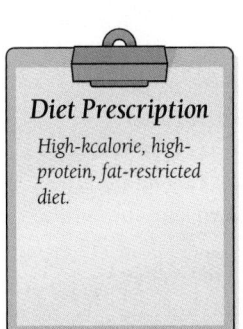

Diet Prescription

High-kcalorie, high-protein, fat-restricted diet.

Short-bowel syndrome may result from surgery in which more than 50 percent of the small intestine is resected. Intestinal resections may be necessary for some people with inflammatory bowel diseases, cancer of the intestine, intestinal obstruction, diverticulitis, or impaired blood supply to the intestine. Resection of a large segment of the small intestine reduces the absorptive surface considerably. Diarrhea, weight loss, muscle wasting, protein and fat malabsorption, hypocalcemia, hypomagnesemia, and anemia often result.

short bowel or short gut syndrome: a complex of symptoms that may include malabsorption, diarrhea, weight loss, hypocalcemia, hypomagnesemia, and anemia; it can occur whenever the absorptive surface of the small bowel is reduced.

People with short bowel syndrome generally absorb carbohydrates and most water-soluble vitamins without difficulty, but their ability to absorb fat, protein, fat-soluble vitamins, calcium, and magnesium is impaired. When the ileum (last portion of the small intestine) has been resected, vitamin B_{12} cannot be absorbed and must be supplemented parenterally. Also, the reabsorption of bile salts normally occurs in the ileum; without their reabsorption, a smaller body pool of bile salts is available for recycling, and this intensifies fat absorption problems (see Figure 21–3 on p. 556).

After a small bowel resection, a remarkable adaptive response occurs in the portion of the intestine that remains intact. The remaining bowel becomes longer, thicker, wider, and better able to absorb nutrients. The presence of nutrients appears to stimulate this adaptation. However, when too much bowel has been resected, even this remarkable adaptation will fail to compensate for the reduced surface area. People with extensive resections may require permanent parenteral nutrition support.

Immediately after surgery, the primary nutrition concern is to replace fluids and electrolytes. TPN is often provided initially to ensure that energy and protein needs are met until adaptation has occurred.[5] However, enteral

FIGURE 21–3 **Nutrient Absorption in the GI Tract**

Absorption of 90 to 95% of nutrients takes place in the first half of the small intestine. After a resection, nutrient absorption is reduced.

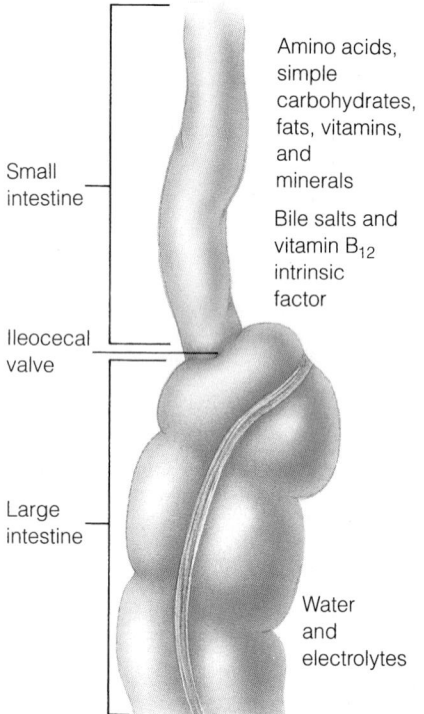

Small intestine

Amino acids, simple carbohydrates, fats, vitamins, and minerals

Bile salts and vitamin B$_{12}$ intrinsic factor

Ileocecal valve

Large intestine

Water and electrolytes

nutrition (usually by tube feeding) is initiated as early as possible to stimulate adaptation. Intact formulas appear to enhance gut adaptation more quickly than do hydrolyzed formulas. Gradually clients receive oral, high-kcalorie, high-protein, fat-restricted diets, as tolerated. Fat intake can be increased if it does not precipitate steatorrhea or diarrhea. MCT can help provide some of the missing food energy, but some regular dietary fat is needed to provide essential fatty acids.

Fat-restricted diets help control the symptoms of disorders that affect the GI tract and interfere with the absorption of fat. Alternatively, as Chapter 22 illustrates, fat-controlled diets serve to alter the metabolism of fat.

CASE STUDY

Crohn's Disease

Sara was first diagnosed with Crohn's disease when she was 18 years old. At that time, she weighed 120 pounds and was 5 feet 7 inches tall. Her normal weight had been 130 pounds until she began having the symptoms of Crohn's disease. Since that time, she has been hospitalized several times and has undergone surgery twice to resect portions of the small bowel. She has an ileostomy. She is now 21, her weight is 123 pounds, and she is in the hospital again with a suspected intestinal obstruction. As anticipated from her weight-loss history, Sara's nutrition assessment shows that she is suffering from severe PEM. Sara is very particular about the foods she eats and often simply does not eat. Sara's physician has ordered a hydrolyzed diet for Sara to be fed through a nasogastric tube.

Review Sara's weight history. What is her ideal body weight? What measures could have been taken earlier to prevent weight loss?

What possible benefits might a hydrolyzed formula diet offer Sara? Give two reasons why the physician might prefer nasogastric over oral feedings for Sara. Under what circumstances would TPN be more appropriate than a tube feeding for Sara?

Consider Sara's long-term dietary management. What type of diet should she eventually follow? Are there any dietary precautions made necessary by the ileostomy (see Chapter 17)? What goals for weight gain should be established?

Study Questions

1. What is the primary use of a fat-restricted diet? Recommend ways to make a low-fat diet palatable and easy to follow.
2. What is pancreatitis? Contrast the dietary treatment of the person with acute pancreatitis with the dietary treatment of the person with chronic pancreatitis.
3. What is cystic fibrosis? Why is fat restriction not recommended for the treatment of malabsorption in people with cystic fibrosis? Describe the dietary treatment of cystic fibrosis.
4. What are inflammatory bowel diseases? How can inflammatory bowel diseases lead to malabsorption?
5. Describe the diet therapy for a person with Crohn's disease. Discuss the possible advantages of TPN and hydrolyzed formulas for people with Crohn's disease.
6. What is the recommended diet for the person with ulcerative colitis?
7. What is the blind loop syndrome and how can it lead to malabsorption? What nutrition considerations are important in the treatment of this syndrome?
8. What is the short bowel syndrome? Describe the nutritional care of the person with short bowel syndrome.

Notes

1. K. A. Kudsk and coauthors, Postoperative jejunal feedings following complicated pancreatitis, *Nutrition in Clinical Practice* 5 (1990): 14–17.
2. J. D. Lloyd-Still, A. E. Smith, and H. U. Wessel, Fat intake is low in cystic fibrosis despite unrestricted dietary practices, *Journal of Parenteral and Enteral Nutrition* 13 (1989): 296–298.
3. Lloyd-Still, Smith, and Wessel, 1989.
4. S. J. D. O'Keefe and coauthors, Steroids and bowel rest versus elemental diet in the treatment of patients with Crohn's disease: The effects on protein metabolism and immune function, *Journal of Parenteral and Enteral Nutrition* 13 (1989): 455–460; C. O'Morain, A. W. Segal, and A. J. Levi, Elemental diet as primary treatment of acute Crohn's disease: A controlled trial, *British Medical Journal* 288 (1984): 1859–1862.
5. P. P. Purdum and D. F. Kirby, Short-bowel syndrome: A review of the role of nutrition support, *Journal of Parenteral and Enteral Nutrition* 15 (1991): 93–101.

21

Best Choices for Fast Foods

The widespread prevalence of fast-food establishments around the world attests to their popularity. People of every age group frequent fast-food establishments, and for many, fast foods are a dietary mainstay. People on special diets, especially fat-restricted diets, may have a difficult time selecting appropriate foods from fast food menus. The answers to the following questions can help people make wise decisions about fast foods.

I really like fast foods, but am wondering how nutritious they are.

Fast foods tempt many consumers because they are convenient and because their flavors and aromas appeal to many people. Part of their appeal comes from their high fat and salt contents. Frying in fat adds flavor and crispness to foods. Salt is an inexpensive flavor enhancer.

If you recall the dietary guidelines presented in Chapter 1, you know that limiting fat and salt are important dietary goals. The fats found in fast foods are often saturated, the type most important to avoid. In moderate amounts, fat and salt contribute necessary nutrients to the diet; but in excess, they are associated with high blood pressure. Fat is also associated with obesity, cardiovascular disease, cancer, and other disorders.

Fast foods provide other nutrients, of course, including protein, carbohydrate, and some vitamins and

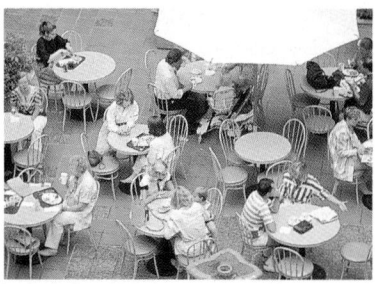

Choosen wisely, fast foods can fit into a balanced diet.

minerals, so they can be part of a healthy diet. The key is to choose the right ones and to eat them at reasonable intervals.

Many fast-food chains are now claiming that their foods are low in kcalories and fat. Are these claims valid, and if so, are these foods better choices?

Fast-food chains have begun to try to meet consumer demands for healthy food choices. Salads, lean products, and skinless grilled or baked chicken are a few examples. Some chains now fry their foods in vegetable oils to help reduce their saturated fat content.

Used appropriately, these products can be better choices, but they may also give the consumer a false sense of security. The person selecting the menu must know enough about foods to make good choices. For example, a nutritious, low-fat salad consisting of lettuce, spinach, carrots, cucumbers, celery, mushrooms, and other low-kcalorie vegetables and topped with a moderate amount of low-kcalorie dressing can be a nutritious choice. However, the same salad smothered in cheese and chopped eggs and topped with a quarter cup or more of salad dressing is a high-kcalorie, high-fat meal.

Can you give an example of how fast foods can fit into a person's well-balanced diet?

An underweight person eating one meal a week that consists of a cheeseburger, a shake, and french fries is getting needed food energy. Other meals, if well chosen, can make up for the lack of fiber, vitamins, and minerals—they need to include whole grains, vegetables, and fruits.

An overweight person, on the other hand, cannot afford the extra food energy the meal described above provides. If the person wanted to enjoy fast foods on occasion, such a person might try substituting a hamburger for the cheeseburger, a salad of low-kcalorie vegetables and low-kcalorie dressing for the french fries, and a diet soft drink for the shake. In addition to the lower fat from this meal, the person would be getting vitamins, minerals, and fiber from the salad, but would still need to include low-fat dairy foods in other meals.

In previous chapters the effects on the body of vitamin and mineral deficiencies were described. A steady diet of hamburgers, fries, and soft drinks could lead to scurvy from a lack of vitamin C, eye problems from a deficiency of vitamin A, rickets in children from a deficiency of vitamin D and calcium, and skin disorders from a lack of B vitamins, to name a few.

Is it possible to eat fast foods, keep a close tab on kcalories, and get the needed vitamins and minerals from supplements?

Even the most nutritionally complete supplements provide only known vitamins and minerals. It is possible that some nutrients have not yet been identified. Complex carbohydrates and protein are also lacking from fast foods, and supplements don't provide them. Furthermore, nutrients are interrelated; the presence of many nutrients found together in natural foods enhances the absorption of other nutrients. When a diet is very restrictive, even some of the nutrients present in it might be so poorly absorbed that deficiencies would occur.

Do you have any other suggestions for eating a balanced diet from fast-food places?

When fast foods are a major part of your diet, it is important to choose them wisely. As mentioned earlier, appropriately selected salads, baked or grilled skinless chicken, and lean meats are better choices. Asian fast-food restaurants often include vegetables with their main dishes.

Instead of choosing sweet-and-sour baked chicken, try chicken stir-fried with vegetables and a side dish of steamed rice. At Mexican fast-food restaurants, chicken fajitas and bean burritos are better choices than fried tortillas.

To improve a fast-food diet, try ordering low-fat milk in place of soft drinks. Orange juice is another commonly available beverage choice. Baked potatoes, beans, rice, coleslaw, and rolls may replace french fries as a side dish.

Always be aware of extras added to burgers, sandwiches, salads, and baked potatoes. In place of catsup and mayonnaise, choose lettuce, tomato, and raw onion.

Fast foods are a part of modern life that appear to be here to stay. As their use increases, making careful fast-food choices is important in maintaining optimal health.

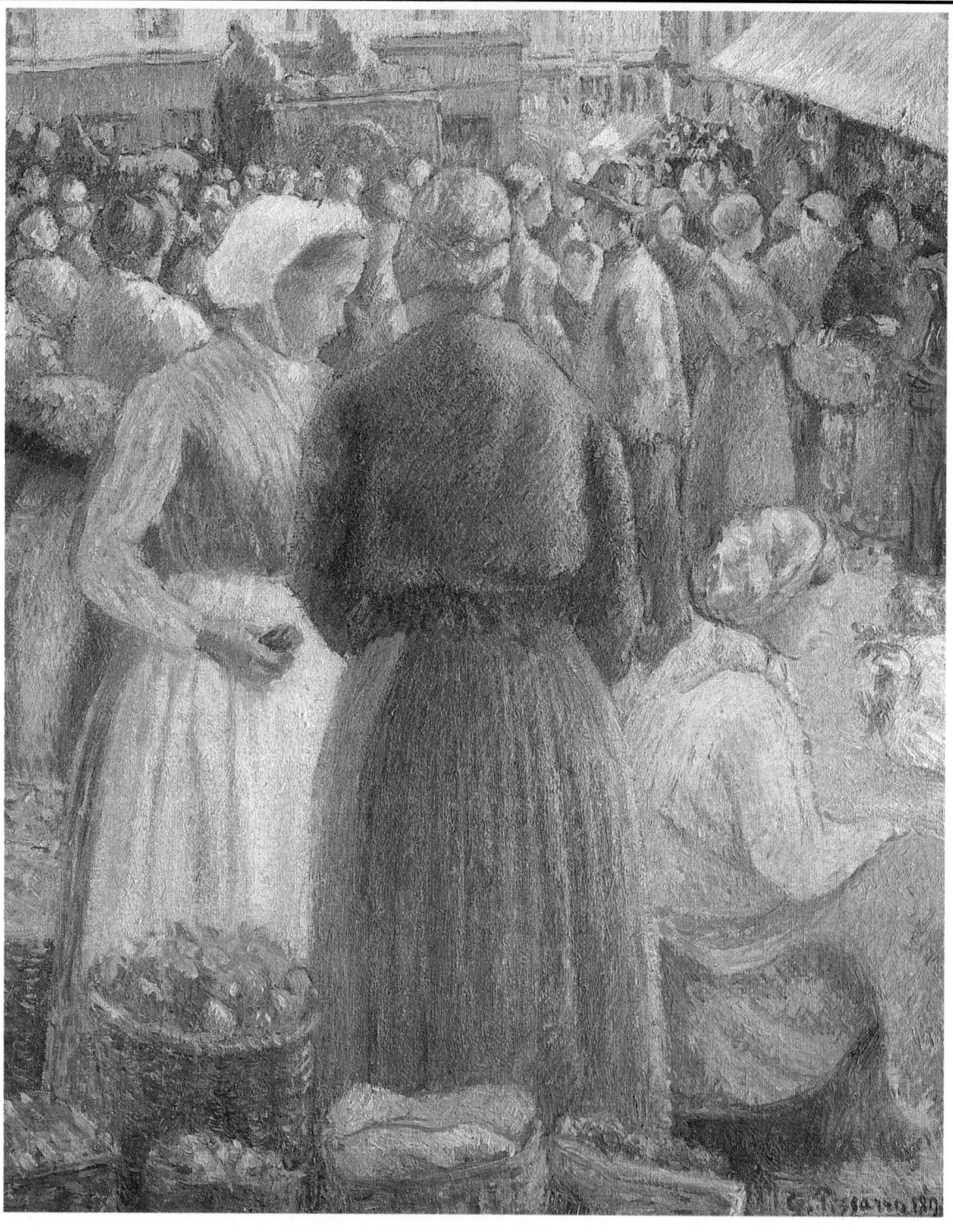

Camille Pissarro, Market at Pontoise, *1895, The Nelson—Atkins Museum of Art, Kansas City, Missouri (Nelson Fund) 33–150.*

22

Diets Modified in Fat: II. Fat-Controlled and Mineral-Modified Diets

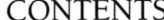

CONTENTS

TABLE 22–1   Indications for the Use of Diets Modified in Fats and Minerals

Atherosclerosis
Diabetes mellitus
Hyperlipidemia
Hypertension
Myocardial infarction
Nephrotic syndrome
Renal failure (chronic)

Saturated fats carry the maximum possible number of hydrogen atoms. **Monounsaturated fats** lack two hydrogen atoms and have one double bond between carbons. **Polyunsaturated fats** lack four or more hydrogen atoms and have two or more double bonds between carbons.

CHAPTER

22

Fat-controlled, mineral-modified diets are most frequently prescribed to prevent and treat cardiovascular diseases, as shown in Table 22–1. Cardiovascular diseases remain the leading cause of adult deaths in the United States, despite the fact that the incidence is decreasing.[1] More than 1 million people suffer heart attacks each year, and half of these people die.

Efforts to fight cardiovascular diseases have led to valuable discoveries and public education awareness. Many people have changed their lifestyles by quitting or refusing to smoke; exercising; and eating less fat, saturated fat, cholesterol, and salt. For some or all of these reasons, the rate of cardiovascular diseases has fallen steadily since 1950.

This chapter examines the diet useful for controlling blood lipid levels and other strategies for reducing the risk of cardiovascular disease. It also describes the nephrotic syndrome, another disorder for which fat-controlled, low-sodium diets are frequently prescribed.

Fat-Controlled Diets

Fat-controlled diets limit both the total amount of fats as well as the amounts of polyunsaturated, monounsaturated, and saturated fats and cholesterol. Taking time to review the information in Chapter 3 (see pp. 52–54) regarding the food sources of various fats and the practical suggestions for identifying fats in foods will serve as a valuable refresher for this chapter. Table 22–2 describes a fat-controlled diet, and the sample menu shows how the diet translates into a day's meals.

The purpose of fat-controlled diets, intended to reduce the risk of heart disease, is to adjust the levels of blood lipids and blood cholesterol. Many people find the diet difficult to follow, and drastic changes cannot be ex-

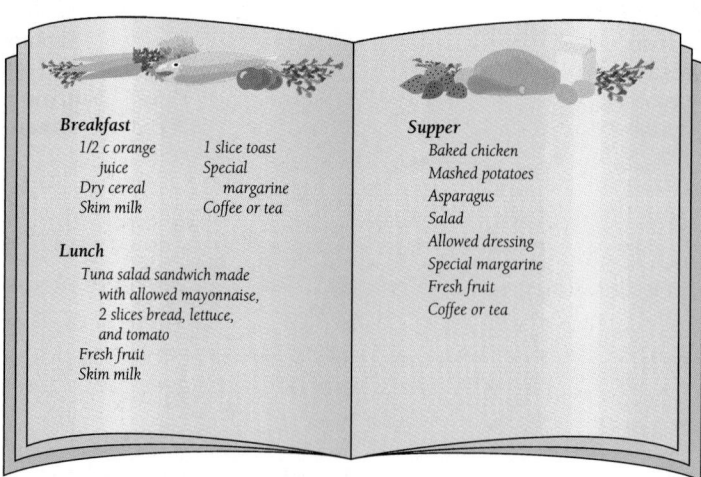

Breakfast
1/2 c orange juice
Dry cereal
Skim milk
1 slice toast
Special margarine
Coffee or tea

Lunch
Tuna salad sandwich made with allowed mayonnaise, 2 slices bread, lettuce, and tomato
Fresh fruit
Skim milk

Supper
Baked chicken
Mashed potatoes
Asparagus
Salad
Allowed dressing
Special margarine
Fresh fruit
Coffee or tea

Sample Fat-Controlled Diet Menu
Note that all foods, including margarine, are prepared with allowed amounts and types of fats.

TABLE 22–2   Foods to Be Avoided on a Fat-Controlled Diet

MEAT AND MEAT ALTERNATES

Canned, cured, salted, or smoked meats, including luncheon meats, sausage, ham, bacon, and frankfurters; highly marbled and fatty meats; organ meats and sweetbreads; caviar; frozen dinners; egg yolks in excess of two per week.

MILK AND MILK PRODUCTS

Whole and 2% milk; buttermilk; milk products made with more than 1% milk fat, including some yogurts and ice cream; half and half; eggnog; nondairy coffee creamer; high-fat cheeses (containing more that 2 g fat per ounce), including American, blue, brick, Brie, Camembert, cheddar, Colby, cream, Edam, feta, Gouda, gruyère, Monterey Jack, Muenster, provolone, Roquefort, and Swiss.

FRUITS AND VEGETABLES

Any prepared with egg, butter, cream, or cheese sauces; fried vegetables.

GRAINS

Butter rolls, egg bread, bagels, cheese bread, biscuits, muffins, doughnuts, sweet rolls, pancakes, French toast, cheese crackers, butter crackers; cereal containing coconut, coconut oil, or nuts; potato chips, corn chips, and other fried snacks; grains prepared with eggs, whole milk, cream, fats, or vegetable shortening.

FATS

Butter, meat fat, lard, ham hocks, salt pork, fat back, bacon drippings; gravy or sauce made from fats to be avoided; margarine made from animal fat; salad dressing made from sour cream or cheese; chocolate; coconut or coconut oil; palm or palm kernel oil; cashews, pistachios, and macadamia nuts; nondairy creamer.

OTHER[a]

Salt; high-salt seasonings or sauces such as Worcestershire or soy; pickles; relish.

[a]Because of the relationship between atherosclerosis and hypertension, a diet moderately restricted in salt is recommended for the individual on a fat-controlled diet. More information on sodium- and salt-restricted diets is given later in this chapter.

pected overnight. However, artificial fats (see Nutrition in Practice 3) and other specially designed foods (cholesterol-free eggs, special cheeses, and polyunsaturated margarines) help considerably. Additional help is available from the American Heart Association (AHA) in the form of its many pamphlets and recipe booklets for both professionals and clients.

People with elevated blood lipids can easily adapt the exchange lists (see Appendix E) for fat-controlled diets. One can carefully adjust the cholesterol and saturated fats in the diet by limiting the use of medium-fat and high-fat meats, whole milk and whole milk products, saturated fats, and bread exchanges high in fat.

Studies of the roles of foods in altering blood lipid levels continue to receive high priority. Thus the advice given today may be outdated tomor-

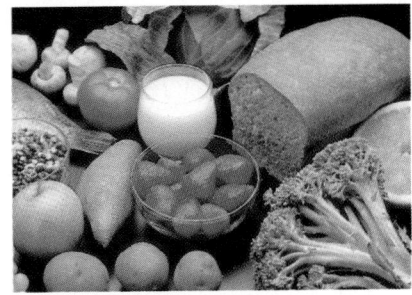

Foods to enjoy on a fat-controlled diet.

row. Nutrition in Practice 22 provides additional information about dietary components that may help lower blood lipid levels.

> The distinction between *blood* cholesterol and the cholesterol in *food* is important here. Everyone agrees that low blood cholesterol levels are desirable, but it is not clear whether one can lower one's cholesterol by reducing cholesterol intake from foods. It is clear that reducing total fats and saturated fats do reduce blood cholesterol levels. Nutrition in Practice 22 address this question more fully.

Atherosclerosis

A general term used to describe thickening and hardening of the arteries is **arteriosclerosis.** When this process is due to the accumulation of lipid plaques within arterial walls, the condition is called **atherosclerosis.**

plaques: mounds of lipid material mixed with smooth muscle cells and calcium that grow in artery walls.

thrombus: a stationary clot. When it has grown enough to block off a blood vessel, it is a **thrombosis.** A **coronary thrombosis** is the closing off of a vessel that feeds the heart muscle. A **cerebral thrombosis** is the closing off of a vessel that feeds the brain.
  coronary = heart
  thrombo = clot
  cerebrum = part of the brain

gangrene (GANG-green): death of tissue caused by lack of blood flow to the area.

embolus (EM-boh-luss): a thrombus that breaks loose. When it causes sudden closure of a blood vessel, it is an **embolism.**
  embol = to insert

heart attack: the event in which an embolus lodges in vessels that feed the heart muscle, causing sudden tissue death. Also called **myocardial infarction.**

stroke: the shuttting off of the blood flow to the brain by a thrombus or embolism.

Diseases of the heart and blood vessels are grouped together and termed cardiovascular diseases (CVD). The two most common disorders responsible for most CVD are atherosclerosis (described here) and hypertension (described later in this chapter).

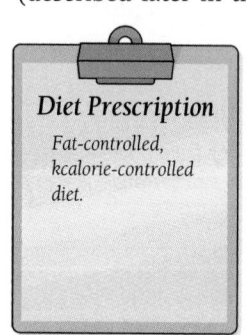

Diet Prescription

Fat-controlled, kcalorie-controlled diet.

Atherosclerosis is characterized by accumulations of lipid plaques in the linings of arterial walls. As each plaque enlarges, the lumen of the artery narrows, and the pressure of the blood against the arterial wall rises (much as water pressure increases in a garden hose that has been pinched). The increased pressure can damage the artery wall, and restrict circulation to all organs in the body. Plaques also cause artery walls to lose their elasticity so that they cannot expand in response to the beats of the heart; this is why atherosclerosis is sometimes called hardening of the arteries. Figure 22–1 illustrates the development of atherosclerosis.

If plaques narrow the lumen of an artery enough, they can completely block the flow of blood. Then if a clot forms in the blood—and they do form and dissolve all the time—they may attach themselves to the plaques and gradually enlarge until they shut off the blood supply to the tissue supplied by that artery. That tissue may die slowly and be replaced by scar tissue.

A clot can also break loose and travel along the system until it reaches an artery too small to allow its passage; there it gets caught. Then the tissues fed by the artery are suddenly robbed of oxygen and nutrients, and they die. Such a clot, lodging in an artery that feeds the heart muscle, results in a heart attack. When the clot lodges in an artery of the brain, a stroke results. Clots lodging in arteries of the kidneys, lungs, and peripheral tissues can also cause death of those tissues.

Table 22–3 lists the risk factors for atherosclerosis. Although it befits a nutrition book to focus on dietary strategies to reduce the risk of atherosclerosis, it is important to note that diet is not the only, and perhaps not even the most important, factor in the development of atherosclerosis. In fact, among the many controversies over diet and nutrition in recent years, one of the noisiest ones has been over the questions of how important diet is in heart disease; whether changes in diet can reduce this risk; and if so,

FIGURE 22–1   **The Formation of Plaques in Atherosclerosis**
When plaques have covered 60% of the coronary artery walls, the critical phase of heart disease begins.

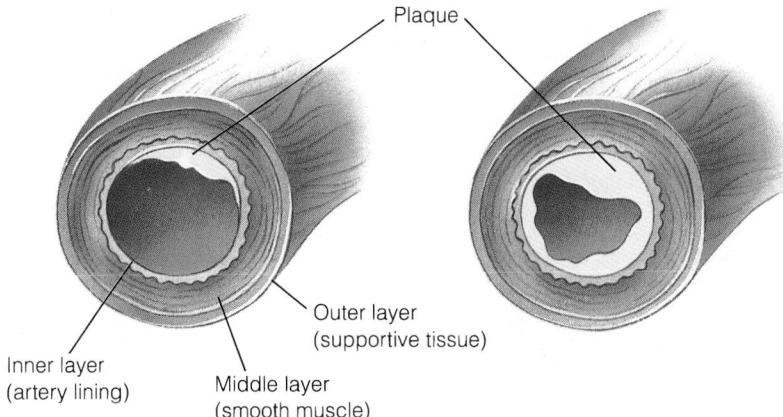

An artery (section) with plaque just beginning to form. Plaques can easily appear in a person as young as 15.

The same artery, years later, half blocked by plaque.

whether such changes should be advocated for everyone or just for selected high-risk individuals. These issues are discussed in more detail in Nutrition in Practice 22.

Far less controversial is the use of fat-controlled diets to treat people who have elevated blood lipids, or hyperlipidemia. Blood cholesterol, triglycerides, or both may be elevated. Since these lipids are carried through the blood in the lipoproteins (see Chapter 3), different lipoproteins are also elevated. For example, when cholesterol levels are high, low-density lipoproteins (LDL) are elevated; when triglycerides are high, very-low-

hyperlipidemia (HIGH-per-LIP-ih-DEE-mee-ah): elevated blood lipids.

TABLE 22–3   **Risk Factors for Atherosclerosis[a]**

- Glucose intolerance (diabetes)
- Heredity (history of CVD prior to age 55 in family members)
- High blood cholesterol, high LDL, and/or low HDL
- Hypertension
- Lack of exercise
- Obesity (30% or more overweight)
- Smoking
- Stress

[a]Women and men suffer from a similar incidence of heart disease. However, women tend to be older and to have a more severe degree of heart disease at diagnosis.

TABLE 22–4   **The Hyperlipidemias**

TYPE	LIPOPROTEIN ABNORMALITY
I	Elevated chylomicrons, triglycerides, and cholesterol
IIa	Elevated LDL and cholesterol
IIb	Elevated LDL, VLDL, cholesterol, and triglycerides
III	Elevated VLDL, cholesterol, and triglycerides
IV	Elevated VLDL; normal or elevated cholesterol and triglycerides
V	Elevated chylomicrons, VLDL, triglycerides, and cholesterol

hyperlipoproteinemia (HIGH-per-LIP-oh-PRO-teen-EE-mee-ah): elevated blood lipoproteins; a term often used interchangeably with hyperlipidemia.

density lipoproteins (VLDL) and/or chylomicrons are elevated. An elevation of any lipid or lipoprotein is called *hyperlipoproteinemia.*

Table 22–4 shows one of the most widely used systems for classifying hyperlipidemias. This system identifies six basic types of hyperlipidemias: Types I, IIa, IIb, III, IV, and V. The table also shows which lipids and lipoproteins are elevated in each type of hyperlipidemia. Table 22–5 provides an overview of the general strategies effective for lowering blood lipids. Table 22–6 shows the specific recommendations of a panel of experts to reduce serum lipids for the most common types of hyperlipidemias using a two-step plan.[2] If step 1 brings high blood cholesterol levels down, good; if not, the therapy goes on to step 2.

Types I and V hyperlipidemias are rare. Because both of these types of hyperlipidemias are associated with elevated chylomicrons, a low-fat diet is recommended. This makes sense because chylomicrons initially transport all dietary fats. Clients with Type I hyperlipidemia who need to increase their energy intakes can benefit from the use of MCT oil, because medium-chain triglycerides enter the blood directly, bypassing the need for a chylomicron carrier. However, MCT oil is not used in Type V hyperlipidemia, because it can cause an even greater elevation in VLDL, which are elevated already. Abstinence from alcohol is also recommended for people with Types I and V hyperlipidemia.

Types IIa and IV hyperlipidemias are by far the most common, and they are associated with an increased risk of CVD. In Type IIa, dietary treatment aims at lowering blood cholesterol primarily by restricting cholesterol and saturated fat intakes and by substituting polyunsaturated fats for saturated

TABLE 22–5   **General Dietary Approaches for Lowering Blood Lipids**

ELEVATED LIPID	MAJOR LIPOPROTEIN INVOLVED	DIETARY APPROACH
Dietary triglycerides	Chylomicrons	Total fat restriction
Triglycerides	VLDL	Weight reduction
		Restriction of total fat
Cholesterol	LDL	Restriction of saturated fat
		Restriction of cholesterol

TABLE 22–6   **Specific Dietary Approaches for Lowering Blood Cholesterol and Triglycerides**

	TOTAL FAT	SATURATED FATTY ACIDS	POLYUN-SATURATED FATTY ACIDS	MONOUN-SATURATED FATTY ACIDS	COMPLEX CARBOHYDRATES	PROTEIN	CHOLESTEROL
Step 1	< 30%	< 10%	Up to 10%	10 to 15%	50 to 60%	10 to 20%	< 300 mg/day
Step 2	< 30%	< 7%	Up to 10%	10 to 15%	50 to 60%	10 to 20%	< 200 mg/day

Note: All but cholesterol are expressed as percentages of total food energy. Total food energy intake should be such as to achieve and maintain desirable weight.
Source: Adapted from N. D. Einst and J. C. LaRosa, Recommendations for treatment of high blood cholesterol: The National Cholesterol Education Program Adult Treatment Panel, *Contemporary Nutrition* 13, no. 1 (1988).

fats. In Type IV, the focus is on lowering blood triglycerides primarily through weight loss. The weight reduction limits the client's total fat intake. In addition, the diet moderately restricts cholesterol, substitutes polyunsaturated fats for saturated fats, and limits concentrated sweets.

As a rule, physicians do not prescribe drugs to treat hyperlipidemias until after a three-month trial period on the recommended diet has proven unsuccessful in lowering blood lipid concentrations. Drugs useful in the treatment of hyperlipidemias and their nutrition-related side effects are shown in Table 22–7.

TABLE 22–7   **Drugs Used to Lower Blood Lipids**

DRUG NAME	TIMING WITH MEALS	COMMON SIDE EFFECTS THAT MAY INFLUENCE NUTRITION STATUS
Cholestyramine	Give with water or other fluids; never give dry or with carbonated beverages.	Nausea, vomiting, abdominal discomfort, gas, diarrhea, constipation, heartburn, steatorrhea, anorexia, altered taste perception. May decrease absorption of calcium; fat; vitamins A, D, K, and B_{12}; folate; and glucose. Depletes iron stores.
Clofibrate	Give with meals.	Nausea, vomiting, abdominal discomfort, loose stools, gas, aftertaste, altered taste perception, increased appetite. May decrease absorption of glucose, iron, and vitamin B_{12}. May induce anemias.
Colestipol	(Same as cholestyramine.)	(Same as cholestyramine.)
Gemfibrozil	Give ½ hour before meals.	Nausea, vomiting, abdominal discomfort, gas, constipation. May induce anemia.
Lovastatin	Give with meals.	Diarrhea, gas, constipation, abdominal pain, heartburn, nausea, indigestion, altered taste perception.
Nicotinic acid	Give with meals.	Nausea, vomiting, abdominal discomfort, diarrhea. Flushing. Decreased glucose tolerance.
Probucol	Give with meals.	Nausea, vomiting, gas, abdominal discomfort, diarrhea, anorexia, altered taste and smell perceptions.

Source: Adapted from D. E. Powers and A. O. Moore, *Food Medication Interactions,* 7th ed. (Phoenix: Food Medication Interactions, 1991); *Nursing 91 Handbook* (Springhouse, Pa.: Springhouse Corporation, 1991).

Evidence is mounting that low serum levels of HDL may be a significant risk factor for the development of CVD. Dietary measures aimed at raising HDL levels include weight reduction (if necessary), correction of hypertriglyceridemia, and moderate alcohol consumption. Frequent and vigorous physical activity and abstinence from cigarette smoking are encouraged.

People with hyperlipidemia are often advised to restrict sodium in addition to controlling fat in their diets, because people with hyperlipidemia often also have high blood pressure (described later in this chapter). Furthermore, since hypertension is another risk factor for the development of atherosclerosis, any measure that might prevent hypertension is warranted. Hyperlipidemia often occurs along with other disorders, including diabetes (Chapter 20), renal disease (Chapter 23), and nephrotic syndrome (discussed later in this chapter). When these disorders are present simultaneously, the diet is adjusted accordingly.

hypertension: high blood pressure. People sometimes confuse hypertension with stress, but hypertension is an internal and stress, an external, condition. Stress may cause hypertension in sensitive people, however.

Sodium-Restricted Diets

People with a variety of disorders (including hypertension, congestive heart failure, some kidney diseases, and cirrhosis), along with people who have suffered heart attacks, often benefit from sodium-restricted diets as a part of their treatment plans. People who have diabetes or CVD or who are on corticosteroids may also be advised to follow sodium-restricted diets. A sample sodium-restricted diet menu is shown in the text.

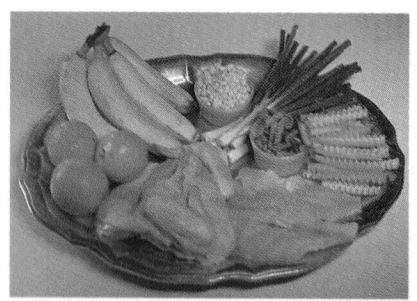

Foods to enjoy on a sodium-restricted diet.

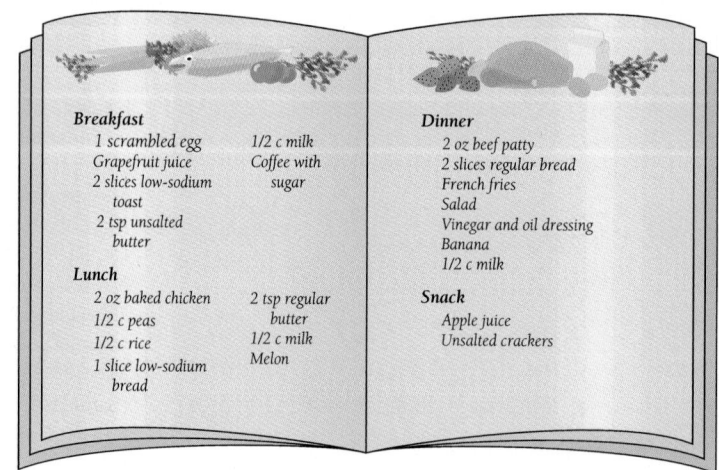

Breakfast
1 scrambled egg   1/2 c milk
Grapefruit juice   Coffee with
2 slices low-sodium   sugar
   toast
2 tsp unsalted
   butter

Lunch
2 oz baked chicken   2 tsp regular
1/2 c peas   butter
1/2 c rice   1/2 c milk
1 slice low-sodium   Melon
   bread

Dinner
2 oz beef patty
2 slices regular bread
French fries
Salad
Vinegar and oil dressing
Banana
1/2 c milk

Snack
Apple juice
Unsalted crackers

Sample 1 Gram Sodium-Restricted Diet Menu

The amount of sodium allowed on a sodium-restricted diet varies from 250 milligrams to about 4 grams of sodium daily. The types and amounts of foods making up the diet depend on the level of sodium prescribed. Table 22–8 shows the foods allowed on several different sodium-restricted diets. Table 22–9 on p. 570 describes a no-added-salt, or 4-grams-sodium, diet.

TABLE 22–8   Sodium-Restricted Diets

FOODS	Number of Servings Allowed on Various Levels of Sodium Restriction				SERVING SIZE	SODIUM PER SERVING (mg)
	250 mg	500 mg	1,000 mg (1G)	2,000 mg (2G)		
Nonfat, whole, and evaporated milk	0	2	2	2	8 oz	120
Low-sodium milk	2	Not restricted	Not restricted	Not restricted	8 oz	7
Meat, fish, poultry, and unsalted cheese	4	4	4	6	1 oz	25
Eggs	1	1	1	1	1	60
Bread and allowed ready-to-eat cereal	0	0	2	5	1 slice or ¾ oz	200
Low-sodium bread, cereal, and cereal products	7	7	7	4 or more	Varies	5
Fresh, frozen, or canned without salt: asparagus, bean sprouts, broccoli, brussels sprouts, cabbage, cauliflower, cucumbers, eggplant, endive, escarole, green pepper, collard and turnip greens, lettuce, mushrooms, okra, onions, radishes, rhubarb, rutabagas, string beans, summer squash, tomatoes, watercress, zucchini, and low-sodium tomato and vegetable juices	2	2	2	Not restricted	½ c	9
Fresh, frozen, or canned without salt: corn, lima beans, parsnips, peas, potatoes, pumpkin, sweet potatoes, winter squash, and yams	1	1	1	Not restricted	½ c	5
Canned vegetables and vegetables frozen with salt	0	0	0	1	½ c	200
Salted butter and margarine	0	0	2	6	1 tsp	50
Regular mayonnaise	0	0	2	6	1 ½ tsp	50

General diet guidelines:

The foods listed below cannot be used unless they have been calculated into the diet. However, allowances can be made, particularly when the higher levels of sodium are allowed. For example, a person on a 2-g sodium diet who does not drink milk can have 240 mg of sodium from any other food source (see Appendix C). With this in mind, the following foods should be avoided:

1. Salt used in cooking or at the table.

2. Highly salted snacks, such as potato chips, corn chips, tortilla chips, salted popcorn, and pretzels.

3. Barbecue sauce; bouillon cubes (except low sodium); catsup; celery salt, seeds, or leaves; chili sauce; garlic salt; horseradish made with salt; meat extracts, sauces, and tenderizers; monosodium glutamate; prepared mustard; olives; onion salt; pickles; relishes; saccharin; soy sauce; and Worcestershire sauce.

4. Commercial foods made with milk: ice cream, sherbet, malted milk, milk mixes, and milk shakes.

5. Artichokes, beets, carrots, Chinese or red cabbage, greens (except those listed with vegetables in the table above), sauerkraut, and spinach.

6. Maraschino cherries, crystallized or glazed fruits, and dried fruit with sodium sulfite added.

7. Brains; kidneys; canned, salted, or smoked meats; bacon; luncheon meats; chopped or corned beef; kosher meats; shellfish; regular cheeses; egg substitutes; and regular peanut butter.

8. Salted butter or margarine, salt pork, commercial salad dressing (except low sodium), and salted nuts.

9. Leavening agents, such as baking powder and baking soda; rennet tablets; pudding mixes; and molasses.

10. Fountain beverages; instant cocoa mixes; prepared beverage mixes (including fruit-flavored powders); and commercial candy, cakes, cookies, sweetened gelatin mixes, pastries, puddings, cakes, and biscuit mixes.

11. Most commercial dry cereals or instant hot cereals; puffed wheat, puffed rice, and shredded wheat are allowed.

Source: Adapted from American Dietetic Association, *Handbook of Clinical Dietetics* (New Haven, Conn.: Yale University Press, 1981).

TABLE 22–9   **No-Added-Salt Diet**

■ You may lightly salt foods during cooking, but do not add salt at the table.
■ Avoid foods high in sodium, including:
Meats—bacon; bologna; cold cuts; chipped or corned beef; frankfurters; smoked meats; sausage; salt pork or codfish; canned, salted, or smoked fish.
Sauces, seasonings, and condiments—regular catsup; celery, garlic, and onion salt; regular chili sauce; commercial meat extracts; meat tenderizers; monosodium glutamate; olives; pickles; prepared mustard; soy and Worcestershire sauce.
Other—regular canned or frozen soups; regular bouillon; soup mixes; pretzels, popcorn, crackers, nuts, potato chips, or other salted snack foods; sauerkraut; regular cheese; regular peanut butter.
■ Low-sodium products can be substituted for regular foods.

The person who normally uses salt liberally may find foods unpalatable without salt. Diet compliance will probably be poor if the person is handed an instruction sheet with no accompanying encouragement or guidance. These suggestions may help clients make the necessary changes:

■ Take time, one-on-one, to thoroughly explain the diet, ensuring that the client becomes familiar with obvious sources of sodium (such as table salt), as well as hidden sources of sodium (such as processed foods and milk). Instruct the client to read labels and to look out for the many food ingredients that contain sodium (see margin).
■ Reduce sodium gradually to allow the person time to adjust to the flavor of unsalted foods. (People whose illnesses require that they be on very-low-sodium diets, however, usually cannot afford to gradually reduce their sodium intakes.)
■ See the person regularly to adjust the sodium level, to give encouragement, and to answer questions.
■ Recommend the use of spices and herbs, as shown in Table 22–10, to replace salt in cooking. Cookbooks with low-sodium recipes can be a big help in making foods tasty.

Local water supplies may have a high sodium content, and when this water is used for preparing and cooking foods, it can significantly contribute to sodium intake. Health departments can supply information on the sodium content of local water supplies.

Medications such as antacids, antibiotics, cough medicines, laxatives, pain relievers, and sedatives may contain sodium. Some toothpastes and mouthwashes also contain large amounts of sodium; recommend that people rinse thoroughly after brushing their teeth or using mouthwash, as well as that they avoid swallowing these compounds.

Many low-sodium products are available for use with sodium-restricted diets, although a palatable diet can be planned without the use of these products. Some people, however, particularly those on diets very low in sodium, like to use low-sodium items to add variety. However, often these products are not sodium-free, and clients using them should be instructed to make the necessary dietary adjustments.

1 tsp salt contains about 2 g sodium. Read labels. Some processed foods that contain no table salt and don't taste salty actually contain sodium. Look for the words *soda* or *sodium* or the symbol *Na* on labels. Examples are *sodium* bicarbonate (baking *soda*), mono*sodium* glutamate, most baking powders, di*sodium* phosphate, *sodium* alginate, *sodium* benzoate, *sodium* hydroxide, *sodium* proprionate, *sodium* sulfite, and *sodium* saccharin.

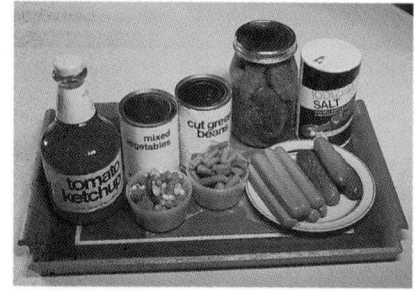

TABLE 22–10   **Sodium-Free Spices and Flavorings**

Allspice	Onion powder
Almond extract	Paprika
Bay leaves	Parsley
Caraway seeds	Pepper
Cinnamon	Peppermint extract
Curry powder	Pimiento
Garlic	Rosemary
Garlic powder	Sage
Ginger	Sesame seeds
Lemon extract	Thyme
Mace	Turmeric
Maple extract	Vanilla extract
Marjoram	Vinegar
Mustard powder	Walnut extract
Nutmeg	

Potassium often replaces the sodium in salt substitutes. Many people don't like the taste of salt substitutes but may find them acceptable if they use them sparingly. Salt substitutes should not be heated, however, because they turn bitter. Some people find food more acceptable without any salt at all. Potassium-containing salt substitutes increase potassium intake. Although this may be good in the treatment of some disorders, in others, such as renal disease, potassium must be restricted, and salt substitutes with potassium are contraindicated. Thus each client should check with the physician before using a salt substitute. Other products are a half-and-half combination of regular table salt and salt substitute. Such products may be more palatable, but they also can contribute significant amounts of salt to the diet. Still other products are composed of herbs to season foods without any sodium or potassium added. These products may be the best alternative, if the client finds them acceptable.

Caution: The person who must limit potassium should not use potassium-containing salt substitutes.

For most people with disorders requiring sodium-restricted diets, all sources of sodium must be restricted. An exception is the person with hypertension (described next) who may benefit more from restricting sodium chloride (salt) than other forms of sodium.

Hypertension

The body' ability to maintain blood pressure is vital to life. Blood pressure pushes the blood through the major arteries into smaller arteries and finally into tiny capillaries, whose thin walls permit exchange of fluids between the blood and the tissues (see Figure 22–2 on p. 572). When the pressure is right, the cells receive a constant supply of nutrients and oxygen and give up their wastes.

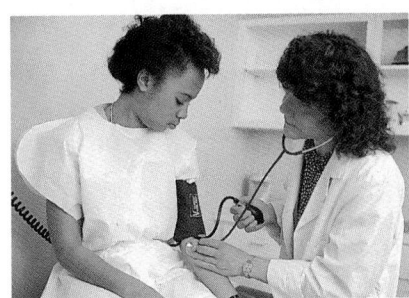

Hypertension, the most prevalent cardiovascular disease, affects some 60 million people in the United States.

FIGURE 22–2 **The Blood Pressure**
Two major contibutors to the pressure
inside an artery are the heart's pushing
blood into it and the small-diameter
arteries and capillaries at its other end
resisting the blood's flow (peripheral
resistance). Another determining factor
is the volume of fluid in the circulatory
system, which depends in turn on the
number of dissolved particles in that
fluid.

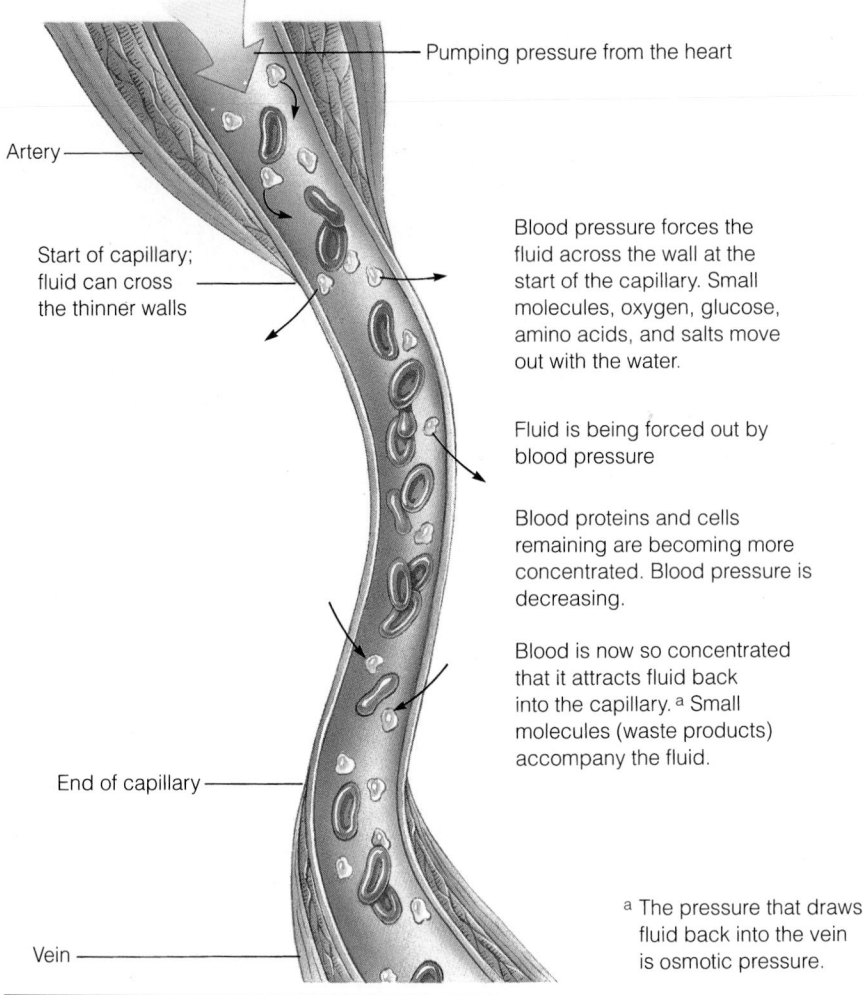

Pumping pressure from the heart

Artery

Start of capillary;
fluid can cross
the thinner walls

Blood pressure forces the
fluid across the wall at the
start of the capillary. Small
molecules, oxygen, glucose,
amino acids, and salts move
out with the water.

Fluid is being forced out by
blood pressure

Blood proteins and cells
remaining are becoming more
concentrated. Blood pressure is
decreasing.

Blood is now so concentrated
that it attracts fluid back
into the capillary. [a] Small
molecules (waste products)
accompany the fluid.

End of capillary

Vein

[a] The pressure that draws
fluid back into the vein
is osmotic pressure.

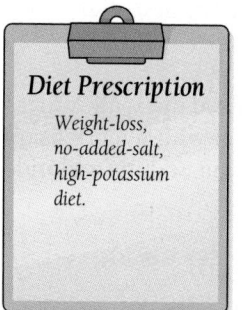

Diet Prescription

Weight-loss,
no-added-salt,
high-potassium
diet.

When the blood pressure falls, the lives of all the
body's cells are threatened. The kidneys detect the
lowered pressure and immediately set in motion a
mechanism to raise the blood pressure again.

Dehydration sets these actions in motion, which is
beneficial, because when the blood volume is low,
higher blood pressure is needed to facilitate the exchange of substances between the tissues and the
capillaries. Sometimes, however, the kidneys are
fooled; they experience dehydration when there is
none. A common culprit is atherosclerosis, which
obstructs the blood vessels so that less fluid reaches the kidneys. In response
to poor circulation of blood fluid, the kidneys raise the blood pressure, and
the heart has to pump extra hard to push the fluid around against resistant
arteries. So although blood pressure might otherwise be normal, atheroscle-
rotic kidneys raise it too high, causing hypertension.

Added body weight (obesity) raises blood pressure further; surplus adipose tissue means miles of additional capillaries through which the blood must be pumped. The combination of high blood pressure, obesity, and atherosclerosis is deadly.

A major national effort has been launched to identify and treat hypertension. Even mild hypertension can be dangerous; however, individuals who have it benefit from treatment, retaining better health and enjoying longer lives.

Epidemiological studies have identified several risk factors to predict the development of hypertension, including:

- *Age.* Blood pressure levels increase with age.
- *Family history.* A family history of hypertension and heart disease raises the risk of developing hypertension.
- *Obesity.* Obese people are more likely to develop hypertension.
- *Race.* Hypertension is twice as common among blacks as whites; it tends to develop earlier and become more severe.

The role of *diet-related* factors in the development of hypertension has been debated extensively. Most of the controversy centers on whether a high-sodium diet causes hypertension and, conversely, whether a sodium-restricted diet can prevent it. Research into sodium's role in hypertension has disappointed investigators who hoped they were on the track to a single answer. Other diet-related factors that appear to play roles in the development of hypertension include:

- *Weight control.* As previously mentioned, a positive link between obesity and hypertension exists. Weight reduction in overweight people with hypertension significantly lowers blood pressure, even if the person does not achieve ideal body weight.
- *Sodium/sodium chloride.* For years, research has seemed to indicate that high sodium intakes were "the" factor responsible for hypertension. However, sodium's partner, chloride, may also be a factor, so it is more helpful to think in terms of salt. And it may *not* be necessary to restrict baking soda (sodium bicarbonate), baking powder (sodium carbonate), and other sodium compounds. It is clear that salt avoidance helps prevent hypertension in some individuals who are sensitive to sodium, but for others—the majority of people with hypertension—it may be an ineffective diet strategy.
- *Exercise.* Moderate exercise of the right kind directly lowers the resting heart rate and blood pressure.[3] The "right kind" of exercise is the aerobic, endurance type, such as walking, swimming, bicycling, or jogging performed regularly (see Chapter 9 for more information).
- *Potassium.* Many authorities believe that potassium might both prevent and treat hypertension. Even in people without high blood pressure, a high potassium intake protects against stroke, and a low intake raises blood pressure.[4]
- *Calcium.* Surveys suggest that people with hypertension consume less calcium than those with normal blood pressure. Researchers estimate that people with the lowest calcium intakes (below 300 milligrams per day) have a two to three times greater risk of developing hypertension than people with the highest calcium intakes (1200 milligrams per day).[5]

■ *Fat.* Fat is well known as a dietary factor contributing to atherosclerosis; less well known is its role in hypertension. Epidemiological studies show that diets high in fat are associated with hypertension. When people restrict their total dietary fat intakes and increase the ratio of polyunsaturated to saturated fatty acids, their blood pressure falls, regardless of whether it was their intent to make it do so.[6] This probably works at least partly by way of eicosanoids (see p. 48) that regulate sodium excretion and peripheral blood vessel contraction and relaxation.

■ *Alcohol.* Alcohol plays several roles in heart disease. In moderate doses (one to two drinks per day), alcohol initially reduces pressure in the peripheral arteries and so reduces blood pressure, but high doses clearly raise blood pressure. In fact, of people with alcoholism, 30 to 60 percent have hypertension.

■ *Other factors.* Research continues to reveal relationships of other dietary factors to hypertension. Magnesium deficiency causes visible changes in the walls of arteries and capillaries and makes them tend to constrict, a possible mechanism for the hypertensive effect of magnesium deficiency.[7] Hypertension may also be an insulin-resistant state, and it is possible that measures preventive of diabetes are also protective against hypertension.[8]

Dietary treatment of hypertension is fairly straightforward. The most effective dietary measure people with hypertension can take is to reduce weight if they are overweight. Because hypertensive people are at greater-than-normal risk for developing CVD, and because dietary fat and body fat contribute to hypertension, many professionals advise them to follow fat-controlled diets. They also usually recommend no-added-salt diets. Salt-sensitive individuals should limit their sodium intakes to 2 to 4 grams per day.

When the body retains sodium, it excretes potassium. When people with normal blood pressure eat foods high in sodium, ultimately their blood pressure rises—and at the same time, their potassium excretion increases. If they receive potassium simultaneously with the sodium, their blood pressure does not rise. Additionally, some diuretics used in the treatment of hypertension (see Table 22–11 on pp. 576–577) can lead to a potassium deficiency. People using these drugs should be encouraged to include good food sources of potassium daily (see Table 22–12 on p. 578); they may also be advised to use potassium supplements. A sample no-added-salt, fat-controlled, high-potassium diet menu is shown in the text, and Appendix C shows the sodium and potassium contents of foods. Blood levels of potassium should be monitored regularly to prevent hypokalemia, and clients should watch for signs of hypokalemia, such as weakness (particularly of the legs), an unexplained numbness or tingling sensation, cramps, irregular heartbeat, and excessive thirst and urination.

Heart Attacks

The heart gets its nutrients and oxygen not from inside its chambers but from arteries that lie on its surface (see Figure 22–3). A heart attack, or myocardial infarction (MI), occurs when the supply of blood to the heart

Drugs used to treat hypertension include diuretics and adrenergic blockers. Diuretics work by increasing fluid loss, thus lowering blood pressure. Adrenergic blockers interfere with a neurotransmitter to alter blood pressure. Side effects including fatigue, sexual complaints, and sleep disturbances are commonly reported.

FIGURE 22–3   **The Coronary Arteries**

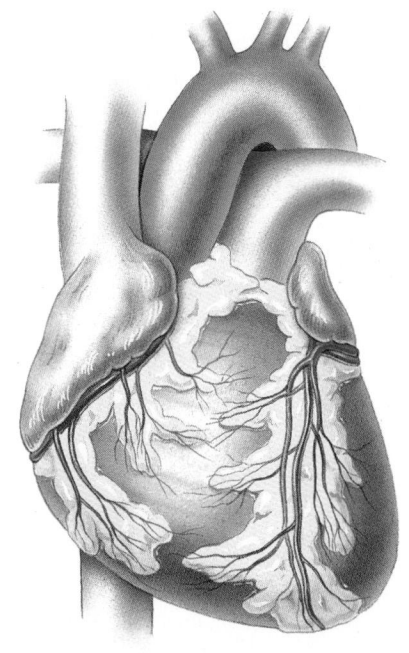

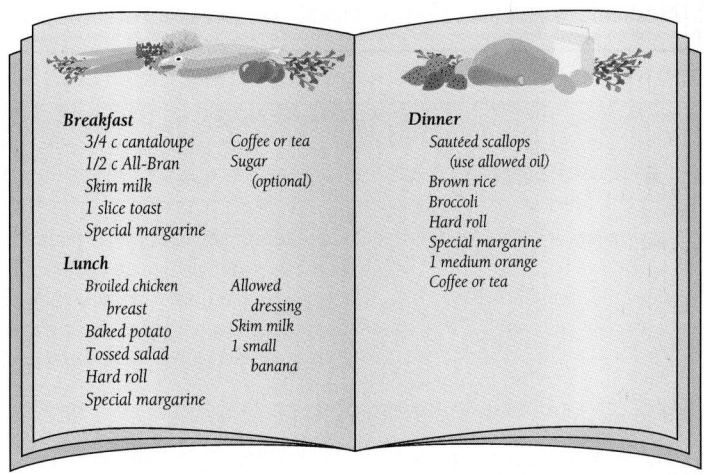

Sample No-Added-Salt, Fat-Controlled, High-Potassium Diet Menu
Foods for this menu are prepared with little or no salt and minimal amounts of fat.
The fats used for cooking or for flavor are monounsaturated or polyunsaturated.

muscle is cut off, causing tissue death. Atherosclerosis often contributes to heart attacks; some other contributors are hypertension, abnormal blood clotting, spasms of the coronary arteries, infection of the membrane covering the heart, and rheumatic heart disease.

rheumatic (roo-MAT-ick) **heart disease:** heart damage (often affecting the heart valves) that follows rheumatic fever (caused by a bacterial infection).

As an area of heart tissue dies, enzymes specific to heart cells leak out into the general circulation, much as digestive enzymes leak out of the pancreas in people with pancreatitis. Physicians use elevated concentrations of these enzymes in the blood to help diagnose heart attacks.

A heart attack victim, like an accident victim, is in shock at first. Fluid leaves the vascular compartment and moves temporarily to the interstitial space. The person experiences this fluid shift as if it came from dehydration and complains of extreme thirst. The body does not need water during shock, however, and increasing its fluid load at such a time is unwise.

shock: sudden, dramatic shift of fluid from the blood to the interstitial space.

Diet Prescription

Progress diet from a liquid, 2-g-sodium diet to a bland, fat-controlled, no-added-salt diet as tolerated.

Do not offer water or food to people immediately after an MI. They commonly experience nausea at this time. If, as shock resolves, a person remains nauseated, start IV infusions to prevent dehydration.

After several hours of observation, the person can usually begin to eat. At this time, provide foods that minimize the work of the heart. The diet is often moderately restricted in sodium (about 2 grams) and is low in kcalories (1000 to 1200). The diet begins with liquid or soft, bland foods that are easy to eat, given in frequent, small meals. Select foods that do not cause gas formation or abdominal distention. Abdominal distention pushes the diaphragm up toward the heart, thus adding stress on the heart muscle. Serve foods neither too hot nor too cold; temperature extremes can stimulate nerves that slow the heart rate. Many practitioners also restrict caffeine-containing beverages during the first few days after an MI, but this measure remains controversial.

TABLE 22–11   **Drugs Used in the Treatment of Hypertension**

DRUG NAME	TIMING WITH MEALS	COMMON SIDE EFFECTS THAT MAY INFLUENCE NUTRITION STATUS
Acebutolol	Give without regard to meals.	Constipation, gas, abdominal pain. May mask signs of hypoglycemia.
Amiloride hydrochloride and hydrochlorothiazide	Give with food at the same time each day.	Anorexia, dry mouth, appetite changes, nausea, diarrhea, GI pain, constipation. May induce electrolyte imbalance and anemias.
Atenolol	Give without regard to meals.	Dry mouth, diarrhea, nausea. May mask signs of hypoglycemia.
Atenolol and chlorothalidone	Give on empty stomach at the same time each day.	Anorexia, diarrhea, nausea, vomiting, GI irritation, constipation. May induce hypokalemia, anemias.
Captopril	Give on empty stomach 1 hr before meals.	Altered taste perception, weight loss, sore mouth. May include hypokalemia, anemias.
Chlorothiazide	Avoid natural licorice.	Nausea, vomiting, diarrhea, constipation, anorexia, dry mouth.
Chlorthalidone	Give with food 6 or more hr before bedtime. Avoid natural licorice.	Anorexia, dry mouth, GI irritation, nausea, vomiting, diarrhea, constipation.
Clonidine hydrochloride	Give without regard to meals.	Dry mouth, weight gain, nausea, vomiting, constipation. May induce edema.
Deserpidine/methyclothiazide	Give with food 6 or more hr before bedtime. Avoid natural licorice.	Dry mouth, weight gain, anorexia, nausea, vomiting, diarrhea, cramps.
Digitalis, digitoxin, digoxin	Give with water ½ hr before or 2 hr after food. Avoid natural licorice.	Nausea, vomiting. May inhibit glucose absorption.
Enalapril maleate	May give with food.	Altered taste perceptions, diarrhea, nausea, vomiting, abdominal pain.
Guanethidine sulfate	Give at the same time each day. Avoid natural licorice.	Dry mouth, weight gain, diarrhea, nausea. May induce edema.
Guanfacine hydrochloride		Constipation, nausea, vomiting, stomach cramps.
Hydralazine hydrochloride	Give with food at the same time each day. Avoid natural licorice.	Anorexia, GI distress, constipation.
Hydrochlorothiazide	Give with food 6 or more hr before bedtime. Avoid natural licorice.	Anorexia, dry mouth, nausea, vomiting, diarrhea, constipation. May alter insulin requirements in diabetes. May induce hypokalemia.
Indapamide	Give with food at the same time each day if GI distress.	Dry mouth, weight loss, anorexia, constipation, GI distress. May alter glucose tolerance.

(continued)

TABLE 22–11 (*continued*)

DRUG NAME	TIMING WITH MEALS	COMMON SIDE EFFECTS THAT MAY INFLUENCE NUTRITION STATUS
Labetalol hydrochloride	Give with food.	Altered taste perception, nausea, vomiting, indigestion. May mask signs of hypoglycemia.
Lisinopril	Give without regard to meals.	Diarrhea, vomiting.
Methyldopa	Avoid natural licorice.	Dry mouth, weight gain, diarrhea, nausea. May induce edema.
Metoprolol tartrate	Give with food.	Dry mouth, diarrhea, GI pain, gas, constipation, heartburn. May mask signs of hypoglycemia.
Minoxidil	Give at the same time each day.	May induce edema.
Nadolol	Give without regard to meals. Avoid natural licorice.	Dry mouth, constipation, GI distress, nausea, gas. May mask signs of hypoglycemia.
Nifedipine	Give with food or milk.	Altered taste perception, nausea, diarrhea, constipation, cramps, gas. May induce edema.
Pindolol	Give without regard to meals.	Diarrhea, vomiting. May mask signs of hypoglycemia. May alter glucose tolerance. May induce edema.
Prazosin hydrochloride	Give without regard to meals.	Dry mouth, nausea, diarrhea, constipation, GI distress. May induce edema.
Propranolol hydrochloride	Give with food. Avoid natural licorice.	Dry mouth, constipation, GI distress, nausea. May mask signs of hypoglycemia.
Rauwolfia serpentina	Give with food or milk to reduce GI irritation.	Anorexia, weight gain, dry mouth, diarrhea, nausea, vomiting, increased GI motility and gastric secretion. May lower glucose tolerance.
Spironolactone with hydrochlorothiazide	Give with food 6 or more hr before bedtime. Avoid natural licorice. Avoid salt substitutes.	Anorexia, cramps, diarrhea, nausea, vomiting. May alter serum glucose.
Terazosin hydrochloride	Give without regard to meals at the same time each day.	Sore throat, nausea. May induce edema.
Timolol maleate	Give with food at the same time each day.	Weight loss, nausea. May mask signs of hypoglycemia. May induce edema.
Triamterene with hydrochlorothiazide	Give with food or milk 6 or more hr before bedtime.	Dry mouth, thirst, dehydration, nausea, vomiting, diarrhea, constipation. May alter glucose levels.

Source: Adapted from D. E. Powers and A. O. Moore, *Food Medication Interactions,* (Phoenix: Food Medication Interactions, 1991); *Nursing 91 Drug Handbook* (Springhouse, Pa.: Springhouse Corporation, 1991).

TABLE 22–12   **Foods High in Potassium**

VEGETABLES	
Artichokes	Potatoes, baked or pared and boiled
Asparagus	Potatoes, sweet
Beets	Pumpkins
Broccoli	Rutabagas
Brussels sprouts	Spinach
Cabbage, common varieties and Chinese	Squash
Dried beans and peas	Tomato juice
Green beans	Tomatoes
Kale	Turnip greens
Mixed vegetables	Vegetable juice
Parsnips	Winter squash
Pinto beans	Yams
FRUITS	
Apricot nectar	Oranges
Apricots	Papayas
Avocados	Peaches
Bananas	Pears
Cantaloupes	Pineapple juice
Dates	Pineapple
Figs	Prune juice
Grapefruit	Prunes
Grapefruit juice	Raisins
Honeydew melon	Rhubarb
Kiwi fruit	Strawberries
Nectarines	Tangerines
Orange juice	
OTHER	
Chocolate	Molasses, dark and light
Cocoa	Peanuts
Meat	Walnuts
Milk	Wheat germ

After the person is out of immediate danger (in about five to ten days), tailor the diet to meet individual needs—for example, to deal with such conditions as hyperlipidemia, hypertension, obesity, or diabetes. Oftentimes, a diet to reduce weight (Chapter 19), control fat, and moderately restrict sodium is appropriate. Such a diet can be planned to include only three meals a day, but people who continue to have chest pain after an MI may benefit from eating small, frequent meals. Advise them to eat slowly and to rest before and after meals.

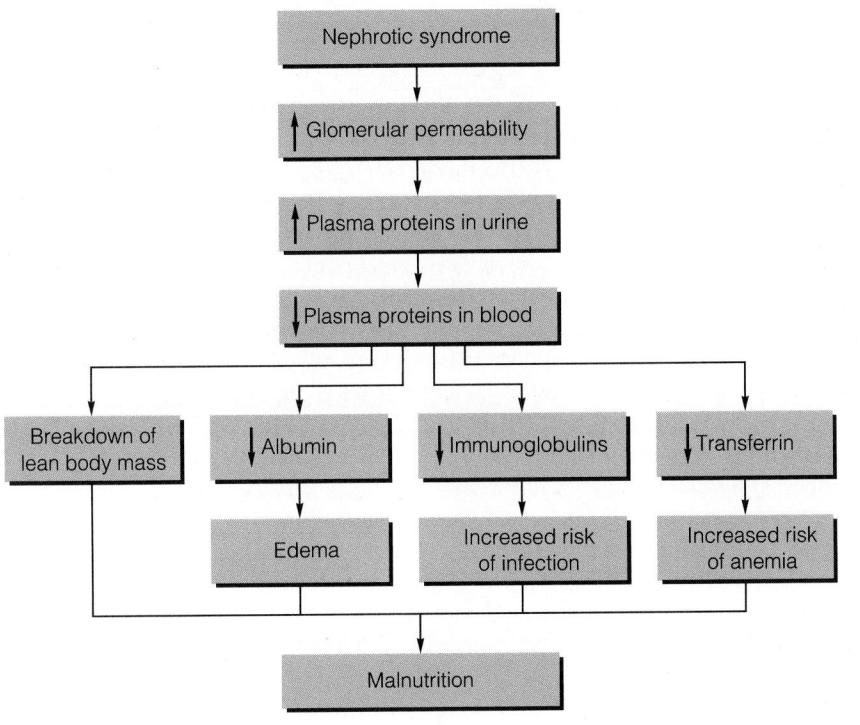

FIGURE 22–4   **Consequences of the Nephrotic Syndrome**

CASE STUDY

Hyperlipidemia and Hypertension

Mr. Garrett, age 45, has just been diagnosed with Type IV hyperlipidemia. He is 5 feet 7 inches tall and weighs 200 pounds. Mr. Garrett has a family history of CVD. His diet history shows excessive intakes of food energy, cholesterol, total fat, saturated fat, and sodium. He smokes a pack of cigarettes a day, and his lifestyle leaves him little room for exercise. Mr. Garrett also has hypertension, for which diuretics have been prescribed. He frequently forgets to take his pills, though, and his blood pressure is often quite high.

Name the risk factors for CVD in Mr. Garrett's history. Which of them can he control? Which can be helped by diet? What complications might you expect if his condition goes untreated?

What type of diet, if any, would you recommend for Mr. Garrett's type of hyperlipidemia? Explain the rationale for each diet change. How will his current diet change? What types of foods should he eat?

What type of diet, if any, would you recommend for Mr. Garrett's hypertension? What suggestions might you offer to help him make the necessary diet changes? Are these diet changes consistent with those you would recommend for Type IV hyperlipidemia? Plan a day's menu for Mr. Garrett based on the diet you would recommend for him.

What laboratory and clinical tests would you expect to see monitored regularly? Why?

Name at least three ways in which Mr. Garrett could benefit from losing weight. How does exercise fit into a weight-loss plan?

Discuss nutrition considerations if Mr. Garrett should have a heart attack, develop congestive heart failure, or have a stroke. Describe the relationships of these disorders to hyperlipidemia and hypertension.

Study Questions

1. How does a fat-controlled diet differ from a fat-restricted diet?
2. What is atherosclerosis? How can atherosclerosis lead to hypertension, thrombosis, heart attacks, and strokes?
3. Describe ways people can alter their diets to lower their blood cholesterol levels. Describe other measures that may be useful for lowering serum lipid levels.
4. What is hypertension? What causes hypertension? Discuss the role of diet in hypertension.
5. What is a myocardial infarction? Describe the diet therapy for a heart attack victim immediately after a heart attack, after several hours, and after a week. State the rationale for each diet modification you list.
6. What is congestive heart failure? Why is malnutrition common in people with CHF? Describe the diet recommended for the person with CHF.

7. What is the nephrotic syndrome? What are the consequences of the nephrotic syndrome? Discuss the dietary treatment of the nephrotic syndrome.

Notes

1. National Center for Health Statistics, as cited in Life expectancy growing for U.S. whites, study says, *Atlanta Constitution,* 8 January 1992, p. A9.

2. National Cholesterol Education Program, Coordinated by the National Heart Lung and Blood Institute, National Institutes of Health, Public Health Service, *Report of the Expert Panel on Detection, Evaluation and Treatment of High Blood Cholesterol in Adults,* U.S. Department of Health and Human Services, October 5, 1987.

3. L. G. Ekelund and coauthors, Physical fitness as a predictor of cardiovascular mortality in asymptomatic North American men, *New England Journal of Medicine* 319 (1988): 1379–1384.

4. G. G. Krishna, E. Miller, and S. Kapoor, Increased blood pressure during potassium depletion in normotensive men, *New England Journal of Medicine* 320 (1989): 1177–1182; L. Tobian, Potassium and hypertension, *Nutrition Reviews* 46 (1988): 273–283; F. C. Luft and M. H. Weinberger, Potassium and blood pressure regulation, *American Journal of Clinical Nutrition* 45 (1987): 1289–1294; K. T. Khaw and E. Barrett-Connor, Dietary potassium and stroke-associated mortality: A 12-year prospective population study, *New England Journal of Medicine* 316 (1987): 235–240.

5. D. A. McCarron and coauthors, Blood pressure and nutrient intake in the United States, *Science* 224 (1984): 1392–1398.

6. R. Weinsier, Recent developments in the etiology and treatment of hypertension: Dietary calcium, fat, and magnesium, *American Journal of Clinical Nutrition* 42 (1985): 1331–1338.

7. M. R. Joffres, D. M. Reed, and K. Yano, Relationship of magnesium intake and other dietary factors to blood pressure: The Honolulu heart study, *American Journal of Clinical Nutrition* 45 (1987): 469–475.

8. P. N. Hopkins and R. R. Williams, Human genetics and coronary heart disease: A public health perspective, *Annual Review of Nutrition* 9 (1989): 303–345.

22

Diet and the Prevention of Atherosclerosis

More than half the people who die in the United States each year die of heart and blood vessel disease, mostly by way of heart attacks and strokes. The underlying condition that contributes to most of these deaths is atherosclerosis, and therefore, much effort has been focused on preventing it. Nutrition in Practice 22 discusses whether people can prevent atherosclerosis by following special diet guidelines.

I'm very concerned about preventing atherosclerosis. Several members of my family have hyperlipidemia, and others have died from heart attacks. What are my chances of having the same problems?

First of all, it's important for you to remember that no one knows the causes of atherosclerosis. The risk factors for cardiovascular diseases (CVD) that have been identified are correlations only. Smoking, high blood cholesterol, and high blood pressure seem to be the most important of these, but clearly there are others, still unknown.

Table NP22–1 (p. 586) shows one way of calculating your risk based on present knowledge. Such a quiz helps you look not only at what your risks may be but also points out areas that you can change to reduce your risk.

Well, after taking the quiz, I see there are areas that I can change to improve

my risk score. How much will changing these areas really help?

Many people, of course, would like to know the answer to your question. Again, there are no absolutes, but many studies are being conducted to try to find out.

In some massive studies conducted during the 1970s, thousands of men were persuaded to give up smoking, take medication to reduce their blood pressure if it was high, and alter their diets to reduce their blood cholesterol levels. These studies were complicated by a curious situation, however: everyone else was doing those same things. Word had gotten around to the whole U.S. population that these measures were beneficial. The studies failed to show significant improvement of the experimental groups over controls, perhaps because there *were* no good controls. An analysis of the impressive downturn in the rate of deaths from CVD between the late 1960s and the late 1970s suggests that a large-scale prevention effort may have been spontaneously mounted by the entire U.S. population.

In any case, something certainly seems to have happened in that ten-year period in which 200,000 lives were saved. At a major conference held in 1979, the experts who had been following the lifestyle changes and trends among people in the United States reported four significant trends:

1. We are smoking less.
2. We are controlling our blood pressure better.
3. Our blood cholesterol levels have fallen slightly.
4. We are exercising more.

In other words, independently of the research studies, people have been taking measures that are lowering mortality. The evidence on associated health benefits suggests that reduction of risk factors is advisable for all members of the population, not just for those most prone to heart attacks.

Fortunately, I don't have high blood pressure, and I quit smoking years ago. Tell me more about blood cholesterol levels.

Let's first clarify one point: we are talking about *blood* cholesterol, not about the cholesterol in foods. In the blood, cholesterol is carried in LDL and HDL. It is the LDL that are associated with heart disease. Changes in diet that reduce serum cholesterol concentrations mostly do so by reducing LDL. The most important dietary factor affecting blood

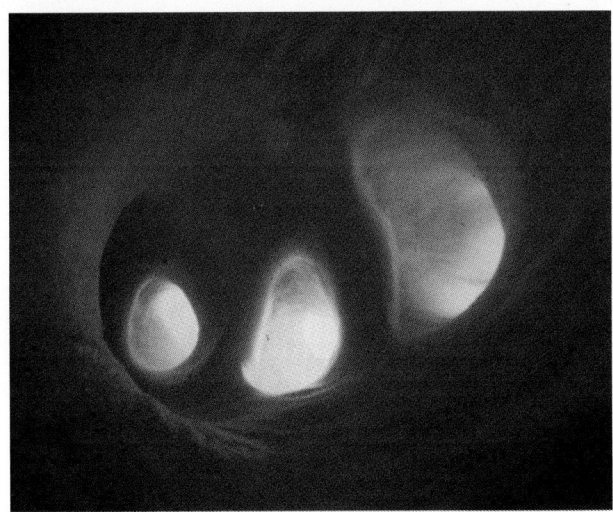

A healthy artery provides an open passage for the flow of blood.

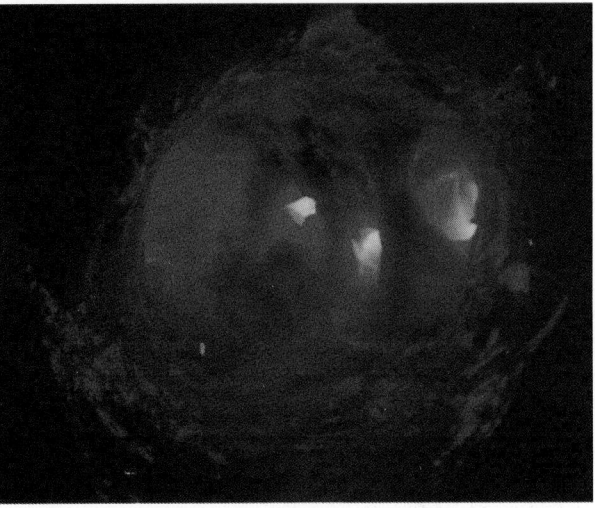

Plaques along an artery narrow its diameter and obstruct blood flow. Clots can form, aggravating the problem.

cholesterol is saturated fat, not the cholesterol in foods.

How can I change my diet, then, to reduce the risk of atherosclerosis?

The most effective dietary measures to lower blood cholesterol are these:

- Keep total fat intake at or below 30 percent of kcalories. Keep saturated fat intake to 10 percent of kcalories.
- Partially substitute monounsaturated and polyunsaturated fats for saturated fats.
- Limit cholesterol intake to 300 milligrams a day or less.
- Balance food intake and physical activity to maintain appropriate body weight.

Saturated fats have received a lot of bad press for raising blood cholesterol concentrations. While this is true for many saturated fats, not all saturated

fats have the same effect on blood cholesterol. The main saturated fats known to cause cholesterol concentrations to climb are palmitic and myristic acids. Those fatty acids having no effect on cholesterol include stearic and lauric acids. The fat in milk is mostly saturated fat—and most of that is palmitic acid—so choose nonfat and low-fat milk and milk products. The fats in meats are mostly saturated, largely stearic acid; those in poultry and fish have a better balance between saturated and polyunsaturated fats. To keep fat intake moderate, select lean cuts of meat and poultry, trim the fat, remove the skin, and bake or broil it.

As for the other fat-contributing components of the diet, olive oil and canola oil are recommended selections among the oils, for these are high in monounsaturated fatty acids—but like all fat, they should be used sparingly.

Periodically, eat meals of fish, especially fatty fish, to help balance intakes of omega-6 fatty acids with the omega-3 type (see pp. 48).

As far as cholesterol is concerned, feel free to use some eggs, but use them in moderation, unless medically advised otherwise. Eggs are an inexpensive source of high-quality protein, and while high in cholesterol, they are not as high as was once thought, and they are not high in saturated fat. Neither are shellfish as high in cholesterol as has been believed, and they do contain eicosapentanoic acid (EPA) and other omega-3 fatty acids. And eat foods high in soluble fiber—oats, oat bran, barley, and legumes—as well as fruits and vegetables, to help lower blood cholesterol.

In addition to taking these positive measures, concentrate on obtaining adequate nutrients from food without excessive food energy, and go easy on protein-rich foods. Body weight has proven, in some studies, to be the most important single determinant of blood cholesterol level, but even if weight control does not reduce blood cholesterol, it will reduce blood pressure. Exercise will also reduce blood pressure. So will eating a low-fat diet. Even if the high-fiber, high-complex-carbohydrate aspect does not reduce cholesterol, it will improve glucose tolerance (diabetes, remember from Chapter 22, is a predictor of CVD). And even if the monounsaturated oils and the omega-3 oils from the fish do not lower blood cholesterol, they may help prevent heart disease by favoring the right eicosanoid balance so that clot formation is unlikely.

Earlier you mentioned that cholesterol is carried in the blood in LDL or HDL. I have heard of HDL in the news and am wondering if they are related to CVD risk.

TABLE NP22–1   **Your Risk of Heart Disease**

What is your heart disease risk score? Some of the following risk factors are powerful predictors of heart disease. Respond to each of the statements below, and give yourself a score in each of the 12 categories listed. Then total your points to determine your degree of risk.

Age	If you are:		
	56 or over	1	_____
	55 or under	0	_____
Sex	If you are:		
	Male	1	_____
	Female	0	_____
Family history	If you have blood relatives who have had a:		
	Heart attack or stroke before age 60	12	_____
	History of heart disease at or before age 60	10	_____
	Heart attack or stroke after age 60	6	_____
	No history of heart disease	0	_____
Personal history	If you are:		
	50 or under and have had a heart attack, stroke, or cardiovascular surgery	20	_____
	51 or over and have had any of the above	10	_____
	None of the above	0	_____
Diabetes	If onset of diabetes appeared:		
	Before age 40 and you take insulin	10	_____
	At or after age 40 and you take insulin or pills	5	_____
	After age 55 and you control it with diet	3	_____
	No diabetes	0	_____
Smoking	If you smoke:		
	2 packs/day	10	_____
	1 to 2 packs/day or quit within past year	6	_____
	Six or more cigars/day or use a pipe regularly	6	_____
	Less than 1 pack/day or quit over a year ago	3	_____
	Never smoked	0	_____
Cholesterol	If your cholesterol level is:		
	240 or higher	10	_____
	200 to 239	5	_____
	199 or lower	0	_____

(continued)

Yes, they are, but in a different way. While most of the blood cholesterol is carried in the LDL and correlates *directly* with CVD risk, some is carried in the HDL and correlates *inversely* with risk. In fact, for men over 50, the most potent single predictor of heart attack risk may be the HDL level—the higher, the better. A word of caution: as with other risk factors, we don't know for sure if raising HDL will have a beneficial effect on reducing CVD risk.

How can I raise my HDL levels?

TABLE NP22–1   **Your Risk of Heart Disease** (*continued*)

If you do not know your cholesterol level, answer the diet question. If you answered the cholesterol question, skip the diet question.

Diet	If you normally eat:		
	Red meat daily; more than seven eggs weekly; and butter, whole milk, and cheese daily	8	_____
	Red meat 4 to 6 times weekly; margarine, low-fat dairy products, and some cheese	4	_____
	Poultry, fish, little or no red meat; three or fewer eggs weekly; some margarine, nonfat milk and milk products	0	_____
Blood pressure	If either number is:		
	160 over 100 or higher	10	_____
	140 over 90 but less than 160 over 100	5	_____
	If both numbers are less than 140 over 90	0	_____
Weight	Using the formula 110 lb + 6 lb/inch over 5 ft for men, or 100 lb + 5 lb/inch over 5 ft for women, if you are:		
	25 lb overweight	4	_____
	10 to 24 lb overweight	2	_____
	Less than 10 lb overweight	0	_____
Exercise	If you engage in aerobic exercise more than 20 minutes:		
	Less than once a week	4	_____
	1 to 2 times a week	2	_____
	3 or more times a week	0	_____
Stress	When waiting, if you are:		
	Frustrated and easily angered	4	_____
	Impatient and occasionally moody	2	_____
	Comfortable and easygoing	0	_____
		TOTAL POINTS	_____

If you answered the blood pressure question:
High risk . . . .   36 and above
Medium risk . . . .   19 to 35
Low risk . . . .   18 and below

If you did not answer the blood pressure question:
High risk . . . .   40 and above
Medium risk . . . .   20 to 30
Low risk . . . .   19 and below

Note: A high score does not mean you will develop heart disease. It should, however, awaken you to the potential risk. Consult your physician if you have questions about your score results.
Source: Adapted from Arizona Heart Institute, Cardiovascular Risk Factor Analysis.

One way to have higher HDL levels is to be female. Women have higher HDL levels than men. Another seems to be to stop smoking. Nonsmokers have uniformly higher HDL levels than smokers. Still another is losing weight.

Investigators report that moderate amounts of red wine appears to raise HDL levels and lower LDL levels. The substance in red wine responsible for this effect is resveratrol, a compound that helps grapes resist fungal diseases. However, research in this area is recent and unconfirmed.

By far the most powerful influence on HDL levels is exercise—prolonged, intense, and frequent. Evidence suggests that HDL levels can be improved in very sedentary people who become only moderately active.

Is there anything else I should know about reducing my risk of heart disease?

Remember that even if you religiously take all the steps discussed here, there is no 100 percent guarantee that you will never have heart trouble. We'd encourage you to do them anyway, though, because they are good health practices.

Although diet and nutrition have been the focus of attention here, it seems important to conclude by taking a broader view of the problem of atherosclerosis. Nutrition is obviously not the only factor involved. Genetics plays a very significant role. The lifestyle of our whole population is that of an urbanized, competitive, industrial society with built-in stresses that have major impacts on health. Society itself may need to change in fundamental ways before we can arrive at ultimate solutions to some health problems.

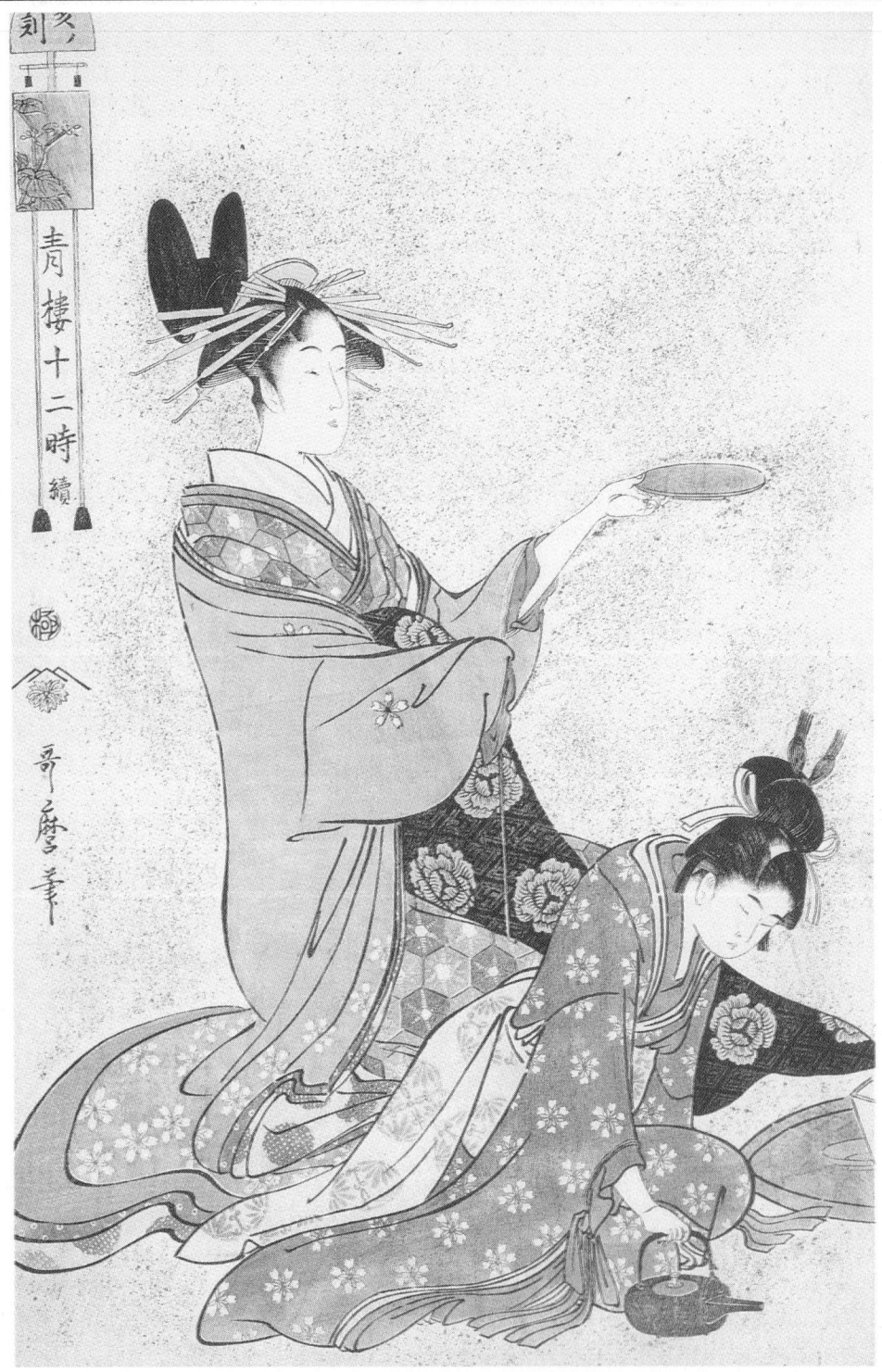

Kitagawa Utamaro, The Hour of the Wild Boar *(9PM–11PM), Japanese, 1753-1806,*
Woodblock print, 1796, 38.1 cm × 25.4 cm, Clarence Buckingham Collection, 1925.
3061, © 1991 The Art Institute of Chicago, All Rights Reserved.

Diets Modified in Protein, Minerals, and Water

CONTENTS

TABLE 23–1　Indications for the Use of Diets Modified in Protein and Fluid

PROTEIN-RESTRICTED DIETS
Acute renal failure
Chronic renal disease
Cirrhosis
Hepatic coma

GLUTEN-RESTRICTED DIETS
Celiac disease

PHENYALANINE-RESTRICTED DIETS
Phenylketonuria

FLUID-RESTRICTED DIETS
Acute renal failure (oliguric phase)
Chronic renal disease
Cirrhosis
Congestive heart failure
Hepatic coma
Myocardial infarction

CHAPTER 23

Diets modified in protein and amino acids are among the most difficult to plan and follow. Likewise, the disorders they are used to treat are complicated and hard to manage. Yet most of these diets are critical, and failure to comply with them can have adverse and sometimes fatal consequences. Table 23–1 shows some disorders for which protein- and fluid-modified diets are indicated.

In most cases, physicians prescribe protein- and amino acid–restricted diets, and skilled dietitians translate the diet prescriptions into meal plans. Although other health care professionals do not plan the diets, they are often called upon by clients and their caretakers to answer questions or communicate information about the diets.

Protein-Restricted Diets

Protein-restricted diets aim to provide enough protein to maintain nutrition status, but not enough to allow the buildup of waste products from protein metabolism. In the disorders for which protein-restricted diets are required, these wastes accumulate and are toxic to the tissues. Protein-restricted diets generally provide from 40 to 60 grams of protein daily. A sample 60-gram protein-restricted diet is shown here.

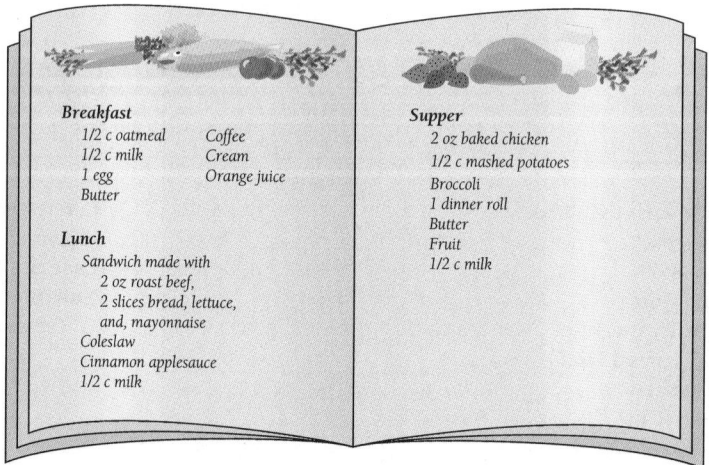

Breakfast
1/2 c oatmeal　　Coffee
1/2 c milk　　Cream
1 egg　　Orange juice
Butter

Lunch
Sandwich made with
2 oz roast beef,
2 slices bread, lettuce,
and, mayonnaise
Coleslaw
Cinnamon applesauce
1/2 c milk

Supper
2 oz baked chicken
1/2 c mashed potatoes
Broccoli
1 dinner roll
Butter
Fruit
1/2 c milk

Sample 60-Gram Protein-Restricted Diet Menu

Protein-restricted diets carefully limit foods from the milk, meat, and bread and starch exchanges. Vegetables and fruits also contain some protein, and for very-low-protein diets, these foods must be calculated into the diet. The lower the amount of protein allowed, the more important it becomes that all the protein included in the diet be of high quality. Milk and eggs are used preferentially to supply protein unless contraindicated for other medical reasons.

An adequate total energy intake is critical for people on protein-restricted diets because, without adequate energy, protein will be used for energy rather than in protein synthesis. To boost energy intake, clients use many fats (margarine, cream, butter) and concentrated sweets (hard candy, jelly, sugar), whenever possible. Special low-protein products (pastas, bread, cookies, wafers, and gelatin) made with wheat starch can improve energy intake and add variety to the diet. Carbohydrate supplements in powdered and liquid forms can also provide additional energy.

Oftentimes, people on protein-restricted diets require other dietary restrictions. For example, a person with renal failure may also need to restrict sodium and potassium, follow a fat-controlled diet for hyperlipidemia, and limit concentrated sweets for diabetes. This situation challenges the individual and the diet planner to plan acceptable meals that ensure an adequate intake of nutrients.

Liver Disease

Treatment for two major disorders affecting the liver, cirrhosis and hepatic coma, frequently involves a protein-restricted diet. A liver disorder for which a protein-restricted diet is not indicated is hepatitis, because the client with hepatitis can handle a normal protein intake, and the liver needs this protein to repair itself. Provide a well-balanced, normal diet to the person with hepatitis who is in good nutrition status. The malnourished person with hepatitis, like any malnourished person, needs a high-kcalorie, high-protein diet (see Chapter 18). People with alcohol-related hepatitis are at high risk for poor nutrition status; malnutrition is a common complication of alcohol abuse, and hepatitis further taxes nutrient stores.

hepatitis (HEP-ah-TIE-tis): inflammation of the liver caused by a virus, alcohol, drugs, or other toxin. Hepatitis can progress to cirrhosis.
hepat = liver
itis = inflammation

The impact of alcohol abuse on nutrition status is the subject of Nutrition in Practice 6.

Anorexia, nausea, vomiting, and fever are common symptoms of hepatitis that can adversely affect nutrition status. The person with malnutrition unable to take foods orally benefits from IV glucose solutions temporarily. Suggest small, frequent meals, liquid supplements, or both for the person who is unable to eat enough food. Persistent anorexia and nausea may make tube feedings necessary. Parenteral nutrition is an alternative for the person who experiences persistent vomiting.

Cirrhosis

Cirrhosis, a serious liver disorder, is characterized by liver cells that become filled with fat or damaged by inflammation. The liver cells die, and scar tissue invades the liver. Chronic alcohol abuse is the most common cause of cirrhosis in the United States, although not all people with cirrhosis are alcohol abusers, and not all alcohol abusers develop cirrhosis. Some other causes of cirrhosis include infections, biliary obstructions, heart disease and exposure to toxic chemicals.

cirrhosis (seer-OH-sis): a disease of the liver characterized by scarring; **Laennec's cirrhosis** is the type associated with alcohol abuse and malnutrition.

portal vein: the blood vessel that carries nutrients from the GI tract to the liver.
port = entrance to an organ

hepatic artery: the blood vessel that brings oxygen-rich blood from the heart to the liver; the **hepatic vein** returns blood from the liver to the heart.

portal hypertension: elevated blood pressure in the portal vein caused by obstructed blood flow through the liver.

ascites (ah-SIGH-teez): a type of edema characterized by the accumulation of fluid in the abdominal cavity.

collaterals: small blood vessels that develop to divert blood flow away from an obstructed organ; also called **shunts.**
shunt = to avoid

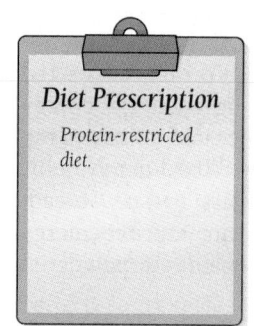

Diet Prescription
Protein-restricted diet.

Unlike normal liver tissue, which is soft and flexible, scar tissue is unyielding, a difference that has major consequences. The portal vein and the hepatic artery carry 1 ½ quarts of blood every minute through the miles of intermeshed capillaries within the liver. This huge volume of blood cannot pulse easily through the mass of scar tissue in the cirrhotic liver, so the blood backs up into the portal vein. Consequently, blood pressure in the portal vein rises sharply, causing portal hypertension. Figure 23–1 provides a diagram of the liver's circulatory system.

The rising pressure in the portal vein forces plasma out of the liver's blood vessels. The plasma fills the abdominal cavity, causing the abdomen to swell. This accumulation of fluid in the abdominal cavity is called ascites. Ascites tends to be a self-aggravating condition. Because the volume of blood in the circulatory system declines, less blood reaches the kidneys. The kidneys respond by calling for more aldosterone, the hormone that enlarges the blood volume by triggering the body's retention of sodium and water. As a result of the body's sodium and water retention, edema spreads to all body compartments. To make matters worse, the diseased liver cannot dispose of aldosterone as it normally does, so aldosterone levels remain high. Figure 23–2 summarizes the sequence of events that lead to edema.

With normal blood flow through the liver blocked, pressure forces some of the blood to take a detour through smaller vessels around the liver and out to the rest of the body. These collaterals, or shunts, often develop in the area around the esophagus. Frequently, the raised pressure enlarges the collaterals so that they bulge into the lumen of the esophagus, much as

FIGURE 23–1   The Liver's Circulatory System
Note that poor circulation in the liver can raise blood pressure in the portal vein, causing portal hypertension. Veins surrounding the intestinal system, including the esophagus, can also enlarge.

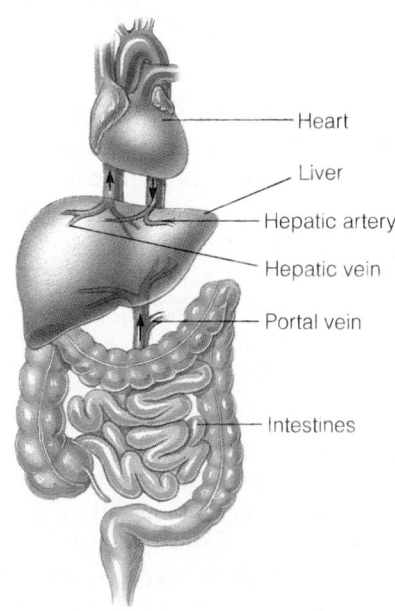

Heart

Liver

Hepatic artery

Hepatic vein

Portal vein

Intestines

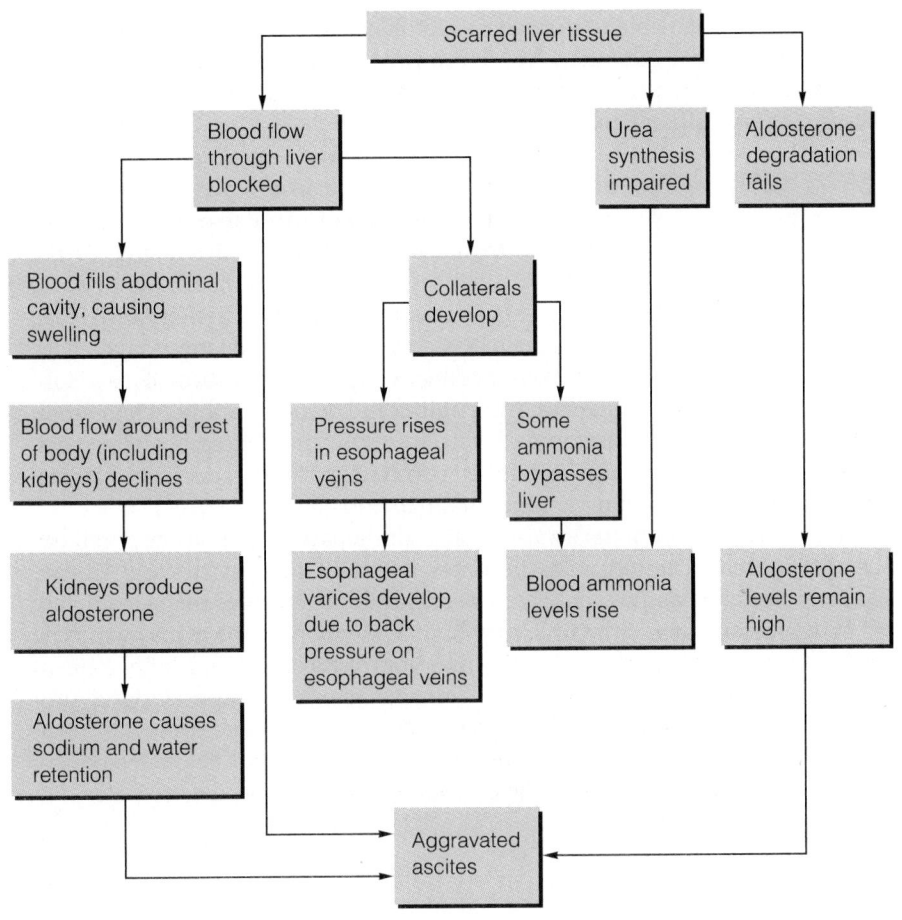

FIGURE 23–2   **The Consequences of Cirrhosis**

varicose veins do in the legs, creating esophageal varices. Eventually, the lining of the esophagus on top of the varices erodes. When the erosion penetrates into the varices themselves, massive bleeding follows. Bleeding esophageal varices tend to recur, and such bleeding episodes can lead to death.

Normally the healthy liver removes ammonia from the circulation and converts it to urea. A seriously diseased liver cannot synthesize urea adequately, and consequently, ammonia levels rise. Even if the liver could handle the ammonia it receives, some ammonia-laden blood bypasses the liver by way of the collaterals. Elevated blood ammonia levels insult the central nervous system, compounding the risk of hepatic coma, discussed next.

Hepatic Coma

Hepatic coma is a dangerous complication of cirrhosis. Typically, the person with impending hepatic coma exhibits mental disturbances such as changes in judgment, personality, or mood. Sometimes sleep patterns change. Such

esophageal varices (ee-SOFF-ah-GEE-al VAIR-ih-seez): tangles of distended blood vessels that protrude into the esophagus.

An elevated blood ammonia level is called **hyperammonemia** (HIGH-per-am-moe-KNEE-mee-uh).

hepatic coma: a state of unconsciousness that results from severe liver disease; also called **hepatic encephalopathy** or **portal systemic encephalopathy.**

flapping tremor: uncontrolled movement of certain muscles, which cause the outstretched arm and hand to flap like a wing; occurs in hepatic coma and other diseases that cause encephalopathy; also called **asterixis.**

Phenylalanine and tyrosine are the aromatic amino acids; they are characterized by a ringlike structure.

Leucine, isoleucine, and valine are the branched-chain amino acids; they are characterized by a branched structure.

Two enteral formulas that are low in aromatic amino acids and high in branched-chain amino acids are Hepatic-Aid II and Travasorb-Hepatic (see Appendix D). These formulas can be given orally or by tube. Parenteral solutions of similar amino acid composition are also available.

a person may be unable to draw even a simple shape, such as a star. A sweet, musty, or pungent odor may develop on the breath. Flapping tremor may also develop in the precoma state. Just before passing into coma, the person becomes very difficult to arouse.

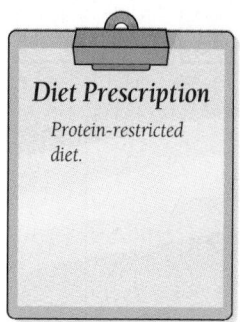

Diet Prescription
Protein-restricted diet.

The exact cause of hepatic coma remains elusive, but high blood ammonia levels play an important role. Most people in hepatic coma have elevated blood ammonia levels, although the degree of the elevation does not correlate with the severity of coma. This poor correlation may exist because *blood* ammonia levels do not reflect *brain* ammonia levels. The body produces greater quantities of two substances (glutamine and ketoglutarate) when brain ammonia levels are high; the degree of their elevation tends to correlate with the degree of coma. Other nitrogen-containing compounds may also be involved.

Blood amino acid patterns also change in hepatic coma. Normal catabolism of aromatic amino acids becomes impaired in liver disease. Consequently, aromatic amino acid levels rise. Hormonal changes that accompany liver disease encourage the uptake of branched-chain amino acids by muscle cells. Therefore, branched-chain amino acid levels fall. The high ratio of aromatic to branched-chain amino acids may cause the production of substances that act like neurotransmitters, and these substances may, in turn, contribute to hepatic coma. Additionally, altered amino acid metabolism generates high blood ammonia levels, which, as already noted, play a role in hepatic coma.

Dietary Treatment of Liver Disease

A diet adequate in energy and restricted in protein sets the cornerstone for diet therapy in cirrhosis. To maintain positive nitrogen balance, clients need a diet that provides 35 to 45 kcalories per kilogram of actual body weight daily (about 2000 to 3000 kcalories) and just enough high-quality protein for liver cells to regenerate, but not enough to aggravate ammonia buildup.[1] The diet should provide 1.0 to 1.5 grams protein per kilogram of body weight.[2]

A person who shows signs of impending coma requires additional dietary modifications. Protein intake must be restricted to 40 to 60 grams of high-quality protein per day. Special enteral and parenteral formulas low in aromatic amino acids and high in branched-chain amino acids can be used to provide additional protein to meet needs. Clients also receive drugs to rid their bodies of excess ammonia. If coma ensues, all protein, including special formulas, must be restricted.[3] As the client's neurological status improves, protein can be gradually increased.

Clients may better tolerate vegetable and milk proteins than meat proteins, perhaps because vegetable and milk proteins have fewer amino acids that readily form ammonia. Vegetable and dairy proteins also have fewer aromatic amino acids than do meat proteins. In addition, diets high in plant foods contain more fiber, which prevents constipation, thereby reducing the time available for the production and absorption of ammonia in the gut.

Because fats help make foods appetizing and deliver energy efficiently, fats serve an important role in the diet of a person with cirrhosis. Fat needs to be restricted only if the cirrhotic person develops steatorrhea, a clear sign of fat malabsorption. Even then, the body can usually handle MCT fat (see Chapter 21).

To protect the liver from further injury, clients with cirrhosis must completely abstain from alcohol use. A cirrhotic liver exposed to the continued onslaught of alcohol cannot manufacture the lipoproteins needed to rid itself of accumulated lipids.

Often, clients receive supplements of water-soluble vitamins in large amounts (up to five times the RDA). Recall from Chapter 7 how the B vitamins serve as coenzymes for the liver's many metabolic reactions and repair work. Deficiencies of folate, thiamin, and vitamin B_{12} occur most frequently.

Fat-soluble vitamins may be malabsorbed when steatorrhea develops. The body's use of vitamin A may be impaired when the diseased liver fails to synthesize adequate amounts of retinol-binding protein—the protein that carries vitamin A through the blood to the tissues that need it. Vitamin D nutrition status may suffer when the diseased liver fails to activate vitamin D for the body's use. Both liver disease and vitamin K deficiency may prolong the time it takes for blood to clot; a person with liver disease and a prolonged prothrombin time should be offered vitamin K supplements.

The diuretics used to correct fluid and electrolyte imbalances associated with liver disease may lead to deficiencies of the minerals potassium, magnesium, and zinc. The GI bleeding that occurs with liver disease can lead to iron deficiencies. Calcium deficiencies can also develop as a consequence of steatorrhea, low albumin levels (albumin, manufactured in the liver, carries calcium in the blood), and impaired vitamin D metabolism.

People with ascites need to restrict their intakes of fluids (see "Fluid-Restricted Diets" later in this chapter) and sodium (see Chapter 22). The level of restriction varies with the severity of the ascites. Sodium amounts may range from 1500 to 2000 milligrams during a day and fluids, from 1500 to 2000 milliliters a day. To assess changes in fluid balance, weigh the person *daily*. A rapid weight gain indicates fluid retention; sudden weight loss, in contrast, indicates successful fluid excretion.

Dietitians face a challenge in providing a diet low in sodium that provides adequate protein and also stimulates the appetite. Many high-protein foods contain significant amounts of sodium. To circumvent this problem, special low-sodium supplements and milk products are valuable.

The person who has bleeding esophageal varices will be unable to consume food by mouth and is often given a simple IV solution to maintain fluid and electrolyte balance. Peripheral or central TPN should be considered if the person is malnourished or unable to resume adequate oral intake for long periods of time.

Diet is vital to liver regeneration and recovery from cirrhosis. Therefore, every effort must be made to ensure a diet's acceptance. The person with anorexia may accept food more willingly in small, frequent meals than in three large ones. Work closely with clients and their families to individualize the diet, and serve foods attractively. Try the tactics suggested in Chapter 15 to encourage the client to eat.

prothrombin time: the time it takes for the blood to clot. Both vitamin K deficiency and liver disease can prolong the prothrombin time.

Fluid-Restricted Diets

Fluid-restricted diets prevent overhydration in people with disorders that cause the body to retain fluids abnormally. Some of these disorders include liver disease, renal disease, myocardial infarction, and congestive heart failure.

All beverages and foods contain some water. Although liquids are carefully restricted on a fluid-restricted diet, generally the only foods that are restricted are those composed largely of water, shown in Table 23–2.

Many people on fluid-restricted diets experience extreme thirst, making compliance with the restriction difficult. Suggestions to help relieve this thirst include:

- Chew gum or suck hard candy.
- Freeze fluids so they take longer to consume.
- Add lemon juice to water to make it more refreshing.
- Garble with refrigerated mouthwash.

Fluid restrictions are often temporary. Sometimes, though, as for renal disease, they are permanent, and monitoring fluid intake becomes crucial—and difficult. One method a person can use to monitor fluid intake is to fill a container with water equal to the total fluid allowance at the start of each day. For example, a person can fill a jar with 1500 milliliters of water if this is the person's fluid allowance. For each liquid food or drink taken, the person discards an equivalent amount of water from the container. A look at the jar at any time shows how much fluid is left for the remainder of the day.

TABLE 23–2   **Foods and Beverages Controlled on Fluid-Restricted Diets**

BEVERAGES	
Alcoholic beverages	Milk
Carbonated beverages	Tea
Coffee	Water
Juices	Any other

FOODS	
Frozen yogurt (melts to ½ initial volume)	Popsicles
Gelatin	Sherbet (melts to ⅔ initial volume)
Ice cream (melts to ½ initial volume)	Soup
Ice milk (melts to ½ initial volume)	

OTHER	
Cream	Liquid medications
Ice (melts to ⁹⁄₁₀ initial volume)	

Note: All foods contain some water, but these foods are considered part of the fluid allowance on a fluid-restricted diet.

Remind the person to save some of the fluid allowance for taking medications, if necessary.

Renal Disease

Like the liver, the kidneys serve a vital role in the maintenance of the body's homeostasis by filtering out substances the body doesn't need and eliminating them in the urine. In so doing, the kidneys maintain fluid, electrolyte, and acid-base balance, and they rid the body of metabolic waste products. Figure 23–3 shows a nephron, the working unit of the kidney, and illustrates how nephrons work.

The kidneys also help regulate blood pressure and produce a hormone that stimulates red blood cell production. Finally, the kidneys convert vitamin D to its most active form.

Because the kidneys perform all these vital functions, their failure results in serious consequences. Renal failure can be caused by damage to the

The **nephron** (NEF-ron), the working unit of the kidney, consists of the glomerulus and a tubule. The **glomerulus** (glow-MARE-you-lus) is a cup-shaped membrane enclosing a tuft of capillaries. The first part of the **tubule** surrounds the glomerulus. A pressure gradient between the glomerulus and the tubule returns needed materials to the blood and sends the wastes to the bladder.

renal failure: failure of the nephrons to maintain normal function.

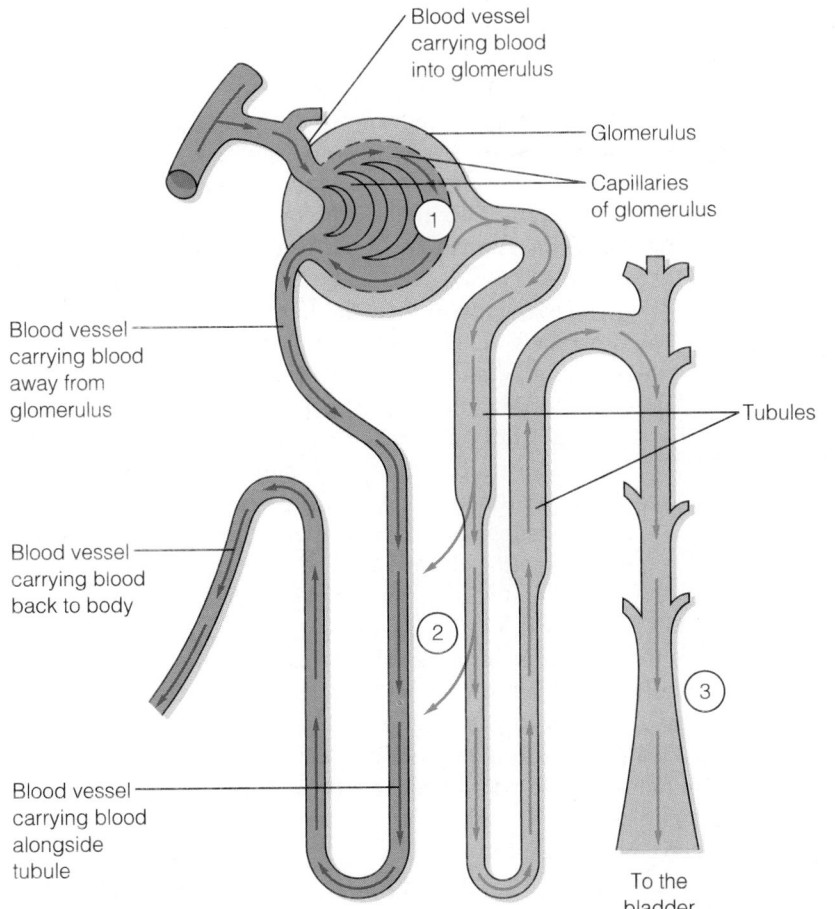

Blood vessel carrying blood into glomerulus

Glomerulus

Capillaries of glomerulus

Blood vessel carrying blood away from glomerulus

Tubules

Blood vessel carrying blood back to body

Blood vessel carrying blood alongside tubule

To the bladder

FIGURE 23–3 **A Nephron, One of the Kidney's Many Functioning Units** Blood flows into the glomerulus, and some of its fluid is filtered into the tubules (1). As the filtrate descends through the tubules, substances the body needs are returned to the blood through the intricate network of capillaries that surround the tubules (2). The waste materials that remain pass from the tubules on to the bladder (3).

kidneys themselves or by other diseases, such as diabetic nephropathy (Chapter 20), hypertension (Chapter 22), or atherosclerosis (Chapter 22). Renal failure can occur suddenly (acute renal failure) or over a period of time (chronic renal failure). Acute renal failure may be temporary; chronic renal failure is irreversible.

In the early stages of renal disease, the nephrons get bigger in an attempt to maintain normal function. The hypertrophied nephrons work so efficiently that about 80 percent of them can be destroyed before renal function is seriously affected.

As nephrons fail, the composition of the blood and urine changes. The body's principal nitrogen-containing metabolic waste products—blood urea nitrogen (BUN), creatinine, and uric acid—accumulate in the blood when renal function is impaired. Consequently, laboratory tests for the person with renal failure show high blood levels of BUN, creatinine, and uric acid.

As renal failure progresses to a severe stage, the buildup of toxic waste products in the blood (uremia) can precipitate a wide array of symptoms in virtually every body system, known collectively as the uremic syndrome. The person experiences fatigue, weakness, diminished mental alertness, muscular twitches, muscle cramps, anorexia, nausea, vomiting, stomatitis, and an unpleasant taste in the mouth. The skin may itch uncomfortably, and in later stages, GI ulcers and bleeding commonly develop.

Chronic Renal Disease

The early stages of renal disease generally go undetected, so dietary restrictions are not imposed. As renal function declines, dietary adjustments assume a critical role in treatment. Eventually, as renal failure progresses still further and uremia threatens, the person must begin dialysis or receive a kidney transplant to survive.

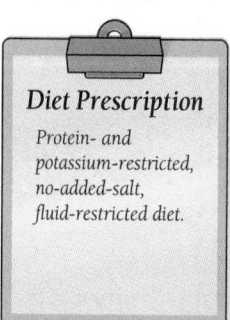

Diet Prescription

Protein- and potassium-restricted, no-added-salt, fluid-restricted diet.

Dialysis works on the principles of diffusion and osmosis across a semipermeable membrane and is used to remove excess fluids and wastes from the blood. The membrane that covers the abdominal organs (the peritoneal membrane) can serve as the semipermeable membrane; fluid can be infused into the peritoneum, can take up wastes from the blood vessels in the peritoneal membrane, and then can be collected again in a procedure called *peritoneal dialysis*. A synthetic semipermeable membrane can also be used. In this case, blood leaves the person's artery and passes through tubing that serves as a semipermeable membrane. The tubes are continually bathed by solutions that selectively remove unwanted material. The blood returns to the body through the person's veins after being cleansed. This procedure is called *hemodialysis*.

Kidney transplants provide an alternative to dialysis in end-stage renal disease. Given a choice, many would prefer transplants; however, a suitable kidney donor can't always be found. Kidney transplants can successfully restore kidney function and promote normal body growth. For this reason, transplants are particularly desirable for children. People who generally are not considered candidates for kidney transplants are the elderly, people with other life-threatening conditions, or people who prefer dialysis.

uremia (you-REE-me-ah): the buildup of toxic waste products in the blood, associated with renal insufficiency.

uremic syndrome: a complex of symptoms seen late in renal failure, caused by uremia.

When urea (which can be excreted through sweat) crystallizes and becomes visible on the skin, the condition is called **uremic frost.**

The severe stage of renal disease in which diet alone is no longer effective in preventing the buildup of toxic waste products is called **end-stage renal disease.**

diffusion and osmosis: the movement of water across a membrane to equalize the concentration of particles on both sides of the membrane. Water moves from the less concentrated to the more concentrated side.

peritoneal (PERR-ee-toe-NEE-al) **dialysis:** removal of wastes from the blood using the peritoneal membrane as a semipermeable membrane.

hemodialysis (HE-mow-die-AL-ih-sis): removal of wastes from the blood by passing it outside the body through tubes made of semipermeable membranes submerged in a water solution.

The objectives of dietary management of chronic renal failure are:

■ To achieve or maintain optimal nutrition status and nitrogen balance.
■ To prevent the buildup of toxic metabolic products, thus minimizing the risk of uremia.
■ To delay the progression of renal failure and to postpone the need for dialysis.
■ To prevent complications, such as growth failure, wasting syndrome, bone disease, hypertension, edema, and congestive heart failure.
■ To foster the client's well-being.

The actual diet is highly individualized; most commonly it restricts protein, sodium, potassium, phosphorus, and fluids and carefully controls total energy intake. A sample renal diet menu is shown on p. 603.

wasting syndrome: the pattern of growth failure in children and reduced muscle mass, fat tissue, and blood protein levels in people of any age that frequently develops as a consequence of renal disease.

In both liver disease and renal disease, protein-restricted diets help prevent the buildup of nitrogen-containing waste products that accumulate as a result of amino acid metabolism; however, there is an important distinction. In liver disease, blood ammonia levels rise because the liver cannot convert ammonia to urea. Thus ammonia is the toxin. In kidney disease, the liver does make urea, but the kidneys can't excrete it in the urine. Blood ammonia levels are normal, blood urea levels rise, and urea is the toxin of concern.

The ideal renal diet provides enough protein to support normal nitrogen balance and not enough to elevate BUN. Diet prescriptions may range from as low as 20 grams protein to as high as 70 grams. A person on dialysis receives a more liberal protein allowance, because the dialysis procedure results in the loss of some protein. Table 23–3 summarizes nutrient needs of people with chronic renal failure and shows how these needs change for the person on hemodialysis or peritoneal dialysis.

Regardless of the protein allowance, all people with renal failure need adequate energy intakes to achieve or maintain desirable body weight and to keep from using protein to meet energy needs. Children with renal disease often fail to grow normally, and people of any age with renal disease may have the wasting syndrome—reduced muscle mass, fat tissue, and blood protein levels, as described earlier.

The little girl beams with pleasure when Charlie, the nurse, comes into the room. This is one of the high points of her day. "Do you have a lollipop for me?" she asks.

"Yep," says Charlie, reaching into his pocket. "Your favorite color, red. Eat it all up, and I'll bring you another one."

Why is this nurse feeding the child candy? Because the child has renal disease and has a hard time getting enough kcalories to protect the protein she eats, the staff has been instructed to keep giving her sugar in whatever form she will accept it. A lollipop is like a clear liquid, because it melts in the mouth; it contains no protein and few or no electrolytes to burden the kidney; but it offers sugar to help spare protein. Nothing could be more appropriate for this growing child's health.

TABLE 23–3   **Typical Nutrient Needs in Chronic Renal Failure**

NUTRIENTS	PREDIALYSIS	HEMODIALYSIS	PERITONEAL DIALYSIS
Energy (kcal/kg)	35–45	35–45	35–45
Protein (g/kg)	0.5–1.0	1.0–1.5	1.5–2.0
Fluid (ml)	1000–1500	800–1000	800–1000
Sodium (g)	0.5–2.0	2.0	2.0–4.0
Potassium (g)	1.5–2.5	1.5–2.5	2.0–4.0
Phosphorus (mg)	a	a	a
Supplements			
Calcium (mg)	1200–1600	1000	1200–1600
Folate (mg)	1	1	1
Vitamin B$_6$ (mg)	5	10	10
Vitamin C (mg)	70–100	100	100
Other water-soluble vitamins	RDA	RDA	RDA
Vitamin D	As appropriate	As appropriate	As appropriate

Note: The actual amounts of these nutrients in the diet must be highly individualized based on each person's responses.
[a]The extent of phosphorus restriction depends on serum levels of phosphorus. Often, phosphate binders are used to help control these levels.

Renal disease disturbs the balance of fluids and electrolytes that bathes the cells. Sodium is one electrolyte that is affected. Early in renal failure, the person can maintain sodium balance with a moderate sodium intake. As renal disease progresses, however, both sodium and water must be restricted to prevent hypertension, edema, and heart failure. A typical diet will contain from 1 to 4 grams of sodium and 500 to 3000 milliliters of fluid daily.

Individual needs vary, so each person's weight, blood pressure, and urine output are carefully monitored to determine exact needs. Body weight and blood pressure increase when the person is retaining sodium (and fluid). Urine output also provides a useful estimation of daily fluid needs. Simply add 500 milliliters for insensible water loss to 24-hour urine output.

Potassium balance may also be disturbed in the person with renal failure. Most people with renal failure do not have problems handling typical intakes of potassium. However, hyperkalemia can develop, and if it does, it can be fatal. Therefore, potassium is often moderately restricted to about 1½ to 3 grams per day. Table 22–12 on p. 578 lists foods high in potassium. A sample renal diet menu is illustrated on p. 603.

People on dialysis who excrete little or no urine need to be careful not to exceed their prescribed sodium, potassium, and fluid allowances. These people often need the lower range of intakes for these nutrients.

Disruption of the normal balance of calcium to phosphorus in the blood frequently occurs in people with chronic renal failure, and bone diseases can result. Dietary control helps prevent the problem. The person is advised to

hyperkalemia: excessive potassium in the blood.

When urine volume is reduced, **oliguria** exists; when no urine is being excreted, **anuria** exists.

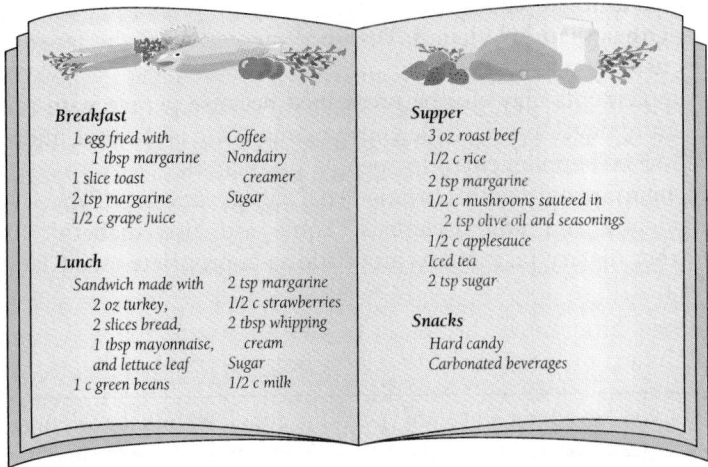

Sample Renal Diet Menu

This diet provides 60 g of protein and controls sodium and potassium intake.
To add kcalories to this diet, prepare food with oil or unsalted margarine (salted
margarine, if allowed), and use additional sugar or syrup whenever possible. For
example, canned fruit packed in heavy syrup, rather than juice, adds kcalories.

restrict phosphorus intake by avoiding foods high in phosphorus, such as
those shown in Table 23–4. Many foods high in phosphorus are also high
in protein, so it is not more difficult to manage this restriction, than to
manage protein restriction alone.

Most people with renal disease receive calcium supplements to help prevent bone disease. Large doses of vitamin D (50,000 to 200,000 IU daily)
may improve the absorption and utilization of calcium. If the active form of
vitamin D is given in supplement form, smaller doses are prescribed.

Vitamin deficiencies frequently develop in people with renal failure. The
restrictive diet is partly responsible, since diets low in potassium also are
low in water-soluble vitamins. Vitamins can be lost in dialysis, and drug
therapy can change nutrient needs. Uremia can affect the metabolism of
nutrients. For these reasons, clients receive generous amounts of vitamin B_6,

TABLE 23–4   **Foods High in Phosphorus**

Canned fish	Milk and milk products
Chocolate	Nuts
Cocoa	Organ meats
Dried beans and peas	Peanut butter
Dried fruit	Whole-grain breads
Game meats	Whole-grain cereals

vitamin C, and folate, along with the RDA of the remaining water-soluble vitamins. Other than for vitamin D, supplementation of the fat-soluble vitamins is usually not necessary.

Iron supplements may also be prescribed because people with renal failure frequently develop iron-deficiency anemia. Zinc is another mineral that may need to be supplemented for people on dialysis.

Lastly, many people with chronic renal failure develop Type IV hyperlipoproteinemia and atherosclerosis. Some are also diabetic. In these cases, further dietary restrictions are made as appropriate (see Chapters 20 and 22).

No doubt you have long since arrived at the conclusion that designing renal diets is a task for a specialist. The complexities pile up, and the diet planners must raise or lower intakes of sodium, potassium, protein, kcalories, liquids, lipids, vitamins, and minerals. They must find food combinations that will deliver the necessary amounts of these nutrients, and these must be foods that *the individual on the diet will accept and enjoy.* The renal dietitian faces these challenges every day.

With all that hard work to do, the diet planner has still another task—communicating with, and especially listening to, the client. Inside that tangled web of grossly altered metabolic processes, dialysis lines, and toxic products is a person, often a frightened or discouraged one. One individual will say she dreams of ice cream sodas, forbidden because of their high-sodium content. She needs to feel understood, at least. Another says he feels guilty because his mother spends so much time preparing special foods for him. He, too, needs support. Another is fighting guilt and resentment because she repeatedly sneaks forbidden foods high in protein in spite of the rules she knows she should follow. If you have ever been "on a diet," even though it wasn't a renal diet, you will appreciate some of the problems these people face.

The person with renal disease has to live a life that involves many frustrations. Successful treatment often hinges on compliance with diet and drug orders. All the members of the health care team need to know what is involved if they are to offer the most effective possible support.

Acute Renal Failure

Acute renal failure occurs suddenly and is the consequence of another medical condition. The typical victim of acute renal failure has a major illness, such as an infection or a burn, or has suffered a cardiac arrest. Suddenly, metabolism becomes hypercatabolic, the glomerular filtration rate drops, urine output declines, blood pressure shoots up, and toxic waste products begin to build in the blood. As the body's cells break down, potassium is released from the intracellular fluid, and the kidneys fail to excrete it. Consequently, blood potassium levels rise sharply. Common clinical symptoms of acute renal failure include hiccups, anorexia, nausea, and vomiting. GI bleeding and diarrhea sometimes occur. Drowsiness, agitation, and confusion are frequently seen.

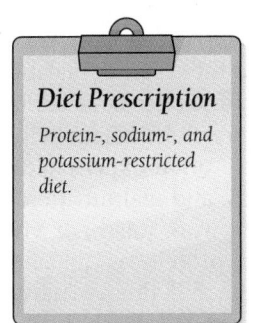

Diet Prescription

Protein-, sodium-, and potassium-restricted diet.

In the early stages of acute renal failure, urine volume often diminishes markedly. Sometimes, though, too much urine is produced. Later in the course of acute renal failure, the kidneys cannot conserve water, and the person begins to excrete large amounts of urine and electrolytes.

In some cases, acute renal failure is reversible. In others, it progresses to chronic renal failure. About one-half of all people with acute renal failure die.

The primary concern in acute renal failure is to treat the underlying disorder in order to prevent permanent or further damage to the kidneys. For example, if severe blood loss is the problem, a blood transfusion is given to restore blood volume. Other measures must be taken to restore fluid and electrolyte balance and minimize levels of toxic waste products. In addition to the nutrition factors mentioned in the following paragraphs, treatment may require diuretics to mobilize fluids in the oliguric phase of acute renal failure. Dialysis (either peritoneal dialysis or hemodialysis) is necessary when blood urea, creatinine, or potassium concentrations are high.

As mentioned, the person in acute renal failure is often hypercatabolic and suffering from another major illness. Add to these conditions nausea, vomiting, and confusion, and you have a person who really needs food energy but is unable to eat. The person's actual kcaloric needs depend on the rate of catabolism; usually 35 to 50 kcalories per kilogram of body weight will meet these needs.

Protein needs also vary, depending on metabolic rate. Generally, the diet restricts protein to about 30 to 40 grams per day. Some practitioners prefer to provide higher protein intakes, even if this will necessitate dialysis, to prevent negative nitrogen balance and its possible consequences (see Chapter 14). If dialysis is instituted, a more liberal protein intake of 70 to 85 grams may be allowed.

Fluid and electrolyte restrictions are also warranted. Sodium may be restricted (500 to 1000 milligrams) in the oliguric phase, but this may change as the person enters the diuretic phase. Likewise, potassium is often restricted to less than 2 grams per day in the oliguric phase, but may need to be supplemented in the diuretic phase.

The total amount of fluid is carefully adjusted to avoid overhydration or dehydration. Fluid requirements can be measured by measuring urine output, as described earlier (see p. 602). Additional fluid is provided if the person experiences vomiting, diarrhea, or high fever. In the oliguric phase, the person will need small volumes of fluids. In the diuretic phase, up to 3 liters of urine may be lost daily, and large amounts of fluids are needed.

The early phase of acute renal failure, when urine volume is reduced, is the **oliguric phase;** the phase characterized by large fluid and electrolyte losses in the urine is the **diuretic phase;** the gradual return of renal function marks the **recovery phase.**

Celiac Disease and the Gluten-Restricted Diet

Celiac disease, a hereditary disorder with an incidence of about 1 in every 2000 to 3000 births, is characterized by malabsorption resulting from a sensitivity to gluten. Gluten is a protein found in wheat, oats, rye, and barley. A fraction of the gluten protein, gliadin, acts as a toxic substance

celiac (SEE-lee-ack) **disease:** a sensitivity to gliadin that causes flattening of the intestinal villi and generalized malabsorption; also called **gluten-sensitive enteropathy** (EN-ter-OP-ah-thee) or **celiac sprue.**

gluten (GLUE-ten): a vegetable protein found in wheat, oats, rye, and barley.

gliadin (GLIGH-ah-din): a fraction of the gluten protein.

causing atrophy of the intestinal villi and seriously reducing the absorptive surface of the intestinal tract. The disaccharidases (including lactase) and carrier molecules normally found on the villi disappear, and the result is malabsorption of many nutrients, including fat, protein, carbohydrate, fat-soluble vitamins, iron, calcium, magnesium, zinc, and some water-soluble vitamins.

Diet Prescription

Gluten-restricted diet.

The person with celiac disease often experiences steatorrhea, diarrhea, weight loss, and malnutrition. Anemia may occur as a result of iron, folate, or vitamin B_{12} deficiency. Because protein is malabsorbed, serum protein levels can fall dramatically, inducing edema. The person may bleed easily because of clotting abnormalities precipitated by a vitamin K deficiency. Furthermore, calcium deficiency can cause tetany and bone pain.

Fortunately, when gluten is removed from the diet, the intestinal changes reverse almost completely. However, lactase deficiency and lactose intolerance may be permanent. If the person fails to follow the diet, the symptoms will return.

The treatment for celiac disease sounds deceptively simple: eliminate gluten. Such a diet prescription is easier to describe than to follow, since wheat, oats, rye, and barley are common in many foods, as you can see from Table 23–5. Processed foods (ice cream, salad dressings, canned foods) often use wheat flour as an extender.

Help people with celiac disease and those who care for them to understand what foods to avoid. Be sure they understand how to read food labels. Suggest the use of arrowroot, corn, potato, rice, and soybean flours as substitutes for wheat flour in recipes. A low-gluten wheat-starch flour is also available. Support groups of people with celiac disease and their families are organized in some parts of the country. They can be a great source of help for the individual with celiac disease.

An easy way to remember the grains that must be restricted in celiac disease is to remember WORB (wheat, oats, rye, and barley).

PKU and the Phenylalanine-Restricted Diet

Phenylketonuria (PKU) is an inherited disorder of metabolism involving the essential amino acid phenylalanine. In PKU, the absence or malfunction of an enzyme, which normally converts excess phenylalanine to tyrosine causes phenylalanine and its metabolites to build up to toxic concentrations in the blood. Left untreated, an infant with PKU suffers severe mental retardation and abnormal growth and development.

phenylketonuria (FEN-ill-KEY-toe-NEW-ree-ah) **(PKU):** an inborn error of metabolism in which phenylalanine cannot be converted to tyrosine. Metabolites of phenylalanine accumulate in the tissues, causing damage and overflow into the urine.

Diet Prescription

Phenylalanine-restricted diet.

Early diagnosis and early dietary treatment of PKU are critical to prevent mental retardation. In most states, infants receive a test for PKU shortly after birth for this reason.

The phenylalanine-restricted diet must provide enough phenylalanine to promote normal growth and development, but not enough to allow excess phenylalanine to accumulate in the blood. The health care team determines the amount of phenylalanine that is appropriate for the client by monitoring blood phenylalanine concentrations.

TABLE 23–5　**Gluten-Restricted Diet**

MEAT AND MEAT ALTERNATES
Any allowed except those that are breaded, prepared with bread crumbs, or creamed.

MILK AND MILK PRODUCTS
Any allowed except milk mixed with Ovaltine, commercial chocolate milk with a cereal additive, pudding thickened with wheat flour, or ice cream or sherbet containing gluten stabilizers.

FRUITS AND VEGETABLES
Any allowed except those that are breaded, prepared with bread crumbs, or creamed.

GRAINS
Allowed: Bread, cereal, or dessert products made from arrowroot, cornmeal, soybean flour, rice flour, potato flour and gluten-free starch; gluten-free macaroni and porridge; tapioca; cornmeal, cornflakes, popcorn, and hominy; rice, cream of rice, puffed rice, and rice flakes; potato chips.   Not allowed: Bread, cereal, or dessert products made from wheat, rye, oats, or barley; commercially prepared mixes for biscuits, cornbread, muffins, pancakes, buckwheat pancakes, cakes, cookies, or waffles; bran; pasta, macaroni, or noodles; malt; pretzels; wheat germ; doughnuts; ice cream cones; matzo.

OTHER
Not allowed: Beer; ale; certain whiskeys (Canadian rye); cereal beverages (Postum); root beer; commercial salad dressings that contain gluten stabilizers; soups containing any ingredient not allowed (such as barley or noodles).

As is true for all diets, the phenylalanine-restricted diet must provide ample energy, protein, and essential nutrients. Because tyrosine (normally not an essential amino acid) is not made from phenylalanine in PKU, tyrosine must be provided in the diet. Infants are fed special formulas low in phenylalanine, and later, solids are introduced gradually. The diet planner uses special exchange lists to plan the diet. The diet excludes high-protein foods such as meat, fish, poultry, cheese, eggs, milk, nuts, dried beans, and peas. Also excluded are commercial breads and pastries made from regular flour, which has a high phenylalanine content. A sample menu is shown here.

People with PKU must also be aware of the phenylalanine contents of products containing the sweetener aspartame. Aspartame contains phenylalanine, and so can be used only if it is specifically planned into the diet.

Some controversy surrounds the issue of whether or not the phenylalanine-restricted diet can be discontinued as the child with PKU gets older. Most clinicians recommend that the diet be continued at least through

Lofenalac is a special formula used in the treatment of PKU that is low in phenylalanine. Another formula, Phenyl-Free, contains no phenylalanine.

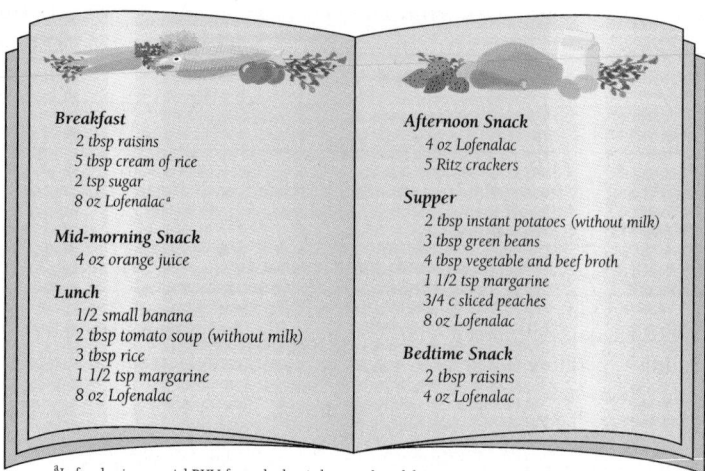

Breakfast
2 tbsp raisins
5 tbsp cream of rice
2 tsp sugar
8 oz Lofenalac[a]

Mid-morning Snack
4 oz orange juice

Lunch
1/2 small banana
2 tbsp tomato soup (without milk)
3 tbsp rice
1 1/2 tsp margarine
8 oz Lofenalac

Afternoon Snack
4 oz Lofenalac
5 Ritz crackers

Supper
2 tbsp instant potatoes (without milk)
3 tbsp green beans
4 tbsp vegetable and beef broth
1 1/2 tsp margarine
3/4 c sliced peaches
8 oz Lofenalac

Bedtime Snack
2 tbsp raisins
4 oz Lofenalac

[a]Lofenalac is a special PKU formula that is low in phenylalanine.

Sample Phenylalanine-Restricted Menu for a Child with PKU

adolescence. A pregnant woman with PKU must follow the diet, or her unborn infant can be seriously affected. Congenital malformations and mental and physical retardation are likely when the fetus is exposed to high phenylalanine levels.

The successful treatment of children with PKU depends on the parents. They must understand the diet and the consequences of poor compliance. As children with PKU grow, responsibility for diet compliance shifts more and more to them. The health care team must provide the parents and children with the help, support, and continuing education that they need to cope with the disorder and to manage their lifestyles appropriately.

Diets restricted in protein and amino acids are complicated and difficult for clients to understand and follow. Yet adherence to these diets can make a livesaving difference. In the case of cirrhosis, failure to adhere to the diet can sometimes lead to hepatic coma and death. In the final stages of renal disease, the consequence of poor dietary compliance is either the early appearance of the uremic syndrome or the need for almost continuous dialysis or a kidney transplant. In celiac disease, failure to adhere to the gluten-restricted diet leads to serious nutrient deficiencies and wasting. In PKU, poor dietary compliance, although not fatal, results in otherwise avoidable mental and physical retardation.

CASE STUDY

Renal Failure

Mrs. Ethan was 42 when she began to have kidney problems. While she was being treated in the hospital for a major burn, she developed acute renal failure. Gradually, the acute renal failure progressed to chronic renal failure. At 5 feet 3 inches tall, she weighs 100 pounds. Up to this point, she has been able to avoid dialysis by following a 50-gram protein-, fluid- and electrolyte-restricted diet.

Describe the two stages of acute renal failure. What nutrients are of concern in each stage? What factors would the physician keep in mind when prescribing Mrs. Ethan's kcalorie, protein, and electrolyte needs during the episode of acute renal failure?

Think about the diet of a person with chronic renal disease. What nutrients are of particular concern? How would the diet change if the person had diabetes or hyperlipidemia?

How does Mrs. Ethan's current weight for height affect her energy needs? What effect would dialysis have on her nutrient needs?

Write down everything you ate yesterday. Now cross out the foods you could not have eaten if you had been on a diet in which sodium, potassium, and phosphorus were restricted. Now use the exchange lists in Chapter 19 to get a rough idea of how much protein you ate. Would you have to cut out many foods to follow a 50-gram-protein diet? If yes, would your diet still be adequate in kcalories? Would it be easy to follow every day?

Study Questions

1. Discuss cirrhosis, and describe how cirrhosis leads to portal hypertension, ascites, formation of collaterals, esophageal varices, and elevated blood ammonia levels.

2. Describe the dietary treatment of the person with cirrhosis and hepatic coma. Consider special dietary concerns of the person with ascites and bleeding esophageal varices.

3. What is renal failure, and why is it difficult to detect in the early stages?

4. When is a special diet instituted in the course of renal failure? When is dialysis or a kidney transplant considered for the person with renal failure?

5. Describe the dietary modifications made in the diet of the person with chronic renal failure, and discuss why these modifications are necessary.

6. What are the differences between acute and chronic renal failure?

7. What are the nutrient needs of the person in acute renal failure, and how do these needs change throughout the course of the disorder?

8. Discuss the basic problem in celiac disease, and describe the diet used in its treatment.
9. What is PKU? What are the consequences of untreated PKU?
10. Describe the diet used in the treatment of PKU.

Notes

1. E. P. Shronts, Nutritional assessment of adults with end-stage hepatic failure, *Nutrition in Clinical Practice* 3 (1988): 108–112.
2. J. E. Fischer, Branched-chain-enriched amino acid solutions in patients with liver failure: An early example of nutritional pharmacology, *Journal of Parenteral and Enteral Nutrition* 14 (Supplement, 1990): 249–256; Shronts, 1988; N. H. Mexhitis, Nutritional management in liver disease, *Nutrition in Clinical Practice* 3 (1988): 108–112.
3. E. P. Shronts and coauthors, Nutrition support of the adult liver transplant candidate, *Journal of the American Dietetic Association* 87 (1987): 441–451.

23

Nutrition in the Prevention and Treatment of Kidney Stones

Chapter 23 described renal failure, a kidney disorder that greatly alters nutrient needs. A far more common kidney disorder, kidney stones, has traditionally included a modified diet as a part of its treatment. In the United States, about one in every ten adults (mostly men over 25 years of age) suffers from kidney stones, a painful, although rarely fatal, condition. A person who has experienced a kidney stone may have a recurrence, but most people with kidney stones report only a single episode each, suggesting that with proper treatment, recurrence may be preventable.

The role of diet in the prevention of kidney stones is the topic of this Nutrition in Practice. Just as the traditional bland diet described in Nutrition in Practice 17 has evolved, the dietary recommendations for people with kidney stones has changed over the years.

What are kidney stones?

Kidney stones are masses of various composition that form in the kidney. Most kidney stones contain calcium oxalate (60 percent of all stones), calcium phosphate (9 percent), or a combination of both (11 percent). Less commonly, stones are composed of uric acid, cystine, or magnesium ammonium phosphate. The accompanying Miniglossary defines terms related to kidney stones.

What causes kidney stones to form?

Calcium stones may form in response to a variety of underlying medical conditions that cause either elevated serum calcium levels, excessive urinary excretion of calcium, or deficiencies of substances in the urine that normally inhibit stone formation. Most frequently, calcium stones are associated with excessive urinary calcium excretion for which no cause can be identified (idiopathic hypercalciuria).

Uric acid stones are associated with the excessive urinary excretion of uric acid, an acid urine, and a low urine volume. Cystine stones occur as the result of a metabolic disorder that is characterized by the abnormal excretion of cystine in the urine (cystinuria). Table NP23–1 summarizes some of the disorders that are associated with stone formation.

The exact mechanisms by which kidney stones form remain undefined. Why is it, for example, that all people pass crystals in the urine routinely, whereas only 10 percent develop kidney stones?[1] Practitioners widely accept three theories that help to explain how kidney stones form. These theories provide the basis for the current treatment and prevention of kidney stones.

One proposed mechanism of stone formation—supersaturation—can be explained by the relative insolubility of stone constituents (such as calcium salts, uric acid, or oxalic acid) in urine. When stone constituents

TABLE NP23–1 Conditions Associated with Kidney Stones

Bowel diseases causing
  malabsorption
Cystinuria
Glucocorticoid excess
Gout
Hyperparathyroidism
Hyperthyroidism
Immobilization
Malignancies (some types)
Osteoporosis
Paget's disease
Recurrent urinary tract infections
Renal tubular acidosis
Vitamin D intoxication

become concentrated, they form crystals that eventually precipitate and grow larger. The more concentrated a mineral is in the urine, the greater the likelihood that a stone will form.

Another proposal holds that a small seed (sometimes called a nucleus or nidus) is responsible for the formation of some stones. Composed of a substance different from that found in the remainder of the stone, the seed develops from the crystallization of a supersaturated compound in the urine. The crystalline structure then provides a matrix upon which less saturated substances can attach. In some cases, calcium oxalate stones have been found to form around a uric acid seed. Treatment of this type of stone focuses on the mineral found in the seed rather than on the minerals that make up most of the stone.

Finally, many practitioners believe that a deficiency of one or more naturally occurring stone inhibitors in the urine may contribute to stone formation. For example, researchers have identified a protein that inhibits the formation of kidney stones; its defective version fails to inhibit stone formation.[2] Other probable inhibitors include citrate, a type of phosphate, a type of polysaccharide, magnesium, zinc, and ribonucleic acid (RNA).[3] All of these substances have been identified as inhibitors of calcium oxalate stone formation. Research has yet to provide enough knowledge about these inhibitors to influence therapy.

What happens to the stones once they form?

Small stones (less than 5 millimeters, or one-fifth of an inch, in diameter) may pass through the ureters and be excreted in the urine; therefore, they may not require treatment. Larger stones cannot exit the body as easily. When a large stone or a large piece of a broken-off stone enters a ureter (see Figure NP23–1, p. 613), the person experiences a severe, stabbing pain, called renal colic. Typically, the pain starts suddenly in the back, just above the ribs, and follows the course of the stone down the abdomen toward the groin. When the stone reaches the bladder, the pain usually subsides. If a stone blocks the flow of urine or causes an infection, a physician must either remove it surgically or, more commonly, use sound waves or shock waves to break up the stone into pieces small enough to pass easily through the urinary tract.

How does diet fit into the picture?

The answer to this question is complicated, because so many

MINIGLOSSARY

cystinuria (SIS-te-NEW-ree-ah): the presence of cystine in the urine; the symptom of an inherited metabolic disorder in which large amounts of the amino acids cystine, lysine, arginine, and ornithine are excreted in the urine. Cystinuria commonly results in kidney stone formation.

dysuria (dis-YOU-ree-ah): painful or difficult urination.

gout: a metabolic disorder that results in excess uric acid in the blood and sometimes in the urine, characterized by acute arthritis and inflammation of the joints.

hematuria (HEME-ah-TOO-ree-ah): blood in the urine.

hypercalciuria (HIGH-per-KAL-see-YOU-ree-ah): excessive urinary excretion of calcium. When the excessive urinary excretion of calcium is not related to a known underlying medical condition, it is known as **idiopathic hypercalciuria**.

hyperoxaluria (HIGH-per-OK-sa-LOO-ree-ah): excessive urinary excretion of oxalate; it may occur when calcium intake is insufficient to bind oxalate in the intestine, thus allowing excessive oxalate absorption. When GI diseases cause excessive oxalate absorption and subsequent excessive oxalate excretion, it is known as **enteric hyperoxaluria**.

nidus (NIGH-dus), **nucleus**: a small bit of crystallized mineral or other substance that serves as a matrix for further crystallization.

renal colic: the severe pain that accompanies the movement of a kidney stone from the kidney through the ureter to the bladder.

struvite: crystals of magnesium ammonium phosphate.

supersaturation: a term that describes the concentration of a substance in a liquid at the moment when it becomes too concentrated to stay in solution and begins to precipitate.

disorders can cause stones to form (see Table NP23–1). Dietary regimens vary according to the type of stone, but all include one bit of advice: increase fluid intake. A high fluid intake raises urine output, thus diluting the concentration of minerals in the urine and reducing the risk of stone formation. People with kidney stones need to drink enough fluid to maintain a urine volume of at least 2 liters per day. This requires a total intake of about 3 to 4 liters taken at regular intervals throughout the day. Other aspects of diet in the treatment of kidney stones have been far more controversial and have changed dramatically in recent years.

What are some of the controversies?

One of the most controversial topics in the treatment of stones concerns the role of dietary calcium restriction for the person with a calcium-containing stone. On the surface, it appears reasonable that a person who is excreting large amounts of calcium in the urine should restrict dietary calcium. For years, people with calcium stones were routinely instructed to reduce their calcium intakes by eliminating milk and milk products from their diets. Such a diet may be advisable for those clients with idiopathic hypercalciuria whose calcium absorption increases significantly when they follow an unrestricted-calcium diet. In these cases, urinary calcium concentration increases, thus increasing the risk of calcium stone formation. For these people, then, a low-calcium diet (600 milligrams of calcium per day) may be beneficial. In addition, they need to refrain from using vitamin-mineral

preparations and medicines containing calcium (such as calcium-containing antacids) or vitamin D (which enhances calcium absorption).

However, for clients who do not absorb calcium excessively, calcium restriction might lead to negative calcium balance and bone loss. They have high urinary calcium levels even when their dietary calcium intakes are not high. This indicates that they are losing calcium from their bones. Calcium loss from bones raises urinary calcium, thus making stone formation more, not less, likely.

Calcium restriction is also contraindicated for people susceptible to developing calcium oxalate stones. Calcium normally binds to oxalate in

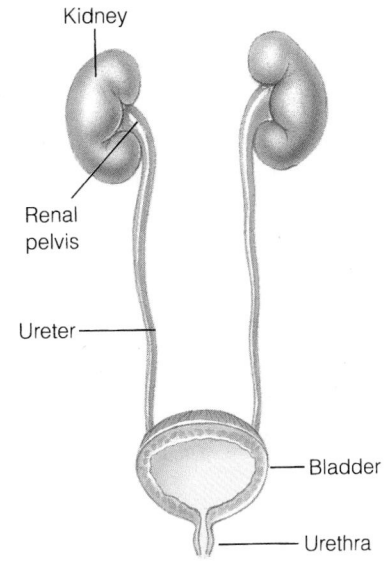

FIGURE NP23–1 **The Urinary Tract**

Kidney

Renal pelvis

Ureter

Bladder

Urethra

the intestinal tract. If dietary calcium is severely limited, oxalate absorption and subsequent excretion may increase, resulting in hyperoxaluria. Hyperoxaluria increases the likelihood of calcium oxalate stone formation. Instead of restricting calcium, then, treatment focuses on oxalate. Of all the oxalate in the urine, only a small percentage derives from the diet. Nevertheless, people with calcium oxalate stones are advised to limit their intakes of foods high in oxalate. Table NP23–2 on p. 614 lists foods containing considerable amounts of oxalate.

Most of the oxalate in the urine comes from the body's synthesis of it. One of the oxalate synthesis pathways in the body begins with vitamin C. Consequently, megadoses of vitamin C over a prolonged time raise urinary oxalate concentrations, which, in some people, can aggravate stone formation. People with hyperoxaluria should steer clear of vitamin C supplements.

While the goal of calcium stone treatment is to reduce urinary calcium excretion, diet alone rarely accomplishes this goal satisfactorily. Certain medications, such as thiazide diuretics, reduce the excretion of calcium, and thus the recurrence of idiopathic calcium stones. However, because thiazide diuretics can precipitate a potassium deficiency, they are generally given along with another type of diuretic that conserves potassium.

Health care professionals advise clients on thiazide diuretics to follow a moderately restricted sodium diet. A high sodium intake can offset the beneficial effects of the diuretic and can cause excessive potassium excretion. Clinicians must monitor potassium levels closely and provide potassium supplements when necessary.

Sodium restriction may offer another benefit: calcium excretion may be linked to sodium excretion.[4] A moderately restricted sodium diet might lower calcium concentrations in the urine, even for calcium stone formers not taking thiazide diuretics.

Other studies have shown that a diet high in animal protein may influence calcium stone formation. Such diets raise the urinary excretion of calcium and oxalate—two risk factors for calcium stones. In addition, diets high in animal protein contain large quantities of purines, which in turn raise uric acid excretion. As mentioned earlier, uric acid may form the seed for the crystallization of a calcium oxalate stone. However, researchers have yet to demonstrate that restricting dietary protein will help prevent calcium stone formation.

In summary, for a person with calcium stones who absorbs excessive amounts of calcium, calcium is restricted to the RDA level. People with calcium oxalate stones are cautioned to limit their intakes of foods high in oxalate. Those on thiazide diuretics may benefit from moderately restricted sodium intakes, and possibly potassium supplements, if potassium becomes deficient. Of course, high fluid intakes are encouraged in all cases.

Can diet be of value in treating or preventing other types of stones?

A common practice in the treatment of kidney stones has been to design diets to alter the acidity of the urine. An acid ash diet, intended to make the urine more acid than usual, centers on meat, cheese, eggs, whole grains, and some fruits. An alkaline ash diet, intended to reduce the acidity of the urine, emphasizes milk, vegetables, and most fruits. Diet can affect the acidity of the urine, it is true, but current methods used to calculate the effects of different foods on the acidity of the urine are inaccurate and difficult to use.[5] Until a better estimate of the effects of dietary components on urine acidity is available, drug therapy remains more reliable and more frequently used for this purpose.

TABLE NP23–2 **Foods High in Oxalate**

VEGETABLES

Baked beans canned in tomato sauce	Mustard greens
Beans (green, wax, or dried)	Okra
Beets	Parsley
Celery	Peppers, green
Chives	Potatoes, sweet
Collards	Rutabagas
Dandelion greens	Spinach
Eggplant	Summer squash
Escarole	Swiss chard
Kale	Watercress
Leeks	

FRUITS

Blackberries	Lemon peel
Blueberries	Lime peel
Currants, red	Orange peel
Dewberries	Raspberries
Fruit cocktail	Rhubarb
Gooseberries	Strawberries
Grapes, Concord	Tangerines

OTHER

Chocolate	Pepper (more than 1 tsp/day)
Cocoa	Soybean crackers
Cola beverages	Soybean curd (tofu)
Draft beer	Tea
Fruit cake	Tomato soup
Grits	Vegetable soup
Peanut butter	Wheat germ

Uric acid stones are commonly treated with low-purine diets to reduce uric acid concentrations in the urine. A low-purine diet restricts foods that consist of large numbers of cells loaded with DNA and RNA, notably red meats (particularly organ meats), anchovies, sardines, and meat extracts. The benefits of such a diet are unproven, but it may be beneficial to limit excessive protein intake; health care professionals recommend a diet containing no more than 120 grams of protein per day.[6] Drug therapy may be prescribed to inhibit uric acid production, thus reducing the uric acid levels and acidity of the urine.

Cystine stones form as a result of a metabolic disorder called cystinuria. In cystinuria, large amounts of the amino acid cystine (in addition to other amino acids) are excreted in the urine.

To reduce cystine in the urine, clinicians prescribe a diet restricted in the amino acid methionine, because the body makes the nonessential amino acid cystine from methionine. Drug therapy to reduce the acidity of the urine may also be beneficial.

As you can see, many connections between diet and kidney stones have been explored. Dramatic advances in the nonsurgical treatment of kidney stones have triggered a renewed interest in this area. Health care professionals will want to keep up with changes such as these to provide the best possible care for their clients.

Notes

1. B. Godwasser, J. L. Weinerth, and C. C. Carson, Calcium stone disease: An overview, *Journal of Urology* 135 (1986): 1–9.
2. Mystery of kidney stone formation is solved, *Journal of the American Dietetic Association* 85 (1985): 1493.
3. S. P. Kanig and R. L. Conn, Kidney stones: Medical management and newer options for stone removal, *Postgraduate Medicine* 78, no. 6 (1985): 38–51.
4. Kanig and Conn, 1985.
5. J. Dwyer and coauthors, Acid/alkaline ash diets: Time for assessment and change, *Journal of the American Dietetic Association* 85 (1985): 841–845.
6. B. Goldwasser, J. L. Weinerth, and C. C. Carson, Calcium stone disease: An overview, *Journal of Urology* 135 (1986): 1–9.

Appendixes

Appendix B

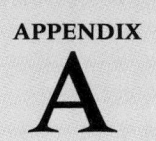

Recommended Nutrient Intakes (RDA, RNI)

Some of the U.S. recommendations for nutrient intakes appear in the RDA table on the inside front cover, left. The remaining RDA are here, in Tables A–1, A–2, and A–3. The U.S. RDA used on food labels are on the inside front cover, right. The Canadian recommendations are in Tables A–4 and A–5.

■ TABLE A–1
Estimated Safe and Adequate Daily Dietary Intakes of Additional Selected Vitamins and Minerals (United States)[a]

Age (years)	Vitamins		
	Biotin (μg)		Pantothenic Acid (mg)
Infants			
0–0.5	10		2
0.5–1	15		3
Children			
1–3	20		3
4–6	25		3–4
7–10	30		4–5
11 +	30–100		4–7
Adults	30–100		4–7

Age (years)	Trace Elements[b]				
	Chromium (μg)	Molybdenum (μg)	Copper (mg)	Manganese (mg)	Fluoride (mg)
Infants					
0–0.5	10–40	15–30	0.4–0.6	0.3–0.6	0.1–0.5
0.5–1	20–60	20–40	0.6–0.7	0.6–1.0	0.2–1.0
Children					
1–3	20–80	25–50	0.7–1.0	1.0–1.5	0.5–1.5
4–6	30–120	30–75	1.0–1.5	1.5–2.0	1.0–2.5
7–10	50–200	50–150	1.0–2.0	2.0–3.0	1.5–2.5
11 +	50–200	75–250	1.5–2.5	2.0–5.0	1.5–2.5
Adults	50–200	75–250	1.5–3.0	2.0–5.0	1.5–4.0

[a]Because there is less information on which to base allowances, these figures are not given in the main table of the RDA and are provided here in the form of ranges of recommended intakes.
[b]Because the toxic levels for many trace elements may be only several times usual intakes, the upper levels for the trace elements given in this table should not be habitually exceeded.

Reprinted with permission from *Recommended Dietary Allowances*, 10th Edition, © 1989 by the National Academy of Sciences. Published by National Academy Press, Washington D.C.

■ TABLE A−2
Estimated Minimum Requirements of Sodium, Chloride, and Potassium

Age (years)	Sodium[a] (mg)	Chloride (mg)	Potassium[b] (mg)
Infants			
0.0−0.5	120	180	500
0.5−1.0	200	300	700
Children			
1	225	350	1,000
2−5	300	500	1,400
6−9	400	600	1,600
Adolescents	500	750	2,000
Adults	500	750	2,000

[a]Sodium requirements are based on estimates of needs for growth and for replacement of obligatory losses. They cover a wide variation of physical activity patterns and climatic exposure but do not provide for large, prolonged losses from the skin through sweat.
[b]Dietary potassium may benefit the prevention and treatment of hypertension and recommendations to include many servings of fruits and vegetables would raise potassium intakes to about 3500 mg/day.

Reprinted with permission from *Recommended Dietary Allowances*, 10th Edition, © 1989 by the National Academy of Sciences. Published by National Academy Press, Washington, D.C.

■ TABLE A–3
Median Heights and Weights and Recommended Energy Intakes (United States)

Age	Weight		Height		Average Energy Allowance			
(years)	(kg)	(lb)	(cm)	(inches)	REE[a] (kcal/day)	Multiples of REE[b]	kcal per kg	kcal per day[c]
Infants								
0.0–0.5	6	13	60	24	320		108	650
0.5–1.0	9	20	71	28	500		98	850
Children								
1–3	13	29	90	35	740		102	1,300
4–6	20	44	112	44	950		90	1,800
7–10	28	62	132	52	1,130		70	2,000
Males								
11–14	45	99	157	62	1,440	1.70	55	2,500
15–18	66	145	176	69	1,760	1.67	45	3,000
19–24	72	160	177	70	1,780	1.67	40	2,900
25–50	79	174	176	70	1,800	1.60	37	2,900
51 +	77	170	173	68	1,530	1.50	30	2,300
Females								
11–14	46	101	157	62	1,310	1.67	47	2,200
15–18	55	120	163	64	1,370	1.60	40	2,200
19–24	58	128	164	65	1,350	1.60	38	2,200
25–50	63	138	163	64	1,380	1.55	36	2,200
51 +	65	143	160	63	1,280	1.50	30	1,900
Pregnant (2nd and 3rd trimesters)								+300
Lactating								+500

[a]REE (resting energy expenditure) represents the energy expended by a person at rest under normal conditions.
[b]Recommended energy allowances assume light to moderate activity and were calculated by multiplying the REE by an activity factor.
[c]Average energy allowances have been rounded.

Reprinted with permission from *Recommended Dietary Allowances*, 10th Edition, © 1989 by the National Academy of Sciences. Published by National Academy Press, Washington, D.C.

■ TABLE A–4
Recommended Nutrient Intakes for Canadians, 1990

Age	Sex	Weight (kg)	Protein (g/day)[a]	Fat-Soluble Vitamins		
				Vitamin A (RE/day)[b]	Vitamin D (μg/day)[c]	Vitamin E (mg/day)[d]
Months						
0–4	Both	6.0	12[b]	400	10	3
5–12	Both	9.0	12	400	10	3
Years						
1	Both	11	13	400	10	3
2–3	Both	14	16	400	5	4
4–6	Both	18	19	500	5	5
7–9	M	25	26	700	2.5	7
	F	25	26	700	2.5	6
10–12	M	34	34	800	2.5	8
	F	36	36	800	2.5	7
13–15	M	50	49	900	2.5	9
	F	48	46	800	2.5	7
16–18	M	62	58	1,000	2.5	10
	F	53	47	800	2.5	7
19–24	M	71	61	1,000	2.5	10
	F	58	50	800	2.5	7
25–49	M	74	64	1,000	2.5	9
	F	59	51	800	2.5	6
50–74	M	73	63	1,000	5	7
	F	63	54	800	5	6
75+	M	69	59	1,000	5	6
	F	64	55	800	5	5
Pregnancy (additional amount needed)						
1st trimester			5	0	2.5	2
2nd trimester			15	0	2.5	2
3rd trimester			24	0	2.5	2
Lactation (additional amount needed)			20	400	2.5	3

Recommended intakes of energy and of certain nutrients are not listed in this table because of the nature of the variables upon which they are based. The figures for energy are estimates of average requirements for expected patterns of activity (see Table A–5). For nutrients not shown, the following amounts are recommended based on at least 2,000 kcal/day and body weights as given: thiamin, 0.4 mg/1,000 kcal (0.48/5,000 kJ); riboflavin, 0.5 mg/1,000 kcal (0.6 mg/5,000 kJ); niacin, 7.2 NE/1,000 kcal (8.6 NE/5,000 kJ); vitamin B_6, 15 μg, as pyridoxine, per gram of protein. Recommended intakes during periods of growth are taken as appropriate for individuals representative of the midpoint in each age group. All recommended intakes are designed to cover individual variations in essentially all of a healthy population subsisting upon a variety of common foods available in Canada.

Source: Health and Welfare Canada, *Nutrition Recommendations: The Report of the Scientific Review Committee,* (Ottawa: Canadian Government Publishing Centre, 1990), Table 20, p. 204.

Water-Soluble Vitamins			Minerals					
Vitamin C (mg/day)[e]	Folate (μg/day)	Vitamin B_{12} (μg/day)	Calcium (mg/day)	Phosphorus (mg/day)	Magnesium (mg/day)	Iron (mg/day)	Iodine (μg/day)	Zinc (mg/day)
20	25	0.3	250	150	20	0.3[g]	30	2[h]
20	40	0.4	400	200	32	7	40	3
20	40	0.5	500	300	40	6	55	4
20	50	0.6	550	350	50	6	65	4
25	70	0.8	600	400	65	8	85	5
25	90	1.0	700	500	100	8	110	7
25	90	1.0	700	500	100	8	95	7
25	120	1.0	900	700	130	8	125	9
25	130	1.0	1,100	800	135	8	110	9
30	175	1.0	1,100	900	185	10	160	12
30	170	1.0	1,000	850	180	13	160	9
40	220	1.0	900	1,000	230	10	160	12
30	190	1.0	700	850	200	12	160	9
40	220	1.0	800	1,000	240	9	160	12
30	180	1.0	700	850	200	13	160	9
40	230	1.0	800	1,000	250	9	160	12
30	185	1.0	700	850	200	13[i]	160	9
40	230	1.0	800	1,000	250	9	160	12
30	195	1.0	800	850	210	8	160	9
40	215	1.0	800	1,000	230	9	160	12
30	200	1.0	800	850	210	8	160	9
0	200	0.2	500	200	15	0	25	6
10	200	0.2	500	200	45	5	25	6
10	200	0.2	500	200	45	10	25	6
25	100	0.2	500	200	65	0	50	6

[a]The primary units are expressed per kilogram of body weight. The figures shown here are examples.
[b]One retinol equivalent (RE) corresponds to the biological activity of 1 μg of retinol, 6 μg of beta-carotene, or 12 μg of other carotenes.
[c]Expressed as cholecalciferol or ergocalciferol.
[d]Expressed as δ-α-tocopherol equivalents, relative to which β- and γ-tocopherol and α-tocotrienol have activities of 0.5, 0.1, and 0.3, respectively.
[e]Cigarette smokers should increase intake by 50 percent.
[f]The assumption is made that the protein is from breast milk or is of the same biological value as that of breast milk, and that between 3 and 9 months, adjustment for the quality of the protein is made.
[g]Based on the assumption that breast milk is the source of iron.
[h]Based on the assumption that breast milk is the source of zinc.
[i]After menopause, the recommended intake is 8 mg/day.

■ TABLE A–5
Average Energy Requirements for Canadians

Age	Sex	Average Height (cm)	Average Weight (kg)	Requirements[a]					
				(kcal/kg)[b]	(MJ/kg)[b]	(kcal/day)	(MJ/day)	(kcal/cm)	(MJ/cm)
Months									
0–2	Both	55	4.5	120–100	0.50–0.42	500	2.0	9	0.04
3–5	Both	63	7.0	100–95	0.42–0.40	700	2.8	11	0.05
6–8	Both	69	8.5	95–97	0.40–0.41	800	3.4	11.5	0.05
9–11	Both	73	9.5	97–99	0.41	950	3.8	12.5	0.05
Years									
1	Both	82	11	101	0.42	1,100	4.8	13.5	0.06
2–3	Both	95	14	94	0.39	1,300	5.6	13.5	0.06
4–6	Both	107	18	100	0.42	1,800	7.6	17	0.07
7–9	M	126	25	88	0.37	2,200	9.2	17.5	0.07
	F	125	25	76	0.32	1,900	8.0	15	0.06
10–12	M	141	34	73	0.30	2,500	10.4	17.5	0.07
	F	143	36	61	0.25	2,200	9.2	15.5	0.06
13–15	M	159	50	57	0.24	2,800	12.0	17.5	0.07
	F	157	48	46	0.19	2,200	9.2	14	0.06
16–18	M	172	62	51	0.21	3,200	13.2	18.5	0.08
	F	160	53	40	0.17	2,100	8.8	13	0.05
19–24	M	175	71	42	0.18	3,000	12.6		
	F	160	58	36	0.15	2,100	8.8		
25–49	M	172	74	36	0.15	2,700	11.3		
	F	160	59	32	0.13	1,900	8.0		
50–74	M	170	73	31	0.13	2,300	9.7		
	F	158	63	29	0.12	1,800	7.6		
75+	M	168	69	29	0.12	2,000	8.4		
	F	155	64	23	0.10	1,500	6.3		

[a]Requirements can be expected to vary within a range of ±30%.
[b]First and last figures are averages at the beginning and at the end of the 3-month period.

Source: Health and Welfare Canada, *Nutrition Recommendations: The Report of the Scientific Review Committee,* (Ottawa: Canadian Government Publishing Centre, 1990), Tables 5 and 6, pp. 25, 27.

Nutrition Assessment: Supplemental Information

Contents

Chapter 10 describes the nutrition assessment techniques health care professionals commonly use to determine clients' nutrition status. From this assessment, they identify clients' nutrition needs and develop care plans for meeting those needs. This Appendix provides additional details and alternative methods of assessing nutrition status to support a complete nutrition assessment.

■ *Drug History: Nutrition and Drug Interactions*

Chapters 17 through 23 include a series of tables listing drugs used in the treatment of the specific diseases being discussed. Those tables provide information on how the drugs are administered with respect to timing of food intake and on common side effects that may influence nutrition status. Table B-1 (A and B) presents an expanded summary of those drug tables for your reference.

■ TABLE B–1A
Guide to Table B–1B*

Drug Name	Drug Classification in Table B–1B
Acebutolol	Antihypertensive Agents
Acetaminophen	Analgesic Agents
Acetohexamide	Antidiabetic Agents
Acetylsalicylic acid	Analgesic Agents
Acyclovir	Anti-Infective Agents
Adrenocorticosteroids	Antineoplastic Agents
Aluminum hydroxide	Antacids
Amiloride HCl	Diuretics
Amphotericin B	Anti-Infective Agents
Ampicillin	Anti-Infective Agents
Asparaginase	Antineoplastic Agents
Atenolol	Antihypertensive Agents
Azathioprine	Immunosuppressants
Azidothymidine (AZT)	Anti-Infective Agents
Belladonna	Antidiarrheal Agents
Bisacodyl	Laxatives
Bleomycin	Antineoplastic Agents
Buspirone HCl	Antianxiety Agents
Busulfan	Antineoplastic Agents
Calcium carbonate	Antacids
Captopril	Antihypertensive Agents
Carmustine	Antineoplastic Agents
Castor oil	Laxatives
Chloramphenicol	Anti-Infective Agents
Chlorothiazide	Diuretics
Chlorpromazine HCl	Antipsychotic Agents
Chlorpropamide	Antidiabetic Agents
Chlorthalidone	Diuretics
Cholestyramine	Antilipemic Agents
Cimetidine	Antiulcer Agents
Cisplatin	Antineoplastic Agents
Clofibrate	Antilipemic Agents
Clonidine HCl	Antihypertensive Agents
Clotrimazole	Anti-Infective Agents
Colchicine	Miscellaneous
Colestipol	Antilipemic Agents
Cyclophosphamide	Antineoplastic Agents
Cyclosporine	Immunosuppressants
Dactinomycin	Antineoplastic Agents
Deserpidine/methyclothiazide	Antihypertensive Agents
Dicumarol	Anticoagulants
Digitalis	Antihypertensive Agents
Digitoxin	Antihypertensive Agents
Digoxin	Antihypertensive Agents
Dihydroxyaluminum sodium carbonate	Antacids
Diphenoxylate	Antidiarrheal Agents
Doxepin HCl	Antidepressant Agents—Other
Doxorubicin	Antineoplastic Agents
Enalapril maleate	Antihypertensive Agents
Erythromycin	Anti-Infective Agents
Estrogen	Antineoplastic Agents
Ethambutol HCl	Anti-Infective Agents
Famotidine	Antiulcer Agents
Fluconazole	Anti-Infective Agents
Fluorouracil	Antineoplastic Agents

■ TABLE B–1A
Guide to Table B–1B* (continued)

Drug Name	Drug Classification in Table B–1B
Ganciclovir	Anti-Infective Agents
Gemfibrozil	Antilipemic Agents
Glipizide	Antidiabetic Agents
Glyburide	Antidiabetic Agents
Guanethidine sulfate	Antihypertensive Agents
Guanfacine HCl	Antihypertensive Agents
Hydralazine HCl	Antihypertensive Agents
Hydrochlorothiazide	Diuretics
Hydroxyurea	Antineoplastic Agents
Ibuprofen	Analgesic Agents
Indapamide	Diuretics
Isocarboxide	Antidepressant Agents—MAO Inhibitors
Isoniazid (INH)	Anti-Infective Agents
Kaolin	Antidiarrheal Agents
Ketoconazole	Anti-Infective Agents
Labetalol HCl	Antihypertensive Agents
Lactulose	Laxatives
Levodopa	Miscellaneous
Lisinopril	Antihypertensive Agents
Lithium carbonate	Miscellaneous
Loperamide	Antidiarrheal Agents
Lovastatin	Antilipemic Agents
Loxapine HCl	Antipsychotic Agents
Magaldrate	Antacids
Magnesium hydroxide	Antacids
Meprobamate	Antianxiety Agents
Mercaptopurine	Antineoplastic Agents
Methotrexate	Antineoplastic Agents
Methyldopa	Antihypertensive Agents
Metoprolol tartrate	Antihypertensive Agents
Metronidazole	Anti-Infective Agents
Mineral oil	Laxatives
Minoxidil	Antihypertensive Agents
Mithramycin	Antineoplastic Agents
Nadolol	Antihypertensive Agents
Neomycin	Anti-Infective Agents
Nicotinic acid	Antilipemic Agents
Nifedipine	Antihypertensive Agents
Nystatin	Anti-Infective Agents
Opium	Antidiarrheal Agents
Oral contraceptives	Miscellaneous; see also estrogen
Paregoric	Antidiarrheal Agents
Pectin	Antidiarrheal Agents
Penicillin	Anti-Infective Agents
Pentamidine isethionate	Anti-Infective Agents
Perphenazine	Antipsychotic Agents
Phenelzine sulfate	Antidepressant Agents—MAO Inhibitors
Phenytoin	Anticonvulsants
Pindolol	Antihypertensive Agents
Prazosin HCl	Antihypertensive Agents
Prednisone	Immunosuppressants
Probucol	Antilipemic Agents
Procarbazine	Antineoplastic Agents
Propranolol HCl	Antihypertensive Agents
Pyrimethamine	Anti-Infective Agents

(continued)

B

■ TABLE B–1A
Guide to Table B–1B*   (continued)

Drug Name	Drug Classification in Table B–1B
Ranitidine	Antiulcer Agents
Rauwolfia serpentina	Antihypertensive Agents
Rifampin	Anti-Infective Agents
Sodium bicarbonate	Antacids
Spironolactone	Diuretics
Sucralfate	Antiulcer Agents
Sulfadiazine	Anti-Infective Agents
Sulfasalazine	Anti-Infective Agents
Terazosin HCl	Antihypertensive Agents
Tetracycline	Anti-Infective Agents
Thioridazine HCl	Antipsychotic Agents
Timolol maleate	Antihypertensive Agents
Tolazamide	Antidiabetic Agents
Tolbutamide	Antidiabetic Agents
Tranylcypromine sulfate	Antidepressant Agents—MAO Inhibitors
Trazodone HCl	Antidepressant Agents—Other
Triamterene	Diuretics
Trimethoprim	Anti-Infective Agents
Valproic acid	Anticonvulsants
Vinblastine	Antineoplastic Agents
Vincristine	Antineoplastic Agents
Warfarin	Anticoagulants

*This table provides an alphabetical listing of the drugs described in Table B–1B and shows where each drug can be found.
Note: The drug classifications shown here have been adapted for use in this text and are not always the formal drug classification. For example, lithium carbonate listed here as "Miscellaneous" is formally a "Miscellaneous Psychotherapeutic Agent." Also, many drugs actually have more than one classification. For example, corticosteroid hormones can be considered to be both "Immunosuppressants" and "Antineoplastic Agents." Only one classification is shown in this table for each drug.

■ TABLE B–1B
Administration and Common Nutrition-Related Side Effects of Selected Drugs

Drug Classification and Name	Administration	Common Side Effects That May Influence Nutrition Status
Analgesic Agents		
Acetaminophen	Give with food to decrease GI distress.	Side effects rarely occur.
Acetylsalicylic acid	Give with water, or with food if GI distress occurs with use.	Stomach upset, vomiting, nausea, GI bleeding, irritation of ulcers. May induce iron deficiency by causing GI bleeding. May enhance effects of anticlotting and antidiabetic medicine. Severe allergic reaction in some people.
Ibuprofen	Give on empty stomach, or with food or milk if GI distress occurs with use.	Nausea, stomach pain, heartburn, anorexia, dry mouth, diarrhea, vomiting, indigestion, constipation, abdominal cramps or pain, bloating, gas. May induce iron deficiency by causing GI bleeding.

■ TABLE B–1B
Administration and Common Nutrition-Related Side Effects of Selected Drugs   (continued)

Drug Classification and Name	Administration	Common Side Effects That May Influence Nutrition Status
Antacids		
Aluminum hydroxide	Give 1 to 3 hr after meals.	Constipation, cramps, bloating, nausea, vomiting, anorexia, chalky taste. Inactivates thiamin; decreases absorption of vitamin A, phosphorous, and calcium.
Calcium carbonate	Give 1 to 3 hr after meals. Give iron supplements 1 to 2 hr before or after use. Do not take with large amounts of dairy products.	Belching, nausea, constipation, steatorrhea, chalky taste. May decrease iron absorption.
Dihydroxyaluminum sodium carbonate	Give 1 to 3 hr after meals.	Constipation, diarrhea, anorexia, weight loss.
Magaldrate	Give on empty stomach.	Chalky taste. May decrease absorption of fat-soluble vitamins, especially vitamin A.
Magnesium hydroxide	Give 1 hr after meals.	Constipation. May decrease absorption of vitamin A, phosphorus, and calcium; inactivates thiamin.
Sodium bicarbonate	Give 1 to 3 hr after meals.	Belching, gas, bloating, weight gain. Decreases iron absorption.
Antianxiety Agents		
Buspirone HCl	Give with food.	Nausea, vomiting, diarrhea, dry mouth.
Meprobamate	Give with food to decrease GI distress.	Anorexia, nausea, vomiting.
Anticoagulant Agents		
Dicumarol	Avoid excessive amounts of foods containing vitamin K (see p. 263).	Anorexia, nausea, vomiting, diarrhea, abdominal pain, mouth ulcers.
Warfarin	Avoid excessive amounts of foods containing vitamin K (see p. 263).	Nausea, vomiting, diarrhea, abdominal pain.
Anticonvulsants		
Phenytoin	Give with food to decrease GI distress. Tube feedings may reduce drug absorption and should be stopped for 2 hours before and after giving the drug, if possible.	Nausea, vomiting, swollen gums. May cause folate and vitamin B_{12} deficiencies.
Valproic acid	Give with food to decrease GI distress. Do not mix liquid form with carbonated beverages.	Anorexia, nausea, vomiting, abdominal pain.
Antidepressant Agents—MAO Inhibitors		
Isocarboxide	Avoid foods containing tyramine and tryptophan. Avoid alcohol and caffeine.	Anorexia, constipation.
Phenelzine sulfate	Avoid foods containing tyramine and tryptophan. Avoid alcohol and caffeine.	Anorexia, constipation.
Tranylcypromide sulfate	Avoid foods containing tyramine and tryptophan. Avoid alcohol and caffeine.	Anorexia.
Antidepressant Agents—Other		
Doxepin HCl	Dilute oral concentrate with water, milk, or juice. Do not mix with carbonated beverages. Avoid alcohol and caffeine.	Dry mouth, constipation.
Trazodone HCl	Give with food.	Nausea, dry mouth, constipation.

(continued)

B

■ TABLE B–1B
Administration and Common Nutrition-Related Side Effects of Selected Drugs (continued)

B

Drug Classification and Name	Administration	Common Side Effects That May Influence Nutrition Status
Antidiabetic Agents		
Acetohexamide	Give with meals. Avoid alcohol.	Diarrhea, nausea, vomiting, heartburn, metallic taste. May induce anemia.
Chlorpropamide	Give with breakfast. Avoid alcohol.	Dyspepsia, nausea, vomiting, metallic taste, anorexia. Water intoxication, edema.
Glipizide	Give 30 min before breakfast. Limit alcohol.	GI distress, nausea, diarrhea, constipation, heartburn, altered taste perceptions.
Glyburide	Give before breakfast. Limit alcohol.	GI distress, nausea, diarrhea, constipation, heartburn.
Tolazamide	Give in morning or divided during day with meals. Avoid alcohol.	Diarrhea, GI distress, nausea, vomiting, dyspepsia, heartburn, altered taste perceptions, anorexia.
Tolbutamide	(same as above)	(same as above)
Antidiarrheal Agents		
Diphenoxylate	May give with food.	Nausea, vomiting, bloating, anorexia, dry mouth, sore or swollen gums.
Kaolin, pectin	Mix at room temperature with milk or juice.	Constipation, dry mouth, altered taste perception.
Loperamide		Abdominal pain, constipation, bloating, dry mouth, vomiting, nausea.
Opium, belladonna, and paregoric	May give with food.	Nausea, vomiting, constipation. Sedation.
Antihypertensive Agents		
Acebutolol	Give without regard to meals.	Constipation, gas, abdominal pain. May mask the signs of hypoglycemia. May induce electrolyte imbalance and anemias.
Atenolol	Give without regard to meals.	Dry mouth, diarrhea, nausea. May mask signs of hypoglycemia.
Atenolol and chlorothalidone	Give on empty stomach same time each day.	Anorexia, diarrhea, nausea, vomiting, GI irritation, constipation. May induce hypokalemia, anemia.
Captopril	Give on empty stomach 1 hr before meals.	Altered taste perception, weight loss, sore mouth. May induce hypokalemia, anemias.
Clonidine HCl		Dry mouth, weight gain, nausea, vomiting, constipation. May induce edema.
Deserpidine/methyclothiazide	Give with food 6 or more hr before bedtime. Avoid natural licorice.	Dry mouth, weight gain, anorexia, nausea, vomiting, diarrhea, cramps. May inhibit glucose absorption.
Digitalis, digitoxin, digoxin	Give with water ½ hr before or 2 hr after food. Avoid natural licorice.	Nausea, vomiting.
Enalapril maleate	May give with food.	Altered taste perceptions. Diarrhea, nausea, vomiting, abdominal pain.

■ TABLE B–1B
Administration and Common Nutrition-Related Side Effects of Selected Drugs (continued)

Drug Classification and Name	Administration	Common Side Effects That May Influence Nutrition Status
Antihypertensive Agents (continued)		
Guanethidine sulfate	Give at same time each day. Avoid natural licorice.	Dry mouth, weight gain, diarrhea, nausea. May induce edema.
Guanfacine HCl		Constipation, nausea, vomiting, stomach cramps.
Hydralazine HCl	Give with food at the same time each day. Avoid natural licorice.	Anorexia, GI distress, constipation.
Labetalol HCl	Give with food.	Altered taste perception, nausea, vomiting, indigestion. May mask signs of hypoglycemia.
Lisinopril		Diarrhea, vomiting.
Methyldopa	Avoid natural licorice.	Dry mouth, weight gain, diarrhea, nausea. May induce edema.
Metoprolol tartrate	Give with food.	Dry mouth, diarrhea, GI pain, gas, constipation, heartburn. May mask the signs of hypoglycemia.
Minoxidil	Give at same time each day.	May induce edema.
Nadolol	Give without regard to meals. Avoid natural licorice.	Dry mouth, constipation, GI distress, nausea, gas. May mask the signs of hypoglycemia.
Nifedipine	Give with food or milk.	Altered taste perception, nausea, diarrhea, constipation, cramps, gas. May induce edema.
Pindolol	Give without regard to meals.	Diarrhea, vomiting. May mask the signs of hypoglycemia. May alter glucose tolerance. May induce edema.
Prazosin HCl		Dry mouth, nausea, diarrhea, constipation, GI distress. May induce edema.
Propranolol HCl	Give with food. Avoid natural licorice.	Dry mouth, constipation, GI distress, nausea. May mask the signs of hypoglycemia.
Rauwolfia serpentina	Give with food or milk to reduce GI irritation.	Anorexia, weight gain, dry mouth, diarrhea, nausea, vomiting, raises GI motility and gastric secretion. May lower glucose tolerance.
Terazosin HCl	Avoid salt substitutes. Give without regard to meals at the same time each day.	May alter serum glucose. Sore throat. Nausea. May induce edema.
Timolol maleate	Give with food at the same time each day.	Weight loss, nausea. May mask signs of hypoglycemia. May induce edema.
Anti-Infective Agents		
Acyclovir	Give parenterally or orally with food.	Nausea, diarrhea, vomiting, anorexia.
Amphotericin B	Give parenterally.	Nausea, vomiting, fever, anemia, kidney dysfunction.
Ampicillin	Give with water 1 hr before or 2 hr after meals; do not give with fruit juice, beer, wine.	Nausea, vomiting, diarrhea, steatorrhea, anemia, inflammation of the mouth and tongue; stomatitis, altered taste perceptions, hypokalemia.

B

■ TABLE B–1B
Administration and Common Nutrition-Related Side Effects of Selected Drugs   (continued)

Drug Classification and Name	Administration	Common Side Effects That May Influence Nutrition Status
Anti-Infective Agents (continued)		
Azidothymidine (AZT)		Anorexia, nausea, vomiting, diarrhea, constipation, altered taste perceptions, mouth ulcers, edema of tongue and lips, abdominal pain, anemia.
Chloramphenicol	Give with water 1 hr before or 2 hr after meals.	Diarrhea, nausea, vomiting, irritation of mouth or tongue. May enhance effects of antidiabetic medicine. May raise requirements of riboflavin, vitamin B_6, and vitamin B_{12}.
Clotrimazole	Dissolve slowly in mouth and swallow saliva.	Nausea, vomiting.
Erythromycin	Give on empty stomach 1 hr before or 2 hr after meals; if GI distress, give with meals, not milk, fruit juice, beer, or wine.	Nausea, vomiting, cramps, abdominal pain, diarrhea, inflammation of the mouth.
Ethambutol HCl		Anorexia, nausea, vomiting, abdominal pain.
Fluconazole	Give orally or parenterally.	Nausea, vomiting, diarrhea, intestinal inflammation.
Ganciclovir	Give parenterally.	Anorexia, nausea, vomiting.
Isoniazid (INH)	Give 1 hr before or 2 hr after meals; may give with food to relieve GI distress.	Anorexia, nausea, vomiting, dry mouth, diarrhea, anemia, cracked lips.
Ketoconazole	Give with food to reduce nausea and vomiting.	Nausea, vomiting, abdominal pain, diarrhea, anemia. Renal and liver dysfunction.
Metronidazole	Give with food.	Anorexia, nausea, vomiting, diarrhea, altered taste perceptions, dry mouth, constipation, stomatitis, abdominal discomfort.
Neomycin		Nausea, vomiting, diarrhea, sore mouth. Decreases absorption of fats, nitrogen, carbohydrates, folate, vitamin B_6, vitamin B_{12}, fat-soluble vitamins, calcium, and iron.
Nystatin	Give orally as directed; retain drug in mouth as long as possible.	Diarrhea, nausea, and vomiting, GI pain (occasionally).
Penicillin	Give penicillin G on an empty stomach; penicillin K with or without meals.	Nausea, vomiting, diarrhea, gas, anemia, sore mouth, altered taste perceptions, anorexia.
Pentamidine isethionate	Give parenterally or as an inhalant.	Nausea, vomiting, taste alterations. Hypoglycemia or hyperglycemia, diabetes, kidney dysfunction.
Pyrimethamine	Give with food.	Anorexia, nausea, vomiting, diarrhea, and anemia.
Rifampin	Give with water on empty stomach.	Anorexia, nausea, vomiting, cramps, diarrhea, altered taste perceptions, abdominal distress.
Sulfadiazine		Anorexia, nausea, vomiting, and diarrhea.
Sulfasalazine	Give with food or milk.	May cause anorexia, nausea, GI distress.

■ TABLE B–1B
Administration and Common Nutrition-Related Side Effects of Selected Drugs   (continued)

Drug Classification and Name	Administration	Common Side Effects That May Influence Nutrition Status
Anti-Infective Agents (continued)		
Tetracycline	Give on an empty stomach; don't give with milk or dairy products; don't give iron-containing supplements within 3 hours of tetracycline ingestion.	Anorexia, nausea, vomiting, diarrhea, altered taste perceptions, sore mouth. Decreases absorption of fat, amino acids, calcium, iron, magnesium, and zinc. Decreases bacterial synthesis of vitamin K in intestines.
Trimethoprim	Give with water on empty stomach.	Nausea, vomiting, anorexia, anemia, diarrhea, stomatitis, GI distress.
Antilipemic Agents		
Cholestyamine	Give with water or other fluids; never give dry or with carbonated beverages.	Nausea, vomiting, abdominal discomfort, gas, diarrhea, constipation, heartburn, steatorrhea, anorexia, altered taste perception. May decrease absorption of calcium, fat, vitamins A, D, K, B_{12}, folate, and glucose. Depletes iron stores.
Colestipol	(same as above)	(same as above)
Clofibrate	Give with meals.	Nausea, vomiting, abdominal discomfort, loose stools, gas, aftertaste, altered taste perception, increased appetite. May decrease absorption of glucose, iron, and vitamin B_{12}. May induce anemia.
Gemfibrozil	Give ½ hour before meals.	Nausea, vomiting, abdominal discomfort, gas, constipation. May induce anemia.
Lovastatin	Give with meals.	Diarrhea, gas, constipation, abdominal pain, heartburn, nausea, indigestion, altered taste perception.
Nicotinic acid	Give with meals.	Nausea, vomiting, abdominal discomfort, diarrhea. Flushing. Decreased glucose tolerance.
Probucol	Give with meals.	Nausea, vomiting, gas, abdominal discomfort, diarrhea, anorexia, altered taste and smell perceptions.
Antineoplastic Agents		
Adrenocorticosteroids	Give with food.	Increased appetite, GI upset. Glucose intolerance, negative nitrogen and calcium balance.
Asparaginase	Give parenterally.	Anorexia, nausea, vomiting. Pancreatitis, hepatitis, glucose intolerance.
Bleomycin	Give parenterally, intramuscularly, or subcutaneously.	Anorexia, nausea, vomiting, mouth ulcers, stomatitis, weight loss, altered taste perceptions.
Busulfan	Give with food.	Nausea, vomiting, diarrhea, cracking at corners of mouth, inflammation of the tongue, anemias, weight loss, dry mouth.

B

■ TABLE B–1B
Administration and Common Nutrition-Related Side Effects of Selected Drugs   (continued)

Drug Classification and Name	Administration	Common Side Effects That May Influence Nutrition Status
Antineoplastic Agents (continued)		
Carmustine	Give parenterally.	Anorexia, nausea, vomiting, esophagitis, diarrhea. Impaired liver function.
Cisplatin	Give parenterally.	Anorexia, nausea, vomiting, altered taste perceptions.
Cyclophosphamide	Give during or after meals.	Anorexia, nausea, vomiting, mouth ulcers, inflammation of the colon, anemia.
Dactinomycin	Give parenterally.	Anorexia, nausea, vomiting, mouth ulcers, heartburn, anemia.
Doxorubicin	Give parenterally.	Anorexia, nausea, vomiting, diarrhea, stomach pain, sore throat, mouth ulcers, mouth blindness, esophagitis.
Estrogen	Give with food at same time each day.	Anorexia, nausea, vomiting, edema, weight changes. Alters glucose tolerance.
Fluorouracil	Give parenterally. If given orally, give with water, not acidic beverages.	Anorexia, nausea, vomiting, stomatitis, diarrhea, heartburn, sore mouth, altered taste perceptions, GI bleeding, esophagitis.
Hydroxyurea	Give with food.	Anorexia, nausea, vomiting, mouth ulcers.
Mercaptopurine	Give with food.	Anorexia, nausea, vomiting, stomatitis, stomach pain, diarrhea, anemia, vitamin B_6 depletion.
Methotrexate	Give on an empty stomach; give with food to reduce gastric distess. Do not give with milk.	Anorexia, nausea, vomiting, diarrhea, GI ulcers, GI inflammation, anemia, stomatitis, steatorrhea, mouth ulcers.
Mithramycin	Give parenterally; slow infusion reduces nausea.	Anorexia, nausea, vomiting, diarrhea, inflammation of the tongue, metallic taste.
Procarbazine	Give with food. Avoid foods containing tyramine.	Anorexia, nausea, vomiting, diarrhea, constipation, anemia, sore throat, dry mouth, difficulty swallowing.
Vinblastine	Give parenterally.	Anorexia, nausea, vomiting, diarrhea, constipation, stomatitis, sore throat, reduced bowel activity, abdominal pain, bowel inflammation.
Vincristine	Give parenterally.	Anorexia, nausea, vomiting, diarrhea, constipation, abdominal pain, mouth ulcers, anemia, thirst, weight loss, altered taste perceptions.
Antipsychotic Agents		
Chlorpromazine HCl	Give with food. Dilute liquid concentrate with milk, fruit juice, or semisolid foods.	Dry mouth, constipation.
Loxapine HCl	Give with food or water. Dilute liquid concentrate with orange or grapefruit juice.	Dry mouth, constipation.
Perphenazine	Give with food. Dilute liquid concentrate with milk, fruit juice, carbonated beverages, or semisolid foods; do not dilute with colas, black coffee, tea, or grape or apple juice.	Dry mouth, constipation.

■ TABLE B–1B
Administration and Common Nutrition-Related Side Effects of Selected Drugs   (continued)

Drug Classification and Name	Administration	Common Side Effects That May Influence Nutrition Status
Antipsychotic Agents (continued)		
Thioridazine HCl	Give with food. Dilute liquid concentrate with fruit juice or water.	Dry mouth, constipation.
Antiulcer Agents		
Cimetidine	Give with meals; caffeine and alcohol reduce effectiveness.	Diarrhea. Reduced gastric secretion. May induce hyperglycemia.
Famotidine		Nausea, diarrhea, constipation, flatulence.
Ranitidine		Constipation, nausea, abdominal discomfort. (Fewer reported side effects and interactions than with cimetidine.)
Sucralfate	Give on empty stomach 1 hour before meals and at bedtime.	Constipation, diarrhea, nausea, cramps, dry mouth. Interferes with absorption of fat-soluble vitamins.
Diuretics		
Amiloride HCl and hydrochlorothiazide	Give with food at the same time each day.	Anorexia, dry mouth, appetite changes, nausea, diarrhea, GI pain, constipation.
Chlorothiazide	Give with food 6 or more hr before bedtime. Avoid natural licorice.	Nausea, vomiting, diarrhea, constipation, anorexia, dry mouth.
Chlorthalidone	Give with food 6 or more hr before bedtime. Avoid natural licorice.	Anorexia, dry mouth, GI irritation, nausea, vomiting, diarrhea, constipation.
Hydrochlorothiazide	Give with food 6 or more hr before bedtime. Avoid natural licorice.	Anorexia, dry mouth, nausea, vomiting, diarrhea, constipation. May alter insulin requirements in diabetes. May induce hypokalemia.
Indapamide	Give with food at the same time each day if GI distress.	Dry mouth, weight loss, anorexia, constipation, GI distress. May alter glucose tolerance.
Spironolactone with hydrochlorothiazide	Give with food 6 or more hr before bedtime. Avoid natural licorice.	Anorexia, cramps, diarrhea, nausea, vomiting.
Triamterene with hydrochlorothiazide	Give with food or milk 6 or more hr before bedtime.	Dry mouth, thirst, dehydration, nausea, vomiting, diarrhea, constipation. May alter glucose levels.
Immunosuppressants		
Azathioprine	Give with meals.	Nausea, vomiting, diarrhea, stomach pain, anorexia, sore throat, altered taste perceptions.
Cyclosporine	Give with water, juice, or milk. Give at same time each day.	Raises blood pressure. Nausea, vomiting, diarrhea, inflamed gums, anorexia. May induce anemia. May induce hyperglycemia.
Prednisone	Give with food or milk.	Fluid retention, stomach upset, peptic ulcers, blood glucose abnormalities, growth inhibition in children, decreased resistance to infection, weight gain. May decrease effects of insulin or antidiabetic medicine. May induce edema.

B

(continued)

■ TABLE B–1B
Administration and Common Nutrition-Related Side Effects of Selected Drugs   (continued)

Drug Classification and Name	Administration	Common Side Effects That May Influence Nutrition Status
Immunosuppressants (continued)		
Prednisone (continued)		Alters protein and carbohydrate metabolism. Decreases absorption of calcium and phosphorus.
Laxatives		
Bisacodyl	Do not give with milk or antacids.	Nausea, vomiting, abdominal cramps.
Castor oil	Give with juice or carbonated beverages to mask taste.	Nausea, abdominal cramps. May reduce absorption of fat-soluble vitamins.
Lactulose		Nausea, constipation, abdominal cramps.
Mineral oil	Give with juice or carbonated beverages to mask taste. Do not give with meals.	Nausea, abdominal cramps. May reduce absorption of fat-soluble vitamins.
Miscellaneous		
Colchicine	Give with meals to decrease GI distress.	Nausea, vomiting, diarrhea, abdominal pain.
Lithium carbonate	Give with food. Maintain consistent sodium intake daily.	Thirst, metallic taste.
Oral contraceptives	Give with food.	Nausea, edema, weight changes. May cause hyperglycemia, hypercalcemia, or folate deficiency.

Sources: *Nursing 91 Drug Handbook*, (Springhouse, PA: Springhouse Corporation, 1991) and D. E. Powers and A. O. Moore, *Food Medication Interaction*, (Phoenix, AR: Food Medication Interactions, 1991).
Note: The multitude of drugs and nutrients that interact are far too numerous to list in a nutrition textbook like this one. Indeed, whole books are available to cover the subject. The side effects shown in this table are common side effects. Other side effects can and do occur. This table provides only a sampling of interactions. More detailed texts should be consulted for the drugs you encounter in clinical practice.

■ *Growth Charts and Anthropometric Data*

Growth charts allow health care professionals to evaluate the growth and development of children from birth to 18 years of age. To evaluate growth in infants, an assessor uses charts such as the ones shown in Figures B–1A through B–6. The assessor follows these steps to plot a weight measurement on a percentile graph:

■ Select the appropriate chart based on age and gender. (When length is measured, use the chart for birth to 36 months; when height is measured, use the chart for 2 to 18 years.)
■ Locate the child's age along the horizontal axis on the bottom or top of the chart.
■ Locate the child's weight in pounds or kilograms along the vertical axis on the lower left or right side of the chart.
■ Mark the chart where the age and weight lines intersect, and read off the percentile.

To assess length, height, or head circumference, the assessor follows the same procedure using the appropriate chart.

■ FIGURE B–1A
Girls: Birth to 36 Months Physical
Growth NCHS Percentiles—Length
and Weight for Age

B

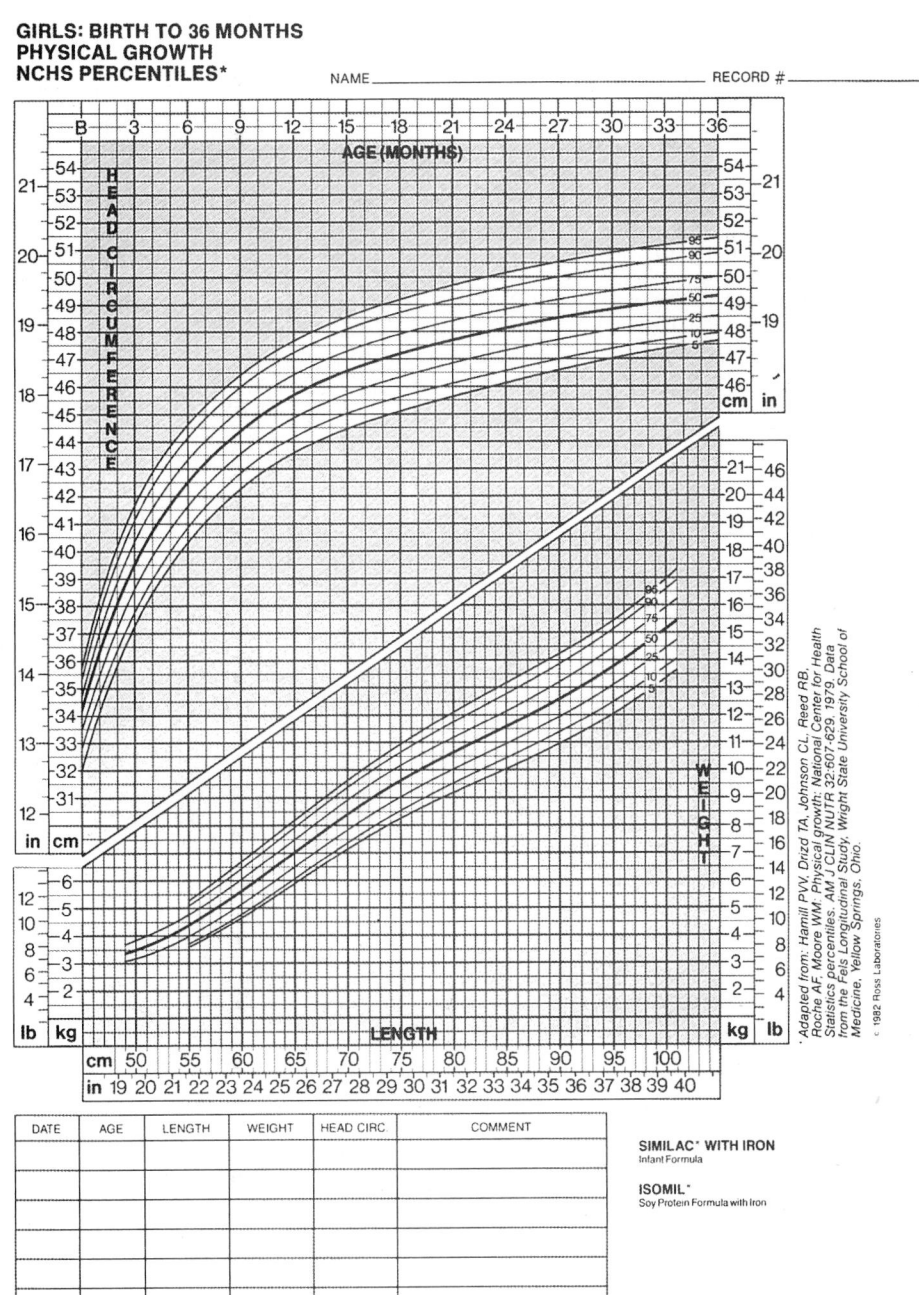

GIRLS: BIRTH TO 36 MONTHS
PHYSICAL GROWTH
NCHS PERCENTILES*

NAME_____ RECORD #_____

* Adapted from: Hamill PVV, Drizd TA, Johnson CL, Reed RB,
Roche AF, Moore WM. Physical growth: National Center for Health
Statistics percentiles. AM J CLIN NUTR 32:607-629, 1979. Data
from the Fels Longitudinal Study, Wright State University School of
Medicine, Yellow Springs, Ohio.

© 1982 Ross Laboratories

DATE	AGE	LENGTH	WEIGHT	HEAD CIRC	COMMENT

SIMILAC* WITH IRON
Infant Formula

ISOMIL*
Soy Protein Formula with Iron

Reprinted with permission
of Ross Laboratories

■ FIGURE B–1B
Girls: Birth to 36 Months Physical
Growth NCHS Percentiles—Head
Circumference for Age and Weight
for Length

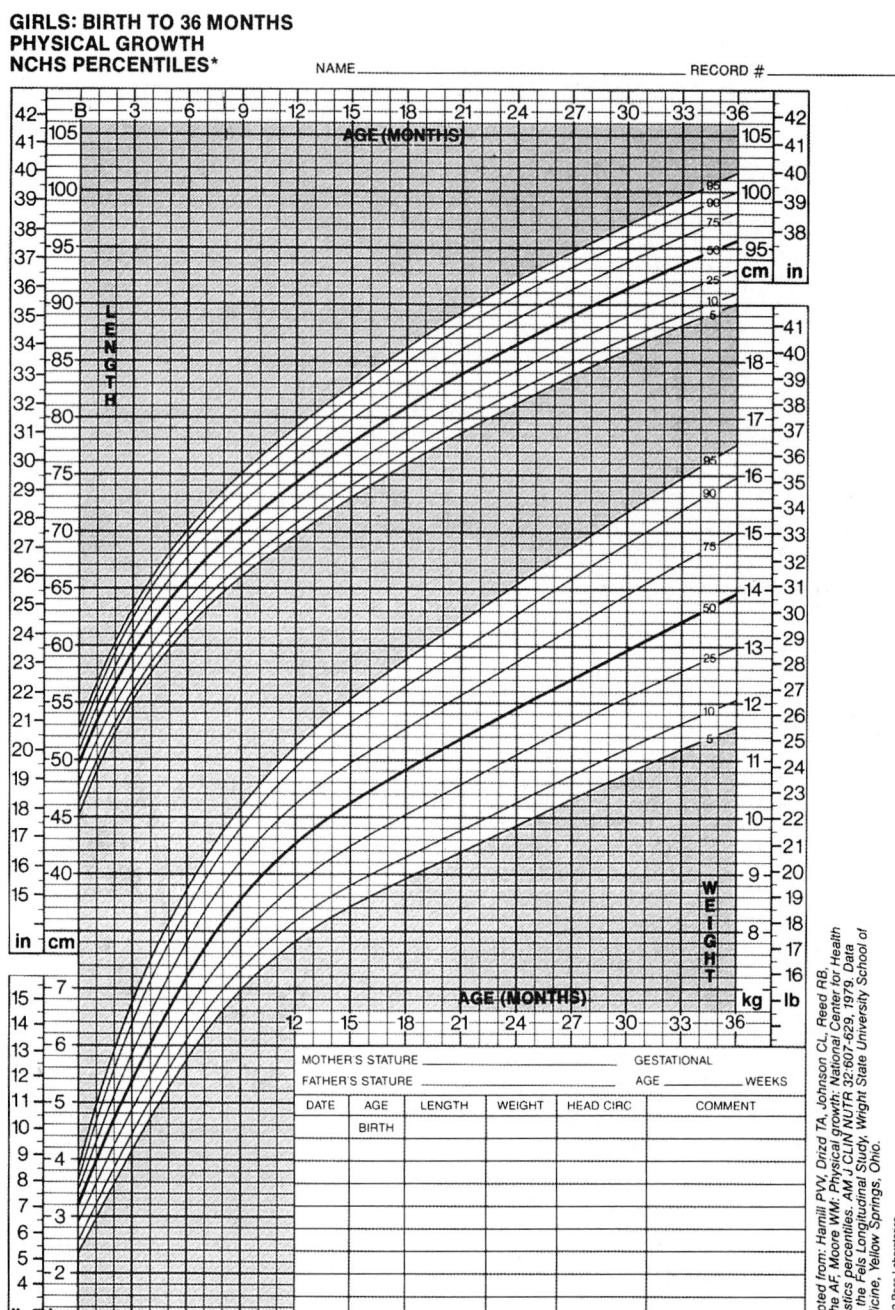

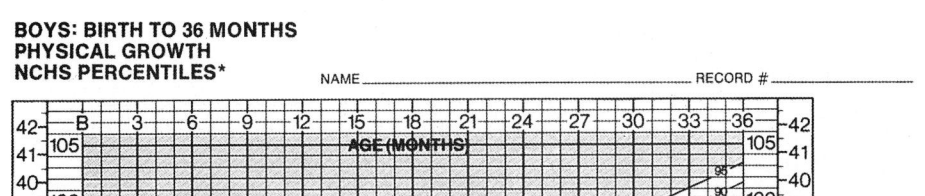

■ FIGURE B–2A
Boys: Birth to 36 Months Physical
Growth NCHS Percentiles—Length
and Weight for Age

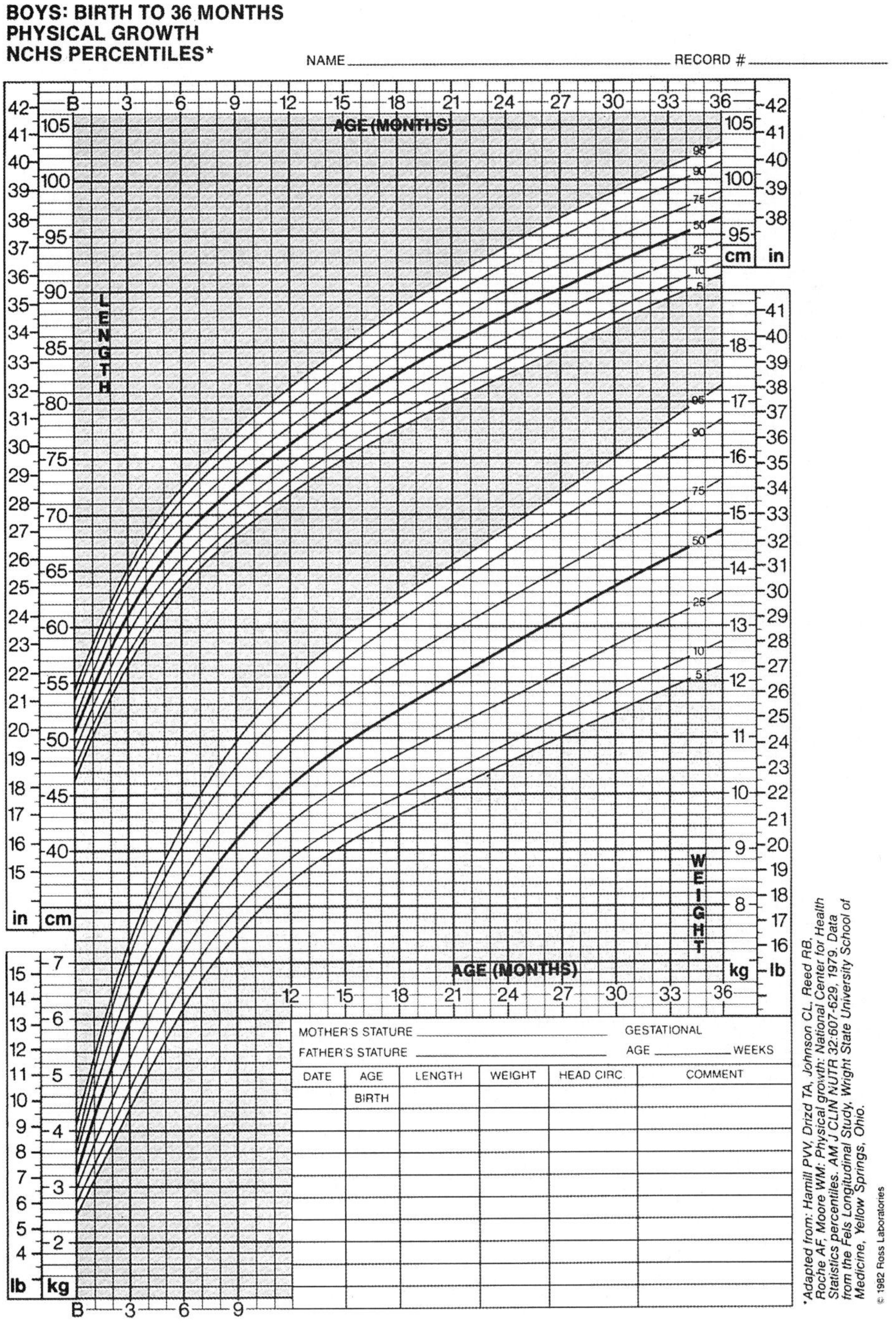

B

■ FIGURE B–2B
Boys: Birth to 36 Months Physical
Growth NCHS Percentiles—Head
Circumference for Age and Weight
for Length

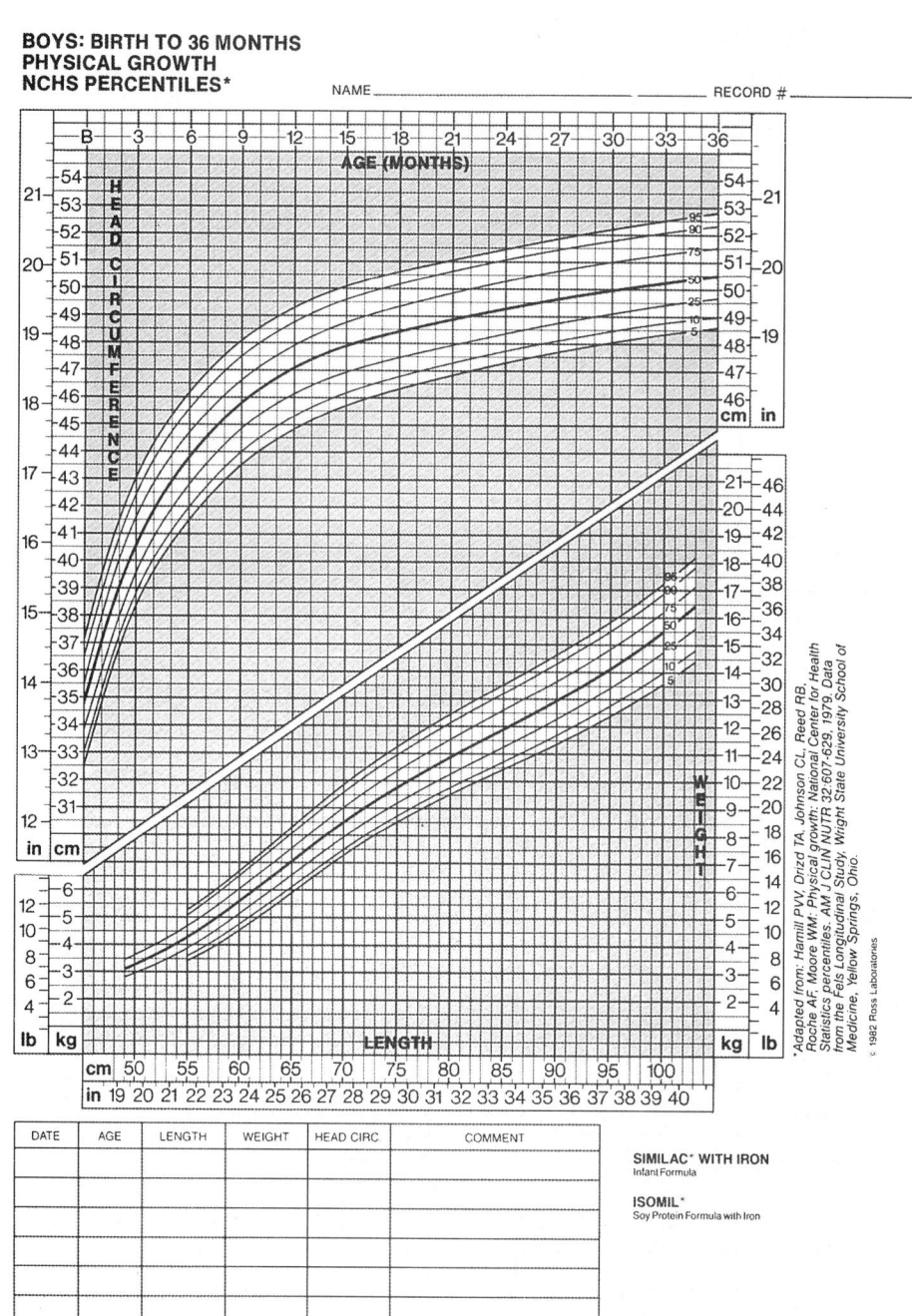

**BOYS: BIRTH TO 36 MONTHS
PHYSICAL GROWTH
NCHS PERCENTILES***

NAME _____ RECORD # _____

*Adapted from: Hamill PVV, Drizd TA, Johnson CL, Reed RB,
Roche AF, Moore WM: Physical growth: National Center for Health
Statistics percentiles. AM J CLIN NUTR 32:607-629, 1979. Data
from the Fels Longitudinal Study, Wright State University School of
Medicine, Yellow Springs, Ohio.

© 1982 Ross Laboratories

DATE	AGE	LENGTH	WEIGHT	HEAD CIRC	COMMENT

SIMILAC® WITH IRON
Infant Formula

ISOMIL®
Soy Protein Formula with Iron

Reprinted with permission
of Ross Laboratories

B

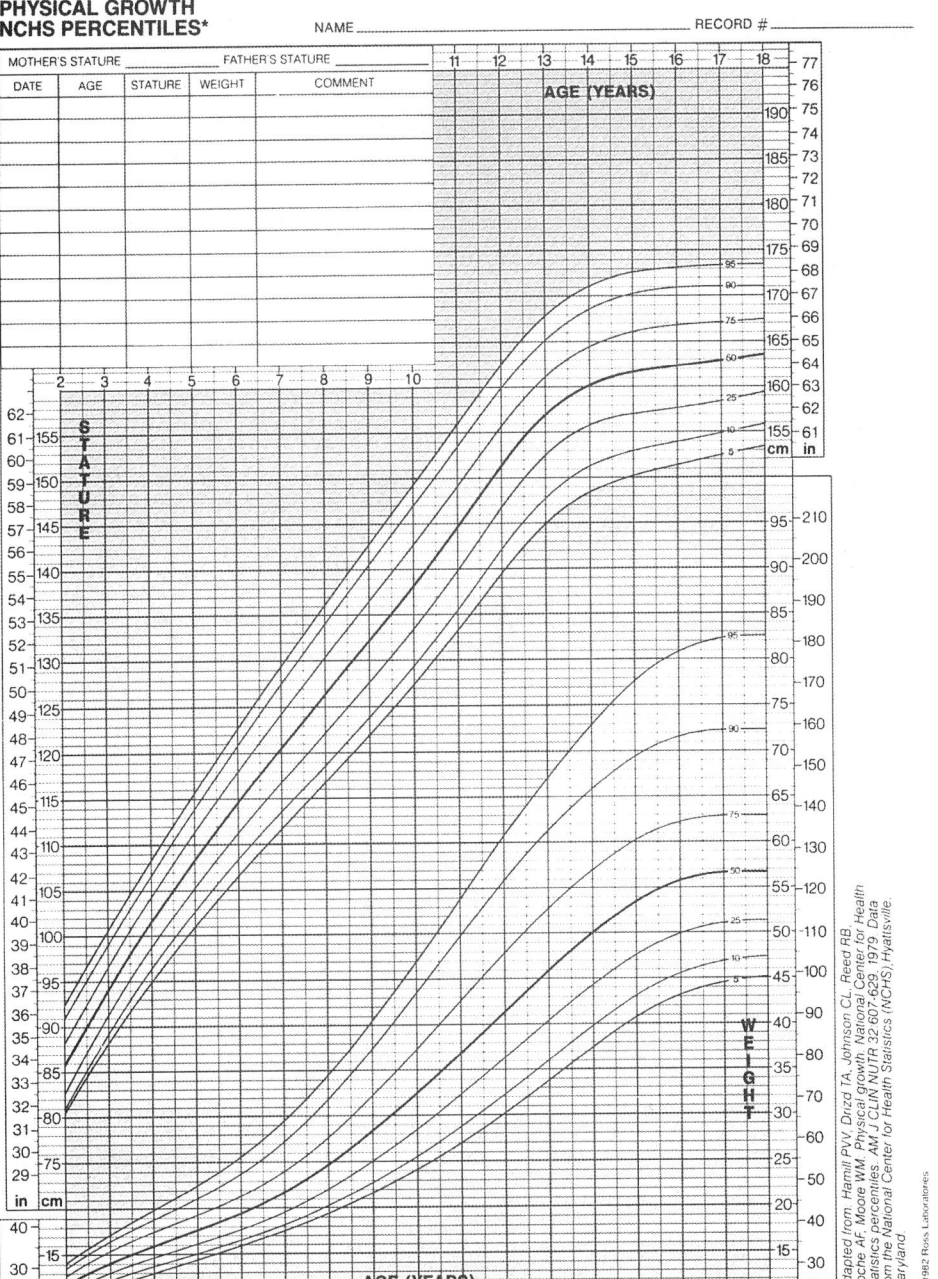

■ FIGURE B–4
Boys: 2 to 18 Years Physical Growth
NCHS Percentiles—Height and
Weight for Age

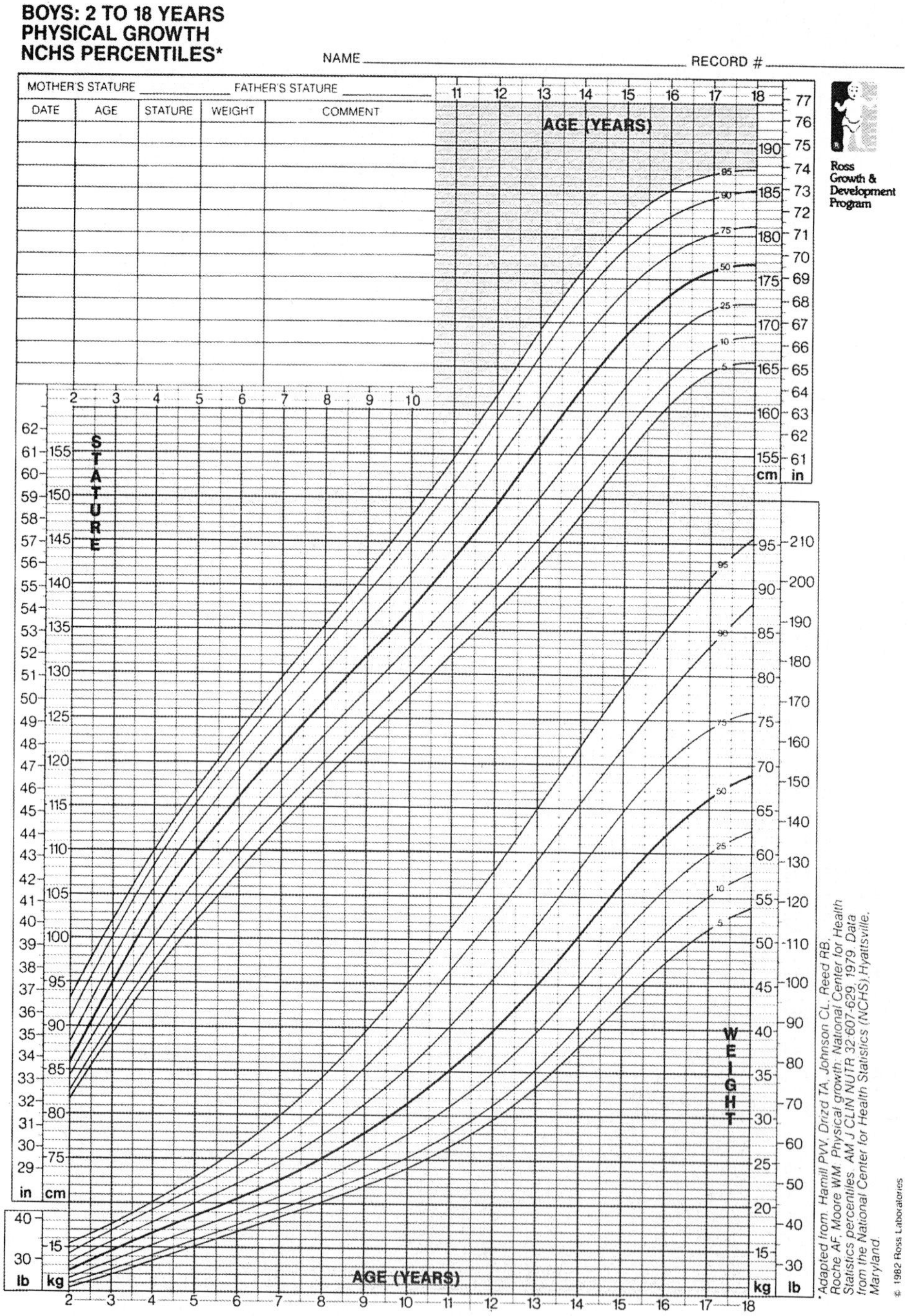

B

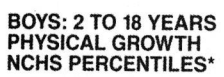

FIGURE B–5
Girls: Prepubescent Physical Growth NCHS Percentiles—Weight for Height

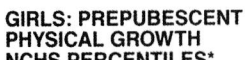

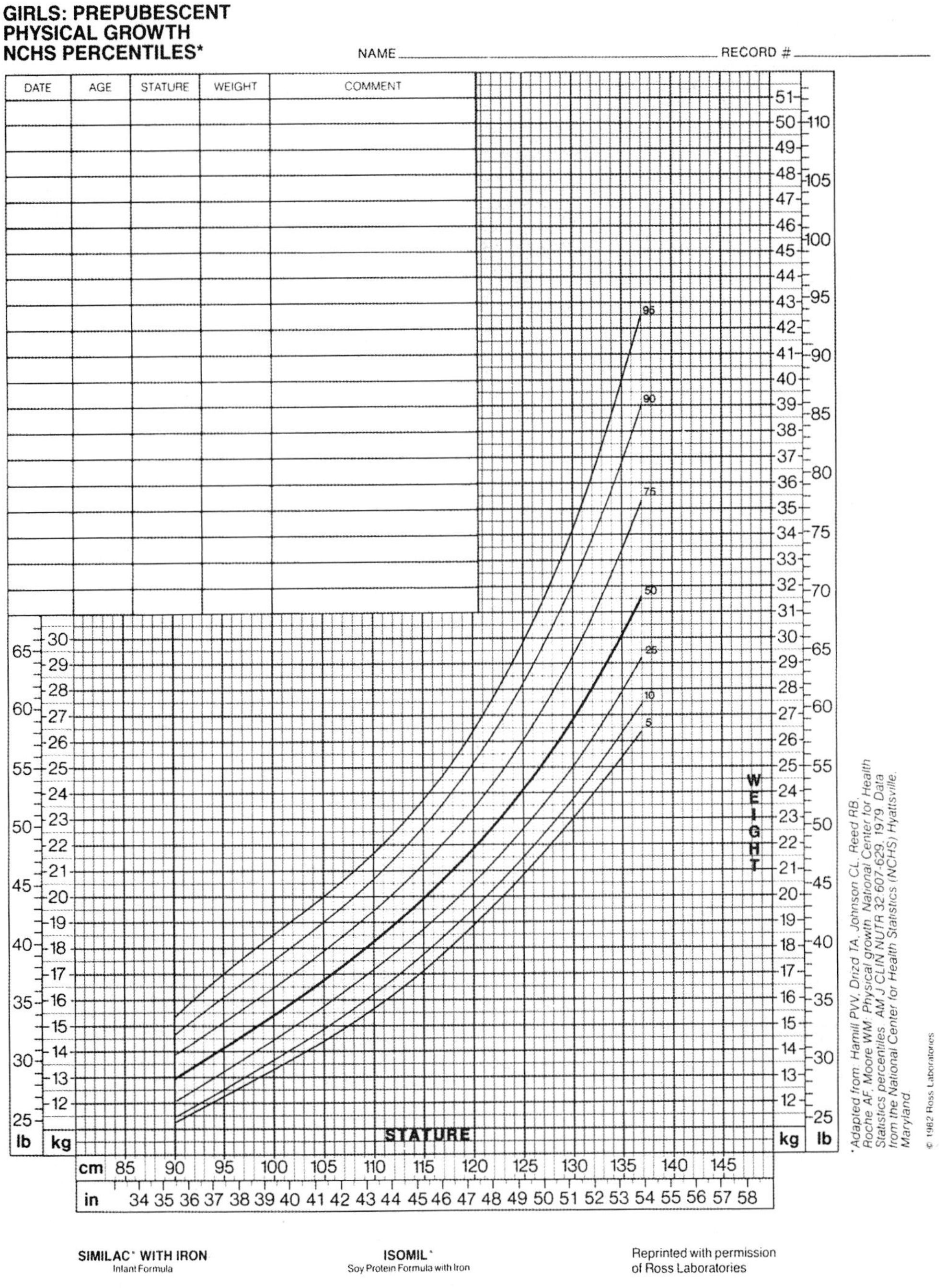
GIRLS: PREPUBESCENT
PHYSICAL GROWTH
NCHS PERCENTILES*
NAME
RECORD #
DATE
AGE
STATURE
WEIGHT
COMMENT
95
90
75
50
25
10
5
WEIGHT
STATURE
lb
kg
cm 85 90 95 100 105 110 115 120 125 130 135 140 145
in 34 35 36 37 38 39 40 41 42 43 44 45 46 47 48 49 50 51 52 53 54 55 56 57 58
*Adapted from: Hamill PVV, Drizd TA, Johnson CL, Reed RB, Roche AF, Moore WM: Physical growth: National Center for Health Statistics percentiles. AM J CLIN NUTR 32:607-629, 1979. Data from the National Center for Health Statistics (NCHS) Hyattsville, Maryland.
© 1982 Ross Laboratories
SIMILAC® WITH IRON
Infant Formula
ISOMIL®
Soy Protein Formula with Iron
Reprinted with permission of Ross Laboratories

■ FIGURE B–6
Boys: Prepubescent Physical Growth
NCHS Percentiles—Weight for Height

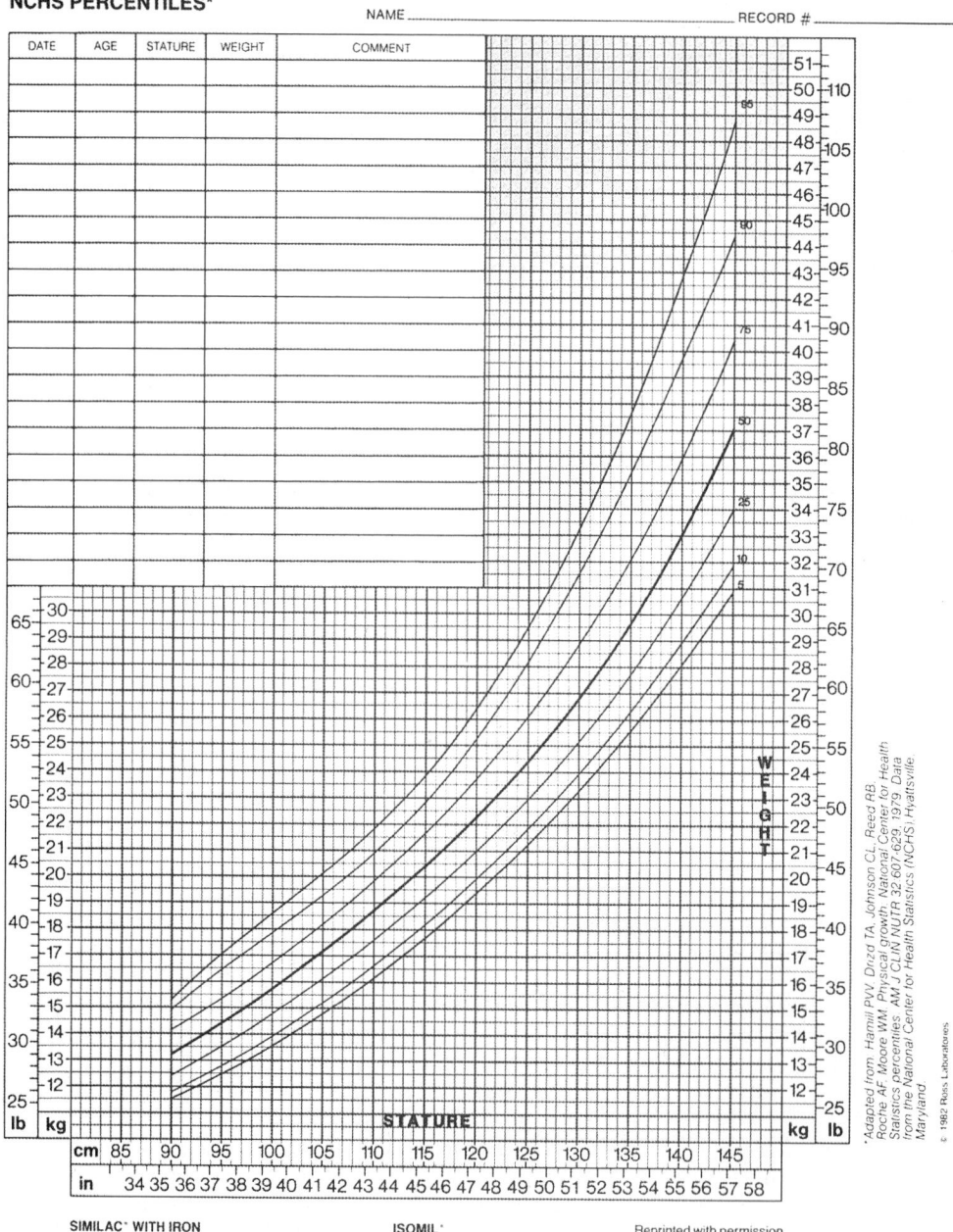

■ TABLE B–2
How to Determine Body Frame by Elbow Breadth

To make a simple approximation of frame size, do the following. Extend the arm, and bend the forearm upward at a 90° angle. Keep the fingers straight, and turn the inside of the wrist away from the body. Place the thumb and index finger on the two prominent bones on *either side* of the elbow. Measure the space between the fingers against a ruler or a tape measure.[a] Compare the measurements with the following standards.

These standards represent the elbow measurements for medium-framed men and women of various heights. Measurements smaller than those listed indicate a small frame, and larger measurements indicate a large frame.

Men		Women	
Height in 1-Inch Heels	Elbow Breadth	Height in 1-Inch Heels	Elbow Breadth
5 ft 2 inches to 5 ft 3 inches	2½ to 2⅞ inches	4 ft 10 inches to 4 ft 11 inches	2¼ to 2½ inches
5 ft 4 inches to 5 ft 7 inches	2⅝ to 2⅞ inches	5 ft 0 inches to 5 ft 3 inches	2¼ to 2½ inches
5 ft 8 inches to 5 ft 11 inches	2¾ to 3 inches	5 ft 4 inches to 5 ft 7 inches	2⅜ to 2⅝ inches
6 ft 0 inches to 6 ft 3 inches	2¾ to 3⅛ inches	5 ft 8 inches to 5 ft 11 inches	2⅜ to 2⅝ inches
6 ft 4 inches and over	2⅞ to 3¼ inches	6 ft 0 inches and over	2½ to 2¾ inches

[a]For the most accurate measurement, measure elbow breadth with a caliper.

Source: Metropolitan Life Insurance Company.

■ TABLE B–3
Frame Size from Height-Wrist Circumference Ratios (r)[a]

Frame Size	Male r Values	Female r Values
Small	>10.4	>11.0
Medium	9.6–10.4	10.1–11.0
Large	<9.6	<10.1

[a]$r = \dfrac{\text{height (cm)}}{\text{wrist circumference (cm)}^b}$.

[b]The wrist is measured where it bends (distal to the styloid process), on the right arm (see Figure E–7).

Source: Adapted from J. P. Grant, Patient selection, *Handbook of Total Parenteral Nutrition* (Philadelphia: Saunders, 1980), p. 15.

■ FIGURE E–7
Wrist Circumference

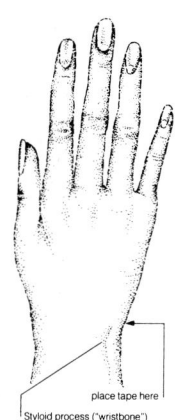

place tape here
Styloid process ("wristbone")

In adults, assessors evaluate weight for height. To use most height-weight tables, the assessor must determine the client's frame size. Tables B-2 and B-3 present two methods of determining frame size, and Figure B-7 shows how to measure the wrist when it is used to determine frame size. Another method of assessing body weight in adults is the body mass index (BMI). Figure B-8 presents a nomogram for BMI.

One of the most important anthropometric measures predictive of the birthweight of a child is the mother's amount and pattern of weight gain or loss during pregnancy. Normal weight gains related to duration of the pregnancy in weeks are shown in Figure B-9. Patterns of weight gain that deviate from these require further investigation.

Fatfold measurements assist health care professionals in evaluating the composition of body weight. Figure B-10 shows how to locate the midpoint of the upper arm and how to measure the triceps fatfold. Figure B-11 shows how to measure the midarm circumference. As already explained in Chapter 10, a lean tissue measure can be computed from the triceps fatfold measurement together with the midarm circumference measurement: the midarm muscle circumference (see Figure B-12). Table B-4 gives triceps fatfold percentile standards, Table B-5 shows the midarm muscle circumference percentile standards, and Figure B-13 illustrates a nomogram method for determining midarm muscle circumference from these two measures.

■ FIGURE B–8

Nomogram for Body Mass Index (BMI)

Weights and heights are without clothing. With clothes, add 5 lb for men or 3 lb for women, and 1 inch in height for shoes. Draw a straight line, or place a ruler, from your height (left) to your weight (right). At the point where it crosses the BMI line, read your BMI. The accompanying table in the margin indicates the BMI used to define cutoff points and the inside back covers present this information graphically.

Source: From the 1983 Metroplitan Life Insurance Company tables, designed by B. T. Burton and W. R. Roster, Health implications of obesity, and NIH Consensus Development Conference, *Journal of the American Dietetic Association* 85 (1985): 1117–1121.

B

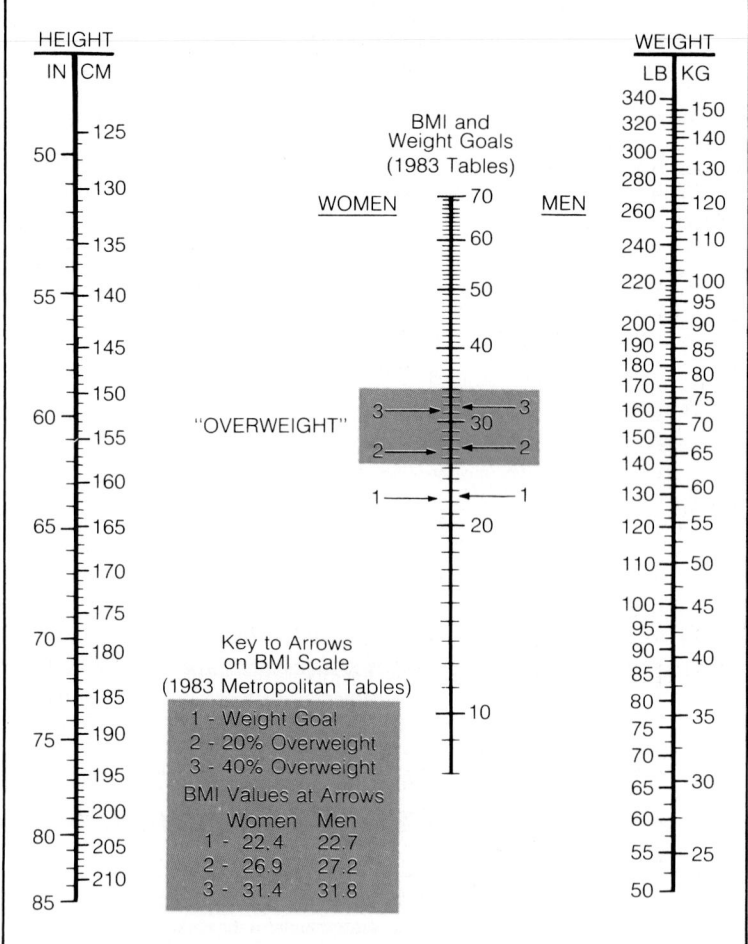

	Men	Women
Underweight	<20.7	<19.1
Acceptable weight	20.7 to 27.8	19.1 to 27.3
Overweight	≥27.8	≥27.3
Severe overweight	≥31.1	≥32.3
Morbid obesity	≥45.4	≥44.8

Prenatal gain in weight

Immediate pregravid weight _____

Height in inches without
shoes (plus one inch) _____

Standard weight _____

(Record weight *with* shoes)

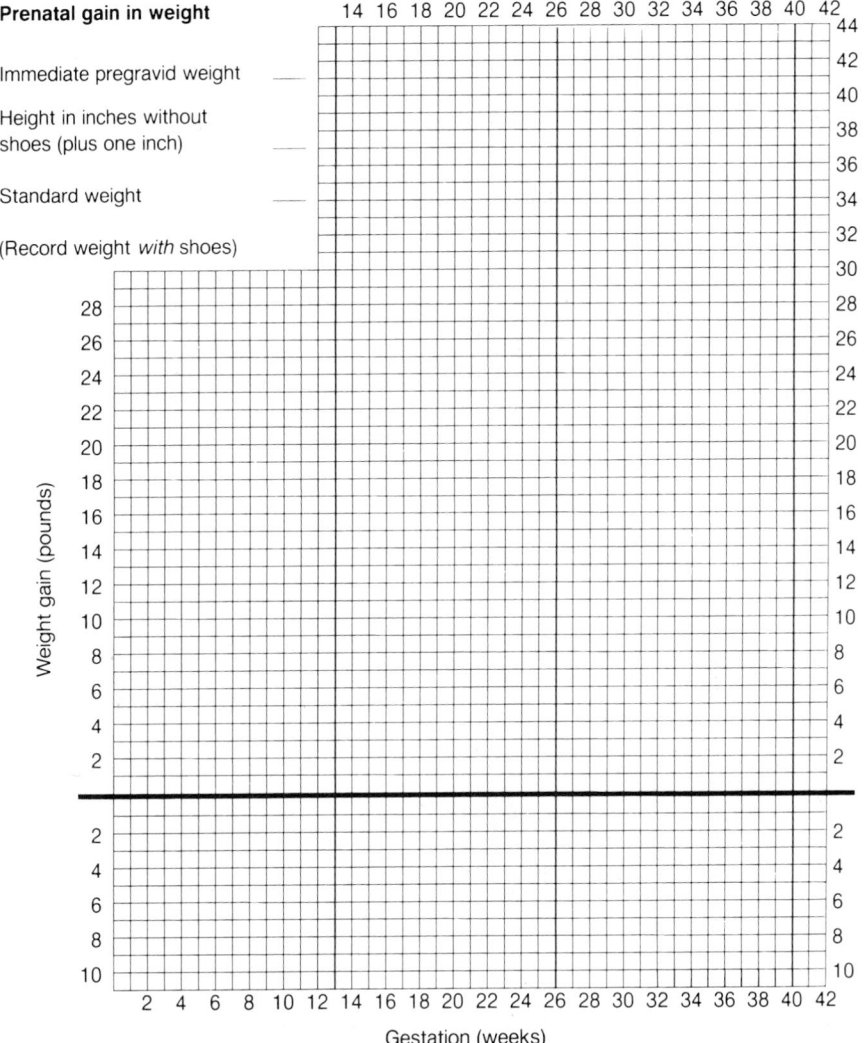

Weight gain (pounds)

Gestation (weeks)

■ FIGURE B–9
Prenatal Weight Gain Grid

■ FIGURE B–10
How to Locate the Midpoint of the
Upper Arm and Measure the Triceps
Fatfold

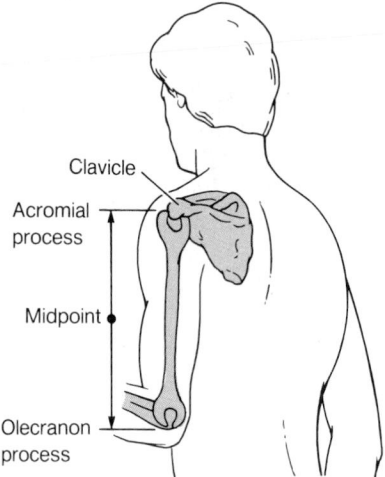

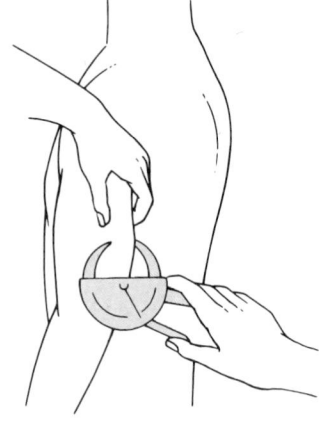

Find the midpoint of the arm:
1. Ask the subject to bend his or her arm
at the elbow and lay the hand across the
stomach. (If he or she is right-handed,
measure the left arm, and vice versa.
2. Feel the shoulder to locate the
acromial process. It helps to slide your
fingers along the clavicle to find the
acromial process. The olecranon process
is the tip of the elbow.
3. Place a measuring tape from the
acromial process to the tip of the elbow.
Divide this measurement by 2, and mark
the midpoint of the arm with a pen.

Measure the flatfold:
1. Ask the subject to let his or her arm
hang loosely to the side.
2. Grasp a fold of skin and subcutaneous
fat between the thumb and forefinger
slightly above the midpoint mark. Gently
pull the skin away from the underlying
muscle. (This step takes a lot of practice.
To be sure you don't have muscle as well
as fat, ask the subject to contract and
relax the muscle. You should be able to
feel if you are pinching muscle.)
3. Place the calipers over the fatfold at
the midpoint mark, and read the
measurement to the nearest 1.0 mm in
two to three seconds. (If using plastic
calipers, align pressure lines, and read the
measurement to the nearest 1.0 mm in
two to three seconds.)
4. Repeat steps 2 and 3 twice more. Add
the three readings, and then divide by 3
to find the average.

■ FIGURE B–11
How to Measure Midarm
Circumference
A nonstretchable measuring tape is placed
around the arm at the midpoint.

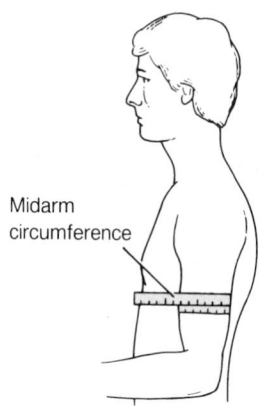

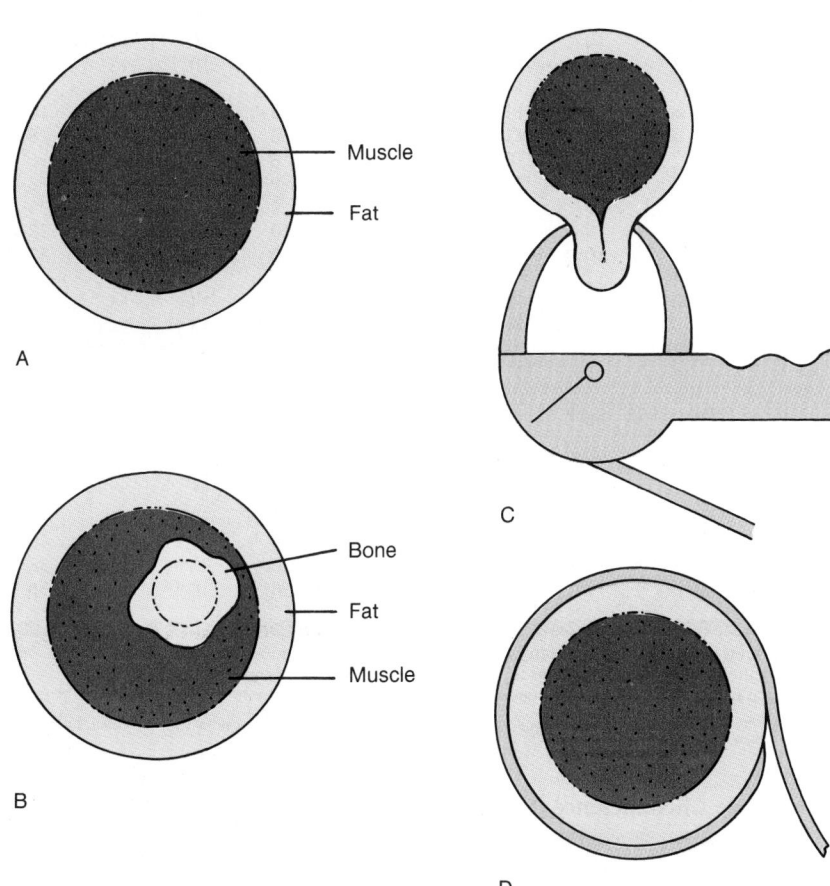

A. The arm is visualized as an inner circle of muscle surrounded by an outer circle of fat.
B. In reality, the arm is not circular, and there is some bone, but the simplified picture is approximately correct.
C. This measurement (the fatfold) gives you two times the thickness of the fat.
D. This measurement (the midarm circumference) gives you the measure of muscle plus fat.
E. An equation then derives the *circumference of the muscle,* an index of the body's total skeletal muscle mass. The equation is:
Midarm muscle circumference (cm) = midarm circumference (cm) − [0.314[a] × triceps fatfold (mm)].

---

[a]This factor converts the fatfold measurement to a circumference measurement and millimeters to centimeters.

■ TABLE B–4
Triceps Fatfold Percentiles (millimeters)

Age	Male					Female				
	5th	25th	50th	75th	95th	5th	25th	50th	75th	95th
1–1.9	6	8	10	12	16	6	8	10	12	16
2–2.9	6	8	10	12	15	6	9	10	12	16
3–3.9	6	8	10	11	15	7	9	11	12	15
4–4.9	6	8	9	11	14	7	8	10	12	16
5–5.9	6	8	9	11	15	6	8	10	12	18
6–6.9	5	7	8	10	16	6	8	10	12	16
7–7.9	5	7	9	12	17	6	9	11	13	18
8–8.9	5	7	8	10	16	6	9	12	15	24
9–9.9	6	7	10	13	18	8	10	13	16	22
10–10.9	6	8	10	14	21	7	10	12	17	27
11–11.9	6	8	11	16	24	7	10	13	18	28
12–12.9	6	8	11	14	28	8	11	14	18	27
13–13.9	5	7	10	14	26	8	12	15	21	30
14–14.9	4	7	9	14	24	9	13	16	21	28
15–15.9	4	6	8	11	24	8	12	17	21	32
16–16.9	4	6	8	12	22	10	15	18	22	31
17–17.9	5	6	8	12	19	10	13	19	24	37
18–18.9	4	6	9	13	24	10	15	18	22	30
19–24.9	4	7	10	15	22	10	14	18	24	34
25–34.9	5	8	12	16	24	10	16	21	27	37
35–44.9	5	8	12	16	23	12	18	23	29	38
45–54.9	6	8	12	15	25	12	20	25	30	40
55–64.9	5	8	11	14	22	12	20	25	31	38
65–74.9	4	8	11	15	22	12	18	24	29	36

Note: Measurements sometimes fall between the percentiles shown here and require you to estimate the percentile given the information provided in this table. For example, a measurement of 7 mm for a 27-year-old male would be about the 20th percentile.

Source: Adapted from A. R. Frisancho, New norms of upper limb fat and muscle areas for assessment of nutritional status, *American Journal of Clinical Nutrition* 34 (1981): 2540–2545.

■ TABLE B–5
Midarm Muscle Circumference Percentiles (centimeters)

Age	Male					Female				
	5th	25th	50th	75th	95th	5th	25th	50th	75th	95th
1–1.9	11.0	11.9	12.7	13.5	14.7	10.5	11.7	12.4	13.9	14.3
2–2.9	11.1	12.2	13.0	14.0	15.0	11.1	11.9	12.6	13.3	14.7
3–3.9	11.7	13.1	13.7	14.3	15.3	11.3	12.4	13.2	14.0	15.2
4–4.9	12.3	13.3	14.1	14.8	15.9	11.5	12.8	13.6	14.4	15.7
5–5.9	12.8	14.0	14.7	15.4	16.9	12.5	13.4	14.2	15.1	16.5
6–6.9	13.1	14.2	15.1	16.1	17.7	13.0	13.8	14.5	15.4	17.1
7–7.9	13.7	15.1	16.0	16.8	19.0	12.9	14.2	15.1	16.0	17.6
8–8.9	14.0	15.4	16.2	17.0	18.7	13.8	15.1	16.0	17.1	19.4
9–9.9	15.1	16.1	17.0	18.3	20.2	14.7	15.8	16.7	18.0	19.8
10–10.9	15.6	16.6	18.0	19.1	22.1	14.8	15.9	17.0	18.0	19.7
11–11.9	15.9	17.3	18.3	19.5	23.0	15.0	17.1	18.1	19.6	22.3
12–12.9	16.7	18.2	19.5	21.0	24.1	16.2	18.0	19.1	20.1	22.0
13–13.9	17.2	19.6	21.1	22.6	24.5	16.9	18.3	19.8	21.1	24.0
14–14.9	18.9	21.2	22.3	24.0	26.4	17.4	19.0	20.1	21.6	24.7
15–15.9	19.9	21.8	23.7	25.4	27.2	17.5	18.9	20.2	21.5	24.4
16–16.9	21.3	23.4	24.9	26.9	29.6	17.0	19.0	20.2	21.6	24.9
17–17.9	22.4	24.5	25.8	27.3	31.2	17.5	19.4	20.5	22.1	25.7
18–18.9	22.6	25.2	26.4	28.3	32.4	17.4	19.1	20.2	21.5	24.5
19–24.9	23.8	25.7	27.3	28.9	32.1	17.9	19.5	20.7	22.1	24.9
25–34.9	24.3	26.4	27.9	29.8	32.6	18.3	19.9	21.2	22.8	26.4
35–44.9	24.7	26.9	28.6	30.2	32.7	18.6	20.5	21.8	23.6	27.2
45–54.9	23.9	26.5	28.1	30.0	32.6	18.7	20.6	22.0	23.8	27.4
55–64.9	23.6	26.0	27.8	29.5	32.0	18.7	20.9	22.5	24.4	28.0
65–74.9	22.3	25.1	26.8	28.4	30.6	18.5	20.8	22.5	24.4	27.9

Source: Adapted from A. R. Frisancho, New norms of upper limb fat and muscle areas for assessment of nutritional status, *American Journal of Clinical Nutrition* 34 (1981): 2540–2545.

B

■ FIGURE B–13
Nomograms for Determination of Midarm Muscle Circumference
To obtain arm muscle circumference using either nomogram, lay a ruler between values of arm circumference and fatfold, and read off arm muscle circumference.

Source: Reproduced with permission from J. Gurney and D. Jelliffe, Arm anthropometry in nutritional assessment; nomogram for rapid calculation of muscle circumference and cross-sectional muscle and fat areas, *American Journal of Clinical Nutrition* 26 (1973): 912, as adapted by A. Grant, *Nutritional Assessment Guidelines*, 2nd ed., 1979 (available from Anne Grant, Box 25057, Northgate Station, Seattle, WA 98125).

■ TABLE B–6
Lower Limits of Acceptable
Grip Strength

Age	Female grip strength (kg)	Male grip strength (kg)
15	28	42
20	29	43
25	30	44
30	30	45
35	30	45
40	30	45
45	30	45
50	29	45
55	28	44
60	27	43
65	25	41
70	23	39
75	20	37
80	18	35
85	15	32
90	11	29
95	8	26

Source: Reprinted by permission of the American Society of Parenteral and Enteral Nutrition, Silver Spring, MD 20879, from A. R. Webb, L.A. Newman, M. Taylor, and J. B. Keogh, Hand grip dynamometry as a predicator of postoperative complications: Reappraisal using age standardized grip strengths, *Journal of Parenteral and Enteral Nutrition* 13 (1989): 30–33.
Note: The figures shown in this table represent 85% of the standard for each age and gender category.

Functional Tests of Nutrition Status

Nutrition assessors sometimes use functional tests of nutrition status to identify nutrient deficiencies. One such test uses a dynamometer (described in Chapter 10) to measure hand grip strength. Like all assessment methods, following instructions carefully helps to ensure accurate measures. To measure hand grip strength, the assessor asks the client to squeeze the dynamometer as tightly as possible, takes three or four measurements, and records the highest value measured. Measurements can be taken on either the dominant or nondominant arm. Table B-6 shows the lower limits of acceptable hand grip strength in males and females based on age.

Laboratory Tests of Nutrition Status

As Chapter 10 pointed out, urine and blood tests provide valuable information in a nutrition assessment. Table B-7 shows how serum proteins relate to undernutrition. The total lymphocyte count, another laboratory test valuable in assessing PEM, is calculated from the number of white blood cells (WBC) and the percentage of lymphocytes:

■ Total lymphocyte count (mm^3) = WBC (mm^3) × % lymphocytes.

A person with a WBC count of 7,500 mm^3 with 15% lymphocytes would have a total lymphocyte count of:

■ Total lymphocyte count (mm^3) = 7,500 mm^3 × 0.15 = 1,125 mm^3.

The standard lymphocyte count is 2,500 mm^3; values below 1,500 mm^3 are considered depleted. A lymphocyte count of 1,125 mm^3, then, suggests a moderate degree of depletion.

Two urine tests—creatinine excretion and urine urea nitrogen—require a 24-hour urine collection, and, therefore, are not routinely used. Collecting a 24-hour urine sample presents many problems. Much effort is wasted if everyone involved does not conscientiously follow proper techniques. The collection of urine and recording of food intake data requires client cooperation. The client must receive thorough instructions on how to collect and save all urine samples, and must be advised to call for help if needed. If even one urine sample is spilled or discarded, the test is invalid.

■ TABLE B–7
Relationship between Degree of Undernutrition and Serum Proteins

Indicator	Mild	Moderate	Severe
Albumin (g/100 ml)	2.8 – 3.4	2.1 – 2.7	<2.1
Transferrin (mg/100 ml)	150–200	100–149	<100
Prealbumin (mg/100 ml)	10 – 15	5–9	<5
Retinol-binding protein[a] (mg/100 ml)	—	—	—

Note: To convert albumin (g/100 ml) to international standard units (nmol/L), multiply by 37.06. To convert transferrin (mg/100 ml) to standard international units (g/L), multiply by 0.01.
[a]Levels of < 3 mg/100 ml suggest compromised protein status. The actual degree of depletion (mild, moderate, and severe) has not been defined.

Most hospitals have a standard time for beginning urinary collections (often, between 6:00 AM and 6:00 PM). For nitrogen balance studies, food intake must also be recorded during the exact same time period. All nurses caring for the client on all shifts must record, or ensure that the client records, food intake data carefully. Each urine sample is added to the collection container and refrigerated until the collection is complete.

To determine nitrogen balance requires knowing the 24-hour nitrogen intake and output. To estimate nitrogen intake from dietary protein use the formula:

$$\text{Nitrogen intake} = \frac{\text{Protein intake (g)}}{6.25}.$$

Nitrogen output per day equals the measured urinary urea nitrogen (UUN) plus a factor of 4 grams to account for nitrogen lost through the lungs, hair, skin, and nails as well as nonurea nitrogen losses in the urine.

$$\text{Nitrogen output} = \text{UUN} + 4 \text{ g.}$$

Calculate nitrogen balance from the nitrogen intake and output:

$$\text{Nitrogen balance} = \text{Nitrogen intake} - \text{nitrogen output.}$$

Using the above equations, calculate nitrogen balance for a person with a protein intake of 45 g/24 hr and a UUN of 10 g/24 hr.

$$\text{Nitrogen balance} = \frac{45 \text{ g}}{6.25} - (10 \text{ g} + 4 \text{ g}).$$

$$\text{Nitrogen balance} = 7 \text{ g} - 14 \text{ g or } - 7 \text{ g.}$$

The person in this example is in negative nitrogen balance; that is, nitrogen intake is inadequate to meet nitrogen needs.

To calculate the creatinine-height index (CHI) from the measured urinary creatinine and the client's height, use the following equation:

$$\text{CHI} = \frac{\text{Measured urinary creatinine (24-hour sample)}}{\text{Standard creatinine excretion for height and sex}} \times 100.$$

For example, to calculate the CHI in a man of medium frame, 5 ft 8 inches tall, who excretes 1,090 mg of creatinine in 24 hours, follow these steps:

■ Look up the standard creatinine excretion (Table B-8).

In this example, the standard creatinine excretion is 1.56 g or 1,560 mg.

■ Use this information to complete the CHI equation:

$$\text{CHI} = \frac{1,090 \text{ mg}}{1,560 \text{ mg}} \times 100 = 70\%.$$

Based on the CHI, the man in this example has a skeletal muscle mass 70 percent of that considered typical for a man of his height. Table B-9 shows the standard creatinine excretions for women.

Other laboratory tests help detect iron deficiency. Chapter 10 describes the tests used in assessing iron status. Tables B-10 through B-15 provide standards for measures of iron status: hemoglobin, hematocrit, serum ferritin, serum iron, transferrin saturation, erythrocyte protoporphyrin, and mean corpuscular volume.

TABLE B–8
Creatinine-Height Index Standards for Men

Height		Small Frame			Medium Frame			Large Frame		
		Ideal Weight	Creatinine		Ideal Weight	Creatinine		Ideal Weight	Creatinine	
in	cm	(kg)	(g/24 h)	(mmol/d)[a]	(kg)	(g/24 h)	(mmol/d)[a]	(kg)	(g/24 h)	(mmol/d)[a]
61	154.9	52.7	1.21	10.7	56.1	1.29	11.4	60.7	1.40	12.4
62	157.5	54.1	1.24	11.0	57.7	1.33	11.8	62.0	1.43	12.6
63	160.0	55.4	1.27	11.2	59.1	1.36	12.0	63.6	1.46	12.9
64	162.5	56.8	1.31	11.6	60.4	1.39	12.3	65.2	1.50	13.3
65	165.1	58.4	1.34	11.8	62.0	1.43	12.6	66.8	1.54	13.6
66	167.6	60.2	1.39	12.3	63.9	1.47	13.0	68.9	1.59	14.1
67	170.2	62.0	1.43	12.6	65.9	1.52	13.4	71.1	1.64	14.5
68	172.7	63.9	1.47	13.0	67.7	1.56	13.8	72.9	1.68	14.9
69	175.3	65.9	1.52	13.4	69.5	1.60	14.1	74.8	1.72	15.2
70	177.8	67.7	1.56	13.8	71.6	1.65	14.6	76.8	1.77	15.6
71	180.3	69.5	1.60	14.1	73.6	1.69	14.9	79.1	1.82	16.1
72	182.9	71.4	1.64	14.5	75.7	1.74	15.4	81.1	1.87	16.5
73	185.4	73.4	1.69	14.9	77.7	1.79	15.8	83.4	1.92	17.0
74	187.9	75.2	1.73	15.3	80.0	1.85	16.4	85.7	1.97	17.4
75	190.5	77.0	1.77	15.6	82.3	1.89	16.7	87.7	2.02	17.9

[a]To convert urinary creatinine measures (g/24 h) to standard international units (mmol/d) multiply by 8.840.

Source: A. Grant and S. DeHoog, *Nutritional Assessment and Support*, 3rd ed., 1985 (available from P.O. Box 25057, Northgate Station, Seattle, WA 98125).

TABLE B–9
Creatinine-Height Index Standards for Women

Height		Small Frame			Medium Frame			Large Frame		
		Ideal Weight	Creatinine		Ideal Weight	Creatinine		Ideal Weight	Creatinine	
in	cm	(kg)	(g/24 h)	(mmol/d)[a]	(kg)	(g/24 h)	(mmol/d)[a]	(kg)	(g/24 h)	(mmol/d)[a]
56	142.2	43.2	0.79	7.0	46.1	0.83	7.3	50.7	0.91	8.0
57	144.8	44.3	0.80	7.1	47.3	0.85	7.5	51.8	0.93	8.2
58	147.3	45.4	0.82	7.2	48.6	0.88	7.8	53.2	0.96	8.5
59	149.8	46.8	0.84	7.4	50.0	0.90	8.0	54.5	0.98	8.7
60	152.4	48.2	0.87	7.7	51.4	0.93	8.2	55.9	1.01	8.9
61	154.9	49.5	0.89	7.9	52.7	0.95	8.4	57.3	1.03	9.1
62	157.5	50.9	0.92	8.1	54.3	0.98	8.7	58.9	1.06	9.4
63	160.0	52.3	0.94	8.3	55.9	1.01	8.9	60.6	1.09	9.6
64	162.5	53.9	0.97	8.6	57.9	1.04	9.2	62.5	1.13	10.0
65	165.1	55.7	1.00	8.8	59.8	1.08	9.5	64.3	1.16	10.3
66	167.6	57.5	1.04	9.2	61.6	1.11	9.8	66.1	1.19	10.5
67	170.2	59.3	1.07	9.5	63.4	1.14	10.1	67.9	1.22	10.8
68	172.7	61.4	1.11	9.8	65.2	1.17	10.3	70.0	1.26	11.1
69	175.2	63.2	1.14	10.1	67.0	1.21	10.7	72.0	1.30	11.5
70	177.8	65.0	1.17	10.3	68.9	1.24	11.0	74.1	1.33	11.8

[a]To convert urinary creatinine measures (g/24 h) to standard international units (mmol/d) multiply by 8.840.

Source: A. Grant and S. DeHoog, *Nutritional Assessment and Support*, 3rd ed., 1985 (available from P.O. Box 25057, Northgate Station, Seattle, WA 98125).

■ TABLE B–10
Standards for Hemoglobin Test Results

< 2 yr	(M-F)	< 9.0	10.0 or >
2–5 yr	(M-F)	< 10.0	11.0 or >
6–12 yr	(M-F)	< 10.0	11.5 or >
13–16 yr	(M)	< 12.0	13.0 or >
	(F)	< 10.0	11.5 or >
> 16 yr	(M)	< 12.0	14.0 or >
	(F)	< 10.0	12.0 or >
trimester 2		< 9.5	11.0 or >
trimester 3		< 9.0	10.5 or >

Note: To convert hemoglobin values (g/100 ml) to international standard units, multiply by 10.

■ TABLE B–11
Standards for Hematocrit Test Results

Age	Sex	Deficient	Acceptable
< 2 yr	(M-F)	< 0.28	0.31 or >
2–5 yr	(M-F)	< 0.30	0.34 or >
6–12 yr	(M-F)	< 0.30	0.36 or >
13–16 yr	(M)	< 0.37	0.40 or >
	(F)	< 0.31	0.36 or >
> 16 yr	(M)	< 0.37	0.44 or >
	(F)	< 0.31	0.38 or >
trimester 2		< 0.30	0.35 or >
trimester 3		< 0.30	0.33 or >

Note: To convert hematocrit values (%) to international standard units, multiply by 0.01.

■ TABLE B–12
Standards for Serum Ferritin

Group	Deficient (ng/ml)
Children (3–14 yr)	<10
Adolescents and adults	<12
Pregnant women	<10

■ TABLE B–13
Standards for Serum Iron

Age	Sex	Deficient (µg/100 ml)	Deficient (µmol/L)	Acceptable (µg/100 ml)	Acceptable (µmol/L)
< 2 yr	(M-F)	< 30	< 5.3	30 or >	5.3 or >
2–5 yr	(M-F)	< 40	< 7.1	40 or >	7.1 or >
6–12 yr	(M-F)	< 50	< 8.9	50 or >	8.9 or >
> 12 yr	(M)	< 60	< 10.7	60 or >	10.7 or >
	(F)	< 40	< 7.1	40 or >	7.1 or >

Note: To convert serum iron values (µg/100 ml) to international standard units, (µmol/L), multiply by 0.1791.

B

■ TABLE B–14
Standards for Percent Transferrin Saturation

Age	Sex	Deficient	Acceptable
< 2 yr	(M-F)	< 15	15 or >
2–12 yr	(M-F)	< 20	20 or >
> 13 yr	(M)	< 20	20 or >
	(F)	< 15	15 or >

■ TABLE B–15
Standards for Erythrocyte Protoporphyrin and Mean Corpuscular Volume

Age	Erythrocyte Protoporphyrin (μg/dL RBC)	MCV (fL)
1–2 yr	> 80	< 73
3–4 yr	> 75	< 75
5–10 yr	> 70	< 76
11–14 yr	> 70	< 78
15–74 yr	> 70	< 80

■ Physical Findings

Finally, the nutrition assessor uses physical examinations to search for signs of nutrient deficiency or toxicity. Table 10–10 in Chapter 10 presents a summary of physical findings organized by body system; Table B-16 presents a summary of symptoms of vitamin and mineral imbalances organized by nutrients.

Nutrition assessments vary in their depth and accuracy. While for some cases, minimal measures may be all that is necessary, but for clients who are very ill or who show signs of nutrition problems, thorough tests must be conducted.

■ TABLE B–16
Symptoms of Vitamin and Mineral Imbalances

Vitamin Name	Deficiency Disease Name	Deficiency Symptoms	Toxicity Symptoms
		Bones/Teeth[a]	
Vitamin A	Hypovitaminosis A	Cessation of bone growth, change in shapes of bones, painful joints; malfunctioning of enamel-forming cells, development of cracks in teeth and tendency to decay, atrophy of dentin-forming cells	Increased activity of osteoclasts[b] causing decalcification, joint pain, fragility, stunted growth, and thickening of long bones; increase of pressure inside skull, mimicking brain tumor; headaches
		Blood	
		Microcytic anemia, often masked by dehydration	Loss of hemoglobin and potassium by red blood cells, cessation of menstruation, slowed clotting time, easily induced bleeding
		Eyes[c]	
		Night blindness, change in epithelial tissue caused by failure to secrete mucopolysaccharide (hyperkeratinization), drying (xerosis), triangular gray spots on eye (Bitot's spots), irreversible drying (keratomalacia), and degeneration of the cornea causing blindness (most severe)	
		Skin[d]	
		Plugging of hair follicles with keratin, forming white lumps (hyperkeratosis)	Dryness; itching; peeling; rashes; dry, scaling lips; cracking and bleeding of lips; nosebleeds; loss of hair; brittle nails
		Digestive System	
		Changes in lining, diarrhea	Nausea, vomiting, abdominal pain, diarrhea, weight loss
		Immune System	
		Depression of immune reactions	Stimulation of immune reactions
		Nervous/Muscular System	
		Brain and spinal cord growth too fast for stunted skull and spine, paralysis caused by injury to brain and nerves	Loss of appetite, irritability, fatigue, insomnia, restlessness, headache, blurred vision, nausea, vomiting, muscle weakness, interference with thyroxin

(continued)

■ **TABLE B–16**
Symptoms of Vitamin and Mineral Imbalances (continued)

Vitamin Name	Deficiency Disease Name	Deficiency Symptoms	Toxicity Symptoms

Respiratory Tract

Vitamin A (continued)		Changes in lining, infections	

Urogenital Tract

Changes in lining that favor calcium deposition, resulting in kidney stones and bladder disorders; infections of bladder and kidney; infections of vagina

Reproductive System

Amenorrhea[e]

Liver[f]

Jaundice,[g] enlargement, massive accumulation of fat and vitamin A

Spleen

Enlargement

Bones/Teeth

| Vitamin D | Rickets, osteomalacia | *Rickets* Faulty calcification, resulting in misshapen bones (bowing of legs) and retarded growth; enlargement of ends of long bones (knees, wrists); deformities of ribs (bowed, with beads or knobs);[h] delayed closing of fontanel, resulting in rapid enlargement of head (see accompanying figure); slow eruption of teeth; teeth not well formed, with a tendency to decay | *Osteomalacia* Softening effect; deformities of limbs, spine, thorax, and pelvis; demineralization; pain in pelvis, lower back, and legs; bone fractures   Increased calcium withdrawal |

Fontanel
A fontanel is the open space in the top of a baby's skull before the bones have grown together. In rickets, closing of the fontanel is delayed.

Posterior fontanel normally closes by the end of the first year.

Anterior fontanel normally closes by the end of the second year.

Blood

		Decreased calcium and/or phosphorus	Decreased calcium and/or phosphorus, increased alkaline phosphatase[i] · Increased calcium and phosphorus concentrations

Nervous/Muscular Systems

		Lax muscles resulting in protrusion of abdomen; muscle spasms	Involuntary twitching, muscle spasms · Loss of appetite, headache, weakness, fatigue, excessive thirst, irritability, apathy

■ TABLE B–16
Symptoms of Vitamin and Mineral Imbalances   (continued)

Vitamin Name	Deficiency Disease Name	Deficiency Symptoms	Toxicity Symptoms
		Excretory System	
Vitamin D (continued)		Increased calcium in stools, decreased calcium in urine	Increased excretion of calcium in urine, kidney stones, irreversible renal damage
		Other	
		Abnormally high secretion of parathormone	Calcification of soft tissues (blood vessels, kidneys, heart, lungs, tissues around joints), death
		Blood/Circulatory System	
Vitamin E		Red blood cell breakage,[j] anemia	Augments effects of anticlotting medication
		Digestive System	
			General discomfort
		Nervous/Muscular Systems	
		Degeneration, weakness, difficulty walking, severe pain in calf muscles	Headache, weakness, dizziness, fatigue, visual abnormalties
		Other	
		Fibrocystic breast disease	
		Blood/Circulatory System	
Vitamin K		Hemorrhaging	Interference with anticlotting medication, possible jaundice caused by vitamin K analogues
		Blood/Circulatory System	
Thiamin	Beriberi	Edema, enlarged heart, abnormal heart rhythms, heart failure	Rapid pulse
		Nervous/Muscular Systems	
		Degeneration, wasting, weakness, painful calf muscles, low morale, difficulty walking, loss of ankle and knee jerk reflexes, mental confusion, paralysis	Weakness, headaches, insomnia, irritability
		Mouth, Gums, Tongue	
Riboflavin	Ariboflavinosis	Cracks at corners of mouth,[k] magenta tongue	
		Nervous System and Eyes	
		Hypersensitivity to light,[l] reddening of cornea	
		Other	
		Skin rash	Interference with anticancer medication

■ TABLE B–16
Symptoms of Vitamin and Mineral Imbalances (continued)

Vitamin Name	Deficiency Disease Name	Deficiency Symptoms	Toxicity Symptoms
		Digestive System	
Niacin	Pellagra	Diarrhea	Diarrhea, heartburn, nausea, ulcer irritation, vomiting
		Mouth, Gums, Tongue	
			Inflamed, swollen, smooth tongue[m]
		Nervous System	
		Irritability, loss of appetite, weakness, dizziness, mental confusion progressing to psychosis or delirium	
		Skin	
		Bilateral symmetrical dermatitis, especially on areas exposed to sun	Painful flush and rash, itching, burning, excessive sweating
		Other	
			Abnormal liver function, low blood pressure
		Blood/Circulatory System	
Vitamin B$_6$		Microcytic anemia	Bloating
		Mouth, Gums, Tongue	
		Smooth tongue,[m] cracked corners of the mouth[k]	
		Nervous/Muscular Systems	
		Abnormal brain wave pattern, irritability, muscle twitching, convulsions	Depression, fatigue, irritability, headaches, numbness, damage to nerves leading to loss of reflexes and sensation, difficulty walking
		Skin	
		Irritation of sweat glands, dermatitis	
		Other	
		Kidney stones	
		Blood/Circulatory System	
Folate		Macrocytic or megaloblastic anemia	
		Digestive System	
		Heartburn, diarrhea (loss of villi and their enzymes), constipation	Diarrhea
		Immune System	
		Suppression, frequent infections	
		Mouth, Gums, Tongue	
		Smooth, red tongue[m]	
		Nervous System	
		Depression, mental confusion, fainting, fatigue	Insomnia, irritability

(continued)

■ TABLE B–16
Symptoms of Vitamin and Mineral Imbalances   (continued)

Vitamin Name	Deficiency Disease Name	Deficiency Symptoms	Toxicity Symptoms
		Other	
Folate (continued)			Masking of vitamin B_{12}– deficiency symptoms
		Blood/Circulatory System	
Vitamin B_{12}	Pernicious anemia[n]	Macrocytic or megaloblastic anemia	
		Mouth, Gums, Tongue	
		Smooth tongue[m]	
		Nervous System	
		Fatigue, degeneration of peripheral nerves progressing to paralysis	
		Skin	
		Hypersensitivity	
		Digestive System	
Pantothenic acid		Vomiting, intestinal distress	Occasional diarrhea
		Nervous System	
		Insomnia, fatigue	
		Other	
			Water retention (infrequent)
		Blood/Circulatory System	
Biotin		Abnormal heart action	
		Digestive System	
		Loss of appetite, nausea	
		Nervous/Muscular Systems	
		Depression, muscle pain, weakness, fatigue	
		Skin	
		Drying, scaly dermatitis, loss of hair	
		Blood/Circulatory System	
Vitamin C	Scurvy	Microcytic anemia, atherosclerotic plaques, pinpoint hemorrhages	Blood cell breakage in certain racial groups[o]
		Digestive System	
			Nausea, abdominal cramps, diarrhea
		Immune System	
		Depression, frequent infections	
		Mouth, Gums, Tongue	
		Bleeding gums, loosened teeth	
		Nervous/Muscular Systems	
		Muscle degeneration and pain, hysteria, depression	Headache, fatigue, insomnia

(continued)

■ TABLE B–16
Symptoms of Vitamin and Mineral Imbalances   (continued)

Vitamin/Mineral Name	Deficiency Symptoms	Toxicity Symptoms
	Skeletal System	
Vitamin C (continued)	Bone fragility, joint pain	
	Skin	
	Rough skin, blotchy bruises	Hot flashes, rashes
	Other	
	Failure of wounds to heal	Interference with medical tests, aggravation of gout symptoms, excessive urination, kidney stones,[p] (deficiency symptoms may appear at first on withdrawal of high doses)
Major Minerals		
Calcium	Stunted growth in children, implicated in bone loss (osteoporosis) in adults	Excess calcium is excreted except in hormonal imbalance states (not caused by nutritional deficiency)
Phosphorus	Deficiency unknown	
Magnesium	Weakness; confusion; depressed pancreatic hormone secretion; if extreme, convulsions, bizarre muscle movements (especially of the eye and facial muscles), hallucinations, and difficulty in swallowing;[q] in children, growth failure	Not known; large doses have been taken in the form of the laxative Epsom salts without ill effects except diarrhea
Sodium	Muscle cramps, mental apathy, loss of appetite	Hypertension[r]
Chloride	Growth failure in children; muscle cramps, mental apathy, loss of appetite	Vomiting
Potassium	Deficiency accompanies dehydration; causes muscular weakness, paralysis, and confusion	Muscular weakness; vomiting; if given into a vein, can stop the heart
Sulfur	None known; protein deficiency would occur first	Would occur only if sulfur amino acids were eaten in excess; this (in animals) depresses growth
Trace Minerals		
	Eyes	
Iron	Blue sclerae	
	GI Tract	
	Lactose intolerance, and possibly intolerance to other sugars; increased risk of lead and cadmium poisoning	
	Immune System	
	Reduced resistance to infection (lowered immunity)	Infections

(continued)

■ TABLE B–16
Symptoms of Vitamin and Mineral Imbalances   (continued)

Mineral Name	Deficiency Symptoms	Toxicity Symptoms
	Nervous/Muscular Systems	
Iron (continued)	Reduced work productivity, tolerance to work, and voluntary work; reduced physical fitness; weakness; fatigue; impaired cognitive function (children); reduced learning ability; increased distractibility (inability to pay attention); impaired visual discrimination; impaired reactivity and coordination (infants)	
	Skin	
	Itching; pale nailbeds, eye membranes, and palm creases; concave nails; impaired wound healing	
	General	
	Reduced resistance to cold, inability to regulate body temperature, pica (clay eating, ice eating)	
	Blood	
Zinc	Tendency to atherosclerosis, elevated ammonia levels, decreased alkaline phosphatase, decreased insulin concentration	Anemia: reduced hemoglobin production
	Bones	
	Growth retardation, abnormal collagen synthesis	Growth in length, but without normal zinc content
	Cells/Metabolism	
	Decreased DNA synthesis, impaired cell division and protein synthesis	Raised LDL, lowered HDL
	Digestive System	
	Diarrhea, vomiting, decreased calcium and copper absorption	Reduced sense of smell, reduced sensitivity to the taste of salt, weight loss, delayed glucose absorption, diarrhea, nausea, impaired folate absorption
	Eyes	
	Night blindness	

B

(continued)

■ TABLE B–16
Symptoms of Vitamin and Mineral Imbalances   (continued)

Mineral Name	Deficiency Symptoms	Toxicity Symptoms
	Glandular System	
Zinc (continued)	Delayed onset of puberty, small gonads in males, decreased synthesis and release of testosterone, abnormal glucose tolerance, reduced synthesis of adrenocortical hormones, altered thyroid function	
	Immune System	
	Altered skin test responses, reduced numbers of white blood cells and antibody-forming cells, thymus atrophy, increased susceptibility to infection	Fever, elevated white blood cell count
	Kidney	
		Renal failure
	Liver/Spleen	
	Enlargement	
	Nervous/Muscular Systems	
	Anorexia (poor appetite), mental lethargy, irritability	Muscular pain and incoordination, heart muscle degeneration, exhaustion, dizziness, drowsiness
	Reproductive System	
	Impaired reproductive function (rats), low sperm counts	Reproductive failure
	Skin	
	Generalized hair loss; lesions; rough, dry appearance; slow healing of wounds and burns	
Iodine	Enlargement of the thyroid gland, weight gain, mental and physical retardation of an infant	Enlargement of the thyroid gland, depressed thyroid activity
Copper	Anemia, bone changes (rare in human beings)	Vomiting, diarrhea
Fluoride	Susceptibility to tooth decay	Fluorosis (discoloration of teeth), nausea, diarrhea, chest pain, itching, vomiting
Selenium	Anemia (rare); heart disease	Digestive system disorders, loss of hair and nails, skin lesions, nervous system disorders, tooth damage

(continued)

■ TABLE B–16
Symptoms of Vitamin and Mineral Imbalances   (continued)

Mineral Name	Deficiency Symptoms	Toxicity Symptoms
Chromium	Diabetes-like condition marked by an inability to use glucose normally; associated with coronary artery disease	Unknown as a nutrition disorder; occupational exposures damage skin and kidneys
Cobalt	Unknown in human beings except in vitamin B_{12} deficiency	Unknown as a nutrition disorder; occupational exposures damage skin and red blood cells
Molybdenum	Unknown	Enzyme inhibition
Manganese	(In animals): poor growth, nervous system disorders, reproductive abnormalities	Nervous system disorders

[a]Chapter 7 describes vitamin A's role in tooth formation in more detail.
[b]Osteoclasts are the cells that destroy bone during its growth. Those that build bone are osteoblasts.
[c]The eyes' symptoms of vitamin A deficiency are collectively known as *xerophthalmia*.
[d]A related toxicity condition, hypercarotenemia, is caused by the accumulation of too much of the vitamin A precursor beta-carotene in the blood, which turns the skin noticeably yellow. Hypercarotenemia is not, strickly speaking, a toxicity symptom.
[e]Elevated serum carotene concentrations are associated with amenorrhea.
[f]If liver impairment is severe, the "classic" signs seen in skin and hair may be masked.
[g]A symptom of liver disease, in which bile and related pigments spill into the bloodstream and the skin yellows, is *jaundice* (JAWN-diss).
[h]Bowing of the ribs causes the symptom known as *pigeon breast*. The beads that form on the ribs resemble rosary beads; thus this symptom is known as *rachitic* (ra-KIT-ik) *rosary* ("the rosary of rickets").
[i]Alkaline phosphatase is an enzyme in the blood that rises during bone resorption.
[j]The breaking of red blood cells is called *erythrocyte hemolysis*.
[k]Cracks at the corners of the mouth are termed *cheilosis* (kee-LOH-sis).
[l]Hypersensitivity to light is *photophobia*.
[m]Smoothness of the tongue is caused by loss of its surface structures and is termed *glossitis* (gloss-EYE-tis).
[n]The name *pernicious anemia* refers to the vitamin B_{12} deficiency caused by lack of intrinsic factor, but not to that caused by inadequate dietary intake.
[o]Groups susceptible to vitamin C toxicity are Sephardic Jews, black Americans and Africans, and Asians.
[p]People who have a tendency toward gout and those who have a genetic abnormality that alters the break down of vitamin C are prone to forming kidney stones. Vitamin C is inactivated and degraded by several routes, and sometimes a product along the way is oxalate, which can form stones in the kidneys (see Nutrition in Practice 23). People can also have oxalate crystals in their kidneys that are not due to vitamin C overdoses.
[q]A still more severe deficiency causes tetany, an extreme, prolonged contraction of the muscles similar to that caused by low blood calcium.
[r]Chapter 22 describes the role of sodium in the development of hypertension.

B

Table of Food Composition

This table of food composition is not the standard table found in most nutrition textbooks. The list of foods chosen is an expanded version of that presented in the 1986 edition of the USDA *Home and Garden Bulletin Number 72, Nutritive Value of Foods*. The *Bulletin*, however, does not contain the values for dietary fiber, vitamin B_6, folate, magnesium, or zinc. Also, many additional foods have been added (such as frozen yogurt, canola oil, and imitation seafood items) to reflect current food patterns. The latest data for beef is also included. It is from the USDA data tapes and reflects the leaner cuts of beef now sold.

To achieve a complete and reliable listing of nutrients for all the foods, many sources of information had to be researched. Government sources of information is the primary base for all of the data: USDA *Handbooks 8–1* through *8–18*; *Handbook 8–21*; prepublication material on cereals, grains, and pasta; current supplemental data on vegetables and other foods; and provisional USDA information on nutrient values—both published and unpublished. Many conversations with professional staff members at the USDA Human Information Service in Hyattsville, Maryland also contributed to the refinement and completion of the data.

Even with all the government sources available, there are still many missing nutrient values; and, as the various government data are updated, conflicting values are often reported from the USDA. To fill in the missing values and resolve discrepancies, other sources of information were used. These reliable sources include referred journal articles, food composition tables from Canada and England, information from other nutrient data banks and publications, unpublished scientific data, and manufacturers' data.

Estimates of nutrient amounts for foods include all possible adjustments. When multiple values are reported for a nutrient, the numbers are averaged and weighted with consideration of the original number of samples in the separate sources. Whenever water percentages are available, estimates of nutrient amounts are adjusted for water content. When no water is given, water percentage is assumed to be that shown in the table. Whenever a reported weight appears inconsistent (cooked eggplant and collards, for example), many kitchen tests are made, and the average weight of the typical product is given as tested.

When estimates of nutrient amounts in cooked foods are derived from reported amounts in raw foods, published retention factors are applied. Some reported data for combination foods are modified in this table to include newer data available for major ingredients. For example, since the "pies" were analyzed and reported, newer data on fruits have been published. Older reported data on certain bakery items are updated for the new enrichment levels for certain nutrients.

Considerable effort has been made to report the most accurate data available and to eliminate missing values. There will always be future changes, and the authors welcome any suggestions or comments from readers.

■ *It is important to know*

that there can be many different values reported for the same nutrient. Many factors influence the amounts of nutrients in foods: the mineral content of the soil, the method of processing, genetics, the diet of the animal or the fertilizer of the plant, the season of the year, methods of analysis, the differences in moisture contents of the samples analyzed, the length and method of storage, and methods of cooking the food.

Even reliable sources report conflicting data. Although each nutrient from USDA government data is presented as a single number in some USDA publications, each number is actually an average of a range of data. In the more detailed reports (Handbook 8 series), the number of samples is identified, and the standard deviation is also noted. USDA data will report different values for foods as well, because old information is being updated in the more recent publications. Therefore, nutrient data should be used only as a guide, a close approximation of nutrient content.

Dietary fiber deserves a special word. It is important to remember that changes will be made to dietary fiber data, as research continues and analytical techniques are modified. Estimates of dietary fiber are included for all the foods in this table. The sources of this information are primarily extensive published and unpublished information from the USDA Human Nutrition Information Service in Hyattsville, Maryland; *Composition of Foods by Southgate* (England); and many journal articles.

Dietary fiber is composed of cellulose, hemicellulose, lignin, pectin, gums, and mucilages. Very little data is available for gum and mucilage, but there is considerable data for the other components.

Many different analytical techniques are used to measure various components of fiber, and these methods are undergoing their own review of accuracy in the scientific community. In this table, either an estimate of the total dietary fiber (a specific analytical technique) or a combination of measures for the insoluble components and pectin, when available, are used.

Vitamin A is reported in retinol equivalents. The amount of this vitamin can vary with the season of the year. Reported values in both dairy products and plants are higher in summer and early fall than in winter. The values reported here represent year-round averages. In the organ meats of all animal products (liver especially), there are large amounts of vitamin A, and these amounts vary widely with the background of the animal. The vitamin is present in very small amounts in regular meat and is often reported as a trace.

Newer reported vitamin A values for some plant foods have increased significantly due to additional information and sometimes to newer plant genetics. New vitamin A values for canned pumpkin, for example, are 3.5 times greater than the previously reported values. This information was used to modify the vitamin A value of pumpkin pie, which had not yet been updated.

The energy and nutrients in recipes and combination foods vary widely, depending on the ingredients. The various fatty acids and cholesterol are influenced by the type of fat used (the specific type of oil, vegetable shortening, butter, margarine, etc.).

Total fat, as well as the breakdown of total fat to saturated, monounsaturated, and polyunsaturated fat, is listed in the table. The fatty acids seldom add up exactly to the total. This is due to rounding and to the existence of small amounts of other fatty acid components that are not included in the three basic categories.

Niacin values are for preformed niacin and do not include additional niacin that may form in the body from the conversion of tryptophan.

The items in this table have been organized into several categories, which are listed at the head of each right-hand page. As the key shows, each group has a number and that number is indicated in the first column. For ease in paging through this table, the category listed on the page you are on is highlighted in color. Thus if 7-GRAIN is colored and you are looking for dairy foods, turn back a few pages; if you are looking for sweets, turn forward.

C

Note: This table has been prepared for West Publishing Company and is copyrighted by ESHA Research in Salem, Oregon—the developer and publisher of "The Food Processor®" computerized nutrition systems. The major sources for the data from the U.S. Department of Agriculture are supplemented by over 450 additional sources of information. Because the list of references is so extensive, it is not provided here, but it is available from the publisher.

Table C–1   Food Composition

Grp	Computer Code No.	Food Description	Measure	Wt (g)	H$_2$O (%)	Ener (kcal)	Prot (g)	Carb (g)	Dietary Fiber (g)	Fat (g)	Fat Breakdown (g)		
											Sat	Mono	Poly
BEVERAGES													
		Alcoholic:											
		Beer:											
1	1	Regular (12 fl oz)	1½ c	356	92	146	1	13	1	0	0	0	0
1	2	Light (12 fl oz)	1½ c	354	95	100[1]	1	5	1	0	0	0	0
		Gin, rum, vodka, whiskey:											
1	3	80 proof	1½ fl oz	42	67	97	0	<.1	0	0	0	0	0
1	4	86 proof	1½ fl oz	42	64	105	0	<.1	0	0	0	0	0
1	5	90 proof	1½ fl oz	42	62	110	0	<.1	0	0	0	0	0
		Liqueur:											
1	1359	Coffee Liqueur, 53 proof	1½ fl oz	52	31	174	0	24	0	<1	.1	t	.1
1	1360	Coffee & cream liqueur, 34 proof	1½ fl oz	47	47	154	1	10	0	7	4.5	2.1	.3
1	1361	Creme de menthe, 72 proof	1½ fl oz	50	28	186	0	21	0	<1	t	t	.1
		Wine:											
1	6	Dessert (4 fl oz)	½ c	118	72	181[2]	<1	14[2]	0	0	0	0	0
1	7	Red	3½ fl oz	103	88	74	<1	2	0	0	0	0	0
1	8	Rosé	3½ fl oz	103	89	73	<1	2	0	0	0	0	0
1	9	White medium	3½ fl oz	103	90	70	<1	1	0	0	0	0	0
		Carbonated[3]:											
1	10	Club soda (12 fl oz)	1½ c	355	100	0	0	0	0	0	0	0	0
1	11	Cola beverage (12 fl oz)	1½ c	370	89	151	0	39	0	0	0	0	0
1	12	Diet cola (12 fl oz)	1½ c	355	100	2	0	<1	0	0	0	0	0
1	13	Diet soda pop–average (12 fl oz)	1½ c	355	100	2	0	<1	0	0	0	0	0
1	14	Ginger ale (12 fl oz)	1½ c	366	91	124	0	32	0	0	0	0	0
1	15	Grape soda (12 fl oz)	1½ c	372	89	161	0	42	0	0	0	0	0
1	16	Lemon-lime (12 fl oz)	1½ c	368	90	149	0	38	0	0	0	0	0
1	17	Orange (12 fl oz)	1½ c	372	88	177	0	46	0	0	0	0	0
1	18	Pepper-type soda (12 fl oz)	1½ c	368	89	151	0	38	0	0	0	0	0
1	19	Root beer (12 fl oz)	1½ c	370	89	152	<1	39	0	0	0	0	0
		Coffee[3]:											
1	20	Brewed	1 c	240	99	2[4]	<1	1	<1	0	0	0	0
1	21	Prepared from instant	1 c	240	99	2[4]	<1	1	0	0	0	0	0
		Fruit drinks, noncarbonated[5]:											
1	22	Fruit punch drink, canned	1 c	253	88	118	<1	30	0	<1	t	t	t
1	1358	Gatorade	1 c	230	99	39	0	11	0	0	0	0	0
1	23	Grape drink, canned	1 c	250	88	112	0	35	<1	<1	t	t	t
1	1304	Koolade, sweetened with sugar	1 c	240	100	100	0	25	0	0	0	0	0
1	1356	Koolade, sweetened with nutrasweet	1 c	240	100	4	0	0	0	0	0	0	0
		Lemonade, frozen:											
1	26	Concentrate (6-oz can)	¾ c	219	52	397	1	103	1	<1	.1	t	.1
1	27	Lemonade prepared from frozen concentrate	1 c	248	89	100	<1	26	<1	<1	t	t	t
		Limeade, frozen:											
1	28	Concentrate (6-oz can)	¾ c	218	50	408	<1	108	1	<1	t	t	.1
1	29	Limeade prepared from frozen concentrate	1 c	247	89	102	<1	27	<1	<1	t	t	t
1	24	Pineapple grapefruit, canned	1 c	250	88	117	1	29	0	<1	t	t	.1
1	25	Pineapple orange, canned	1 c	250	87	125	3	29	0	<1	t	t	.1
		Fruit and vegetable juices: see Fruit and Vegetable sections											

[1]kCalories can vary from 78 to 131 for 12 fl oz.
[2]Values are for sweet dessert wine. Dry dessert wines contain 149 kcal and 5 g of carbohydrate.
[3]Mineral content varies depending on water source.
[4]kCalorie values from USDA vary from 1 to 4 kcalories per cup.
[5]Usually less than 10% fruit juice.

(Computer code number is for West Diet Analysis program)

GRP KEY: 1 = BEV 2 = DAIRY 3 = EGGS 4 = FAT/OIL 5 = FRUIT 6 = BAKERY 7 = GRAIN 8 = FISH 9 = BEEF 10 = POULTRY
11 = SAUSAGE 12 = MIXED/FAST 13 = NUTS/SEEDS 14 = SWEETS 15 = VEG/LEG 16 = MISC 22 = SOUP/SAUCE

Chol (mg)	Calc (mg)	Iron (mg)	Magn (mg)	Phos (mg)	Pota (mg)	Sodi (mg)	Zinc (mg)	VT-A (RE)	Thia (mg)	Ribo (mg)	Niac (mg)	V-B6 (mg)	Fola (μg)	VT-C (mg)
0	18	.11	23	44	89	19	.07	0	.02	.09	1.61	.18	21	0
0	18	.14	18	43	64	10	.11	0	.03	.11	1.39	.12	15	0
0	0	.02	0	2	1	<1	.02	0	<.01	<.01	<.01	t	0	0
0	0	.02	0	2	1	<1	.02	0	<.01	<.01	<.01	0	0	0
0	0	.02	0	2	1	<1	.02	0	<.01	<.01	<.01	0	0	0
0	1	.03	1	3	15	4	.01	0	<.01	.01	.08	—	0	0
—	7	.06	1	23	15	43	.08	—	0	.03	.04	—	0	0
0	0	.04	0	0	0	3	—	0	0	0	<.01	0	0	—
0	9	.24	11	11	109	11	.08	0	.02	.02	.25	0	<1	0
0	8	.44	13	14	115	6	.10	0	<.01	.03	.08	.04	2	0
0	9	.39	10	15	102	5	.06	0	<.01	.02	.08	.03	1	0
0	9	.33	11	14	82	5	.07	0	<.01	<.01	.07	.01	<1	0
0	17	.15	4	0	6	75	.36	0	0	0	0	0	0	0
0	9	.13	3	46	4	15	.05	0	0	0	0	0	0	0
0	12	.11	4	30	0	21[6]	.28	0	.02	.08	0	0	0	0
0	14	.14	3	38	7	21[6]	.10	0	0	0	0	0	0	0
0	12	.66	3	1	5	25	.18	0	0	0	0	0	0	0
0	12	.31	4	0	3	57	.26	0	0	0	0	0	0	0
0	9	.25	2	1	4	41	.18	0	0	0	.06	0	0	0
0	19	.23	4	4	9	46	.38	0	0	0	0	0	0	0
0	12	.14	1	41	2	38	.15	0	0	0	0	0	0	0
0	19	.19	4	2	3	49	.26	0	0	0	0	0	0	0
0	4	.12	14	3	130	5	.08	0	0	.02	.53	0	<1	0
0	8	.12	9	8	87	8	.07	0	0	<.01	.69	0	0	0
0	19	.52	5	3	64	56	.31	4	.06	.06	.05	0	3	75
0	23	—	—	0	23	123	—	0	—	—	—	—	—	—
0	3	.41	5	3	13	16	.28	<1	.08	.02	.07	.02	1	85
0	0	0	0	0	0	0	0	0	0	0	0	0	0	6
0	0	0	0	0	0	0	0	0	0	0	0	0	0	6
0	15	1.58	11	19	148	8	.17	21	.06	.21	.16	.06	22	39[7]
0	4	.41	3	5	38	8	.05	5	.02	.05	.04	.02	6	10[7]
0	11	.22	60	13	129	<1	.11	<1	.02	.02	.22	.11	25	26
0	3	.06	15	3	33	<1	.03	<1	<.01	<.01	.05	.03	6	7
0	18	.77	15	14	154	34	.15	9	.08	.04	.67	.10	26	115
0	13	.67	14	10	116	9	.14	133	.08	.05	.52	.12	27	56

[6] Value for product sweetened with aspartame only; sodium is 32 mg if a blend of aspartame and sodium saccharin is used; 75 mg if just sodium saccharin is used.

[7] Vitamin C can range from 5 to 72 mg in a small can of frozen concentrate, and from 1 to 18 mg in 1 c of prepared lemonade.

(For purposes of calculations, use "0" for t, <1, <.1, <.01, etc.)

Table C–1   Food Composition

Grp	Computer Code No.	Food Description	Measure	Wt (g)	H₂O (%)	Ener (kcal)	Prot (g)	Carb (g)	Dietary Fiber (g)	Fat (g)	Fat Breakdown (g) Sat	Mono	Poly
		BEVERAGES—Con.											
1	1357	Perrier® bottled water, 6.5 fl oz bottle	1 ea	192	100	0	0	0	0	0	0	0	0
		Tea[8]:											
1	30	Brewed	1 c	240	100	2	<.01	1	0	0	0	0	0
1	31	From instant, unsweetened	1 c	237	100	2	0	<1	0	0	0	0	0
1	32	From instant, sweetened	1 c	262	91	86	0	22	0	0	0	0	0
		DAIRY											
		Butter: see Fats and Oils, #158, 159, 160											
		Cheese, natural:											
2	33	Blue	1 oz	28	42	100	6	1	0	8	5.3	2.2	.2
2	34	Brick	1 oz	28	41	105	6	1	0	8	5.3	2.4	.2
2	35	Brie	1 oz	28	48	95	6	<1	0	8	5.0	2.3	.3
2	36	Camembert	1 oz	28	52	85	6	<1	0	7	4.3	2.0	.2
		Cheddar:											
2	37	Cut pieces	1 oz	28	37	114	7	<1	0	9	6.0	2.7	.3
2	38	1″ cube	1 ea	17	37	69	4	<1	0	6	3.6	1.6	.2
2	39	Shredded	1 c	113	37	455	28	1	0	37	24	11	1
		Cottage:											
2	40	Creamed, large curd	1 c	225	79	235	28	6	0	10	6.4	3.0	.3
2	41	Creamed, small curd	1 c	210	79	215	26	6	0	9	6.0	2.7	.3
2	42	With fruit	1 c	226	72	279	22	30	0	8	4.9	2.2	.3
2	43	Low fat 2%	1 c	226	79	205	31	8	0	4	2.8	1.2	.1
2	44	Low fat 1%	1 c	226	82	164	28	6	0	2	1.5	.7	.1
2	45	Dry curd	1 c	145	80	123	25	3	0	1	.4	.2	<.1
2	46	Cream	1 oz	28	54	99	2	1	0	10	6.2	2.8	.4
2	47	Edam	1 oz	28	42	101	7	<1	0	8	5.0	2.3	.2
2	48	Feta	1 oz	28	55	75	5	1	0	6	4.2	1.3	.2
2	49	Gouda	1 oz	28	42	101	7	1	0	8	5.0	2.2	.2
2	50	Gruyère	1 oz	28	33	117	8	<1	0	9	5.4	2.9	.5
2	51	Gorgonzola	1 oz	28	39	111	7	0	0	9	5.5	2.4	.5
2	52	Liederkranz	1 oz	28	53	87	5	0	0	8	5.3	2.2	.2
2	53	Monterey jack	1 oz	28	41	106	7	<1	0	9	5.4	2.4	.2
		Mozzarella, made with:											
2	54	Whole milk	1 oz	28	54	80	5	1	0	6	3.7	1.9	.2
2	55	Part skim milk, low moisture	1 oz	28	49	80	8	1	0	5	3.1	1.4	.1
2	56	Muenster	1 oz	28	42	104	6	<1	0	8	5.4	2.5	.2
		Parmesan, grated:											
2	57	Cup, not pressed down	1 c	100	18	455	42	4	0	30	19	8.7	.7
2	58	Tablespoon	1 tbsp	5	18	23	2	<1	0	2	1	.4	<.1
2	59	Ounce	1 oz	28	18	129	12	1	0	9	5.4	2.5	.2
2	60	Provolone	1 oz	28	41	100	7	1	0	8	4.8	2.1	.2
		Ricotta, made with:											
2	61	Whole milk	1 c	246	72	428	28	7	0	32	20	8.9	1
2	62	Part skim milk	1 c	246	74	340	28	13	0	19	12	5.7	.6
2	63	Romano	1 oz	28	31	110	9	1	0	8	4.9	2.2	.2
2	64	Swiss	1 oz	28	37	107	8	1	0	8	5.0	2.1	.3
		Pasteurized processed cheese products:											
2	65	American	1 oz	28	39	106	6	<1	0	9	5.6	2.5	.3
2	66	Swiss	1 oz	28	42	95	7	1	0	7	4.6	2.0	.2
2	67	American cheese food	1 oz	28	44	93	6	2	0	7	4.4	2.0	.2
2	68	American cheese spread	1 oz	28	48	82	5	2	0	6	3.8	1.8	.2

[8]Mineral content varies depending on water source.

(Computer code number is for West Diet Analysis program)

GRP KEY: 1 = BEV 2 = DAIRY 3 = EGGS 4 = FAT/OIL 5 = FRUIT 6 = BAKERY 7 = GRAIN 8 = FISH 9 = BEEF 10 = POULTRY
11 = SAUSAGE 12 = MIXED/FAST 13 = NUTS/SEEDS 14 = SWEETS 15 = VEG/LEG 16 = MISC 22 = SOUP/SAUCE

Chol (mg)	Calc (mg)	Iron (mg)	Magn (mg)	Phos (mg)	Pota (mg)	Sodi (mg)	Zinc (mg)	VT-A (RE)	Thia (mg)	Ribo (mg)	Niac (mg)	V-B6 (mg)	Fola (µg)	VT-C (mg)
0	26	0	1	0	0	3	0	0	0	0	0	0	0	0
0	0	.05	7	1	89	7	.05	0	0	.03	.1	0	12	0
0	5	.05	5	3	47	8	.07	0	0	<.01	<.01	<.09	1	0
0	1	.04	3	3	49	1	.06	0	0	.04	.09	0	5	0
21	150	.09	7	110	73	396	.75	65	.01	.11	.29	.05	10	0
27	191	.13	7	128	38	159	.73	86	<.01	.1	.03	.02	6	0
28	52	.14	6	53	43	178	.7	57	.02	.15	.11	.07	18	0
20	110	.09	6	98	53	236	.68	71	.01	.14	.18	.06	18	0
30	204	.20	8	146	28	176	.92	86	.01	.11	.02	.02	5	0
18	124	.12	5	88	17	107	.54	52	<.01	.07	.01	.01	3	0
119	815	.77	31	579	111	701	3.51	342	.03	.42	.09	.08	21	0
34	135	.26	11	297	190	911	.8	108	.05	.37	.30	.14	27	<1
31	126	.30	11	277	177	850	.8	101	.04	.34	.27	.14	26	<1
25	108	.25	9	236	151	915	.66	81	.04	.29	.23	.12	22	<1
19	155	.36	14	340	217	918	.95	45	.05	.42	.33	.17	30	0
10	138	.32	12	302	193	918	.86	25	.05	.37	.29	.15	28	t
10	46	.33	6	151	47	19	.68	12	.04	.21	.23	.12	21	0
31	23	.34	2	30	34	84	.33	124	<.01	.06	.03	.01	4	0
25	207	.13	8	152	53	274	1.06	72	.01	.11	.02	.02	5	0
25	140	.18	5	96	18	316	.81	36	.04	.23	.29	.02	3	0
32	198	.07	8	155	34	232	1.1	49	<.01	.10	.02	.02	6	0
31	287	.06	4	172	23	95	1	98	.02	.08	.03	.02	3	0
25	149	.12	8	121	26	513	.57	103	.01	.09	.2	.04	9	0
21	110	.12	7	100	68	390	.7	91	.01	.18	.1	.04	34	0
26	212	.2	8	126	23	152	.85	81	<.01	.11	.02	.02	3	0
22	147	.05	5	105	19	106	.7	68	<.01	.07	.02	.02	2	0
15	207	.08	8	149	27	150	.83	54	<.01	.1	.03	.02	3	0
27	203	.13	8	133	38	178	.84	90	<.01	.09	.03	.02	3	0
79	1376	.95	51	807	107	1862	3.19	173	.04	.39	.32	.11	8	0
4	69	.05	3	40	5	93	.16	9	<.01	.02	.02	<.01	<1	0
22	390	.27	14	229	30	528	1	49	.01	.11	.09	.03	2	0
20	214	.15	8	141	39	248	.89	75	<.01	.09	.04	.02	3	0
124	509	.94	28	389	257	207	2.85	330	.03	.48	.26	.11	14	0
76	669	1.09	4	449	307	307	3.29	278	.05	.46	.19	.05	14	0
29	302	.23	12	215	26	340	1	40	.01	.11	.02	.03	2	0
26	272	.05	10	171	31	74	1.1	72	<.01	.1	.03	.02	2	0
27	174	.11	6	211	46	406	.93	82	.01	.1	.02	.02	2	0
24	219	.17	8	216	61	388	1.02	65	<.01	.08	.01	.01	2	0
18	163	.24	9	130	79	337	.85	62	.01	.13	.04	.02	2	0
16	159	.09	8	201	69	381	.78	54	.01	.12	.04	.03	2	0

(For purposes of calculations, use "0" for t, <1, <.1, <.01, etc.)

Table C–1 Food Composition

Grp	Computer Code No.	Food Description	Measure	Wt (g)	H₂O (%)	Ener (kcal)	Prot (g)	Carb (g)	Dietary Fiber (g)	Fat (g)	Fat Breakdown (g) Sat	Mono	Poly
		DAIRY—Con.											
		Cream, sweet:											
		Half and half (cream and milk):											
2	69	Cup	1 c	242	81	315	7	10	0	28	17	8	1
2	70	Tablespoon	1 tbsp	15	81	20	<1	1	0	2	1.1	.5	.1
		Light, coffee or table:											
2	71	Cup	1 c	240	74	469	6	9	0	46	29	13	1.7
2	72	Tablespoon	1 tbsp	15	74	30	<1	1	0	3	1.8	.8	.1
		Light whipping cream, liquid:											
2	73	Cup	1 c	239	64	699	5	7	0	74	46	22	2.1
2	74	Tablespoon	1 tbsp	15	64	44	<1	<1	0	5	2.9	1.4	.1
		Heavy whipping cream, liquid[9]:											
2	75	Cup	1 c	238	58	821	5	7	0	88	55	25	3.3
2	76	Tablespoon	1 tbsp	15	58	51	<1	<1	0	6	3.5	1.6	.2
		Whipped cream, pressurized[9]:											
2	77	Cup	1 c	60	61	154	2	7	0	13	8.3	3.9	.5
2	78	Tablespoon	1 tbsp	4	61	10	<1	<1	0	1	.5	.2	<.1
		Cream, sour, cultured:											
2	79	Cup	1 c	230	71	493	7	10	0	48	30	14	1.8
2	80	Tablespoon	1 tbsp	14	71	30	<1	1	0	3	1.8	.9	.1
		Cream products—imitation and part dairy:											
		Coffee whitener:											
2	81	Frozen or liquid	1 tbsp	15	77	20	<1	2	0	2	1.4	t	t
2	82	Powdered	1 tsp	2	2	11	<1	1	0	1	.6	t	t
		Dessert topping, frozen:											
2	83	Cup	1 c	75	50	239	1	17	0	19	16	1.2	.4
2	84	Tablespoon	1 tbsp	5	50	15	<1	1	0	1	1.0	.1	t
		Dessert topping from mix:											
2	85	Cup	1 c	80	67	151	3	13	0	10	8.6	.7	.2
2	86	Tablespoon	1 tbsp	5	67	9	<1	1	0	1	.5	<.1	t
		Dessert topping, pressurized:											
2	87	Cup	1 c	70	60	185	1	11	0	16	13	1.4	.2
2	88	Tablespoon	1 tbsp	4	60	11	<1	1	0	1	.8	.1	t
		Sour cream imitation:											
2	91	Cup	1 c	230	71	479	6	15	0	45	41	1.4	.1
2	92	Tablespoon	1 tbsp	14	71	29	<1	1	0	3	2.5	.1	t
		Sour dressing, part dairy:											
2	89	Cup	1 c	235	75	416	8	11	0	39	31	4.6	1.1
2	90	Tablespoon	1 tbsp	15	75	25	<1	1	0	2	2.0	.3	.1
		Milk, fluid:											
2	93	Whole milk	1 c	244	88	150	8	11	0	8	5.1	2.4	.3
2	94	2% low-fat milk	1 c	244	89	121	8	12	0	5	2.9	1.4	.2
2	95	2% milk solids added[10]	1 c	245	89	125	9	12	0	5	2.9	1.4	.2
2	96	1% low-fat milk	1 c	244	90	102	8	12	0	3	1.6	.8	.1
2	97	1% milk solids added[10]	1 c	245	90	105	9	12	0	2	1.5	.7	.1
2	98	Skim milk	1 c	245	91	86	8	12	0	<1	.3	.1	t
2	99	Skim milk solids added[10]	1 c	245	90	91	9	12	0	1	.4	.2	t
2	100	Buttermilk	1 c	245	90	99	8	12	0	2	1.3	.6	.1

[9]For whipped cream, (non-pressurized), double the liquid cream volume of codes 75,76 or 73,74. One tablespoon liquid cream becomes 2 tablespoons when "whipped".
[10]Milk solids added, label claims less than 10 g protein per cup.

(Computer code number is for West Diet Analysis program)

GRP KEY: 1 = BEV 2 = DAIRY 3 = EGGS 4 = FAT/OIL 5 = FRUIT 6 = BAKERY 7 = GRAIN 8 = FISH 9 = BEEF 10 = POULTRY
11 = SAUSAGE 12 = MIXED/FAST 13 = NUTS/SEEDS 14 = SWEETS 15 = VEG/LEG 16 = MISC 22 = SOUP/SAUCE

Chol (mg)	Calc (mg)	Iron (mg)	Magn (mg)	Phos (mg)	Pota (mg)	Sodi (mg)	Zinc (mg)	VT-A (RE)	Thia (mg)	Ribo (mg)	Niac (mg)	V-B6 (mg)	Fola (µg)	VT-C (mg)
89	254	.17	25	230	314	98	1.23	259	.09	.36	.19	.09	6	2
6	16	.01	2	14	20	6	.08	16	.01	.02	.01	<.01	<1	<1
159	231	.1	21	192	292	95	.65	437	.08	.36	.14	.08	6	2
10	14	.01	1	12	18	6	.04	27	<.01	.02	.01	<.01	<1	<1
265	166	.07	17	146	231	82	.60	705	.06	.30	.1	.07	9	1
17	10	<.01	1	9	15	5	.04	44	<.01	.02	.01	<.01	1	<1
326	154	.07	17	149	179	89	.55	1002	.05	.26	.09	.06	10	1
20	10	<.01	1	9	11	6	.03	63	<.01	.02	.01	<.01	1	<1
46	61	.03	6	54	88	78	.22	124	.02	.04	.04	.03	1	0
3	4	<.01	<1	3	5	5	.01	8	<.01	<.01	<.01	<.01	<1	0
102	268	.14	26	195	331	123	.69	448	.08	.34	.15	.04	25	2
6	16	.01	2	12	20	7	.04	27	<.01	.02	.01	<.01	2	<1
0	1	<.01	<1	10	29	12	<.01	1^{10}	0	0	0	0	0	0
0	<1	.02	<1	8	16	4	.01	$<1^{10}$	0	<.01	0	0	0	0
0	5	.09	1	6	14	19	.03	65^{11}	0	0	0	0	0	0
0	<1	.01	<1	<1	1	1	<.01	4^{11}	0	0	0	0	0	0
8	72	.03	8	69	121	53	.22	39^{11}	.02	.09	.05	.02	3	1
<1	5	<.01	<1	4	8	3	.14	3^{11}	<.01	<.01	<.01	<.01	<1	<1
0	4	.01	1	13	13	43	.01	33^{11}	0	0	0	0	0	0
0	<1	<.01	<1	1	1	3	<.01	2^{11}	0	0	0	0	0	0
0	6	.01	—	102	369	235	0	0	0	0	0	0	0	0
0	<1	<.01	—	6	23	14	0	0	0	0	0	0	0	0
213	266	.07	23	205	381	113	.87	5^{11}	.09	.38	.17	.04	28	2
1	17	<.01	2	13	24	7	.05	$<1^{11}$	.01	.02	.01	<.01	2	<1
33	291	.12	33	228	370	120	.94	76	.09	.4	.2	.1	12	2
22	297	.12	33	232	377	122	.96	140	.1	.4	.21	.1	12	2
18	314	.12	35	245	397	128	.98	140	.1	.42	.22	.11	12	2
10	300	.12	34	235	381	123	.96	145	.1	.41	.21	.11	12	2
10	314	.12	35	245	397	128	.98	145	.1	.42	.22	.11	12	2
4	302	.1	28	247	406	126	.92	149	.09	.34	.22	.1	14	2
5	316	.12	37	255	419	130	1	149	.1	.43	.22	.11	12	2
9	285	.12	26	219	371	257	1.03	20	.08	.38	.14	.08	12	2

[11]Vitamin A value is from beta-carotene used for coloring.

(For purposes of calculations, use "0" for t, <1, <.1, <.01, etc.)

Table C–1   Food Composition

Grp	Computer Code No.	Food Description	Measure	Wt (g)	H₂O (%)	Ener (kcal)	Prot (g)	Carb (g)	Dietary Fiber (g)	Fat (g)	Fat Breakdown (g)		
											Sat	Mono	Poly
		DAIRY—Con.											
		Milk, canned:											
2	101	Sweetened condensed	1 c	306	27	982	24	166	0	27	17	7.4	1
2	102	Evaporated, whole	1 c	252	74	340	17	25	0	20	12	5.9	.6
2	103	Evaporated, skim	1 c	255	79	200	19	29	0	1	.3	.2	t
		Milk, dried:											
2	104	Buttermilk	1 c	120	3	464	41	59	0	7	4.3	2.0	.3
		Instant, nonfat:											
2	105	Envelope[12]	1 ea	91	4	326	32	48	0	1	.4	.2	t
2	106	Cup	1 c	68	4	244	24	36	0	1	.3	.1	t
2	107	Goat milk	1 c	244	87	168	9	11	0	10	6.5	2.7	.4
2	108	Kefir[13]	1 c	233	82	122	9	9	0	5	2.9	1.2	.1
		Milk beverages and powdered mixes:											
		Chocolate:											
2	109	Whole	1 c	250	82	210	8	26	4	8	5.3	2.5	.3
2	110	2% fat	1 c	250	84	180	8	26	4	5	3.1	1.5	.2
2	111	1% fat	1 c	250	84	160	8	26	4	3	1.5	.8	.1
		Chocolate-flavored beverages:											
2	112	Powder containing nonfat dry milk:	1 oz	28	1	100	4	23	<1	1	.7	.4	t
2	113	Drink prepared with water	¾ c	206	86	100	4	23	<1	1	.7	.4	t
2	114	Powder without nonfat dry milk:	¾ oz	22	<1	75	1	20	<1	1	.4	.2	t
2	115	Drink prepared with whole milk	1 c	266	81	226	9	31	<1	9	5.5	2.6	.3
2	116	Eggnog, commercial	1 c	254	74	342	10	34	0	19	11	5.7	.9
		Instant Breakfast:											
2	1027	Envelope, dry powder only	1 ea	37	3	130	7	23	0	0	0	0	0
2	1028	Prepared with whole milk	1 c	281	87	280	15	34	0	8	5.1	2.4	.3
2	1029	Prepared with 2% milk	1 c	281	88	251	15	35	0	5	2.9	1.4	.2
2	1283	Prepared with 1% milk	1 c	281	89	232	15	35	0	3	1.5	.7	.1
2	1284	Prepared with skim milk	1 c	282	89	216	15	35	0	<1	.3	.1	t
		Malted milk, chocolate flavor:											
2	117	Powder[14], 3 heaping tsp:	¾ oz	21	1	79	1	18	<1	1	.5	.2	.1
2	118	Drink prepared with whole milk	1 c	265	81	229	9	30	<1	9	5.2	2.6	.4
		Malted milk, natural flavor:											
2	119	Powder[14], 3 heaping tsp:	¾ oz	21	2	87	2	16	<1	2	.9	.4	.3
2	120	Drink prepared with whole milk	1 c	265	81	237	10	27	<1	10	6.0	2.8	.6
		Milk shakes:											
2	121	Chocolate (10 fl oz)	1¼ c	283	72	360	10	58	<1	11	6.6	3.0	.4
2	122	Vanilla (10 fl oz)	1¼ c	283	75	314	10	51	<1	8	5.3	2.4	.3
		Milk desserts:											
2	134	Custard, baked	1 c	265	77	305	14	29	0	15	6.8	5.4	.7
		Ice cream, regular vanilla (about 11% fat):											
		Hardened:											
2	123	½ gallon	½ gal	1064	61	2153	38	254	0	115	71	33	4
2	124	Cup	1 c	133	61	269	5	32	0	14	8.3	4.1	.5
2	125	Fluid ounces	3 oz	50	61	101	2	12	0	5	3.3	1.6	.2
2	126	Soft serve	1 c	173	60	377	7	38	0	22	14	6.7	1.0
		Ice cream, rich vanilla (about 16% fat):											
		Hardened:											
2	127	½ gallon	½ gal	1188	59	2805	33	256	0	190	118	55	7
2	128	Cup	1 c	148	59	349	4	32	0	24	15	6.8	.9

[12]Yields 1 qt fluid milk when reconstituted according to package directions.
[13]Most values provided by product labeling.
[14]The latest USDA data from *Handbook 8–14* on beverages updates previous USDA data.

(Computer code number is for West Diet Analysis program)

GRP KEY: 1 = BEV   2 = DAIRY   3 = EGGS   4 = FAT/OIL   5 = FRUIT   6 = BAKERY   7 = GRAIN   8 = FISH   9 = BEEF   10 = POULTRY
           11 = SAUSAGE   12 = MIXED/FAST   13 = NUTS/SEEDS   14 = SWEETS   15 = VEG/LEG   16 = MISC   22 = SOUP/SAUCE

Chol (mg)	Calc (mg)	Iron (mg)	Magn (mg)	Phos (mg)	Pota (mg)	Sodi (mg)	Zinc (mg)	VT-A (RE)	Thia (mg)	Ribo (mg)	Niac (mg)	V-B6 (mg)	Fola (µg)	VT-C (mg)
104	868	.58	78	775	1136	389	2.88	248	.28	1.27	.64	.16	34	8
74	657	.48	60	510	764	267	1.94	136	.12	.8	.49	.13	18	5
10	738	.7	68	497	845	293	2.18	300	.11	.8	.4	.14	22	3
83	1421	.36	131	1119	1910	621	4.82	65	.47	1.9	1.05	.41	57	7
16	1120	.28	107	896	1552	500	4.01	646[15]	.38	1.59	.81	.31	45	5
12	837	.21	80	670	1160	373	3.06	483[15]	.28	1.19	.61	.24	34	4
28	326	.12	34	270	499	122	.73	137	.12	.34	.68	.11	2	3
10	350	.5	28	319	205	50	.9	155	.45	.44	.3	.09	20	6
31	280	.6	33	251	417	149	1.02	73	.09	.41	.31	.1	12	2
17	284	.6	33	254	422	151	.91	143	.09	.41	.32	.1	12	2
7	287	.6	33	256	425	152	1.02	148	.1	.42	.32	.1	12	2
1	89	.29	23	88	223	139	1.26	1	.03	.17	.18	.04	3	1
1	89	.29	23	88	223	139	1.26	1	.03	.17	.18	.04	3	1
0	8	.68	21	28	128	45	.33	1	.01	.03	.11	<.01	4	<1
33	300	.8	54	256	498	165	1.26	76	.1	.43	.32	.1	12	3
149	330	.51	47	278	420	138	1.17	203	.09	.48	.27	.13	2	4
0	10	7.9	80	15	0	166	3.00	175	.30	.07	5.00	.40	100	27
33	301	8.0	113	243	370	286	3.95	251	.39	.46	5.20	.50	112	29
18	307	8.0	113	247	377	289	3.96	315	.40	.47	5.21	.51	112	29
10	310	8.0	124	250	381	289	3.96	315	.40	.48	5.21	.51	112	29
4	312	8.0	108	262	406	292	3.96	327	.39	.41	5.22	.50	113	29
1	13	.48	15	37	130	53	.17	4	.04	.04	.42	.03	4	<1
34	304	.6	47	265	499	172	1.09	80	13	.44	.63	.14	16	3
4	63	.16	20	75	159	103	.21	19	.11	.19	1.1	.09	10	1
37	354	.27	52	303	529	223	1.14	94	.2	.59	1.31	.19	22	3
37	319	.88	47	288	567	273	1.15	64	.16	.69	.46	.14	10	1
32	344	.26	35	289	492	232	1.01	90	.13	.52	.52	.15	9	2
213	297	1.1	37	310	387	209	1.53	146	.11	.5	.3	.13	24	1
478	1405	.96	149	1075	2053	926	11.3	1064	.42	2.63	1.08	.49	22	6
59	176	.12	18	134	257	116	1.41	133	.05	.33	.13	.06	3	1
23	66	.05	7	50	97	44	.53	50	.02	.12	.05	.02	1	<1
153	236	.43	25	199	338	153	1.99	199	.08	.45	.18	.1	9	1
701	1212	.83	131	927	1770	867	9.74	1758	.36	2.27	.93	.43	23	5
88	151	.1	16	115	221	108	1.21	219	.04	.28	.12	.05	2	1

[15]With added vitamin A.

C

(For purposes of calculations, use "0" for t, <1, <.1, <.01, etc.)

Table C–1 Food Composition

Grp	Computer Code No.	Food Description	Measure	Wt (g)	H₂O (%)	Ener (kcal)	Prot (g)	Carb (g)	Dietary Fiber (g)	Fat (g)	Fat Breakdown (g) Sat	Mono	Poly
		DAIRY—Con.											
		Milk Desserts—Con.											
		Ice milk, vanilla (about 4% fat):											
		Hardened:											
2	129	½ gallon	½ gal	1048	69	1467	41	232	0	45	28	13	1.7
2	130	Cup	1 c	131	69	184	5	29	0	6	3.5	1.6	.2
2	131	Soft serve (about 3% fat)	1 c	175	70	223	8	38	0	5	2.9	1.3	.2
		Pudding, canned, 5 oz can = .55 cup:											
2	135	Chocolate	1 ea	142	68	205	3	30	<1	11	9.5	.5	.1
2	136	Tapioca	1 ea	142	74	160	3	28	0	5	4.8	t	t
2	137	Vanilla	1 ea	142	69	220	2	33	0	10	9.5	.3	.1
		Puddings, prepared from dry mix with whole milk:											
2	138	Chocolate, instant	1 c	260	71	310	8	54	<1	8	4.6	2.2	.4
2	139	Chocolate, regular, cooked	½ c	130	73	150	4	25	<1	4	2.4	1.1	.1
2	140	Rice, cooked	½ c	132	73	155	4	27	<1	4	2.3	1.1	.1
2	141	Tapioca, cooked	½ c	130	75	145	4	25	0	4	2.3	1.1	.1
2	142	Vanilla, instant	½ c	130	73	150	4	27	0	4	2.2	1.1	.2
2	143	Vanilla, regular, cooked	½ c	130	74	145	4	25	0	4	2.3	1	.1
		Sherbet (2% fat):											
2	132	½ gallon	½ gal	1542	66	2158	17	469	0	31	19	8.8	1.1
2	133	Cup	1 c	193	66	270	2	59	0	4	2.4	1.1	.1
2	144	Soy milk	1 c	240	93	79	7	4	0	5	.5	.8	2.0
2	1584	Yogurt, frozen, low fat[16]	½ c	87	70	110	4	17	0	2	1.1	.5	<1
		Yogurt, low fat:											
2	145	Fruit added[17]	1 c	227	74	231	10	43	<1	2	1.6	.7	.1
2	146	Plain	1 c	227	85	144	12	16	0	3	2.3	1.0	.1
2	147	Vanilla or coffee flavor	1 c	227	79	193	11	31	0	3	1.8	.8	.1
2	148	Yogurt, made with nonfat milk	1 c	227	85	127	13	17	0	<1	.3	.1	t
2	149	Yogurt, made with whole milk	1 c	227	88	138	8	11	0	7	4.8	2.0	.2
		EGGS[18]											
		Raw, large:											
3	150	Whole, without shell	1 ea	50	75	75	6	1	0	5	1.6	1.6	.7
3	151	White	1 ea	33.4	88	17	4	<1	0	0	0	0	0
3	152	Yolk	1 ea	16.6	49	59	3	<1	0	5	1.6	1.9	.7
		Cooked:											
3	153	Fried in margarine	1 ea	46	69	91	6	1	0	7	1.9	2.7	1.3
3	154	Hard-cooked, shell removed	1 ea	50	75	79	6	1	0	5	1.6	2.0	.7
3	155	Hard-cooked, chopped	1 c	136	75	211	17	2	0	14	4.5	5.5	2.0
3	156	Poached, no added salt	1 ea	50	75	75	6	1	0	5	1.5	1.9	.7
3	157	Scrambled with milk and margarine	1 ea	61	73	100	7	1	0	7	2.2	2.9	1.3
		FATS and OILS											
		Butter:											
4	158	Stick	½ c	113	16	813	1	<1	0	92	57	27	3.4
4	159	Tablespoon	1 tbsp	14	16	100	<1	<1	0	12	7.2	3.3	.4
4	160	Pat (about 1 tsp)[19]	1 ea	5	16	34	<1	<1	0	4	2.5	1.2	.2

[16] Data is a composite of USDA information and several manufacturers.
[17] Carbohydrate and kcalories vary widely—consult label if more precise values are needed.
[18] This data is newest revised information from the USDA with 24% less cholesterol.
[19] Pat is 1″ square, ⅓″ thick; about 1 tsp; 90 per lb.

(Computer code number is for West Diet Analysis program)

GRP KEY: 1 = BEV 2 = DAIRY 3 = EGGS 4 = FAT/OIL 5 = FRUIT 6 = BAKERY 7 = GRAIN 8 = FISH 9 = BEEF 10 = POULTRY 11 = SAUSAGE 12 = MIXED/FAST 13 = NUTS/SEEDS 14 = SWEETS 15 = VEG/LEG 16 = MISC 22 = SOUP/SAUCE

Chol (mg)	Calc (mg)	Iron (mg)	Magn (mg)	Phos (mg)	Pota (mg)	Sodi (mg)	Zinc (mg)	VT-A (RE)	Thia (mg)	Ribo (mg)	Niac (mg)	V-B6 (mg)	Fola (μg)	VT-C (mg)
146	1404	1.47	147	1035	2117	838	4.40	419	.61	2.78	.94	.68	21	6
18	176	.18	19	129	265	105	.55	52	.08	.35	.12	.09	3	1
13	274	.28	29	202	412	163	.86	44	.12	.54	.18	.13	5	1
1	74	1.2	24	117	254	285	.70	31	.04	.17	.6	.03	3	<1
1	119	.3	24	113	212	252	.70	<1	.03	.14	.4	.03	3	<1
1	79	.2	24	94	155	305	.70	<1	.03	.12	.6	.03	3	<1
28	260	.6	48	658	352	880	1.18	66	.08	.36	.22	.13	10	2
15	146	.2	24	120	190	167	.59	34	.05	.2	.13	.06	4	1
15	133	.5	16	110	165	140	.60	33	.10	.18	.6	.05	6	1
15	131	.1	16	103	167	152	.50	34	.04	.18	.1	.05	6	1
15	129	.1	16	273	164	375	.50	33	.04	.17	.1	.05	6	1
15	132	.1	16	102	166	178	.50	34	.04	.18	.1	.05	6	1
113	827	2.47	124	594	1588	709	10.6	308	.26	.71	1.05	.2	108	31
14	103	.31	15	74	198	88	1.33	39	.03	.09	.13	.03	14	4
0	10	1.38	45	117	338	30	.54	8	.39	.17	.35	.10	4	0
7	120	.05	5	980	148	45	.56	17	.03	.14	.07	.03	7	<1
10	345	.16	31	325	442	125	1.68	25	.08	.4	.22	.09	21	2
14	415	.18	40	326	531	159	2.02	36	.10	.49	.26	.11	25	2
11	388	.16	36	306	497	150	1.88	30	.10	.46	.24	.10	23	2
4	452	.2	43	354	579	173	2.20	5	.11	.53	.28	.12	28	2
30	275	.11	27	216	352	104	1.34	68	.07	.32	.17	.07	16	1
213	25	.72	5	89	60	61	.55	97	.03	.25	.04	.07	25	0
0	2	.01	4	4	48	55	<.1	0	<.01	.15	.03	<.01	1	0
213	23	.7	1	81	16	7	.54	97	.03	.11	.01	.07	24	0
211	25	.72	5	89	61	162	.55	114	.03	.24	.04	.07	18	0
215	25	.72	5	86	63	62	.55	84	.03	.26	.03	.06	22	0
574	68	1.95	14	233	171	169	1.5	227	.09	.70	.09	.16	61	0
212	25	.72	5	89	60	61	.55	95	.03	.22	.03	.06	18	0
215	44	.72	7	104	84	171	.6	119	.03	.26	.05	.07	18	0
247	27	.18	2	26	29	933[20]	.06	852[21]	.01	.04	.05	<.01	3	0
31	3	.02	<1	3	4	116[20]	.01	106[21]	<.01	<.01	.01	t	<1	0
11	1	.01	<1	1	1	41[20]	<.01	38[21]	t	<.01	<.01	t	<1	0

[20] For salted butter; unsalted butter contains 12 mg sodium per stick or ½ c, 1.5 mg/tbsp, or .5 mg/pat.

[21] Values for vitamin A are a year-round average.

(For purposes of calculations, use "0" for t, <1, <.1, <.01, etc.)

Table C–1 Food Composition

Grp	Computer Code No.	Food Description	Measure	Wt (g)	H$_2$O (%)	Ener (kcal)	Prot (g)	Carb (g)	Dietary Fiber (g)	Fat (g)	Fat Breakdown (g)		
											Sat	Mono	Poly
FATS and OILS—Con.													
		Fats, cooking:											
4	1363	Bacon fat	1 tbsp	14	<1	126	0	0	0	14	5.0	6.7	1.7
4	1362	Beef fat/tallow	1 c	205	0	1837	0	0	0	205	102	85.6	8.2
4	1364	Chicken fat	1 c	205	<1	1846	0	0	0	205	61.2	92.0	43.0
		Vegetable shortening:											
4	161	Cup	1 c	205	0	1812	0	0	0	205	51	91	54
4	162	Tablespoon	1 tbsp	13	0	15	0	0	0	13	3.3	5.8	3.4
		Lard:											
4	163	Cup	1 c	205	0	1849	0	0	0	205	80	93	23
4	164	Tablespoon	1 tbsp	13	0	115	0	0	0	13	5.1	5.9	1.5
		Margarine:											
		Imitation (about 40% fat), soft:											
4	165	8-oz container	8 oz	227	58	785	1	1	0	88	18	36	31
4	166	Tablespoon	1 tbsp	14	58	50	<.1	<.1	0	6	1.1	2.2	2.0
		Regular, hard (about 80% fat):											
4	167	Cup	½ c	113	16	812	1	1	0	91	18	41	29
4	168	Tablespoon	1 tbsp	14	16	100	<1	<1	0	11	2.3	5.1	3.6
4	169	Pat[19]	1 ea	5	16	36	<.1	<.1	0	4	.8	1.8	1.3
		Regular, soft (about 80% fat):											
4	170	8-oz container	8 oz	227	16	1626	2	1	0	183	31	65	79
4	171	Tablespoon	1 tbsp	14	16	100	1	<.1	0	11	2.0	4.0	4.9
		Spread (about 60% fat), hard:											
4	172	Cup	½ c	113	37	610	1	0	0	69	16	29	20
4	173	Tablespoon	1 tbsp	14	37	75	<.1	0	0	9	2.0	3.6	2.5
4	174	Pat[19]	1 ea	5	37	25	<.1	0	0	3	.7	1.3	.9
		Spread (about 60% fat), soft:											
4	175	8 oz container	8 oz	227	37	1225	1	0	0	138	29	72	31
4	176	Tablespoon	1 tbsp	14	37	75	<.1	0	0	9	1.8	4.4	1.9
		Oils:											
		Canola:											
4	1585	Cup	1 c	218	0	1927	0	0	0	218	13.1	128	65
4	1586	Tablespoon	1 tbsp	14	0	125	0	0	0	14	.8	8.2	4.1
		Corn:											
4	177	Cup	1 c	218	0	1927	0	0	0	218	28	53	128
4	178	Tablespoon	1 tbsp	14	0	125	0	0	0	14	1.8	3.4	8.2
		Olive:											
4	179	Cup	1 c	216	0	1909	0	0	0	216	29	159	18
4	180	Tablespoon	1 tbsp	14	0	125	0	0	0	14	1.9	10	1.2
		Peanut:											
4	181	Cup	1 c	216	0	1909	0	0	0	216	36	100	69
4	182	Tablespoon	1 tbsp	14	0	125	0	0	0	14	2.4	6.5	4.5
		Safflower:											
4	183	Cup	1 c	218	0	1927	0	0	0	218	20	26	162
4	184	Tablespoon	1 tbsp	14	0	125	0	0	0	14	1.3	1.7	10
		Soybean:											
4	185	Cup	1 c	218	0	1927	0	0	0	218	33	94	82
4	186	Tablespoon	1 tbsp	14	0	125	0	0	0	14	2	6	5
		Soybean/cottonseed:											
4	187	Cup	1 c	218	0	1927	0	0	0	218	39	64	105
4	188	Tablespoon	1 tbsp	14	0	125	0	0	0	14	2.5	4	7

[19]Pat is 1″ square, ⅓″ thick; about 1 tsp; 90 per lb.

(Computer code number is for West Diet Analysis program)

C

GRP KEY: 1=BEV   2=DAIRY   3=EGGS   4=FAT/OIL   5=FRUIT   6=BAKERY   7=GRAIN   8=FISH   9=BEEF   10=POULTRY
11=SAUSAGE   12=MIXED/FAST   13=NUTS/SEEDS   14=SWEETS   15=VEG/LEG   16=MISC   22=SOUP/SAUCE

C

Chol (mg)	Calc (mg)	Iron (mg)	Magn (mg)	Phos (mg)	Pota (mg)	Sodi (mg)	Zinc (mg)	VT-A (RE)	Thia (mg)	Ribo (mg)	Niac (mg)	V-B6 (mg)	Fola (μg)	VT-C (mg)
84	–	–	–	–	–	140	–	<1	–	–	–	0	–	–
223	2	.41	–	27	0	0	–	<1	<.01	<.01	<.01	<.01	<1	0
174	–	–	–	–	–	–	–	350	–	–	–	0	0	0
0	0	0	0	0	0	0	.10	0	0	0	0	0	0	0
0	0	0	0	0	0	0	0	0	0	0	0	0	0	0
195	<1	0	<1	6	<1	<1	.23	0	0	0	0	0	0	0
12	<1	0	<1	<1	<1	<1	.01	0	0	0	0	0	0	0
0	40	0	3	31	57	2178[22]	.23	2254[23]	.01	.05	.03	.01	2	<1
0	3	0	<1	2	4	136[22]	.03	141[23]	<.01	<.01	<.01	<.01	<1	<1
0	34	.07	3	26	48	1066[22]	.23	1122[23]	.01	.04	.03	.01	1	<1
0	4	.01	<1	3	6	133[22]	.03	139[23]	<.01	<.01	<.01	<.01	<1	<1
0	2	.01	<1	1	2	47[22]	.01	50[23]	t	<.01	<.01	t	<1	<1
0	60	0	5	46	86	2448[22]	.46	2254[23]	.02	.07	.05	.02	2	<1
0	4	0	<1	3	5	153[22]	.03	140[23]	<.01	<.01	<.01	<.01	<1	<1
0	24	0	2	18	34	1123[22]	.17	1122[23]	<.01	.03	.02	.01	1	<1
0	3	0	<1	2	4	139[22]	.02	139[23]	<.01	<.01	<.01	<.01	<1	<1
0	1	0	<1	1	2	50[22]	.01	50[23]	t	<.01	<.01	t	<1	<1
0	47	0	4	37	68	2256[22]	.35	2254[23]	.16	.06	.04	.01	2	<1
0	3	0	<1	2	4	139[22]	.02	139[23]	.01	<.01	<.01	<.01	<1	<1
0	0	0	0	0	0	0	–	0	0	0	0	0	0	0
0	0	0	0	0	0	0	–	0	0	0	0	0	0	0
0	0	.01	0	2	0	0	.02	0	0	0	0	0	<1	0
0	0	0	0	0	0	0	.03	0	0	0	0	0	0	0
0	<1	.83	<1	3	0	0	.13	0	0	0	0	0	<1	0
0	<1	.05	<1	<1	0	0	.01	0	0	0	0	0	0	0
0	t	.06	<1	0	0	0	.02	t	0	0	0	0	<1	0
0	t	<.01	<1	0	0	0	<.01	t	0	0	0	0	0	0
0	0	0	–	0	0	0	.41	0	0	0	0	0	0	0
0	0	0	–	0	0	0	.03	0	0	0	0	0	0	0
0	<1	.05	<1	1	0	0	.4	0	0	0	0	0	<1	0
0	t	0	<1	t	0	0	.03	0	0	0	0	0	t	0
0	0	0	–	0	0	0	.4	0	0	0	0	0	<1	0
0	0	0	–	0	0	0	.03	0	0	0	0	0	0	0

[22] For salted margarine.
[23] Based on average vitamin A content of fortified margarine. Federal specifications require a minimum of 15,000 IU/lb.

(For purposes of calculations, use "0" for t, <1, <.1, <.01, etc.)

Table C–1 Food Composition

Grp	Computer Code No.	Food Description	Measure	Wt (g)	H₂O (%)	Ener (kcal)	Prot (g)	Carb (g)	Dietary Fiber (g)	Fat (g)	Fat Breakdown (g) Sat	Mono	Poly
		FATS and OILS—Con.											
		Oils—Con.											
		Sunflower:											
4	189	Cup	1 c	218	0	1927	0	0	0	218	23	43	143
4	190	Tablespoon	1 tbsp	14	0	125	0	0	0	14	1.4	2.7	9.2
		Salad dressings/ sandwich spreads:											
4	191	Blue cheese salad dressing	1 tbsp	15	32	75	1	1	<1	8	1.5	1.9	4.3
		French salad dressing:											
4	192	Regular	1 tbsp	16	35	85	<.1	1	<1	9	1.4	4	3.5
4	193	Low calorie	1 tbsp	16	75	24	<.1	2	<1	2	.2	.3	1
		Italian salad dressing:											
4	194	Regular	1 tbsp	14	34	80	<1	1	<1	9	1.3	3.7	3.2
4	195	Low calorie	1 tbsp	15	86	5	<.1	1	<1	1.5	.2	.3	.9
		Mayonnaise:											
4	196	Regular	1 tbsp	14	15	100	<1	<1	0	11	1.7	3.2	5.8
4	197	Imitation, low calorie	1 tbsp	15	63	35	0	2	0	3	.5	.7	1.6
4	198	Ranch style salad dressing	½ c	119	35	435	4	6	0	45	6.7	19	17
		Mayo type salad dressing:											
4	199	Regular	1 tbsp	15	40	58	<1	4	0	5	.7	1.4	2.7
4	1030	Low calorie	1 tbsp	15	63	35	<1	2	0	3	.5	.8	1.4
4	200	Tartar sauce	1 tbsp	14	34	74	<1	1	<1	8	1.2	2.6	3.9
		Thousand Island salad dressing:											
4	201	Regular	1 tbsp	16	46	60	<1	2	<1	6	1.0	1.3	3.2
4	202	Low calorie	1 tbsp	15	69	25	<1	2	<1	2	.2	.4	.9
		Salad dressings, prepared from home recipe:											
4	203	Cooked type[24]	1 tbsp	16	69	25	1	2	0	2	.5	.6	.3
4	204	Vinegar and oil	1 tbsp	16	47	70	0	0	0	8	1.5	2.4	3.9
		FRUITS and FRUIT JUICES											
		Apples:											
		Fresh, raw, with peel:											
5	205	2¾″ diam (about 3 per lb with cores)	1 ea	138	84	80	<1	21	3	<1	.1	t	.1
5	206	3¼″ diam (about 2 per lb with cores)	1 ea	212	84	125	<1	32	5	1	.1	t	.2
5	207	Raw, peeled slices	1 c	110	84	65	<1	16	3	<1	.1	t	.1
5	208	Dried, sulfured	10 ea	64	32	155	1	42	8	<1	t	t	.1
5	209	Apple juice, bottled or canned	1 c	248	88	116	<1	29	<1	<1	.1	t	.1
		Applesauce:											
5	210	Sweetened	1 c	255	80	195	<1	51	4	<1	<.1	t	.1
5	211	Unsweetened	1 c	244	88	106	<1	28	4	<1	<.1	t	<.1
		Apricots:											
5	212	Raw, without pits (about 12 per lb with pits)	3 ea	106	86	51	1	12	2	<1	t	.2	.1
		Canned (fruit and liquid):											
5	213	Heavy syrup	1 c	258	78	214	1	55	4	<1	t	.1	t
5	214	Halves	3 ea	85	78	70	<1	18	1	<.1	t	t	t
5	215	Juice pack	1 c	248	87	119	2	31	4	<.1	t	t	t
5	216	Halves	3 ea	84	87	40	1	10	1	<.1	t	t	t
		Dried:											
5	217	Dried halves	10 ea	35	31	83	1	22	3	<1	t	.1	t
5	218	Cooked, unsweetened, with liquid	1 c	250	75	210	3	55	7	<1	t	.2	.1
5	219	Apricot nectar, canned	1 c	251	85	141	1	36	2	<1	t	.1	t

[24] Fatty acid values apply to product made with regular margarine.

(Computer code number is for West Diet Analysis program)

GRP KEY: 1 = BEV   2 = DAIRY   3 = EGGS   4 = FAT/OIL   5 = FRUIT   6 = BAKERY   7 = GRAIN   8 = FISH   9 = BEEF   10 = POULTRY
11 = SAUSAGE   12 = MIXED/FAST   13 = NUTS/SEEDS   14 = SWEETS   15 = VEG/LEG   16 = MISC   22 = SOUP/SAUCE

Chol (mg)	Calc (mg)	Iron (mg)	Magn (mg)	Phos (mg)	Pota (mg)	Sodi (mg)	Zinc (mg)	VT-A (RE)	Thia (mg)	Ribo (mg)	Niac (mg)	V-B6 (mg)	Fola (µg)	VT-C (mg)
0	0	0	0	0	0	0	—	0	0	0	0	0	0	0
0	0	0	0	0	0	0	—	0	0	0	0	0	0	0
3	12	.03	11	11	6	164	.04	10	<.01	.02	.01	<.01	4	t
0	2	.06	<1	1	2	188	.01	t	t	t	t	<.01	0	t
0	6	.07	—	5	3	306	.03	t	t	t	t	0	t	t
0	1	.03	<1	1	5	162	.02	3	t	t	t	.03	0	t
0	1	.03	<1	1	4	136	0	t	t	t	t	0	t	t
8	2	.07	<1	4	5	80	.02	12	<.01	<.01	<.01	<.01	<1	0
4	0	0	—	0	2	75	—	0	0	0	0	0	t	0
47	119	.31	12	100	158	522	.43	86	.04	.17	.08	.05	6	1
4	2	.03	<1	4	1	105	0	13	<.01	<.01	t	<.01	t	0
4	3	.03	—	4	1	75	.02	10	.03	t	t	—	t	—
4	3	.1	<1	4	11	182	.02	9	<.01	<.01	<.01	<.01	<1	t
4	2	.09	<1	3	18	110	.03	15	<.01	<.01	.03	<.01	6	t
2	2	.09	<1	3	17	153	0	14	<.01	<.01	.03	<.01	<1	t
9	13	.08	—	14	19	117	0	20	.01	.02	.04	0	<1	t
0	0	0	—	0	1	0	—	0	0	0	0	0	—	0
0	10	.25	6	10	159	1	.05	7	.02	.02	.11	.07	4	8
0	15	.38	9	23	244	1	.08	11	.04	.03	.16	.1	6	12
0	4	.1	3	8	124	1	.04	5	.02	.01	.1	.05	<1	4
0	9	.9	10	24	288	56[25]	.13	0	0	.1	.59	.08	1	3
0	17	.92	8	17	295	7	.07	<1	.05	.04	.25	.07	1	2[26]
0	10	1	7	18	156	8	.1	3	.03	.07	.50	.07	2	4[26]
0	7	.29	7	18	183	5	.06	7	.03	.06	.46	.06	2	3[26]
0	15	.58	8	21	313	1	.28	166	.03	.04	.64	.06	9	11
0	23	.77	18	33	361	10	.27	317	.05	.06	.97	.14	4	8
0	7	.26	6	10	119	3	.09	105	.02	.02	.32	.05	1	3
0	30	.74	24	50	409	9	.27	419	.05	.05	.85	.18	5	12
0	10	.25	8	17	139	3	.1	142	.02	.02	.29	.06	2	4
0	16	1.65	16	41	482	4	.26	253	<.01	.05	1.05	.06	4	1
0	40	4.2	42	103	1222	8	.66	591	.02	.08	2.36	.28	0	4
0	18	.96	13	23	286	8	.23	330	.02	.04	.65	.16	3	2[27]

[25] Sodium bisulfite used to preserve color; unsulfured product would contain lower levels of sodium.
[26] Value based on products without added vitamin C. Bottled apple juice with added vitamin C usually contains 41.6 mg/100 g, or 103 mg per cup. Check label for specific vitamin C values.
[27] Without added vitamin C. Products with added vitamin C contain 136 mg per cup. Check label.

(For purposes of calculations, use "0" for t, <1, <.1, <.01, etc.)

Table C–1   Food Composition

Grp	Computer Code No.	Food Description	Measure	Wt (g)	H₂O (%)	Ener (kcal)	Prot (g)	Carb (g)	Dietary Fiber (g)	Fat (g)	Fat Breakdown (g) Sat	Mono	Poly
		FRUITS and FRUIT JUICES—Con.											
		Avocados, raw, edible part only:											
5	220	California (½ lb with refuse)	1 ea	173	73	305	4	12	17	30	4.5	19	3.5
5	221	Florida (1 lb with refuse)	1 ea	304	80	340	5	27	29	27	5	15	5
5	222	Mashed, fresh, average	1 c	230	74	370	5	17	22	35	6	22	5
		Bananas, raw, without peel:											
5	223	Whole, 8¾″ long (weighs 175 g w/peel)	1 ea	114	74	105	1	27	2	1	.2	<.1	.1
5	224	Slices	1 c	150	74	138	2	35	3	1	.3	.1	.1
5	1285	Bananas, dehydrated slices	1 c	100	3	346	4	88	8	2	.7	.2	.3
5	225	Blackberries, raw	1 c	144	86	74	1	18	10	1	.3	.1	.1
		Blueberries:											
5	226	Fresh	1 c	145	85	82	1	21	4	1	<.1	.2	.3
		Frozen, sweetened:											
5	227	10-oz container	10 oz	284	77	230	1	62	7	<1	.1	.1	.2
5	228	Cup	1 c	230	77	185	1	51	5	<1	.1	.1	.2
		Cherries:											
5	229	Sour, red pitted, canned water pack	1 c	244	90	90	2	22	3	<1	.1	.1	.1
5	230	Sweet, raw, without pits	10 ea	68	81	49	1	11	1	1	.1	.2	.2
5	231	Cranberry juice cocktail[28]	1 c	253	85	145	<1[29]	36	1	<1	t	t	.1
5	232	Cranberry-apple juice	1 c	253	86	169	<1	43	1	1[30]	.2	.1	.4
5	233	Cranberry sauce, canned, strained	1 c	277	61	419	1	108	6	<1	<.1	.1	.2
		Dates:											
5	234	Whole, without pits	10 ea	83	22	228	2	61	7	<1	.2	.1	t
5	235	Chopped	1 c	178	22	489	4	131	15	1	.3	.2	.1
5	236	Figs, dried	10 ea	187	28	477	6	122	21	2	.4	.5	1.1
		Fruit cocktail, canned, fruit and liquid:											
5	237	Heavy syrup pack	1 c	255	80	185	1	48	3	<1	<.1	<.1	.1
5	238	Juice pack	1 c	248	87	115	1	29	3	<1	t	t	t
		Grapefruit:											
		Raw 3¾″ diam-weight with rind is 241 g for one-half											
5	239	Pink/red, half fruit, edible part	1 half	123	91	37	1	9	2	<1	t	t	<.1
5	240	White, half fruit, edible part	1 half	118	90	39	1	10	2	<1	t	t	<.1
5	241	Canned sections with liquid	1 c	254	84	152	1	39	3	<1	<.1	<.1	.1
		Grapefruit juice:											
5	242	Fresh, raw	1 c	247	90	96	1	23	1	<1	<.1	<.1	.1
		Canned:											
5	243	Unsweetened	1 c	247	90	93	1	22	1	<1	<.1	<.1	.1
5	244	Sweetened	1 c	250	87	115	1	28	1	<1	<.1	<.1	.1
		Frozen concentrate, unsweetened:											
5	245	Undiluted, 6-fl-oz can	¾ c	207	62	300	4	72	3	1	.2	.2	.3
5	246	Diluted with 3 cans water	1 c	247	89	102	1	24	1	<1	<.1	<.1	.1
		Grapes, raw, European type (adherent skin):											
5	247	Thompson seedless	10 ea	50	81	35	<1	9	1	<1	.1	t	.1
5	248	Tokay/Emperor, seeded types	10 ea	57	81	40	<1	10	1	<1	.1	t	.1
		Grape juice:											
5	249	Bottled or canned	1 c	253	84	155	1	38	1	<1	.1	t	.1
		Frozen concentrate, sweetened:											
5	250	Undiluted, 6-fl-oz can	¾ c	216	54	385	1	96	4	1	.2	<.1	.2
5	251	Diluted with 3 cans water	1 c	250	87	128	<1	32	1	<1	.1	t	.1

[28]Data here are from the newest USDA *Handbook 8–14* on beverages. These data are somewhat different from that presented in *Handbook 8–9* on fruits and fruit juices.

[29]The newest USDA *Handbook 8–14* data on beverages indicates "0" for protein.

[30]The newest USDA *Handbook 8–14* data on beverages indicates "0" for fat.

(Computer code number is for West Diet Analysis program)

GRP KEY: 1 = BEV   2 = DAIRY   3 = EGGS   4 = FAT/OIL   5 = FRUIT   6 = BAKERY   7 = GRAIN   8 = FISH   9 = BEEF   10 = POULTRY
   11 = SAUSAGE   12 = MIXED/FAST   13 = NUTS/SEEDS   14 = SWEETS   15 = VEG/LEG   16 = MISC   22 = SOUP/SAUCE

Chol (mg)	Calc (mg)	Iron (mg)	Magn (mg)	Phos (mg)	Pota (mg)	Sodi (mg)	Zinc (mg)	VT-A (RE)	Thia (mg)	Ribo (mg)	Niac (mg)	V-B6 (mg)	Fola (µg)	VT-C (mg)
0	19	2.04	70	73	1097	21	.73	106	.19	.21	3.32	.48	113	14
0	33	1.6	104	119	1484	14	1.28	186	.33	.37	5.84	.85	162	24
0	25	2.3	90	95	1378	24	.97	141	.25	.28	4.42	.64	142	18
0	7	.35	32	22	451	1	.19	9	.05	.11	.62	.66	24	10
0	9	.46	43	29	593	1	.25	12	.07	.15	.81	.87	31	14
0	22	1.15	108	74	1491	3	.61	31	.18	.24	2.80	.54	40	7
0	46	.8	29	30	282	0	.39	24	.04	.06	.58	.08	49	30
0	9	.24	7	15	129	9	.16	15	.07	.07	.7	.05	9	20
0	16	1.11	7	20	169	4	.14	12	.06	.15	.72	.17	19	3
0	13	.9	6	16	138	3	.14	10	.05	.12	.58	.14	16	2
0	27	3.34	15	25	240	17	.17	184	.04	.1	.43	.11	20	5
0	10	.3	8	13	152	0	.04	15	.03	.04	.3	.02	3	5
0	8	.38	5	5	45	5	.18	1	.02	.02	.09	.05	<1	90[31]
0	18	.15	5	7	68	5	.1	<1	.01	.05	.15	.06	<1	81[31]
0	11	.61	8	17	72	80	.09	6	.04	.06	.28	.05	3	6
0	27	1	29	33	541	2	.24	4	.08	.08	1.83	.16	14	0
0	58	2.14	63	70	1161	5	.52	9	.16	.18	3.92	.34	29	0
0	269	4.18	111	128	1331	21	.94	25	.13	.17	1.3	.42	16	1
0	16	.73	14	28	224	15	.21	52	.05	.05	.95	.11	1	5
0	20	.53	17	34	235	10	.21	76	.03	.04	0	.13	2	7
0	13	.15	10	11	158	0	.09	32[32]	.04	.03	.24	.05	15	47
0	14	.07	11	9	175	0	.08	1	.04	.02	.32	.05	12	39
0	36	1.02	25	25	328	4	.21	0	.1	.05	.62	.05	22	54
0	22	.49	30	37	400	2	.13	2[33]	.1	.05	.49	.11	52	94
0	17	.49	24	27	378	2	.22	2	.1	.05	.57	.05	26	72
0	20	.9	24	28	405	5	.15	2	.1	.06	.8	.05	26	67
0	56	1.02	78	101	1002	6	.38	6	.3	.16	1.6	.32	26	248
0	20	.34	26	34	337	2	.12	2	.1	.05	.54	.11	52	83
0	5	.13	3	7	92	1	.03	4	.05	.03	.15	.06	4	5
0	6	.15	4	8	105	1	.03	4	.05	.03	.17	.06	4	6
0	22	.61	24	27	334	8	.13	2	.07	.09	.66	.16	7	<1
0	28	.78	32	32	160	15	.28	6	.11	.2	.93	.32	9	179[34]
0	10	.26	11	11	53	5	.10	2	.04	.07	.31	.11	4	60[34]

[31] Nutrient added.
[32] Vitamin A in Texas red grapefruit would be 74 RE.
[33] This is vitamin A for white grapefruit juice; pink or red grapefruit juice = 109 RE per cup.
[34] With added vitamin C (ascorbic acid).

(For purposes of calculations, use "0" for t, <1, <.1, <.01, etc.)

Table C–1   Food Composition

Grp	Computer Code No.	Food Description	Measure	Wt (g)	H₂O (%)	Ener (kcal)	Prot (g)	Carb (g)	Dietary Fiber (g)	Fat (g)	Fat Breakdown (g) Sat	Mono	Poly
		FRUITS and FRUIT JUICES—Con.											
5	252	Kiwi fruit, raw, peeled (88 g with peel)	1 ea	76	83	46	1	11	3	<1	t	.2	.2
5	253	Lemons, raw, without peel and seeds (about 4 per lb whole)	1 ea	58	89	17	1	5	1	<1	t	t	.1
		Lemon juice:											
		Fresh:											
5	254	Cup	1 c	244	91	60	1	21	1	t	t	t	t
5	255	Tablespoon	1 tbsp	15	91	4	<.1	1	<1	t	t	t	t
		Canned or bottled, unsweetened:											
5	256	Cup	1 c	244	92	52	1	16	1	<1	.1	<.1	.2
5	257	Tablespoon	1 tbsp	15	92	3	<1	1	<1	<.1	t	t	t
		Frozen, single strength, unsweetened:											
5	258	Cup	1 c	244	92	54	1	16	1	<1	.1	<.1	.2
5	259	Tablespoon	1 tbsp	15	92	3	<1	1	<1	<.1	t	t	t
		Lime juice:											
		Fresh:											
5	260	Cup	1 c	246	90	65	1	22	1	<1	<.1	<.1	.1
5	261	Tablespoon	1 tbsp	15	90	4	<1	1	<1	<.1	t	t	t
5	262	Canned or bottled, unsweetened	1 c	246	92	50	1	16	1	1	.1	.1	.2
5	263	Mangos, raw, edible part (weighs 300 g with skin and seeds)	1 ea	207	82	135	1	35	7	1	.1	.2	.1
		Melons, raw, without rind and cavity contents:											
5	264	Cantaloupe, 5″ diam (2⅓ lb whole with refuse), orange flesh	½ ea	267	90	94	2	22	3	1	.1	.1	.2
5	265	Honeydew, 6½″ diam (5¼ lb whole with refuse), slice = ⅒ melon	1 slice	129	90	45	1	12	1	<1	t	t	<.1
5	266	Nectarines, raw, without pits, 2½″ diam	1 ea	136	86	67	1	16	3	1	t	.2	.3
		Oranges, raw:											
5	267	Whole without peel and seeds, 2⅝″ dm. (weighs 180 g with peel and seeds)	1 ea	131	87	60	1	15	3	<1	t	<.1	<.1
5	268	Sections, without membranes	1 c	180	87	85	2	21	4	<1	<.1	<.1	<.1
		Orange juice:											
5	269	Fresh, all varieties	1 c	248	88	111	2	26	1	<1	.1	.1	.1
5	270	Canned, unsweetened	1 c	249	89	105	1	25	<1	<1	<.1	.1	.1
5	271	Chilled	1 c	249	88	110	2	25	<1	1	.1	.1	.2
		Frozen concentrate:											
5	272	Undiluted (6-oz can)	¾ c	213	58	339	5	81	2	<1	.1	.1	.1
5	273	Diluted with 3 parts water by volume	1 c	249	88	110	2	27	<1	<1	t	<.1	<.1
5	1345	Orange juice, from dry crystals	1 c	248	89	114	2	27	0	<1	.1	.1	.1
5	274	Orange and grapefruit juice, canned	1 c	247	89	105	1	25	<1	<1	<.1	<.1	.1
		Papayas, raw:											
5	275	½″ slices	1 c	140	89	60	1	14	2	<1	.1	.1	<.1
5	276	Whole fruit, 3½″ diam by 5⅛″, without seeds and skin (1 lb with refuse)	1 ea	304	89	117	2	30	5	<1	.1	.1	.1
5	1031	Papaya nectar, canned	1 c	250	85	142	<1	36	2	<1	.1	.1	.1
		Peaches:											
5	277	Raw, whole, 2½″ diam, peeled, pitted (about 4 per lb whole)	1 ea	87	88	37	1	10	2	<1	t	<.1	<.1

(Computer code number is for West Diet Analysis program)

GRP KEY: 1 = BEV 2 = DAIRY 3 = EGGS 4 = FAT/OIL 5 = FRUIT 6 = BAKERY 7 = GRAIN 8 = FISH 9 = BEEF 10 = POULTRY
11 = SAUSAGE 12 = MIXED/FAST 13 = NUTS/SEEDS 14 = SWEETS 15 = VEG/LEG 16 = MISC 22 = SOUP/SAUCE

Chol (mg)	Calc (mg)	Iron (mg)	Magn (mg)	Phos (mg)	Pota (mg)	Sodi (mg)	Zinc (mg)	VT-A (RE)	Thia (mg)	Ribo (mg)	Niac (mg)	V-B6 (mg)	Fola (µg)	VT-C (mg)
0	20	.3	23	30	252	4	.08[35]	13	.02	.04	.4	.05[35]	17[35]	75
0	15	.35	2	9	80	1	.06	2	.02	.01	.06	.05	7	31
0	18	.08	16	14	303	2	.12	5	.07	.02	.24	.12	32	112
0	1	<.01	1	1	19	<1	.01	<1	<.01	<.01	.02	.01	2	7
0	26	.31	22	21	248	50[36]	.15	4	.10	.02	.48	.11	25	61
0	2	.02	1	1	15	3[36]	.01	<1	.01	<.01	.03	.01	2	4
0	19	.30	20	20	218	4	.12	4	.14	.03	.33	.15	23	77
0	1	.02	1	1	14	<1	.01	<1	.01	<.01	.02	.01	1	5
0	22	.08	14	18	268	2	.15	3	.05	.03	.25	.11	21	72
0	1	<.01	1	1	17	<1	.01	<1	<.01	<.01	.02	.08	1	5
0	30	.6	16	25	185	39[36]	.15	4	.08	.01	.4	.07	20	16
0	21	2.6	18	22	323	4	.07	806	.12	.12	1.21	.28	39	57
0	29	.56	19	45	825	24	.43	861	.1	.06	1.53	.31	80	113
0	8	.09	9	13	350	13	.11	5	.1	.02	.77	.08	39	32
0	6	.21	11	22	288	0	.12	100	.02	.06	1.35	.03	5	7
0	52	.14	13	18	237	<1	.09	27	.11	.05	.37	.08	40	70
0	72	.19	18	25	326	<1	.4	37	.16	.07	.51	.11	83	96
0	27	.50	27	42	496	2	.12	50	.22	.07	.99	.1	109	124
0	20	1.1	27	35	436	5	.17	44	.15	.04	.4	.1	15	86
0	25	.42	28	27	473	2	.11	19[37]	.28	.05	.7	.13	45[37]	82[37]
0	68	.75	73	121	1436	6	.38	59	.6	.14	1.53	.33	331	294
0	22	.27	24	40	474	2	.13	19	.2	.04	.5	.11	109	97
0	40	.02	5	31	50	1	—	.50	.20	.07	1.00	0	0	80
0	20	1.1	24	35	390	7	.18	29	.14	.07	.83	.06	20	72
0	33	.3	14	12	247	9	.10	282	.04	.05	.47	.03	26	92
0	72	.3	31	16	780	8	.22	612	.08	.10	1.03	.06	48	188
0	24	.86	8	1	78	14	.38	28	.02	.01	.38	.02	5	8
0	4	.1	6	10	171	0	.12	47	.02	.04	.86	.02	3	6

[35] Data are estimated from other fruit data.
[36] Sodium benzoate and sodium bisulfite added as preservatives.
[37] Values for juice from California oranges indicate the following values for 1 c: 36 RE of vitamin A, 72 µg of folacin, and 106 mg of vitamin C.

(For purposes of calculations, use "0" for t, <1, <.1, <.01, etc.)

Table C–1 Food Composition

Grp	Computer Code No.	Food Description	Measure	Wt (g)	H_2O (%)	Ener (kcal)	Prot (g)	Carb (g)	Dietary Fiber (g)	Fat (g)	Fat Breakdown (g) Sat	Mono	Poly
		FRUITS and FRUIT JUICES—Con.											
		Peaches—Con.											
5	278	Raw, sliced	1 c	170	88	73	1	19	3	<1	t	.1	.1
		Canned, fruit and liquid:											
		Heavy syrup pack:											
5	279	Cup	1 c	256	79	190	1	51	3	<1	<.1	.1	.1
5	280	Half	1 ea	81	79	60	<1	16	1	<1	t	<.1	<.1
		Juice pack:											
5	281	Cup	1 c	248	88	109	2	29	3	<1	t	<.1	<.1
5	282	Half	1 ea	77	88	34	<1	9	1	<1	t	t	t
		Dried:											
5	283	Uncooked	10 ea	130	32	311	5	80	11	1	.1	.4	.5
5	284	Cooked, fruit and liquid	1 c	258	78	200	3	51	4	1	.1	.2	.3
		Frozen, sliced, sweetened:											
5	285	10-oz package	1 ea	284	75	267	2	68	6	<1	<.1	.1	.2
5	286	Cup, thawed measure	1 c	250	75	235	2	60	4	<1	<.1	.1	.2
5	1032	Peach nectar, canned	1 c	249	86	134	1	35	1	<1	t	<.1	<.1
		Pears:											
		Fresh, with skin, cored:											
5	287	Bartlett, 2½″ diam (about 2½ per lb)	1 ea	166	84	98	1	25	5[38]	1	<.1	.1	.2
5	288	Bosc, 2½″ diam (about 3 per lb)	1 ea	141	84	85	1	21	4[38]	1	<.1	.1	.1
5	289	D'Anjou, 3″ diam (about 2 per lb)	1 ea	200	84	120	1	30	6[38]	1	<.1	.2	.2
		Canned, fruit and liquid:											
		Heavy syrup pack:											
5	290	Cup	1 c	255	80	188	1	49	4[38]	<1	t	.1	.1
5	291	Half	1 ea	79	80	59	<1	15	1[38]	<1	t	t	t
		Juice pack:											
5	292	Cup	1 c	248	86	123	1	32	4[38]	<1	t	<.1	<.1
5	293	Half	1 ea	77	86	38	<1	10	1[38]	<1	t	t	t
5	294	Dried halves	10 ea	175	27	459	3	122	19	1	.1	.2	.3
5	1033	Pear nectar, canned	1 c	250	84	149	<1	39	2	<1	t	t	t
		Pineapple:											
5	295	Fresh chunks, diced	1 c	155	86	76	1	19	2	1	<.1	<.1	.2
		Canned, fruit and liquid:											
		Heavy syrup pack:											
5	296	Crushed, chunks, tidbits	1 c	255	79	199	1	52	2	<1	t	<.1	.1
5	297	Slices	1 ea	58	79	45	<1	12	1	<.1	t	t	<.1
		Juice Pack:											
5	298	Crushed, chunks, tidbits	1 c	250	84	150	1	39	2	<1	t	<.1	.1
5	299	Slices	1 ea	58	84	35	<1	9	1	<.1	t	t	t
5	300	Pineapple juice, canned, unsweetened	1 c	250	86	140	1	34	1	<1	t	t	.1
		Plantains, without peel:											
5	301	Raw slices (one whole plantain weighs 179 g without peel)	1 c	148	65	181	2	47	7[39]	1	.2	.1	.1
5	302	Cooked, boiled, sliced	1 c	154	67	179	1	48	7	<1	.1	<.1	.1
		Plums, canned:											
		Fresh:											
5	303	Medium 2⅛″ diam	1 ea	66	85	36	1	9	1	<1	<.1	.3	.1
5	304	Small, 1½″ diam	1 ea	28	85	15	<1	4	1	<1	t	.1	<.1

(38) Dietary fiber data vary 2.4 to 3.4 g/100 g for fresh pears; 1.6 to 2.6 g/100 g for canned pears.

(39) Dietary fiber value partially derived from data for bananas.

C

GRP KEY: 1 = BEV 2 = DAIRY 3 = EGGS 4 = FAT/OIL 6 = BAKERY 7 = GRAIN 8 = FISH 9 = BEEF 10 = POULTRY
11 = SAUSAGE 12 = MIXED/FAST 13 = NUTS/SEEDS 14 = SWEETS 15 = VEG/LEG 16 = MISC 22 = SOUP/SAUCE

Chol (mg)	Calc (mg)	Iron (mg)	Magn (mg)	Phos (mg)	Pota (mg)	Sodi (mg)	Zinc (mg)	VT-A (RE)	Thia (mg)	Ribo (mg)	Niac (mg)	V-B6 (mg)	Fola (µg)	VT-C (mg)
0	9	.19	11	20	335	1	.18	91	.03	.07	1.68	.03	6	11
0	8	.69	13	29	235	16	.22	85	.03	.06	1.57	.05	8	7
0	3	.22	4	9	75	5	.07	27	.01	.02	.5	.01	3	2
0	15	.72	18	43	317	11	.26	94	.02	.04	1.44	.05	8	9
0	5	.21	6	13	98	3	.09	29	.01	.01	.45	.02	3	3
0	37	5.28	54	155	1295	9	.74	281	<.01	.28	5.69	.09	6	6
0	23	3.37	35	99	825	6	.46	51	.01	.05	3.92	.1	<1	10
0	9	1.05	14	31	369	17	.14	81	.04	.10	1.9	.05	9	268[40]
0	8	.93	12	28	325	16	.13	71	.03	.09	1.63	.04	8	236[40]
0	13	.47	11	16	101	10	.20	64	.01	.04	.72	.03	2	13
0	19	.42	9	18	208	1	.20	3	.03	.07	.17	.03	12	7
0	16	.40	8	16	176	<1	.17	3	.03	.06	.1	.03	10	6
0	22	.50	11	22	250	<1	.24	4	.04	.08	.2	.04	14	8
0	13	.56	11	18	166	13	.21	1	.03	.06	.62	.04	3	3
0	4	.17	3	5	51	4	.06	<1	.01	.02	.19	.01	1	1
0	22	.71	17	29	238	10	.22	1	.03	.03	.5	.04	5	4
0	7	.22	5	9	74	3	.07	<1	.01	.01	.15	.01	2	1
0	59	3.68	58	103	932	10	.68	1	.01	.25	2.4	.01	21	12
0	11	.65	6	7	33	8	.16	<1	<.01	.03	.32	.03	2	3
0	11	.57	21	11	175	2	.12	4	.14	.06	.65	.14	16	24
0	36	.97	40	18	265	3	.31	4	.23	.06	.73	.19	12	19
0	8	.22	9	4	60	1	.70	1	.05	.02	.17	.04	3	4
0	35	.70	35	15	305	3	.25	10	.24	.05	.71	.19	12	24
0	8	.16	8	4	71	1	.06	2	.06	.02	.17	.04	3	6
0	43	.65	34	20	335	3	.28	1	.14	.06	.64	.24	58	27[41]
0	4	.89	55	50	739	6	.27	167[42]	.08	.08	1.02	.44	33	27
0	3	.89	49	43	716	8	.21	140	.07	.08	1.16	.37	40	17
0	3	.07	4	7	114	<1	.07	21	.03	.06	.33	.05	3	6
0	1	.03	2	3	48	<1	.03	9	.01	.03	.14	.02	1	3

[40] With added vitamin C (ascorbic acid).
[41] If vitamin C is added, it contains 96 mg per cup.
[42] Vitamin A values range from 1.5 RE for white-fleshed varieties to 178 RE for yellow-fleshed varieties.

(For purposes of calculations, use "0" for t, <1, <.1, <.01, etc.)

Table C-1   Food Composition

Grp	Computer Code No.	Food Description	Measure	Wt (g)	H$_2$O (%)	Ener (kcal)	Prot (g)	Carb (g)	Dietary Fiber (g)	Fat (g)	Fat Breakdown (g) Sat	Mono	Poly
		FRUITS—Con.											
		Plums—Con.											
		Canned, purple, with liquid:											
		Heavy Syrup pack:											
5	305	Cup	1 c	258	76	230	1	60	4	<1	t	.2	.1
5	306	Plums	3 ea	110	76	98	<1	25	2	<1	t	.1	t
		Juice pack:											
5	307	Cup	1 c	252	84	146	1	38	4	<.1	t	<.1	t
5	308	Plums	3 ea	95	84	55	<1	14	2	<.1	t	t	t
		Prunes, dried, pitted:											
5	309	Uncooked (10 prunes weigh	10 ea	84	32	201	2	53	8[43]	<1	<.1	.3	.1
		97 g with pits, 84 g without pits.)											
5	310	Cooked, unsweetened, fruit and liquid	1 c	212	70	227	2	60	9	<1	<.1	.3	.1
		(250 g with pits)											
5	311	Prune juice, bottled or canned	1 c	256	81	181	2	45	3	<.1	t	<.1	t
		Raisins, seedless:											
5	312	Cup, not pressed down	1 c	145	15	435	5	115	9	1	.2	<.1	.2
5	313	One packet, ½ oz	½ oz	14	15	41	<1	11	1	<.1	t	t	t
		Raspberries:											
5	314	Fresh	1 c	123	87	60	1	14	8	1	t	.1	.4
		Frozen, sweetened:											
5	315	10-oz container	10 oz	284	73	293	2	74	15	<1	t	<.1	.3
5	316	Cup, thawed measure	1 c	250	73	255	2	65	12	<1	t	<.1	.2
5	317	Rhubarb, cooked, added sugar	1 c	240	68	279	1	75	5	<1	t	t	.1
		Strawberries:											
5	318	Fresh, whole, capped	1 c	149	92	45	1	11	4	1	<.1	.1	.3
		Frozen, sliced, sweetened:											
5	319	10-oz container	10 oz	284	73	273	2	74	6	<1	t	.1	.2
5	320	Cup, thawed measure	1 c	255	73	245	1	66	8	<1	t	.1	.2
		Tangerines, without peel and seeds:											
5	321	Fresh (2⅜″ whole) 116 g with refuse	1 ea	84	88	37	1	9	2	<1	t	<.1	<.1
5	322	Canned, light syrup, fruit and liquid	1 c	252	83	154	1	41	4	<1	<.1	<.1	.1
5	323	Tangerine juice, canned, sweetened	1 c	249	87	125	1	30	1	<1	<.1	<.1	.1
		Watermelon, raw, without rind and seeds:											
5	324	Piece, 1″ thick by 10″ diam (weighs 2 lb	1 pce	482	92	152	3	35	2	2	.3	.2	1
		with refuse or 926 g)											
5	325	Diced	1 c	160	92	50	1	12	1	1	.1	.1	.4
		BAKED GOODS:											
		BREADS, CAKES, COOKIES, CRACKERS, PIES, PANCAKES, TORTILLAS											
6	326	Bagels, plain, enriched, 3½″ diam	1 ea	68	32	180	7	35	1	1	.2	.3	.4
		Biscuits:											
6	327	From home recipe	1 ea	28	28	100	2	13	1	5	1.2	2	1.3
6	328	From mix	1 ea	28	29	94	2	14	1	3	.8	1.4	.9
6	329	From refrigerated dough	1 ea	20	30	65	1	10	<1	2	.6	.9	.6
6	330	Bread crumbs, dry grated (see 364, 365	1 c	100	7	390	13	73	4	5	1.5	1.6	1
		for soft crumbs)											
		Breads:											
6	331	Boston brown bread, canned, 3¼″ slice	1 pce	45	45	95	2	21	2	1	.26	.13	.14
		Cracked wheat bread (¼ cracked-wheat											
		flour, ¾ enr wheat flour):											
6	332	1-lb loaf	1 ea	454	35	1190	42	227	23	16	3.1	4.3	5.7
6	333	Slice (18 per loaf)	1 pce	25	35	65	2	13	1	1	.2	.2	.3
6	334	Slice, toasted	1 pce	21	26	65	2	13	1	1	.2	.2	.3

[43]Dietary fiber data can vary between 8 and 13 g for 10 prunes.

(Computer code number is for West Diet Analysis program)

GRP KEY: 1 = BEV   2 = DAIRY   3 = EGGS   4 = FAT/OIL   5 = FRUIT   6 = BAKERY   7 = GRAIN   8 = FISH   9 = BEEF   10 = POULTRY
            11 = SAUSAGE   12 = MIXED/FAST   13 = NUTS/SEEDS   14 = SWEETS   15 = VEG/LEG   16 = MISC   22 = SOUP/SAUCE

Chol (mg)	Calc (mg)	Iron (mg)	Magn (mg)	Phos (mg)	Pota (mg)	Sodi (mg)	Zinc (mg)	VT-A (RE)	Thia (mg)	Ribo (mg)	Niac (mg)	V-B6 (mg)	Fola (µg)	VT-C (mg)
0	23	2.17	13	34	235	49	.18	67	.04	.1	.75	.07	7	1
0	10	.92	6	14	100	21	.08	29	.02	.04	.32	.03	3	<1
0	25	.86	20	38	388	3	.28	254	.06	.15	1.19	.1	8	7
0	10	.32	8	15	147	1	.11	96	.02	.06	.45	.04	3	3
0	43	2.08	38	66	626	3	.45	167	.07	.14	1.65	.22	3	3
0	49	2.35	43	74	708	4	.51	65	.05	.21	1.53	.46	<1	6
0	31	3.02	36	64	707	10	.54	1	.04	.18	2.01	.56	1	11
0	71	3.02	48	140	1089	17	.46	1	.23	.13	1.19	.36	5	5
0	7	.29	5	14	105	2	.05	<1	.02	.01	.12	.04	1	<1
0	27	.7	22	15	187	0	.57	16	.04	.11	1.11	.07	32	31
0	43	1.85	37	48	324	3	.51	17	.05	.13	.65	.1	74	47
0	38	1.62	32	43	285	3	.45	15	.05	.11	1.5	.09	65	41
0	348	.5	30	19	230	2	.19	17	.04	.06	.48	.05	13	8
0	21	.57	16	28	247	2	.19	4	.03	.1	.34	.09	28	85
0	31	1.7	20	37	278	9	.17	7	.05	.14	1.1	.09	47	118
0	28	1.5	18	33	250	8	.15	6	.04	.13	1.02	.08	42	106
0	12	.08	10	8	132	1	.38	77	.09	.02	.13	.06	17	26
0	18	.93	19	25	197	15	.60	212	.13	.11	1.1	.11	34	50
0	45	.5	20	35	443	2	.08	105	.15	.05	.25	.08	8	55
0	38	.82	52	41	560	10	.34	176	.39	.1	.96	.69	10	47
0	13	.27	17	14	186	3	.11	59	.13	.03	.32	.23	3	15
0	20	2.1	15	61	65	300	.61	0	.26	.20	2.4	.03	16	0
t	48	.7	6	36	32	195	.15	3	.08	.08	.8	.01	2	t
t	59	.58	7	129	57	265	.18	4	.12	.11	.85	.01	2	t
1	4	.47	4	78	18	249	.09	0	.08	.05	.67	.01	1	0
5	122	4.1	31	141	152	736	.50	0	.35	.35	4.8	.02	28	0
3	41	.90	40	72	131	113	.35	0	.06	.04	.7	.06	8	0
0	295	12.1	218	581	608	1966	6.36	0	1.73	1.73	15.3	.42	218	t
0	16	.67	12	32	34	106	.35	0	.1	.1	.84	.02	12	t
0	16	.67	12	32	34	106	.35	0	.07	.1	.84	.02	9	t

(For purposes of calculations, use "0" for t, <1, <.1, <.01, etc.)

Table C–1   Food Composition

Grp	Computer Code No.	Food Description	Measure	Wt (g)	H₂O (%)	Ener (kcal)	Prot (g)	Carb (g)	Dietary Fiber (g)	Fat (g)	Fat Breakdown (g)		
											Sat	Mono	Poly
		BAKED GOODS—Con.											
		Breads—Con.											
		French/Vienna bread, enriched:											
6	335	1-lb loaf	1 ea	454	34	1270	43	230	8	18	4	6	6
6	336	French, slice, 5 × 2½ × 1″	1 pce	35	34	100	3	18	1	1	.3	.4	.5
6	337	Vienna, slice 4¾ × 4 × ½″	1 pce	25	34	70	2	13	1	1	.2	.3	.3
		French toast: see Mixed Dishes, and Fast Foods, code # 691											
		Italian bread, enriched:											
6	338	1-lb loaf	1 ea	454	32	1255	41	256	5	4	.6	.3	1.6
6	339	Slice, 4½ × 3¼ × ¾″	1 pce	30	32	83	3	17	<1	<1	<.1	t	.1
		Mixed grain bread, enriched:											
6	340	1-lb loaf	1 ea	454	37	1165	45	212	18	17	3	4	7
6	341	Slice (18 per loaf)	1 pce	25	37	65	2	12	2	1	.2	.2	.4
6	342	Slice, toasted	1 pce	23	27	65	2	12	2	1	.2	.2	.4
		Oatmeal bread, enriched:											
6	343	1-lb loaf	1 ea	454	37	1145	38	212	16	20	4	7	8
6	344	Slice (18 per loaf)	1 pce	25	37	65	2	12	1	1	.2	.4	.5
6	345	Slice, toasted	1 pce	23	30	65	2	12	1	1	.2	.4	.5
6	346	Pita pocket bread, enr, 6½″ round	1 ea	60	31	165	6	33	1	1	.1	.1	.4
		Pumpernickel bread (⅔ rye flour, ⅓ enr. wheat flour):											
6	347	1-lb loaf	1 ea	454	37	1160	42	218	19	16	3	4	6
6	348	Slice, 5 × 4 × ⅜″	1 pce	32	37	80	3	15	2	1	.2	.3	.5
6	349	Slice, toasted	1 pce	29	28	80	3	15	1	1	.2	.3	.5
		Raisin bread, enriched:											
6	350	1-lb loaf	1 ea	454	33	1260	37	239	12	18	4	7	7
6	351	Slice (18 per loaf)	1 pce	25	33	68	2	13	1	1	.2	.4	.4
6	352	Slice, toasted	1 pce	21	24	68	2	13	1	1	.2	.4	.4
		Rye bread, light (⅓ rye flour, ⅔ enr. wheat flour):											
6	353	1-lb loaf	1 ea	454	37	1190	38	218	30	17	3.3	5.2	5.5
6	354	Slice, 4¾ × 3¾ × ⁷⁄₁₆″	1 pce	25	37	65	2	12	2	1	.2	.3	.3
6	355	Slice, toasted	1 pce	22	28	65	2	12	2	1	.2	.3	.3
		Wheat bread (blend of enr. wheat flour and whole-wheat flour):[44]											
6	356	1-lb loaf	1 ea	454	37	1160	43	213	25	19	3.9	7.3	4.5
6	357	Slice (18 per loaf)	1 pce	25	37	65	2	12	1	1	.2	.4	.3
6	358	Slice, toasted	1 pce	23	28	65	2	12	1	1	.2	.4	.3
		White bread, enriched:											
6	359	1-lb loaf	1 ea	454	37	1210	38	222	12	18	5.6	6.5	4.2
6	360	Slice (18 per loaf)	1 pce	25	37	65	2	12	<1	1	.3	.4	.2
6	361	Slice, toasted	1 pce	22	28	65	2	12	<1	1	.3	.4	.2
6	362	Slice (22 per loaf)	1 pce	20	37	55	2	10	<1	1	.2	.3	.2
6	363	Slice, toasted	1 pce	17	28	55	2	10	<1	1	.2	.3	.2
		White bread cubes, crumbs:											
6	364	Cubes, soft	1 c	30	37	80	2	15	1	1	.4	.4	.3
6	365	Crumbs, soft	1 c	45	37	120	4	22	1	2	.6	.6	.4
		Whole-wheat bread:											
6	366	1-lb loaf	1 ea	454	38	1110	44	206	51	20	6	7	5
6	367	Slice (16 per loaf)	1 pce	28	38	70	3	13	2	1	.4	.4	.3
6	368	Slice, toasted	1 pce	25	29	70	3	13	2	1	.4	.4	.3

[44]A blend of white and whole-wheat flour—no official ratio specified.

(Computer code number is for West Diet Analysis program)

GRP KEY: 1 = BEV   2 = DAIRY   3 = EGGS   4 = FAT/OIL   5 = FRUIT   6 = BAKERY   7 = GRAIN   8 = FISH   9 = BEEF   10 = POULTRY   11 = SAUSAGE   12 = MIXED/FAST   13 = NUTS/SEEDS   14 = SWEETS   15 = VEG/LEG   16 = MISC   22 = SOUP/SAUCE

Chol (mg)	Calc (mg)	Iron (mg)	Magn (mg)	Phos (mg)	Pota (mg)	Sodi (mg)	Zinc (mg)	VT-A (RE)	Thia (mg)	Ribo (mg)	Niac (mg)	V-B6 (mg)	Fola (µg)	VT-C (mg)
0	499	14	91	386	409	2633	2.9	0	2.09	1.59	18.2	.24	168	t
0	39	1.08	7	30	32	203	.22	0	.16	.12	1.4	.02	13	t
0	28	.77	5	21	23	145	.16	0	.12	.09	1	.01	9	t
0	77	12.7	106	350	336	2656	3.1	0	1.86	1.06	15.1	.24	160	0
0	5	.8	7	23	22	176	.21	0	.12	.07	1	.02	11	0
0	472	14.8	222	962	990	1870	5.45	t	1.77	1.73	18.9	.47	295	0
0	27	.8	12	55	56	106	.3	t	.1	.1	1.1	.03	16	t
0	27	.8	12	55	56	106	.3	t	.08	.1	1.1	.02	12	t
0	267	12	154	563	707	2231	4.45	0	2.09	1.2	15.4	.07	15	0
0	15	.7	9	31	39	124	.25	0	.12	.07	.85	<.01	1	0
0	15	.7	9	31	39	124	.25	0	.09	.07	.85	<.01	1	0
0	49	1.45	16	60	71	339	.50	0	.27	.13	2.32	.01	12	0
0	322	12.4	309	990	1966	2461	5.18	0	1.54	2.36	15	.72	222	0
0	23	.88	22	71	141	177	.4	0	.11	.17	1.06	.05	16	0
0	23	.88	22	71	141	177	.4	0	.09	.17	1.06	.05	12	0
0	463	14.1	114	395	1058	1657	2.81	1	1.5	2.81	18.6	.15	159	t
0	25	.78	6	22	59	92	.16	t	.08	.16	1.02	.01	9	t
0	25	.80	6	22	59	92	.16	t	.06	.16	1.02	.01	8	t
0	363	12.3	109	658	926	3164	5.77	0	1.86	1.45	15	.43	177	0
0	20	.68	8	36	51	175	.38	0	.1	.08	.83	.02	10	0
0	20	.68	6	36	51	175	.38	0	.08	.08	.83	.02	8	0
0	572	15.8	209	835	627	2447	4.77	t	2.09	1.45	20.5	.50	204	t
0	32	.87	12	47	35	135	.26	t	.12	.08	1.13	.03	11	t
0	32	.87	12	47	35	135	.26	t	.10	.08	1.20	.02	8	t
0	572	12.9	95	490	508	2334	2.81	t	2.13	1.41	17.0	.15	159	t
0	32	.71	5	27	28	129	.16	t	.12	.08	.94	.01	9	t
0	32	.71	5	27	28	129	.16	t	.09	.08	.94	.01	9	t
0	25	.57	4	22	22	103	.12	t	.09	.06	.75	.01	7	t
0	25	.6	4	21	22	103	.12	t	.07	.06	.75	.01	7	t
0	38	.85	6	32	34	154	.19	t	.14	.09	1.13	.01	11	t
0	57	1.28	9	49	50	231	.28	t	.21	.14	1.69	.02	16	t
0	327	15.5	422	1180	799	2887	7.63	t	1.59	.95	17.4	.85	250	t
0	20	.97	26	74	50	180	.50	t	.10	.06	1.09	.05	16	t
0	20	.97	26	74	50	180	.50	t	.08	.06	1.08	.05	12	t

(For purposes of calculations, use "0" for t, <1, <.1, <.01, etc.)

Table C–1   Food Composition

Grp	Computer Code No.	Food Description	Measure	Wt (g)	H$_2$O (%)	Ener (kcal)	Prot (g)	Carb (g)	Dietary Fiber (g)	Fat (g)	Fat Breakdown (g)		
											Sat	Mono	Poly
		BAKED GOODS—Con.											
		Bread stuffing, prepared from mix:											
6	369	Dry type	1 c	140	33	500	9	50	4	31	6	13	10
6	370	Moist type, with egg	1 c	203	61	420	9	40	4	26	5	11	8
		Cakes, prepared from mixes:[45]											
		Angel food cake:											
6	371	Whole cake, 9¾″ diam tube	1 ea	635	38	1510	38	342	3	2	.4	.2	1
6	372	Piece, ¹⁄₁₂ of cake	1 pce	53	38	125	3	29	<1	<1	t	t	.1
6	373	Boston cream pie, ⅛ of cake	1 pce	120	35	260	3	44	1	8	2.8	3.1	1.5
		Coffee cake:											
6	374	Whole cake, 7¾ × 5⅛ × 1¼″	1 ea	430	30	1385	27	225	3	41	12	17	10
6	375	Piece, ⅙ of cake	1 pce	72	30	230	5	38	2	7	2.0	2.8	1.6
		Devil's food with chocolate frosting:											
6	376	Whole cake, 2 layer, 8 or 9″ diam	1 ea	1107	24	3755	49	645	5	136	56	51	20
6	377	Piece, ¹⁄₁₆ of cake	1 pce	69	24	235	3	40	1	8	3.5	3.2	1.2
6	378	Cupcake, 2½″ diam	1 ea	42	24	143	2	25	<1	5	2.1	2.0	.7
		Gingerbread:											
6	379	Whole cake, 8″ square	1 ea	570	37	1575	18	291	3	39	10	16	11
6	380	Piece, ⅑ of cake	1 pce	63	37	174	2	32	2	4	1.1	1.8	1.2
		Yellow, with chocolate frosting, 2 layer:											
6	381	Whole cake, 8 or 9″ diam	1 ea	1108	26	3735	45	638	5	125	48	49	22
6	382	Piece, ¹⁄₁₆ of cake	1 pce	69	26	235	3	40	<1	8	3	3.1	1.4
		Cakes from home recipes with enriched flour:											
		Carrot cake, cream cheese frosting:[46]											
6	383	Whole, 9 × 13″ cake	1 ea	1792	23	6496	63	832	20	328	69	135	114
6	384	Piece, ¹⁄₁₆ of 9 × 13″ cake 2¼ × 3¼″	1 pce	112	23	406	4	52	1	21	4.3	8.5	7.1
		Fruitcake, dark, 7½″ diam tube, 2¼″ high:[46]											
6	385	Whole cake	1 ea	1361	18	5185	74	783	38	228	48	113	52
6	386	Piece, ¹⁄₃₂ of cake, ⅔″ arc	1 pce	43	18	165	2	25	2	7	1.5	3.6	1.6
		Sheet cake, plain, no frosting:[47]											
6	387	Whole cake, 9″ square	1 ea	777	25	2830	35	434	3	108	30	45	26
6	388	Piece, ⅑ of cake	1 pce	86	25	315	4	48	<1	12	3.3	5	2.8
		Sheet cake, plain, uncooked white frosting:[48]											
6	389	Whole cake, 9″ square	1 ea	1096	21	4020	37	694	3	129	42	50	26
6	390	Piece, ⅑ of cake	1 pce	121	21	445	4	77	<1	14	5	6	3
		Pound cake:[48]											
6	391	Loaf, 8½ × 3½ × 3¼″	1 ea	514	22	2025	33	265	4	94	21	41	27
6	392	Piece, ¹⁄₁₇ of loaf, ½″ slice	1 pce	30	22	120	2	15	<1	5	1.2	2.4	1.6
		Cakes, commercial:											
		Pound cake:											
6	393	Loaf, 8½ × 3½ × 3″	1 ea	500	24	1935	26	257	4	94	52	30	4
6	394	Slice, ¹⁄₁₇ of loaf, ½″ slice	1 pce	29	24	110	2	15	<1	5	3.0	1.7	.2
		Snack cakes:											
6	395	Chocolate w/creme filling, 2 small cakes per package	1 ea	28	20	105	1	17	<1	4	1.7	1.5	.6
6	396	Sponge cake w/creme filling, 2 small cakes per package	1 ea	42	19	155	1	27	<1	5	2.3	2.1	.5

[45] Excepting angel food cake, cakes were made from mixes containing vegetable shortening, and frostings were made with margarine. All mixes use enriched flour.
[46] Made with vegetable oil.
[47] Cake made with vegetable shortening.
[48] Made with margarine.

(Computer code number is for West Diet Analysis program)

GRP KEY: 1=BEV 2=DAIRY 3=EGGS 4=FAT/OIL 5=FRUIT 6=BAKERY 7=GRAIN 8=FISH 9=BEEF 10=POULTRY
11=SAUSAGE 12=MIXED/FAST 13=NUTS/SEEDS 14=SWEETS 15=VEG/LEG 16=MISC 22=SOUP/SAUCE

Chol (mg)	Calc (mg)	Iron (mg)	Magn (mg)	Phos (mg)	Pota (mg)	Sodi (mg)	Zinc (mg)	VT-A (RE)	Thia (mg)	Ribo (mg)	Niac (mg)	V-B6 (mg)	Fola (µg)	VT-C (mg)
0	92	2.2	30	136	126	1254	.55	273	.17	.20	2.50	.02	14	0
67	81	2.03	45	134	118	1023	.78	256	.10	.18	1.62	.04	20	t
0	527	2.73	51	1086	845	3226	.82	0	.32	1.27	1.6	.08	51	0
0	44	.23	4	91	71	269	.07	0	.03	.11	.13	.01	4	0
20	26	.6	11	70	40	225	.23	70	.01	.18	.7	.05	7	0
279	262	7.30	27	748	469	1853	3.70	194	.82	.90	7.70	.12	30	1
47	44	1.22	5	125	78	310	.62	32	.14	.15	1.29	.02	5	t
598	653	22.1	200	1162	1439	2900	7.95	498	1.11	1.66	10	.32	82	1
37	41	1.40	12	72	90	181	.53	31	.07	.1	.6	.02	1	t
23	25	.85	7	44	55	110	.40	19	.04	.06	.37	.01	3	t
6	513	10.8	41	570	1562	1733	5.52	0	.86	1.03	7.4	.07	36	1
1	57	1.20	5	63	173	192	.61	0	.10	.11	.82	.01	4	t
576	1008	15.5	72	2017	1208	2515	3.31	465	1.22	1.66	11.1	.45	80	1
36	63	.97	5	126	75	157	.21	29	.08	.10	.69	.03	5	t
912	440	20	185	1040	1856	2336	7.2	10,600	1.92	1.97	15.0	1.12	192	23
57	27	1.2	12	65	116	146	.45	663	.11	.14	1.0	.06	12	1
640	1293	37.6	340	1592	6138	2123	6.8	422	2.41	2.55	17	1.72	54	504
20	41	1.2	11	50	194	67	.22	13	.08	.08	.5	.05	2	16
552	497	11.7	108	793	614	2331	2.75	373	1.24	1.40	10.1	.26	54	2
61	55	1.3	12	88	68	258	.31	41	.14	.15	1.1	.03	15	t
636	548	11	108	822	669	2488	2.90	647	1.21	1.42	9.9	.27	110	2
70	61	1.2	12	91	74	275	.32	71	.13	.16	1.1	.03	12	t
555	339	9.3	48	473	483	1645	2.69	1033	.93	1.08	7.8	.39	55	1
32	20	.5	3	28	28	98	.16	60	.05	.06	.5	.02	3	t
1100	146	9.3	48	517	443	1857	1.95	715	.96	1.12	8.1	.38	55	1
64	8	.5	3	30	26	108	.11	41	.06	.06	.5	.02	3	t
15	21	1.0	3	26	34	105	.17	4	.06	.09	.7	.01	3	0
7	14	.6	3	44	37	155	.21	9	.07	.06	.6	.02	4	0

C

(For purposes of calculations, use "0" for t, <1, <.1, <.01, etc.)

Table C–1   Food Composition

Grp	Computer Code No.	Food Description	Measure	Wt (g)	H₂O (%)	Ener (kcal)	Prot (g)	Carb (g)	Dietary Fiber (g)	Fat (g)	Fat Breakdown (g) Sat	Mono	Poly
		BAKED GOODS—Con.											
		Cakes—Con.											
		White cake with white frosting, 2-layer:											
6	397	Whole cake, 8 or 9″ diam	1 ea	1140	24	4170	43	670	5	148	33	62	42
6	398	Piece, 1/16 of cake	1 pce	71	24	260	3	42	<1	9	2.1	3.8	2.6
		Yellow cake with chocolate frosting, 2-layer:											
6	399	Whole cake, 8 or 9″ diam	1 ea	1108	23	3895	40	620	5	175	92	59	10
6	400	Piece, 1/16 of cake	1 pce	69	23	245	3	39	<1	11	5.7	3.7	.6
		Cheesecake:											
6	401	Whole cake, 9″ diam	1 ea	1110	46	3350	60	317	5	213	120	66	15
6	402	Piece, 1/12 of cake	1 pce	92	46	278	5	26	1	18	9.9	5.4	1.2
6	1035	Cheese puffs/Cheetos®	1 oz	28.4	1	158	2	14	<1	10	4.8	3.4	.6
		Cookies made with enriched flour:											
		Brownies with nuts:											
6	403	Commercial with frosting, 1½ × 1¾ × ⅞	1 ea	25	13	100	1	16	<1	4	1.6	2	.8
6	404	Home recipe, 1¾ × 1¾ × ⅞″[49]	1 ea	20	10	95	1	11	<1	6	1.4	2.8	1.2
		Chocolate chip cookies:											
6	405	Commercial, 2¼″ diam	4 ea	42	4	180	2	28	<1	9	2.9	3.1	2.6
6	406	Home recipe, 2¼″ diam[50]	4 ea	40	3	185	2	26	1	11	3.9	4.3	2
6	407	From refrigerated dough, 2¼″ diam	4 ea	48	5	225	2	32	1	11	4	4.4	2
6	408	Fig bars	4 ea	56	12	210	2	42	3	4	1	1.5	1
6	409	Oatmeal raisin cookies, 2⅝″ diam	4 ea	52	4	245	3	36	1	10	2.5	4.5	2.8
6	410	Peanut butter cookies, home recipe, 2⅝″ diam[50]	4 ea	48	3	245	4	28	1	14	4	5.8	2.8
6	411	Sandwich-type cookies, all	4 ea	40	2	195	2	29	<1	8	2	3.6	2.2
		Shortbread cookies:											
6	412	Commercial, small	4 ea	32	6	155	2	20	1	8	2.9	3	1.1
6	413	From home recipe, large[51]	2 ea	28	3	145	2	17	1	8	1.3	2.7	3.4
6	414	Sugar cookies from refrigerated dough, 2½″ diam	4 ea	48	4	235	2	31	<1	12	2.3	5	3.6
6	415	Vanilla wafers	10 ea	40	4	185	2	29	<1	7	1.8	3	1.8
6	416	Corn chips	1 oz	28	1	155	2	16	1	9	1.8	3.4	3.7
		Crackers:[52]											
6	1034	Armenian cracker bread	4 pce	28.4	4	117	5	19	4	2	.4	.7	1.1
6	417	Cheese crackers	10 ea	10	4	50	1	5	<1	3	.9	1.2	.3
6	418	Cheese crackers with peanut butter	4 ea	30	3	150	4	19	<1	8	1.6	3.2	1.2
6	419	Graham crackers	2 ea	14	4	60	1	11	<1	1	.4	.6	.4
6	420	Melba toast, plain	1 pce	5	4	20	1	4	<1	<1	.1	.1	.1
6	421	Rye wafers, whole grain	2 ea	14	5	55	1	10	2	1	.3	.4	.3
6	422	Saltine® crackers[53]	4 ea	12	4	50	1	9	<1	1	.5	.4	.2
6	423	Snack-type crackers, round	3 ea	9	3	45	1	6	<1	3	.6	1.2	.3
6	424	Wheat crackers, thin	4 ea	8	3	35	1	5	1	1	.4	.5	.4
6	425	Whole wheat wafers	2 ea	8	4	35	1	5	1	2	.5	.6	.4
6	426	Croissants, 4½ × 4 × 1¾″	1 ea	57	22	235	5	27	1	12	3.5	6.7	1.4
		Danish pastry:											
6	427	Packaged ring, plain, 12 oz	1 ea	340	27	1305	21	152	3	71	22	29	16
6	428	Round piece, plain, 4¼″ diam 1″ high	1 ea	57	27	220	4	26	1	12	3.6	4.8	2.6

[49] Made with vegetable oil.
[50] Made with vegetable shortening.
[51] Made with margarine.
[52] Crackers made with enriched white (wheat) flour except for rye wafers and whole-wheat wafers.
[53] Made with lard.

(Computer code number is for West Diet Analysis program)

GRP KEY: 1 = BEV   2 = DAIRY   3 = EGGS   4 = FAT/OIL   5 = FRUIT   6 = BAKERY   7 = GRAIN   8 = FISH   9 = BEEF   10 = POULTRY
11 = SAUSAGE   12 = MIXED/FAST   13 = NUTS/SEEDS   14 = SWEETS   15 = VEG/LEG   16 = MISC   22 = SOUP/SAUCE

Chol (mg)	Calc (mg)	Iron (mg)	Magn (mg)	Phos (mg)	Pota (mg)	Sodi (mg)	Zinc (mg)	VT-A (RE)	Thia (mg)	Ribo (mg)	Niac (mg)	V-B6 (mg)	Fola (µg)	VT-C (mg)
46	536	15.5	60	1585	832	2827	1.77	194	3.19	2.05	27.6	.16	64	0
3	33	1	4	99	52	176	.11	12	.2	.13	1.7	.01	4	0
609	366	19.9	72	1884	1972	3080	3.3	488	.78	2.22	10	.45	80	0
38	23	1.24	5	117	123	192	.21	30	.05	.14	.62	.03	5	0
2053	622	5.33	111	977	1088	2464	4.66	833	.33	1.44	5.11	.71	200	56
170	52	.44	9	81	90	204	.39	69	.03	.12	.42	.06	17	5
5	18	.20	7	29	23	344	—	26	.01	.03	.20	—	—	0
14	13	.61	14	26	50	59	.36	18	.08	.07	.33	.04	5	t
18	9	.40	11	26	35	51	.31	6	.05	.05	.3	.04	4	t
5	16	.8	10	41	56	140	.3	15	.1	.23	.9	.02	4	t
18	13	1	14	34	82	82	.22	5	.06	.06	.58	.03	4	0
22	13	1.04	10	34	62	173	.24	8	.06	.10	.89	.01	4	0
27	40	1.36	15	34	162	180	.36	6	.08	.07	.73	.07	4	t
2	18	1.1	26	58	90	148	.53	12	.09	.08	1	.03	6	0
22	21	1.1	19	60	110	142	.36	5	.07	.07	1.9	.04	12	0
0	12	1.4	15	40	66	189	.21	0	.09	.07	.8	.01	1	0
27	13	.8	4	39	38	123	.15	8	.10	.09	.9	.01	3	0
0	6	.55	4	31	18	125	.13	89	.08	.06	.71	.01	2	t
29	50	.9	8	91	33	261	.24	11	.09	.06	1.1	.02	4	0
25	16	.8	6	36	50	150	.12	14	.07	.1	1	.01	4	0
0	35	.5	21	52	52	233	.44	11	.04	.05	.4	.04[54]	3[55]	1
0	21	.45	41	1	77	—	.90	1	.06	.04	1.05	.03	12	2
6	11	.35	3	17	17	112	.07	5	.05	.04	.4	.01	—	0
4	26	1.2	2	94	64	338	.06	3	.16	.12	2.4	.03	—	0
0	6	.37	6	20	36	86	.11	0	.02	.03	.6	.01	2	0
0	6	.1	1	10	11	44	—	0	.01	.01	.1	.01	.7	0
0	7	.5	16	44	65	115	1.60	0	.06	.03	.5	.03	10	0
4	3	.5	3	12	17	165	.09	0	.06	.05	.6	<.01	2	0
0	9	.3	2	18	12	90	.05	t	.03	.03	.3	<.01	1	0
.6	3	.25	6[56]	15	17	69	.24[56]	t	.04	.03	.4	.01	3[55]	0
0	3	.24	8[56]	22	31	59	.23	0	.02	.03	.4	.01	3[55]	0
13	20	2.1	9	64	68	452	.32	13	.17	.13	1.3	.03	18	0
292	360	6.5	68	347	316	1302	2.86	99	.95	1.02	8.5	.12	84	t
49	60	1.1	11	58	53	218	.48	17	.16	.17	1.4	.02	14	t

[54] Vitamin B$_6$ values vary from 0 to .04 g between various brands—check label.
[55] Folacin values estimated and derived from values for cornmeal and corn tortillas.
[56] Values derived from whole-wheat recipes and retention values.

(For purposes of calculations, use "0" for t, <1, <.1, <.01, etc.)

Table C–1   Food Composition

	Computer Code								Dietary		Fat Breakdown (g)		
Grp	No.	Food Description	Measure	Wt (g)	H₂O (%)	Ener (kcal)	Prot (g)	Carb (g)	Fiber (g)	Fat (g)	Sat	Mono	Poly
BAKED GOODS—Con.													
		Danish Pastry—Con.											
6	429	Ounce, plain	1 oz	28	28	110	2	13	<1	6	1.8	2.4	1.3
6	430	Round piece with fruit	1 pce	65	30	235	4	28	1	13	3.9	5.2	2.9
		Desserts, 3 × 3 inch piece:											
6	1348	Apple crisp	1 pce	78	58	146	1	25	1	5	1.0	2.3	1.7
6	1353	Apple cobbler	1 pce	104	56	201	2	35	2	6	1.4	2.7	1.9
6	1349	Cherry crisp	1 pce	138	73	157	2	27	2	5	1.0	2.3	1.7
6	1352	Cherry cobbler	1 pce	129	65	199	2	34	1	6	1.4	2.7	1.9
6	1350	Peach crisp	1 pce	139	72	166	2	30	2	5	1.0	2.3	1.7
6	1351	Peach cobbler	1 pce	130	64	130	2	37	2	6	1.4	2.7	1.9
		Doughnuts:											
6	431	Cake type, plain, 3¼″ diam	1 ea	50	21	210	2	25	1	12	3.4	5.8	2
6	432	Yeast-leavened, glazed, 3¾″ diam	1 ea	60	27	235	4	26	1	13	5.2	5.5	.9
		English muffins:											
6	433	Plain, enriched	1 ea	57	42	140	5	26	2	1	.3	.2	.3
6	434	Toasted	1 ea	50	29	140	5	26	2	1	.3	.2	.3
		Muffins, 2½″ diam, 1½″ high:											
		From home recipe:											
6	435	Blueberry[57]	1 ea	45	37	135	3	20	2	5	1.5	2.1	1.2
6	436	Bran, wheat[58]	1 ea	45	35	125	3	19	3	6	1.4	1.6	2.3
6	437	Cornmeal	1 ea	45	33	145	3	21	2	5	1.5	2.2	1.4
		From commercial mix:											
6	438	Blueberry	1 ea	45	33	140	3	22	2	5	1.4	2	1.2
6	439	Bran	1 ea	45	28	140	3	24	3	4	1.3	1.6	1
6	440	Cornmeal	1 ea	45	30	145	3	22	2	6	1.7	2.3	1.4
		Pancakes, 4″ diam:											
6	441	Buckwheat, from mix with egg and milk	1 ea	27	58	55	2	6	1	2	.9	.9	.5
6	442	Plain, from home recipe	1 ea	27	50	60	2	9	1	2	.5	.8	.5
6	443	Plain, from mix; egg, milk, oil added	1 ea	27	54	60	2	8	1	2	.5	.9	.5
		Piecrust, with enriched flour, vegetable shortening, baked:											
6	444	Home recipe, 9″ shell	1 ea	180	15	900	11	79	4	60	15	26	16
		From mix:											
6	445	Piecrust for 2-crust pie	1 ea	320	19	1485	21	141	6	93	23	41	25
6	446	1 pie shell	1 ea	180	19	835	12	79	4	52	13	23	14
		Pies, 9″ diam; pie crust made with vegetable shortening, enriched flour:											
		Apple pie:[59]											
6	447	Whole pie	1 ea	945	48	2420	22	360	19	105	25	46	29
6	448	Piece, ⅙ of pie	1 pce	158	48	405	4	60	3	18	4.1	7.6	4.9
		Banana cream pie:[60]											
6	449	Whole pie	1 ea	1190	66	1915	38	282	10	77	27	29	15
6	450	⅙ of pie	1 pce	198	66	319	6	47	2	13	4.5	4.9	2.5
		Blueberry pie:[59]											
6	451	Whole pie	1 ea	945	51	2285	23	330	22	102	24	45	28
6	452	Piece, ⅙ of pie	1 pce	158	51	380	4	55	4	17	4.0	7.5	4.7

[57]Made with vegetable shortening.
[58]Made with vegetable oil.
[59]Recipes updated for latest USDA values for fruits/nuts/fruit juice.
[60]Recipe based on pie crust, cooked vanilla pudding, 2 bananas.

(Computer code number is for West Diet Analysis program)

GRP KEY: 1 = BEV   2 = DAIRY   3 = EGGS   4 = FAT/OIL   5 = FRUIT   6 = BAKERY   7 = GRAIN   8 = FISH   9 = BEEF   10 = POULTRY
        11 = SAUSAGE   12 = MIXED/FAST   13 = NUTS/SEEDS   14 = SWEETS   15 = VEG/LEG   16 = MISC   22 = SOUP/SAUCE

Chol (mg)	Calc (mg)	Iron (mg)	Magn (mg)	Phos (mg)	Pota (mg)	Sodi (mg)	Zinc (mg)	VT-A (RE)	Thia (mg)	Ribo (mg)	Niac (mg)	V-B6 (mg)	Fola (µg)	VT-C (mg)
24	30	.55	6	29	27	109	.24	9	.08	.09	.7	.01	7	t
56	17	1.3	13	80	57	233	.55	11	.16	.14	1.4	.02	16	t
0	20	.77	12	15	112	66	.09	65	.05	.04	.41	.03	3	4
1	32	.76	7	42	86	305	.17	76	.08	.07	.70	.04	3	<1
0	29	2.16	16	22	163	73	.14	144	.06	.08	.56	.05	10	3
1	39	1.78	10	46	113	311	.21	135	.09	.10	.81	.05	9	2
0	24	.00	18	30	197	71	.19	104	.05	.05	1.01	.03	5	5
1	35	.90	11	52	139	309	.24	105	.08	.08	1.15	.03	5	3
20	23	.8	12	111	58	192	.25	5	.12	.12	1.1	.02	4	t
21	17	1.4	13	55	64	222	.30	<1	.28	.12	1.8	.28	13	0
0	96	1.7	11	67	331	378	.41	0	.26	.18	2.14	.02	18	0
0	96	1.7	11	67	331	378	.41	0	.23	.18	2.14	.02	15	0
19	54	.9	11	46	47	198	.29	9	.10	.11	.9	<.01	12	1
24	60	1.4	34	125	99	189	.37	30	.11	.13	1.3	.01	9	3
23	66	.9	11	59	57	169	.31	15	.11	.11	.9	.04	5	t
45	15	.9	7	90	54	225	.21	11	.11	.13	1.17	<.01	14	<1
28	27	1.7	28	182	50	385	.95	14	.08	.12	1.9	.12	19	0
42	30	1.3	11	128	31	291	.34	16	.09	.09	.8	.04	5	t
20	59	.4	18	91	66	125	.5	17	.04	.05	.2	.06	6	t
16	27	.5	7	38	33	115	.23	10	.06	.07	.5	.02	4	t
16	36	.7	7	71	43	160	.23	7	.09	.12	.8	.01	3	t
0	25	4.5	31	90	90	1100	1.50	0	.54	.40	5.0	.17	32	0
0	131	9.3	44	272	179	2600	1.19	0	1.07	.79	9.89	.27	57	0
0	74	5.23	25	153	101	1462	.79	0	.60	.44	5.57	.15	32	0
0	170	10	69	300	600	2844	1.6	28	1.04	.76	9.5	.5	48	2
0	28	1.67	12	50	100	476	.27	5	.18	.13	1.6	.08	8	<1
90	880	6.54	186	809	2000	2532	4.17	222	.94	1.75	7.40	1.77	116	26
15	147	1.09	31	135	333	422	.69	37	.16	.29	1.23	.30	19	4
0	155	12.3	60	274	756	2533	1.68	85	1.04	.85	10.4	.43	84	36
0	26	2.1	10	46	126	423	.28	14	.17	.14	1.73	.07	14	6

C

(For purposes of calculations, use "0" for t, <1, <.1, <.01, etc.)

Table C–1   Food Composition

Grp	Computer Code No.	Food Description	Measure	Wt (g)	H₂O (%)	Ener (kcal)	Prot (g)	Carb (g)	Dietary Fiber (g)	Fat (g)	Fat Breakdown (g)		
											Sat	Mono	Poly
		BAKED GOODS—Con.											
		Pies—Con.											
		Cherry pie:[59]											
6	453	Whole pie	1 ea	945	47	2465	26	363	15	107	25	47	30
6	454	Piece, ⅙ of pie	1 pce	158	47	410	4	61	2	18	4.2	7.8	4.9
		Chocolate cream pie:[61]											
6	455	Whole pie	1 ea	1051	63	1863	45	255	4	76	27	30	15
6	456	Piece, ⅙ of pie	1 pce	175	63	311	7	42	1	13	4.5	5.0	2.5
		Custard pie:											
6	457	Whole pie	1 ea	910	58	1760	46	204	4	84	28	35	17
6	458	Piece, ⅙ of pie	1 pce	152	58	293	8	34	1	13	.9	5.8	2.8
		Lemon meringue pie:[59]											
6	459	Whole Pie	1 ea	840	47	2140	31	317	5	84	21	37	22
6	460	Piece, ⅙ of pie	1 pce	140	47	355	5	53	1	14	3.5	6.2	3.7
		Peach pie:[59]											
6	461	Whole pie	1 ea	945	48	2410	24	361	17	105	25	46	29
6	462	Piece, ⅙ of pie	1 pce	158	48	405	4	61	3	17	4.1	7.7	4.8
		Pecan pie:[59]											
6	463	Whole pie	1 ea	825	20	3500	38	551	10	142	24	75	34
6	464	Piece, ⅙ of pie	1 pce	138	20	583	6	92	5	24	3.9	13	5.7
		Pumpkin pie:[59]											
6	465	Whole Pie	1 ea	910	59	2200	54	308	15	94	34	37	17
6	466	Piece, ⅙ of pie	1 pce	152	59	367	9	51	5	16	5.7	6.1	2.8
		Pies, fried, commercial:											
6	467	Apple	1 ea	85	43	255	2	32	2	14	5.8	6.6	.6
6	468	Cherry	1 ea	85	43	250	2	32	1	14	5.8	6.7	.6
		Pretzels, made with enriched flour:											
6	469	Thin sticks, 2¼″ long	10 ea	3	2	10	<1	2 (	<1	<1	t	<.1	<.1
6	470	Dutch twists, 2¾ × 2⅝″	1 ea	16	2	65	2	13	<1	1	.1	.2	.2
6	471	Thin twists, 3¼ × 2¼ × ¼″	10 ea	60	3	240	6	48	2	2	.4	.8	.6
		Rolls and buns, enriched:											
		Commercial:											
6	472	Cloverleaf rolls, 2½″ diam, 2″ high	1 ea	28	32	85	2	14	1	2	.5	.8	.6
6	473	Hotdog buns	1 ea	40	34	115	3	20	1	2	.5	.8	.6
6	474	Hamburger buns	1 ea	45	34	129	4	23	1	2	.6	.9	.7
6	475	Hard rolls, white, 3¾″ diam, 2″ high	1 ea	50	25	155	5	30	1	2	.4	.5	.6
6	476	Submarine rolls or hoagies, 11½ × 3 × 2½″	1 ea	135	31	400	11	72	2	8	1.8	3	2.2
		From home recipe:											
6	477	Dinner rolls 2½″ diam, 2″ high	1 ea	35	26	120	3	20	1	3	.8	1.2	.9
6	478	Toaster pastries, fortified	1 ea	54	13	210	2	38	1	6	1.7	3.6	.4
		Tortilla chips:											
6	1271	Plain	1 oz	28	4	139	2	17	1	8	1.1	3.1	3.1
6	1036	Nacho flavor	1 oz	28	1	139	2	18	1	7	1.4	2.5	2.8
6	1037	Taco flavor	1 oz	28	1	140	3	18	1	7	1.4	2.5	2.7
		Tortillas:											
6	479	Corn, enriched, 6″ diam	1 ea	30	45	65	2	13	2	1	.1	.3	.6
6	480	Flour, 8″ diam	1 ea	35	27	105	3	19	1	3	.4	1.2	1.0
6	1301	Flour tortilla, 10.5″ diam.	1 ea	57	27	168	4	31	2	4	.6	1.9	1.6
6	481	Taco shells	1 ea	14	4	59	1	9	1	2	.2	.6	1.2

[59]Recipes updated for latest USDA values for fruits/nuts/fruit juice.
[61]Based on value for pie crust, cooked chocolate pudding with meringue.

(Computer code number is for West Diet Analysis program)

GRP KEY: 1 = BEV 2 = DAIRY 3 = EGGS 4 = FAT/OIL 5 = FRUIT 6 = BAKERY 7 = GRAIN 8 = FISH 9 = BEEF 10 = POULTRY
11 = SAUSAGE 12 = MIXED/FAST 13 = NUTS/SEEDS 14 = SWEETS 15 = VEG/LEG 16 = MISC 22 = SOUP/SAUCE

Chol (mg)	Calc (mg)	Iron (mg)	Magn (mg)	Phos (mg)	Pota (mg)	Sodi (mg)	Zinc (mg)	VT-A (RE)	Thia (mg)	Ribo (mg)	Niac (mg)	V-B6 (mg)	Fola (µg)	VT-C (mg)
0	220	19	91	350	920	2873	1.87	416	1.13	.85	9.50	.50	93	5
0	37	3.17	15	58	153	480	.31	70	.19	.14	1.58	.08	16	1
90	958	6.46	176	881	1332	2565	4.46	204	.91	1.80	6.38	.54	66	3
15	160	1.08	29	147	222	427	.74	34	.15	.30	1.06	.09	11	<1
705	742	8.64	110	880	1040	2000	4.75	573	.82	1.60	5.50	.51	91	1
118	124	1.44	18	147	173	333	.79	96	.14	.27	.92	.08	15	4
822	150	8.4	54	412	420	2369	3.06	395	.59	.84	.50	.30	78	25
137	25	1.4	9	69	70	395	.51	66	.10	.14	.83	.05	13	4
0	160	11.3	98	332	1408	2533	2.11	690	1.04	.93	13.9	.39	72	28
0	27	1.90	16	55	235	423	.35	115	.18	.16	2.30	.07	12	5
822	210	12.0	192	777	781	1823	8.8	248	1.63	.99	6.6	.51	110	0
137	35	1.85	32	130	130	304	1.47	41	.22	.17	1.1	.08	18	0
655	1273	15.8	240	1269	2400	2029	5.96	11,170[62]	.82	1.76	7.3	.64	120	6
109	212	2.63	40	211	400	338	.99	1861[62]	.14	.29	1.22	.11	20	1
14	12	.94	6	34	42	326	.14	3	.09	.06	1.0	.03	4	1
13	11	.70	7	41	61	371	.15	19	.06	.06	.60	.04	8	1
0	1	.06	1	3	3	48	.03	0	.01	.01	.13	<.01	<1	0
0	4	.32	4	15	16	258	.17	0	.05	.04	.70	<.01	3	0
0	16	1.2	15	55	61	966	.42	0	.19	.15	2.6	.01	10	0
t	33	.81	6	44	36	155	.22	t	.14	.09	1.10	.01	11	<1
0	54	1.19	8	44	56	241	.36	t	.20	.13	1.58	.01	15	<1
0	61	1.34	9	50	63	271	.41	t	.22	.15	1.78	.02	17	<1
0	24	1.40	14	46	49	313	.44	0	.20	.12	1.70	.02	17	0
0	100	3.80	31	115	128	683	1.17	0	.54	.33	4.50	.09	49	0
12	16	1.10	10	36	41	98	.32	8	.12	.12	1.20	.01	12	0
0	104	2.16	10	104	91	248	.31	150[63]	.17	.18	2.27	.2	43	4
0	82	1.00	22	74	30	140	.42	1	.01	.02	.20	.08	<1	<1
0	17	.40	13	98	109	107	.42	13	.04	.03	.40	.10	—	0
0	45	.70	27	91	72	191	.42	15	.08	.09	.80	.10	—	0
0	42	.60	19	55	43	1	.36	8	.05	.03	.40	.09	6	0
0	21	.55	12	59	35	134	.27	0	.13	.08	1.20	.01	16	0
0	34	.88	19	94	56	215	.43	0	.21	.13	1.93	.02	25	0
0	26	.26	9	33	25	62	.22	1	<.01	.01	.25	.02	2	0

[62] Latest USDA values of vitamin A for canned pumpkin are almost 3.5 times greater than previously published values. Canned pumpkin is usually a blend of pumpkin and winter squash.

[63] Vitamin A values from label declaration varies from 100 to 150 RE for major brands.

(For purposes of calculations, use "0" for t, <1, <.1, <.01, etc.)

Table C–1　Food Composition

Grp	Computer Code No.	Food Description	Measure	Wt (g)	H₂O (%)	Ener (kcal)	Prot (g)	Carb (g)	Dietary Fiber (g)	Fat (g)	Fat Breakdown (g) Sat	Mono	Poly
BAKED GOODS—Con.													
		Waffles, 7″ diam:											
6	482	From home recipe	1 ea	75	37	245	7	26	1	13	4	4.9	2.6
6	483	From mix, egg/milk added	1 ea	75	42	205	7	27	1	8	2.7	2.9	1.5
GRAIN PRODUCTS: CEREAL, FLOUR, GRAIN, PASTA and NOODLES, POPCORN													
		Barley, pearled:											
7	484	Dry, uncooked	1 c	200	11	700	16	158	31	2	.4	.3	1.1
7	485	Cooked	1 c	157	69	193	4	44	4	1	.1	.1	.3
		Breakfast cereals, hot, cooked:											
		Corn grits (hominy) enriched cooked:											
7	486	Regular and quick, prepared	1 c	242	85	146	4	31	5	<1	t	.1	.3
7	487	Instant, prepared from packet, white	1 pkt	137	85	80	2	18	3	<1	t	.1	.1
		Cream of Wheat®, cooked:											
7	488	Regular, quick, instant	1 c	244	86	140	4	29	3	1	.1	.1	.2
7	489	Mix and eat, plain, packet	1 ea	142	82	100	3	21	2	<1	<.1	<.1	.1
7	490	Malt-O-Meal® cereal, cooked	1 c	240	88	122	4	26	3	<1	<.1	<.1	.1
		Oatmeal or rolled oats, cooked:											
7	491	Regular, quick, instant, nonfortified	1 c	234	85	145	6	25	4	2	.4	.8	1
		Instant, fortified:											
7	492	Plain, from packet	¾ c	177	86	104	4	18	3	2	.3	.6	.7
7	493	Flavored, from packet	¾ c	164	76	160	5	31	3	2	.3	.7	.8
7	494	Whole wheat cereal, cooked	1 c	242	84	150	5	33	4	1	.1	.1	.3
		Breakfast cereals, ready to eat:											
7	495	All-Bran®	⅓ c	28	3	70	4	22	9	<1	.1	.1	.3
7	1306	Alpha Bits®	1 c	28	1	111	2	25	1	1	.1	.2	.3
7	1307	Apple Jacks®	1 c	28	2	110	2	26	<1	<1	<.1	<.1	<.1
7	1308	Bran Buds®	1 c	84	3	217	12	64	23	2	.4	.3	1.1
7	1305	Bran Chex®	1 c	49	2	156	5	39	9	1	.2	.2	.8
7	1309	Buc Wheats®	¾ c	28	3	110	2	24	2	1	.1	.1	.5
7	1310	C.W. Post® plain	1 c	97	2	432	9	69	2	15	11.3	1.7	1.4
7	1311	C.W. Post® with raisins	1 c	103	4	446	9	74	2	15	11.0	1.7	1.4
7	496	Cap'n Crunch®	1 c	37	2	156	2	30	1	3	2.2	.4	.5
7	1312	Cap'n Crunchberries®	1 c	35	3	146	2	29	<1	3	1.9	.4	.5
7	1313	Cap'n Crunch®, peanut butter	1 c	35	2	154	3	27	<1	5	1.9	1.4	1.0
7	497	Cheerios®	1 c	23	5	89	3	16	2	1	.3	.5	.6
7	1314	Cocoa Krispies®	1 c	36	3	139	2	32	<1	<1	.2	.2	.2
7	1316	Cocoa Pebbles®	⅔ c	21	2	87	1	18	<1	1	<.1	<.1	<.1
7	1315	Corn Bran®	1 c	36	3	124	3	30	7	1	.2	.3	.7
7	1317	Corn Chex®	1 c	28	2	111	2	25	<1	<1	.1	.3	.6
7	498	Corn Flakes, Kellogg's®	1¼ c	28	3	110	2	24	1	<1	t	t	.1
7	499	Corn Flakes, Post Toasties®	1¼ c	28	3	110	2	24	1	<1	t	t	.1
7	1318	Cracklin' Oat Bran®	1 c	60	4	229	6	41	9	9	2.1	2.3	3.5
7	1038	Crispy Wheat 'N Raisins®	1 c	43	7	150	3	35	2	1	.1	.1	.4
7	1319	Fortified oat flakes	1 c	48	3	177	9	35	1	1	.1	.3	.3
7	500	40% Bran Flakes, Kellogg's®	1 c	39	3	125	5	35	5	1	.14	.14	.4
7	501	40% Bran Flakes, Post®	1 c	47	3	152	5	37	6	1	.2	.2	.3
7	502	Froot Loops®	1 c	28	2	111	2	25	<1	1	.2	.1	.1

(Computer code number is for West Diet Analysis program)

GRP KEY: 1 = BEV 2 = DAIRY 3 = EGGS 4 = FAT/OIL 5 = FRUIT 6 = BAKERY 7 = GRAIN 8 = FISH 9 = BEEF 10 = POULTRY
11 = SAUSAGE 12 = MIXED/FAST 13 = NUTS/SEEDS 14 = SWEETS 15 = VEG/LEG 16 = MISC 22 = SOUP/SAUCE

Chol (mg)	Calc (mg)	Iron (mg)	Magn (mg)	Phos (mg)	Pota (mg)	Sodi (mg)	Zinc (mg)	VT-A (RE)	Thia (mg)	Ribo (mg)	Niac (mg)	V-B6 (mg)	Fola (µg)	VT-C (mg)
102	154	1.50	17	135	129	445	.65	39	.18	.24	1.50	.03	13	t
59	179	1.20	14	257	146	515	.52	49	.14	.23	.90	.03	4	t
0	32	4.2	51	378	320	6	4.47	0	.24	.1	7.9	.45	40	0
0	17	2.1	35	85	146	5	1.29	0	.13	.1	3.2	.18	25	0
0	1	1.55[64]	11	29	54	0[65]	.18	15[66]	.24[64]	.15[64]	1.96[64]	.06	2	0
0	7	1[64]	5	16	29	343	.08	0	.18[64]	.08[64]	1.3[64]	.03	1	0
0	54[64]	10.9[64]	12	43[67]	46	5[67,68]	.35	0	.24[64]	.07[64]	1.5[64]	.02	9	0
0	20[64]	8.10[64]	7	20[64]	38	241	.20	376[64]	.43[64]	.28[64]	5.0[64]	.01	5	0
0	5	9.6[64]	14	24[64]	31	2[68]	.17	0	.48[64]	.24[64]	5.8[64]	.02	5	0
0	19	1.59	56	178	131	2[68]	1.15	5	.26	.05	.3	.05	9	0
0	163[64]	6.32[64]	51	133	99	285[64]	1	453[64]	.53[64]	.29[64]	5.49[64]	.74	150	0
0	168[64]	6.7[64]	51	148	137	254[64]	1	460[64]	.53[64]	.38[64]	5.9[64]	.77	150	<1
0	17	1.5	53	168	171	3	1.16	0	.17	.12	2.13	.07	25	0
0	23	4.5[64]	106	264	320	260	3.7	375[64]	.37[64]	.43[64]	5.0[64]	.5	100	15[64]
0	8	1.80	17	51	100	219	1.50	375	.40	.40	5.0	.50	100	—
0	3	4.50	6	30	23	125	3.70	375	.40	.40	5.0	.50	100	15
0	56	13.4	267	729	930	516	11.1	1112	1.10	1.30	14.8	1.50	297	45
0	29	7.80	126	327	394	455	2.14	11	.60	.26	8.6	.90	173	26
0	60	8.10	24	60	—	235	.30	682	.68	.77	9.0	.90	—	27
0	47	15.4	67	224	198	167	1.64	1284	1.30	1.50	17.1	1.70	342	—
0	51	16.4	74	232	260	160	1.64	1364	1.30	1.50	18.1	1.90	364	—
0	6	9.83[64]	15	47	48	278	4.01	5[64]	.66[64]	.71[64]	8.64[64]	1	238	0
0	11	9.04	14	47	49	243	3.56	0	.59	.67	8.14	.93	128	—
0	7	9.10	19	49	57	268	3.79	0	.60	.70	8.97	1.04	244	—
0	38	3.6[64]	31	109	82	246	.63	304[64]	.32[64]	.32[64]	4.0[64]	.4	5	12[64]
0	6	2.30	12	47	53	275	1.90	477	.50	.50	6.3	.60	127	19
0	4	1.30	9	16	35	102	1.10	282	.30	.30	3.7	.40	75	—
0	41	12.2	18	52	70	310	4.00	—	.38	.70	10.9	.86	232	—
0	3	1.80	4	11	23	271	.10	14	.40	.07	5.0	.50	100	15
0	1	1.8[64]	3	18	26	351	.06	375[64]	.37[64]	.43[64]	5.0[64]	.51	100	15[64]
0	1	.7[64]	3	12	33	297	.06	375[64]	.37[64]	.43[64]	5.0[64]	.51	100	0
0	40	3.80	116	241	355	402	3.20	794	.80	.90	10.6	1.10	212	32
0	71	6.80	35	117	174	204	.51	569	.60	.60	7.6	.80	40	—
0	68	13.7	58	176	343	429	1.50	636	.60	.70	.39	.90	169	—
0	19	11.2[64]	71	192	248	363	5.15	522[64]	.51[64]	.59[64]	6.86[64]	.7	138	0
0	21	7.47[64]	102	296	251	431	2.5	629[64]	.62[64]	.72[64]	8.3[64]	.85	166	0
0	3	4.5[64]	9	28	30	125	3.7	225[64]	.4[64]	.4[64]	5.0[64]	.5	100	15[64]

[64] Nutrient added (values sometimes based on label declaration).
[65] Cooked without salt. If salt is added according to label recommendation, sodium content is 540 mg.
[66] Value for yellow corn grits; cooked white corn grits contain 0 RE of vitamin A.
[67] Values for regular and instant cereal. For quick cereal, phosphorus is 102 mg, and sodium is 142 mg.
[68] Cooked without salt. If added according to label recommendations, sodium content is 390 mg for Cream of Wheat; 324 mg for Malt-O-Meal; 374 mg for oatmeal.

(For purposes of calculations, use "0" for t, <1, <.1, <.01, etc.)

Table C–1   Food Composition

Grp	Computer Code No.	Food Description	Measure	Wt (g)	H₂O (%)	Ener (kcal)	Prot (g)	Carb (g)	Dietary Fiber (g)	Fat (g)	Fat Breakdown (g)		
											Sat	Mono	Poly
GRAIN PRODUCTS—Con.													
		Cereals—Con.											
7	1320	Frosted Mini-Wheats®	4 ea	31	5	111	3	26	2	<1	.1	<.1	.2
7	1321	Frosted Rice Krispies®	1 c	28	3	109	1	26	1	<1	<.1	<.1	<.1
7	1323	Fruit & Fiber® w/apples	½ c	28	2	90	3	22	4	1	.2	.2	.6
7	1324	Fruit & Fiber® w/dates	½ c	28	2	90	3	21	4	1	.2	.2	.6
7	1325	Fruitful Bran® cereal	¾ c	34	3	110	3	27	5	0	0	0	0
7	1322	Fruity Pebbles® cereal	⅞ c	28	3	113	1	24	<1	2	.3	.2	.4
7	503	Golden Grahams®	1 c	39	2	156	2	33	2	2	1.0	.1	.2
7	504	Granola, homemade	1 c	122	3	595	15	67	13	33	5.8	9.4	17
7	505	Grape Nuts®	½ c	57	3	210	6	46	5	<1	t	t	.2
7	1326	Grape Nuts® flakes	⅞ c	28	3	102	3	23	2	<1	<.1	<.1	.1
7	1327	Honey & Nut Corn flakes	¾ c	28	4	113	2	23	<1	2	.2	.5	.7
7	506	Honey Nut Cheerios®	1 c	33	3	127	4	27	1	1	.2	.4	.5
7	1328	Honey Bran	1 c	35	3	119	3	29	4	1	.1	.1	.4
7	1329	Honeycomb®	1 c	22	1	86	1	20	<1	<1	.1	.1	.2
7	1330	King Vitamin® cereal	1 c	21	2	85	1	18	<1	1	.7	.2	.2
7	1039	Kix®	1 c	19	3	73	2	16	<1	<1	.1	.1	.2
7	1331	Life®	1 c	44	5	162	8	32	1	1	.1	.2	.4
7	507	Lucky Charms®	1 c	32	3	125	3	26	1	1	.2	.4	.5
7	508	Nature Valley® Granola	1 c	113	4	503	12	76	12	20	13	2.8	2.8
7	1332	Nutri-Grain™—Barley	1 c	41	3	153	5	34	2	<1	<.1	<.1	.1
7	1333	Nutri-Grain™—Corn	1 c	42	3	160	3	36	3	1	.1	.3	.6
7	1334	Nutri-Grain™—Rye	1 c	40	3	144	4	34	3	<1	.1	.1	.1
7	1335	Nutri-Grain™—Wheat	1 c	44	3	158	4	37	3	<1	.1	.1	.3
7	1336	100% Bran	1 c	66	3	178	8	48	20	3	.6	.6	1.9
7	509	100% Natural® cereal, plain	¼ c	28	2	135	3	18	3	6	4.1	1.2	.5
7	1337	100% Natural® with apples	1 c	104	2	478	11	70	5	20	15.5	1.8	1.3
7	1338	100% Natural® with raisins & dates	1 c	100	4	496	11	72	4	20	13.7	3.7	1.7
7	510	Product 19®	1 c	33	3	126	3	27	<1	<1	t	t	.1
7	1339	Quisp®	1 c	30	2	124	2	25	<1	2	1.5	.3	.3
7	511	Raisin Bran, Kellogg's®	1 c	49	8	158	5	37	6	1	.2	.1	.4
7	512	Raisin Bran, Post®	1 c	56	9	170	5	42	6	1	.2	.2	.4
7	1040	Raisins, Rice & Rye™	1 c	46	9	155	3	39	<1	<1	<.1	<.1	<.1
7	1041	Rice Chex®	¾ c	19	3	75	1	17	1	1	.2	.2	.3
7	513	Rice Krispies, Kellogg's®	1 c	29	2	112	2	25	<1	<1	t	t	.1
7	514	Rice, puffed	1 c	14	3	55	1	13	<1	<1	t	t	<.1
7	515	Shredded Wheat®	¾ c	32	5	115	3	25	4	1	.1	.1	.3
7	516	Special K®	1½ c	32	2	125	6	24	<1	<1	t	t	t
7	1340	Sugar Corn Pops®	1 c	28	3	108	1	26	<1	<1	t	<.1	.1
7	518	Sugar Frosted Flakes®	1 c	35	3	133	2	32	1	<1	t	t	t
7	517	Super Sugar Crisp®	1 c	33	2	123	2	30	<1	<1	t	t	.1
7	519	Sugar Smacks®	¾ c	28	3	106	2	25	<1	<1	.1	.1	.2
7	1341	Tasteeos®	1 c	24	2	94	3	19	1	1	.2	.2	.3
7	1342	Team®	1 c	42	4	164	3	36	<1	1	.2	.2	.3
7	520	Total®, wheat, with added calcium	1 c	33	4	122	3	26	2	1	.1	.1	.4
7	521	Trix®	1 c	28	2	109	1	25	<1	1	.2	.1	.1
7	1042	Wheat & Raisin Chex®	1 c	54	7	185	5	43	4	<1	.1	.1	.2
7	1344	Wheat Chex®	1 c	46	3	169	5	38	3	1	.2	.2	.6
7	1043	Wheat, puffed	1 c	12	3	44	2	10	2	<1	t	t	.1
7	522	Wheaties®	1 c	29	5	101	3	23	3	1	.1	.1	.2

(Computer code number is for West Diet Analysis program)

GRP KEY: 1 = BEV 2 = DAIRY 3 = EGGS 4 = FAT/OIL 5 = FRUIT 6 = BAKERY 7 = GRAIN 8 = FISH 9 = BEEF 10 = POULTRY
11 = SAUSAGE 12 = MIXED/FAST 13 = NUTS/SEEDS 14 = SWEETS 15 = VEG/LEG 16 = MISC 22 = SOUP/SAUCE

Chol (mg)	Calc (mg)	Iron (mg)	Magn (mg)	Phos (mg)	Pota (mg)	Sodi (mg)	Zinc (mg)	VT-A (RE)	Thia (mg)	Ribo (mg)	Niac (mg)	V-B6 (mg)	Fola (μg)	VT-C (mg)
0	10	2.00	26	81	106	9	1.60	410	.40	.50	5.5	.60	109	16
0	1	1.80	5	27	21	240	.31	375	.40	.40	5.0	.50	100	15
0	10	4.50	60	150	168	195	1.50	375	.38	.43	5.0	.50	100	0
0	10	4.50	60	100	168	170	1.50	378	.38	.43	5.0	.50	100	0
0	10	8.10	60	150	150	240	3.75	378	.38	.43	5.0	.50	100	0
0	4	1.80	6	16	22	157	2	375	.40	.40	5.0	.50	100	0
0	24	6.2[64]	16	56	82	476	.34	521[64]	.5[64]	.6[64]	6.9[64]	.7	136	21[64]
0	76	4.84	141	494	612	12	4.47	4	.73	.31	2.14	.43	99	1
0	20	16	52	153	183	341	2	753[64]	.7[64]	.9[64]	10.0[64]	1	200	0
0	11	4.50	31	84	99	218	.57	375	.40	.40	5.0	.50	100	—
0	3	1.80	6	13	36	225	.11	375	.40	.40	5.0	.50	100	15
0	23	5.2[64]	39	122	115	299	.87	437[64]	.4[64]	.5[64]	5.8[64]	.6	4	17[64]
0	16	5.60	46	132	151	202	.90	463	.50	.50	6.2	.60	23	19
0	4	1.40	8	22	70	166	1.20	291	.30	.30	3.9	.40	78	—
0	—	12.7	7	—	26	161	.16	717	.09	1.06	12.9	1.18	286	33
0	23	5.40	8	26	29	226	.17	250	.27	.27	3.33	.33	2	10
0	154	11.6	55	238	197	229	1.55	0	.95	1.00	11.6	.05	37	—
0	36	5.1[64]	27	88	66	227	.56	424[64]	.4[64]	.5[64]	5.6[64]	.6	—	17[64]
0	71	3.78	116	354	389	232	2.19	8	.39	.19	.83	.32	85	0
0	11	1.45	32	126	108	277	5.40	540	.50	.60	7.2	.70	145	22
0	1	.89	27	120	98	276	5.50	556	.50	.60	7.4	.75	148	22
0	8	1.13	31	104	72	272	5.30	530	.50	.60	7.0	.70	141	21
0	12	1.24	34	164	120	299	5.80	583	.60	.70	7.7	.80	155	23
0	46	8.12	312	801	824	457	5.74	0	1.60	1.80	20.9	2.10	200	63
0	49	.83	34	104	138	12	.63	2	.09	.15	.6	.64	8	0
0	157	2.89	71	350	513	52	2.00	8	.33	.58	1.88	.11	17	—
0	160	3.12	124	347	538	47	2.11	8	.30	.64	2.08	.17	45	—
0	4	21[64]	12	47	51	378	.5	1769[64]	1.7[64]	2[64]	23.3[64]	2.3	466	70[64]
0	9	6.31	12	25	45	241	.18	—	.54	.76	5.80	.91	8	—
0	25	24[64]	73	200	307	293	5.0	500[64]	.51[64]	.57[64]	6.67[64]	.67	133	0
0	27	9.01[64]	96	237	349	370	3.01	750[64]	.74[64]	.85[64]	10[64]	1.02	200	0
0	10	5.60	20	50	144	350	4.70	467	.50	.60	6.30	.60	125	0
0	3	1.20	5	19	22	158	.26	1	.27	.20	3.34	.33	67	10
0	4	1.8[64]	10	34	30	340	.48	388[64]	.4[64]	.4[64]	5.0[64]	.5	100	15[64]
0	1	.15[64]	4	14	16	<1	.14	0	.02[64]	.01[64]	.42[64]	.01	3	0
0	12	1.35	42	112	115	3	1.05	0	.08	.09	1.67	.08	16	0
0	9	5.06[64]	18	62	55	298	4.16	429[64]	.45[64]	.45[64]	5.63[64]	.56	112	17[64]
0	2	1.80	2	8	20	90	1.50	225	.40	.40	5.00	.50	100	15
0	1	2.2[64]	3	26	22	284	.05	463[64]	.5[64]	.5[64]	6.2[64]	.6	124	19[64]
0	7	2.1[64]	20	60	123	29	1.7	437[64]	.4[64]	.5[64]	5.8[64]	.6	116	0
0	3	1.8[64]	13	31	42	75	.28	375[64]	.37[64]	.43[64]	5[64]	.5	100	15[64]
0	11	3.80	26	96	71	183	.69	318	.30	.40	4.20	.40	9	13
0	6	2.57	19	65	71	259	.58	556	.55	.63	7.40	.80	—	22
0	200	21[64]	34	137	123	330	.15	1769[64]	1.7[64]	2[64]	23.3[64]	2.3	400	70[64]
0	6	4.5[64]	6	22	27	169	.13	379[64]	.4[64]	.4[64]	4.9[64]	.5	99	15[64]
0	—	7.70	53	163	174	306	1.19	<1	.50	.60	7.10	.70	143	2
0	18	7.30	58	182	174	308	1.23	0	.60	.17	8.10	.80	162	24
0	3	.57	17	43	42	0	.30	0	.02	.03	1.30	.02	4	0
0	44	4.6[64]	32	100	108	363	.65	388[64]	.4[64]	.4[64]	5.1[64]	.5	9	15[64]

[64] Nutrient added (values sometimes based on label declaration).

(For purposes of calculations, use "0" for t, <1, <.1, <.01, etc.)

Table C–1   Food Composition

Grp	Computer Code No.	Food Description	Measure	Wt (g)	H₂O (%)	Ener (kcal)	Prot (g)	Carb (g)	Dietary Fiber (g)	Fat (g)	Sat	Mono	Poly
		GRAIN PRODUCTS—Con.											
		Buckwheat:											
		Flour:											
7	523	Dark	1 c	98	12	338	12	71	8	3	.5	.8	.9
7	524	Light	1 c	98	12	340	6	78	6	1	.2	.4	.4
7	525	Whole grain, dry	1 c	175	11	586	23	128	16	4	.8	1.4	1.5
		Bulgar:											
7	526	Dry, uncooked	1 c	140	9	479	17	106	31	2	.3	.2	.8
7	527	Cooked	1 c	182	78	151	6	34	11	<1	.1	.1	.2
		Cornmeal:											
7	528	Whole-ground, unbolted, dry	1 c	122	10	442	10	94	13	4	.6	1.2	2
7	529	Bolted, nearly whole, dry	1 c	122	10	441	10	91	12	4	.6	1.2	2
7	530	Degermed, enriched, dry	1 c	138	12	505	12	107	10	2	.3	.6	1
7	531	Degermed, enriched, cooked	1 c	240	88	120	3	26	3	<1	.1	.1	.3
		Macaroni, cooked:											
7	532	Enriched	1 c	140	66	197	7	40	2	1	.1	.1	.4
7	533	Vegetable, enriched	1 c	134	68	172	6	36	2	.1	<.1	<.1	<.1
7	534	Whole wheat	1 c	140	67	174	8	37	2	1	.1	.1	.3
7	535	Millet, cooked	½ c	120	71	143	4	28	1	1	.2	.2	.6
		Noodles:											
7	536	Egg noodles, cooked	1 c	160	69	213	8	40	4	2	.5	.7	.6
7	537	Chow mein, dry	1 c	45	.73	237	4	26	2	14	2	4	8
7	538	Spinach noodles, dry	3½ oz	100	8	372	13	75	7	2	1.0	1.1	1.1
7	1343	Oat bran, dry	¼ c	25	6	61	4	17	4	2	.3	.6	.7
		Popcorn:											
7	539	Air popped, plain	1 c	8	4	30	1	6	1	<1	t	.1	.2
7	540	Popped in veg oil/salted	1 c	11	3	55	1	6	1	3	.5	1.4	1.2
7	541	Sugar-syrup coated	1 c	35	4	135	2	30	1	1	.1	.3	.6
		Rice:											
7	542	Brown rice, cooked	1 c	195	73	217	5	45	3	2	.3	.6	.6
		White, enriched, all types:											
7	543	Regular/long grain, dry	1 c	185	12	675	13	148	2	1	.3	.4	.3
7	544	Regular/long grain, cooked	1 c	205	69	264	6	57	1	<1	.2	.2	.2
7	545	Instant, prepared without salt	1 c	165	76	162	3	35	1	<1	.1	.1	.1
		Parboiled/converted rice:											
7	546	Raw, dry	1 c	185	10	686	13	151	4	1	.3	.3	.3
7	547	Cooked	1 c	175	73	200	4	43	1	<1	.1	.2	<.1
7	548	Wild rice, cooked	1 c	164	74	166	4	35	3	<1	.1	.1	<.1
7	549	Rye flour, medium	1 c	102	10	361	10	79	15	2	.2	.2	.8
7	1044	Soy flour, low fat	1 c	88	3	370	51	34	12	6	.9	1.3	3.3
		Spaghetti, cooked:											
7	550	without salt, enriched	1 c	140	66	197	7	40	2	1	.5	.1	.4
7	551	with salt, enriched	1 c	140	66	197	7	40	2	1	.5	.1	.4
7	552	Whole wheat spaghetti, cooked	1 c	140	94	174	7	37	5	1	.1	.1	.3
7	1302	Tapioca, dry	1 c	152	11	518	.3	135	2	<.1	<.1	<.1	<.1
7	553	Wheat bran	½ c	30	10	65	5	19	8	1	.2	.2	.7
		Wheat germ:											
7	554	Raw	1 c	100	11	360	23	52	12	10	1.7	1.4	6
7	555	Toasted	1 c	113	6	432	33	56	16	12	2.1	1.7	7.5
7	556	Rolled wheat, cooked	1 c	240	80	142	4	32	5	1	.1	.1	.3
7	557	Whole-grain wheat, cooked	⅓ c	50	86	28	1	7	1	<1	<.1	<.1	.1

(Computer code number is for West Diet Analysis program)

GRP KEY: 1=BEV 2=DAIRY 3=EGGS 4=FAT/OIL 5=FRUIT 6=BAKERY 7=GRAIN 8=FISH 9=BEEF 10=POULTRY
11=SAUSAGE 12=MIXED/FAST 13=NUTS/SEEDS 14=SWEETS 15=VEG/LEG 16=MISC 22=SOUP/SAUCE

Chol (mg)	Calc (mg)	Iron (mg)	Magn (mg)	Phos (mg)	Pota (mg)	Sodi (mg)	Zinc (mg)	VT-A (RE)	Thia (mg)	Ribo (mg)	Niac (mg)	V-B6 (mg)	Fola (µg)	VT-C (mg)
0	32	2.5	135	298	490	1	2.65	0	.58	.16	2.75	.41	125	0
0	11	1	47	86	314	1	2.56	0	.09	.05	.47	.09	100	0
0	200	6.7	335	560	740	3	4.4	0	1.05	.26	7.7	.37	53	0
0	49	3.4	230	420	574	24	2.7	0	.33	.16	7.2	.48	38	0
0	18	1.8	58	73	124	9	1.04	0	.1	.05	1.8	.15	33	0
0	7	4.2	155	294	350	43	2.22	57	.47	.25	4.4	.37	31	0
0	21	4.2	154	272	303	43	2.22	57	.37	.1	2.3	.56	29	0
0	7	5.7	55	116	224	4	1	57	1	1	7	.35	66	0
0	2	1.48	17	34	38	1	.23	14	.14	.1	1.2	.06	6	0
0	10	2	25	76	43	1	.74	0	.29	.14	2.34	.05	10	0
0	15	1	26	67	42	8	.59	7	.15	.08	1.4	.03	4	0
0	21	1.5	42	125	62	4	1.1	0	.2	.1	1	.11	7	0
0	4	1	53	120	74	2	1.1	0	.1	.1	1.6	.13	23	0
50	19	2.5	30	110	45	11	1	10	.3	.13	2.4	.06	11	0
0	14	2.1	23	72	54	197	1	4	.3	.2	3	.05	10	0
0	58	2.1	174	322	376	36	2.8	46	.37	.2	4.6	.32	48	0
0	15	1.4	59	184	142	1	.78	0	.29	.05	.23	.04	13	—
0	1	.2	23	22	20	<1	.22	1	.03	.01	.2	.02	3	0
0	3	.27	25	31	19	86	.28	2	.01	.02	.1	.02	3	0
0	2	.5	29	47	90	<1	.29	3	.13	.02	.4	.03	3	0
0	20	1	84	162	84	10	1.23	0	.19	.05	3	.28	8	0
0	52	8	46	213	213	9	2.02	0	1	1	7.76	.3	15	0
0	23	2.3	27	96	80	4	.94	0	.33	.03	3.03	.19	6	0
0	13	1.04	8	23	6.6	5[69]	.4	0	.12	.08	1.45	.017	6.6	0
0	111	7	57	252	222	9.3	1.78	0	1.1	.13	6.7	.65	32	0
0	33	2	21	74	65	5	.54	0	.44	.03	2.5	.03	7	0
0	5	1	53	135	166	5	2.2	0	.1	.14	2.1	.221	43	0
0	25	2.16	77	211	347	3	2	0	.29	.11	1.76	.273	38	0
0	165	5.27	202	522	2262	16	1.04	4	.33	.25	1.90	.46	361	0
0	10	2.00	25	76	43	1	.74	0	.29	.14	2.34	.05	10	0
0	10	2	25	76	43	140	.74	0	.29	.14	2.34	.05	10	0
0	21	1.5	42	125	62	4	1.14	0	.15	.06	1	.11	7	0
0	30	2.4	1.5	10.6	17	2	.182	0	.01	.15	0	0	6	0
0	22	3.2	183	304	355	.6	2.18	0	.16	.17	4.07	.39	24	0
0	39	6.3	239	842	892	12	12	0	1.88	.5	6	1.3	281	0
0	51	10.3	362	1295	1070	5	18.9	0	1.89	.93	6.32	1.11	398	0
0	17	1.5	58	130	165	2	1.22	0	.17	.06	2.2	.08	27	0
0	3	.3	12	26	33	<1	.24	0	.04	.01	.5	.03	4	0

[69]If prepared with salt according to label recommendation, sodium would be 608 mg.

(For purposes of calculations, use "0" for t, <1, <.1, <.01, etc.)

Table C–1 Food Composition

Grp	Computer Code No.	Food Description	Measure	Wt (g)	H₂O (%)	Ener (kcal)	Prot (g)	Carb (g)	Dietary Fiber (g)	Fat (g)	Fat Breakdown (g) Sat	Mono	Poly
		GRAIN PRODUCTS—Con.											
		Wheat flour (unbleached):											
		All-purpose white flour, enriched:											
7	558	Sifted	1 c	115	12	419	12	88	3	1	.2	.1	.5
7	559	Unsifted	1 c	125	12	455	13	95	3	1	.2	.1	.5
7	560	Cake or pastry flour, enriched, sifted	1 c	96	12	348	8	75	3	1	.1	.1	.4
7	561	Self-rising, enriched, unsifted	1 c	125	11	442	12	93	3	1	.2	.1	.5
7	562	Whole wheat, from hard wheats	1 c	120	10	407	16	87	15	2	.4	.3	1
		MEATS: FISH and SHELLFISH											
8	1045	Bass, baked or broiled	3.5 oz.	100	70	125	24	0	0	4	.9	1.6	1.2
		Bluefish:											
8	1046	Baked or broiled	3.5 oz.	100	68	159	26	0	0	5	1.1	2.1	1.3
8	1047	Fried in bread crumbs	3.5 oz.	100	61	205	23	5	0	10	2.1	4.3	2.5
		Clams:											
8	563	Raw meat only	3 oz	85	82	63	11	2	<1	1	.1	.1	.2
8	564	Canned, drained	3 oz	85	64	126	22	4	t	2	.2	.2	.5
8	1290	Steamed, meat only	20 ea	90	64	133	23	5	<1	2	.2	.2	.5
		Cod:											
8	565	Baked with butter	3½ oz	100	75	132	23	0	0	3	.4	.3	.5
8	566	Batter fried	3½ oz	100	61	199	20	8	0	10	3.9	5.5	.9
8	567	Poached, no added fat	3½ oz	100	76	102	22	0	0	1	.2	.1	.3
		Crab, meat only:											
8	1048	Blue crab, cooked	1 c	135	77	138	27	0	0	2	.3	.4	.9
8	1049	Dungeness Crab, cooked	.75 c	101	74	85	18	<1	0	2	.3	.6	1.1
8	568	Canned	1 c	135	76	133	28	0	0	2	.3	.3	.6
8	1587	Crab, imitation, from surimi	3 oz	85	74	87	10	9	0	1	—	—	—
8	569	Fish sticks, breaded pollock	2 ea	57	46	155	9	14	<1	7	1.8	2.9	1.8
		Flounder/sole, baked with lemon juice:											
8	570	With butter	3 oz	85	73	120	16	<1	0	6	3.2	1.5	.5
8	571	With margarine	3 oz	85	73	120	16	<1	0	6	1.2	2.3	1.9
8	572	Without added fat	3 oz	85	78	99	21	0	0	1	.3	.3	.4
		Haddock:											
8	573	Breaded, fried[70]	3 oz	85	61	175	17	7	<1	9	2.4	3.9	2.4
8	1050	Smoked	3.5 oz	100	72	116	25	0	0	1	.2	.2	.3
8	574	Broiled with butter and lemon juice	3 oz	85	72	140	23	0	0	6	3.3	1.6	.7
8	1051	Smoked	3.5 oz	100	49	224	21	0	0	15	2.5	4.8	6.9
8	1054	Raw	3.5 oz	100	78	110	21	0	0	2	.3	.7	.8
8	575	Herring, pickled	3 oz	85	55	223	12	8	0	15	2.0	10	1.4
8	1052	Lobster meat, cooked w/ moist heat	1 c	145	77	142	30	2	0	1	.2	.2	1
8	576	Ocean perch, breaded/fried	3 oz	85	59	185	16	7	<1	11	3	5	3
8	1056	Octopus, raw	3.5 oz.	100	80	82	15	2	0	1	.2	.2	.2
		Oysters:											
8	577	Raw, Eastern	1 c	248	85	170	18	10	0	6	1.6	.6	1.8
8	578	Raw, Pacific	1 c	248	82	200	23	12	0	6	1.3	.9	2.2
		Cooked:											
8	579	Eastern, breaded, fried, medium	6 ea	88	65	173	8	10	<1	11	2.8	4.1	2.9
8	580	Western, simmered	3½ oz	100	71	135	19	7	0	2	.5	.4	.9
		Pollock, cooked:											
8	581	Baked or broiled	3 oz	85	74	96	20	0	0	1	.2	.1	.6
8	1055	Moist heat, poached	3.5 oz	100	72	128	23	0	0	1	.2	.1	.6

[70]Dipped in egg, milk and bread crumbs; fried in vegetable shortening.

(Computer code number is for West Diet Analysis program)

GRP KEY: 1 = BEV 2 = DAIRY 3 = EGGS 4 = FAT/OIL 5 = FRUIT 6 = BAKERY 7 = GRAIN 8 = FISH 9 = BEEF 10 = POULTRY
11 = SAUSAGE 12 = MIXED/FAST 13 = NUTS/SEEDS 14 = SWEETS 15 = VEG/LEG 16 = MISC 22 = SOUP/SAUCE

Chol (mg)	Calc (mg)	Iron (mg)	Magn (mg)	Phos (mg)	Pota (mg)	Sodi (mg)	Zinc (mg)	VT-A (RE)	Thia (mg)	Ribo (mg)	Niac (mg)	V-B6 (mg)	Fola (µg)	VT-C (mg)
0	17	5.34	25	124	123	2	.8	0	.90	.57	6.8	.05	30	0
0	19	5.8	28	135	134	3	.88	0	1.0	.62	7.4	.06	33	0
0	13	7	15	82	101	2	.6	0	.90	.41	6.5	.032	18	0
0	423	5.8	24	744	155	1587	.78	0	.80	.50	7.29	.06	53	0
0	41	4.7	166	415	486	6	3.52	0	.54	.26	7.6	.41	53	0
80	86	1.61	32	216	385	75	.70	35	.10	.03	2.40	.35	9	0
63	9	.62	42	290	477	77	1.04	127	.08	.11	7.78	.53	2	<1
60	8	.53	37	285	413	67	.90	120	.06	.08	5.50	.37	2	<1
29	39	11.9	8	144	267	47	1.16	77	.09	.18	1.5	.07	13	9
57	78	23.8	16	287	534	95	2.32	145	.01	.36	2.85	.07	4	3
60	83	25.2	17	304	565	100	2.46	154	.01	.38	3.02	.08	4	4
60	20	.49	42	140	245	224	.58	30	.09	.08	2.51	.28	10	<1
55	80	.5	36	200	370	100	.5	26	.04	.04	2.2	.24	9	<1
55	14	.49	42	138	244	78	.58	14	.09	.08	2.51	.28	11	<1
135	140	1.22	45	278	437	376	5.70	20	.14	.12	3.00	.33	20	2
64	46	.37	46	184	359	299	4.33	14	.04	.16	2.92	.33	20	2
120	137	1.13	52	351	505	450	5.42	14	.11	.11	1.85	.41	22	0
17	11	.33	—	—	77	715	—	—	—	.02	.15	—	—	—
64	11	.42	14	103	149	332	.38	18	.07	.1	1.21	.03	10	0
68	16	.28	50	187	272	145	.53	54	.07	.1	1.85	.20	10	1
55	16	.28	50	187	273	151	.53	69	.07	.1	1.85	.20	10	1
58	16	.28	50	246	292	89	.53	10	.07	.1	1.85	.20	10	1
55	34	1.15	26	183	270	123	.85	20	.06	.1	2.9	.13	14	0
77	49	1.40	54	251	415	763	.50	22	.05	.05	5.07	.40	3	<1
45	51	.91	91	242	490	100	.43	174	.06	.08	6.06	.34	6	<1
100	48	.84	83	222	450	480	.42	45	.05	.07	5.80	.33	5	<1
32	47	.84	83	222	450	54	.42	47	.06	.08	5.85	.34	12	<1
11	65	1.04	8	76	59	740	.45	219	.03	.12	2.8	.11	2	0
104	88	.57	51	268	510	551	4.23	38	<1	1	1.55	.112	16	t
46	92	1.2	26	191	241	138	.41	20	.10	.11	2	.22	6	0
48	53	5.30	—	186	—	—	1.68	<1	.03	.04	2.10	.36	—	<1
136	111	16.6	135	344	568	277	226[71]	223	.34	.41	3.3	.12	25	24
136	20	12.7	55	402	417	262	41.2[71]	223	.17	.58	5	.12	25	72
72	54	6.12	51	140	215	367	76.7[71]	86	.13	.18	1.45	.06	12	7
48	16	10.2	44	322	334	210	33[71]	81	.14	.46	3.82	.10	17	7
82	5	.24	31	250	329	98	.51	19	.06	.07	1.4	.06	4	t
70	60	.53	1	252	400	98	.54	9	.04	.18	3.14	.27	12	0

[71]Value varies widely.

(For purposes of calculations, use "0" for t, <1, <.1, <.01, etc.)

Table C–1   Food Composition

Grp	Computer Code No.	Food Description	Measure	Wt (g)	H₂O (%)	Ener (kcal)	Prot (g)	Carb (g)	Dietary Fiber (g)	Fat (g)	Fat Breakdown (g) Sat	Mono	Poly
MEATS: FISH and SHELLFISH—Con.													
		Salmon:											
8	582	Canned pink, solids and liquid	3 oz	85	69	118	17	0	0	5	1.3	1.5	1.7
8	583	Broiled or baked	3 oz	85	62	183	23	0	0	9	1.6	4.5	2.1
8	584	Smoked	3 oz	85	72	99	16	0	0	4	.8	1.7	.8
8	585	Atlantic sardines, canned, drained, 2 = 24 g	3 oz	85	60	177	21	0	0	11	1.4	3.6	4.7
8	586	Scallops, breaded, cooked from frozen	6 ea	93	59	200	17	9	<1	10	2.5	4.2	2.7
8	1588	Scallops, imitation, from surimi	3 oz	85	74	84	11	9	0	<1	—	—	—
		Shrimp:											
8	587	Cooked, boiled, 18 large shrimp	3½ oz	100	77	99	21	0	0	1	.3	.2	.4
8	588	Canned, drained	⅔ c	85	73	102	20	1	0	2	.3	.3	.6
8	589	Fried, 4 large = 30 g[70]	12 ea	90	53	218	19	10	<1	11	1.9	3.4	4.6
8	1057	Raw, large, about 7 g each	14 ea	100	76	106	20	1	0	2	.3	.3	.7
8	1589	Shrimp, imitation, from surimi	3 oz	85	75	86	11	8	0	1	—	—	—
8	1053	Snapper, baked or broiled	3.5 oz	100	70	128	26	0	0	2	.4	.3	.6
8	1060	Squid, fried in flour[72]	3 oz	85	65	149	15	7	<1	6	1.6	2.3	1.8
8	1590	Surimi[73]	3 oz	85	76	84	13	6	0	1	—	—	—
		Swordfish:											
8	1058	Baked or broiled	3.5 oz	100	76	121	20	0	0	4	1.1	1.6	.9
8	1059	Raw	3.5 oz	100	69	155	25	0	0	5	1.4	2.0	1.2
8	590	Trout, baked or broiled	3 oz	85	63	129	22	<1	0	4	.7	1.1	1.3
		Tuna, light, canned, drained solids:											
8	591	Oil pack	3 oz	85	60	163	25	0	0	7	1.2	1.4	3.1
8	592	Water pack	3 oz	85	71	111	25	0	0	1	.2	.1	.3
8	1061	Tuna, raw, average	3.5 oz	100	68	144	23	0	0	5	1.3	1.4	1.7
MEATS: BEEF, LAMB, PORK and others													
		BEEF, cooked:[74]											
		Braised, simmered, pot roasted:											
		Relatively fat, like choice chuck blade:											
9	593	Lean and fat, piece 2½ × 2½ × ¾″	3 oz	85	47	295	23	0	0	22	9	9	.8
9	594	Lean only	3 oz	85	55	223	26	0	0	12	5	5	.4
		Relatively lean, like choice round:											
9	595	Lean and fat, piece 4⅛ × 2¼ × ¾″	3 oz	85	52	233	24	0	0	14	5	6	.5
9	596	Lean only	3 oz	85	57	187	27	0	0	8	2.7	3.5	.3
		Ground beef, broiled, patty 3 × ⅝″:											
9	597	Extra lean, about 16% fat	3 oz	85	57	225	24	0	0	13	5.3	6.0	.5
9	598	Lean, 21% fat	3 oz	85	53	238	24	0	0	15	6	6.7	.6
		Roasts, oven cooked, no added liquid:											
		Relatively fat, prime rib:											
9	601	Lean and fat, piece 4⅛ × 2¼ × ½″	3 oz	85	46	319	19	0	0	27	11	11	1
9	602	Lean only	3 oz	85	58	204	23	0	0	12	5	5	.4
		Relatively lean, choice round:											
9	603	Lean and fat, piece 2½ × 2½ × ¾″	3 oz	85	59	204	23	0	0	12	5	5	.4
9	604	Lean only	3 oz	85	65	148	25	0	0	5	2	2	.15
		Steak, broiled, relatively lean, choice sirloin:											
9	605	Lean and fat, piece 2½ × 2½ × ¾″	3 oz	85	52	240	23	0	0	16	7	7	.6
9	606	Lean only	3 oz	85	62	171	26	0	0	7	3.0	3	.3

[70] Dipped in egg, bread crumbs, and flour; fried in vegetable shortening.
[72] Recipe is 94.6% squid, 4.9% flour, and 0.6% salt.
[73] Surimi is processed from Walleye (Alaska) pollock. Also see Imitation crab, shrimp, scallops.
[74] Outer layer of fat removed to about 1/2″ of the lean. Deposits of fat within the cut remain.

(Computer code number is for West Diet Analysis program)

GRP KEY: 1 = BEV 2 = DAIRY 3 = EGGS 4 = FAT/OIL 5 = FRUIT 6 = BAKERY 7 = GRAIN 8 = FISH 9 = BEEF 10 = POULTRY
11 = SAUSAGE 12 = MIXED/FAST 13 = NUTS/SEEDS 14 = SWEETS 15 = VEG/LEG 16 = MISC 22 = SOUP/SAUCE

Chol (mg)	Calc (mg)	Iron (mg)	Magn (mg)	Phos (mg)	Pota (mg)	Sodi (mg)	Zinc (mg)	VT-A (RE)	Thia (mg)	Ribo (mg)	Niac (mg)	V-B6 (mg)	Fola (μg)	VT-C (mg)
37	181[75]	.72	29	279	277	471	.78	14	.02	.16	5.6	.10	13	0
74	6	.47	26	234	319	56	.43	53	.18	.14	5.67	.19	14	0
20	9	.72	15	139	149	666	.26	22	.02	.09	4.01	.24	2	0
121	325[75]	2.5	33	417	337	429	1.11	57	.07	.19	4.5	.14	10	0
57	39	.76	55	219	310	431	.99	21	.04	.10	1.4	.18	11	0
18	7	.26	—	—	88	676	—	—	.01	.01	.26	—	—	—
195	39	3.09	34	137	182	224	1.56	18	.03	.03	2.59	.13	4	<1
147	50	2.32	35	198	179	143	1.07	15	.02	.03	2.34	.09	2	0
159	60	1.13	36	196	213	310	1.24	50	.12	.12	2.76	.09	7	1.4
152	52	2.41	37	205	185	148	1.11	3	.03	.03	2.55	.10	3	2
31	16	.51	—	—	76	599	—	—	.02	.03	.15	—	—	—
47	40	.24	37	201	522	57	.44	12	.05	.08	3.46	.27	9	<1
221	33	.86	33	213	237	260	1.5	0	.05	.39	2.21	.05	—	4
25	7	.22	—	—	95	122	—	—	.02	.02	.19	—	—	—
39	4	.81	27	263	288	90	1.15	36	.04	.10	9.68	.33	14	1
50	6	1.04	34	337	369	115	1.47	41	.04	.12	11.8	.38	16	1
62	73	2.07	33	272	539	29	1.18	19	.07	.19	2.3	.42	6	3
27	11	1.2	26	265	176	301	.77	20	.03	.09	10.1	.32	5	0
28	10	2.7	26	158	267	303	.77	20	.03	.10	13.2	.32	5	0
38	16	1.02	38	191	252	39	.60	18	.24	.25	8.65	.46	25	0
84	9	2.6	16	183	206	50	5.7	0	.06	.20	2.0	.24	8	0
90	11	3.13	20	199	223	60	8.73	0	.07	.24	2.27	.25	5	0
82	5	2.65	19	208	239	43	4.18	0	.06	.21	3.17	.28	9	0
82	4	2.94	21	231	262	43	4.66	0	.06	.22	3.47	.31	9	0
84	8	2.36	21	162	314	70	5.47	0	.06	.27	5	.27	9	0
86	10	2.08	20	155	297	76	5.27	0	.05	.2	5	.27	9	0
72	9	2	16	146	251	54	4.5	0	.06	.15	2.9	.22	6	0
69	9	2.2	21	181	319	63	5.90	0	.07	.18	3.5	.26	7	0
61	5	1.6	20	175	305	50	3.7	0	.07	.14	2.95	.3	5	0
58	4	3	23	192	335	53	4	0	.08	.15	3.2	.31	6	0
77	9	2.6	24	185	305	53	5	0	1	.22	3.3	.34	8	0
76	9	3	27	208	343	56	6	0	.1	.25	3.6	.38	9	0

[75]If bones are discarded, calcium value is greatly reduced.

(For purposes of calculations, use "0" for t, <1, <.1, <.01, etc.)

Table C–1   Food Composition

Grp	Computer Code No.	Food Description	Measure	Wt (g)	H₂O (%)	Ener (kcal)	Prot (g)	Carb (g)	Dietary Fiber (g)	Fat (g)	Fat Breakdown (g)		
											Sat	Mono	Poly
MEATS: BEEF, LAMB, PORK and others—Con.													
		BEEF, cooked—Con.											
		Steak, broiled, relatively fat, choice T-bone:											
9	1063	Lean and fat	3 oz	85	50	253	21	0	0	18	7	7.5	.7
9	1064	Lean only	3 oz	85	60	182	24	0	0	9	3.5	3.5	.3
		Variety meats:											
9	1086	Brains, pan fried	3 oz	85	71	167	11	0	0	13	3.2	3.4	2.0
9	599	Heart, simmered	3 oz	85	64	149	25	<1	0	5	1.4	1.1	1.2
9	600	Liver, fried	3 oz	85	56	185	23	7	0	7	2.3	1.4	1.5
9	1062	Tongue, cooked	3 oz	85	56	241	19	<1	0	18	7.6	8.1	.7
9	607	Beef, canned, corned	3 oz	85	58	213	23	0	0	13	5	5	.5
9	608	Beef, dried, cured	1 oz	28	57	47	8	<1	0	1	.4	.5	.1
		LAMB, domestic, cooked:											
		Chop, arm, braised (5.6 oz raw with bone):											
9	609	Lean and fat	2.5 oz	70	44	244	21	0	0	17	7	7	1
9	610	Lean part of #609	1.9 oz	55	49	152	19	0	0	8	2.8	3.4	.5
		Chop, loin, broiled (4.2 oz raw with bone):											
9	611	Lean and fat	2.3 oz	64	52	201	16	0	0	15	6	6	1
9	612	Lean part of #611	1.6 oz	46	61	100	14	0	0	5	1.6	2.0	.3
9	1067	Cutlet, avg of lean cuts, cooked	3 oz	85	62	175	24	0	0	8	2.9	3.6	.5
		Leg, roasted, 3 oz piece = 4⅛ × 2¼ × ½″:											
9	613	Lean and fat	3 oz	85	57	219	22	0	0	14	5.9	5.9	1.0
9	614	Lean only	3 oz	85	64	162	24	0	0	7	2.4	2.9	.4
		Rib, roasted, 3 oz piece = 2½ × 2½ × ¾″:											
9	615	Lean and fat	3 oz	85	48	305	18	0	0	25	11	11	1.9
9	616	Lean only	3 oz	85	60	197	22	0	0	11	4	5	1
		Shoulder, roasted:											
9	1065	Lean and fat	3 oz	85	56	235	19	0	0	17	7.4	7.1	1.4
9	1066	Lean only	3 oz	85	64	163	22	0	0	8	3.1	3.2	.7
		Variety meats:											
9	1069	Brains, pan-fried	3 oz	85	61	232	14	0	0	19	4.8	3.4	1.9
9	1068	Heart, braised	3 oz	85	64	158	22	2	0	7	2.7	1.9	.66
9	1070	Sweetbreads, cooked	3 oz	85	62	196	16	0	0	13	6.3	5.1	.7
9	1071	Tongue, cooked	3 oz	85	58	234	18	0	0	17	6.7	8.5	1.1
		PORK, CURED, cooked (see also #669–672):											
9	617	Bacon, medium slices	3 pce	19	13	109	6	<1	0	9	3.3	4.5	1.1
9	1087	Breakfast strips, cooked	3 pce	34	27	156	10	<1	0	13	4.3	5.6	1.9
9	618	Canadian-style bacon	2 pce	47	62	86	11	1	0	4	1.3	1.9	.4
		Ham, roasted:											
9	619	Lean and fat, 2 pieces 4⅛ × 2¼ × ¼″	3 oz	85	58	207	18	0	0	14	5.1	7	2
9	620	Lean only	3 oz	85	66	133	21	0	0	5	1.6	2.2	.5
9	621	Ham, canned, roasted	3 oz	85	66	140	18	<1	0	7	2.4	3.5	.8
		PORK, fresh, cooked:											
		Chops, loin (cut 3 per lb with bone):											
		Braised:											
9	1291	Lean and fat	1 ea	71	44	261	19	0	0	20	7.2	9.1	2.2
9	1292	Lean only	1 ea	55	51	150	18	0	0	8	2.8	3.6	.0
		Broiled:											
9	622	Lean and fat	3.1 oz	87	50	275	24	0	0	19	7	9	2
9	623	Lean only from #622	2.5 oz	72	57	166	23	0	0	8	2.6	3.4	.9

(Computer code number is for West Diet Analysis program)

GRP KEY: 1 = BEV 2 = DAIRY 3 = EGGS 4 = FAT/OIL 5 = FRUIT 6 = BAKERY 7 = GRAIN 8 = FISH 9 = BEEF 10 = POULTRY
11 = SAUSAGE 12 = MIXED/FAST 13 = NUTS/SEEDS 14 = SWEETS 15 = VEG/LEG 16 = MISC 22 = SOUP/SAUCE

Chol (mg)	Calc (mg)	Iron (mg)	Magn (mg)	Phos (mg)	Pota (mg)	Sodi (mg)	Zinc (mg)	VT-A (RE)	Thia (mg)	Ribo (mg)	Niac (mg)	V-B6 (mg)	Fola (µg)	VT-C (mg)
71	7	2.3	21	156	302	52	3.98	<1	.09	.19	3.47	.29	6	0
68	6	2.55	25	177	346	56	4.59	<1	.09	.21	3.94	.33	7	0
1697	8	1.89	12	328	301	134	1.15	0	.11	.22	3.21	.33	5	3
164	5	6.39	21	213	198	54	2.66	0	.12	1.31	3.46	.18	2	1
410	9	5.34	20	392	310	90	4.63	9126[76]	.18	3.52	12.3	1.22	187	20
91	6	2.88	14	121	153	51	4.08	0	.03	.30	1.83	.14	4	<1
73	10	1.77	12	94	116	856	3.04	0	.02	.13	2.07	.11	8	1
12	2	1.28	9	49	126	984	1.49	0	.02	.06	1.6	1	3	4.2
84	18	1.7	18	145	216	51	4.28	2	.05	.18	4.7	.08	13	0
66	14	1.5	16	127	185	41	4.0	1	.04	.15	3.5	.07	12	0
64	13	1.15	15	125	209	49	2.22	2	.07	.16	4.5	.08	12	0
44	9	.93	13	105	175	39	1.91	1	.05	.13	3.2	.07	11	0
78	13	1.74	22	179	293	64	4.48	<1	.09	.24	5.37	.14	19	0
79	9	1.69	20	162	266	56	3.74	2	.09	.23	5.6	.13	17	0
76	7	1.81	22	175	287	58	4.2	1	.09	.25	5.4	.14	20	0
82	19	1.4	17	141	231	62	2.96	2	.07	.18	5.7	.10	13	0
74	18	1.5	20	165	268	69	3.8	<1	.08	.20	5.24	.13	19	0
78	15	1.72	19	155	220	55	3.81	<1	.08	.21	5.66	.10	17	0
73	14	1.9	22	172	236	57	4.46	<1	.08	.23	5.39	.12	21	0
2128	18	1.73	18	421	304	133	1.70	0	.14	.31	3.87	.20	6	20
212	12	4.70	21	216	160	54	3.13	0	.14	1.01	3.71	.25	2	6
347	29	1.53	20	357	221	179	1.79	0	.03	.2	1.79	.02	12	15
161	8	2.24	14	114	134	57	2.54	0	.07	.36	3.14	.14	2	6
16	2	.32	5	64	92	303	.62	0	.13	.05	1.39	.05	1	6[77]
36	5	.67	9	90	158	714	1.25	0	.25	.13	2.58	.12	1	15
27	5	.38	10	138	181	719	.79	0	.38	.09	3.22	.21	2	10[77]
53	6	.74	16	182	243	1009	1.97	0	.51	.19	3.8	.32	3	0
47	6	.8	19	193	269	1128	2.19	0	.58	.22	4.27	.4	3	0
35	6	.91	16	188	298	908	1.97	0	.82	.21	4.27	.33	4	19[77]
73	6	.82	14	141	245	46	2.15	2	.43	.21	4.24	.26	3	<1
58	5	.77	13	131	230	41	2.05	2	.38	.20	3.82	.25	3	<1
84	4	.71	22	184	312	61	1.68	3	.87	.24	4.35	.35	4	<1
71	4	.66	22	176	302	56	1.61	2	.83	.22	3.99	.34	4	<1

[76] Value varies widely.

[77] Values based on products containing added ascorbic acid or sodium ascorbate. If none added, ascorbic acid content would be negligible.

(For purposes of calculations, use "0" for t, <1, <.1, <.01, etc.)

Table C–1   Food Composition

Grp	Computer Code No.	Food Description	Measure	Wt (g)	H$_2$O (%)	Ener (kcal)	Prot (g)	Carb (g)	Dietary Fiber (g)	Fat (g)	Fat Breakdown (g) Sat	Mono	Poly
		MEATS: BEEF, LAMB, PORK and others—Con.											
		PORK, fresh cooked—Con.											
		Pan fried:											
9	624	Lean and fat	3.1 oz	89	45	334	21	0	0	27	10	13	3
9	625	Lean only from #624	2.4 oz	67	54	178	19	0	0	11	3.7	4.8	1.3
		Leg, roasted:											
9	626	Lean and fat, piece 2½ × 2½ × ¾″	3 oz	85	53	250	21	0	0	18	6	8	2
9	627	Lean only from #626	3 oz	85	60	187	24	0	0	9	3.2	4.2	1.1
		Rib, roasted:											
9	628	Lean and fat, piece 2½ × 2½ × ¾″	3 oz	85	51	270	21	0	0	20	7	9	2
9	629	Lean only	3 oz	85	57	210	24	0	0	12	4.1	5.3	1.4
		Shoulder, braised:											
9	630	Lean and fat, 3 pieces 2½ × 2½ × ¼″	3 oz	85	47	293	23	0	0	22	8	10	2
9	631	Lean only	3 oz	85	54	208	27	0	0	10	4	5	1.3
9	1088	Spareribs, cooked, yield from 1 lb raw with bone	6.25 oz	177	40	703	51	0	0	54	20.8	25.1	6.2
9	1095	Rabbit, roasted (1 cup meat = 140g)	3 oz	85	59	175	26	0	0	7	2.1	1.9	1.4
		VEAL, cooked:											
9	632	Veal cutlet, braised or broiled, 4⅛ × 2¼ × ½″	3 oz	85	60	166	27	0	0	6	1.6	2.0	.5
9	633	Veal rib roasted, lean, 2 pieces 4⅛ × 2¼ × ¼″	3 oz	85	65	151	22	0	0	6	1.8	2.3	.6
9	634	Veal liver, pan-fried	3 oz	85	53	208	25	3	0	10	3.6	1.6	1.5
9	1096	Venison (Deer meat) roasted	3.5 oz	100	65	158	30	0	0	3	1.3	.9	.6
		MEATS: POULTRY and POULTRY PRODUCTS											
		CHICKEN, cooked:											
		Fried, batter dipped:[78]											
10	635	Breast (5.6 oz with bones)	1 ea	140	52	364	35	13	<1	19	5	8	4
10	636	Drumstick (3.4 oz with bones)	1 ea	72	53	193	16	6	<1	11	3	5	3
10	637	Thigh	1 ea	86	52	238	19	8	<1	14	4	6	3
10	638	Wing	1 ea	49	46	159	10	5	<1	11	3	4	3
		Fried, flour coated:[78]											
10	639	Breast (4.2 oz with bones)	1 ea	98	57	218	31	2	<1	9	2.4	3.4	1.9
10	1212	Breast, without skin	1 ea	86	60	161	29	<1	0	4	1.1	1.5	.9
10	640	Drumstick (2.6 oz with bones)	1 ea	49	57	120	13	1	<1	7	1.8	2.7	1.6
10	641	Thigh	1 ea	62	54	162	17	2	<1	9	2.5	3.6	2.1
10	1099	Thigh, without skin	1 ea	52	59	113	15	1	<1	5	1.5	2.0	1.3
10	642	Wing	1 ea	32	49	103	8	1	<1	7	1.9	2.8	1.6
		Roasted:											
10	643	All types of meat	1 c	140	64	266	41	0	0	10	2.9	3.7	2.4
10	644	Dark meat	1 c	140	63	286	38	0	0	14	3.7	5.0	3.2
10	645	Light meat	1 c	140	65	242	43	0	0	6	1.8	2.2	1.4
10	646	Breast, without skin	½ ea	86	65	142	27	0	0	3	.9	1.1	.7
10	647	Drumstick	1 ea	44	67	76	13	0	0	2	.7	.8	.6
10	648	Thigh	1 ea	62	59	153	16	0	0	10	2.9	3.8	2.1
10	1100	Thigh, without skin	1 ea	52	63	109	14	0	0	6	1.6	2.2	1.3
10	649	Stewed, all types:	1 c	140	67	248	38	0	0	9	2.6	3.3	2.2
10	656	Canned, boneless chicken	5 oz	142	69	235	31	0	0	11	3.1	4.5	2.5
10	1102	Chicken gizzards, simmered	1 ea	22	67	34	6	<1	0	1	.2	.2	.2
10	1101	Chicken hearts, simmered	1 ea	3.3	65	6	1	<1	0	<1	.1	.1	.1
10	650	Chicken liver, simmered	1 ea	20	68	30	5	2	0	1	.4	.3	.2

[78]Fried in vegetable shortening.

(Computer code number is for West Diet Analysis program)

GRP KEY: 1 = BEV   2 = DAIRY   3 = EGGS   4 = FAT/OIL   5 = FRUIT   6 = BAKERY   7 = GRAIN   8 = FISH   9 = BEEF   10 = POULTRY
        11 = SAUSAGE   12 = MIXED/FAST   13 = NUTS/SEEDS   14 = SWEETS   15 = VEG/LEG   16 = MISC   22 = SOUP/SAUCE

Chol (mg)	Calc (mg)	Iron (mg)	Magn (mg)	Phos (mg)	Pota (mg)	Sodi (mg)	Zinc (mg)	VT-A (RE)	Thia (mg)	Ribo (mg)	Niac (mg)	V-B6 (mg)	Fola (µg)	VT-C (mg)
92	4	.75	23	190	323	64	1.74	3	.91	.25	4.58	.35	4	<1
71	3	.67	21	178	305	57	1.61	2	.84	.22	4.03	.34	4	<1
79	5	.85	18	210	280	50	2.43	2	.54	.27	3.89	.33	9	<1
80	6	.95	21	239	317	54	2.77	2	.59	.3	4.2	.38	10	<1
69	9	.76	16	190	313	37	1.67	3	.5	.24	4.17	.3	7	<1
67	10	.85	18	218	360	40	1.9	3	.54	.26	4.6	.34	7	<1
93	6	1.4	16	162	286	74	3.43	3	.46	.26	4.43	.23	3	<1
95	6	1.64	19	189	339	85	4.16	3	.5	.3	5	.35	4	<1
214	83	3.27	43	462	566	165	8.14	5	.72	.68	9.69	.62	7	0
73	17	2.02	17	192	255	31	2.02	2	.05	.14	6.09	.29	8	0
100	20	.99	24	213	288	76	4.33	t	.05	.29	7.16	.28	13	0
97	10	.82	20	176	264	82	3.81	t	.05	.25	6.4	.23	12	0
280	10	4.45	22	373	372	112	6.69	4784[79]	.21	2.86	14.4	.73	272	18
112	7	4.47	24	226	335	54	2.75	0	.18	.60	6.71	.32[80]	4[80]	0
119	28	1.75	34	258	282	385	1.33	28	.16	.2	14.7	.6	8	0
62	12	.97	14	106	134	194	1.67	19	.08	.16	3.67	.2	6	0
80	16	1.24	18	134	165	248	1.75	25	.1	.2	4.92	.23	8	0
39	10	.63	8	59	68	157	.67	17	.05	.07	2.58	.15	3	0
88	16	1.17	29	228	253	74	1.07	15	.08	.13	13.5	.57	4	0
78	14	.98	27	212	237	68	.93	6	.07	.11	12.7	.55	4	0
44	6	.66	11	86	112	44	1.42	12	.04	.11	2.96	.17	4	0
60	8	.93	15	116	147	55	1.56	18	.06	.15	4.31	.21	5	0
53	7	.76	14	103	134	49	1.45	11	.05	.13	3.70	.20	4	0
26	5	.4	6	48	57	25	.56	12	.02	.04	2.14	.13	1	0
125	21	1.69	35	273	340	120	2.94	22	.1	.25	12.8	.65	8	0
130	21	1.86	33	250	336	130	3.92	30	.1	.32	9.17	.5	11	0
118	21	1.49	38	302	345	108	1.73	12	.09	.16	17.4	.84	5	0
73	13	.89	25	196	220	64	.86	5	.06	.1	11.8	.52	3	0
41	5	.57	11	81	108	42	1.4	8	.03	.1	2.67	.17	4	0
58	8	.83	14	108	137	52	1.46	30	.04	.13	3.95	.19	4	0
49	6	.68	12	95	124	46	1.34	10	.04	.12	3.39	.18	4	0
116	20	1.63	29	210	252	98	2.79	21	.07	.23	8.56	.37	8	0
88	20	2.2	17	158	196	714	2.13	48	.02	.18	8.99	.5	4	3
43	2	.91	4	34	39	15	.96	12	.01	.05	.87	.03	12	<1
8	1	.30	1	7	4	2	.24	<1	<.01	.02	.09	.01	3	<1
126	3	1.7	2	62	28	10	.87	983	.03	.35	.89	.12	154	3

[79] Value varies widely.
[80] Values estimated from other game meat.

(For purposes of calculations, use "0" for t, <1, <.1, <.01, etc.)

Table C–1   Food Composition

Grp	Computer Code No.	Food Description	Measure	Wt (g)	H$_2$O (%)	Ener (kcal)	Prot (g)	Carb (g)	Dietary Fiber (g)	Fat (g)	Fat Breakdown (g) Sat	Mono	Poly
MEATS: POULTRY and POULTRY PRODUCTS—Con.													
		DUCK, roasted:											
10	1293	Meat with skin, about 2.7 cups	½ duck	382	52	1287	73	0	0	108	37	49	14
10	651	Meat only, about 1.5 cups	½ duck	221	64	445	52	0	0	25	9.2	8.2	3.2
		GOOSE, domesticated, roasted:											
10	1294	Meat only, 4.2 cups	½ goose	591	57	1406	171	0	0	75	27	26	9
10	1295	Meat w/skin, about 5.5 cups	½ goose	774	52	2362	195	0	0	170	53	79	20
		TURKEY, roasted, meat only:											
10	652	Dark meat	3 oz	85	63	159	24	0	0	6	2.1	1.4	1.8
10	653	Light meat	3 oz	85	66	133	25	0	0	3	.9	.5	.7
10	654	All types, chopped or diced	1 c	140	65	238	41	0	0	7	2.3	1.5	2.0
10	655	All types, sliced	3 oz	85	65	145	25	0	0	4	1.4	.9	1.2
10	1103	Ground turkey, cooked	3.5 oz	100	60	229	24	0	0	14	3.8	5.0	3.3
		Turkey breast:											
10	1104	Barbecued	1 oz	28	70	40	6	0	0	1	.4	.5	.3
10	1105	Hickory smoked	1 oz	28	70	35	6	1	0	1	.3	.3	.3
10	1106	Gizzard, cooked	1 ea	67	65	109	20	<1	0	3	.7	.5	.7
10	1107	Heart, cooked	1 ea	16	64	28	4	<1	0	1	.3	.2	.3
10	1108	Liver, cooked	1 ea	75	66	127	18	3	0	4	1.4	1.1	1.1
		Poultry food products (see also items in sausages and lunchmeats section):											
10	658	Chicken roll, light meat	2 pce	57	69	90	11	1	0	4	1.2	1.7	.9
10	659	Gravy and turkey, frozen package	5 oz	142	85	95	8	7	<1	4	1.2	1.4	.7
10	660	Turkey loaf, breast meat	2 pce	42	72	46	10	0	0	1	.2	.2	.1
10	661	Turkey patties, breaded, fried	1 ea	64	50	181	9	10	<1	12	3	4.8	3
10	662	Turkey, frozen, roasted, seasoned	3 oz	85	68	130	18	3	0	5	1.6	1	1.4
MEATS: SAUSAGES and LUNCHMEATS (see also Poultry food products)													
		Beerwurst/beer salami:											
11	1072	Beef	1 pce	23	54	75	3	<1	0	7	2.8	3.3	.2
11	1074	Pork	1 pce	23	62	55	3	<1	0	4	1.4	2.1	.5
11	1075	Berliner	1 pce	23	61	53	4	1	0	4	1.4	1.8	.4
		Bologna:											
11	1297	Beef	1 pce	23	55	72	3	<1	0	7	2.7	3.1	.2
11	663	Beef and pork	1 pce	28	54	89	3	1	0	8	3.0	3.8	.7
11	1298	Pork	1 pce	23	61	57	4	<1	0	5	1.6	2.3	.5
11	664	Turkey	1 pce	28	66	56	4	<1	0	4	1.5	1.9	1.2
11	665	Braunschweiger sausage	2 pce	57	48	205	8	2	0	18	6.2	8.5	2.1
11	1073	Brotwurst, link	1 ea	70	51	226	10	2	0	20	7.0	9.3	2.0
11	666	Brown-and-serve sausage links, cooked	1 ea	13	45	50	2	<1	0	5	1.7	2.2	.5
11	1089	Cheesefurter/cheese smokie	1 ea	43	53	141	6	1	0	13	4.5	5.9	1.3
11	1090	Corned beef loaf, jellied	1 pce	28	67	46	7	0	0	2	.8	.9	.1
		Frankfurters (see also #657):											
11	1077	Beef, large link, 8/pkg.	1 ea	57	54	184	6	1	0	17	6.8	8.2	.7
11	1078	Beef and pork, large link, 8/pkg.	1 ea	57	54	183	6	1	0	17	6.1	7.8	1.6
11	667	Beef and pork, smaller link, 10/pkg.	1 ea	45	54	145	5	1	0	13	4.8	6.2	1.2
10	657	Chicken frankfurter, 10/pkg.	1 ea	45	58	115	6	3	0	9	2.5	3.8	1.8
11	668	Turkey, smaller link, 10/pkg.	1 ea	45	63	102	6	1	0	8	2.7	3.3	2.1
		Ham:											
11	669	Ham lunchmeat, canned, 3 x 2 x ½"	1 pce	21	52	70	3	<1	0	6	2.3	3.0	.8
11	670	Chopped ham, packaged	2 pce	22	61	98	7	<1	0	8	2.6	3.9	.9

(Computer code number is for West Diet Analysis program)

GRP KEY: 1 = BEV   2 = DAIRY   3 = EGGS   4 = FAT/OIL   5 = FRUIT   6 = BAKERY   7 = GRAIN   8 = FISH   9 = BEEF   10 = POULTRY
11 = SAUSAGE   12 = MIXED/FAST   13 = NUTS/SEEDS   14 = SWEETS   15 = VEG/LEG   16 = MISC   22 = SOUP/SAUCE

Chol (mg)	Calc (mg)	Iron (mg)	Magn (mg)	Phos (mg)	Pota (mg)	Sodi (mg)	Zinc (mg)	VT-A (RE)	Thia (mg)	Ribo (mg)	Niac (mg)	V-B6 (mg)	Fola (µg)	VT-C (mg)
320	43	10.3	62	595	780	227	7.12	241	.67	1.03	18.4	.70	25	0
198	26	5.97	44	449	557	143	5.75	51	.57	1.04	11.3	.55	22	0
569	84	17.0	148	1828	2291	447	16.0	71	.54	2.31	24.1	2.75	13	0
708	104	21.9	169	2091	2546	543	16.0	162	.60	2.50	32.3	2.89	17	0
72	27	1.99	21	174	247	67	3.8	0	.05	.21	3.1	.3	8	0
59	16	1.14	24	186	259	54	1.73	0	.05	.12	5.81	.46	5	0
107	35	2.49	37	298	418	99	4.34	0	.09	.26	7.62	.64	10	0
64	21	1.51	23	181	254	60	2.64	0	.05	.16	4.63	.39	6	0
69	25	1.93	24	196	270	83	2.86	0	.05	.17	4.82	.39	7	0
16	2	.12	7	74	57	156	.35	0	.01	.03	2.73	.11	1	<1
13	1	.20	7	79	59	208	.30	0	.01	.03	2.75	.11	1	<1
155	10	3.64	13	86	141	37	2.79	37	.02	.22	2.06	.08	36	1
36	2	1.10	4	33	29	9	.84	1	.01	.14	.52	.05	13	<1
469	8	5.85	11	204	146	48	2.32	2806	.04	1.07	4.46	.39	499	1
28	24	.55	10	89	129	331	.41	14	.04	.07	3	.31	2	0
26	20	1.32	11	115	87	787	.99	18	.03	.18	2.55	.14	2	0
17	3	.17	9	97	118	608	.48	0	.02	.05	3.54	.15	2	0[81]
40	9	1.41	12	173	176	512	1.5	7	.06	.12	1.47	.13	3	0
45	4	1.4	20	207	253	578	2.37	0	.04	.14	5.3	.24	5	0
13	2	.31	3	24	42	214	.61	0	.03	.03	.66	.05	1	3
13	2	.17	3	24	58	285	.40	0	.13	.04	.75	.08	1	7
11	3	.27	3	30	65	298	.57	0	.09	.05	.72	.05	1	2
13	3	.32	2	19	36	230	.46	0	.01	.03	.61	.04	1	4
16	3	.43	3	26	51	289	.55	0	.05	.04	.73	.05	1	6[82]
14	3	.18	3	33	65	272	.47	0	.12	.04	.90	.06	1	8
28	23	.43	4	37	56	248	.49	0	.02	.05	1.04	.05	1	<1
89	6	5.32	6	96	113	652	1.62	2406	.14	.87	4.78	.19	57	5[82]
44	34	.72	11	94	197	778	1.47	0	.18	.16	2.31	.09	2	20
9	1	.1	2	14	25	105	.15	0	.05	.02	.40	.03	1	0
29	25	.46	5	76	89	465	.97	3	.11	.07	1.25	.05	1	8
12	3	.58	3	18	25	294	1.08	0	<.01	.03	.46	.04	1	2
27	7	.76	7	47	90	584	1.21	0	.03	.06	1.44	.06	2	14
29	6	.66	7	49	95	639	1.05	0	.11	.07	1.50	.08	2	15
23	5	.52	6	39	75	504	.83	0	.09	.05	1.18	.06	2	12[82]
45	43	.9	8	48	38	616	1	17	.03	.05	1.39	.09	2	0
39	58	.77	8	83	88	454	1	17	.04	.08	1.7	.10	2	<1
13	1	.15	2	17	45	271	.31	0	.08	.04	.66	.04	1	<1
21	3	.4	5	58	119	573	.77	0	.23	.07	1.4	.13	2	1[82]

[81] If sodium ascorbate is added, product contains 11 mg ascorbic acid.
[82] Values based on products containing added ascorbic acid or sodium ascorbate. If none added, ascorbic acid content would be negligible.

(For purposes of calculations, use "0" for t, <1, <.1, <.01, etc.)

Table C–1   Food Composition

Grp	Computer Code No.	Food Description	Measure	Wt (g)	H$_2$O (%)	Ener (kcal)	Prot (g)	Carb (g)	Dietary Fiber (g)	Fat (g)	Fat Breakdown (g)		
											Sat	Mono	Poly
MEATS: SAUSAGES and LUNCHMEATS—Con.													
		Ham—Con.											
11	671	Ham lunchmeat, regular	2 pce	57	65	103	10	2	0	6	1.9	2.8	.7
11	672	Ham lunchmeat, extra lean	2 pce	57	70	75	11	1	0	3	.9	1.3	.3
11	673	Turkey ham	2 pce	57	72	73	11	1	0	3	1.0	.8	.8
11	1091	Keilbasa sausage	1 pce	26	54	81	3	1	0	7	2.6	3.4	.8
11	1092	Knockwurst sausage-link	1 ea	68	56	209	8	1	0	19	6.9	8.7	2.0
11	1093	Mortadella lunchmeat	1 pce	15	52	47	2	<1	0	4	1.4	1.7	.5
11	1097	Olive loaf lunchmeat	2 pce	57	58	133	7	5	<1	9	3.3	4.5	1.1
11	1080	Pastrami, turkey	2 pce	57	72	74	11	1	0	4	1.0	1.2	.9
11	1081	Pepperoni sausage, small slices	4 pce	22	27	109	5	1	0	10	3.6	4.6	1
11	1094	Pickle & pimento loaf	2 pce	57	57	149	7	3	<1	12	4.5	5.4	1.5
11	1082	Polish sausage	1 oz.	28	53	92	4	<1	0	8	2.9	3.8	.9
		Pork sausage, cooked:[83]											
11	674	Link, small	1 ea	13	45	48	3	<1	0	4	1.4	1.8	.5
11	1079	Patty	1 pce	27	45	100	5	<1	0	8	2.9	3.8	1.0
		Salami:											
11	675	Pork and beef	2 pce	57	60	143	8	1	0	11	4.6	5.2	1.1
11	676	Turkey	2 pce	57	66	111	9	<1	0	8	2.3	2.6	2.0
11	677	Dry, beef and pork	2 pce	20	35	85	5	1	0	7	2.4	3.4	.6
		Sandwich spreads:											
11	1300	Ham salad	1 c	240	63	518	21	26	<1	37	12.1	17.3	6.5
11	678	Pork and beef	1 tbsp	15	60	35	1	2	0	3	.9	1.1	.4
10	1296	Poultry sandwich spread	1 tbsp	13	60	25	2	1	0	2	.5	.4	.8
		Smoked link sausage:											
11	1083	Beef and pork	1 ea	68	39	265	15	1	0	22	7.7	10.0	2.6
11	1084	Pork	1 ea	68	52	229	9	1	0	21	7.2	9.7	2.2
11	1085	Summer sausage	1 pce	23	48	80	4	1	0	7	2.8	3.2	.4
11	1076	Turkey breakfast sausage	1 pce	28	60	65	6	0	0	4	1.6	1.8	1.2
11	679	Vienna sausage, canned	1 ea	16	60	45	2	<1	0	4	1.5	2.0	.3
MIXED DISHES and FAST FOODS													
		MIXED DISHES:											
		Beef stew with vegetables:											
12	680	Homemade	1 c	245	82	220	16	15	3	11	4.4	4.5	.5
12	1109	Canned	1 c	245	83	194	14	18	1	8	3.1	3.1	.4
12	1116	Beef, macaroni & tomato sauce casserole	1 c	226	80	189	10	25	2	6	2.1	2.3	.4
12	681	Beef pot pie, homemade[84]	1 pce	210	55	515	21	39	1	30	8	13	7
12	682	Chicken à la king, home recipe	1 c	245	68	470	27	12	1	34	13	13	6
12	683	Chicken and noodles, home recipe	1 c	240	71	365	22	26	1	18	5	7	4
12	684	Chicken chow mein, canned	1 c	250	89	95	7	18	5	1	.1	.1	.8
12	685	Chicken chow mein, home recipe	1 c	250	78	255	23	10	4	11	4	4	3
12	686	Chicken pot pie, home recipe[84]	1 pce	232	57	545	23	42	2	31	10	16	7
12	1112	Chicken salad w/celery	.5 c	78	53	266	11	1	<1	25	4.1	7.2	12.0
12	687	Chili with beans, canned	1 c	255	76	286	15	30	8	14	6	6	1
12	688	Chop suey with beef and pork	1 c	250	75	300	26	13	2	17	4	7	4
12	689	Corn pudding[85]	1 c	250	76	271	11	32	9	13	6.3	4.3	1.7
12	690	Cole slaw[86]	1 c	120	82	84	2	15	2	3	.5	.9	1.6
12	1110	Corned beef hash-canned	1 c	220	67	382	18	22	1	10	4.2	4.9	.5
12	1113	Egg salad	1 c	183	66	438	19	3	<1	39	8.4	13.2	13.5

[83] Cooked weight is half the weight of raw sausage.

[84] Crust made with vegetable shortening and enriched flour.

[85] Recipe: 55% yellow corn, 23% whole milk, 14% egg, 4% sugar, 3% salt, and 1% pepper.

[86] Recipe: 41% cabbage; 12% celery; 12% table cream; 12% sugar; 7% green pepper; 6% lemon juice; 4% onion; 3% pimento; 3% vinegar; 2% each for salt, dry mustard, and white pepper.

(Computer code number is for West Diet Analysis program)

GRP KEY: 1 = BEV 2 = DAIRY 3 = EGGS 4 = FAT/OIL 5 = FRUIT 6 = BAKERY 7 = GRAIN 8 = FISH 9 = BEEF 10 = POULTRY
11 = SAUSAGE 12 = MIXED/FAST 13 = NUTS/SEEDS 14 = SWEETS 15 = VEG/LEG 16 = MISC 22 = SOUP/SAUCE

Chol (mg)	Calc (mg)	Iron (mg)	Magn (mg)	Phos (mg)	Pota (mg)	Sodi (mg)	Zinc (mg)	VT-A (RE)	Thia (mg)	Ribo (mg)	Niac (mg)	V-B6 (mg)	Fola (µg)	VT-C (mg)
32	4	.56	11	140	188	746	1.21	0	.49	.14	2.98	.19	2	16[82]
27	4	.43	10	124	198	810	1.09	0	.53	.13	2.74	.26	2	15[82]
32	5	1.56	12	138	163	548	1.58	0	.04	.15	2.72	.16	4	0
17	11	.38	4	38	70	280	.52	0	.06	.06	.75	.05	1	6
39	7	.62	8	67	136	687	1.13	0	.23	.10	1.86	.11	2	18
8	3	.21	2	15	24	187	.32	0	.02	.02	.40	.02	<1	4
22	62	.31	11	72	169	842	.78	0	.17	.15	1.04	.13	1	5
30	5	.81	10	142	155	569	1.46	0	.05	.15	2.48	.16	4	<1
8	2	.31	4	26	76	449	.55	0	.07	.06	1.09	.06	—	<1
21	54	.58	10	79	193	787	.79	<1	.17	.14	1.16	.11	1	8
20	3	.41	4	39	67	248	.55	0	.14	.04	.98	.05	1	0
11	4	.16	2	24	47	168	.33	0	.1	.03	.59	.04	1	<1
22	9	.34	5	50	97	349	.68	0	.20	.07	1.22	.09	2	<1
37	7	1.51	9	65	112	604	1.21	0	.14	.21	2.02	.12	1	7[82]
46	11	.93	9	73	125	535	1.25	0	.06	.15	2.23	.14	5	<1
16	2	.3	4	28	76	372	.64	0	.12	.06	.97	.1	0	6[82]
88	19	1.42	23	286	359	2187	2.64	42	1.04	.29	5.02	.36	3	14
6	2	.12	1	9	16	152	.15	1	.03	.02	.26	.02	<1	0
4	1	.08	3	4	24	49	.25	6	<.01	.01	.22	.01	1	<1
46	20	.79	13	110	228	1020	1.92	0	.48	.18	3.08	.24	2	1
48	7	.99	8	73	129	642	1.44	0	.18	.12	2.19	.12	2	13
16	2	.47	3	23	53	334	.47	0	.04	.07	.94	.07	1	5
23	5	.52	6	52	76	191	.97	0	.03	.08	1.42	.08	1	—
8	2	.14	1	8	16	152	.26	0	.01	.02	.26	.02	<1	0
71	29	2.9	40	184	613	292	5.3	569	.15	.17	4.7	.28	37	17
15	23	3.18	39	56	417	992	4.23	262	.07	.12	2.43	.20	31	7
22	30	2.39	37	118	562	974	2.07	111	.19	.17	3.51	.30	23	16
42	29	3.8	6	149	334	596	3.17	517	.29	.29	4.8	.24	29	6
221	127	2.5	20	358	404	760	1.8	272	.1	.42	5.4	.23	11	12
103	26	2.4	37	247	211	600	2.14	130	.05	.17	4.3	.16	9	1
8	45	1.3	14	85	418	725	1.3	28	.05	.1	1	.09	12	13
75	58	2.50	28	293	473	718	2.12	50	.08	.23	4.3	.41	19	10
56	70	3.0	25	232	343	594	2.0	735	.32	.32	4.9	.46	29	5
48	16	.66	11	80	137	199	.80	31	.03	.08	3.25	.17	4	1
43	119	8.75	115	393	932	1330	5.10	86	.12	.27	.91	.34	41	4
68	60	4.80	32	248	425	1053	3.58	60	.28	.38	5.0	.32	22	33
230	100	1.40	38	143	402	138	1.26	89	1.03	.32	2.47	.30	63	7
10[87]	54	.70	12	38	218	28	.24	98	.08	.07	.33	.18	32	39
132	29	4.40	3	147	440	1354	4.38	0	.12	.40	4.60	.41	15	8
629	94	3.39	21	282	211	428	2.24	300	.12	.45	.16	.18	74	0

[82] Values based on products containing added ascorbic acid or sodium ascorbate. If none added, ascorbic acid content would be negligible.
[87] From dairy cream in recipe.

(For purposes of calculations, use "0" for t, <1, <.1, <.01, etc.)

Table C–1 Food Composition

Grp	Computer Code No.	Food Description	Measure	Wt (g)	H₂O (%)	Ener (kcal)	Prot (g)	Carb (g)	Dietary Fiber (g)	Fat (g)	Fat Breakdown (g) Sat	Mono	Poly
MIXED DISHES and FAST FOODS—Con.													
		MIXED DISHES—Con.											
12	691	French toast, home recipe[88]	1 pce	65	53	123	5	15	1	4	1.1	1.4	1.1
12	1355	Green pepper, stuffed	1 ea	172	76	217	10	16	1	13	5.3	5.2	.6
		Lasagna:											
12	1346	With meat	1 pce	245	64	398	26	30	2	20	9.2	7.2	1.5
12	1111	Without meat	1 pce	218	64	316	20	30	2	14	6.9	4.7	1.3
12	1117	Frozen entree	1 pce	205	73	275	17	19	1	12	6.3	4.2	1.2
		Macaroni and cheese:											
12	692	Canned[89]	1 c	240	80	230	9	26	1	10	5	3	1
12	693	Home recipe[90]	1 c	200	58	430	17	40	1	22	10	7	4
12	1115	Macaroni salad-no cheese	1 c	141	61	371	3	18	1	33	5.1	9.5	17.2
		Meat loaf:											
12	1120	Beef	1 pce	87	62	193	16	4	<1	12	4.8	5.2	.6
12	1119	Beef and pork (1/3)	1 pce	87	59	212	15	5	<1	15	5.5	6.3	1.2
12	1303	Moussaka (lamb and eggplant)	1 c	250	79	250	21	16	6	11	3.6	4.3	1.9
12	715	Potato salad with mayonnaise and egg[91]	1 c	250	76	358	7	28	4	21	4	6	9
12	694	Quiche lorraine, ⅛ of 8″ quiche[84]	1 pce	176	47	600	13	29	1	48	23	18	4
		Spaghetti (enriched) in tomato sauce:											
		With cheese:											
12	695	Canned	1 c	250	80	190	6	39	3	2	.4	.4	.5
12	696	Home recipe	1 c	250	77	260	9	37	3	9	3	3.6	1.2
		With meatballs:											
12	697	Canned	1 c	250	78	260	12	39	3	10	2	4	3
12	698	Home recipe	1 c	248	70	330	19	39	3	12	4	4	2
12	716	Spinach soufflé[92]	1 c	136	74	218	11	3	4	18	7	7	3
12	717	Tuna salad[93]	1 c	205	63	383	33	19	2	19	3	6	9
12	1121	Tuna noodle casserole, recipe	1 c	202	73	251	21	24	<1	7	2.0	1.5	3.2
12	1270	Waldorf salad	1 c	142	58	424	4	13	4	42	5.6	11.2	23.1
		FAST FOODS and SANDWICHES: see end of this appendix for additional Fast Foods.											
		Burrito:[94]											
12	699	Beef and bean	1 ea	175	54	390	21	40	5	18	7	7	2
12	700	Bean	1 ea	174	55	322	13	47	8	10	4	3	2
		Cheeseburger:											
12	701	Regular	1 ea	112	46	300	15	28	1	15	7	6	1
12	702	4-oz patty	1 ea	194	46	524	30	40	2	31	15	12	1
12	703	Chicken patty sandwich	1 ea	157	52	436	25	34	1	22	6	10	5
12	704	Corn dog	1 ea	111	45	330	10	27	<1	20	8	10	1
12	705	Enchilada, cheese	1 ea	163	63	320	10	29	3	19	11	6	.8
12	706	English muffin with egg, cheese, bacon	1 ea	138	49	360	18	31	2	18	8	8	.7
		Fish sandwich:											
12	707	Regular, with cheese	1 ea	140	43	420	16	39	1	23	6	7	8
12	708	Large, without cheese	1 ea	170	48	470	18	41	1	27	6	9	10

[84]Crust made with vegetable shortening and enriched flour.
[88]Recipe: 35% whole milk, 32% white bread, 29% egg, and cooked in 4% margarine.
[89]Made with corn oil.
[90]Made with margarine.
[91]Recipe: 62% potatoes; 12% egg; 8% mayonnaise; 7% celery; 6% sweet pickle relish; 2% onion; 1% each for green pepper, pimiento, salt, and dry mustard.
[92]Recipe: 29% whole milk, 26% spinach, 13% egg white, 13% cheddar cheese, 7% egg yolk, 7% butter, 4% flour, 1% salt and pepper.
[93]Made with drained chunk light tuna, celery, onion, pickle relish, and mayonnaise-type salad dressing.
[94]Made with a 10½″-diameter flour tortilla.

(Computer code number is for West Diet Analysis program)

GRP KEY: 1 = BEV 2 = DAIRY 3 = EGGS 4 = FAT/OIL 5 = FRUIT 6 = BAKERY 7 = GRAIN 8 = FISH 9 = BEEF 10 = POULTRY
11 = SAUSAGE 12 = MIXED/FAST 13 = NUTS/SEEDS 14 = SWEETS 15 = VEG/LEG 16 = MISC 22 = SOUP/SAUCE

Chol (mg)	Calc (mg)	Iron (mg)	Magn (mg)	Phos (mg)	Pota (mg)	Sodi (mg)	Zinc (mg)	VT-A (RE)	Thia (mg)	Ribo (mg)	Niac (mg)	V-B6 (mg)	Fola (μg)	VT-C (mg)
73	79	1.08	12	82	96	189	.47	57	.15	.17	1.09	.04	18	<1
38	15	2.32	23	91	227	210	2.58	29	.11	.10	2.96	.22	14	83
56	460	3.08	41	393	507	783	3.23	168	.22	.33	3.64	.35	16	7
30	457	2.38	35	345	424	760	1.93	168	.21	.28	2.01	.22	14	7
90	246	2.48	52	253	437	967	1.25	97	.19	.33	2.70	.29	25	6
24	199	1.0	31	182	139	730	1.20	72	.12	.24	1.0	.02	8	<1
24	27	1.14	23	50	162	315	.34	40	.10	.07	.67	.07	7	3
98	29	1.90	19	123	227	340	3.50	26	.06	.18	3.19	.18	8	1
97	33	1.39	18	128	238	392	2.86	26	.19	.19	3.07	.19	8	1
143	129	2.75	44	245	695	485	3.29	125	.25	.32	4.78	.35	44	7
170	48	1.63	39	130	635	1323	.78	83	.19	.15	2.23	.35	17	25
44	362	1.8	37	322	240	1086	1.20	232	.20	.40	1.8	.05	10	1
285	211	1.4	23	276	283	653	1.95	454	.11	.32	1.2	.15	17	<1
3	40	2.8	21	88	303	955	1.12	120	.35	.28	4.5	.13	6	10
8	80	2.3	26	135	408	955	1.3	140	.25	.18	2.3	.20	8	13
23	53	3.3	20	113	245	1220	2.39	100	.15	.18	2.3	.12	5	5
89	124	3.7	40	236	665	1009	2.45	159	.25	.30	.4	.20	10	22
184	230	1.34	37	231	202	763	1.29	675	.09	.31	.48	.12	62	3
27	35	2.0	40	365	365	824	1.15	55	.06	.14	13.3	.17	15	5
52	37	1.94	31	182	224	869	.97	34	.14	.17	8.59	.24	13	1
22	44	.98	41	88	279	246	.69	41	.10	.06	.37	.16	19	6
52	165	2.7	61	274	388	516	3.30	58	.26	.29	4.36	.73	48	5
15	181	2.53	76	243	427	1030	2.37	58	.26	.23	2.40	1.01	55	5
44	135	2.30	22	174	219	672	2.53	65	.26	.24	3.70	.11	20	1
104	236	4.45	43	320	407	1224	5.27	128	.33	.49	7.37	.23	23	3
68	44	1.87	30	173	194	2732	1.00	16	.29	.26	9.21	.37	18	4
37	34	1.94	22	303	164	1252	1.44	<1	.28	.17	3.27	.11	2	3
44	324	1.31	50	133	240	784	2.51	186	.09	.42	1.91	.39	34	1
213	197	3.10	28	290	201	832	1.86	160	.46	.50	3.71	.15	35	1
56	132	1.85	29	223	274	667	.95	25	.32	.27	3.30	.10	24	3
90	61	2.23	34	246	375	621	.88	15	.35	.24	3.52	.12	43	1

C

(For purposes of calculations, use "0" for t, <1, <.1, <.01, etc.)

Table C–1   Food Composition

Grp	Computer Code No.	Food Description	Measure	Wt (g)	H$_2$O (%)	Ener (kcal)	Prot (g)	Carb (g)	Dietary Fiber (g)	Fat (g)	Fat Breakdown (g) Sat	Mono	Poly
		MIXED DISHES and FAST FOODS—Con.											
		FAST FOODS and SANDWICHES—Con.											
		Hamburger with bun:											
12	709	Regular	1 ea	98	46	245	12	28	1	11	4	5	1
12	710	4-oz patty	1 ea	174	50	445	25	38	1	21	7	12	1
12	711	Hotdog/frankfurter and bun	1 ea	85	53	260	8	21	1	15	5	7	2
12	712	Cheese pizza, ⅛ of 15″ round[95]	1 pce	120	46	290	15	39	2	9	4	3	1
		SANDWICHES:											
		Avocado, cheese, tomato & lettuce:											
12	1276	On white bread, firm	1 ea	205	59	464	15	39	7	29	9.1	11.8	6.0
12	1278	On part whole wheat	1 ea	195	60	432	14	33	8	29	8.7	11.8	6.0
12	1277	On whole wheat	1 ea	209	58	459	16	39	13	29	9.1	11.9	6.2
		Bacon, lettuce & tomato sandwich:											
12	1137	On white bread, soft	1 ea	135	54	333	11	30	2	19	5.2	7.4	5.5
12	1139	On part whole wheat	1 ea	135	54	327	12	28	3	19	4.9	7.5	5.5
12	1138	On whole wheat	1 ea	149	53	355	13	34	8	20	5.4	7.7	5.7
		Cheese sandwich, grilled:											
12	1140	On white bread, soft	1 ea	117	37	399	17	28	1	24	12.7	7.6	2.3
12	1142	On part whole wheat	1 ea	117	37	393	18	27	3	24	12.5	7.7	2.3
12	1141	On whole wheat	1 ea	131	38	420	20	33	7	25	12.9	7.9	2.6
		Chicken salad sandwich:											
12	1143	On white bread, soft	1 ea	99.7	44	300	10	28	1	16	3.0	4.9	7.5
12	1145	On part whole wheat	1 ea	99.7	44	294	11	27	3	16	2.8	5.0	7.5
12	1144	On whole wheat	1 ea	114	44	321	12	33	8	17	3.2	5.2	7.8
12	1146	Corned beef & swiss cheese on rye	1 ea	147	45	429	27	25	5	24	9.4	8.2	5.0
		Egg salad sandwich:											
12	1147	On white bread, soft	1 ea	111	47	325	9	28	1	19	3.9	6.2	7.7
12	1149	On part whole wheat	1 ea	111	47	319	10	27	3	19	3.7	6.3	7.7
12	1148	On whole wheat	1 ea	125	47	346	12	33	7	20	4.1	6.4	8.0
		Ham sandwich:											
12	1279	On rye bread	1 ea	116	55	242	16	25	5	9	1.9	3.2	2.8
12	1151	On white bread, soft	1 ea	122	54	262	16	28	1	9	2.2	3.4	2.7
12	1153	On part whole wheat	1 ea	122	54	256	17	27	3	9	2.0	3.5	2.7
12	1152	On whole wheat	1 ea	136	53	283	18	33	7	10	2.4	3.7	3.0
		Ham & cheese sandwich:											
12	1280	On soft white bread	1 ea	151	51	369	22	29	1	18	7.8	6.0	3.0
12	1282	On part whole wheat bread	1 ea	151	51	363	23	28	3	18	7.6	6.1	3.0
12	1281	On whole wheat	1 ea	165	50	390	25	33	7	19	8.0	6.2	3.3
12	1150	Ham & swiss on rye	1 ea	145	51	350	24	26	5	17	7.0	5.3	3.1
		Ham salad sandwich:											
12	1154	On white bread, soft	1 ea	125	48	345	10	34	1	19	4.8	7.2	5.9
12	1156	On part whole wheat	1 ea	125	48	339	11	33	3	19	4.6	7.3	6.0
12	1155	On whole wheat	1 ea	139	47	366	12	38	7	20	5.0	7.5	6.2
12	1157	Patty melt sandwich: ground beef & cheese on rye:	1 ea	177	45	567	32	25	5	38	14.1	13.9	6.5
		Peanut butter & jam sandwich:											
12	1158	On soft white bread	1 ea	100	27	347	12	45	3	15	2.8	6.8	4.3
12	1160	On part whole wheat	1 ea	100	27	341	12	44	5	15	2.5	6.9	4.3
12	1159	On whole wheat	1 ea	114	29	368	14	50	9	16	3.0	7.1	4.6
12	1161	Reuben sandwich, grilled: corned beef, swiss cheese, sauerkraut on rye:	1 ea	233	61	480	28	29	7	28	10.2	10.0	6.2
		Roast beef sandwich:											
12	713	On a bun	1 ea	150	52	345	22	34	1	13	4	7	2
12	1162	On soft white bread	1 ea	122	51	286	17	28	1	11	2.5	3.7	4.4

[95]Crust made with vegetable shortening and enriched flour.

(Computer code number is for West Diet Analysis program)

GRP KEY: 1 = BEV 2 = DAIRY 3 = EGGS 4 = FAT/OIL 5 = FRUIT 6 = BAKERY 7 = GRAIN 8 = FISH 9 = BEEF 10 = POULTRY
         11 = SAUSAGE 12 = MIXED/FAST 13 = NUTS/SEEDS 14 = SWEETS 15 = VEG/LEG 16 = MISC 22 = SOUP/SAUCE

C

Chol (mg)	Calc (mg)	Iron (mg)	Magn (mg)	Phos (mg)	Pota (mg)	Sodi (mg)	Zinc (mg)	VT-A (RE)	Thia (mg)	Ribo (mg)	Niac (mg)	V-B6 (mg)	Fola (µg)	VT-C (mg)
32	56	2.20	19	107	202	463	2.0	14	.23	.24	3.80	.12	16	1
71	75	4.84	38	225	404	763	5.01	28	.38	.38	7.85	.28	24	2
23	59	1.71	13	83	113	745	1.19	<1	.29	.19	2.48	.07	17	12
56	220	1.60	36	216	230	699	1.81	106	.34	.29	4.20	.04	40	2
32	312	3.02	54	242	557	556	1.69	160	.41	.43	3.98	.25	74	11
32	299	3.09	66	274	562	518	1.87	160	.36	.40	4.02	.29	76	11
32	279	3.52	105	353	608	660	2.46	160	.35	.37	4.18	.36	91	11
21	81	2.22	22	138	253	647	1.06	50	.42	.25	3.71	.10	35	13
21	80	2.57	36	181	269	661	1.30	50	.42	.26	4.13	.15	41	13
21	60	3.00	76	260	315	803	1.89	50	.41	.23	4.29	.21	55	13
55	424	1.82	25	489	158	1155	2.24	214	.28	.38	2.14	.06	25	<1
55	424	2.17	39	531	174	1169	2.49	214	.28	.38	2.56	.10	30	<1
55	404	2.61	78	610	219	1311	3.07	214	.26	.35	2.72	.17	45	<1
25	80	1.94	18	102	136	401	.76	18	.28	.21	3.73	.11	22	1
25	79	2.30	32	144	152	415	.00	18	.28	.22	4.15	.15	28	1
25	59	2.73	71	223	197	557	1.59	18	.27	.19	4.31	.22	43	1
85	331	3.98	32	310	174	1045	4.37	85	.23	.41	3.65	.14	25	0
164	96	2.49	17	133	119	447	.92	90	.29	.29	2.14	.07	38	<1
164	95	2.85	31	176	135	461	1.16	90	.29	.29	2.56	.11	44	<1
164	75	3.28	71	255	180	603	1.75	90	.28	.26	2.72	.18	59	<1
29	49	1.94	25	203	311	1261	1.91	4	.74	.30	4.50	.32	23	14
29	80	2.17	25	191	271	1199	1.50	4	.80	.31	4.94	.29	23	14
29	79	2.52	39	234	287	1213	1.74	4	.80	.32	5.36	.33	29	14
29	59	2.96	78	313	333	1355	2.33	4	.79	.29	5.52	.40	44	14
56	256	2.28	31	405	318	1610	2.44	88	.81	.42	4.96	.31	26	14
56	256	2.64	45	447	334	1624	2.69	88	.81	.42	5.38	.35	31	14
56	236	3.07	84	526	379	1766	3.27	88	.79	.39	5.54	.42	46	14
55	325	1.99	35	376	342	1336	3.03	77	.75	.40	4.52	.34	25	14
27	77	2.00	18	134	156	887	1.02	19	.52	.25	3.36	.11	21	4
27	77	2.36	32	177	172	901	1.26	19	.52	.25	3.78	.15	26	4
27	57	2.79	71	256	217	1043	1.85	19	.51	.22	3.94	.22	41	4
107	228	3.33	40	423	410	923	6.63	139	.25	.45	6.08	.31	26	<1
0	83	2.23	55	153	246	403	1.06	1	.30	.21	5.39	.12	42	<1
0	82	2.59	69	195	262	417	1.30	1	.30	.21	5.81	.16	47	<1
0	62	3.02	108	274	308	559	1.89	1	.28	.18	5.97	.23	62	<1
85	358	5.20	44	328	313	1642	4.55	133	.25	.43	3.80	.24	27	12
55	60	4.04	38	222	338	757	3.66	32	.39	.33	6.02	.28	42	2
30	80	2.86	23	157	298	757	2.63	8	.31	.29	5.10	.21	23	<1

(For purposes of calculations, use "0" for t, <1, <.1, <.01, etc.)

Table C–1   Food Composition

Grp	Computer Code No.	Food Description	Measure	Wt (g)	H₂O (%)	Ener (kcal)	Prot (g)	Carb (g)	Dietary Fiber (g)	Fat (g)	Fat Breakdown (g) Sat	Mono	Poly
MIXED DISHES and FAST FOOD—Con.													
		SANDWICHES—Con.											
		Roast Beef—Con.											
12	1164	On part whole wheat bread	1 ea	122	51	280	18	27	3	11	2.3	3.8	4.4
12	1163	On whole wheat bread	1 ea	136	50	307	19	32	7	12	2.7	3.9	4.7
		Tuna salad sandwich:											
12	1165	On soft white	1 ea	116	47	309	13	32	2	14	2.6	4.1	6.6
12	1167	On part whole wheat bread	1 ea	116	47	303	14	31	3	14	2.4	4.2	6.7
12	1166	On whole wheat bread	1 ea	130	47	331	15	37	8	15	2.8	4.4	6.9
		Turkey sandwich:											
12	1168	On soft white bread	1 ea	122	52	277	18	28	1	10	2.1	3.2	4.5
12	1170	On part whole wheat	1 ea	122	52	271	18	26	3	11	1.9	3.3	4.5
12	1169	On whole wheat	1 ea	136	51	298	20	32	7	11	2.3	3.4	4.8
		Turkey ham sandwich:											
12	1272	On rye bread	1 ea	116	55	239	15	25	5	9	1.9	2.6	3.3
12	1273	On soft white bread	1 ea	122	55	259	16	29	1	9	2.2	2.8	3.2
12	1275	On part whole wheat	1 ea	122	54	253	16	28	3	9	2.0	2.9	3.2
12	1274	On whole wheat	1 ea	136	53	281	18	33	7	10	2.4	3.1	3.5
12	714	Taco, corn tortilla, beef filling	1 ea	78	52	207	14	10	1	13	5	5	2
		Tostada:											
12	1114	With refried beans	1 ea	157	69	212	10	26	7	9	3.6	2.5	2.3
12	1118	With beans & beef	1 ea	192	67	332	18	20	4	21	9.4	7.2	2.6
12	1354	With beans & chicken	1 ea	157	67	249	19	19	4	11	4.4	3.5	2.9
		Vegetarian Foods:											
12	1175	Nuteena	1 ea	34	52	89	7	3	1	6	—	—	—
12	1171	Proteena	1 pce	67	58	160	8	5	1	12	—	—	—
12	1172	Redi-burger	1 pce	71	56	140	17	5	2	6	—	—	—
12	1173	Vege-Burger	1 pce	68	57	130	14	5	1	6	—	—	—
12	1174	Breakfast links	.5 c	108	73	110	22	4	1	1	—	—	—
NUTS, SEEDS and PRODUCTS													
		Almonds:											
13	1365	Dry roasted, salted	1 c	138	3	810	23	33	18	71	6.8	46.2	15.0
13	718	Slivered, packed, unsalted	1 c	135	4	795	27	28	15[96]	70	7	46	15
		Whole, dried, unsalted:											
13	719	Cup	1 c	142	4	837	28	29	17[96]	74	7	48	16
13	720	Ounce	1 oz	28	4	167	6	6	3[96]	15	1	10	3
13	721	Almond butter	1 tbsp	16	1	101	2	3	1	9	1	6	2
13	722	Brazil nuts, dry (about 7)	1 oz	28	3	186	4	4	3	19	5	7	7
		Cashew nuts:											
		Dry roasted, salted											
13	723	Cup	1 c	137	2	787	21	45	8	63	13	37	11
13	724	Ounce	1 oz	28	2	163	4	9	2	13	3	8	2
		Oil roasted, salted:											
13	725	Cup	1 c	130	4	748	21	37	8	63	12	37	11
13	726	Ounce	1 oz	28	4	163	5	8	2	14	3	8	2

[96] Values reported for dietary fiber in almonds vary from 7.0 to 14.3 g/100 g.

(Computer code number is for West Diet Analysis program)

GRP KEY: 1 = BEV 2 = DAIRY 3 = EGGS 4 = FAT/OIL 5 = FRUIT 6 = BAKERY 7 = GRAIN 8 = FISH 9 = BEEF 10 = POULTRY
11 = SAUSAGE 12 = MIXED/FAST 13 = NUTS/SEEDS 14 = SWEETS 15 = VEG/LEG 16 = MISC 22 = SOUP/SAUCE

Chol (mg)	Calc (mg)	Iron (mg)	Magn (mg)	Phos (mg)	Pota (mg)	Sodi (mg)	Zinc (mg)	VT-A (RE)	Thia (mg)	Ribo (mg)	Niac (mg)	V-B6 (mg)	Fola (µg)	VT-C (mg)
30	79	3.22	37	200	314	771	2.87	8	.31	.29	5.52	.25	29	<1
30	59	3.65	76	279	359	912	3.46	8	.29	.26	5.68	.32	44	<1
25	80	2.27	23	133	199	559	.65	22	.28	.21	5.43	.14	30	2
25	80	2.63	37	176	215	573	.89	22	.28	.22	5.85	.19	36	2
25	60	3.06	76	255	260	715	1.48	22	.26	.19	6.01	.25	51	2
29	76	1.87	23	192	223	1151	1.00	8	.29	.24	6.82	.23	23	<1
29	76	2.23	37	235	239	1165	1.24	8	.28	.24	7.24	.27	28	<1
29	56	2.66	77	314	285	1307	1.83	8	.27	.21	7.40	.34	43	<1
35	50	3.04	27	214	273	986	2.37	4	.25	.32	4.46	.21	24	0
35	81	3.28	26	203	233	924	1.96	5	.31	.34	4.90	.18	24	<1
35	80	3.63	40	245	249	938	2.20	5	.30	.34	5.32	.23	29	<1
35	60	4.06	80	324	295	1080	2.79	5	.29	.31	5.48	.29	44	<1
45	85	1.29	23	141	183	141	2.89	27	.03	.13	2.49	.16	13	1
15	177	1.93	62	195	422	618	1.55	74	.06	.14	.85	1.01	47	6
62	186	2.16	52	247	442	483	3.57	132	.08	.24	2.94	.67	37	6
53	162	1.69	48	242	358	474	1.94	81	.07	.19	4.53	.73	34	3
<1	11	1.96	—	—	43	203	—	<1	1.65	.17	3.77	.20	—	<1
0	21	1.20	40	111	200	120	.87	10	.47	.58	.14	.45	60	—
0	22	1.60	31	99	280	460	1.20	26	.64	.50	7.80	.50	23	—
0	19	1.40	13	56	120	370	1.20	10	.60	.40	6.70	.80	17	—
0	32	2.70	24	105	110	190	1.10	10	.53	.68	5.00	.56	27	—
0	389	5.25	419	756	1063	1076	6.76	0	.18	.83	3.89	.10	88	1
0	359	4.94	400	702	988	15	3.94	0	.28	1.05	4.54	.15	79	1
0	378	5.20	420	738	1034	15[97]	4.15	0	.30	1.11	4.77	.16	83	1
0	75	1.04	84	147	208	3[97]	.83	0	.06	.22	.96	.03	17	<1
0	43	.59	49	84	121	2[98]	.49	0	.02	.1	.46	.01	0	<1
0	50	.97	64	170	170	<1	1.30	t	.28	.04	.46	.07	1	<1
0	62	8.22	356	671	774	877[99]	7.67	0	.27	.27	1.92	.35	95	0
0	13	1.70	74	139	160	181[99]	1.59	0	.06	.06	.4	.07	20	0
0	53	5.33	332	554	689	814[100]	6.18	0	.55	.23	2.34	.33	88	0
0	12	1.16	72	121	151	177[100]	1.35	0	.12	.05	.51	.07	19	0

[97] Salted almonds contain 1108 mg sodium per cup, 221 mg per ounce.
[98] Salted almond butter contains 72 mg sodium per tablespoon.
[99] Dry-roasted cashews without salt contain 21 mg sodium per cup, or 4 mg per ounce.
[100] Oil-roasted cashews without salt contain 22 mg sodium per cup, or 5 mg per ounce.

(For purposes of calculations, use "0" for t, <1, <.1, <.01, etc.)

Table C–1   Food Composition

Grp	Computer Code No.	Food Description	Measure	Wt (g)	H$_2$O (%)	Ener (kcal)	Prot (g)	Carb (g)	Dietary Fiber (g)	Fat (g)	Fat Breakdown (g)		
											Sat	Mono	Poly
		NUTS, SEEDS and PRODUCTS—Con.											
		Cashew nuts, unsalted:											
13	1366	Dry roasted	1 c	137	2	787	21	45	8	64	12.6	37.4	10.7
13	1367	Oil roasted	1 c	130	4	748	21	37	8	63	12.4	36.9	10.6
13	727	Cashew butter	1 tbsp	16	3	94	3	4	1	8	2	5	1
13	728	European chestnuts, roasted, 1 c = approx 17 kernels	1 c	143	40	350	5	76	19	3	.6	1.1	1.2
		Coconut:											
		Raw:											
13	729	Piece 2 × 2 × ½″	1 pce	45	47	159	2	7	5	15	13	.6	.2
13	730	Shredded/grated, unpacked[101]	1 c	80	47	283	3	12	9	27	24	1	.3
		Dried, shredded/grated:											
13	731	Unsweetened	1 c	78	3	515	5	19	12	50	45	2	.6
13	732	Sweetened	1 c	93	16	466	3	44	9	33	29	1	.4
		Filberts (hazelnuts), chopped:											
13	733	Cup	1 c	115	5	727	15	18	7	72	5	57	7
13	734	Ounce	1 oz	28	5	179	4	4	2	18	1	14	2
		Macadamia nuts, oil roasted:											
		Salted:											
13	735	Cup	1 c	134	2	962	10	17	7	103	15	81	2
13	736	Ounce	1 oz	28	2	204	2	4	1	22	3	17	.4
13	1368	Unsalted	1 c	134	2	962	10	17	7	103	15.4	80.9	1.8
		Mixed nuts:											
13	737	Dry roasted, salted	1 c	137	2	814	24	35	12	70	10	43	15
13	738	Oil roasted, salted	1 c	142	2	876	24	30	13	80	12	45	19
13	1369	Oil roasted, unsalted	1 c	142	2	876	24	30	13	80	12.4	45.0	18.9
		Peanuts:											
		Oil roasted, salted:											
13	739	Cup	1 c	144	2	837	38	27	13	71	10	35.2	22.4
13	740	Ounce	1 oz	28	2	163	7	5	2	14	2	7	4
13	1370	Oil roasted, unsalted	1 c	144	2	837	38	27	13	71	9.9	35.2	22.4
		Dried, unsalted:											
13	741	Cup	1 c	146	7	827	38	24	13	72	10	36	23
13	742	Ounce	1 oz	28	7	161	7	5	3	14	2	7	4
13	743	Peanut butter	1 tbsp	16	2	94	4	3	1	8	1.5	4.0	2.3
		Pecans, halves:											
		Dried, unsalted:											
13	744	Cup	1 c	108	5	720	8	20	7[102]	73	6	46	18
13	745	Ounce	1 oz	28	5	190	2	5	2[102]	19	1.5	12	5
13	1372	Dry roasted, salted	¼ c	28	1	187	2	6	2	18	1.5	11.5	4.6
13	746	Pine nuts/piñons, dried	1 oz	28	6	161	3	5	2	17	3	7	7
		Pistachio nuts:											
13	747	Dried, shelled	1 oz	28	4	164	6	7	1	14	2	9	2
13	1373	Dry roasted, salted, shelled	1 c	128	2	776	19	35	14	68	8.6	45.7	10.3

[101]1 c packed = 130 g.

[102]Dietary fiber data calculated/derived from data on other nuts.

(Computer code number is for West Diet Analysis program)

GRP KEY: 1 = BEV 2 = DAIRY 3 = EGGS 4 = FAT/OIL 5 = FRUIT 6 = BAKERY 7 = GRAIN 8 = FISH 9 = BEEF 10 = POULTRY
11 = SAUSAGE 12 = MIXED/FAST 13 = NUTS/SEEDS 14 = SWEETS 15 = VEG/LEG 16 = MISC 22 = SOUP/SAUCE

Chol (mg)	Calc (mg)	Iron (mg)	Magn (mg)	Phos (mg)	Pota (mg)	Sodi (mg)	Zinc (mg)	VT-A (RE)	Thia (mg)	Ribo (mg)	Niac (mg)	V-B6 (mg)	Fola (µg)	VT-C (mg)
0	62	8.22	356	671	774	21	7.67	0	.27	.27	1.92	.35	95	0
0	53	5.33	332	554	689	22	6.18	0	.55	.23	2.34	.33	88	0
0	7	.09	41	73	87	2[103]	.83	0	.05	.03	.26	.04	11	0
0	42	1.30	47	153	846	3	.82	4	.35	.25	1.92	.71	100	37
0	6	1.09	14	51	160	9	.50	0	.03	.01	.24	.02	12	2
0	12	1.94	26	90	285	16	.88	0	.05	.02	.43	.04	21	3
0	20	2.59	70	161	423	29	1.57	0	.05	.08	.47	2.34	7	1
0	14	1.79	47	100	313	244	1.69	0	.03	.02	.44	.29	9	1
0	216	3.76	328	359	512	3	2.76	8	.57	.13	1.31	.7	83	1
0	53	.93	81	89	126	1	.68	2	.14	.03	.32	.17	20	<1
0	60	2.41	157	268	441	348[104]	1.47	1	.28	.15	2.71	.33	79	0
0	13	.51	33	57	94	74[104]	.31	<1	.06	.03	.57	.07	17	0
0	60	2.41	157	268	441	9	1.47	1	.28	.15	2.71	.33	79	0
0	96	5.07	308	596	817	917[105]	5.21	2	.27	.27	6.44	.41	69	1
0	153	4.56	334	659	825	926[105]	7.22	3	.71	.32	7.19	.34	118	1
0	153	4.56	334	659	825	16	7.22	3	.71	.32	7.19	.34	118	1
0	126	2.63	266	744	982	624[106]	9.55	0	.364	.156	20.6	.367	181	0
0	24	.51	52	145	191	121[106]	1.86	0	.07	.03	4	.07	35	0
0	126	2.63	266	744	982	8.6	9.55	0	.364	.156	20.6	.367	181	0
0	85	4.72	263	559	1047	23	4.78	0	.97	.19	20.7	.43	153	0
0	17	.92	51	109	204	5	.93	0	.19	.04	4.02	.08	30	0
0	5.5	.27	25	52	115	77[107]	.4	0	.02	.02	2.1	.06	13	0
0	39	2.30	138	314	423	1[108]	5.91	14	.92	.14	.96	.20	42	1
0	10	.61	36	83	111	<1	1.55	4	.24	.04	.25	.05	11	1
0	10	.62	38	86	105	221	1.61	4	.09	.04	.26	.05	12	1
0	2	.87	67	10	178	20	1.22	1	.35	.06	1.24	.08	19	<1
0	38	1.93	45	143	310	2[109]	.38	7	.22	.05	.31	.06	17	<1
0	90	4.06	166	609	1242	998	1.74	30	.54	.32	1.80	.27	74	0

[103] Salted cashew butter contains 98 mg sodium per tablespoon.
[104] Macadamia nuts without salt contain 9 mg sodium per cup, or 2 mg per ounce.
[105] Mixed nuts without salt contain about 15 mg sodium per cup.
[106] Peanuts without salt contain 22 mg sodium per cup, or 4 mg per ounce.
[107] Peanut butter without added salt contains 3 mg sodium per tablespoon.
[108] Salted pecans contain 816 mg sodium per cup, or 214 mg per ounce.
[109] Salted pistachios contain approx 221 mg sodium per ounce.

(For purposes of calculations, use "0" for t, <1, <.1, <.01, etc.)

Table C–1   Food Composition

Grp	Computer Code No.	Food Description	Measure	Wt (g)	H₂O (%)	Ener (kcal)	Prot (g)	Carb (g)	Dietary Fiber (g)	Fat (g)	Sat	Mono	Poly
											Fat Breakdown (g)		

NUTS, SEEDS and PRODUCTS—Con.

Grp	No.	Food Description	Measure	Wt (g)	H₂O (%)	Ener (kcal)	Prot (g)	Carb (g)	Fiber (g)	Fat (g)	Sat	Mono	Poly
		Pumpkin kernels:											
13	748	Dried, unsalted	1 oz	28	7	154	7	5	2	13	2.5	4	6
13	1374	Roasted, salted	1 c	227	7	1185	75	31	9	96	18.1	29.7	43.6
13	749	Sesame seeds, hulled, dried	¼ c	38	5	221	10	4	6	21	3	8	9
		Sunflower seed kernels:											
13	750	Dry	¼ c	36	5	205	8	7	2	18	2	3	12
13	751	Oil roasted	¼ c	34	3	208	7	5	2	19	2	4	13
13	752	Tahini (sesame butter)	1 tbsp	15	3	91	3	3	2	8	1	3	4
		Black walnuts, chopped:											
13	753	Cup	1 c	125	4	759	30	15	7	71	5	16	47
13	754	Ounce	1 oz	28	4	172	7	3	2	16	1	4	11
		English walnuts, chopped:											
13	755	Cup	1 c	120	4	770	17	22	7	74	7	17	47
13	756	Ounce	1 oz	28	4	182	4	5	2	18	2	4	11

SWEETENERS and SWEETS: see also Dairy (milk desserts) and Baked Goods

Grp	No.	Food Description	Measure	Wt (g)	H₂O (%)	Ener (kcal)	Prot (g)	Carb (g)	Fiber (g)	Fat (g)	Sat	Mono	Poly
14	757	Apple butter	2 tbsp	35	52	66	<1	17	<1	<1	.1	<.1	.1
14	1124	Butterscotch topping	3 tbsp	50	33	156	1	41	0	<1	—	—	—
		Cake frosting:											
14	1127	Canned, average of all types	2.5 tbsp	39	15	160	0	24	0	7	1.7	2.9	1.7
14	1123	Prepared from mix	2.5 tbsp	39	15	167	0	28	0	6	—	—	—
		Candy:											
14	1128	Almond Joy® candy bar	1 oz	28	7	151	2	19	1.9	8	6.7	.6	.1
14	758	Caramel, plain or chocolate	1 oz	28	8	115	1	22	<1	3	2.2	.3	.1
		Chocolate (see also, #784, 785, 971):											
		Milk chocolate:											
14	759	Plain	1 oz	28	1	145	2	16	1	9	5.4	3	.3
14	760	With almonds	1 oz	28	2	150	3	15	1	10	4.4	4.7	1.0
14	761	With peanuts	1 oz	28	1	155	5	10	2	12	3.5	5.2	2.7
14	762	With rice cereal	1 oz	28	2	140	2	18	1	7	4.4	2.5	.2
14	763	Semisweet chocolate chips	1 c	170	1	860	7	97	5	61	36	20	2
14	764	Sweet dark chocolate	1 oz	28	1	150	1	16	1	10	5.9	3.3	.3
14	1133	English toffee candy bar	1 ea	32	2	220	1	11	<1	19	7	7	2
14	765	Fondant candy, uncoated (mints, candy corn, other)	1 oz	28	3	105	0	27	0	0	0	0	0
14	766	Fudge, chocolate	1 oz	28	8	115	1	21	2	3	2.1	1	.1
14	767	Gum drops	1 oz	28	12	98	0	25	0	<1	t	t	.1
14	768	Hard candy, all flavors	1 oz	28	1	109	0	28	0	0	0	0	0
14	769	Jelly beans	1 oz	28	6	104	t	26	0	<.1	t	t	.1
14	1134	M&M's Plain choc. candies®	48 grm	48	1	237	3	33	<1	10	5	3	3
14	1135	M&M's Peanut choc. candies®	47 grm	47.3	2	240	5	28	1	12	5	5	2
14	1130	MARS® bar	1 ea	50	7	240	4	30	1	11	4.8	4.4	.8
14	1129	MILKY WAY® candy bar	1 ea	60	7	260	3	43	<1	9	5.4	3.0	.3
14	1132	REESE's® peanut butter cup	2 ea	45	4	240	6	22	2	14	5.2	5.4	2.4
14	1131	SNICKERS® candy bar, 2.2oz size	1 ea	61.2	7	290	7	37	2	14	—	—	—
14	1125	Caramel topping	3 tbsp	50	31	155	1	39	<1	—	—	—	—
14	771	Gelatin salad/dessert	½ c	120	84	70	2	17	<1	0	0	0	0
		Honey:											
14	772	Cup	1 c	339	17	1030	1	279	0	0	0	0	0
14	773	Tablespoon	1 tbsp	21	17	65	<.1	17	0	0	0	0	0

(Computer code number is for West Diet Analysis program)

GRP KEY: 1=BEV 2=DAIRY 3=EGGS 4=FAT/OIL 5=FRUIT 6=BAKERY 7=GRAIN 8=FISH 9=BEEF 10=POULTRY
11=SAUSAGE 12=MIXED/FAST 13=NUTS/SEEDS 14=SWEETS 15=VEG/LEG 16=MISC 22=SOUP/SAUCE

Chol (mg)	Calc (mg)	Iron (mg)	Magn (mg)	Phos (mg)	Pota (mg)	Sodi (mg)	Zinc (mg)	VT-A (RE)	Thia (mg)	Ribo (mg)	Niac (mg)	V-B6 (mg)	Fola (µg)	VT-C (mg)
0	12	4.25	152	333	229	5[110]	2.12	11	.06	.09	.50	.03	26	<1
0	98	33.9	1212	2600	1830	1305	16.9	88	.25	.66	3.60	.20	115	0
0	49	2.93	130	291	153	15	2.23	<1	.27	.03	1.76	.30	38	0
0	42	2.44	128	254	248	1	1.82	2	.83	.10	1.62	.46	85	<1
0	19	2.26	43	385	163	205[111]	1.76	2	.11	.10	1.40	.40	79	<1
0	21	.83	53	119	69	5	1.57	1	.24	.02	.85	.06	15	1
0	73	3.84	253	580	655	1	4.28	37	.27	.14	.86	.70	83	1
0	16	.87	57	132	149	0	.97	8	.06	.03	.20	.16	19	<1
0	113	2.93	203	380	602	12	3.28	15	.46	.18	1.25	.67	79	4
0	27	.69	48	90	142	3	.78	4	.11	.04	.30	.16	19	1
0	5	.25	2	13	89	1	.01	0	<.01	.01	.08	.01	<1	1
14	56	.10	3	23	34	66	.12	<1	0	.04	0	<.01	.06	0
0	—	—	—	—	—	91	—	0	—	—	—	—	—	—
0	—	—	—	—	—	84	—	0	—	—	—	—	—	—
0	20	.5	16	42	92	48	.43	3	.01	.05	.14	.05	2.1	.1
1	42	.4	6	35	54	64	.15	<1	.01	.05	.1	<.01	0	t
6	50	.4	16	61	96	23	.37	10	.02	.1	.1	.02	<1	t
5	61	.56	33	77	125	23	.48	8	.03	.13	.31	.02	4	t
3	32	.68	35	87	155	19	.68	8	.11	.07	2.2	.05	16	t
6	48	.2	13	57	100	46	.29	8	.01	.08	.1	.01	<1	t
0	51	5.8	230	178	593	24	2.39	3	.1	.14	.9	.04	22	t
0	7	.6	32	41	86	5	.42	1	.01	.04	.1	.01	5	t
0	0	.20	11.5	0	50	90	.24	5	.053	.05	.10	.04	1	0
0	2	.1	—	2	1	57	.1	0	<.01	<.01	.01	.01	0	0
1	22	.3	14	24	42	54	.16	16	.01	.03	.1	.01	2	t
0	2	.1	—	—	1	10	0	5	0	<.01	.01	0	0	0
0	6	.1	<1	2	1	7	0	0	0	0	0	0	0	0
0	1	.30	—	1	11	7	0	0	0	<.01	.01	—	0	0
0	79	.76	30	65	171	41	.57	13	.03	.12	.27	.01	5	—
0	59	.67	38	64	162	29	.66	<1	.03	.09	1.48	.03	5	—
0	85	.55	37	63	176	85	.59	<1	.02	.16	.48	.01	5	—
14	86	.49	22	80	167	140	.45	25	.03	.15	.20	.01	7	1
3	35	.68	47	87	168	92	.9	8	.03	.05	2.12	.06	17	—
0	70	.49	39	75	209	170	.69	5	.03	.11	1.84	.02	6	—
0	28	.10	3	23	33	152	—	<1	0	.05	0	—	—	0
0	2	.10	<1	23	91	55	.03	0	.01	.01	.20	<.01	0	0
0	17	1.70	7	20	173	17	.40	0	.02	.14	1.0	.06	32	3
0	1	.11	<1	1	11	1	.02	0	<.01	.01	.06	<.01	2	<1

[110]Salted pumpkin/squash kernels contain approximately 163 mg sodium per ounce.
[111]Unsalted sunflower seeds contain 1 mg sodium per ¼ cup.

(For purposes of calculations, use "0" for t, <1, <.1, <.01, etc.)

Table C-1　Food Composition

Grp	Computer Code No.	Food Description	Measure	Wt (g)	H₂O (%)	Ener (kcal)	Prot (g)	Carb (g)	Dietary Fiber (g)	Fat (g)	Fat Breakdown (g) Sat	Mono	Poly
		SWEETENERS and SWEETS—Con.											
		Jams or preserves:											
14	774	Tablespoon	1 tbsp	20	29	54	<1	14	<1	<.1	0	t	t
14	775	Packet	1 ea	14	29	38	<.1	10	<1	<.1	0	t	t
		Jellies:											
14	776	Tablespoon	1 tbsp	18	28	49	<.1	13	<1	<.1	t	t	t
14	777	Packet	1 ea	14	28	39	<.1	10	<1	<.1	t	t	t
14	1136	Marmalade	1 tbsp	20	29	52	<1	14	<1	0	0	0	0
14	770	Marshmallows	4 ea	28	17	90	t	23	0	0	0	0	0
14	1126	Marshmallow creme topping	3 tbsp	50	20	158	<1	40	0	0	0	0	0
14	778	Popsicles, 3 oz when fluid	1 ea	95	80	70	0	18	0	0	0	0	0
		Sugars:											
14	779	Brown sugar	1 c	220	2	820	0	212	0	0	0	0	0
		White sugar, granulated:											
14	780	Cup	1 c	200	1	770	0	199	0	0	0	0	0
14	781	Tablespoon	1 tbsp	12	1	45	0	12	0	0	0	0	0
14	782	Packet	1 ea	6	1	25	0	6	0	0	0	0	0
14	783	White sugar, powdered, sifted	1 c	100	<1	385	0	99	0	0	0	0	0
		Syrups:											
		Chocolate:											
14	784	Thin type	2 tbsp	38	37	85	1	22	1	<1	.2	.1	.1
14	785	Fudge type	2 tbsp	38	25	125	2	21	1	5	3	2	.2
14	786	Molasses, blackstrap[112]	2 tbsp	40	24	85	0	22	0	0	0	0	0
14	787	Pancake table syrup (corn and maple)	¼ c	84	25	244	0	64	0	0	0	0	0
		VEGETABLES and LEGUMES											
15	788	Alfalfa seeds, sprouted	1 c	33	91	10	1	1	1	<1	t	t	.1
15	789	Artichokes, cooked globe (300 g with refuse)	1 ea	120	84	60	4	13	10	<1	<.1	t	.1
		Artichoke hearts:											
15	1177	Cooked from frozen	9 oz	240	87	108	7	22	18	1	.3	<.1	.5
15	1176	Marinated	6 oz	170	59	168	4	13	11	14	2.0	3.0	7.7
		Asparagus, green, cooked:											
		From raw:											
15	790	Cuts and tips	½ c	90	92	23	2	4	2	<1	.1	t	.1
15	791	Spears, ½″ diam at base	4 spears	60	92	15	2	3	1	<1	<.1	t	.1
		From frozen:											
15	792	Cuts and tips	1 c	180	91	50	5	9	3	1	.2	t	.3
15	793	Spears, ½″ diam at base	4 spears	60	91	17	2	3	1	<1	.1	t	.1
15	794	Canned, spears, ½″ diam at base	4 spears	80	95	11	2	2	1	1	.1	t	.2
15	795	Bamboo shoots, canned, drained slices	1 c	131	94	25	2	4	3	1	.1	t	.2
		Beans (see also Great northern, #855; Kidney beans, #860; Navy beans, #876; Pinto beans, #898; Refried beans, #921; Soybeans, #925):											
15	796	Black beans, cooked	1 c	172	66	227	15	41	15	1	.2	.1	.4
		Canned beans (white/navy):											
15	803	Beans w/pork and tomato sauce	1 c	253	73	247	13	49	14	3	1.0	1.1	.3
15	804	Beans w/pork and sweet sauce	1 c	253	71	282	13	53	14	4	1.4	1.6	.5
15	805	Beans with frankfurters	1 c	257	70	366	17	40	18	17	6	7	2
		Lima beans:											
15	797	Thick seeded (Fordhooks), cooked from frozen	½ c	85	74	85	5	16	5	<1	.1	t	.1

[112]Light molasses would contain about 66 mg calcium, 2.1 mg iron, 18 mg magnesium, and 366 mg potassium for 2 tbsp.

(Computer code number is for West Diet Analysis program)

GRP KEY: 1 = BEV   2 = DAIRY   3 = EGGS   4 = FAT/OIL   5 = FRUIT   6 = BAKERY   7 = GRAIN   8 = FISH   9 = BEEF   10 = POULTRY
11 = SAUSAGE   12 = MIXED/FAST   13 = NUTS/SEEDS   14 = SWEETS   15 = VEG/LEG   16 = MISC   22 = SOUP/SAUCE

Chol (mg)	Calc (mg)	Iron (mg)	Magn (mg)	Phos (mg)	Pota (mg)	Sodi (mg)	Zinc (mg)	VT-A (RE)	Thia (mg)	Ribo (mg)	Niac (mg)	V-B6 (mg)	Fola (µg)	VT-C (mg)
0	4	.20	1	2	18	2	.01	t	<.01	.01	.04	<.01	2	<1
0	3	.14	<1	1	13	1	<.01	t	<.01	.01	.03	<.01	1	<1
0	2	.12	<1	1	16	4	0	t	<.01	<.01	.04	<.01	2	1
0	1	.09	<1	1	12	3	0	t	<.01	<.01	.03	<.01	2	1
0	7	.12	1	3	12	4	—	1	<.01	<.01	.02	<.01	1	1.2
0	1	.45	1	2	2	25	<.01	0	0	<.01	.01	<.01	0	0
0	16	.8	2	6	16	29	<.01	0	0	<.01	.02	—	0	2
0	0	.01	—	0	4	11	0	0	0	0	0	0	0	0
0	187	4.80	135	56	757	97	.08	0	.02	.07	.20	0	0	0
0	3	.10	<1	.1	7	5	.04	0	0	0	0	0	0	0
0	<1	.01	<1	t	t	t	<.01	0	0	0	0	0	0	0
0	<1	<.01	<1	t	t	t	<.01	0	0	0	0	0	0	0
0	0	.08	<1	0	4	2	<.01	0	0	0	0	0	0	0
0	6	.75	26	49	85	36	.39	1	.02	.02	.11	<.01	3	0
0	38	.50	18	60	82	42	.39	13	.08	.08	.08	<.01	3	0
0	274[112]	10.1[112]	103[112]	34	1171[112]	38	0	0	.08	.08	.80	.11	6	0
0	2	.06	2	8	14	38	.08	0	0	0	0	t	<1	0
0	11	.32	9	23	26	2	.30	5	.03	.04	.16	.01	12	3
0	54	1.55	72	103	425	114	.59	22	.08	.08	1.20	.13	61	12
0	50	1.34	74	146	634	127	.86	39	.15	.38	2.20	.21	285	12
0	39	1.62	48	102	438	900	.54	28	.06	.17	1.38	.15	149	52
0	22	.59	17	55	279	4	.43	75	.09	.11	.95	.13	88	25
0	14	.4	11	37	186	2	.29	50	.06	.07	.63	.09	59	16
0	41	1.15	23	99	392	7	1.01	147	.12	.19	1.87	.16	176	44
0	14	.38	8	33	131	2	.34	49	.04	.06	.62	.06	59	15
0	11	.5	8	30	122	278[113]	.32	38	.05	.07	.7	.04	69	13
0	10	.42	6	33	105	9	.30	1	.03	.03	.18	—	40	1
0	47	3.60	121	241	611	1	1.92	1	.42	.10	.87	.12	256	0
17	141	8.30	88	297	759	45	2.60	31	.13	.12	1.26	.18	57	8
17	155	4.20	87	266	673	1113	3.80	29	.12	.15	.89	.22	95	8
15	123	4.45	71	267	604	849	4.79	40	.15	.14	2.32	.12	77	6
0	19	1.16	29	54	347	1105	.37	16	.06	.05	.91	.10	55	11

[112] Light molasses would contain about 66 mg calcium, 2.1 mg iron, 18 mg magnesium, and 366 mg potassium for 2 tbsp.
[113] Special dietary pack contains 3 mg sodium.

(For purposes of calculations, use "0" for t, <1, <.1, <.01, etc.)

Table C-1   Food Composition

Grp	Computer Code No.	Food Description	Measure	Wt (g)	H₂O (%)	Ener (kcal)	Prot (g)	Carb (g)	Dietary Fiber (g)	Fat (g)	Fat Breakdown (g) Sat	Mono	Poly
VEGETABLES and LEGUMES—Con.													
		Lima Beans—Con.											
15	798	Thin seeded (baby), cooked from frozen	½ c	90	72	94	6	18	8	<1	.1	t	.1
15	799	Cooked from dry, drained	1 c	188	70	217	15	39	18	1	.2	.1	.3
		Snap beans/green beans, cuts and french style:											
15	800	Cooked from raw	1 c	125	89	44	2	10	3	<1	.1	t	.2
15	801	Cooked from frozen	1 c	135	92	36	2	8	4	<1	<.1	t	.1
15	802	Canned, drained	1 c	136	93	26	2	6	2	<1	<.1	t	.1
		Bean sprouts (mung):											
15	806	Raw	1 c	104	90	31	3	6	3	<1	<.1	t	.1
15	807	Cooked, stir fried	1 c	124	84	62	5	13	3	<1	<.1	.1	.1
15	808	Cooked, boiled, drained	1 c	124	93	26	3	5	3	<1	<.1	t	<.1
		Beets:											
		Cooked from fresh:											
15	809	Sliced or diced	½ c	85	91	26	1	6	2	<.1	t	t	t
15	810	Whole beets, 2″ diam	2 beets	100	91	31	1	7	2	<.1	t	t	t
		Canned:											
15	811	Sliced or diced	½ c	85	91	27	1	6	2	<1	t	t	<.1
15	812	Pickled slices	½ c	114	82	74	1	19	2	<1	t	t	<.1
15	813	Beet greens, cooked, drained	1 c	144	89	40	4	8	3	<1	<.1	.1	.1
		Black-eyed peas: see Peas											
		Broccoli:											
15	817	Raw, chopped	1 c	88	91	24	3	5	3	<1	.1	t	.1
15	818	Raw, spears	1 spear	151	91	42	5	8	6	1	.1	<.1	.3
		Cooked from raw:											
15	819	Spears	1 spear	180	91	50	5	9	7	<1	.1	<.1	.3
15	820	Chopped	1 c	156	91	44	5	8	6	<1	.1	<.1	.3
		Cooked from frozen:											
15	821	Spear, small piece	1 spear	30	91	8	1	2	1	<.1	t	t	t
15	822	Chopped	1 c	184	91	51	6	10	6	<1	<.1	t	<.1
		Brussels sprouts:											
15	823	Cooked from raw	1 c	156	87	60	6	14	6	1	.2	.1	.4
15	824	Cooked from frozen	1 c	155	87	65	6	13	5	1	.1	.1	.3
		Cabbage, common varieties:											
15	825	Raw, shredded or chopped	1 c	70	92	16	1	4	2	<1	t	t	.1
15	826	Cooked, drained	1 c	150	94	32	1	7	4	<1	.1	<.1	.2
		Chinese cabbage:											
15	1178	Bok-choy, raw, shredded	1 c	70	95	9	1	2	1	<1	t	t	.1
15	827	Bok choy, cooked, drained	1 c	170	96	20	3	3	3	<1	<.1	t	.1
15	828	Pe-Tsai, raw, chopped	1 c	76	94	11	1	2	2	<1	<.1	t	.1
		Cabbage, red, coarsely chopped:											
15	829	Raw	1 c	70	92	19	1	4	2	<1	t	t	.1
15	830	Cooked	½ c	75	94	16	1	3	4	<1	t	t	.1
15	831	Savoy cabbage, coarsely chopped, raw	1 c	70	91	20	1	4	2	<.1	t	t	<.1

(Computer code number is for West Diet Analysis program)

GRP KEY: 1=BEV 2=DAIRY 3=EGGS 4=FAT/OIL 5=FRUIT 6=BAKERY 7=GRAIN 8=FISH 9=BEEF 10=POULTRY
11=SAUSAGE 12=MIXED/FAST 13=NUTS/SEEDS 14=SWEETS 15=VEG/LEG 16=MISC 22=SOUP/SAUCE

Chol (mg)	Calc (mg)	Iron (mg)	Magn (mg)	Phos (mg)	Pota (mg)	Sodi (mg)	Zinc (mg)	VT-A (RE)	Thia (mg)	Ribo (mg)	Niac (mg)	V-B6 (mg)	Fola (μg)	VT-C (mg)
0	25	1.76	50	101	370	26	.50	15	.06	.05	.69	.11	58	5
0	32	4.50	82	208	955	4	1.79	0	.30	.10	.79	.30	156	0
0	58	1.60	32	48	373	4	.45	83[114]	.09	.12	.77	.07	42	12
0	61	1.11	29	33	151	17	.84	71[115]	.07	.10	.56	.08	42	11
0	36	1.22	18	26	147	339[116]	.39	47[117]	.02	.08	.27	.05	43	6
0	14	.95	22	56	154	6	.43	2	.09	.13	.78	.09	63	14
0	16	2.40	38	70	200	14	1.12	3	.17	.22	1.49	.10	72	20
0	15	.81	18	34	125	12	.58	2	.06	.13	1.01	.05	35	14
0	9	.53	31	26	266	42	.21	1	.03	.01	.23	.03	49	5
0	11	.62	37	31	312	49	.25	1	.03	.01	.27	.03	86	6
0	13	1.55	13	15	126	233[118]	.18	1	.01	.04	.15	.05	22	4
0	13	.47	17	19	169	301	.30	1	.03	.06	.29	.03	35	3
0	165	2.74	97	58	1308	346	.72	734	.17	.42	.72	.19	47	36
0	42	.78	22	58	286	24	.36	136[119]	.06	.10	.56	.14	62	82
0	72	1.33	38	99	490	41	.60	233[119]	.10	.18	.96	.24	107	141
0	83	1.51	43	106	525	47	.68	250[119]	.10	.2	1.03	.26	90	134
0	72	1.24	37	92	456	40	.59	217[119]	.09	.18	.90	.22	78	116
0	15	.18	6	16	54	7	.09	57[119]	.02	.02	.14	.04	9	12
0	94	1.12	37	101	331	44	.55	348[119]	.10	.15	.84	.19	55	74
0	56	1.88	32	87	491	17	.50	112	.17	.12	.95	.31	94	97
0	38	1.15	37	84	504	36	.55	91	.16	.18	.83	.27	157	71
0	32	.40	10	16	172	12	.12	9	.04	.02	.21	.07	40	33
0	50	.59	23	38	308	29	.24	13	.09	.08	.34	.10	31	36
0	74	.56	13	26	176	<1	.29	210	.03	.05	.35	.07	57	32
0	158	1.77	18	49	630	57	.43	437	.05	.11	.73	.30	32	44
0	59	.23	10	22	181	7	.17	91	.03	.04	.30	.18	60	21
0	36	.35	11	29	144	8	.15	3	.05	.02	.21	.15	19	40
0	28	.27	8	21	105	6	.11	2	.03	.01	.15	.11	9	26
0	25	.28	20	29	161	20	.26	70	.05	.02	.21	.13	32	22

[114]Data is for green varieties; yellow beans contain 10 RE per cup.
[115]Data is for green varieties; yellow beans contain 15 RE per cup.
[116]Dietary pack contains 3 mg sodium per cup.
[117]For green varieties; yellow beans contain 14 RE per cup.
[118]Dietary pack contains 39 mg sodium.
[119]Vitamin A for whole plant: leaves are 1600 RE/100 g raw; flower clusters are 300/100 g raw; stalks are 40 RE/100 g raw.

(For purposes of calculations, use "0" for t, <1, <.1, <.01, etc.)

Table C–1　Food Composition

Grp	Computer Code No.	Food Description	Measure	Wt (g)	H₂O (%)	Ener (kcal)	Prot (g)	Carb (g)	Dietary Fiber (g)	Fat (g)	Fat Breakdown (g) Sat	Mono	Poly
		VEGETABLES and LEGUMES—Con.											
		Carrots:											
		Raw:											
15	832	Whole, 7½ × 1⅛″	1 carrot	72	88	31	1	7	2	<1	t	t	.1
15	833	Grated	½ c	55	88	24	1	6	2	<1	t	t	<.1
		Cooked, sliced, drained:											
15	834	Cooked from raw	½ c	78	87	35	1	8	3	<1	<.1	t	.1
15	835	Cooked from frozen	½ c	73	90	26	1	6	3	<.1	t	t	<.1
15	836	Canned, sliced, drained	½ c	73	93	17	<1	4	1	<1	<.1	t	.1
15	837	Carrot juice	½ c	123	89	49	1	11	2	<1	<.1	t	.1
		Cauliflower:											
15	838	Raw, flowerets	½ c	50	92	12	1	2	1	<.1	t	t	<.1
		Cooked, drained, flowerets:											
15	839	From raw	½ c	62	92	15	1	3	1	<1	t	t	.1
15	840	From frozen	1 c	180	94	34	3	7	3	<1	.1	<.1	.2
		Celery, pascal type, raw:											
15	841	Large outer stalk, 8 × 1½″ (at root end)	1 stalk	40	95	6	<1	1	1	<.1	t	t	t
15	842	Diced	½ c	60	95	11	<1	2	1	<.1	t	t	<.1
		Chard, swiss:											
15	1179	Raw, chopped	1 c	36	93	7	1	1	1	<1	t	t	<.1
15	1180	Cooked	1 c	175	93	35	3	7	4	<1	<.1	t	.1
		Chick-peas (see Garbanzo, #854)											
		Collards, cooked, drained:											
15	843	From raw	1 c	128	92	35	2	8	4	<1	.1	<.1	.1
15	844	From frozen	1 c	170	88	63	3	14	6	1	.1	.1	.3
		Corn:											
		Cooked, drained:											
15	845	From raw, on cob, 5″ long	1 ear	77	70	83	3	19	3	1	.2	.3	.5
15	846	From frozen, on cob, 3½″ long	1 ear	63	73	59	2	14	3	<1	.1	.1	.2
15	847	Kernels, cooked from frozen	½ c	82	76	67	2	17	3	<.1	t	t	<.1
		Canned:											
15	848	Cream style	½ c	128	79	93	2	23	2	<1	.1	.2	.3
15	849	Whole kernel, vacuum pack	1 c	210	77	166	5	41	3	1	.2	.3	.5
		Cowpeas; (see Black-eyed peas, #814–816)											
15	850	Cucumbers with peel, ⅛″ thick, 2⅛″ diam	6 slices	28	96	4	<1	1	<1	<.1	t	t	t
		Dandelion greens:											
15	851	Raw	1 c	55	86	25	1	5	1	<1	<.1	<.1	.2
15	852	Chopped, cooked, drained	1 c	105	90	35	2	7	1	1	.2	<.1	.4
15	853	Eggplant, cooked	1 c	160	92	45	1	11	6	<1	.1	<.1	.2
15	854	Garbanzo beans (chick-peas), cooked	1 c	164	60	269	15	45	11	4	.4	1.0	2.0
15	855	Great northern beans, cooked	1 c	177	69	210	15	37	11	1	.3	<.1	.3
15	856	Escarole/curly endive, chopped	1 c	50	94	9	1	2	1	<1	t	t	<.1
15	857	Jerusalem artichokes, raw slices	1 c	150	78	114	3	26	2	<.1	—	t	t
		Kale, cooked, drained:											
15	858	From raw	1 c	130	91	42	3	7	4	1	.1	<.1	.3
15	859	From frozen	1 c	130	90	39	4	7	3	1	.1	<.1	.3
15	860	Kidney beans, canned	1 c	256	77	216	13	39	19	<1	.1	.1	.4
		Kohlrabi:											
15	1181	Raw slices	1 c	140	91	38	2	9	2	<1	t	t	.1
15	861	Cooked	1 c	165	90	48	3	11	2	<1	t	t	.1

(Computer code number is for West Diet Analysis program)

GRP KEY: 1 = BEV 2 = DAIRY 3 = EGGS 4 = FAT/OIL 5 = FRUIT 6 = BAKERY 7 = GRAIN 8 = FISH 9 = BEEF 10 = POULTRY
11 = SAUSAGE 12 = MIXED/FAST 13 = NUTS/SEEDS 14 = SWEETS 15 = VEG/LEG 16 = MISC 22 = SOUP/SAUCE

Chol (mg)	Calc (mg)	Iron (mg)	Magn (mg)	Phos (mg)	Pota (mg)	Sodi (mg)	Zinc (mg)	VT-A (RE)	Thia (mg)	Ribo (mg)	Niac (mg)	V-B6 (mg)	Fola (µg)	VT-C (mg)
0	19	.36	11	32	233	25	.14	2025	.07	.04	.67	.11	10	7
0	15	.28	8	24	178	19	.11	1547	.05	.03	.51	.08	8	5
0	24	.48	10	24	177	52	.23	1915	.03	.04	.40	.19	11	2
0	21	.35	7	19	115	43	.18	1292	.02	.03	.32	.09	8	2
0	19	.47	6	17	131	176[120]	.19	1006	.01	.02	.40	.08	7	2
0	29	.56	17	51	358	36	.22	3159	.11	.07	.47	.27	5	11
0	14	.29	7	23	178	7	.09	1	.04	.03	.32	.12	33	36
0	17	.26	7	22	200	4	.15	1	.04	.04	.34	.13	32	34
0	31	.74	16	43	250	33	.23	4	.07	.10	.56	.16	74	56
0	16	.16	5	10	115	35	.05	5	.02	.02	.13	.04	11	3
0	25	.25	7	15	170	55	.08	8	.03	.03	.19	.06	13	4
0	18	.65	29	17	136	77	.16	259	.01	.03	.14	.03	20	11
0	102	3.96	150	58	961	313	.59	1198	.06	.15	.63	.12	57	32
0	29	.21	9	10	168	21	.14	349	.03	.07	.37	.07	8	16
0	54	.38	16	19	307	37	.26	638	.05	.12	.68	.12	129	28
0	2	.47	25	79	192	13	.37	17[121]	.17	.06	1.24	.18	36	5
0	2	.38	18	47	158	3	.40	13[121]	.11	.04	.96	.14	19	3
0	2	.25	15	39	114	4	.29	20[121]	.06	.06	1.05	.18	19	2
0	4	.49	22	65	172	365[122]	.68	12[121]	.03	.07	1.23	.08	57	6
0	11	.88	48	134	390	572[123]	.97	51[121]	.09	.15	2.46	.12	104	17
0	4	.08	3	5	42	1	.07	1	.01	.01	.09	.02	4	1
0	103	1.71	20	36	218	42	.62	770	.11	.14	.39	.02	64	19
0	147	1.89	26	44	244	46	.80	1229	.14	.18	.50	.04	82	19
0	10	.56	21	35	397	5	.24	10	.12	.03	.96	.14	23	2
0	80	4.74	78	275	477	11	2.51	4	.19	.10	.86	.23	282	2
0	121	3.77	88	293	692	4	1.55	<1	.28	.10	1.21	.21	181	2
0	26	.42	8	14	157	11	.40	103	.04	.04	.20	.01	71	3
0	21	5.10	26	117	644	6	.11	3	.30	.09	1.95	.11	15	6
0	94	1.17	23	36	296	30	.31	962	.07	.09	.70	.18	30	53
0	179	1.22	23	36	417	20	.23	826	.06	.15	.87	.11	31	33
0	62	3.22	73	240	658	873	1.41	0	.27	.23	1.17	.06	129	3
0	34	.56	27	64	490	28	.32	5	.07	.03	.56	.21	14	87
0	41	.66	31	74	561	34	.32	6	.07	.03	.64	.18	13	89

[120] Dietary pack contains 31 mg sodium.
[121] For yellow varieties; white varieties contain only a trace of vitamin A.
[122] Dietary pack contains 4 mg sodium per ½ cup.
[123] Dietary pack contains 6 mg sodium per cup.

(For purposes of calculations, use "0" for t, <1, <.1, <.01, etc.)

Table C–1   Food Composition

Grp	Computer Code No.	Food Description	Measure	Wt (g)	H₂O (%)	Ener (kcal)	Prot (g)	Carb (g)	Dietary Fiber (g)	Fat (g)	Fat Breakdown (g)		
											Sat	Mono	Poly
VEGETABLES and LEGUMES—Con.													
		Leeks:											
15	1183	Raw, chopped	1 c	104	83	63	2	15	2	<1	.1	<.1	.4
15	1182	Cooked, chopped	.5 c	52	91	16	<1	4	2	<1	t	t	.1
15	862	Lentils, cooked from dry	1 c	198	70	230	18	40	10	1	.1	.1	.4
		Lentils, sprouted:											
15	1288	Stir fried	3.5 oz	100	69	101	9	21	4	<1	.1	.1	.2
15	1289	Raw	1 c	77	67	81	7	17	3	<1	<.1	.1	.2
		Lettuce:											
		Butterhead/Boston types:											
15	863	Head, 5″ diam	1 head	163	96	21	2	4	3	<1	<.1	t	.2
15	864	Leaves, 2 inner or outer	2 leaves	15	96	2	<1	<1	<1	<.1	t	t	t
		Iceberg/crisphead:											
15	865	Head, 6″ diam	1 head	539	96	70	5	11	9	1	.1	<.1	.5
15	866	Wedge, ¼ of head	1 wedge	135	96	18	1	3	2	<1	<.1	t	.1
15	867	Chopped or shredded	1 c	56	96	7	1	1	1	<1	t	t	.1
15	868	Loose leaf, chopped	1 c	56	94	10	1	2	1	<1	t	t	.1
		Romaine:											
15	869	Chopped	1 c	56	95	9	1	1	1	<1	t	t	.1
15	870	Inner leaf	1 leaf	10	95	2	<1	<1	<1	<.1	t	t	t
		Mushrooms:											
15	871	Raw, sliced	½ c	35	92	9	1	2	1	<1	t	t	.1
15	872	Cooked from raw, pieces	½ c	78	91	21	2	4	2	<1	<.1	t	.1
15	873	Canned, drained	½ c	78	91	19	1	4	2	<1	<.1	t	.1
		Mustard greens:											
15	874	Cooked from raw	1 c	140	94	21	3	3	3	<1	t	.2	.1
15	875	Cooked from frozen	1 c	150	94	29	3	5	3	<1	t	.2	.1
15	876	Navy beans, cooked from dry	1 c	182	63	259	16	43	16	1	.3	.1	.4
		Okra, cooked:											
15	877	From fresh pods	8 pods	85	90	27	2	6	2	<1	<.1	t	<.1
15	878	From frozen slices	½ c	92	91	34	2	8	2	<1	.1	.1	.1
		Onions:											
15	879	Raw, chopped	1 c	160	90	61	2	14	3	<1	<.1	<.1	.1
15	880	Raw, sliced	1 c	115	90	44	1	10	2	<1	<.1	<.1	.1
15	881	Cooked, drained, chopped	½ c	105	88	46	1	11	2	<1	<.1	<.1	.1
15	882	Dehydrated flakes	¼ c	14	4	45	1	12	1	<.1	t	t	<.1
		Spring onions:											
15	883	Chopped, bulb and top	½ c	50	90	16	1	4	1	.1	t	t	<.1
15	1185	Green tops only, chopped	1 c	100	92	34	2	6	3	<1	.1	.1	.2
15	1184	White part only, chopped	1 c	100	92	50	1	10	3	<1	<.1	t	.1
15	884	Onion rings, breaded, prepared f/frozen	2 rings	20	29	81	1	8	<1	5	1.7	2.2	1
		Parsley:											
15	885	Raw, chopped	½ c	30	88	10	1	2	2	<.1	t	t	<.1
15	886	Raw, sprigs	10 sprigs	10	88	3	<1	1	1	<.1	t	t	t
15	887	Freeze dried	¼ c	1	2	4	<1	1	1	<.1	t	t	<.1
15	888	Parsnips, sliced, cooked	1 c	156	78	125	2	30	5	1	.1	.2	.1
		Peas:											
		Black-eyed peas, cooked:											
15	814	From dry, drained	1 c	171	70	198	13	36	21	1	.2	.1	.4
15	815	From fresh, drained	1 c	165	76	160	5	33	12	1	.2	<.1	.3
15	816	From frozen, drained	1 c	170	66	224	14	40	14	1	.3	.1	.5
15	889	Edible-pod, peas, cooked	1 c	160	89	67	5	11	4	<1	.1	<.1	.2

(Computer code number is for West Diet Analysis program)

GRP KEY: 1 = BEV   2 = DAIRY   3 = EGGS   4 = FAT/OIL   5 = FRUIT   6 = BAKERY   7 = GRAIN   8 = FISH   9 = BEEF   10 = POULTRY
11 = SAUSAGE   12 = MIXED/FAST   13 = NUTS/SEEDS   14 = SWEETS   15 = VEG/LEG   16 = MISC   22 = SOUP/SAUCE

Chol (mg)	Calc (mg)	Iron (mg)	Magn (mg)	Phos (mg)	Pota (mg)	Sodi (mg)	Zinc (mg)	VT-A (RE)	Thia (mg)	Ribo (mg)	Niac (mg)	V-B6 (mg)	Fola (μg)	VT-C (mg)
0	61	2.18	29	36	187	21	.17	10	.06	.03	.42	.24	67	13
0	16	.57	7	9	45	5	.12	2	.01	.01	.10	.08	16	2
0	37	6.59	71	356	731	4	2.50	2	.34	.14	2.10	.35	358	3
0	14	3.10	35	153	284	9	1.60	4	.22	.09	1.20	.16	84	13
0	19	2.47	28	133	248	8	1.16	4	.18	.10	.87	.15	77	13
0	52	.49	18	38	419	8	.42	158	.10	.10	.49	.11	119	13
0	5	.05	2	3	39	1	.04	15	.01	.01	.05	.01	11	1
0	102	2.70	49	108	852	48	1.19	178	.25	.16	1.01	.22	302	21
0	26	.68	12	27	213	12	.30	45	.06	.04	.25	.05	76	5
0	11	.28	5	11	89	5	.12	19	.03	.02	.11	.02	31	2
0	38	.78	6	14	148	5	.19	106	.03	.04	.22	.03	60	10
0	20	.62	3	25	162	4	.19	146	.06	.06	.28	.03	76	13
0	4	.11	1	5	29	1	.03	26	.01	.01	.05	.06	14	2
0	2	.43	4	36	130	1	.30	0	.04	.16	1.44	.03	7	1
0	5	1.36	9	68	278	2	.68	0	.06	.23	3.48	.07	14	3
0	9	.62	6	52	101	332	.56	0	.05	.17	1.25	.06	10	0
0	104	1.56	21	57	283	22	.30	424	.06	.09	.61	.18	20	35
0	152	1.68	20	36	209	38	.30	671	.06	.08	.39	.16	20	21
0	128	4.5	107	285	669	2	1.93	<1	.37	.11	.97	.30	255	1
0	54	.38	48	48	274	4	.47	49	.11	.05	.74	.16	39	14
0	88	.62	47	42	215	3	.57	47	.09	.11	.72	.04	134	11
0	32	.35	16	53	251	5	.30	0	.07	.03	.24	.19	30	10
0	23	.25	12	38	181	3	.22	0	.05	.02	.17	.13	22	7
0	23	.25	12	37	174	3	.22	0	.04	.02	.17	.14	16	5
0	36	.22	13	42	227	3	.26	0	.01	.01	.03	.22	23	11
0	36	.74	10	19	138	8	.20	20	.03	.04	.26	.03	32	9
0	56	2.20	21	39	260	7	.22	400	.07	.10	.60	0	80	51
0	40	.89	16	40	230	7	.25	<1	.07	.03	.33	.10	36	27
0	6	.34	4	16	26	75	.08	5	.06	.03	.72	.02	3	<1
0	39	1.86	13	12	161	12	.22	156	.02	.03	.21	.05	55	27
0	13	.62	4	4	54	4	.07	52	.01	.01	.07	.02	18	9
0	2	.75	5	8	88	5	.09	89	.02	.03	.15	.02	22	2
0	58	.90	46	108	573	16	.40	0	.13	.08	1.10	.15	91	20[124]
0	42	4.30	91	266	476	6	2.20	3	.35	.1	.85	.17	356	1
0	211	1.85	86	84	690	7	1.7	131	.17	.24	2.3	.11	210	4
0	40	3.60	85	208	638	9	2.42	13	.42	.11	1.24	.16	240	5
0	67	3.15	42	89	383	6	.60	30	.21	.12	.86	.23	48	77

[124] Value for vitamin C is highest right after harvest and drops after that.

(For purposes of calculations, use "0" for t, <1, <.1, <.01, etc.)

Table C–1 Food Composition

Grp	Computer Code No.	Food Description	Measure	Wt (g)	H$_2$O (%)	Ener (kcal)	Prot (g)	Carb (g)	Dietary Fiber (g)	Fat (g)	Fat Breakdown (g) Sat	Mono	Poly
		VEGETABLES and LEGUMES—Con.											
		Peas—Con.											
		Green peas:											
15	890	Canned, drained	½ c	85	82	59	4	11	4	<1	.1	<.1	.1
15	891	Cooked from frozen	½ c	80	80	63	4	11	4	<1	<.1	t	.1
15	892	Split, green, cooked from dry	1 c	196	69	231	16	41	10	1	.1	.2	.3
		Peas and carrots:											
15	1187	Cooked from frozen	½ c	80	86	38	2	8	3	<1	.1	<.1	.2
15	1186	Canned, with liquid	½ c	128	88	48	3	11	4	<1	.1	<.1	.2
		Peppers, hot:											
15	893	Hot green chili, canned	½ c	68	92	17	1	4	1	<.1	t	t	<.1
15	894	Hot green chili, raw	1 pepper	45	88	18	1	4	1	<.1	t	t	<.1
15	895	Jalapenos, chopped, canned	½ c	68	90	17	1	3	2	<1	.4	t	.2
		Peppers, sweet, green:											
15	896	Whole pod (90 g with refuse), raw	1 pod	74	92	20	1	5	1	<1	.1	t	.1
15	897	Cooked, chopped (1 pod cooked = 73 g)	½ c	68	92	19	1	5	1	<1	<.1	t	.1
		Peppers, sweet, red:											
15	1286	Raw, chopped	½ c	50	92	14	<1	3	1	<1	<.1	t	.1
15	1287	Cooked, chopped	½ c	68	92	19	1	5	1	<1	<.1	t	.1
15	898	Pinto beans, cooked from dry	1 c	171	64	235	14	44	20	1	.2	.2	.3
15	1191	Poi - two finger	1 c	240	72	269	1	65	6	<1	.1	<.1	.1
		Potatoes:[125]											
		Baked in oven, 4¾ × 2⅓″ diam:											
15	899	With skin	1 potato	202	71	220	5	51	5	<1	.1	t	.1
15	900	Flesh only	1 potato	156	75	145	3	34	2	<1	<.1	t	.1
15	901	Skin only	1 ea	58	47	115	2	27	2	<.1	t	t	<.1
		Baked in microwave, 4¾ × 2⅓″ diam:											
15	902	With skin	1 potato	202	72	212	5	49	5	<1	.1	t	.1
15	903	Flesh only	1 potato	156	74	156	3	36	2	<1	<.1	t	.1
15	904	Skin only	1 ea	58	64	77	3	17	2	<.1	t	t	<.1
		Boiled, about 2½″ diam:											
15	905	Peeled after boiling	1 potato	136	77	119	3	27	2	<1	<.1	t	.1
15	906	Peeled before boiling	1 potato	135	78	116	2	27	2	<1	<.1	t	.1
		French fried, strips 2-3½″ long, frozen:											
15	907	Oven heated	10 strips	50	53	111	2	17	1	4	2.1	1.8	.3
15	908	Fried in veg oil	10 strips	50	38	158	2	20	1	8	2.5	1.6	3.8
15	1188	Fried in veg. and animal oil	10 strips	50	38	158	2	20	1	8	3.4	4.0	.5
15	909	Hashed brown, from frozen	1 c	156	56	340	5	44	3	18	7	8	2
		Mashed:											
15	910	Home recipe with milk[126]	1 c	210	78	162	4	37	3	1	.7	.3	.1
15	911	Home recipe with milk and margarine	1 c	210	76	222	4	35	3	9	2.2	3.7	2.5
15	912	Prepared from flakes; water, milk, margarine, salt added	1 c	215	76	239	4	28	2	13	3.0	5.4	3.7
		Potato products, prepared:											
		Au gratin:											
15	913	From dry mix	1 c	245	79	228	6	32	4	10	6.3	3	.3
15	914	From home recipe[127]	1 c	245	74	322	12	28	4	19	12	5	1

[125]Vitamin C varies with length of storage. After 3 months of storage approximately two-thirds of the ascorbic acid remains; after 6 to 7 months, about one-third remains.

[126]Recipe: 84% potatoes, 15% whole milk, 1% salt.

[127]Recipe: 55% potatoes, 30% whole milk, 9% cheddar cheese, 3% butter, 2% flour, 1% salt.

(Computer code number is for West Diet Analysis program)

GRP KEY: 1 = BEV 2 = DAIRY 3 = EGGS 4 = FAT/OIL 5 = FRUIT 6 = BAKERY 7 = GRAIN 8 = FISH 9 = BEEF 10 = POULTRY
11 = SAUSAGE 12 = MIXED/FAST 13 = NUTS/SEEDS 14 = SWEETS 15 = VEG/LEG 16 = MISC 22 = SOUP/SAUCE

Chol (mg)	Calc (mg)	Iron (mg)	Magn (mg)	Phos (mg)	Pota (mg)	Sodi (mg)	Zinc (mg)	VT-A (RE)	Thia (mg)	Ribo (mg)	Niac (mg)	V-B6 (mg)	Fola (µg)	VT-C (mg)
0	17	.81	15	57	147	186[128]	.60	65	.10	.07	.62	.05	38	8
0	19	1.25	23	72	134	70	.75	77	.23	.14	1.18	.09	47	8
0	26	2.52	71	195	710	4	1.96	1	.37	.11	1.74	.09	127	1
0	18	.75	13	39	127	55	.36	621	.18	.06	.92	.07	21	7
0	29	.97	18	58	128	332	.74	739	.10	.07	.74	.11	24	8
0	5	.34	8	12	143	10	.02	42[129]	.01	.03	.54	.08	35	46
0	8	.54	11	21	153	3	.14	35[129]	.04	.04	.43	.13	11	109
0	18	1.90	8	12	92	995	.13	116	.02	.03	.34	.14	35	9
0	7	.34	7	14	131	1	.09	47	.05	.02	.38	.18	16	66
0	6	.31	7	12	113	1	.08	40	.04	.02	.32	.16	10	51
0	5	.23	5	10	89	1	.06	285	.03	.02	.26	.12	11	95
0	6	.31	7	12	113	1	.08	256	.04	.02	.32	.16	11	116
0	82	4.47	95	273	800	3	1.85	<1	.32	.16	.68	.27	294	4
0	37	2.11	58	94	439	28	2.04	5	.31	.10	2.64	—	—	10
0	20	2.75	55	115	844	16	.65	0	.22	.07	3.32	.70	22	26
0	8	.55	39	78	610	8	.45	0	.16	.03	2.18	.47	14	20
0	20	2.20	25	59	332	12	.28	0	.07	.07	1.78	.35	13	8
0	22	2.50	54	212	903	16	.73	0	.24	.07	3.46	.70	24	31
0	8	.64	39	170	641	11	.51	0	.20	.04	2.54	.50	19	24
0	27	3.44	22	48	377	9	.30	0	.04	.04	1.29	.28	10	9
0	7	.42	30	60	515	6	.41	0	.14	.03	1.96	.41	14	18
0	10	.42	26	54	443	7	.37	0	.13	.03	1.77	.36	12	10
0	4	.67	11	43	229	15	.21	0	.06	.02	1.15	.12	8	6
0	10	.38	17	47	366	108	.19	0	.09	.01	1.63	.12	15	5
0	10	.38	17	47	366	108	.19	0	.09	.01	1.63	.12	15	5
0	24	2.36	27	112	680	53	.50	0	.17	.03	3.78	.20	26	10
4	55	.57	39	100	628	636	.60	12	.19	.08	2.35	.49	17	14
4[130]	54	.55	37	97	607	619	.58	41	.18	.11	2.27	.47	17	13
4[130]	92	.40	30	108	428	733	.51	176	.30	.14	1.91	.26	15	25
12	203	.78	37	233	537	1076	.59	76	.05	.20	2.30	.10	3	8
56[131]	292	1.56	48	277	970	1064	1.69	93	.16	.28	2.43	.43	25	24

[128] Dietary pack contains 1.7 mg sodium.
[129] Data is for green chili peppers; red varieties contain 809 RE vitamin A per ½ cup; 484 RE per whole pepper.
[130] Data is for margarine; if butter is used, cholesterol = 25 mg for 29 total mg.
[131] Data is for butter; if margarine is used, cholesterol = 37 mg.

(For purposes of calculations, use "0" for t, <1, <.1, <.01, etc.)

Table C–1　Food Composition

Grp	Computer Code No.	Food Description	Measure	Wt (g)	H₂O (%)	Ener (kcal)	Prot (g)	Carb (g)	Dietary Fiber (g)	Fat (g)	Fat Breakdown (g)		
											Sat	Mono	Poly
		VEGETABLES and LEGUMES—Con.											
		Potato Products—Con.											
		Potato salad (see Mixed Dishes #715)											
		Scalloped:											
15	915	From dry mix	1 c	245	79	228	5	31	3	11	6.5	3.0	.5
15	916	Home recipe[132]	1 c	245	81	210	7	26	3	9	5.5	2.6	.4
15	1192	Potato puffs, cooked from frozen	.5 c	62	53	138	2	19	1	7	3.2	2.7	.5
15	917	Potato chips (14 chips = about 1 oz)	14 chips	28	2	148	2	15	1	10	2.6	1.8	5.2
		Pumpkin:											
15	918	Cooked from raw, mashed	1 c	245	94	50	2	12	4	<1	.1	t	t
15	919	Canned	1 c	245	90	83	3	20	5	1	.4	.1	<.1
15	920	Red radishes	10 radishes	45	95	7	<1	2	1	<1	t	t	t
15	921	Refried beans, canned	1 c	253	72	270	16	47	22	3	1	1.2	.4
15	1375	Rutabaga, cooked cubes	.5 c	85	90	29	1	7	1	<1	<.1	<.1	.1
15	922	Sauerkraut, canned with liquid	1 c	236	92	44	2	10	4	<1	.1	<.1	.1
		Seaweed:											
15	923	Kelp, raw	1 oz	28	82	12	1	3	1	<1	.1	<.1	t
15	924	Spirulina, dried	1 oz	28	5	82	16	7	1	2	.8	.2	.6
15	925	Soybeans, cooked from dry	1 c	172	63	298	29	17	5	15	2.2	3.4	8.7
		Soybean products:											
15	926	Miso	½ c	138	46	283	16	39	7	8	1.2	1.9	4.7
15	927	Tofu	½ c	124	85	94	10	2	2	6	.9	1.3	3.4
		Spinach:											
15	928	Raw, chopped	1 c	56	92	12	2	2	2	<1	<.1	t	.1
		Cooked, drained:											
15	929	From raw	1 c	180	91	41	5	7	4	<1	.1	t	.2
15	930	From frozen (leaf)	1 c	190	90	53	6	10	5	<1	.1	t	.2
15	931	Canned, drained solids	1 c	214	92	50	6	7	6	1	.2	<.1	.5
		Spinach soufflé (Mixed Dishes)											
		Squash, summer varieties, cooked slices:											
15	932	Varieties averaged	1 c	180	94	36	2	8	3	1	.1	<.1	.2
15	933	Crookneck	1 c	180	94	36	2	8	3	1	.1	<.1	.2
15	934	Zucchini	1 c	180	95	29	1	7	4	<.1	t	t	<.1
		Squash, winter varieties, cooked:											
		Average of all varieties, baked:											
15	935	Mashed	1 c	245	89	96	2	21	7	2	.3	.1	.7
15	936	Baked cubes	1 c	205	89	79	2	18	6	1	.3	.1	.5
		Acorn squash:											
15	937	Baked, mashed	1 c	245	83	137	3	36	7	<1	<.1	t	.1
15	1218	Boiled, mashed	1 c	245	90	83	2	22	6	<1	<.1	t	.1
15	938	Butternut, baked cubes	1 c	205	88	83	2	22	6	<1	<.1	t	.1
		Butternut squash:											
15	1219	Baked, mashed	1 c	245	88	99	2	26	7	<1	<.1	t	.1
15	1193	Cooked from frozen	1 c	240	88	94	3	24	7	<1	<.1	t	.1
		Hubbard squash:											
15	1194	Baked, mashed	1 c	240	85	120	6	26	6	1	.3	.1	.6
15	1195	Boiled, mashed	1 c	236	91	70	4	15	7	1	.2	.1	.4
15	1196	Spaghetti squash, baked or boiled	1 c	155	92	45	1	10	4	<1	.1	<.1	.2
15	1189	Succotash, cooked from frozen	1 c	170	74	158	7	34	9	2	.3	.3	.7

[132]Recipe: 59% potatoes, 36% whole milk, 2% butter, 2% flour, 1% salt.

(Computer code number is for West Diet Analysis program)

GRP KEY: 1 = BEV 2 = DAIRY 3 = EGGS 4 = FAT/OIL 5 = FRUIT 6 = BAKERY 7 = GRAIN 8 = FISH 9 = BEEF 10 = POULTRY 11 = SAUSAGE 12 = MIXED/FAST 13 = NUTS/SEEDS 14 = SWEETS 15 = VEG/LEG 16 = MISC 22 = SOUP/SAUCE

Chol (mg)	Calc (mg)	Iron (mg)	Magn (mg)	Phos (mg)	Pota (mg)	Sodi (mg)	Zinc (mg)	VT-A (RE)	Thia (mg)	Ribo (mg)	Niac (mg)	V-B6 (mg)	Fola (µg)	VT-C (mg)
27	88	.93	34	137	497	835	.61	51	.05	.14	2.52	.10	3	8
29[133]	140	1.41	46	154	926	821	.98	46	.17	.23	2.58	.44	21	26
0	19	.97	12	30	236	462	.19	1	.12	.05	1.34	.14	.10	4
0	7	.34	17	43	369	133[134]	.30	0	.04	.01	1.19	.14	13	12
0	37	1.40	22	74	564	3	.45	265	.08	.19	1.01	.16	33	12
0	64	3.41	56	85	504	12	.42	5404	.06	.13	.9	.14	30	10
0	9	.13	4	8	104	11	.13	t	<.01	.02	.14	.03	12	10
0	118	4.5	99	214	994	1071	3.45	0	.12	.14	1.23	.28	150	15
0	36	.40	18	42	244	15	.26	0	.06	.03	.54	.08	13	19
0	72	3.47	31	46	401	1561	.44	4	.05	.05	.34	.31	4	35
0	48	.81	34	12	25	66	.35	3	.01	.04	.13	—	51	—
0	34	8.08	55	33	386	297	—	16	.68	1.04	3.63	.10	—	3
0	175	8.84	148	421	886	1	1.98	2	.27	.49	.69	.40	93	3
0	92	3.78	58	211	226	5032	4.58	12	.13	.35	1.19	.3	46	0
0	130	6.65	127	120	150	9	1.00	11	.10	.06	.24	.06	19	<1
0	55	1.52	44	27	312	44	.30	448	.04	.11	.41	.11	109	16
0	244	6.42	157	100	838	126	1.37	1750	.17	.43	.88	.44	262	40
0	277	2.89	131	91	566	163	1.33	1756	.11	.32	.80	.28	204	23
0	271	4.92	162	94	740	683[135]	.99	1878	.03	.30	.83	.21	209	31
0	48	.64	44	69	346	2	.71	52[136]	.08	.07	.92	.12	36	9
0	48	.64	44	69	346	2	.71	52[136]	.09	.09	.92	.17	36	10
0	23	.63	40	72	455	5	.32	43[136]	.07	.07	.77	.14	30	8
0	34	.81	20	49	1071	2	.64	872	.21	.06	1.72	.18	69	24
0	28	.67	16	41	895	3	.54	730	.17	.05	1.43	.15	57	20
0	108	2.28	104	111	1071	11	.42	105	.41	.03	2.16	.48	46	26
0	65	1.37	63	67	645	6	.27	63	.25	.02	1.30	.29	28	16
0	84	1.23	59	55	582	7	.27	1435	.15	.04	1.99	.25	39	31
0	100	1.47	71	66	697	8	.32	1715	.18	.04	2.38	.30	47	37
0	46	1.40	22	34	319	4	.29	801	.12	.09	1.11	.17	29	8
0	41	1.13	53	55	859	19	.36	1450	.18	.11	1.34	.41	39	23
0	23	.67	32	33	504	12	.22	945	.10	.07	.79	.24	23	15
0	33	.52	17	21	182	28	.31	17	.06	.03	1.26	.15	12	6
0	25	1.51	39	119	451	77	.76	39	.13	.12	2.22	.16	57	10

[133] Data is for butter; if margarine is used cholesterol = 15 mg.

[134] If no salt added, sodium = 2 mg.

[135] Dietary pack contains 58 mg sodium.

[136] Applies to squash including skin; flesh has no appreciable vitamin A value.

(For purposes of calculations, use "0" for t, <1, <.1, <.01, etc.)

Table C–1   Food Composition

Grp	Computer Code No.	Food Description	Measure	Wt (g)	H$_2$O (%)	Ener (kcal)	Prot (g)	Carb (g)	Dietary Fiber (g)	Fat (g)	Fat Breakdown (g)		
											Sat	Mono	Poly
VEGETABLES and LEGUMES—Con.													
		Sweet potatoes:											
		Cooked, 5 × 2″ diam:											
15	939	Baked in skin, peeled	1 potato	114	73	118	2	28	3	<1	<.1	t	.1
15	940	Boiled without skin	1 potato	151	73	160	2	37	5	<1	.1	t	.2
15	941	Candied, 2½ × 2″	1 pce	105	67	144	1	29	2	3	1.4	.7	.2
		Canned:											
15	942	Solid pack, mashed	1 c	265	74	258	5	59	6	<1	.1	t	.2
15	943	Vacuum pack, mashed	1 c	255	76	233	4	54	5	1	.1	t	.2
15	944	Vacuum pack, 2¾ × 1″	1 pce	40	76	36	1	8	1	<1	t	t	<.1
		Tomatoes:											
15	945	Raw, whole, 2⅗″ diam	1 tomato	123	94	26	1	6	2	<1	<.1	<.1	.2
15	946	Raw, chopped	1 c	180	94	38	2	8	3	<1	.1	.1	.2
15	947	Cooked from raw	1 c	240	92	65	3	14	4	1	.1	.2	.4
15	948	Canned, solids and liquid	1 c	240	94	47	2	10	3	1	.1	.1	.2
15	949	Tomato juice, canned	1 c	244	94	42	2	10	2	<1	t	t	.1
		Tomato products, canned:											
15	950	Paste	1 c	262	74	220	10	49	11	2	.3	.4	.9
15	951	Puree	1 c	250	87	102	4	25	6	<1	<.1	<.1	.1
15	952	Sauce	1 c	245	89	74	3	18	4	<1	.1	.1	.2
15	953	Turnips, cubes, cooked from raw	½ c	78	94	14	1	4	2	<1	t	t	<.1
		Turnip greens, cooked:											
15	954	From raw (leaves and stems)	1 c	144	94	29	2	6	4	<1	.1	t	.1
15	955	From frozen (chopped)	½ c	82	90	24	3	4	4	<1	.1	t	.1
15	956	Vegetable juice cocktail, canned	1 c	242	94	46	2	11	2	<1	<.1	<.1	.1
		Vegetables, mixed:											
15	957	Canned, drained	1 c	163	87	77	4	15	6	<1	.1	<.1	.2
15	958	Frozen, cooked, drained	1 c	182	83	107	5	24	7	<1	.1	t	.1
		Water chestnuts, canned:											
15	959	Slices	½ c	70	86	35	1	9	2	<.1	t	t	t
15	960	Whole	4 ea	28	86	14	<1	4	1	<1	t	t	t
15	1190	Watercress, fresh, chopped	.5 c	17	95	2	<1	<1	<1	<1	t	t	t
MISCELLANEOUS													
		Baking powders for home use:											
		Sodium aluminum sulfate:											
16	962	With monocalcium phosphate monohydrate	1 tsp	3	2	5	t	1	0	0	0	0	0
16	963	With monocalcium phosphate monohydrate, calcium sulfate	1 tsp	3	1	5	t	1	0	0	0	0	0
16	964	Straight phosphate	1 tsp	4	2	5	t	1	0	0	0	0	0
16	965	Low sodium	1 tsp	4	1	5	t	1	0	0	0	0	0
16	1204	Baking soda	1 tsp	3	1	0	0	0	0	0	0	0	0
16	966	Basil, ground	1 tbsp	5	6	11	1	3	1	<1	—	—	—
16	961	Carob flour	1 c	103	3	185	5	92	34	1	.1	.2	.2

(Computer code number is for West Diet Analysis program)

GRP KEY: 1=BEV 2=DAIRY 3=EGGS 4=FAT/OIL 5=FRUIT 6=BAKERY 7=GRAIN 8=FISH 9=BEEF 10=POULTRY
11=SAUSAGE 12=MIXED/FAST 13=NUTS/SEEDS 14=SWEETS 15=VEG/LEG 16=MISC 22=SOUP/SAUCE

Chol (mg)	Calc (mg)	Iron (mg)	Magn (mg)	Phos (mg)	Pota (mg)	Sodi (mg)	Zinc (mg)	VT-A (RE)	Thia (mg)	Ribo (mg)	Niac (mg)	V-B6 (mg)	Fola (µg)	VT-C (mg)
0	32	.52	23	63	397	12	.33	2488	.08	.14	.7	.28	26	28
0	32	.8	15	41	278	20	.4	2575	.08	.21	1	.36	22	26
0[137]	27	1.2	12	27	198	73	.16	440	.02	.04	.41	.17	12	7
0	77	3.4	61	133	536	191	.54	3857	.07	.23	2.4	.48	42	13
0	56	2.27	57	125	796	136	.46	2036	.09	.14	1.89	.49	42	67
0	9	.36	9	20	125	21	.07	319	.02	.02	.3	.08	7	11
0	6	.55	14	30	273	11	.11	77	.07	.06	.77	.10	18	22[138]
0	9	.81	20	43	400	16	.16	112	.11	.09	1.13	.14	27	34[138]
0	14	1.34	34	74	670	26	.26	178	.17	.14	1.80	.23	31	55
0	63[139]	1.45	29	46	529	390[140]	.38	145	.11	.07	1.76	.22	35	36
0	22	1.41	27	46	537	881[141]	.34	136	.12	.08	1.64	.27	49	45
0	92	7.84	134	207	2442	170[142]	2.1	647	.41	.5	8.44	1	40	111
0	37	2.32	60	99	1051	49[143]	.54	340	.18	.14	4.29	.38	39	88
0	34	1.88	46	78	908	1481[144]	.6	240	.16	.14	2.82	.33	39	32
0	18	.17	6	15	106	39	.16	0	.02	.02	.23	.05	7	9
0	198	1.15	32	41	293	41	.29	792	.07	.1	.59	.26	171	40
0	125	1.59	21	27	184	12	.34	654	.04	.06	.38	.06	32	18
0	27	1.02	27	41	467	883	.48	283	.1	.07	1.76	.34	38	67
0	44	1.71	26	68	474	243	.67	1899	.07	.08	.94	.13	39	8
0	46	1.49	40	93	308	64	.89	779	.13	.22	1.55	.14	35	6
0	3	.61	3	14	82	6	.27	t	.01	.02	.25	—	8	1
0	1	.25	1	5	33	2	.11	t	<.01	.01	.1	—	3	<1
0	20	.03	4	10	56	7	.03	80	.02	.02	.03	.02	34	7
0	58	0	t	87	5	329	0	0	0	0	0	0	0	0
0	183	0	—	45	4	290	0	0	0	0	0	0	0	0
0	239	0	—	359	6	312	0	0	0	0	0	0	0	0
0	207	0	—	314	891	t	0	0	0	0	0	0	0	0
0	0	—	—	—	—	821	—	0	0	0	0	0	0	0
0	95	1.89	18	22	154	2	.26	42	.01	.01	.31	—	—	3
0	359	3.03	56	81	852	36	.94	2	.06	.48	1.95	.38	30	<1

[137]For recipe using margarine; if butter is used, cholesterol = 8 mg.

[138]Year-round average. From June through October, ascorbic acid is approximately 32 mg and 47 mg, respectively, for one tomato and 1 c chopped tomato. From November through May, market samples average around 12 and 18 mg, respectively.

[139]Calcium is added as a firming agent.

[140]Dietary pack contains 31 mg sodium.

[141]If no salt is added, sodium content is 24 mg.

[142]If salt is added, sodium content is 2070 mg.

[143]If salt is added, sodium content is 998 mg.

[144]With salt added.

(For purposes of calculations, use "0" for t, <1, <.1, <.01, etc.)

Table C–1   Food Composition

Grp	Computer Code No.	Food Description	Measure	Wt (g)	H₂O (%)	Ener (kcal)	Prot (g)	Carb (g)	Dietary Fiber (g)	Fat (g)	Fat Breakdown (g) Sat	Mono	Poly
		MISCELLANEOUS—Con.											
		Catsup:											
16	967	Cup	1 c	245	67	255	4	67	4	1	.2	.2	.4
16	968	Tablespoon	1 tbsp	15	67	16	<1	4	<1	<.1	t	t	t
16	1200	Cayenne (red pepper)	1 tbsp	5.3	8	17	1	3	2	1	.2	.2	.4
16	969	Celery seed	1 tsp	2	6	9	<1	1	<1	1	<.1	.3	.1
16	970	Chili powder	1 tsp	3	8	8	<1	1	1	<1	.1	.1	.2
		Chocolate:											
16	971	Baking, unsweetened For other chocolate items, see Sweeteners and Sweets	1 oz	28	2	145	4	7	4	15	9	5	.5
16	972	Coriander, fresh	¼ c	4	93	<1	<1	<1	<1	<.1	<.01	<.01	.01
16	1197	Cornstarch	1 tbsp	8	8	20	<.1	5	<.1	<.1	t	t	t
16	973	Cinnamon	1 tsp	2	10	6	<1	2	1	<.1	t	t	t
16	974	Curry powder	1 tsp	2	10	6	<1	1	<1	<1	t	.2	<.1
16	1202	Dill weed, dried	1 tbsp	3.1	7	8	1	2	<1	<1	—	—	—
		Garlic:											
16	975	Cloves	4 cloves	12	59	18	1	4	<1	<.1	t	t	<.1
16	976	Powder	1 tsp	3	6	9	<1	2	<1	<.1	t	t	t
16	977	Gelatin, dry, plain	1 envelope	7	13	25	6	0	1	0	0	0	0
16	978	Ginger root, raw, sliced	5 slices	11	87	8	<1	2	<1	<1	t	t	t
16	1198	Horseradish, prepared	1 tbsp	15	87	6	<1	1	<1	<1	t	t	t
16	1199	Hummous/Humous	1 c	246	65	420	33	50	4	21	3.1	8.8	7.8
16	979	Mustard, prepared, (1 packet =1 tsp) Miso (see #926 under Vegetables and Legumes, Soybean products)	1 tsp	5	80	4	<1	<1	<1	<1	t	.2	t
		Olives:											
16	980	Green	10 olives	39	78	45	<1	<1	1	6	.6	3.6	.3
16	981	Ripe, pitted	10 olives	45	80	52	<1	3	1.5	5	.6	3.6	.4
16	982	Onion powder	1 tsp	2.1	5	5	<1	2	<1	<.1	t	t	t
16	983	Oregano, ground	1 tsp	2	7	5	<1	1	<1	<1	t	t	.1
16	984	Paprika	1 tsp	2	10	6	<1	1	<1	<1	t	t	.2
16	985	Pepper, black	1 tsp	2	11	5	<1	1	<1	<.1	<.1	<.1	<.1
		Pickles:											
16	986	Dill, medium, 3¾ × 1¼″ diam	1 pickle	65	92	12	<1	3	1	<1	<.1	t	<.1
16	987	Fresh pack, slices, 1½″ diam × ¼″	4 slices	30	79	20	<1	5	<1	<.1	t	t	t
16	988	Sweet, medium	1 pickle	35	65	41	<1	11	<1	.1	t	t	<.1
16	989	Pickle relish, sweet	1 tbsp	15	63	20	<.1	5	<1	<.1	t	t	<.1
16	1201	Sage, ground Popcorn (see Grain Products, #539–541)	1 tbsp	2	8	6	<1	1	<1	<1	.1	<.1	<.1
22	1347	Salsa, from recipe	.85 c	184	91	79	2	9	3	5	.7	3.4	.5
16	990	Salt	1 tsp	6	0	0	0	0	0	0	0	0	0
		Salt substitute:											
16	1205	Morton Salt Substitute	1 tbsp	6	0	0	0	<1	0	0	0	0	0
16	1206	No Salt, packet, Norcliff Thayer	1 packet	.75	0	0	0	0	0	0	0	0	0
16	1207	Light Salt, Morton	1 tsp	6	0	0	0	0	0	0	0	0	0
16	991	Vinegar, cider	1 tbsp	15	94	2	0	1	0	0	0	0	0
		Yeast:											
16	992	Baker's, dry, active, package	1 package	7	5	20	3	3	2	<1	t	.1	t
16	993	Brewer's, dry	1 tbsp	8	5	25	3	3	3	<.1	t	t	0

(Computer code number is for West Diet Analysis program)

GRP KEY: 1 = BEV   2 = DAIRY   3 = EGGS   4 = FAT/OIL   5 = FRUIT   6 = BAKERY   7 = GRAIN   8 = FISH   9 = BEEF   10 = POULTRY
11 = SAUSAGE   12 = MIXED/FAST   13 = NUTS/SEEDS   14 = SWEETS   15 = VEG/LEG   16 = MISC   22 = SOUP/SAUCE

Chol (mg)	Calc (mg)	Iron (mg)	Magn (mg)	Phos (mg)	Pota (mg)	Sodi (mg)	Zinc (mg)	VT-A (RE)	Thia (mg)	Ribo (mg)	Niac (mg)	V-B6 (mg)	Fola (µg)	VT-C (mg)
0	47	1.72	54	96	1178	2906	.56	250	.22	.18	3.3	.44	37	37
0	3	.11	3	6	72	178	.04	15	.01	.01	.21	.03	2	2
0	8	.41	8	16	107	7	.13	221	.02	.05	.46	—	—	4
0	38	.90	10	11	30	4	.14	<1	.01	.01	.1	—	—	<1
0	7	.37	4	8	50	26	.07	91	.01	.02	.21	—	1	2
0	22	1.9	82	109	235	1	1.01	1	.02	.1	.38	.01	18	0
0	4	.08	1	1	22	1	—	11	<.01	<.01	.03	<.01	.4	<1
0	.12	.08	.16	.7	.16	.5	<.01	0	0	0	0	0	0	0
0	28	.86	1	1	11	1	.05	1	<.01	<.01	.03	.02	—	1
0	10	.59	5	7	31	1	.08	2	<.01	<.01	.07	—	—	<1
0	50	1.50	13	16	110	6	.10	—	.01	.01	.09	.05	—	—
0	22	.2	3	18	48	2	1.06	0	.02	.01	.08	.40	<1	4
0	2	.08	2	12	31	1	.07	0	.01	<.01	.02	.57	2	<1
0	1	0	2	0	2	6	0	0	0	0	0	<.01	0	0
0	2	.05	5	3	46	1	.22	0	<.01	<.01	.08	.02	2	1
0	9	.10	4	5	44	14	.18	0	.01	<.01	.06	.01	2	1
0	124	3.87	71	275	427	599	2.70	6	.23	.13	1.01	.98	146	19
0	4	.1	3	4	7	63	.03	0	<.01	<.01	.07	<.01	0	<1
0	24	.6	9	6	21	936	.03	12	<.01	<.01	.01	.01	<1	<1
0	40	1.49	2	1	4	392	.10	18	<.01	<.01	.02	<.01	.3	.4
0	8	.06	3	7	20	1	.05	0	.01	<.01	.01	.03	3	<1
0	24	.66	4	3	25	<1	.07	10	<.01	t	.09	—	—	1
0	4	.50	4	7	49	1	.09	127	.01	.04	.32	—	—	2
0	9	.61	4	4	26	1	.03	<1	<.01	<.01	.02	0	—	0
0	6	.34	7	14	199	833	.09	21	.01	.02	.04	<.01	1	1
0	3	.20	2	6	20	201	.02	4	t	.01	.02	<.01	0	1
0	1	.21	1	4	11	329	.03	4	<.01	.01	.06	.01	<1	<1
0	3	.13	1	2	30	107	.01	2	t	t	<.01	0	0	1
0	33	.56	9	2	21	0	.09	12	.02	.01	.11	—	—	1
0	18	.86	19	41	347	191	.20	150	.09	.07	.93	.16	28	39
0	14	<.01	2	3	.3	2132	t	0	0	0	0	0	0	0
0	30	0	t	28	2800	t	0	0	0	0	0	0	0	0
0	—	—	—	—	385	0	—	0	0	0	0	0	0	0
0	<1	0	4	0	1500	1100	0	0	0	0	0	0	0	0
0	1	.09	<1	1	15	t	.02	0	0	0	0	0	0	0
0	4	1.1	16	90	140	4	.43	t	.17	.38	2.7	.14	266	t
0	17[145]	1.39	18	140	152	10	.63	t	1.25	.34	3.16	.4	313	t

[145] Value varies from 6 to 60 mg.

(For purposes of calculations, use "0" for t, <1, <.1, <.01, etc.)

Table C-1   Food Composition

Grp	Computer Code No.	Food Description	Measure	Wt (g)	H$_2$O (%)	Ener (kcal)	Prot (g)	Carb (g)	Dietary Fiber (g)	Fat (g)	Fat Breakdown (g) Sat	Mono	Poly
SOUPS, SAUCES, AND GRAVIES													
		SOUPS, canned, condensed:											
		Unprepared, condensed:											
22	1210	Cream of celery	1 c	251	85	180	3	18	1	11	2.8	2.6	5.0
22	1215	Cream of chicken	1 c	251	82	233	7	19	<1	15	4.2	.8	3.0
22	1216	Cream of mushroom	1 c	251	81	257	4	19	<1	19	5.2	3.6	8.9
22	1220	Onion	1 c	246	86	114	8	16	1	3	.5	1.5	1.3
		Prepared with equal volume of whole milk:											
22	994	Clam chowder, New England	1 c	248	85	163	9	17	1	7	3.0	2.3	1.1
22	1209	Cream of celery	1 c	248	87	165	6	15	<1	10	4.0	2.5	2.7
22	995	Cream of chicken	1 c	248	85	191	7	15	<1	12	5	4	2
22	996	Cream of mushroom	1 c	248	85	205	6	15	<1	14	5	3	5
22	1214	Cream of potato	1 c	248	87	148	6	17	<1	6	3.8	1.7	.6
22	1213	Oyster stew	1 c	245	89	134	6	10	0	8	5.1	2.1	.3
22	997	Tomato	1 c	248	85	160	6	22	<1	6	2.9	1.6	1.1
		Prepared with equal volume of water:											
22	998	Bean with bacon	1 c	253	84	173	8	23	3	6	1.5	2.2	1.8
22	999	Beef broth, bouillon, consommé	1 c	240	98	16	3	<1	0	1	.3	.2	t
22	1000	Beef noodle	1 c	244	92	84	5	9	<1	3	1.2	1.2	.5
22	1001	Chicken noodle	1 c	241	92	75	4	9	1	2	.7	1.1	.6
22	1002	Chicken rice	1 c	241	94	60	4	7	1	2	.5	.9	.4
22	1208	Chili beef soup	1 c	250	85	169	7	22	1	7	3.3	2.8	.3
22	1003	Clam chowder, Manhatten	1 c	244	92	78	2	12	1	2	.4	.4	1.3
22	1004	Cream of chicken	1 c	244	91	115	3	9	<1	7	2.1	3.3	1.5
22	1005	Cream of mushroom	1 c	244	90	130	2	9	1	9	2.4	1.7	4.2
22	1006	Minestrone	1 c	241	91	80	4	11	1	3	.5	.7	1.1
22	1211	Onion soup	1 c	241	93	57	4	8	<1	2	.3	.8	.7
22	1007	Split pea with ham	1 c	253	82	189	10	28	1	4	1.8	1.8	.6
22	1008	Tomato	1 c	244	90	86	2	17	<1	2	.4	.4	1.0
22	1009	Vegetable beef	1 c	244	92	79	6	10	1	2	.9	.8	.1
22	1010	Vegetarian vegetable	1 c	241	92	70	2	12	2	2	.3	.8	.7
		SOUPS, dehydrated:											
		Unprepared, dry products:											
22	1011	Bouillon	1 packet	6	3	14	1	1	<1	1	.3	.2	t
22	1012	Onion	1 packet	7	4	20	1	4	<1	<1	.1	.2	.1
		Prepared with water:											
22	1299	Beef broth/bouillon	1 c	244	97	20	1	2	<1	1	.3	.3	<.1
22	1376	Chicken broth/bouillon	1 c	244	97	21	1	1	<1	1	.3	.4	.4
22	1013	Chicken noodle	¾ c	188	94	40	2	6	<1	1	.2	.4	.3
22	1122	Cream of chicken	1 c	261	91	107	2	13	1	5	3.4	1.2	.4
22	1014	Onion	¾ c	184	96	20	1	4	<1	<1	.1	.3	.1
22	1217	Split pea	1 c	255	87	133	8	23	1	2	.4	.7	.3
22	1015	Tomato vegetable	¾ c	189	94	41	1	8	<1	1	.3	.3	.1
		SAUCES											
		From dry mixes, prepared with milk:											
22	1016	Cheese sauce	1 c	279	77	305	16	23	<1	17	9	5	2
22	1017	Hollandaise	1 c	259	84	240	5	14	—	20	12	6	1
22	1019	White sauce	1 c	264	81	240	10	21	<1	13	6	5	2
		From home recipe:											
22	1019	White sauce, medium[146]	1 c	250	73	395	10	24	<1	30	9	12	7
		Ready to serve:											
22	1020	Barbeque sauce	1 tbsp	16	81	10	<1	2	<1	<1	<.1	.1	.1
22	1021	Soy sauce	1 tbsp	18	71	9	1	2	0	t	0	0	0

[146] Made with enriched flour, margarine, and whole milk.

(Computer code number is for West Diet Analysis program)

GRP KEY: 1 = BEV 2 = DAIRY 3 = EGGS 4 = FAT/OIL 5 = FRUIT 6 = BAKERY 7 = GRAIN 8 = FISH 9 = BEEF 10 = POULTRY
11 = SAUSAGE 12 = MIXED/FAST 13 = NUTS/SEEDS 14 = SWEETS 15 = VEG/LEG 16 = MISC 22 = SOUP/SAUCE

Chol (mg)	Calc (mg)	Iron (mg)	Magn (mg)	Phos (mg)	Pota (mg)	Sodi (mg)	Zinc (mg)	VT-A (RE)	Thia (mg)	Ribo (mg)	Niac (mg)	V-B6 (mg)	Fola (μg)	VT-C (mg)
28	80	1.25	13	75	246	1899	.30	61	.06	.10	.67	.03	5	<1
20	68	1.21	5	75	174	1973	1.26	112	.06	.12	1.64	.03	3	<1
3	64	1.05	9	84	167	2032	1.19	0	.06	.17	1.62	.03	7	2
0	53	1.35	5	22	138	2116	1.23	0	.07	.05	1.21	.10	31	3
22	187	1.48	23	157	300	992	1.3	40	.07	.24	1.03	.13	12	4
32	186	.69	22	151	309	1010	.20	68	.07	.25	.44	.06	9	1
27	180	.67	18	152	273	1046	.68	94	.07	.26	.92	.07	8	1
20	178	.59	20	156	270	1076	.64	38	.08	.28	.81	.06	15	2
22	166	.54	17	160	323	1060	.68	67	.08	.24	.64	.09	9	1
32	167	1.04	21	162	235	1040	10.3	45	.07	.23	.34	.06	7	4
17	159	1.82	23	148	450	932	.29	109	.13	.25	1.52	.16	21	68
3	81	2.05	44	132	403	952	1.03	89	.09	.03	.57	.04	32	2
1	15	.41	9	31	130	782	.6	0	<.01	.05	1.87	.07	2	0
5	15	1.1	6	46	100	952	1.54	63	.07	.06	1.07	.04	4	<1
7	17	.78	7	36	55	900	.55	71	.05	.06	1.39	.01	2	<1
7	17	.75	1	22	101	815	.26	66	.02	.02	1.13	.02	1	<1
12	43	2.40	30	148	525	1035	1.40	503	.06	.08	1.07	.16	10	4
2	27	1.64	10	41	188	578	.98	98	.03	.04	.82	.10	10	4
10	34	.61	3	37	88	986	.63	56	.03	.06	.82	.02	2	<1
2	46	.5	5	49	100	1032	.59	0	.05	.09	.7	.02	3	1
2	34	.92	7	56	312	911	.74	234	.05	.04	.94	.10	16	1
0	26	.67	2	11	69	1053	.61	0	.03	.02	.60	.05	15	1
8	22	2.28	48	213	399	1008	1.32	44	.15	.08	1.48	.07	3	1
0	13	1.76	8	34	263	872	.24	69	.09	.05	1.42	.11	15	67
5	17	1.11	6	41	173	956	2	189	.04	.05	1.03	.08	11	2
0	21	1.08	7	35	209	823	.46	301	.05	.05	.92	.06	11	1
1	4	.06	3	19	27	1019	0	<1	<.01	.02	.27	.01	2	0
<1	10	.14	3	23	47	627	.06	<1	.02	.04	.4	.01	2	<1
0	10	.02	7	24	37	1362	.07	.5	<.01	.02	.36	0	0	.01
1	15	.08	4	13	25	1484	.01	4	.01	.03	.20	.02	—	<1
2	24	.37	5	24	23	957	.15	5	.05	.04	.66	.01	1	<1
3	76	—	—	96	215	1184	—	—	—	.20	—	.05	—	—
0	9	.14	6	22	48	635	.06	<1	.02	.04	.36	<.01	2	<1
3	22	1.01	46	134	238	1220	.59	5	.22	.15	1.34	.05	15	—
0	6	.47	15	23	78	856	.13	15	.04	.03	.59	.04	2	5
53	569	.3	32	438	552	1565	.95	117	.15	.56	.3	.1	12	2
52	124	.9	—	127	124	1564	—	220	.05	.18	.1	.5	—	t
34	425	.3	30	256	444	797	1.15	92	.08	.45	.5	.06	16	3
32	292	.9	35	238	381	888	1.05	340	.15	.43	.8	.1	12	2
0	3	.13	1	3	27	128	.03	14	<.01	<.01	.06	.02	1	1
0	3	.36	6	20	32	1029	.07	0	.01	.02	.61	.03	3	0

(For purposes of calculations, use "0" for t, <1, <.1, <.01, etc.)

Table C-1   Food Composition

Grp	Computer Code No.	Food Description	Measure	Wt (g)	H₂O (%)	Ener (kcal)	Prot (g)	Carb (g)	Dietary Fiber (g)	Fat (g)	Fat Breakdown (g)		
											Sat	Mono	Poly
		SOUPS, SAUCES and GRAVIES—Con.											
		SAUCES—Con.											
		Spaghetti sauce: canned:											
22	1377	Plain	1 c	249	75	272	5	40	3	12	1.7	6.1	3.3
22	1378	With meat	.8 c	206	75	220	8	27	1	10	2.5	4.5	1.5
22	1379	With mushrooms	.75 c	185	75	162	2	9	2	5	.6	2.3	1.2
22	1380	Teriyaki sauce	1 tbsp	18	84	15	1	3	0	<1	t	t	<.1
		GRAVIES:											
		Canned:											
22	1022	Beef	1 c	233	87	123	9	11	<1	5	2.7	2.2	.2
22	1023	Chicken	1 c	238	85	189	5	13	<1	14	3.4	6.1	3.6
22	1024	Mushroom	1 c	238	89	120	3	13	<1	6	1	3	2.4
		From dry mix:											
22	1025	Brown	1 c	258	92	75	2	13	<1	2	.8	.7	.1
22	1026	Chicken	1 c	260	91	85	3	14	<1	2	.5	.9	.4

(Computer code number is for West Diet Analysis program)

GRP KEY: 1 = BEV 2 = DAIRY 3 = EGGS 4 = FAT/OIL 5 = FRUIT 6 = BAKERY 7 = GRAIN 8 = FISH 9 = BEEF 10 = POULTRY
11 = SAUSAGE 12 = MIXED/FAST 13 = NUTS/SEEDS 14 = SWEETS 15 = VEG/LEG 16 = MISC 22 = SOUP/SAUCE

Chol (mg)	Calc (mg)	Iron (mg)	Magn (mg)	Phos (mg)	Pota (mg)	Sodi (mg)	Zinc (mg)	VT-A (RE)	Thia (mg)	Ribo (mg)	Niac (mg)	V-B6 (mg)	Fola (µg)	VT-C (mg)
0	70	1.62	60	90	957	1236	.53	306	.14	.15	3.75	.40	39	28
17	36	2.80	15	106	444	1045	1.05	189	.20	.16	3.40	.27	13	2
0	22	1.50	22	45	500	744	.51	362	.12	.12	1.40	.24	19	14
0	4	.31	11	28	41	690	.02	0	<.01	.01	.23	.02	4	0
7	14	1.63	5	70	189	1305	2.33	0	.07	.08	1.54	.02	5	0
5	48	1.1	5	69	260	1375	1.91	264	.04	.1	1.06	.02	3	0
0	17	1.6	—	36	252	1357	1.66	0	.08	.15	1.6	.05	0	0
3	67	.2	10	44	57	1076	.31	0	.04	.09	.8	0	0	0
3	39	.3	—	47	62	1134	.32	0	.05	.15	.8	.03	—	3

C

(For purposes of calculations, use "0" for t, <1, <.1, <.01, etc.)

Table C–1   Food Composition

Grp	Computer Code No.	Food Description	Measure	Wt (g)	H₂O (%)	Ener (kcal)	Prot (g)	Carb (g)	Dietary Fiber (g)	Fat (g)	Fat Breakdown (g)		
											Sat	Mono	Poly
ARBY'S													
12	1402	Bac'n Cheddar, deluxe	1 ea	229	56	532	29	35	<1	33	8	14	11
		Roast beef sandwiches:											
12	1403	Regular	1 ea	147	51	353	22	32	<1	15	7	5	2
12	1404	Junior	1 ea	85	48	218	13	21	<1	11	4	5	2
12	1405	Super	1 ea	246	58	529	33	46	<1	28	3	11	9
12	1406	Deluxe	1 ea	247	62	486	26	43	<1	23	9	8	5
12	1407	Beef 'n Cheddar	1 ea	198	57	451	25	42	<1	20	7	8	4
		Chicken sandwiches:											
12	1408	Chicken breast sandwich	1 ea	184	52	489	23	48	<1	26	4	8	14
12	1409	Chicken salad sandwich	1 ea	156	53	386	18	33	<1	20	–	–	–
12	1410	Chicken salad & croissant	1 ea	150	50	472	22	16	<1	36	–	–	–
12	1411	Roast Chicken club sandwich	1 ea	234	44	513	31	40	<1	29	5	8	14
12	1412	Hot ham and cheese sandwich	1 ea	162	62	330	23	33	<1	15	4	7	3
12	1413	Turkey deluxe sandwich	1 ea	221	61	399	27	36	<1	20	4	4	12
		Baked potatoes:											
12	1414	Plain	1 ea	241	75	240	6	50	6	2	0	.5	1
12	1415	Deluxe, w/butter & sour cream	1 ea	312	74	463	8	53	6	25	12	8	3
12	1416	W/broccoli & cheese	1 ea	340	70	417	11	55	6	18	7	7	8
12	1417	W/mushrooms & cheese	1 ea	347	70	515	15	58	6	27	6	11	9
12	1418	Taco	1 ea	425	70	619	23	73	6	27	11	9	3
		Milkshakes:											
12	1419	Chocolate	1 ea	340	74	451	10	77	<1	12	3	7	2
12	1420	Jamocha	1 ea	326	75	368	9	59	0	11	3	6	2
12	1421	Vanilla	1 ea	312	75	330	11	46	0	12	4	5	2

Source: Arby's Inc., Atlanta Georgia for the basic nutrients. Values for dietary fiber, magnesium, phosphorus, potassium, zinc, vitamin A (in RE's), vitamin B6, folacin, some of the fatty acids, and percent water are estimates calculated from known values for major ingredients.

Grp	No.	Food Description	Measure	Wt (g)	H₂O (%)	Ener (kcal)	Prot (g)	Carb (g)	Dietary Fiber (g)	Fat (g)	Sat	Mono	Poly
BURGER KING													
		Croissant sandwiches:											
12	1422	With egg, bacon & cheese	1 ea	119	49	335	15	20	<1	24	13	8	2
12	1423	With egg, sausage & cheese	1 ea	163	49	538	19	20	<1	41	20	12	3
12	1424	With egg, ham & cheese	1 ea	145	58	335	18	20	<1	20	12	7	1
		Whopper sandwiches:											
12	1425	Whopper	1 ea	265	57	640	27	42	<1	41	16	19	4
12	1426	Whopper w/cheese	1 ea	289	57	723	31	43	<1	48	20	20	3
12	1427	Double beef	1 ea	351	56	850	46	52	<1	52	20	24	5
12	1428	Double w/cheese	1 ea	374	55	950	51	54	<1	60	24	28	4
12	1429	Whopper, Junior	1 ea	136	52	370	15	31	<1	17	6	8	1
12	1430	Whopper, Junior w/cheese	1 ea	158	55	420	17	32	<1	20	9	8	1
12	1431	Hamburger	1 ea	109	46	275	15	29	<1	12	5	6	<1
12	1432	Cheeseburger	1 ea	120	45	317	17	30	<1	15	7	6	1
12	1433	Bacon double cheeseburger	1 ea	159	41	510	33	27	<1	31	14	15	2
12	1434	Chicken sandwich	1 ea	230	46	688	26	56	<1	40	11	17	10
12	1435	Chicken tenders	1 ea	95	50	204	20	10	0	10	3	4	2
12	1436	Ham & cheese sandwich	1 ea	230	59	471	24	44	<1	23	10	8	4
12	1437	Whaler fish sandwich	1 ea	189	45	488	19	45	<1	27	6	9	10
12	1438	Whaler sandwich w/cheese	1 ea	201	45	530	21	46	<1	30	7	9	10
12	1439	French fries, regular	1 svg	74	37	227	3	24	<1	13	5	4	1
12	1440	Onion rings, regular	1 svg	79	37	274	4	28	<1	16	5	7	4
		Milkshakes:											
12	1441	Chocolate, medium	1 ea	273	76	320	8	46	<1	12	–	–	–
12	1442	Vanilla, medium	1 ea	273	74	321	9	49	<1	10	–	–	–

(Computer code number is for West Diet Analysis program)

GRP KEY: 1=BEV 2=DAIRY 3=EGGS 4=FAT/OIL 5=FRUIT 6=BAKERY 7=GRAIN 8=FISH 9=BEEF 10=POULTRY
11=SAUSAGE 12=MIXED/FAST 13=NUTS/SEEDS 14=SWEETS 15=VEG/LEG 16=MISC 22=SOUP/SAUCE

Chol (mg)	Calc (mg)	Iron (mg)	Magn (mg)	Phos (mg)	Pota (mg)	Sodi (mg)	Zinc (mg)	VT-A (RE)	Thia (mg)	Ribo (mg)	Niac (mg)	V-B6 (mg)	Fola (µg)	VT-C (mg)
83	120	2.5	—	—	422	1672	3	85	.4	.48	7	—	—	1
39	32	2	16	120	368	588	3	t	.27	.43	6.23	.20	14	0
23	16	1	8	60	197	345	1.5	t	.13	.24	4	.10	7	0
47	48	2.5	25	190	503	798	3.8	60	.34	.4	7	.30	21	1.2
59	100	6.30	25	190	500	1288	3.8	10	.30	.34	5	.30	22	t
52	76	2	24	260	335	955	3	60	.27	.4	6	.22	19	0
45	64	2	30	180	330	1099	1.5	0	.20	.5	7	.38	18	5
30	—	—	—	—	—	630	—	—	—	—	—	—	—	—
12	—	—	—	—	—	725	—	—	—	—	—	—	—	—
75	120	2	—	—	430	1423	2.3	—	.47	.57	8	—	—	0
45	80	1.5	31	405	312	1350	.9	60	.4	.32	4	.31	26	24
39	64	1.5	30	250	346	1047	1.5	91	.27	.4	7	.52	20	5
0	0	1.80	80	175	1333	58	0	0	.08	.13	2.7	1.08	30	33
40	520	1.5	83	200	1420	203	0	60	.08	.13	2.7	1.10	33	33
22	80	1.5	97	400	1455	361	0	60	.08	.16	2.7	1.15	60	45
47	200	1.5	91	440	1445	923	.9	227	.13	.24	2.7	1.25	36	33
145	450	3.60	105	530	1425	1065	4.7	860	.38	.26	8	1.40	38	63
36	200	.4	48	350	410	341	1.5	91	.11	.65	.7	.14	14	0
35	200	0	36	350	525	262	1.5	91	.11	.65	.7	.14	14	0
32	240	0	36	350	686	281	1.5	91	.11	.65	0	.14	37	0
249	136	2.00	20	249	182	762	1.5	150	.32	.30	2	.06	24	t
293	145	2.90	19	292	284	1042	2.4	150	.36	.32	4	.06	24	t
262	136	2.20	24	317	256	987	1.9	150	.49	.32	3	.06	24	t
94	80	4.90	43	237	547	842	4.5	60	.33	.41	7	.40	35	14
117	210	4.90	47	360	570	1126	5.1	85	.34	.48	7	.40	35	14
188	91	7.30	60	387	760	1080	8.5	60	.34	.56	10	.50	45	14
211	222	7.30	65	510	730	1535	9.1	85	.35	.63	10	.50	45	14
41	40	2.80	24	127	275	486	2.3	30	.23	.25	4	.20	17	6
52	105	2.80	27	189	287	628	2.6	85	.23	.29	4	.20	17	6
37	37	2.70	23	124	235	509	2.4	15	.23	.25	4	.12	18	3
48	102	3.80	26	186	247	651	2.6	70	.23	.29	4	.13	24	3
104	168	3.80	37	328	363	728	5.1	85	.31	.42	6	.30	30	t
82	79	3.30	54	274	375	1423	1.2	13	.45	.31	10	.40	18	t
47	18	.70	24	236	200	636	.6	5	.08	.08	7	.34	10	t
70	195	3.20	42	384	419	1534	2.4	85	.87	.42	6	.31	25	7
84	t	2.20	40	249	366	592	.1	20	.28	.21	4	.13	3	t
95	112	2.20	43	311	378	734	1.1	40	.27	.24	4	.13	3	t
14	t	.50	21	114	360	160	.3	0	.10	.30	7.5	.23	20	t
0	124	.80	18	195	173	665	.4	—	t	t	t	.07	8	t
—	260	1.60	46	262	567	202	1.0	—	.13	.55	t	—	—	t
—	295	t	32	284	505	205	1.0	—	.11	.57	t	—	—	t

(For purposes of calculations, use "0" for t, <1, <.1, <.01, etc.)

(For purposes of calculations, use "0" for t, <1, <.1, <.01, etc.)

Table C–1   Food Composition

Grp	Computer Code No.	Food Description	Measure	Wt (g)	H₂O (%)	Ener (kcal)	Prot (g)	Carb (g)	Dietary Fiber (g)	Fat (g)	Fat Breakdown (g) Sat	Mono	Poly
BURGER KING—Con.													
		Pies:											
12	1443	Apple pie	1 ea	125	51	305	3	44	<1	12	—	—	—
12	1444	Cherry pie	1 ea	128	42	357	4	55	<1	13	—	—	—
12	1445	Pecan pie	1 ea	113	20	459	5	64	1	20	3	11	5

Source: Burger King Corporation for basic nutrients. Values for dietary fiber and percent water, calculated from known values for major ingredients.

Grp	Computer Code No.	Food Description	Measure	Wt (g)	H₂O (%)	Ener (kcal)	Prot (g)	Carb (g)	Dietary Fiber (g)	Fat (g)	Sat	Mono	Poly
DAIRY QUEEN													
		Ice cream cones:											
12	1446	Small	1 ea	85	65	140	3	22	0	4	2	1	<1
12	1447	Regular	1 ea	142	65	240	6	38	0	7	—	—	—
12	1448	Large	1 ea	213	65	340	9	57	0	10	—	—	—
		Dipped ice cream cones:											
12	1449	Small	1 ea	92	58	190	3	25	<1	9	—	—	—
12	1450	Regular	1 ea	156	58	340	6	42	<1	16	—	—	—
12	1451	Large	1 ea	234	58	510	9	64	<1	24	—	—	—
		Sundaes:											
12	1452	Small	1 ea	106	60	190	3	33	<1	4	—	—	—
12	1453	Regular	1 ea	177	60	310	5	56	<1	8	—	—	—
12	1454	Large	1 ea	248	60	440	8	78	<1	10	—	—	—
12	1455	Banana split	1 ea	383	67	540	9	103	<1	11	—	—	—
12	1456	Peanut buster parfait	1 ea	305	52	740	16	94	<1	34	—	—	—
12	1457	Hot fudge brownie delight	1 ea	266	55	600	9	85	<1	25	—	—	—
12	1458	Strawberry shortcake	1 ea	312	61	540	10	100	<1	11	—	—	—
12	1459	Buster bar	1 ea	149	45	460	10	41	<1	29	—	—	—
12	1460	Dilly bar	1 ea	85	55	210	3	21	<1	13	—	—	—
12	1461	DQ ice cream sandwich	1 ea	60	47	140	3	24	<1	4	—	—	—
		Milkshakes:											
12	1462	Small	1 ea	291	63	490	10	82	<1	13	—	—	—
12	1463	Regular	1 ea	418	63	710	14	120	<1	19	—	—	—
12	1464	Large	1 ea	489	63	831	16	140	<1	22	—	—	—
		Malted milkshakes:											
12	1465	Small	1 ea	291	60	520	10	91	<1	13	—	—	—
12	1466	Regular	1 ea	418	60	760	14	134	<1	18	—	—	—
12	1467	Large	1 ea	489	60	889	16	157	<1	21	—	—	—
12	1468	Float	1 ea	397	76	410	5	82	0	7	—	—	—
12	1469	Freeze	1 ea	397	72	500	9	89	0	12	—	—	—
		Mr. Misty:											
12	1470	Regular	1 ea	330	81	250	0	63	0	0	0	0	0
12	1471	Kiss	1 ea	89	81	70	0	17	0	0	0	0	0
12	1472	Freeze	1 ea	411	72	500	9	91	0	12	—	—	—
12	1473	Float	1 ea	411	78	390	5	74	0	7	—	—	—
12	1474	Chicken sandwich	1 ea	202	46	608	27	46	<1	34	8	15	17
12	1475	Fish fillet sandwich	1 ea	177	52	430	20	45	<1	18	4	6	6
12	1476	Fish fillet sandwich w/cheese	1 ea	191	51	483	23	46	<1	22	7	7	6
		Hamburgers:											
12	1477	Single	1 ea	148	51	360	21	33	<1	16	6	7	1
12	1478	Double	1 ea	210	52	530	36	33	<1	28	10	13	2
12	1479	Triple	1 ea	272	52	710	51	33	<1	45	17	21	4
		Cheeseburgers:											
12	1480	Single	1 ea	162	51	410	24	33	<1	20	8	8	1
12	1481	Double	1 ea	239	51	650	43	34	<1	37	15	14	2
12	1482	Triple	1 ea	301	52	820	58	34	<1	50	20	20	3

(Computer code number is for West Diet Analysis program)

GRP KEY: 1=BEV 2=DAIRY 3=EGGS 4=FAT/OIL 5=FRUIT 6=BAKERY 7=GRAIN 8=FISH 9=BEEF 10=POULTRY
11=SAUSAGE 12=MIXED/FAST 13=NUTS/SEEDS 14=SWEETS 15=VEG/LEG 16=MISC 22=SOUP/SAUCE

Chol (mg)	Calc (mg)	Iron (mg)	Magn (mg)	Phos (mg)	Pota (mg)	Sodi (mg)	Zinc (mg)	VT-A (RE)	Thia (mg)	Ribo (mg)	Niac (mg)	V-B6 (mg)	Fola (µg)	VT-C (mg)
4	t	1.20	t	31	122	412	.2	4	.27	.16	.6	.03	7	5
6	t	1.10	12	37	166	204	.2	15	.24	.16	.5	.03	4	8
4	24	1.10	16	84	204	374	<1	16	.28	.18	.6	.06	15	t
10	100	.40	13	100	134	45	.47	25	.03	.17	t	.04	2	t
15	150	.70	20	200	220	80	.49	49	.06	.34	t	.06	3	t
25	250	1.40	30	300	330	115	1.0	98	.12	.51	t	.09	4	t
10	100	.40	13	100	134	55	.47	25	.03	.17	t	.04	2	t
20	150	.70	20	200	220	100	.70	49	.06	.34	t	.06	3	t
30	250	1.40	30	300	330	145	1.0	98	.12	.51	t	.09	4	t
10	100	.40	13	150	145	75	.45	25	.03	.17	.17	.03	2	t
20	200	1.10	26	200	290	120	.90	49	.06	.34	.3	.06	4	t
30	250	1.40	40	300	435	165	1.35	98	.12	.43	.4	.09	6	t
30	250	1.80	60	350	670	150	2.1	160	.15	.51	.4	.80	9	15
30	250	1.80	50	450	500	250	1.5	74	.15	.43	2	.10	7	t
20	200	1.80	30	300	300	225	.90	74	.12	.34	.3	.06	4	t
25	250	1.80	—	300	—	215	—	98	.23	.51	t	—	—	12
10	100	1.10	—	250	—	175	—	25	.12	.17	2	—	—	t
10	100	.40	—	100	—	50	—	25	.03	.17	t	—	—	t
5	60	.04	—	60	—	40	—	15	.03	.07	.4	—	—	t
35	350	1.80	30	400	480	180	.10	123	.15	.60	.3	.14	3	t
50	450	2.70	43	500	690	260	.14	184	.23	.77	.4	.20	4	t
60	550	3.60	60	600	960	304	.20	200	.30	.94	.4	.28	6	t
35	350	2.70	30	400	480	180	.10	123	.15	.60	.4	.14	3	t
50	450	4.50	43	600	690	260	.14	184	.30	.85	.8	.20	4	t
60	550	5.40	60	700	960	304	.20	200	.37	.90	.8	.28	6	t
20	200	1.10	—	200	—	85	—	40	.06	.26	t	—	—	t
30	300	1.80	—	350	—	180	—	98	.15	.51	t	—	—	t
0	t	t	—	t	—	10	—	0	t	t	t	—	—	t
0	t	t	—	t	—	10	—	—	t	t	t	—	—	t
30	300	1.40	—	200	—	140	—	98	.12	.51	t	—	—	t
20	200	.70	—	200	—	95	—	49	.06	.26	t	—	—	t
78	150	5.4	15	250	200	725	.5	20	.6	.59	.8	.16	9	2.4
40	150	3.6	20	150	370	674	.3	<1	.6	.42	8	.16	40	<1
49	250	3.6	22	200	370	870	.3	100	.67	.51	8	.16	20	<1
45	100	3.60	33	150	290	630	4.5	10	.30	.17	5	.18	16	t
85	100	6.30	45	300	410	660	6.4	20	.45	.34	9	.28	23	t
135	100	9.00	60	450	532	690	8.2	28	.60	.51	14	.33	29	t
50	200	3.60	35	250	300	790	5.0	110	.30	.17	5	.20	20	t
95	350	6.30	50	500	443	980	7.3	160	.45	.43	9	.30	30	t
145	350	9.00	65	700	550	1010	9.2	200	.60	.60	14	.55	37	t

(For purposes of calculations, use "0" for t, <1, <.1, <.01, etc.)

(For purposes of calculations, use "0" for t, <1, <.1, <.01, etc.)

Table C–1   Food Composition

Grp	Code No.	Food Description	Measure	Wt (g)	H$_2$O (%)	Ener (kcal)	Prot (g)	Carb (g)	Dietary Fiber (g)	Fat (g)	Sat	Mono	Poly
		DAIRY QUEEN—Con.											
		Hotdogs:											
12	1483	Regular	1 ea	100	50	280	11	21	<1	16	6	7	2
12	1484	With cheese	1 ea	114	49	330	15	21	<1	21	8	8	2
12	1485	With chili	1 ea	128	55	320	13	23	2	20	8	8	2
		Super hotdogs:											
12	1486	Regular	1 ea	175	48	520	17	44	<1	27	9	12	3
12	1487	With cheese	1 ea	196	48	580	22	45	<1	34	11	13	3
12	1488	With chili	1 ea	218	53	570	21	47	2	32	11	13	3
12	1489	French fries, small	1 svg	71	47	200	2	25	<1	10	4	3	<1
12	1490	French fries, large	1 svg	113	47	320	3	40	<1	16	7	5	1
12	1491	Onion Rings	1 svg	85	28	280	4	31	<1	16	5	7	4

Source: International Dairy Queen Inc., Minneapolis, MN for basic nutrients. Values for dietary fiber, magnesium, potassium, zinc, fatty acids, vitamin A (RE's), vitamin B6, folacin and percent water, calculated from known values for the major ingredients.

Grp	Code No.	Food Description	Measure	Wt (g)	H$_2$O (%)	Ener (kcal)	Prot (g)	Carb (g)	Dietary Fiber (g)	Fat (g)	Sat	Mono	Poly
		JACK IN THE BOX											
12	1492	Breakfast Jack sandwich	1 ea	126	49	307	18	30	<1	13	—	—	—
12	1493	Canadian crescent	1 ea	134	42	472	19	25	<1	31	—	—	—
12	1494	Sausage crescent	1 ea	156	38	584	22	28	<1	43	—	—	—
12	1495	Supreme crescent	1 ea	146	38	547	20	27	<1	40	—	—	—
12	1496	Pancakes breakfast platter	1 ea	231	45	612	15	87	<1	22	8.6	7.6	3.5
12	1497	Scrambled egg breakfast platter	1 ea	249	51	662	24	52	<1	40	17.1	16	4.7
12	1498	Hamburger	1 ea	98	44	276	13	30	<1	12	—	—	—
12	1499	Cheeseburger	1 ea	113	44	323	16	32	<1	15	—	—	—
12	1500	Jumbo Jack	1 ea	205	57	485	26	38	<1	26	—	—	—
12	1501	Jumbo Jack w/cheese	1 ea	246	56	630	32	45	<1	35	—	—	—
12	1502	Bacon cheeseburger supreme	1 ea	231	45	724	34	44	<1	46	—	—	—
12	1503	Swiss & baconburger	1 ea	231	52	643	33	31	<1	43	—	—	—
12	1504	Ham & swiss burger	1 ea	203	44	638	36	37	<1	39	—	—	—
12	1505	Chicken supreme	1 ea	228	52	601	31	39	<1	36	—	—	—
12	1506	Moby Jack sandwich	1 ea	137	40	444	16	39	<1	25	—	—	—
12	1583	Double cheeseburger	1 ea	149	64	467	21	33	—	27	12.3	11.6	3.1
		Tacos:											
12	1508	Regular	1 ea	81	57	191	8	16	<1	11	—	—	—
12	1509	Super	1 ea	135	63	288	12	21	<1	17	—	—	—
12	1513	Taco salad	1 ea	358	81	377	31	10	1	24	—	—	—
12	1516	French fries	1 svg	68	40	221	2	27	<1	12	—	—	—
12	1517	Hash brown potatoes	1 svg	62	60	116	2	11	<1	7	3.6	3.2	.4
12	1518	Onion rings	1 svg	108	28	382	5	39	<1	23	—	—	—
		Milkshakes:											
12	1519	Chocolate	1 ea	322	77	330	11	55	0	7	—	—	—
12	1520	Strawberry	1 ea	328	77	320	10	55	0	7	—	—	—
12	1521	Vanilla	1 ea	317	76	320	10	57	0	6	—	—	—
12	1522	Apple turnover	1 ea	119	38	410	4	45	<1	24	—	—	—

Source: Jack in the Box Restaurants, Foodmaker, Inc., San Diego, CA for basic nutrients. Some values for dietary fiber, magnesium, phosphorus, potassium, zinc, vitamin A (RE's), vitamin B6, folacin, and fatty acids calculated from known values for major ingredients.

(Computer code number is for West Diet Analysis program)

GRP KEY: 1 = BEV 2 = DAIRY 3 = EGGS 4 = FAT/OIL 5 = FRUIT 6 = BAKERY 7 = GRAIN 8 = FISH 9 = BEEF 10 = POULTRY
11 = SAUSAGE 12 = MIXED/FAST 13 = NUTS/SEEDS 14 = SWEETS 15 = VEG/LEG 16 = MISC 22 = SOUP/SAUCE

Chol (mg)	Calc (mg)	Iron (mg)	Magn (mg)	Phos (mg)	Pota (mg)	Sodi (mg)	Zinc (mg)	VT-A (RE)	Thia (mg)	Ribo (mg)	Niac (mg)	V-B6 (mg)	Fola (μg)	VT-C (mg)
45	80	1.40	21	100	130	830	1.4	t	.12	.14	3	.08	20	<1
55	150	1.40	24	200	140	990	1.9	85	.12	.17	3	.08	24	<1
55	80	1.80	38	150	170	985	1.8	60	.15	.26	4	.17	30	<1
80	150	2.70	24	150	210	1365	2.8	t	.23	.26	5	.14	35	<1
100	250	1.40	38	300	220	1605	2.5	100	.23	.26	5	.16	39	<1
100	150	2.70	48	250	250	1595	2.5	60	.23	.43	6	.25	45	<1
10	t	.34	16	60	450	115	t	0	.06	t	.8	.16	15	9
15	t	1.08	24	100	700	185	.3	0	.09	.03	1.2	.30	25	15
15	20	.72	16	60	110	140	.3	15	.09	t	.4	.08	10	2
203	170	3.10	24	310	190	871	1.8	120	.47	.41	3	.11	—	<1
226	125	3.40	—	—	—	851	—	135	.50	.40	3.6	—	—	3
187	170	2.90	—	—	—	1012	—	—	.60	.51	4.6	—	—	t
178	150	2.70	—	—	—	1053	—	—	.64	.54	4.2	—	—	t
99	100	1.8	36	633	237	888	1.9	69	.03	.75	7	.19	3	6
354	200	5.4	55	483	635	1188	3.0	252	.3	.77	5	.34	30	4.8
29	70	2.70	20	115	165	521	1.8	9	.36	.24	3.2	.10	—	1
42	160	2.70	22	194	177	749	2.3	57	.36	.27	3.3	.10	—	1
64	97	6.90	35	208	390	905	3.7	—	.51	.21	7	.25	—	5
110	250	4.50	49	411	499	1665	4.8	—	.53	.34	12	.31	—	5
70	310	4.90	—	—	—	1307	—	—	.56	.51	8.8	—	—	3
99	230	4.70	—	—	—	1354	—	—	.45	.41	6.8	—	—	3
117	268	6.10	—	—	—	1330	—	—	.76	.48	7.6	—	—	10
60	240	3.00	—	—	—	1582	—	—	.52	.37	10.6	—	—	4
47	160	2.20	30	263	246	820	1.1	—	.40	.25	2.8	.08	—	<1
72	400	2.7	—	—	—	842	—	—	.15	.34	6	—	—	—
21	100	1.10	35	146	257	460	1.2	—	.07	.17	1.0	.13	—	<1
37	150	1.60	45	198	347	765	1.8	—	.12	.08	1.4	.18	—	2
102	280	4.30	—	—	—	1436	—	141	.18	.53	6	—	—	7
8	10	.50	23	75	360	164	.26	<1	.07	.03	1.20	.18	—	3
3	40	.36	—	—	—	211	—	0	.06	.03	1.2	—	—	4
27	30	1.40	16	69	109	407	.40	<1	.21	.12	1.80	.06	—	3
25	350	.70	55	330	650	270	1.20	—	.15	.59	.60	.18	—	3
25	350	.40	40	328	613	240	1.10	—	.15	.43	.40	.16	—	3
25	350	.30	38	312	599	230	1.00	<1	.15	.34	.40	.20	—	<1
15	11	1.40	10	33	69	350	.20	—	.23	.12	2.50	.03	—	<1

(For purposes of calculations, use "0" for t, <1, <.1, <.01, etc.)

(For purposes of calculations, use "0" for t, <1, <.1, <.01, etc.)

Table C–1   Food Composition

Grp	Computer Code No.	Food Description	Measure	Wt (g)	H₂O (%)	Ener (kcal)	Prot (g)	Carb (g)	Dietary Fiber (g)	Fat (g)	Fat Breakdown (g) Sat	Mono	Poly
KENTUCKY FRIED CHICKEN													
		Original Recipe:											
12	1253	Center breast	1 ea	95	52	236	24	7	<1	14	4	7	2
12	1251	Side breast	1 ea	69	39	199	16	7	<1	12	3	5	3
12	1250	Drumstick	1 ea	47	53	117	12	3	<1	7	2	3	2
12	1252	Thigh	1 ea	88	49	257	18	7	<1	18	4	7	4
12	1249	Wing	1 ea	42	44	136	10	4	<1	9	2	4	2
		Dinners:											
12	1254	2 pce dinner, white	1 ea	322	64	604	30	48	1	32	7	12	10
12	1255	2 pce dinner, dark	1 ea	346	65	643	35	46	1	35	8	13	11
12	1256	2 pce dinner, combination	1 ea	341	63	661	33	48	1	38	8	14	11
		Extra crispy recipe:											
12	1261	Center breast	1 ea	104	39	297	24	14	<1	16	4	7	4
12	1259	Side breast	1 ea	84	39	286	17	14	<1	18	5	7	4
12	1258	Drumstick	1 ea	58	51	155	13	5	<1	9	2	4	2
12	1260	Thigh	1 ea	107	45	343	20	13	<1	23	6	10	6
12	1257	Wing	1 ea	53	36	201	11	9	<1	14	4	6	3
		Dinners:											
12	1262	2 pce dinner, white	1 ea	348	60	755	33	60	1	43	10	16	12
12	1263	2 pce dinner, dark	1 ea	375	62	765	38	55	1	54	11	16	13
12	1264	2 pce dinner, combination	1 ea	371	60	902	36	58	1	48	12	18	14
12	1265	Mashed potatoes	⅓ c	80	81	60	2	12	<1	1	<1	<1	<1
12	1266	Chicken gravy	⅓ c	78	76	59	2	4	<1	4	1	2	<1
12	1267	Dinner roll	1 ea	21	31	61	2	11	<1	1	<1	<1	<1
12	1268	Corn on the cob	1 ea	143	70	176	5	32	2	3	<1	1	1
12	1269	Coleslaw	⅓ c	79	76	103	1	12	<1	6	1	2	3
12	1381	Kentucky nuggets	1 ea	16	44	46	3	2	<1	3	1	2	<1
		Kentucky nugget sauces:											
12	1382	Barbeque	2 tbsp	30	51	35	<1	7	—	1	<1	<1	<1
12	1383	Sweet & sour	2 tbsp	30	50	58	<1	13	—	1	<1	<1	<1
12	1384	Honey	1 tbsp	15	50	49	0	12	—	<1	—	—	—
12	1385	Mustard	2 tbsp	30	52	36	1	6	—	1	—	—	—
12	1386	Kentucky fries	1 svg	119	45	268	5	33	<1	13	3	8	1
12	1387	Mashed potatoes & gravy	⅓ c	86	80	62	2	10	<1	1	<1	<1	<1
12	1388	Buttermilk biscuit	1 ea	75	27	269	5	32	<1	14	4	8	1
12	1389	Potato salad	⅓ c	90	76	141	2	13	1	9	1	3	5
12	1390	Baked beans	⅓ c	89	71	105	5	18	6	1	<1	<1	<1
12	1391	Chicken Little sandwich	1 ea	57	52	177	6	17	1	9	2	3	3

Source: Kentucky Fried Chicken Corporation

Grp	No.	Food Description	Measure	Wt (g)	H₂O (%)	Ener (kcal)	Prot (g)	Carb (g)	Dietary Fiber (g)	Fat (g)	Sat	Mono	Poly
LONG JOHN SILVER'S													
		Fish, batter fried:											
12	1523	Fish & fryes, 3 pce	1 ea	350	55	853	43	64	<1	48	—	—	—
12	1524	Fish & fryes, 2 pce	1 ea	260	53	651	30	53	<1	36	—	—	—
12	1525	Fish dinner, 3 pce	1 ea	540	60	1180	47	93	<1	70	—	—	—
		Fish, breaded & fried:											
12	1526	Fish dinner, 3 pce	1 ea	450	60	940	35	84	<1	52	—	—	—
12	1527	Fish dinner, 2 pce	1 ea	400	60	818	26	76	<1	46	—	—	—
		Chicken:											
12	1528	Chicken plank dinner, 3 pce	1 ea	370	60	885	32	72	<1	51	—	—	—
12	1529	Chicken plank dinner, 4 pce	1 ea	440	60	1037	41	82	<1	59	—	—	—
12	1530	Chicken nugget dinner, 6 pce	1 ea	300	60	699	23	54	<1	45	—	—	—
12	1531	Clam chowder	1 svg	185	85	128	7	15	<1	5	—	—	—
12	1532	Clam dinner	1 ea	460	60	955	22	100	<1	58	—	—	—
12	1533	Fish & chicken dinner	1 ea	460	60	935	36	73	<1	55	—	—	—

(Computer code number is for West Diet Analysis program)

GRP KEY: 1 = BEV   2 = DAIRY   3 = EGGS   4 = FAT/OIL   5 = FRUIT   6 = BAKERY   7 = GRAIN   8 = FISH   9 = BEEF   10 = POULTRY
          11 = SAUSAGE   12 = MIXED/FAST   13 = NUTS/SEEDS   14 = SWEETS   15 = VEG/LEG   16 = MISC   22 = SOUP/SAUCE

Chol (mg)	Calc (mg)	Iron (mg)	Magn (mg)	Phos (mg)	Pota (mg)	Sodi (mg)	Zinc (mg)	VT-A (RE)	Thia (mg)	Ribo (mg)	Niac (mg)	V-B6 (mg)	Fola (µg)	VT-C (mg)
87	30	1.17	28	205	267	631	.72	6	.08	.11	7.57	.31	8	2
70	50	.98	19	151	176	558	.77	4	.06	.08	5.66	.20	6	1
63	12	.80	13	95	122	207	1.29	3	.04	.09	2.38	.09	4	1
109	34	1.45	22	169	217	566	1.65	5	.08	.16	4.03	.17	9	2
55	22	.68	10	76	86	302	.58	3	.03	.04	2.28	.10	4	1
133	142	3.31	61	326	643	1528	1.88	77	.22	.19	10.0	.50	39	37
180	116	3.90	66	363	720	1441	3.47	77	.25	.32	8.46	.46	42	37
172	126	3.78	64	344	684	1536	2.76	77	.24	.27	8.36	.47	41	37
79	62	1.29	29	218	244	584	.77	6	.11	.11	7.89	.30	11	2
65	57	1.12	21	157	188	564	.88	5	.12	.13	5.37	.24	9	2
66	11	.95	14	100	147	263	1.32	4	.07	.11	3.07	.16	6	1
109	49	1.49	24	185	228	549	1.73	7	.12	.19	5.35	.17	11	2
59	16	.65	12	77	100	312	.67	3	.06	.09	2.94	.11	5	1
132	143	6.03	65	333	689	1544	2.08	77	.31	.29	10.4	.56	43	37
183	130	4.09	70	383	776	1480	3.58	77	.32	.38	10.4	.54	46	37
176	135	6.40	68	361	729	1529	2.93	77	.31	.35	10.3	.49	45	37
<1	21	.28	14	41	218	228	.16	5	.01	.04	.96	.11	7	5
2	9	.48	2	10	21	398	.04	1	.01	.03	.47	<.01	2	<1
1	21	.53	6	28	29	118	.20	1	.10	.04	.98	.01	7	<1
<1	7	.79	53	134	323	12	.99	27	.14	.11	1.80	.22	71	2
4	29	.19	9	20	115	171	.13	28	.03	.03	.20	.07	10	19
12	2	.13	4	29	33	140	.22	30	.02	.03	1.00	.04	1	2
1	6	.24	5	10	75	450	.05	37	.01	.01	.19	.02	3	<1
1	5	.16	2	5	39	148	.02	6	.01	.02	.04	.01	1	<1
t	1	.11	<1	<1	6	10	<.01	0	.01	<.01	.04	t	1	3
1	10	.26	6	15	23	346	.09	1	.02	.01	.16	.02	3	1
1	24	.94	28	78	606	81	.31	0	.17	.06	2.70	.18	20	3
1	19	.35	9	28	137	297	.11	5	.01	.04	1.00	.08	8	1
1	77	1.22	9	264	95	521	.29	30	.28	.13	1.80	.03	8	<1
11	10	.32	15	32	256	396	.29	27	.07	.02	.60	.19	7	3
1	54	1.43	29	90	229	387	1.29	10	.06	.04	.50	.07	32	2
20	39	1.40	10	105	114	398	.93	6	.15	.14	1.65	.07	11	<1
106	—	—	—	—	—	2025	—	—	—	—	—	—	—	—
75	—	—	—	—	—	1352	—	—	—	—	—	—	—	—
119	—	—	—	—	—	2797	—	—	—	—	—	—	—	—
101	—	—	—	—	—	1900	—	—	—	—	—	—	—	—
76	—	—	—	—	—	1526	—	—	—	—	—	—	—	—
25	—	—	—	—	—	1918	—	—	—	—	—	—	—	—
25	—	—	—	—	—	2433	—	—	—	—	—	—	—	—
25	—	—	—	—	—	853	—	—	—	—	—	—	—	—
17	—	—	—	—	—	611	—	—	—	—	—	—	—	—
27	—	—	—	—	—	1543	—	—	—	—	—	—	—	—
56	—	—	—	—	—	2076	—	—	—	—	—	—	—	—

(For purposes of calculations, use "0" for t, <1, <.1, <.01, etc.)

(For purposes of calculations, use "0" for t, <1, <.1, <.01, etc.)

Table C–1 Food Composition

Grp	Computer Code No.	Food Description	Measure	Wt (g)	H$_2$O (%)	Ener (kcal)	Prot (g)	Carb (g)	Dietary Fiber (g)	Fat (g)	Fat Breakdown (g) Sat	Mono	Poly
LONG JOHN SILVER'S—Con.													
12	1534	Oyster dinner	1 ea	360	60	789	17	78	<1	45	—	—	—
12	1535	Scallop dinner	1 ea	320	60	747	17	66	<1	45	—	—	—
12	1536	Seafood platter	1 ea	410	60	976	29	85	<1	58	—	—	—
12	1537	Batter fried shrimp dinner	1 ea	300	60	711	17	60	<1	45	—	—	—
12	1538	Fish sandwich platter	1 ea	400	60	835	30	84	<1	42	—	—	—
		Salads:											
12	1539	Ocean chef	1 ea	320	85	229	27	13	2	8	—	—	—
12	1540	Seafood	1 ea	480	85	426	19	22	2	30	—	—	—
12	1541	Cole slaw	1 svg	98	70	182	1	11	<1	15	—	—	—
12	1542	Fries	1 svg	85	42	247	4	31	<1	12	—	—	—
12	1543	Hush puppies	1 ea	47	37	145	3	18	<1	7	—	—	—

Source: Long John Silver's Inc., Lexington, KY.

Grp	Computer Code No.	Food Description	Measure	Wt (g)	H$_2$O (%)	Ener (kcal)	Prot (g)	Carb (g)	Dietary Fiber (g)	Fat (g)	Sat	Mono	Poly
McDONALD'S													
		Sandwiches:											
12	1221	Big Mac	1 ea	215	48	560	25	43	1	32	10	21	2
12	1591	McDLT Sandwich	1 ea	234	59	580	26	36	1.4	37	12	17	9
12	1222	Quarter Pounder	1 ea	166	49	410	23	34	1	21	8	11	1
12	1223	Quarter Pounder w/cheese	1 ea	194	48	520	29	35	1	29	11	16	1
12	1224	Filet-O-Fish sandwich	1 ea	142	44	440	14	38	<1	26	5	10	11
12	1225	Hamburger	1 ea	102	46	260	12	31	<1	10	4	5	1
12	1226	Cheeseburger	1 ea	116	45	310	15	31	<1	14	5	8	1
12	1227	French fries	1 svg	68	37	220	4	26	1	12	3	8	.5
12	1228	Chicken McNuggets	6 ea	112	49	270	20	17	<1	15	4	10	2
		Sauces:											
12	1229	Hot Mustard	1 ea	30	53	70	.5	8	<1	4	<1	1	1
12	1230	Barbecue	1 ea	30	51	50	.3	12	<1	<1	<1	<1	<1
12	1231	Sweet & sour	1 ea	32	50	60	<1	14	<1	<1	<1	<1	<1
		Lowfat Milkshakes:											
12	1232	Chocolate	10 fl oz	293	70	320	12	66	<1	2	.8	.9	<1
12	1233	Strawberry	10 fl oz	293	72	320	11	67	<1	1	.6	.6	<1
12	1234	Vanilla	10 fl oz	293	73	290	11	60	<1	1	.63	.67	<1
		Sundaes:											
12	1235	Hot fudge	1 ea	169	60	240	7	51	<1	3	2	1	<1
12	1236	Strawberry	1 ea	171	62	210	6	49	<1	1	1	4	<1
12	1237	Hot Caramel	1 ea	174	57	270	7	59	<1	3	2	1	<1
12	1238	Vanilla cone	1 ea	80	65	100	4	22	<1	1	<1	<1	<1
		Pies:											
12	1239	Apple pie	1 ea	83	45	260	2	30	<1	15	5	9	1
12	1240	Apple Bran Muffin	1 ea	85	44	190	5	46	3	0	0	0	0
		Cookies, package:											
12	1241	McDonaldland cookies	1 pkg	56	3	290	4	47	<1	9	2	7	<1
12	1242	Chocolate chip cookies	1 pkg	56	3	330	4	42	2	16	5	10	<1
		Breakfast items:											
12	1243	English muffin, w/butter	1 ea	59	42	170	5	27	<1	5	2	2	1
12	1244	Egg McMuffin	1 ea	138	51	290	8.2	28	<1	11	4	6	1
12	1245	Hot cakes w/butter & syrup	1 ea	176	46	410	8	74	<1	9	4	3	3
12	1246	Scrambled eggs	1 ea	100	70	140	12	1	<1	10	3	5	1
12	1247	Pork Sausage	1 svg.	48	43	180	8	0	<1	16	6	9	2
12	1248	Hash brown potato patty	1 ea	53	56	130	1	15	1	7	3	4	<1
12	1392	Sausage McMuffin	1 ea	117	38	370	17	27	<1	22	8	12	2
12	1393	Sausage McMuffin w/egg	1 ea	167	47	440	23	28	<1	27	9	15	3
12	1394	Biscuit with spread	1 ea	75	27	260	5	32	<1	13	3	9	1

(Computer code number is for West Diet Analysis program)

GRP KEY: 1 = BEV   2 = DAIRY   3 = EGGS   4 = FAT/OIL   5 = FRUIT   6 = BAKERY   7 = GRAIN   8 = FISH   9 = BEEF   10 = POULTRY
11 = SAUSAGE   12 = MIXED/FAST   13 = NUTS/SEEDS   14 = SWEETS   15 = VEG/LEG   16 = MISC   22 = SOUP/SAUCE

Chol (mg)	Calc (mg)	Iron (mg)	Magn (mg)	Phos (mg)	Pota (mg)	Sodi (mg)	Zinc (mg)	VT-A (RE)	Thia (mg)	Ribo (mg)	Niac (mg)	V-B6 (mg)	Fola (µg)	VT-C (mg)
55	—	—	—	—	—	763	—	—	—	—	—	—	—	—
37	—	—	—	—	—	1579	—	—	—	—	—	—	—	—
95	—	—	—	—	—	2161	—	—	—	—	—	—	—	—
127	—	—	—	—	—	1297	—	—	—	—	—	—	—	—
75	—	—	—	—	—	1402	—	—	—	—	—	—	—	—
64	—	—	—	—	—	986	—	—	—	—	—	—	—	—
113	—	—	—	—	—	1086	—	—	—	—	—	—	—	—
12	—	—	—	—	—	367	—	—	—	—	—	—	—	—
13	—	—	—	—	—	.6	—	—	—	—	—	—	—	—
—	—	—	—	—	—	405	—	—	—	—	—	—	—	—
103	256	4	41	338	268	950	5.04	88	.48	.41	6.81	.285	23	2
109	225	4	45	321	414	990	6	188	.39	.36	7	.26	30	7
86	142	4	38	258	334	660	5.3	45	.36	.29	6.7	.28	24	3
118	296	3.7	42	315	356	1150	6	190	.37	.39	6.7	.24	24	3
50	165	1.8	27	227	149	1030	.88	36	.30	.15	3.00	.10	20	.1
37	122	2.29	20	129	145	500	2.13	15	.28	.16	3.84	.12	17	2
53	197	2.3	23	205	157	750	2.60	112	.30	.21	3.86	.12	21	2
0	9	.61	27	101	564	70	.32	0	.13	0	1.8	.22	19	2
56	14	1	27	293	313	580	.923	0	.12	.12	8.3	.394	11	0
5	15	.22	6	15	23	250	.09	1.6	.01	.01	.15	.01	3	.45
0	13	.31	5	10	75	340	.05	15	.01	.01	.17	.02	3	2.34
0	11	.17	2	5	39	190	.02	32	0	.01	.08	.01	.6	.64
10	322	.84	47	319	555	240	1.21	92	.13	.52	.41	.148	15	0
10	327	.1	36	302	509	170	1.07	92	.13	.48	.31	.148	11	0
10	327	.10	35	339	521	170	1.09	92	.13	.48	.31	.148	36	0
6	235	.48	36	243	422	170	1.01	65	.08	.35	.30	.138	11	0
5	191	.16	29	188	302	95	.838	65	.07	.29	.25	.056	21	1
13	222	.1	31	243	356	180	.916	88	.08	.35	.26	.054	14	0
3	112	.23	13	120	136	70	.482	87	.04	.18	.37	.046	2	0
0	11	.71	6	26	38	240	.16	0	.06	.02	.32	.02	5	11
0	31	.6	—	—	—	230	—	.7	.02	.08	.4	—	—	.7
0	9	2.1	11	72	50	300	.325	0	.25	.18	2.54	.03	6	0
4	24	2.2	27	102	160	280	.50	0	.18	.21	2.47	.03	6	0
9	151	1.61	13	69	66	270	.50	31	.33	.14	2.47	.04	16	0
226	256	2.77	26	322	168	740	1.92	151	.47	.33	3.71	.21	30	0
21	114	2.08	23	412	154	640	.56	52	.32	.33	2.82	.099	7	0
399	57	2.08	13	269	138	290	1.69	157	.07	.26	.05	.20	66	0
48	8	.67	8	86	115	350	1.33	0	.27	.10	2.31	.165	1	0
9	6	.27	13	65	238	330	.164	0	.06	.02	.85	.124	6	2
64	235	2.3	24	189	219	830	1.71	72	.60	.29	4.8	.15	23	0
263	263	3.34	30	291	298	980	2.39	150	.64	.42	4.8	.20	33	0
1	75	1.31	9	264	95	730	.292	0	.23	.11	1.65	.03	8	0

(For purposes of calculations, use "0" for t, <1, <.1, <.01, etc.)

(For purposes of calculations, use "0" for t, <1, <.1, <.01, etc.)

Table C–1   Food Composition

Grp	Computer Code No.	Food Description	Measure	Wt (g)	H₂O (%)	Ener (kcal)	Prot (g)	Carb (g)	Dietary Fiber (g)	Fat (g)	Fat Breakdown (g) Sat	Mono	Poly
McDONALD'S—Con.													
		Breakfast Items—Con.											
12	1395	Biscuit w/sausage	1 ea	123	32	440	13	32	<1	29	9	17	3
12	1396	Biscuit w/sausage & egg	1 ea	180	43	529	20	33	<1	35	11	20	3
12	1397	Biscuit w/bacon, egg & cheese	1 ea	156	41	440	18	33	<1	26	8	16	2
		Salads:											
12	1398	Chef salad	1 ea	283	84	230	21	8	2	13	6	7	1
12	1399	Shrimp salad	1 ea	262	88	104	14	6	2	3	1	2	<1
12	1400	Garden salad	1 ea	213	91	110	7	6	2	7	3	3	<1
12	1401	Chunky Chicken salad	1 ea	250	88	140	23	5	2	3	1	2	1

Source: McDonald's Corporation, Oak Brook, Illinois. Some values for salads estimated from known values for major ingredients.

Grp	Computer Code No.	Food Description	Measure	Wt (g)	H₂O (%)	Ener (kcal)	Prot (g)	Carb (g)	Dietary Fiber (g)	Fat (g)	Sat	Mono	Poly
TACO BELL													
		Burritos:											
12	1544	Bean	1 ea	191	58	357	13	54	8	10	3	5	2
12	1545	Beef	1 ea	191	58	403	22	39	2	17	7	7	2
12	1546	Bean & beef	1 ea	191	58	381	17	46	5	14	7	6	1
12	1547	Burrito supreme	1 ea	241	66	413	18	46	5	18	8	8	2
12	1548	Double beef supreme	1 ea	255	66	457	24	42	2	22	10	10	2
12	1549	Enchirito	1 ea	213	61	382	20	31	5	20	9	8	1
12	1550	Fajita (steak taco)	1 ea	135	65	234	15	20	2	11	5	4	1
		Tacos:											
12	1551	Regular	1 ea	78	55	183	10	11	1	11	5	3	1
12	1552	Taco bellgrande	1 ea	163	63	355	18	18	2	23	11	6	1
12	1553	Taco light	1 ea	170	59	410	19	18	2	29	12	8	5
12	1554	Soft taco	1 ea	92	52	228	12	18	2	12	5	4	1
		Tostadas:											
12	1555	Regular	1 ea	156	67	243	10	27	7	11	4	4	1
12	1556	Beefy tostada	1 ea	198	69	322	15	22	4	20	10	8	1
12	1557	Bellbeefer	1 ea	177	63	312	17	32	<1	13	6	4	2
12	1558	Mexican pizza	1 ea	223	55	575	21	40	5	48	31	14	2
12	1559	Taco salad with salsa	1 ea	595	73	941	36	63	5	61	19	18	12
		Nachos:											
12	1560	Regular	1 ea	106	40	356	7	38	<1	19	12	5	1
12	1561	Bellgrande	1 ea	287	58	649	22	61	6	35	12	20	3
12	1562	Pintos & cheese	1 ea	128	69	190	9	19	7	9	4	4	1
12	1563	Taco sauce	1 ea	3.7	96	2	<1	<1	<1	<1	<1	<1	<1
12	1564	Salsa	1 ea	9.7	95	18	1	4	1	<1	<1	<1	<1
12	1565	Cinnamon Crispas	1 ea	47.3	1	259	3	27	<1	15	4	2	1

Source: Taco Bell Corporation, California for most nutrient values. Values for Dietary fiber, monounsaturated fat, magnesium, phosphorus, zinc, folacin, vitamin B6, vitamin A in REs, and percentage water are estimates calculated from known values of major ingredients.

Grp	Computer Code No.	Food Description	Measure	Wt (g)	H₂O (%)	Ener (kcal)	Prot (g)	Carb (g)	Dietary Fiber (g)	Fat (g)	Sat	Mono	Poly
WENDY's													
		Hamburgers:											
12	1566	Single, on white bun, no toppings	1 ea	119	41	350	21	29	<1	16	7	9	1
12	1568	Double, on white bun, no toppings	1 ea	197	44	560	41	32	<1	34	7	13	8
12	1569	Big classic	1 ea	241	63	470	26	36	2	25	7	10	5
		Cheeseburgers:											
12	1570	Bacon cheeseburger	1 ea	147	46	460	29	23	<1	28	13	13	2
12	1571	Single, w/all toppings	1 ea	215	50	548	30	32	2	33	13	12	5
12	1572	Double, w/all toppings	1 ea	291	50	735	48	27	2	48	18	18	6

(Computer code number is for West Diet Analysis program)

GRP KEY: 1 = BEV   2 = DAIRY   3 = EGGS   4 = FAT/OIL   5 = FRUIT   6 = BAKERY   7 = GRAIN   8 = FISH   9 = BEEF   10 = POULTRY
11 = SAUSAGE   12 = MIXED/FAST   13 = NUTS/SEEDS   14 = SWEETS   15 = VEG/LEG   16 = MISC   22 = SOUP/SAUCE

Chol (mg)	Calc (mg)	Iron (mg)	Magn (mg)	Phos (mg)	Pota (mg)	Sodi (mg)	Zinc (mg)	VT-A (RE)	Thia (mg)	Ribo (mg)	Niac (mg)	V-B6 (mg)	Fola (μg)	VT-C (mg)
49	83	1.98	18	359	235	1080	1.33	0	.49	.21	3.96	.12	12	0
275	116	3.16	25	490	321	1250	3.16	88	.53	.35	3.99	.199	36	0
253	185	2.56	21	496	250	1230	1.67	162	.36	.33	2.47	.11	47	0
128	256	1.51	35	200	400	490	1.40	514	.31	.29	3.6	.04	60	14
193	65	1.33	60	180	420	480	1.90	372	.13	.10	1.08	.06	60	13
83	149	1.26	18	80	280	160	.40	391	.10	.16	.59	.06	60	14
78	24	1	20	140	350	230	.66	458	.22	.17	8.5	.34	61	20
9	147	3.47	65	210	428	888	2.05	65	.037	2.02	1.98	1.00	55	53
57	114	3.73	35	225	313	1051	4.00	100	.398	2.14	3.44	.23	27	2
36	111	2.15	50	220	370	958	2.67	80	.49	.42	3.09	.59	38	2
33	153	3.6	50	227	432	921	3.00	185	.41	2.12	2.89	.52	40	27
57	145	4	52	230	431	1053	4.00	200	.43	2.2	3.68	.30	30	9
54	269	2.84	61	263	423	1243	3.51	157	.256	.418	2.3	.61	29	28
14	117	3.03	24	150	207	485	3.18	133	.403	.341	3.71	.17	15	3
32	84	1.10	16	100	159	276	2.12	42	.05	.142	1.07	.12	10	1
56	182	1.91	18	100	334	472	2.12	132	.11	.29	2.02	.12	13	5
56	155	2.4	18	100	316	594	2.12	128	.2	.33	2.5	.12	13	5
32	116	2.27	18	100	178	516	2.12	42	.39	.22	2.74	.12	10	1
16	179	1.53	62	195	401	596	1.55	84	.061	.169	.626	1.01	47	45
40	185	1.96	43	206	408	764	2.97	152	.24	.29	1.61	.56	31	6
39	174	2.36	22	125	299	855	2.10	121	.16	.30	1.73	.12	<1	5
81	453	3.08	80	400	449	1364	5.40	355	.36	.39	2.00	1.11	60	7
80	398	7.1	130	460	1212	1662	5.59	450	.51	.75	4.8	1.30	140	77
9	178	.99	40	200	158	423	.80	27	.03	.16	.09	.14	4	2
36	297	3.48	100	400	674	997	4.30	280	.104	.34	2.17	.98	33	58
16	156	1.42	110	156	385	642	2.17	87	.05	.146	.396	.21	68	52
0	2	.07	—	—	13	126	—	19	<.01	<.01	.06	—	—	<1
0	36	.60	—	—	376	376	—	112	.02	.14	—	—	—	2
1	37	1.26	—	—	36	127	—	<1	.138	.084	.966	—	—	<1
65	100	4.50	20	118	265	420	2.10	—	.38	.34	6	.12	<1	<1
125	48	6.30	42	339	431	575	8.35	—	.22	.43	9.00	.47	29	<1
80	40	4.55	34	200	470	900	5.11	60	.26	.25	4.80	.25	30	12
65	136	3.60	33	296	332	860	5.14	82	.27	.28	5.70	.24	25	1
84	177	4.00	33	339	430	864	4.41	111	.34	.35	5.29	.25	28	6
165	180	5.40	50	470	620	883	8.80	112	.36	.53	10.0	.46	31	6

(For purposes of calculations, use "0" for t, <1, <.1, <.01, etc.)

(For purposes of calculations, use "0" for t, <1, <.1, <.01, etc.)

Table C–1   Food Composition

	Computer Code				Wt	H₂O	Ener	Prot	Carb	Dietary Fiber	Fat	Fat Breakdown (g)		
Grp	No.	Food Description	Measure		(g)	(%)	(kcal)	(g)	(g)	(g)	(g)	Sat	Mono	Poly
WENDY'S—Con.														
		Baked potatoes:												
12	1573	Plain	1 ea		250	75	250	6	52	5	<1	<1	<1	<1
12	1574	W/bacon & cheese	1 ea		350	71	570	19	57	5	30	12	11	6
12	1575	W/broccoli & cheese	1 ea		365	74	500	13	54	5	25	9	8	5
12	1576	W/cheese	1 ea		350	71	590	17	55	5	34	13	13	7
12	1577	W/chili & cheese	1 ea		400	72	510	22	63	8	20	13	7	<1
12	1578	W/sour cream & chives	1 ea		310	71	460	7	53	5	24	10	8	3
12	1579	Chili	1 c		256	77	230	21	16	5	9	3	4	<1
12	1580	French fries	1 svg		106	43	306	4	38	<1	15	7	5	2
12	1581	Frosty dairy dessert	1 c		216	35	354	7	53	0	13	5	3	2
12	1582	Chocolate chip cookie	1 ea		64	5	320	3	40	1	17	6	6	5

Source: Wendy's International, for most nutrient values. Some of the values for dietary fiber, the types of fatty acids, magnesium, phosphorus, zinc, vitamin B6, vitamin A in REs, and percentage water for estimates calculated from known values of major ingredients.

(Computer code number is for West Diet Analysis program)

GRP KEY: 1 = BEV 2 = DAIRY 3 = EGGS 4 = FAT/OIL 5 = FRUIT 6 = BAKERY 7 = GRAIN 8 = FISH 9 = BEEF 10 = POULTRY
11 = SAUSAGE 12 = MIXED/FAST 13 = NUTS/SEEDS 14 = SWEETS 15 = VEG/LEG 16 = MISC 22 = SOUP/SAUCE

Chol (mg)	Calc (mg)	Iron (mg)	Magn (mg)	Phos (mg)	Pota (mg)	Sodi (mg)	Zinc (mg)	VT-A (RE)	Thia (mg)	Ribo (mg)	Niac (mg)	V-B6 (mg)	Fola (µg)	VT-C (mg)
0	40	2.7	67	169	1360	60	.65	0	.28	.10	3.82	.70	68	36
22	200	3.7	80	406	1380	180	2.53	150	.225	.17	4.64	.866	33	36
22	250	3.6	83	373	1550	2.19	.865	350	.31	.255	4	.861	66	90
22	350	3.6	78	49.7	1380	2.22	.609	200	.225	.255	3.3	.80	33	36
22	250	6.1	111	498	1590	810	3.78	172	.32	.26	4.1	.9	50	36
15	40	2.7	70	185	1420	230	.9	100	.225	.13	3	.79	32	36
30	60	4.50	60	320	565	960	3.78	200	.12	.17	3.00	.26	40	9
15	13	1.02	45	197	689	105	.51	0	.15	.04	2.96	.27	33	12
45	257	.86	43	238	518	194	.92	143	.11	.45	.31	.12	17	<1
5	10	1.09	15	62	100	235	.46	0	.06	.07	.4	.03	6	0

C

(For purposes of calculations, use "0" for t, <1, <.1, <.01, etc.)

(For purposes of calculations, use "0" for t, <1, <.1, <.01, etc.)

Enteral Formulas

The availability of a staggering number of enteral formulas complicates the decision of selecting an appropriate formula. The formulas shown in this Appendix provide some examples, but the list is by no means complete. Furthermore, be aware that the composition of formulas changes periodically. Health care providers must consult with manufacturers' current literature before selecting a formula.

D

■ TABLE D-1
Enteral Formulas

Product	Manufacturer	Form	Volume to meet 100% U.S. RDA	kCal/ml	Protein g/1,000 ml	Carbohydrate g/1,000 ml	Fat g/1,000 ml	mOsm/kg	Notes
Intact Formulas: Isotonic or Near-Isotonic Formulas									
Compleat® Modified	Sandoz Nutrition	liquid	1,500 ml	1.07	43	140	37	300	Lactose-free
Entrition®	aBiosearch	liquid	2,000 ml	1.00	35	136	35	300	Lactose-free, low-residue
Fortison®	Sherwood Medical	liquid	2,000 ml	1.00	35	125	40	300	Lactose-free
Isocal®	Mead Johnson	liquid	1,900 ml	1.06	34	135	44	270	Lactose-free, low-residue
Isocal® HN	Mead Johnson	liquid	1,800 ml	1.06	44	124	45	270	Lactose-free, 40% fat from MCT oil
Isosource®	Sandoz Nutrition	liquid	1,500 ml	1.20	43	170	41	360	Lactose-free, low-residue, 50% fat from MCT oil
Isosource® HN	Sandoz Nutrition	liquid	1,500 ml	1.20	53	160	41	360	Lactose-free, low-residue, 50% fat from MCT oil
Isotein® HN	Sandoz Nutrition	powder	1,770 ml	1.20	68	160	34	300	Lactose-free
Jevity®	Ross	liquid	1,325 ml	1.00	42	144	35	300	Lactose-free, 14 g fiber/1,000 ml, 50% fat from MCT
Osmolite®	Ross	liquid	2,000 ml	1.00	35	137	36	300	Lactose-free, low-residue
Osmolite® HN	Ross	liquid	1,400 ml	1.06	44	141	37	300	Lactose-free, low-residue, 50% fat from MCT
PediaSure®	Ross	liquid	1,100	1.00	30	110	50	325	Intended for use with children; nearly lactose-free
Travasorb® MCT	Travenol	powder, liquid	2,000	1.00	49	123	33	312	Lactose-free, low-residue, 80% fat from MCT oil
Ultracal®	Mead Johnson	liquid	1,180	1.06	44	123	45	310	Lactose-free, 13.6 g fiber/1,000 ml, 40% fat from MCT.
Intact Formulas: Standard, Low- to Moderate-Residue Formulas[a]									
Ensure®	Ross	liquid	2,000	1.06	37	145	37	470	Lactose-free
Meritene®	Sandoz Nutrition	liquid	1,250	0.96	58	110	32	510[b]	Contains lactose

(continued)

TABLE D–1
Enteral Formulas   (continued)

Product	Manufacturer	Form	Volume to meet 100% U.S. RDA	kCal/ ml	Protein g/ 1,000 ml	Carbohydrate g/ 1,000 ml	Fat g/ 1,000 ml	mOsm/ kg	Notes
Nutrex Besure®	Nutrex	powder	1,900	1.06	37	144	35	450	Lactose-free
Resource®	Sandoz Nutrition	liquid	1,900	1.06	37	140	37	430	Lactose-free
Sustacal®	Mead Johnson	liquid	1,100	1.01	61	140	23	650[c]	Lactose-free
Intact Formulas: Standard, Fiber-Containing Formulas									
Compleat® Regular	Sandoz Nutrition	liquid	1,500	1.07	43	130	43	450	Blenderized formula, contains lactose, 4.3 g fiber/1,000 ml
Enrich®	Ross	liquid	1,530	1.10	40	162	37	480	Lactose-free, 14 g fiber/1,000 ml
Fibersource®	Sandoz Nutrition	liquid	1,500	1.20	43	170	41	390	Lactose-free, 10 g fiber/1,000 ml
Fibersource® HN	Sandoz Nutrition	liquid	1,500	1.20	53	160	41	390	Lactose-free, 7 g fiber/1,000 ml
Jevity® (see "Intact Formulas: Isotonic or Near-Isotonic Formulas")									
Nutrex Encare with Fiber®	Nutrex	powder	1,200	1.46	40	241	37	460	Lactose-free, 17 g fiber/1,000 ml
Sustacal with Fiber®	Mead Johnson	liquid	1,400	1.06	46	140	35	480	Lactose-free, 8 g fiber/1,000 ml
Ultracal® (see "Intact Formulas: Isotonic or Near-Isotonic Formulas")									
Hydrolyzed Formulas[d]									
Criticare HN®	Mead Johnson	liquid	1,900	1.06	38	220	53	650	Lactose free, low-residue
Stresstein®	Sandoz Nutrition	powder	2,000	1.20	70	170	28	910	Lactose-free, low-residue
Traum-Aid HBC®	Kendall McGaw	powder	3,000	1.00	56	166	12.4	675	Lactose-free, low-residue, 50% of protein from branched-chain amino acids
Travasorb Standard®	Travenol	liquid	1,900	1.06	35	136	35	488	Lactose-free, low-residue

(continued)

TABLE D–1
Enteral Formulas (continued)

Product	Manufacturer	Form	Volume to meet 100% U.S. RDA	kCal/ml	Protein g/1,000 ml	Carbohydrate g/1,000 ml	Fat g/1,000 ml	mOsm/kg	Notes
Hydrolyzed Formulas[d]									
Vital HN®	Ross	powder	1,500	1.00	42	185	11	500	Lactose-free, low-residue
Vivonex®	Norwich Eaton	powder	1,800	1.00	20	231	2	550	Lactose-free, low-residue
Vivonex HN®	Norwich Eaton	powder	3,000	1.00	46	210	1	810	Lactose-free, low-residue
Vivonex T.E.N.®	Norwich Eaton	powder	2,000	1.00	38	206	3	630	Lactose-free, low-residue, 33% of protein from branched-chain amino acids
Special-Use Formulas: High-kCalorie Formulas (see also "Special Use Formulas: High-kCalorie, High-Protein Formulas")									
Ensure Plus®	Ross	liquid	1,400	1.50	55	200	53	690	Lactose-free
Resource Plus®	Sandoz Nutrition	liquid	1,600	1.50	55	200	53	600	Lactose-free
Sustacal HC®	Mead Johnson	liquid	1,800	1.50	61	190	58	650	Lactose-free
Special-Use Formulas: High-Nitrogen (Protein) Formulas									
Ensure HN®	Ross	liquid	1,400	1.06	44	139	35	470	Lactose-free
Fibersource HN®	Sandoz Nutrition	liquid	1,500	1.20	53	160	41	390	Lactose-free, 7 g fiber/1,000 ml
Isocal HN®	Mead Johnson	liquid	1,250	1.06	44	124	45	270	Lactose-free
Isosource HN®	Sandoz Nutrition	liquid	1,500	1.20	43	170	41	360	Lactose-free
Isotein HN	Sandoz Nutrition	powder	1,800	1.20	68	160	34	300	Lactose-free
Special-Use Formulas: High-kCalorie, High-Protein Formulas									
Isocal HCN®	Mead Johnson	liquid	1,000	2.00	75	200	102	640	Lactose-free
Magnacal®	Sherwood Medical	liquid	1,000	2.00	70	250	80	590	Lactose-free
TraumaCal®	Mead Johnson	liquid	1,500	1.50	82	142	68	490	Lactose-free
TwoCal HN®	Ross	liquid	1,000	2.00	84	217	91	690	Lactose-free
Special-Use Formulas: Other									
Amin-Aid®	Kendall McGaw	powder	—	2.00	19	366	46	700	Hydrolyzed formula, lactose-free, no added vitamins or electrolytes; intended for use in renal failure

(continued)

TABLE D–1
Enteral Formulas (continued)

Product	Manufacturer	Form	Volume to meet 100% U.S. RDA	kCal/ ml	Protein g/ 1,000 ml	Carbohydrate g/ 1,000 ml	Fat g/ 1,000 ml	mOsm/ kg	Notes
Hepatic-Aid II®	Kendall McGaw	powder	—	1.10	44	169	36	560	Hydrolyzed formula with 46% of protein as branched-chained amino acids, lactose-free, no added vitamins or electrolytes; intended for use in liver failure
Impact®	Sandoz Nutrition	liquid	1,500	1.00	56	132	28	375	Lactose-free: enriched with arginine, RNA, and omega-3 fatty acids; intended to improve immune competence
Pediasure	Ross	liquid	1,100	1.00	30	108	49	310	Virtually lactose-free; intended for use with children ages 1 to 6
Pulmocare®	Ross	liquid	950	1.50	63	106	92	490	Lactose-free; intended for use in respiratory insufficiency
Replena®	Ross	liquid	—	2.00	30	253	95	615	Lactose-free: low in electrolytes; intended for use in renal disease before dialysis is instituted
Travasorb Hepatic®	Travenol	powder	2,100	1.10	29	209	14	690	Hydrolyzed formula with 50% of protein from branched-chained amino acids; lactose-free; intended for use in liver failure

(continued)

D

■ TABLE D–1
Enteral Formulas   (continued)

Product	Manufacturer	Form	Volume to meet 100% U.S. RDA	kCal/ml	Protein g/1,000 ml	Carbohydrate g/1,000 ml	Fat g/1,000 ml	mOsm/kg	Notes
Travasorb Renal®	Travenol	powder	—	1.35	23	271	18	590	Hydrolyzed formula; lactose-free; does not contain fat-soluble vitamins or electrolytes; intended for use in renal failure

aWith the exception of Ultracal, all formulas listed under "Intact Formulas: Isotonic or Near-Isotonic Formulas" can be used as a standard, low- to moderate-residue formula.
bVanilla flavor.
cVanilla and strawberry flavors.
dMany special-use formulas are also hydrolyzed (see "Special Use Formulas: Other").

■ TABLE D–2
Enteral Formulas—Protein Modules

Product	Manufacturer	Form	Major Protein Source	kCal/g	Protein (g/100 kcal)	Carbohydrate (g/100 kcal)	Fat (g/100 kcal)	Notes
Casec®	Mead Johnson	powder	Calcium caseinate	3.7	23.8	—	2.0	
Nutrisource Amino Acids®	Sandoz Nutrition	powder	Free amino acids	3.9	24.9	—	—	
Nutrisource Amino Acids-High Branched Chain®	Sandoz Nutrition	powder	Free amino acids	3.8	24.9	—	—	44% branched-chain amino acids
Nutrisource Protein®	Sandoz Nutrition	powder	Delactosed lactalbumin, egg white solids	4.0	18.8	1.7	2.1	
Pro Mod®	Ross	powder	Whey protein and soy lecithin	5.6	18.9	2.4	2.0	
Propac®	Sherwood Medical	powder	Whey protein	4.0	19.2	1.3	20	

TABLE D–3
Enteral Formulas—Carbohydrate Modules

Produt	Manufacturer	Form	Major Carbohydrate Source	kCal/ml or g	Protein (g/100 kcal)	Carbohydrate (g/100 kcal)	Fat (g/100 kcal)
Moducal®	Mead Johnson	powder	Hydrolyzed corn starch	3.8 kcal/g	—	25	—
Nutrisource Carbohydrate®	Sandoz Nutrition	liquid	Deionized corn syrup solids	3.2 kcal/ml	—	25	—
Polycose Liquid®	Ross	liquid	Hydrolyzed corn starch	2.0 kcal/ml	—	25	—
Polycose Powder®	Ross	powder	Hydrolyzed corn starch	3.8 kcal/g	—	25	—
Sumacal®	Sherwood Medical	powder	Maltodextrins	3.8 kcal/g	—	25	—

TABLE D–4
Enteral Formulas—Fat Modules

Product	Manufacturer	Form	Major Fat Source	kCal/ml	Protein (g/100 kcal)	Carbohydrate (g/100 kcal)	Fat (g/100 kcal)	Notes
MCT Oil®	Mead Johnson	liquid	Coconut oil	7.7	—	—	12	84% fat as MCT
Microlipid®	Sherwood Medical	liquid	Soy, corn, or Safflower oil	4.5	—	—	11	
Nutrisource Lipid®—Long Chain Triglycerides	Sandoz Nutrition	liquid	Soybean oil	2.2	—	—	11	
Nutrisource Lipid®—Medium Chain Triglycerides	Sandoz Nutrition	liquid	Coconut oil	2.0	—	—	12	92% fat as MCT

D

■ TABLE D–5
Enteral Vitamin Modules

Product	Manufacturer	Form	Protein (g/packet)	Fat (g/packet)	Carbohydrate (g/packet)	Kcalories/packet	Vitamin A (IU)	Vitamin D (IU)	Vitamin E (IU)	Vitamin C (mg)	Folate (µg)	Thiamin (mg)	Riboflavin (mg)	Niacin (mg)	Vitamin B₆ (mg)	Vitamin B₁₂ (µg)	Biotin (mg)	Pantothenic Acid (mg)	Vitamin K (µg)	Choline (g)
							Nutrient Analysis Per 10 g Packet													
Nutrisource® Vitamins	Sandoz Nutrition	powder	0	0	9	36	5,000	200	10	60	400	1.4	1.6	18	2.2	3.0	0.15	5.5	70	0.10

■ TABLE D–6
Enteral Mineral Modules

Product	Manufacturer	Form	Protein (g/packet)	Fat (g/packet)	Carbohydrate (g/packet)	kCalories/packet	Calcium (g)	Phosphorus (g)	Iodine (µg)	Iron (mg)	Magnesium (mg)	Copper (mg)	Zinc (mg)	Potassium g (mEq)	Sodium g (mEq)	Chloride g (mEq)	Manganese (mg)	Selenium (µg)	Chromium (µg)	Molybdenum (µg)
							Nutrient Analysis Per 24 g Packet													
Nutrisource® Minerals for Amino Acid Formulas	Sandoz Nutrition	powder	0	0	3	12	0.80	0.80	150	18	350	2	15	2.2 (56.3)	1.3 (56.5)	2.0 (56.4)	4	125	125	325
Nutrisource® Minerals for Amino Acid Formulas-Electrolyte Restricted	Sandoz Nutrition	powder	0	0	12	48	0.80	0.80	150	18	350	2	15	0.005 (0.2)	0.015 (0.7)	0.025 (0.7)	4	125	125	325
Nutrisource® Minerals for ProteinFormulas	Sandoz Nutrition	powder	0	0	6	24	0.65	0.65	150	18	350	2	15	1.75 (44.8)	1.0 (43.5)	1.8 (50.8)	4	125	125	325
Nutrisource® Minerals for Protein Formulas-Electrolyte Restriced	Sandoz Nutrition	powder	0	0	13	52	0.65	0.65	150	18	350	2	15	0.005 (0.2)	0.015 (0.7)	0.025 (0.7)	4	125	125	325

The U.S. Exchange System[1]

The U.S. Exchange System divides the foods suitable for use in planning a healthy diet into six lists—the starch/bread, meat/meat alternate, vegetable, fruit, milk, and fat lists.[1] These lists are shown in Tables E–1 through E–6. Following these lists are three other sets of foods: free foods, combination foods, and foods for occasional use (Tables E–7, E–8, and E–9).

The Exchange Lists are the basis of a meal planning system designed by a committee of the American Diabetes Association and the American Dietetic Association. While designed primarily for people with diabetes and others who must follow special diets, the Exchange Lists are based on principles of good nutrition that apply to everyone.

■ TABLE E–1
Starch/Bread List

(15 g carbohydrate, 3 g protein, trace fat, 80 kcal)

Amount	Food
Cereals/Grains/Pasta	
⅓ c	Bran cereals, concentrated[a]
½ c	Bran cereals, flaked[a]
½ c	Bulgur, cooked
½ c	Cooked cereals
2½ tbsp	Cornmeal, dry
3 tbsp	Grape-Nuts
½ c	Grits, cooked
¾ c	Other ready-to-eat unsweetened cereals
½ c	Pasta, cooked
1½ c	Puffed cereals
⅓ c	Rice, white or brown, cooked
½ c	Shredded wheat
3 tbsp	Wheat germ[a]
Dried Beans/Peas/Lentils	
¼ c	Baked beans[a]
⅓ c	Beans and peas, cooked, such as kidney, white, split, black-eyed[a]
⅓ c	Lentils, cooked[a]
Starchy Vegetables	
½ c	Corn[a]
1 cob	Corn, on the cob, 6″ long[a]
½ c	Lima beans[a]
½ c	Peas, green, canned or frozen[a]
½ c	Plantains[a]
1 small (3 oz)	Potatoes, baked
½ c	Potatoes, mashed
¾ c	Squash, winter (acorn, butternut)[a]
⅓ c	Yams, sweet potatoes, plain

■ TABLE E–1
Starch/Bread List   (continued)

Amount	Food
Bread	
½ (1 oz)	Bagels
2 (⅔ oz)	Bread sticks, crisp, 4″ × ½″
1 c	Croutons, low-fat
½	English muffin
½ (1 oz)	Frankfurter or hamburger bun
½	Pita, 6″ across
1 (1 oz)	Plain roll, small
1 slice (1 oz)	Raisin, unfrosted
1 slice (1 oz)	Rye, pumpernickel
1	Tortillas, 6″ across
1 slice (1 oz)	White (including French, Italian)
1 slice (1 oz)	Whole-wheat
Crackers/Snacks	
8	Animal crackers
3	Graham crackers, 2½″ square
¾ oz	Matzoth
5 slices	Melba toast
24	Oyster crackers
3 c	Popcorn, popped, no fat added
¾ oz	Pretzels
4	Rye crisp, 2″ × 3½″[a]
6	Saltine-type crackers
2 to 4 (¾ oz)	Whole-wheat crackers, no fat added (crisp breads such as Finn®, Kavli®, Wasa®)[a]
Starch Foods Prepared with Fat	
(Count as 1 starch/bread exchange, plus 1 fat exchange.)	
1	Biscuit, 2½″ across
½ c	Chow mein noodles
1 (2 oz)	Corn bread, 2″ cube
6	Crackers, round butter type
10 (1½ oz)	French fries, 2″ to 3½″ long
1	Muffin, plain, small
2	Pancakes, 4″ across
¼ c	Stuffing, bread, prepared
2	Taco shells, 6″ across
1	Waffles, 4½″ square
4 to 6 (1 oz)	Whole-wheat crackers, fat added (such as Triscuit®)[a]

[a]3 g or more dietary fiber per exchange. Average fiber contents of whole-grain products is 2 g/exchange. For starch foods not on this list, the general rule is that ½ c cereal, grain, or pasta is 1 exchange; 1 oz of a bread product is 1 exchange.

E

■ TABLE E–2
Meat/Meat Alternate Lists

(Lean meat = 7 g protein, 3 g fat, 55 kcal. Medium-fat meat = 7 g protein, 5 g fat, 75 kcal. High-fat meat = 7 g protein, 8 g fat, 100 kcal.)

Lean Meat and Alternates

Category	Amount	Food
Beef:	1 oz	USDA Select or Choice grades of lean beef, such as round, sirloin, and flank steak; tenderloin; chipped beef[b]
Pork:	1 oz	Lean pork, such as fresh ham; canned, cured, or boiled ham[b]; Canadian bacon[b], tenderloin
Veal:	1 oz	All cuts are lean except for veal cutlets (ground or cubed); examples of lean veal: chops and roasts
Poultry:	1 oz	Chicken, turkey, Cornish hen (without skin)
Fish:	1 oz	All fresh and frozen fish
	2 oz	Crab, lobster, scallops, shrimp, clams (fresh or canned in water)[s]
	6 medium	Oysters
	¼ c	Tuna[c], canned in water
	1 oz	Herring[c], uncreamed or smoked
	2 medium	Sardines, canned
Wild Game:	1 oz	Venison, rabbit, squirrel
	1 oz	Pheasant, duck, goose (without skin)
Cheese:	¼ c	Any cottage cheese[c]
	2 tbsp	Grated Parmesan
	1 oz	Diet cheeses[b] (with less than 55 kcal/oz)
Other:	1½ oz	95% fat-free lunch meats[b]
	3 whites	Egg whites
	½ c	Egg substitutes with less than 55 kcal per ½ c

Medium-Fat Meat and Alternates

Category	Amount	Food
Beef:	1 oz	Most beef products fall into this category; examples: all ground beef, roasts (rib, chuck, rump), steak (cubed, porterhouse, T-bone), meatloaf
Pork:	1 oz	Most pork products fall into this category; examples: chops, loin roast, Boston butt, cutlets
Lamb:	1 oz	Most lamb products fall into this category; examples: chops, leg, roast
Veal:	1 oz	Cutlet, ground or cubed, unbreaded
Poultry:	1 oz	Chicken (with skin), domestic duck or goose (well drained of fat), ground turkey[c]
Fish:	¼ c	Tuna[c], canned in oil and drained
	¼ c	Salmon[c], canned
Cheese:		Skim or part-skim milk cheeses, such as:
	¼ c	Ricotta
	1 oz	Mozzarella
	1 oz	Diet cheeses[b] (with 56 to 80 kcal/oz)

■ TABLE E–2
Meat/Meat Alternate Lists   (continued)

Category	Amount	Food
Other:	1 oz	86% fat-free lunch meat[c]
	1	Eggs (high in cholesterol, limit to 3 per week)
	¼ c	Egg substitutes with 56 to 80 kcal per ¼ c
	4 oz	Tofu, 2 ½″ × 2¾″ × 1″
	1 oz	Liver, hearts, kidneys, sweetbreads (high in cholesterol)

High-Fat Meat and Alternates[d]

Category	Amount	Food
Beef:	1 oz	Most USDA Prime cuts of beef, such as ribs, corned beef[c]
Pork:	1 oz	Spareribs, ground pork, pork sausages[b] (patties or links)
Lamb:	1 oz	Patties, ground lamb
Fish:	1 oz	Any fried fish product
Cheese:	1 oz	All regular cheeses, such as American[b], blue[b], cheddar[c], Monterey[c], Swiss
Other:	1 oz	Lunch meats[b], such as bologna, salami, pimento loaf
	1 oz	Sausage[b], such as Polish, Italian, smoked
	1 oz	Knockwurst[b]
	1 oz	Bratwurst[c]
	1 (10/lb)	Frankfurters[b] (turkey or chicken)
	1 tbsp	Peanut butter (contains unsaturated fat)

Count as 1 high-fat meat plus 1 fat exchange:

	1 (10/lb)	Frankfurters[b] (beef, pork, or combination)

[b]400 mg or more sodium per exchange.
[c]400 mg or more sodium if two or more exchanges are eaten.
[d]These items are high in saturated fat, cholesterol, and kcalories, and should be used no more than three times per week.

■ TABLE E-3
Vegetable List[e]

(5 g carbohydrate, 2 g protein, 25 kcal)
All portion sizes, except as otherwise noted, are ½ c of any cooked vegetable or vegetable juice, 1 c of any raw vegetable

Artichokes, ½ medium	Mushrooms, cooked
Asparagus	Okra
Bean sprouts	Onions
Beans (green, wax, Italian)	Pea pods
Beets	Rutabagas
Broccoli	Sauerkraut[b]
Brussels sprouts	Spinach, cooked
Cabbage, cooked	Summer squash (crookneck)
Carrots	Tomatoes, 1 large
Cauliflower	Tomato/vegetable juice[b]
Eggplant	Turnips
Green peppers	Water chestnuts
Greens (collard, mustard, turnip)	Zucchini, cooked
Kohlrabi	
Leeks	

Starchy vegetables such as corn, peas, and potatoes are found on the Starch/Bread List.
For free vegetables, see the Free Food List (Table E-7).

[b]400 mg or more sodium per exchange.
[e]Vegetables contain 2-3 grams dietary fiber per exchange.

■ TABLE E-4
Fruit List[f]

(15 g carbohydrate, 60 kcal)
All portion sizes, unless otherwise noted, are ½ c fresh fruit or fruit juice, ¼ c dried fruit.

Amount	Food
Fresh, Frozen, and Unsweetened Canned Fruit	
1	Apples, raw, 2" across
½ c	Applesauce, unsweetened
4	Apricots, medium, raw
½ c (4 halves)	Apricots, canned
½	Bananas, 9" long
¾ c	Blackberries[a], raw
¾ c	Blueberries[a], raw
⅓	Cantaloupe, 5" across
1 c	Cantaloupe, cubes
12	Cherries, large, raw
½ c	Cherries, canned
2	Figs, raw, 2" across
½ c	Fruit cocktail, canned
½	Grapefruit, medium
¾ c	Grapefruit, segments
15	Grapes, small
⅛	Honeydew melon, medium
1 c	Honeydew melon, cubes
1	Kiwis, large
¾ c	Mandarin oranges
½	Mangoes, small
1	Nectarines[a], 2½" across
1	Oranges, 2½" across
1 c	Papayas
1 peach (¾ c)	Peaches, 2¾" across
½ c (2 halves)	Peaches, canned
½ large or 1 small	Pears

■ TABLE E-4
Fruit List   (continued)

Amount	Food
½ c (2 halves)	Pears, canned
2	Persimmons, medium, native
¾ c	Pineapple, raw
⅓ c	Pineapple, canned
2	Plums, raw, 2" across
½	Pomegranates[a]
1 c	Raspberries[a], raw
1¼ c	Strawberries[a], raw, whole
2	Tangerines[a], 2½" across
1¼ c	Watermelon, cubes
Dried Fruit	
4 rings	Apples[a]
7 halves	Apricots[a]
2½ medium	Dates
1½	Figs[a]
3 medium	Prunes[a]
2 tbsp	Raisins
Fruit Juice	
½ c	Apple juice/cider
⅓ c	Cranberry juice cocktail
⅓ c	Grape juice
½ c	Grapefruit juice
½ c	Orange juice
½ c	Pineapple juice
⅓ c	Prune juice

[a]3 g or more dietary fiber per exchange.
[f]Fresh, frozen, and dried fruits have about 2 g of dietary fiber per exchange.

■ TABLE E-5
Milk List

(Nonfat and very low-fat milk = 12 g carbohydrate, 8 g protein, trace fat, 90 kcal. Low-fat milk = 12 g carbohydrate, 8 g protein, 5 g fat, 120 kcal. Whole milk = 12 g carbohydrate, 8 g protein, 8 g fat, 150 kcal.)

Amount	Food
Nonfat and Very Low-Fat Milk	
1 c	Nonfat milk
1 c	½% milk
1 c	1% milk
⅓ c	Dry nonfat milk
½ c	Evaporated nonfat milk
1 c	Low-fat buttermilk
8 oz	Plain nonfat yogurt
Lowfat Milk	
1 c fluid	2% milk
8 oz	Plain low-fat yogurt, with added nonfat milk solids
Whole Milk	
1 c	Whole milk
½ c	Evaporated whole milk
8 oz	Whole plain yogurt

E

■ TABLE E–6
Fat List (5 g fat, 45 kcal)

Amount	Food
Unsaturated Fats	
1/8 medium	Avocados
1 tsp	Margarine
1 tbsp	Margarine, diet[c]
1 tsp	Mayonnaise
1 tbsp	Mayonnaise, reduced kcalorie[c]
	Nuts and seeds:
6 whole	Almonds, dry roasted
1 tbsp	Cashews, dry roasted
20 small or 10 large	Peanuts
2 whole	Pecans
2 tsp	Pumpkin seeds
1 tbsp	Other nuts
1 tbsp	Seeds, pine nuts, sunflower seeds (without shells)
2 whole	Walnuts
1 tsp	Oil (corn, cottonseed, safflower, soybean, sunflower, olive, peanut)
10 small or 5 large	Olives[c]
1 tbsp	Salad dressing, all varieties[c]
2 tsp	Salad dressing, mayonnaise type
1 tbsp	Salad dressing, mayonnaise type, reduced kcalorie
2 tbsp	Salad dressing, reduced kcalorie[b]

(Two tablespoons of low-kcalorie salad dressing is a free food.)

Amount	Food
Saturated Fats	
1 slice	Bacon[c]
1 tsp	Butter
1/2 oz	Chitterlings
2 tbsp	Coconut, shredded
2 tbsp	Coffee whitener, liquid
4 tsp	Coffee whitener, powder
1 tbsp	Cream (heavy, whipping)
2 tbsp	Cream (light, coffee, table)
2 tbsp	Cream (sour)
1 tbsp	Cream cheese
1/4 oz	Salt pork[c]

[b]400 mg or more sodium per serving.
[c]400 mg or more sodium if two or more exchanges are eaten.

■ TABLE E–7
Free Foods

A free food is any food or drink that contains less than 20 kcal/serving. People with diabetes are advised to eat as much as they want of those items that have no serving size specified. They may eat two or three servings per day of those items that have a specific serving size. It is suggested that they spread them out through the day.

Amount	Food
Drinks	Bouillon, low-sodium
	Bouillon or broth without fat[b]
	Carbonated drinks, sugar-free
	Carbonated water
	Club soda
1 tbsp	Cocoa powder, unsweetened
	Coffee/tea
	Drink mixes, sugar-free
	Tonic water, sugar-free
Nonstick Pan Spray	
Fruit:	
1/2 c	Cranberries, unsweetened
1/2 c	Rhubarb, unsweetened
Vegetables (raw, 1 c)	Cabbage
	Celery
	Chinese cabbage[a]
	Cucumbers
	Green onions
	Hot peppers
	Mushrooms
	Radishes
	Zucchini[a]
Salad Greens	Endive
	Escarole
	Lettuce
	Romaine
	Spinach
Sweet Substitutes	Candy, hard, sugar-free
	Gelatin, sugar-free
	Gum, sugar-free (with less than 20 kcal/2 tsp)
2 tsp	Jam/jelly, sugar-free (with less than 20 kcal/2 tsp)
1 to 2 tbsp	Pancake syrup, sugar-free
	Sugar substitutes (saccharin, aspartame)
2 tbsp	Whipped topping
Condiments	
1 tbsp	Catsup
	Horseradish
	Mustard
	Pickles[b], dill, unsweetened
2 tbsp	Salad dressing, low-kcalorie
3 tbsp	Taco sauce
	Vinegar

■ TABLE E-7
Free Foods   (continued)

Amount	Food
Seasonings	Basil, fresh
	Celery seeds
	Chili powder
	Chives
	Cinnamon
	Curry
	Dill
	Flavoring extracts (almond, butter, lemon, peppermint, vanilla, walnut, etc.)
	Garlic
	Garlic powder
	Herbs
	Hot pepper sauce
	Lemon
	Lemon juice
	Lemon pepper
	Lime
	Lime juice
	Mint
	Onion powder
	Oregano
	Paprika
	Pepper
	Pimento
	Soy sauce[b]
	Soy sauce[b], low-sodium ("lite")
	Spices
¼ c	Wine, used in cooking
	Worcestershire sauce

[a]3 g or more dietary fiber per serving.
[b]400 mg or more sodium per serving.

■ TABLE E-8
Combination Foods

Much of the food we eat is mixed together in various combinations. These combination foods do not fit into only one exchange list. It can be quite hard to tell what is in a certain casserole dish or baked food item. This is a list of average values for some typical combination foods. This list will help you fit these foods into your meal plan. Ask your dietitian for information about any other foods you'd like to eat. The *American Diabetes Association/American Dietetic Association Family Cookbooks* and the *American Diabetes Association Holiday Cookbook* have many recipes and further information about many foods, including combination foods. Check your library or local bookstore.

Food	Amount	Exchanges
Casseroles, homemade	1 c (8 oz)	2 starch, 2 medium-fat meat, 1 fat
Cheese pizza[b], thin crust	¼ of 15 oz, or ¼ of 10″	2 starch, 1 medium-fat meat, 1 fat
Chili with beans[a,b], commercial	1 c (8 oz)	2 starch, 2 medium-fat meat, 2 fat

■ TABLE E-8
Combination Foods   (continued)

Food	Amount	Exchanges
Chow mein[b], without noodles or rice	2 c (16 oz)	1 starch, 2 vegetable, 2 lean meat
Macaroni and cheese[b]	1 c (8 oz)	2 starch, 1 medium-fat meat, 2 fat
Soups:		
Bean[a,b]	1 c (8 oz)	1 starch, 1 vegetable, 1 lean meat
Chunky[b], all varieties	10¾-oz can	1 starch, 1 vegetable, 1 medium-fat meat
Cream[b], made with water	1 c (8 oz)	1 starch, 1 fat
Vegetable[b] or broth[b]	1 c (8 oz)	1 starch
Spaghetti and meatballs[b], canned	1 c (8 oz)	2 starch, 1 medium-fat meat, 1 fat
Sugar-free pudding, made with nonfat milk	½ c	1 starch

If beans are used as a meat substitute:

Food	Amount	Exchanges
Dried beans[a], peas[a], lentils[a]	1 c (cooked)	2 starch, 1 lean meat

[a]3 g or more dietary fiber per exchange
[b]400 mg or more sodium per exchange.

■ TABLE E-9
Foods for Occasional Use

Moderate amounts of some foods can be used in your meal plan, in spite of their sugar or fat content, as long as you can maintain blood glucose control. The following list includes average exchange values for some of these foods. Because they are concentrated sources of carbohydrate, you will notice that the portion sizes are very small. Check with your dietitian for advice on how often and when you can use them.

Food	Amount	Exchanges
Angel food cake	1/12 cake	2 starch
Cake, no icing	1/12 cake, or a 3″ square	2 starch, 2 fat
Cookies	2 small, 1¾″ across	1 starch, 1 fat
Frozen fruit yogurt	⅓ c	1 starch
Gingersnaps	3	1 starch
Granola	¼ c	1 starch, 1 fat
Granola bars	1 small	1 starch, 1 fat
Ice cream, any flavor	½ c	1 starch, 2 fat
Ice milk, any flavor	½ c	1 starch, 1 fat
Sherbet, any flavor	¼ c	1 starch
Snack chips[c], all varieties	1 oz	1 starch, 2 fat
Vanilla wafers	6 small	1 starch[c]

[c]400 mg or more sodium if two or more exchanges are eaten.

INDEX

The boldfaced page numbers are the pages on which margin definitions appear. Page numbers followed by *n* refer to footnotes. Page numbers preceded by A through E are appendix pages.

A

Abdominal cavity edema,   594, 595, 597
Abdominal fat,   495
Abdominal girth measurement,   233
Absorptive system,   85–87
Abusive drugs,   269, 273, 309–310
Accent (monosodium glutamate),   300
Acebutolol,   576, B6
Acesulfame potassium,   **541**
Acetaminophen,   B4
Acetohexamide,   B6
Acetone,   515
Acetone breath,   514, 515
Acetyl CoA,   **99**, 98–100
Acetylsalicylic acid,   B4
Achalasia,   **435**
Acid ash diet,   614
Acid-base balance,   **62**, 156, 404
Acid indigestion,   83
Acid rain,   255, 257
Acidosis,   **62**, 406, 515
Acne and vitamin A relatives,   119
Acquired immune deficiency syndrome. *See*
    AIDS
Acquired (specific) immunity,   **347**
ACSM (American College of Sports Medicine),
    194, 196
Acute, defined,   **550**
Acute (flow) phase of stress response,   **344**,
    345
Acute renal disease,   xv, 373
Acute renal failure,   592, 600, 604–605, 609
Acyclovir,   475, B7
ADA (American Dietetic Association),   **369**
Adaptive phase of stress response,   **344**, 345
Addictive drugs,   309–310. *See also* Abusive
    drugs
ADH (antidiuretic hormone),   **155**
Administrative dietitian,   **369**

Adolescence
    alcohol use in,   310
    breastfeeding in,   317
    drug use in,   309–310
    energy needs and intakes in,   A3, A6
    food choices and eating habits in,
        308–309, 317
    growth in,   307–308
    height in,   B17–B18
    iron-deficiency anemia in,   296
    nutrient needs and intakes in, *inside front
        cover*,   169, 264, 294–295, 307–309,
        315–317, A1–A6
    pregnancy in,   169, 264, 315–317
    smoking in,   310–311
    weight in,   308, B17–B18
Adrenergic blockers,   574
Adrenocorticosteroids,   468, B9
Adult-onset (Type II) diabetes,   31, **514**–516,
    525–527. *See also* Diabetes (diabetes
    mellitus)
Adult rickets (osteomalacia),   121, 127, 158,
    B34
Adverse reactions to food, 300. *See also* Food
    allergies
Aerobic activity,   **192**. *See also* Exercise
Agility,   **190**
Aging process, retarding,   320–323. *See also*
    Longevity
Agroforestry,   255
AHA (American Heart Association),   563
AIDS (acquired immune deficiency syndrome),
    473
    and breastfeeding,   273
    diet modifications for,   xv, 373, 423, 458,
        473–478, 512, 546
    and nutrition,   480
AIDS-related complex (ARC),   **474**
Air, supply of,   254, 256, 257
Air pollution,   123, 255, 257, 258

Alanine,   60
Albumin,   168, 243, 407, 465. *See also*
    Prealbumin
Albuminuria,   **580**
Alcohol. *See also* Fetal alcohol syndrome; Sugar
    alcohols
    in adolescence,   310
    bland diet exclusion of,   436, 437
    in breast milk,   272–273
    and cancer,   484, 485
    and cirrhosis,   597
    in Daily Food Choices pattern,   11
    and diabetes,   521
    energy from,   7, 21*n*
    and hypertension,   112, 574
    and peptic ulcers,   440, 452
    during pregnancy,   269
    and premenstrual syndrome,   181
    recommended intake of,   13
Alcohol abuse,   110–113, 166–167, 550,
    593
Alcohol addiction (alcoholism),   110–111,
    132, 329
Aldosterone,   594, 595
Alimentary hypoglycemia,   **530**–533
Alka-Seltzer,   329–330
Alkaline ash diet,   614
Alkaline phosphatase, B41*n*
Alkalosis,   **62**
Allergies,   **299**
    to food. *See* Food allergies; Milk allergy
    and vitamin C,   135
Alpha-lactalbumin,   **275**
Aluminum contamination of foods,   359
Aluminum hydroxide,   441, B5
Alveoli,   **478**
Alzheimer's disease,   **354**
Amenorrhea,   508
American College of Sports Medicine (ACSM),
    194, 196

Acceptable Weight for Height Based on Body Mass Index (BMI)

To determine your acceptable weight range, find your height in the top line. Look down the column below it and find the range represented by the color blue. Look to the left column to see what weights are acceptable for you.

Men
Height, m (in)

Key:
- ☐ Underweight
- ■ Acceptable weight
- ■ Marginal overweight
- ■ Overweight
- ■ Severe overweight
- ■ Morbid obesity

Note: For more information on the body mass index, see Appendix B (see Figure B–8).

Source: Reprinted with permission of Ross Laboratories, Columbus, OH 43216 from *Dietetic Currents*, vol. 16, p. 9, 1989 Ross Laboratories.